CLINICAL GASTROINTESTINAL ENDOSCOPY

THIRD EDITION

Vinay Chandrasekhara, MD
Senior Associate Consultant
Division of Gastroenterology & Hepatology
Mayo Clinic
Rochester, Minnesota

B. Joseph Elmunzer, MD, MSc
The Peter B. Cotton Endowed Chair in Endoscopic Innovation
Associate Professor of Internal Medicine
Division of Gastroenterology and Hepatology
Medical University of South Carolina
Charleston, South Carolina

Mouen A. Khashab, MD
Associate Professor of Medicine
Director of Therapeutic Endoscopy
Division of Gastroenterology and Hepatology
Johns Hopkins Hospital
Baltimore, Maryland

V. Raman Muthusamy, MD, MAS
Director of Endoscopy, UCLA Health System
Professor of Clinical Medicine
Vatche and Tamar Manoukian Division of Digestive Diseases
David Geffen School of Medicine at UCLA
Los Angeles, California

ELSEVIER

ELSEVIER

1600 John F. Kennedy Blvd.
Ste 1800
Philadelphia, PA 19103-2899

Notices

Knowledge and best practice in this field are constantly changing. As new research and experience broaden our understanding, changes in research methods, professional practices, or medical treatment may become necessary.

Practitioners and researchers must always rely on their own experience and knowledge in evaluating and using any information, methods, compounds, or experiments described herein. In using such information or methods they should be mindful of their own safety and the safety of others, including parties for whom they have a professional responsibility.

With respect to any drug or pharmaceutical products identified, readers are advised to check the most current information provided (i) on procedures featured or (ii) by the manufacturer of each product to be administered, to verify the recommended dose or formula, the method and duration of administration, and contraindications. It is the responsibility of practitioners, relying on their own experience and knowledge of their patients, to make diagnoses, to determine dosages and the best treatment for each individual patient, and to take all appropriate safety precautions.

To the fullest extent of the law, neither the Publisher nor the authors, contributors, or editors, assume any liability for any injury and/or damage to persons or property as a matter of products liability, negligence or otherwise, or from any use or operation of any methods, products, instructions, or ideas contained in the material herein.

Previous editions copyrighted 2012 and 2005.

Library of Congress Cataloging-in-Publication Data
Names: Chandrasekhara, Vinay, editor. | Elmunzer, B. Joseph, editor. | Khashab, Mouen, editor. | Muthusamy, V. Raman, editor.
Title: Clinical gastrointestinal endoscopy / [edited by] Vinay Chandrasekhara, B. Joseph Elmunzer, Mouen A. Khashab, V. Raman Muthusamy.
Description: Third edition. | Philadelphia, PA : Elsevier, [2019] | Includes bibliographical references and index.
Identifiers: LCCN 2017056974 | ISBN 9780323415095 (hardcover : alk. paper)
Subjects: | MESH: Endoscopy, Gastrointestinal | Gastrointestinal Diseases–therapy | Biliary Tract Diseases–therapy | Pancreatic Diseases–therapy
Classification: LCC RC804.E64 | NLM WI 190 | DDC 616.3/407545–dc23 LC record available at https://lccn.loc.gov/2017056974

Executive Content Strategist: Dolores Meloni
Senior Content Development Specialist: Rae Robertson
Publishing Services Manager: Catherine Jackson
Project Manager: Tara Delaney
Design Direction: Renee Duenow

Printed in the United States of America

Last digit is the print number: 9 8 7 6 5 4 3

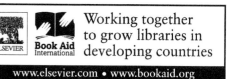

To my parents Bina and Kota and my sister Sheila, who provided a nurturing environment and encouraged me to dream big. The values that you instilled from an early age will forever remain with me.

To my wife Meghana and our children Siddhant and Adya, who have allowed me to pursue my dreams even if it meant being away from home. Every professional accomplishment is only possible because of your love and support.

To my colleagues, friends, trainees, and professional acquaintances: I appreciate everything you have taught me over the years. I am especially ever grateful to Drs. Gregory Ginsberg and Michael Kochman for providing me with unbelievable opportunities, including serving as an editor for this textbook.

—Vinay Chandrasekhara

To my parents, Carol and Hadi, for showing me the right path and to my wife, Alli, for taking it with me. To our patients, without whom there would be no progress.

—B. Joseph Elmunzer

This book is dedicated to my family, trainees, nurses, colleagues and mentors. It took a tremendous effort and commitment to put this comprehensive endoscopy book together. I am grateful to both my personal family and my work family who allowed me to have the focus, dedication, and time to be a coeditor of this book.

—Mouen A. Khashab

I dedicate this book to my teachers, colleagues, and trainees who continue to challenge me to question what is felt to already be known. To my patients for their inspiration in motivating me to continually improve on the care we deliver. To my entire family, I thank you for your constant love and support. Specifically, to my mother, who has always encouraged me to follow my own path, and to my father, who left a medical school faculty position in India 45 years ago to start over as a resident in the USA with nothing other than $20 in his pocket and the American Dream, for the many opportunities I have had in my life and to whom I owe everything. Finally, to my wife Nanda and daughter Sonali for your substantial patience, compassion, warmth, and most importantly for bringing so much joy and laughter into my life.

—V. Raman Muthusamy

CONTRIBUTORS

James L. Achord, MD
Professor Emeritus
University of Mississippi Medical Center
Jackson, Misssissippi
1: The History of Gastrointestinal
    Endoscopy

Michelle J. Alfa, BSc, MSc, PhD
Principal Investigator
St. Boniface Research Centre;
Professor
Department of Medical Microbiology
University of Manitoba
Winnipeg, Manitoba, Canada
4: Cleaning and Disinfecting Gastrointestinal
    Endoscopy Equipment

**Mohammad Al-Haddad, MD, MSc,
FASGE, FACG, AGAF**
Associate Professor of Medicine
Division of Gastroenterology and
    Hepatology
Indiana University School Medicine
Indianapolis, Indiana
62: Evaluation and Staging of
    Pancreaticobiliary Malignancy

Andrea Anderloni, MD, PhD
Digestive Endoscopy Unit
Division of Gastroenterology
Humanitas Research Hospital
Milan, Italy
28: Palliation of Malignant Dysphagia and
    Esophageal Fistulas

Joseph C. Anderson, MD
Associate Professor of Medicine
Department of Veterans Affairs Medical
    Center
White River Junction, Vermont;
The Geisel School of Medicine at Dartmouth
Hanover, New Hampshire;
Division of Gastroenterology and
    Hepatology
University of Connecticut School of
    Medicine
Farmington, Connecticut
36: Colorectal Cancer Screening and
    Surveillance

Anna Baiges, MD
Hepatic Hemodynamic Laboratory
Liver Unit, Hospital Clínic
Barcelona, Spain
15: Portal Hypertensive Bleeding

John Baillie, MD
Professor
Division of Gastroenterology and
    Hepatology
Department of Medicine
Virginia Commonwealth University School
    of Medicine
Richmond, Virginia
3: How Endoscopes Work

Alan N. Barkun, MD, MSc
Division of Gastroenterology
McGill University Health Center
Montreal, Québec, Canada
14: Nonvariceal Upper Gastrointestinal
    Bleeding

Todd H. Baron, MD, FASGE
Professor of Medicine
Division of Gastroenterology and
    Hepatology
University of North Carolina
Chapel Hill, North Carolina
20: Endoscopic Diagnosis and Management
    of Zenker's Diverticula

Omer Basar, MD
Pancreas Biliary Center, Gastrointestinal
    Unit
Massachusetts General Hospital
Boston, Massachusetts;
Professor of Medicine
Department of Gastroenterology
Hacettepe University
Ankara, Turkey
61: Pancreatic Cystic Lesions

Mark Benson, MD
Assistant Professor
Division of Gastroenterology and
    Hepatology
University of Wisconsin School of Medicine
    and Public Health
Madison, Wisconsin
22: Ingested Foreign Objects and Food Bolus
    Impactions

Lyz Bezerra Silva, MD, MSC
Associate Professor of Surgery
Department of Surgery
Federal University of Pernambuco
Recife, Brazil
45: Intramural and Transmural Endoscopy

Stas Bezobchuk, MD
Institute of Gastroenterology, Hepatology,
    and Nutrition
Emek Medical Center
Afula, Israel
17: Middle Gastrointestinal Bleeding

Kenneth F. Binmoeller, MD
Director, Interventional Endoscopy Services
Paul May and Frank Stein Interventional
    Endoscopy Center
California Pacific Medical Center
San Francisco, California
58: Pancreatic Fluid Collections and Leaks

Sarah Blankstein, AB, JD
Boston, Massachusetts
10: Legal Concepts for Gastroenterologists

Daniel Blero, MD, PhD
Department of Gastroenterology
Chu Charleroi
Charleroi, Belgium;
Hôpital Erasme
Brussels, Belgium
43: Endoscopic Techniques for Weight Loss

Michael J. Bourke, BSc, MD
Department of Gastroenterology and
    Hepatology
Westmead Hospital
Sydney, Australia
34: Duodenal and Papillary Adenomas

William R. Brugge, MD
Chief
Division of Gastroenterology
Mount Auburn Hospital
Cambridge, Massachusetts
61: Pancreatic Cystic Lesions

Marco J. Bruno, MD, PhD
Department of Gastroenterology and
    Hepatology
Erasmus Medical Center
University of Rotterdam
Rotterdam, The Netherlands
63: Palliation of Malignant Pancreaticobiliary
    Obstruction

Anna M. Buchner, MD, PhD
Assistant Professor of Medicine
Division of Gastroenterology
University of Pennsylvania
Philadelphia, Pennsylvania
38: Endoscopic Diagnosis and Staging of
    Inflammatory Bowel Disease

Andrés Cárdenas, MD, MMSc, PhD, AGAF, FAASLD
Faculty Member/Consultant
Institute of Digestive Diseases and Metabolism Hospital Clinic
University of Barcelona
Barcelona, Spain
15: Portal Hypertensive Bleeding
54: Postoperative Biliary Strictures and Leaks

David Carr-Locke, MD, FRCP, FASGE, AGAF, NYSGEF
Clinical Director
Center for Advanced Digestive Care
Gastroenterology & Hepatology
Weill Cornell Medical College
Cornell University
New York, New York
55: Infections of the Biliary Tract

Kenneth Chang, MD
Professor and Chief
Division of Gastroenterology and Hepatology
University of California—Irvine
Orange, California
51: Endoscopic Ultrasound and Fine-Needle Aspiration for Pancreatic and Biliary Disorders

Saurabh Chawla, MD, FACG
Director of Endoscopy
Grady Memorial Hospital;
Assistant Professor of Medicine
Emory University School of Medicine
Atlanta, Georgia
48: Preparation for Pancreaticobiliary Endoscopy

John O. Clarke, MD
Clinical Associate Professor
Department of Medicine
Stanford University
Stanford, California
19: Esophageal Motility Disorders
29: Endoscopic Approaches for Gastroparesis

Jonathan Cohen, MD
Clinical Professor
Department of Medicine
New York University Langone School of Medicine
New York, New York
13: Endoscopic Simulators

Andrew P. Copland, MD
Assistant Professor of Medicine
Division of Gastroenterology and Hepatology
University of Virginia Health Systems
Charlottesville, Virginia
40: Colonic Strictures

Guido Costamagna, MD, FACG
Digestive Endoscopy Unit
Catholic University
Gemelli University Hospital
Rome, Italy
54: Postoperative Biliary Strictures and Leaks

Peter B. Cotton, MD, FRCS, FRCP
Professor of Medicine
Digestive Disease Center
Medical University of South Carolina
Charleston, South Carolina
56: Sphincter of Oddi Disorders

Amit P. Desai, MD
Texas Digestive Diseases Consultants
Texas Health Presbyterian Hospital
Dallas, Texas
47: Extraintestinal Endosonography

Jacques Devière, MD, PhD
Professor of Medicine
Chairman, Department of Gastroenterology, Hepatopancreatology, and Digestive Oncology
Erasme Hospital
Université Libre de Bruxelles
Brussels, Belgium
43: Endoscopic Techniques for Weight Loss

Christopher J. DiMaio, MD
Director of Therapeutic Endoscopy
Associate Professor of Medicine
Division of Gastroenterology
Icahn School of Medicine at Mount Sinai
New York, New York
53: Gallstone Disease: Choledocholithiasis, Cholecystitis, and Gallstone Pancreatitis

Peter Draganov, MD
Professor of Medicine
Department of Internal Medicine
University of Florida
Gainesville, Florida
37: Colonoscopic Polypectomy, Mucosal Resection, and Submucosal Dissection

Jérôme Dumortier, MD
Department of Hepatogastroenterology and Digestive Endoscopy
Edouard Herriot Hospital
Lyon, France
11: Small-Caliber Endoscopy

Jeffrey J. Easler, MD
Assistant Professor of Medicine
Division of Gastroenterology and Hepatology
Indiana University School of Medicine;
Richard L. Roudebush VA Medical Center
Indianapolis, Indiana
49: Cholangiography and Pancreatography

Gary W. Falk, MD, MS
Professor of Medicine
Department of Medicine, Division of Gastroenterology
University of Pennsylvania Perelman School of Medicine
Philadelphia, Pennsylvania
25: Barrett's Esophagus: Diagnosis, Surveillance, and Medical Management

Francis A. Farraye, MD, MSc
Clinical Director
Section of Gastroenterology
Boston Medical Center;
Professor of Medicine
Department of Medicine
Boston University School of Medicine
Boston, Massachusetts
39: Dysplasia Surveillance in Inflammatory Bowel Disease

Andrew Feld, MD, JD
Program Chief, Group Health Cooperative
Clinical Professor
University of Washington
Seattle, Washington
10: Legal Concepts for Gastroenterologists

Kayla Feld, JD
Quinn Emanuel Urquhart & Sullivan
Washington, D.C.
10: Legal Concepts for Gastroenterologists

Paul Fockens, MD, PhD, FASGE
Professor and Chair
Department of Gastroenterology and Hepatology
Academic Medical Center
Amsterdam, The Netherlands
33: Palliation of Gastric Outlet Obstruction

Evan L. Fogel, MD, MSc, FRCP(C)
Professor of Medicine
Department of Gastroenterology and Hepatology
Indiana University School of Medicine
Indianapolis, Indiana
49: Cholangiography and Pancreatography

Kyle J. Fortinsky, MD, BSc
Division of Gastroenterology
University of Toronto
Toronto, Ontario, Canada
14: Nonvariceal Upper Gastrointestinal
   Bleeding

Martin L. Freeman, MD
Professor of Medicine
Division of Gastroenterology, Hepatology,
   and Nutrition
University of Minnesota
Minneapolis, Minnesota
57: Recurrent Acute Pancreatitis

Juan Carlos García-Pagán, MD, PhD
Head
Barcelona Hepatic Hemodynamic Lab;
Senior Consultant in Hepatology
Associate Professor
University of Barcelona;
Liver Unit, Hospital Clínic
Barcelona, Spain
15: Portal Hypertensive Bleeding

Hans Gerdes, MD
Attending Physician
Department of Medicine
Memorial Sloan Kettering Cancer Center;
Professor of Clinical Medicine
Weill Cornell Medical College of Cornell
   University
New York, New York
30: Gastric Polyps and Thickened Gastric
   Folds

Joanna A. Gibson, MD, PhD
Assistant Professor of Pathology
Yale University School of Medicine
New Haven, Connecticut
5: Tissue Sampling, Specimen Handling, and
   Laboratory Processing

Gregory G. Ginsberg, MD
Professor of Medicine
Department of Medicine, Division of
   Gastroenterology
Hospital of the University of Pennsylvania
Philadelphia, Pennsylvania
50: Difficult Cannulation and
   Sphincterotomy

Marc Giovannini, MD
Head, Gastroenterology and Endoscopy
   Department
Paoli-Calmettes Institute
Marseille, France
52: Endoscopic Ultrasound-Guided Access
   and Drainage of the Pancreaticobiliary
   Ductal Systems

Ian M. Gralnek, MD, MSHS, FASGE
Clinical Associate Professor of Medicine/
   Gastroenterology
Rappaport Faculty of Medicine Technion
Israel Institute of Technology;
Chief, Institute of Gastroenterology,
   Hepatology and Nutrition
Emek Medical Center
Afula, Israel
17: Middle Gastrointestinal Bleeding

Frank G. Gress, MD
Professor of Medicine
Chief, Interventional Endoscopy
Division of Digestive & Liver Diseases
Columbia University Medical Center
New York, New York
47: Extraintestinal Endosonography

Robert H. Hawes, MD
Professor
Department of Medicine
University of Central Florida College of
   Medicine;
Medical Director
Florida Hospital Institute for Minimally
   Invasive Therapy
Florida Hospital Orlando
Orlando, Florida
59: Chronic Pancreatitis

Virginia Hernández-Gea, MD, PhD
Hepatic Hemodynamic Laboratory
Liver Unit, Hospital Clínic
Barcelona, Spain
15: Portal Hypertensive Bleeding

Ikuo Hirano, MD
Professor of Medicine
Department of Medicine, Division of
   Gastroenterology
Northwestern University Feinberg School of
   Medicine;
Director, Northwestern Esophageal Center
Northwestern Medicine
Chicago, Illinois
23: Eosinophilic Esophagitis

Juergen Hochberger, MD, PhD
Chairman
Department of Gastroenterology
Vivantes Klinikum im Friedrichshain
Berlin, Germany
50: Difficult Cannulation and
   Sphincterotomy

Douglas A. Howell, MD
Director, Advanced Interventional
   Endoscopy Fellowship
Director, Pancreaticobiliary Center
Maine Medical Center
Portland, Maine;
Associate Clinical Professor
Tufts University School of Medicine
Boston, Massachusetts
60: The Indeterminate Biliary Stricture

Chin Hur, MD, MPH
Associate Director, Institute for Technology
   Assessment
Director, GI Health Outcomes Research
Massachusetts General Hospital;
Associate Professor of Medicine
Harvard Medical School
Boston, Massachusetts
26: Screening for Esophageal Squamous Cell
   Carcinoma

Joo Ha Hwang, MD, PhD
Professor of Medicine
Department of Medicine
Division of Gastroenterology and
   Hepatology
Stanford University
Stanford, California
6: Electrosurgery in Therapeutic Endoscopy

Maite Betés Ibáñez, PhD, MD
Department of Gastroenterology
University Clinic of Navarra
Pamplona, Navarra, Spain
18: Occult and Unexplained Chronic
   Gastrointestinal Bleeding

Takao Itoi, MD, PhD, FASGE, FACG
Chair and Professor
Department of Gastroenterology and
   Hepatology
Tokyo Medical University
Tokyo, Japan
52: Endoscopic Ultrasound-Guided Access
   and Drainage of the Pancreaticobiliary
   Ductal Systems

Prasad G. Iyer, MD, MS
Professor and Consultant
Department of Gastroenterology and
   Hepatology
Mayo Clinic
Rochester, Minnesota
27: Endoscopic Treatment of Early
   Esophageal Neoplasia

David A. Johnson, MD, MACG, FASGE, FACP
Professor of Medicine and Chief
Division of Gastroenterology and
    Hepatology
Department of Internal Medicine
Eastern Virginia Medical School
Norfolk, Virginia
9: Bowel Preparation for Colonoscopy

Sreeni Jonnalagadda, MD
Professor of Medicine
Director of Therapeutic and Biliary
    Endoscopy
Saint Luke's Hospital
University of Missouri—Kansas City
Kansas City, Missouri
12: Postsurgical Endoscopic Anatomy

Charles J. Kahi, MD, MS, FACP, FACG, AGAF, FASGE
Professor of Clinical Medicine
Indiana University School of Medicine;
Gastroenterology Section Chief
Richard L. Roudebush VA Medical Center
Indianapolis, Indiana
36: Colorectal Cancer Screening and
    Surveillance

Tonya Kaltenbach, MD, MAS
Associate Professor of Clinical Medicine
Division of Gastroenterology, Department of
    Medicine
University California San Francisco;
Director of Advanced Endoscopy
San Francisco Veterans Affair Medical Center
San Francisco, California
37: Colonoscopic Polypectomy, Mucosal
    Resection, and Submucosal Dissection

Leila Kia, MD
Assistant Professor of Medicine
Department of Medicine, Division of
    Gastroenterology
Northwestern University Feinberg School of
    Medicine
Chicago, Illinois
23: Eosinophilic Esophagitis

Michael B. Kimmey, MD
Franciscan Digestive Care Associates
Gig Harbor, Washington
35: Acute Colonic Pseudo-Obstruction

Amir Klein, MD
Department of Gastroenterology and
    Hepatology
Rambam Health Care Campus
Haifa, Israel
34: Duodenal and Papillary Adenomas

Michael L. Kochman, MD
Wilmott Family Professor of Medicine
Division of Gastroenterology, Department of
    Medicine
Perelman School of Medicine
University of Pennsylvania
Philadelphia, Pennsylvania
21: Benign Esophageal Strictures

Divyanshoo R. Kohli, MD
Division of Gastroenterology and
    Hepatology
Department of Medicine
Virginia Commonwealth University School
    of Medicine
Richmond, Virginia
3: How Endoscopes Work

Andrew Korman
Division of Gastroenterology and
    Hepatology
Saint Peter's University Hospital
New Brunswick, New Jersey
55: Infections of the Biliary Tract

Wilson T. Kwong, MD, MS
Assistant Professor
Department of Gastroenterology
University of California San Diego
La Jolla, California
16: Lower Gastrointestinal Bleeding

Ryan Law, DO
Clinical Lecturer
Division of Gastroenterology and
    Hepatology
University of Michigan
Ann Arbor, Michigan
20: Endoscopic Diagnosis and Management
    of Zenker's Diverticula

David A. Leiman, MD, MSHP
Assistant Professor of Medicine
Division of Gastroenterology
Duke University School of Medicine
Durham, North Carolina
24: Gastroesophageal Reflux Disease

Anne Marie Lennon, MB, PhD, FRCPI
Benjamin Baker Scholar
Associate Professor of Medicine and Surgery
The Johns Hopkins Hospital
Baltimore, Maryland
61: Pancreatic Cystic Lesions

Michael Levy, MD
Professor of Medicine
Division of Gastroenterology and
    Hepatology
Mayo Clinic
Rochester, Minnesota
62: Evaluation and Staging of
    Pancreaticobiliary Malignancy

David Lichtenstein, MD
Director of Endoscopy
Department of Gastroenterology
Boston Medical Center
Boston University School of Medicine
Boston, Massachusetts
4: Cleaning and Disinfecting Gastrointestinal
    Endoscopy Equipment

Gary R. Lichtenstein, MD
Professor of Medicine
Director, Center for Inflammatory Bowel
    Disease
Division of Gastroenterology
University of Pennsylvania
Philadelphia, Pennsylvania
38: Endoscopic Diagnosis and Staging of
    Inflammatory Bowel Disease

Alisa Likhitsup, MD
Gastroenterology Fellow
Department of Gastroenterology
University of Missouri—Kansas City
Kansas City, Missouri
12: Postsurgical Endoscopic Anatomy

Jimmy K. Limdi, MBBS, FRCP, FRCPE, FACG
Consultant Gastroenterologist
Department of Gastroenterology
The Pennine Acute Hospitals NHS Trust;
Honorary Senior Lecturer
Institute of Inflammation and Repair
University of Manchester
Manchester, United Kingdom
39: Dysplasia Surveillance in Inflammatory
    Bowel Disease

Gianluca Lollo, MD
Department of Surgical Oncology and
    Gastroenterological Sciences
University of Padua
Padua, Italy
28: Palliation of Malignant Dysphagia and
    Esophageal Fistulas

Fauze Maluf-Filho, MD, PhD, FASGE
Professor
Department of Gastroenterology
Medical School of University of São Paulo;
Chief
Endoscopy Unit
Institute of Cancer of Univeristy of São
    Paulo
63: Palliation of Malignant Pancreaticobiliary
    Obstruction

Jennifer Maranki, MD, MSc
Associate Professor of Medicine
Director of Endoscopy
Division of Gastroenterology and
    Hepatology
Penn State Hershey Medical Center
Hershey, Pennsylvania
46: Endoscopic Full-Thickness Resection of
    Subepithelial Lesions of the GI Tract

**Richard W. McCallum, MD, FACP,
FRACP (Aust), FACG, AGAF**
Professor of Medicine and Founding Chair
Department of Internal Medicine
Texas Tech University
El Paso, Texas;
Honorary Professor
University of Queensland
Queensland, Australia
29: Endoscopic Approaches for Gastroparesis

Stephen A. McClave, MD
Professor of Medicine
Department of Medicine
University of Louisville School of Medicine
Louisville, Kentucky
42: Techniques in Enteral Access

Klaus Mergener, MD, PhD, MBA
Partner
Digestive Health Specialists
Tacoma, Washington
2: Setting Up an Endoscopy Facility

David C. Metz, MD
Professor of Medicine
Division of Gastroenterology
Perelman School of Medicine
University of Pennsylvania
Philadelphia, Pennsylvania
24: Gastroesophageal Reflux Disease

Volker Meves, MD
Department of Gastroenterology
Vivantes Klinikum im Friedrichshain
Berlin, Germany
50: Difficult Cannulation and
    Sphincterotomy

Marcia L. Morris, MS
Electrosurgery Consultant
St. Paul, Minnesota
6: Electrosurgery in Therapeutic Endoscopy

Daniel K. Mullady, MD
Associate Professor of Medicine
Director, Interventional Endoscopy
Department of Gastroenterology
Washington University in St. Louis School of
    Medicine
St. Louis, Missouri
53: Gallstone Disease: Choledocholithiasis,
    Cholecystitis, and Gallstone Pancreatitis

Miguel Muñoz-Navas, PhD, MD
Professor of Medicine
University of Navarra School of Medicine;
Director
Department of Gastroenterology
University of Navarra Clinic
Pamplona, Navarra, Spain
18: Occult and Unexplained Chronic
    Gastrointestinal Bleeding

V. Raman Muthusamy, MD, MAS
Director of Endoscopy, UCLA Health System
Professor of Clinical Medicine
Vatche and Tamar Manoukian Division of
    Digestive Diseases
David Geffen School of Medicine at UCLA
Los Angeles, California
1: The History of Gastrointestinal
    Endoscopy

Zaheer Nabi, MD, DNB
Consultant Gastoenterologist
Asian Institute of Gastroenterology
Hyderabad, India
55: Infections of the Biliary Tract

Andrew Nett, MD
Paul May and Frank Stein Interventional
    Endoscopy Center
California Pacific Medical Center;
Department of Medicine
University of California San Francisco
San Francisco, California
58: Pancreatic Fluid Collections and Leaks

**Nam Q. Nguyen, MBBS (Hons), FRACP,
PhD**
Associate Professor
Head, Education and Research
Department of Gastroenterology and
    Hepatology
Royal Adelaide Hospital
University of Adelaide
Adelaide, South Australia, Australia
8: Patient Preparation and
    Pharmacotherapeutic Considerations

Nicholas Nickl, MD
Professor of Medicine
University of Kentucky Medical Center
Lexington, Kentucky
31: Subepithelial Tumors of the Esophagus
    and Stomach

Satoru Nonaka, MD, PhD
Endoscopy Division
National Cancer Center Hospital
Tokyo, Japan
32: Diagnosis and Treatment of Superficial
    Gastric Neoplasms

Ichiro Oda, MD
Endoscopy Division
National Cancer Center Hospital
Tokyo, Japan
32: Diagnosis and Treatment of Superficial
    Gastric Neoplasms

Robert D. Odze, MD, FRCPC
Professor of Pathology
Department of Pathology
Brigham and Women's Hospital
Boston, Massachusetts
5: Tissue Sampling, Specimen Handling, and
    Laboratory Processing

Edward C. Oldfield IV, MD
Department of Internal Medicine
Eastern Virginia Medical School
Norfolk, Virginia
9: Bowel Preparation for Colonoscopy

Parth J. Parekh, MD
Department of Internal Medicine
Division of Gastroenterology and
    Hepatology
Tulane University
New Orleans, Louisiana
9: Bowel Preparation for Colonoscopy

Patrick R. Pfau, MD
Professor of Medicine, Chief of Clinical
    Gastroenterology
Division of Gastroenterology and
    Hepatology
University of Wisconsin School of Medicine
    and Public Health
Madison, Wisconsin
22: Ingested Foreign Objects and Food Bolus
    Impactions

Mathieu Pioche, MD, PhD
Department of Hepatogastroenterology and
    Digestive Endoscopy
Edouard Herriot Hospital
Lyon, France
11: Small-Caliber Endoscopy

Heiko Pohl, MD
Associate Professor of Medicine
Geisel School of Medicine at Dartmouth
Hanover New Hampshire;
Department of Gastroenterology
Veterans Affair Medical Center
White River Junction, Vermont
37: Colonoscopic Polypectomy, Mucosal
    Resection, and Submucosal Dissection

Thierry Ponchon, MD, PhD
Department of Hepatogastroenterology and
    Digestive Endoscopy
Edouard Herriot Hospital
Lyon, France
11: Small-Caliber Endoscopy

Robert J. Ponec, MD
Consulting Gastroenterologist and
    Therapeutic Endoscopist
Department of Gastroenterology and
    Hepatology
Salem Gastroenterology Consultants
Salem, Oregon
35: Acute Colonic Pseudo-Obstruction

Michael W. Rajala, MD, PhD
Assistant Professor of Clinical Medicine
Division of Gastroenterology, Department of
    Medicine
Perelman School of Medicine
University of Pennsylvania
Philadelphia, Pennsylvania
21: Benign Esophageal Strictures

Nageshwar Reddy, MBBS, MD, DM
Chairman and Chief of Gastroenterology
Asian Institute of Gastroenterology
Hyderabad, India
55: Infections of the Biliary Tract

Alessandro Repici, MD
Professor of Gastroenterology
Director of Endoscopy
Humanitas Research Hospital & Humanitas
    University
Milan, Italy
28: Palliation of Malignant Dysphagia and
    Esophageal Fistulas

Jérôme Rivory, MD
Department of Hepatogastroenterology and
    Digestive Endoscopy
Edouard Herriot Hospital
Lyon, France
11: Small-Caliber Endoscopy

Marvin Ryou, MD
Division of Gastroenterology, Hepatology,
    and Endoscopy
Brigham and Womens' Hospital;
Instructor
Harvard Medical School
Boston, Massachusetts
44: Management of Post-Bariatric
    Complications

Yutaka Saito, MD, PhD, FASGE, FACG
Chief, Director
Endoscopy Division
National Cancer Center Hospital
Tokyo, Japan
32: Diagnosis and Treatment of Superficial
    Gastric Neoplasms

Jason B. Samarasena, MD
Associate Clinical Professor of Medicine
Division of Gastroenterology and
    Hepatology
University of California—Irvine
Orange, California
51: Endoscopic Ultrasound and Fine-Needle
    Aspiration for Pancreatic and Biliary
    Disorders

Thomas J. Savides, MD
Professor of Clinical Medicine
Division of Gastroenterology
University of California San Diego
La Jolla, California
16: Lower Gastrointestinal Bleeding

Mark Schoeman, MBBS, PhD, FRACP
Head, Gastrointestinal Investigation Unit
Department of Gastroenterology and
    Hepatology
Royal Adelaide Hospital
Adelaide, South Australia, Australia
8: Patient Preparation and
    Pharmacotherapeutic Considerations

Allison R. Schulman, MD, MPH
Physician
Division of Gastroenterology, Hepatology,
    and Endoscopy
Brigham and Women's Hospital;
Harvard Medical School
Boston, Massachusetts
44: Management of Post-Bariatric
    Complications

Amrita Sethi, MD, MSc
Associate Professor of Medicine
Director of Pancreaticobiliary Endoscopy
    Services
Columbia University Medical Center
New York, New York
60: The Indeterminate Biliary Stricture

Pari M. Shah, MD, MSCE
Assistant Attending Physician
Department of Medicine
Memorial Sloan Kettering Cancer Center;
Assistant Professor of Clinical Medicine
Weill Cornell Medical College of Cornell
    University
New York, New York
30: Gastric Polyps and Thickened Gastric
    Folds

Stuart Sherman, MD
Glen A. Lehman Professor of
    Gastroenterology
Professor of Medicine
Division of Gastroenterology and
    Hepatology
Indiana University School of Medicine
Indianapolis, Indiana
49: Cholangiography and Pancreatography

Uzma D. Siddiqui, MD
Center for Endoscopic Research and
    Therapeutics
University of Chicago School of Medicine
Chicago, Illinois
59: Chronic Pancreatitis

Vikesh K. Singh, MD, MSc
Director, Pancreatitis Center
Associate Professor of Medicine
John Hopkins University School of Medicine
Baltimore, Maryland
48: Preparation for Pancreaticobiliary
    Endoscopy

Roy Soetikno, MD, MS
Veterans Affairs Palo Alto Health Care
    System
Stanford University School of Medicine
Palo Alto, California
37: Colonoscopic Polypectomy, Mucosal
    Resection, and Submucosal Dissection

Stavros N. Stavropoulos, MD, FASGE
Chief, GI Endoscopy
Director, Program in Advanced GI
    Endoscopy (P.A.G.E.)
Winthrop University Hospital
Mineola, New York;
Adjunct Professor of Clinical Medicine
Columbia University
New York, New York
46: Endoscopic Full-Thickness Resection of
    Subepithelial Lesions of the GI Tract

Tyler Stevens, MD
Associate Professor
Department of Gastroenterology and
    Hepatology
Cleveland Clinic
Cleveland, Ohio
57: Recurrent Acute Pancreatitis

Christina Surawicz, MD
Professor
Division of Gastroenterology
Department of Medicine
University of Washington
Seattle, Washington
41: Infections of the Luminal Digestive Tract

Barry Tanner, CPA
Chief Executive Officer
Physicians Endoscopy
Jamison, Pennsylvania
2: Setting Up an Endoscopy Facility

Paul Tarnasky, MD
Digestive Health Associates of Texas
Dallas, Texas
56: Sphincter of Oddi Disorders

**Christopher C. Thompson, MD, MSc,
FACG, FASGE, AGAF**
Director of Therapeutic Endoscopy
Division of Gastroenterology, Hepatology,
    and Endoscopy
Brigham and Women's Hospital;
Assistant Professor of Medicine
Harvard Medical School
Boston, Massachusetts
44: Management of Post-Bariatric
    Complications

Mark Topazian, MD
Professor of Medicine
Division of Gastroenterology & Hepatology
Mayo Clinic
Rochester, Minnesota
51: Endoscopic Ultrasound and Fine-Needle
    Aspiration for Pancreatic and Biliary
    Disorders

George Triadafilopoulos, MD, DSc
Clinical Professor of Medicine
Stanford Multidimensional Program for
    Innovation and Research in the
    Esophagus (S-MPIRE)
Division of Gastroenterology and
    Hepatology
Stanford University School of Medicine
Stanford, California
19: Esophageal Motility Disorders

Emo E. van Halsema, MD
Department of Gastroenterology and
    Hepatology
Academic Medical Center
Amsterdam, The Netherlands
33: Palliation of Gastric Outlet Obstruction

Jeanin E. van Hooft, MD, PhD, MBA
Department of Gastroenterology and
    Hepatology
Academic Medical Center
Amsterdam, The Netherlands
33: Palliation of Gastric Outlet Obstruction

John Joseph Vargo II, MD, MPH
Vice Chair, Digestive Disease Institute Chair
Department of Gastroenterology and
    Hepatology
Cleveland Clinic
Cleveland, Ohio
7: Sedation and Monitoring in Endoscopy

Kavel Visrodia, MD
Fellow
Department of Internal Medicine, Division
    of Gastroenterology and Hepatology
Mayo Clinic
Rochester, Minnesota
27: Endoscopic Treatment of Early
    Esophageal Neoplasia

Vaibhav Wadhwa, MD
Clinical Fellow
Department of Gastroenterology and
    Hepatology
Cleveland Clinic Florida
Weston, Florida
7: Sedation and Monitoring in Endoscopy

Kristian Wall, MD
Fellow
Division of Digestive Diseases and Nutrition
University of Kentucky
Lexington, Kentucky
31: Subepithelial Tumors of the Esophagus
    and Stomach

**Catharine M. Walsh, MD, MEd, PhD,
FAAP, FRCPC**
Division of Gastroenterology, Hepatology,
    and Nutrition and the Learning and
    Research Institutes
Department of Paediatrics
Hospital for Sick Children;
The Wilson Centre
University of Toronto
Toronto, Ontario, Canada
13: Endoscopic Simulators

**Andrew Y. Wang, MD, AGAF, FACG,
FASGE**
Associate Professor of Medicine
Chief, Section of Interventional Endoscopy
Division of Gastroenterology and
    Hepatology
University of Virginia Health System
Charlottesville, Virginia
40: Colonic Strictures

Kenneth K. Wang, MD
Kathy and Russ VanCleve Professor of
    Gastroenterology Research
Department of Gastroenterology and
    Hepatology
Mayo Clinic
Rochester, Minnesota
27: Endoscopic Treatment of Early
    Esophageal Neoplasia

Sachin Wani, MD
Associate Professor of Medicine
Department of Medicine, Division of
    Gastroenterology
University of Colorado School of Medicine
Aurora, Colorado
25: Barrett's Esophagus: Diagnosis,
    Surveillance, and Medical Management

C. Mel Wilcox, MD, MSPH
Director
Division of Gastroenterology and
    Hepatology
University of Alabama at Birmingham
Birmingham, Alabama
41: Infections of the Luminal Digestive Tract

Field F. Willingham, MD, MPH, FASGE
Director of Endoscopy
Associate Professor of Medicine
Emory University School of Medicine
Atlanta, Georgia
48: Preparation for Pancreaticobiliary
    Endoscopy

Patrick S. Yachimski, MD, MPH, FASGE
Associate Professor of Medicine
Vanderbilt University School of Medicine
Nashville, Tennessee
26: Screening for Esophageal Squamous Cell
    Carcinoma

Ricardo Zorron, MD, PhD
Professor of Surgery, University UNIRIO,
    UENF;
Director, Center for Innovative Surgery-ZIC,
    Center for Bariatric and Metabolic
    Surgery;
Department of Surgery, Campus Charité
    Mitte/Campus Virchow-Klinikum
Charité-Universitätsmedizin Berlin
Berlin, Germany
45: Intramural and Transmural Endoscopy

Welcome to the third edition of *Clinical Gastrointestinal Endoscopy*. Gastrointestinal endoscopy is a continuously evolving field with the advent of new technologies, refined techniques, and new applications. The prior editions of this book have been universally regarded as a comprehensive guide to the latest endoscopic techniques. Understanding and adoption of such practices leads to optimal outcomes with endoscopy. This text is unique because of the breadth of topics covered by experts in every discipline of gastrointestinal endoscopy from across the globe. *Clinical Gastrointestinal Endoscopy* has been an essential resource for anyone interested in learning about endoscopic procedures, as one can access a variety of topics in succinct, easily understood chapters from content specialists.

This edition marks the transition to a new editorial team and builds on the success of the two prior editions. The previous editions achieved great accolade due to the efforts of the editorial board lead by Gregory Ginsberg and coedited by Michael Kochman, Ian Norton, and Christopher Gostout. The new editorial team was selected due to their expertise in gastrointestinal endoscopy, enthusiasm for disseminating best practices to a worldwide audience, and diverse background of training and experience from different premiere institutions. Commensurate with the change in the editors, we were excited to invite a new set of content experts who share their insights into recent advances in endoscopy and the impact these innovations have had on improving patient care. This has led to an exciting, comprehensive textbook from today's most prestigious specialists.

Clinical Gastrointestinal Endoscopy, third edition, is divided into three main sections covering Equipment and General Principles of Endoscopy, Luminal Gastrointestinal Disorders, and Pancreaticobiliary Disorders. Section I elegantly describes the history of gastrointestinal endoscopy and then provides primers on how endoscopes, endoscopic devices, and endoscopy units function. There are many applicable practice-changing pearls of wisdom in this section. Section II: Luminal Gastrointestinal Disorders covers both benign and malignant disorders as well as emerging endoscopic areas. Section III: Pancreaticobiliary Disorders details standard and advanced techniques in ERCP and EUS for the diagnosis and management of benign and malignant disorders of the pancreaticobiliary systems.

Each chapter has been meticulously crafted to present relevant updates to the topic in a manner that is easy to read and readily retained. These chapters are filled with tips that will help deliver optimal care for your patients. In addition, the content has been enhanced with new images and illustrations to highlight recent major advances in endoscopic techniques and applications for the latest technologies. These images and pictures can be downloaded from the book's website so that you can use them in your presentations. Furthermore, most topics have accompanying videos demonstrating the diagnostic and therapeutic endoscopic procedures. This media platform allows the reader to experience endoscopic procedures firsthand when accessing the content from their handheld device or computer. Each video clip has been meticulously edited to maximize the educational value.

The authors and editors draw upon their collective experience to provide you with the most current, authoritative, and impactful content for the sole purpose of enhancing the education of gastrointestinal endoscopy for years to come.

Vinay Chandrasekhara, MD

CONTENTS

VIDEO CONTENTS

Equipment and General Principles of Endoscopy

The History of Gastrointestinal Endoscopy

James L. Achord and V. Raman Muthusamy

CHAPTER OUTLINE

INTRODUCTION

The role of the physician is to observe, detect anatomic abnormalities or disease, and conceive ways and means by which discovered deficiencies in function can be corrected or ameliorated. To extend the physical examination to areas hidden from external view, such as within body orifices, presents a problem of safe and effective access. In insatiable attempts to accomplish these goals, there is no human orifice along with its recesses that has not been inspected, probed, prodded, and otherwise examined over the centuries. It was a compelling necessity to develop safe, nonsurgical methods to accomplish this purpose. Before the 20th century, numerous attempts to access these hidden cavities were plagued by instrumentation that was inadequate and dangerous. The history of every science or technical development is invariably a series of small discoveries or innovations, often in fields remote from those under investigation. Small improvements, each resulting in incremental gains, lead toward the idealized goal. Often, changes that appear to be an advance are found to be an impediment by further discoveries, and we recognize that a different way is better. Therefore, the task is never ending.

The term *endoscopy* comes from the Greek prefix *endo-* ("within") and the verb *skopein* ("to view or observe"). In this chapter, we summarize major developments over the years in gastrointestinal (GI) endoscopy to the present. As in any summary, the contributions of some individuals inevitably are not cited, and we offer our apologies to these individuals.

SEQUENTIAL HISTORY OF ENDOSCOPY

The visual exploration and examination of body orifices date to at least Egyptian and later Greco-Roman times, during which mechanical specula for viewing the vagina and anus were developed and used to a limited extent. Further progress was delayed by lack of sufficiently strong metals and the ability to form them into usable instruments, as well as the lack of adequate illumination. These initial efforts were directed at the genitourinary (GU) tract, with cavities that were only a short and relatively straight distance from the exterior.

Bozini (1805) is credited with the earliest known attempt to visualize the interior of a body cavity with a primitive endoscope (Fig. 1.1).[1-3] Bozini devised a tin tube illuminated by a candle from which light was reflected by a mirror; this was a device he called a *lichtleiter* (light conductor). He used this device to examine the urethra, urinary bladder, and vagina, but it was an impractical instrument that never gained wide acceptance. Although there were multiple attempts to develop more usable instruments, all directed toward the GU tract, none were widely used. The most notable efforts were by Segalas in France in 1826 and Fisher in Boston in 1827,[2] both using straight metal tubes, but the lack of a satisfactory light source remained a major impediment.

The next significant development was the instrument of Desormeaux in France.[2] Desormeaux's contribution in 1855 was a better, although still inadequate, light source using a lamp fueled with alcohol and turpentine ("gazogene") (Fig. 1.2). His instrument was based on that of Segalas. Others continued with efforts to improve the light source and the means to deliver it, but the devices were unsatisfactory for the more inaccessible areas of the GI tract.

Rigid Gastrointestinal Endoscopes

Kussmaul is credited as being the first to perform a gastroscopy in 1868, using a straight rigid metal tube passed over a flexible obturator and a cooperative sword swallower (Fig. 1.3).[1-4] For a light source, he used a mirror reflecting light from the

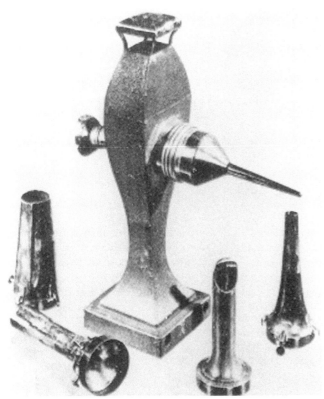

FIG 1.1 Bozzini's lichtleiter, 1805. (From Edmonson JM: History of the instruments for gastrointestinal endoscopy. *Gastrointest Endosc* 37[Suppl 2]:S27–S56, 1991.)

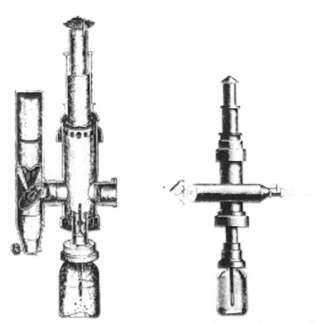

FIG 1.2 Desormeaux's endoscope, 1853. (From Edmonson JM: History of the instruments for gastrointestinal endoscopy. *Gastrointest Endosc* 37[Suppl 2]:S27–S56, 1991.)

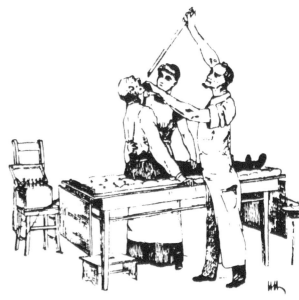

FIG 1.3 Kussmaul's gastroscope, 1868. (From Edmonson JM: History of the instruments for gastrointestinal endoscopy. *Gastrointest Endosc* 37[Suppl 2]:S27–S56, 1991.)

Desormeaux device but found it inadequate. He also quickly discovered that gastric secretions were a problem, despite using a flexible tube he had developed earlier to empty the stomach before the procedure. The value of his efforts was the demonstration that the curves and bends of the esophagus and esophago-

gastric junction could be traversed with careful manipulation and that the gastric pouch could be visualized. Kussmaul apparently demonstrated his "gastroscope" several times, but the illumination was too poor to allow a clinically useful image,[4] and he abandoned his efforts.

Encouraged by the efforts of Kussmaul, others switched their attention to developing esophagoscopes because the esophagus is much easier to visualize, and a less complex design than the gastroscope was required. The problems of perforation, at that time usually fatal, and of illumination, remained major obstacles. Before the late 19th century, illumination of light reflected by a mirror into a straight metal tube continued to be used. As noted earlier, several light sources were developed, but the intensity left much to be desired. Several innovations were developed to solve this problem, including a burning magnesium wire, which produced a brilliant light but unacceptable heat and smoke. The most promising device seemed to be the brilliant light from a loop of platinum wire charged with direct current, introduced simultaneously by Bruck in Breslau and Milliot of Paris in 1882.[2] Although the illumination was adequate, major difficulties were encountered with the considerable heat generated, necessitating a water cooling system and the cumbersome batteries used for a power source. Nevertheless, the platinum wire device was an encouraging development and was used in several instruments that saw relatively widespread use.

These instruments were made obsolete just a few years later by Edison's incandescent electric light bulb, introduced in 1879. In 1886, Leiter, an instrument maker, was the first to use the electric incandescent light bulb in a cystoscope just 7 years after Edison introduced it. With a few short-lived exceptions, all instruments used Edison's invention after 1886. Working with Leiter, von Mikulicz developed an unsuccessful gastroscope but a practical esophagoscope that he used extensively until distracted by his many other medical interests.

At the turn of the 20th century, Jackson, an otolaryngologist, also examined the esophagus and the stomach using a straight rigid tube and a distal electric light bulb, but few could match his talents in the GI tract. Under his influence, esophagoscopy was considered the exclusive province of ear, nose, and throat (ENT) departments in many community hospitals in the United States as late as the 1950s. The design of the esophagoscope remained a straight rigid tube, usually with a rubber finger-tipped obturator to make insertion safer. With the later addition of a 4 × power lens on the proximal end and a distal incandescent bulb, various models were popular until the introduction of fiberoptics in 1961. The Eder-Hufford rigid esophagoscope (Fig. 1.4), introduced in 1949, was popular and still in use in the early 1960s.

It was not until after 1900 that persistent efforts to develop a usable gastroscope were successful. All attempts to build a flexible instrument using a multiplicity of lenses were designed to be straightened after introduction and were fragile, easily damaged, and cumbersome. Straight tubes with simpler optics were useful, but perforations were still a problem.[1] In 1911, Elsner introduced a rigid gastroscope with an outer tube through which a separate inner optical tube with a flexible rubber tip and side-viewing portal could be passed (Fig. 1.5). The rubber tip, previously used in the esophagoscope obturator, was more crucial than it might appear, for it seemed to be, along with the later

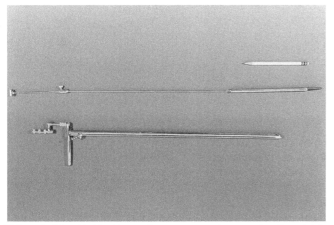

FIG 1.4 Eder-Hufford esophagoscope, the result of multiple attempts to develop a clinically useful instrument, 1949.

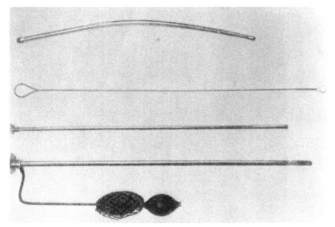

FIG 1.5 Elsner's gastroscope, 1911. (From Edmonson JM: History of the instruments for gastrointestinal endoscopy. *Gastrointest Endosc* 37[Suppl 2]:S27–S56, 1991.)

addition of a flexible metal coil proximal to it, the single feature that reduced the rate of perforation. Elsner's instrument worked as designed and was widely used, especially by Schindler, then in his native Germany, who called it the "mother of all instruments until 1932."[5]

In 1922, Schindler introduced his own version of the Elsner gastroscope, the major innovation of which was the important addition of an air channel to clear the lens of secretions. With the Elsner gastroscope, Schindler examined the stomachs of several hundred patients and meticulously recorded his findings in each procedure. He published *Lehrbuch und Atlas der Gastreoskopie* in 1923, with descriptions and remarkably accurate drawings. He trained others in the technique and was responsible for wide acceptance of gastroscopy. The procedure began with emptying the stomach using a nasogastric tube, followed by sedation. The patient was placed on the left side, and an assistant held the head rigidly extended to produce a straight path into the esophagus and the stomach (the "sword swallower's technique"). The role of the assistant was crucial. Schindler's effort was impressive and convinced many of the value of an expert examination of the stomach.

Semiflexible Gastroscopes

It became apparent that straight, rigid tubes were not ideal for examination of the stomach. Fatal perforations continued to the detriment of acceptance of the procedure. Visualization of the surface of the stomach was incomplete at best, with many consistent blind spots. These problems stimulated investigation of methods to manufacture safer, "flexible" instruments. The use of the term *flexible* here is problematic in view of what we think of today as flexible instruments. Although these early instruments were not flexible by our standards, they were more flexible than the straight, rigid instruments that came before. *Semiflexible*, with passive angulation of the distal portion of 34 degrees and sometimes more, was a more appropriate term.

In 1911, Hoffman showed that an image could be transmitted through a curved line by linking several short-focus prisms. Using this principle, several instruments were constructed, but these were unsatisfactory or were not widely accepted. Schindler, working with Wolf, the renowned instrument maker, constructed a semiflexible instrument with a rigid proximal portion and a distal portion made elastic by coiled copper wire and terminating with first a rubber finger and later a small rubber ball. Illumination was with a distal incandescent light bulb. Air insufflation was made possible with a rubber bulb, expanding the stomach wall to beyond the focal length of the prisms, which were manufactured by Zeiss. In 1932, the sixth and final version was patented. This instrument, known as the Wolf-Schindler gastroscope, greatly improved the safety and efficacy of gastroscopy and was used throughout the world (Fig. 1.6).

Thanks to the published meticulous work and enthusiasm of Schindler, whose designation as the "father of gastroscopy" is well deserved, the procedure was finally widely accepted as a valuable extension of the physical examination. The era of the semiflexible gastroscope from 1932 to 1957 has been called *the Schindler era*. Schindler was chiefly responsible for transforming gastroscopy from a dangerous and seldom used procedure to one that was relatively safe and indispensable for evaluation of known or suspected disease of the stomach. He insisted that all clinicians who planned to use the instrument be properly trained and that "… no manipulation inside of the body is without danger; therefore no endoscopic examination should be done

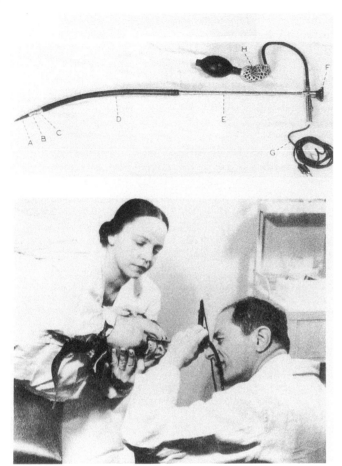

FIG 1.6 Wolf-Schindler "flexible" gastroscope *(top)* being used by Schindler *(bottom)* with his wife as the head holder. (From Edmonson JM: History of the instruments for gastrointestinal endoscopy. *Gastrointest Endosc* 37[Suppl 2]:S27–S56, 1991.)

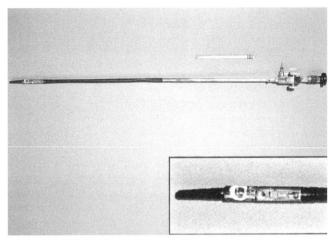

FIG 1.7 Benedict operating gastroscope.

without reasonable indication."[6] In today's vernacular, the risk approaches infinity if the benefit approaches zero.

Schindler was born in Berlin in 1888. He gained considerable experience as an Army physician in World War I, where he became convinced that gastritis, then an often-disparaged cause of symptoms, was a bona fide disease. His interest in gastritis lasted throughout his career and undoubtedly stimulated his interest in gastroscopy. The Wolf-Schindler endoscope of 1932 and Schindler's publications with drawings further enhanced what thereafter rapidly became a discipline. His enthusiasm for and talent in using the gastroscope led to what has been called his *gospel of gastroscopy*, which he and others spread throughout academia and to the community of practicing physicians. Because of his Jewish background, Schindler was put in "protective custody" by the Nazis, but with the help of the physicians Ortmeyer and Palmer and philanthropists in Chicago, he was able to immigrate to the United States in 1934.[1–4,7]

Chicago became the hub of GI endoscopy, and it was here, in Schindler's home, that the first discussions were held about forming a new organization for GI endoscopy, now known, after several name changes, as the *American Society of Gastrointestinal Endoscopy*. In 1943, just 9 years after his arrival in the United States, Schindler left Chicago for Loma Linda University. In 1958, he accepted an appointment as Professor of Medicine at the

University of Minas Gerais in Belo Horizonte, Brazil. He came back to the United States in 1960 because of an eventually fatal illness of his wife and returned to his native Berlin in 1964, where he died in 1968 at the age of 80.[1] Despite his acclaim in endoscopy, Schindler insisted that one must be a physician first and an endoscopist second. He was very knowledgeable in the field of general gastroenterology and published, without coauthors, a synopsis of the entire field in 1957.[6]

The Wolf-Schindler endoscope was introduced into the United States by Benedict, Borland, and many others. Schindler's immigration to Chicago inspired a surge of interest in the United States, but with the outbreak of war in Europe, the German source of instruments disappeared. Several US companies working with Schindler and others produced many popular gastroscopes that were significant variations on the Wolf-Schindler model, including Cameron Co., which produced its first instrument in 1940.[8] The Eder-Hufford semiflexible gastroscope followed in 1946,[9] and American Cystoscope Makers, Inc. (ACMI) produced a gastroscope in 1950. A combination of the Eder-Hufford esophagoscope with a semiflexible gastroscope to be passed through it was the Eder-Palmer transesophagoscopic flexible gastroscope produced by the Eder Company in 1953. Each gastroscope had its proponents.

Biopsy

With the availability of instruments for visualization, it became apparent that tissue must be obtained to identify the nature of the observed abnormalities. Instruments for blind biopsies were used early on, but a device was needed that would allow the operator to obtain a biopsy specimen of abnormal tissue directly when seen at endoscopy. The Benedict Operating Gastroscope was produced in 1948 based on a 1940 model by Kenamore (Fig. 1.7).[10] The Benedict instrument was a popular instrument that was widely used. In the debates about the necessity for biopsy, Benedict, a surgeon who switched entirely to endoscopy, stated that gastroscopy was not a routine procedure and should be reserved for those with a complex differential diagnosis, but "gastroscopic examination is not complete unless the gastroscopist has some means of biopsy readily available."[11] It soon became clear that the correlation between histology and a diagnosis based on visualization alone was often widely discrepant, and certain diagnoses could not be reliably made without tissue examination.

Efforts such as wash and brush cytology continued and have persisted in various forms to the present time.

Fiberoptics

By the 1950s, the ideal of a totally flexible GI endoscope with good visualization that could withstand the rigors of clinical use had not been realized, although the semi-flexible instruments with their biopsy capabilities were satisfactory for most clinical purposes. In fact, these instruments were not rapidly abandoned by all with the introduction of the remarkably flexible fiberscope. The development of the science of fiberoptics and its application to endoscopes truly revolutionized the diagnostic and, later, the therapeutic abilities of endoscopy. Its importance in the development of this field cannot be overstated.

The principle of internal reflection of light along a conduction pathway was used by Lamm in October 1930.[1] The image was severely degraded by light escaping from the thin fibers of quartz he used, although the potential for total flexibility was present. Lamm could not interest Schindler or others in his efforts, and the experiment was discontinued. Almost 25 years later, in 1954, Hirschowitz, in fellowship training at the University of Michigan, visited Hopkins and Kapany in London to review their work[12] with glass fibers, which totally confirmed the work of Lamm and his predecessors. Hirschowitz became convinced that application of this principle could be used to develop a totally new and superior endoscope. He began work with a graduate student, Curtiss, who developed a technique of coating glass fibers with glass of a different optical density, preventing the escape of light and degradation of the image. This was the critical discovery that made the principle of internal reflection through glass fibers workable.

In 1957, Hirschowitz demonstrated his fiberscope, and he published his work in 1958 (Fig. 1.8).[13] His audience was not impressed, and it took another 3 years, working with ACMI, to produce a marketable scope, which he called the *Hirschowitz*

Gastroduodenal Fiberscope. This was a very flexible side-viewing instrument with an electric light on its distal end, an air channel, and an adjustable focusing lens proximally. The tip lacked what was by then the "obligatory" rubber finger, and this omission was a source of criticism; one was added on a later model. Although some individuals criticized the quality of the image, most believed the size and brightness were superior to the semiflexible scopes. This model, the ACMI 4990, was introduced to the market late in 1960 after being tested by Hirschowitz on himself and numerous patients. In 1961, the senior author of this chapter was in a gastroenterology fellowship at the Emory University Clinic with Schroder. He vividly recalls Schroder's reaction after the first use of the new fiberscope around March 1962 (Fig. 1.9). Upon finishing the initial examination using the new device, he turned to him and said, "Anybody want to buy a used Benedict operating scope?" The senior author does not recall it ever being used again, as the Hirschowitz Gastroduodenal Fiberscope was clearly superior in his view, and he finished his training with that instrument.

There were problems with the fiberscope noted by users. The distal light source would become so heated that thermal injury to the gastric mucosa was possible unless the tip was continuously moved. In prolonged procedures, protein in gastric secretions would coagulate on the bulb and the adjacent visualizing port, totally obscuring the lens. As the number of procedures with a single instrument increased, some glass fibers would break, producing small black dots in the visual field. This was a persistent problem with fiberscopes during their entire history and especially apparent in training programs where a single scope was used by several trainees on many patients. The side-viewing lens prevented visualization of the esophagus, and the scope had to be passed blindly through the pharyngeal orifice. The previous semiflexible scopes in use shared this problem, and it was not considered a defect at the time. The flexibility itself resulted in some difficulty in advancing because attempts to push the instrument through the pylorus and into the gut resulted in more bowing in the gastric pouch (Fig. 1.10). Although one could sometimes visualize the duodenum, this was done by overinflating the stomach and looking through the pylorus without actually entering it. If one managed to introduce the tip into the duodenum, as occasionally happened, the visual field was inside the focal length of the instrument, and only a "red-out" was observed.[4]

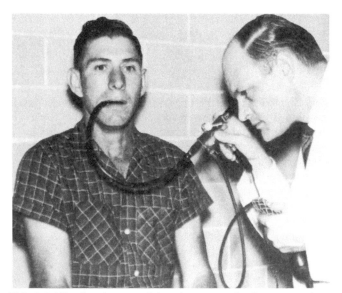

FIG 1.8 Hirschowitz examining the stomach of an outpatient. (From Hirschowitz BI: Endoscopic examination of the stomach and duodenal cap with the fiberscope. *Lancet* 277[7186]:1074–1078, 1961.)

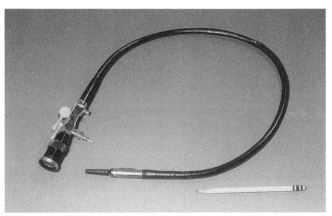

FIG 1.9 ACMI fiberscope, 1962.

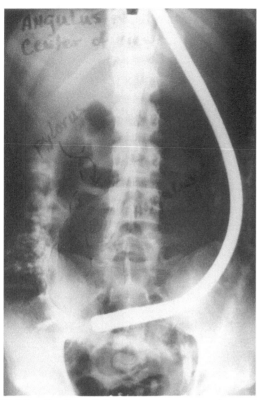

FIG 1.10 Visualization of duodenum was sometimes obtained by overinflating the stomach.

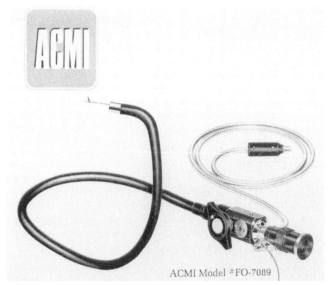

FIG 1.11 LoPresti forward-viewing esophagogastroscope. (From advertisement in *Gastrointest Endosc* 16:79, 1970.)

Many clinicians did not believe the additional expense of replacing the older, beloved instruments with which they had been successful for many years was warranted. Even ACMI officials did not see the fiberscope as totally replacing the instruments with a lens system.[2] Despite reservations, comparison and experiential studies showed the advantages of the new fiberscopes.[14–17] Following the flagship ACMI model 4990, several models of the fiberscope were introduced by ACMI and other companies, each with significant improvements, including the controllable tip in the side-viewing ACMI model 5004. Visualization of the gastric pouch, including retroflexed views of the cardia, was now complete. The major objection to these instruments was the inability to pass the instrument under direct vision and examine the esophagus; in addition, the area beyond the pylorus could not be consistently examined.

Most clinicians were already fully trained in use of the Eder-Hufford esophagoscope, and in the absence of a forward-viewing fiberscope, use of the Eder-Hufford esophagoscope continued. A forward-viewing scope was mandatory. LoPresti modified the tip of the fiberscope to create the foroblique fiberoptic esophagoscope in 1964.[18] Passing the instrument under direct vision was possible, and clinicians immediately discovered that they could examine not only the esophagus, but also a large portion of the proximal stomach. At a length of 90 cm, however, one could not reach the duodenum. Working with ACMI, LoPresti produced the longer Panview Mark "87" gastroesophageal endoscope in 1970. By about 1971, the instrument had been lengthened to 105 cm with a four-way controllable tip capable of 180 degrees of deflection (Fig. 1.11).

The aptly named *panendoscope* was now a reality. Japanese and American manufacturers began to produce new models with such rapidity that endoscopists hardly had time to become thoroughly familiar with one before another, significantly improved (and more expensive) model was on the market. Patient comfort was greatly improved, and the relative safety of the fiberoptic endoscopes rapidly became apparent. By 1970, most gastroscopic examinations were done with fiberscopes. The development of a "teaching head" fiberoptic bundle with a light splitter and attached eyepiece and attachment to the eyepiece of the scope allowed two people to visualize the image. Dividing the light from the endoscope considerably diminished the brightness of the image, however, to both the operator and the observer. This device saw limited use and was utilized primarily in teaching institutions.

Endoscopic Retrograde Cholangiopancreatography (ERCP)

With access to the duodenum, the ampulla of Vater became visible. It followed that one should be able to inject contrast material into the bile and pancreatic ducts and increase diagnostic capabilities. Initial attempts in 1968 by McCune et al[19] to modify an existing scope were only partially successful, but did show that endoscopic visualization by injection of radiologic contrast agents into ducts was possible. In 1970, Machida and Olympus in Japan produced usable, side-viewing scopes with controllable tips and elevators to move the injection tube to the ampulla.

Japanese endoscopists[20] developed the technique of endoscopic retrograde cholangiopancreatography (ERCP) with an 80% success rate. Vennes and Silvis[21] showed the utility of ERCP in the United States and taught many physicians to use it.[4] It was immediately apparent that if clinicians could visualize the biliary and pancreatic ducts endoscopically (i.e., nonsurgically), they should be able to apply by some means long-established surgical techniques for treatment of choledocholithiasis and pancreatitis, such as sphincterotomy and stone removal. In 1974, just 4 years after the demonstration of the diagnostic utility of the new ERCP scopes, Kawai et al in Japan[22] and Classen and Demling in Germany[23] independently developed methods of endoscopic electrosurgical sphincterotomy for extraction of biliary calculi in the common duct. This procedure requires great skill; in 1976, Geenen[24] reported that only 62 operative procedures had been done by four endoscopists, and seven of the procedures were failures. In 1983, Schuman[4] reported that several thousands of patients had undergone ERCP, and by now, hundreds of thousands of ERCP procedures have been done. Because of advances in radiologic techniques, ERCP is now seldom used for purely diagnostic purposes.

Photography

It is one thing to describe to others what one may see through any device and another to be able to show them. The large impact of Schindler's early publications was related, in part, to the excellent color drawings he presented. Early on, neither cameras nor photographic films were advanced enough to allow good color reproduction or sharp, accurate images in relatively poor lighting. Such documentation is essential for widespread appreciation of endoscopy by individuals who do not perform the procedure. The first clinically useful photography came with improvements in film by Kodak and the construction of an external integrated camera by Segal and Watson in 1948.[25,26] Although these authors reported that approximately 61% of the images were of good quality, this was not the experience of all clinicians.[4]

Although an intragastric camera was developed as early as 1848 by Lange and Meltzung, a clinically useful device was not available until 1950, when Uji, Sugiura, and Fukami, working with Olympus Corp. (Center Valley, PA),[27] developed the Gastrocamera with synchronized flash, which took good intragastric pictures and had a controllable distal portion. By following a prescribed pattern of rotation and flexion, a series of pictures was obtained that included the entire surface of the stomach. The big disadvantage was that the operator could not see through the instrument and had to await development of the very narrow (5-mm) film before the results could be seen. Photographs for demonstration required additional time in the photo laboratory while enlargements were made.

After the introduction of fiberoptic scopes in 1961, Olympus introduced a combination Gastrocamera fiberscope (GTF-A) in 1964, but, as Schuman[4] commented, "it was *just* a gastroscope" and never attained popularity. Simultaneously, rapid development and physician acceptance of fiberscopes with the ability to use technically advanced 35-mm cameras with an external adapter made the Gastrocamera obsolete, and it was abandoned.

Sigmoidoscopy and Colonoscopy

The problems presented by examination of the anus and rectum were relatively easy. Straight metal tubes were used and found in the ruins of Pompeii.[2] The basic design of the anoscope has not changed in the past century or more except that it is now made of disposable plastic. It remains a tapering short tube with an obturator that is removed after introduction through the anal sphincter. Examination of the rectum and sigmoid required a longer tube, but no truly satisfactory device was available until 1894, when Kelly[28] at Johns Hopkins developed a 30-cm rigid tube with light reflected down the tube from a head lamp. Tuttle[29] incorporated a distal light source in his proctosigmoidoscope of 25 cm in 1903. These instruments have remained the basic design for the past 100 years. For the past 25 years or so, disposable

clear plastic tubes have been widely used. These are essentially a plastic version of the Kelly and Tuttle tubes with a distal electric light source, but visualization is possible through the clear plastic. With the application of fiberoptics to sigmoidoscopy in the late 1960s, examination of the sigmoid colon became not only satisfactory, but also much more comfortable for the patient.

Overholt,[30] who later went on to be the principal developer of colonoscopy using similar technology, presented his results of flexible sigmoidoscopy in 250 patients in 1968. Although early flexible sigmoidoscopes were made in variable lengths, the current length of 60 cm came to be the preferred one. Examination of the colon above the sigmoid presents obvious additional problems of multiple curves and angulations amenable only to highly flexible instruments and trained operators. Attempts, all unsuccessful, were made using semiflexible instruments, and these are reviewed by Edmonson.[2] Satisfactory examination of the length of the colon was impossible until the introduction of the flexible fiberscope. Attempts to use forward-viewing gastroscopes were not technically satisfactory, although several clinicians tried. Turell[31] presented his attempts in 1967 using a modified gastroscope, but he concluded that the instrument was not ready for routine clinical use. By 1970, several manufacturers produced instruments specifically designed for colonoscopy, including ACMI working with Overholt in the United States and Olympus Corporation in Japan.

The primary problem with regularly completing examinations to the cecum was not the instruments so much as it was the techniques necessary for passage of the scopes into the more proximal portions of the colon. Earlier pioneers in developing successful techniques still in use include, among others, Overholt, Wolf, Shinya, and Waye in the United States; Niwa and colleagues in Japan; Salmon and Williams in England; and Dehyle in Germany.[4] Many of these early efforts were accomplished with the guidance of fluoroscopy to negotiate the more difficult turns and to identify the actual area being observed, but, as experience was gained, fluoroscopy was no longer required. Learning under expert guidance and experience continues to be more necessary in colonoscopy (and ERCP) than in upper endoscopy. By 1971, the diagnostic advantage of fiberoptic colonoscopy over single-contrast barium enema was firmly established,[32] and the efficacy and safety of polypectomy were established by 1973.[33]

Digital Endoscopy (Videoendoscopy)

In 1984, barely 20 years after introduction of the endoscopic fiberscope, Welch Allyn, Inc. (Skaneateles Falls, NY), replaced the coherent fiberoptic image bundle in a colonoscope with a light-sensitive computer chip or charge-coupled device on which the image was focused by a small lens (see Chapter 3).[34] The digital signal was fed to a video processor, which generated an image to a television monitor. The image did not occupy the entire screen, leaving space for information to be typed in by a keyboard. The resolution of the image was at least equal to that of the fiberscope.

It was unnecessary to change the basic mechanics of the fiberscope. The fiberoptic light bundle remained unchanged, as did water, suction, and biopsy channels; in addition, the deflection and locking mechanisms were the same. The basic elements of the videoendoscope have not changed, although a magnified image is now available. Since the original introduction of the videoendoscope by Welch Allyn, which no longer produces the Video Endoscope, the market has been supplied by Olympus, Pentax, and Fujinon. The technology was rapidly adapted to

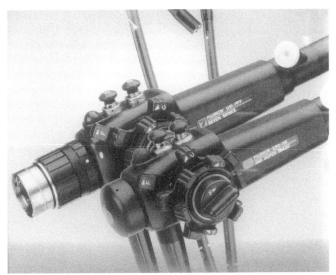

FIG 1.12 Fujinon fiberoptic panendoscope *(top)* and its successor, the Videopanendoscope *(bottom),* 1990, showing the two kinds of operating heads. (From advertisement in *Gastrointest Endosc* 36:240–241, 1990.)

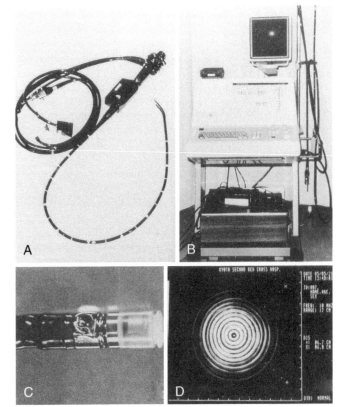

FIG 1.13 **A** to **D,** Ultrasonic endoscope system, model IV, made by Olympus Corp., 1986. (From Yasuda K, Mukai H, Fujimoto S, et al: The diagnosis of pancreatic cancer by endoscopic ultrasonography. *Gastrointest Endosc* 34:1–8, 1988.)

all endoscopes, used not only in gastroenterology but also in other fields.

Advantages of the electronic instruments include an image that can be seen not only by the operator, but also by anyone with access to a connected monitor in the same or another room. This feature greatly enhanced the ability to teach others about the procedure and to inform other interested physicians about the findings in the individual patient. If desired, recording of procedures could be accomplished with videotape machines, and good-quality pictures of individual frames could be made immediately with externally integrated digital equipment. Individual endoscopists found that no adjustment of techniques was necessary when videoendoscopes were used, although they had to become accustomed to looking at the monitor screen rather than through an optical system with one eye (Fig. 1.12). This feature added to the useful length of the instrument because the whole scope could be held at the waist rather than being brought to eye level.

More recent innovations in colonoscopy instruments by Olympus include the ability to make a portion less flexible to facilitate navigation of difficult bends and turns. In addition, an enlarged image is now available that is an improvement in vision and ease of manipulation. A major disadvantage of videoendoscopes is cost. Fiberoptic endoscopes, when they were still in use, could be purchased for less than $6000 and did not require processors or monitors, whereas the latest videoendoscopes are priced at more than $20,000, and initial purchase of the entire package of endoscope, processing computer, monitors, and attachments may exceed $30,000. Initially, many questioned the wisdom of this added cost, which is passed on to the patient and their insurance companies.

Endoscopic Ultrasonography (EUS)

Although the improvements in GI endoscopy are remarkable in the synthesis of diverse but complementary technologies, the information gained remains confined to what one can see from within the lumen of the gut. Simultaneous with these developments were those of computed tomography and external ultrasonographic tomograms. Conceptually, it was not only logical but also compelling to look beneath the mucosa of the gut by incorporating miniaturized models of ultrasonographic transducers already in use into GI endoscopes. The ability to noninvasively explore tissue and organs in proximity to the gut had exciting implications for diagnosis and therapy.

In Germany in 1976, working with Siemens Co., (Berlin, Germany) Lutz and Rosch[35] reported the use of a 1-cm ultrasonographic 4-MHz probe that could be passed through the biopsy channel of an Olympus TGF. They used it in two patients to successfully differentiate between pancreatic pseudocysts and tumors.[7] In 1980, Classen's group in Germany[36] and DiMagno et al[37] at the Mayo Clinic reported EUS devices that were incorporated onto the tip of conventional fiberscopes, one using a 5-MHz transducer and the other using a 10-MHz transducer. These probes had good resolution at an acoustic focus depth of 3 cm. Others incorporated the transducer in the distal shaft of fiberoptic scopes and primarily explored the gut wall.[33,38] By 1985, ultrasonic transducers with variable frequencies incorporated into videoendoscopes were readily available, although expensive (> $100,000 for initial setup) (Fig. 1.13). It was immediately apparent that this procedure could accurately evaluate known or suspected intramural lesions of the gut,[39,40] and it was rapidly expanded to include the esophagus; problems of diagnosis and recurrence of neoplasia, especially in the pancreas; portal hypertension; the colon and rectum; and bile ducts.[41] In 1991, Wiersema et al[42,43] showed that EUS could be used to obtain fine-needle aspiration cytology of mediastinal nodes and of nodes and lesions of the upper and lower GI tract. The addition of Doppler technology has now made possible the study of the flow through various structures, including the thoracic duct and blood vessels. EUS is increasingly being used to provide therapy, leading to the development of "interventional EUS." EUS-guided interventions include celiac plexus block/neurolysis, placement of fiducial markers to facilitate radiotherapy, direct injection of alcohol or chemotherapeutic agents for the treatment of tumors or cystic lesions, drainage of the pancreatic or biliary ductal systems, and the creation of gastrojejunal anastomoses using lumen-apposing metal stents. The techniques of using EUS instruments differ only slightly from using videoendoscopes, but dedicated training is necessary to interpret the sonographic images obtained accurately. EUS is not amenable to self-instruction. EUS training centers have been established in academic centers, but retraining of practicing physicians is challenging due to the duration of training necessary to achieve competence.[44]

Capsule Endoscopy (Wireless Endoscopy)

In 2000, Iddan et al[45] reported the development of a capsule containing a tiny CMOS camera that could be swallowed, obtain images (at 2 frames per second), and transmit the images over 7 hours to a receiving digital storage unit worn by the patient as he or she goes about his or her normal activities. These frames are downloaded to a computer from which they are projected onto a monitor at a rate that can be controlled by the observer. Pictures can be printed of areas of interest. Gastroenterologists in Israel conducted randomized trials comparing the efficacy of the wireless capsule with push enteroscopy and obtained superior results with the capsule.[46–48]

Wireless capsule endoscopy caught the imagination of gastroenterologists over the world, and capsule endoscopy has been adopted as a part of standard practice for small bowel imaging. The findings are virtually unanimous in demonstrating better results in identifying lesions in the small bowel with capsule endoscopy when compared to push enteroscopy.[49] The capsule avoids the discomfort and need for sedation inherent with push enteroscopy. In addition to lack of biopsy capability, an additional disadvantage is the time needed to review the study, but this has been overcome by a variety of methods including software advancements, improved training techniques, and utilizing non-physician personnel to initially review the obtained images. The major use of the capsule to date has been in elucidating the cause of occult bleeding from small bowel sources, where it seems to be superior to other methods. Future applications, such as in the colon, are continuing to be investigated in large, multicenter comparative studies. The future of wireless capsule endoscopy is bright. It will be interesting to see how the principle of wireless endoscopy is incorporated into videoendoscopes, such as the potential for a wireless connection between the endoscope and the image processor.

Enteroscopy

The small intestine has traditionally been regarded as the final frontier of GI endoscopy. Although capsule endoscopy provides remarkable images of the small bowel mucosa, tissue acquisition

and therapy with a capsule-based instrument is many years away. Surgically assisted small bowel enteroscopy may be performed via either the transoral or anal route or via a mid–small bowel enterotomy incision. The disadvantage of this technique is its invasive nature.[50] Endoscopic examination of the small intestine has remained technically difficult. The many loops of the small intestine prevent progression of the instrument tip by simple pushing. This problem was overcome initially with the use of the Sonde enteroscope,[51] which is a very fine, floppy instrument with a balloon at the tip. The Sonde enteroscope progressed through much of the small bowel under peristalsis, and then the proceduralist would slowly withdraw the instrument, assessing the mucosa while pulling back. This technique was thought to visualize 50% to 70% of the mucosal surface.[52] However, the procedure was uncomfortable, time-consuming, and did not permit therapeutics, all of which limited its use.

The concept of small bowel enteroscopy was revolutionized by Yamamoto with the introduction of the double-balloon enteroscope in 2001.[53] This technique uses traction between a balloon at the tip of the enteroscope and another balloon on a flexible overtube to fix the loops of small bowel and provide traction for forward movement. The procedure requires peroral and anal procedures to examine the entire small intestine, and even then only in a minority of Western patients is the whole small bowel visualized. Nonetheless, double-balloon–assisted enteroscopy permits endoscopic therapeutics to most of the small bowel without the need for surgical assistance. A single balloon version is also available.

Natural Orifice Transluminal Endoscopic Surgery (NOTES) and Peroral Endoscopy Myotomy (POEM)

A new development in endoscopy is natural orifice transluminal endoscopic surgery (NOTES), in which the endoscope is inserted into the abdominal cavity via an incision in an accessible organ. The first report appeared in 2002. Incisions have been made in the stomach, vagina, and colon with successful tubal ligation, liver biopsies, biopsy of peritoneal metastases, oophorectomy, cholecystectomy, and nephrectomy procedures having been performed. Most published articles report experimental use in animals, but more recent reports have described the simultaneous use of NOTES with laparoscopic techniques. Comparative studies are ongoing. A difficulty with the technique has been overcoming the lack of instrument "triangulation"; that is, approaching a surgical site from two or more directions to create countertraction, tie sutures, and so forth. Although NOTES is an exciting development, its remarkable potential will have to await the development of new instruments and the acquisition of additional expertise. At a minimum, it appears the development of NOTES will result in marked improvements in mucosal and transmural closure devices. Recently, flexible endoscopes have also been used to tunnel into the submucosal space of the esophagus and perform a myotomy, resulting in a treatment for achalasia termed peroral endoscopy myotomy, or POEM. First performed by Inoue in 2008 and reported by Inoue in 2010, this procedure has gained widespread popularity worldwide and has been performed thousands of times to date with impressive short- and long-term results and an excellent safety profile.[54,55] Additional applications of "submucosal" endoscopy include performing a similar procedure in the antrum to treat gastroparesis (G-POEM) and to perform resection of intramural lesions of the GI tract.[56,57]

SUMMARY

The development of endoscopy is a testimony to human ingenuity. Instruments have evolved from dangerous straight tubes illuminated by light reflected from candles, to more flexible and safer instruments with an image transmitted through a series of prism lenses and illumination by an electric light bulb, to images transmitted through fiberoptic bundles with illumination transmitted by fiber bundles from an external source, to our present remarkably safe electronic instruments with digital images transmitted to a video screen through wires and processed by computers. Most recently, we can visualize the lumen of the gut without touching the patient. Now we can not only visualize, biopsy tissue, and perform surgical procedures within the hidden cavities of the body, but also directly and indirectly see beneath the mucosa and into immediately adjacent organs. The evolution of gastrointestinal endoscopy is a truly remarkable story, and advances in the diagnostic and therapeutic capabilities of these instruments continue to be made at a rapid pace. To know and understand what has occurred previously lends strength to efforts toward achieving what is to come.

KEY REFERENCES

1. Modlin IM: *A brief history of endoscopy*, Milano, 2000, MultiMed.
2. Edmonson JM: History of the instruments for gastrointestinal endoscopy. *Gastrointest Endosc* 37:S27–S56, 1991.
6. Schindler R: *Synopsis of gastroenterology*, Philadelphia, 1957, Grune & Stratton.
7. Kirsner JB: American gastroscopy—yesterday and today. *Gastrointest Endosc* 37:643–648, 1991.
11. Benedict EB: Gastroscopic biopsy. *Gastroenterology* 37:447–448, 1959.
12. Hopkins HH, Kapany NS: A flexible fiberscope using static scanning. *Nature* 173:39–41, 1954.
13. Hirschowitz BI, Curtiss LE, Pollard HM: Demonstration of the new gastroscope, the "fiberscope." *Gastroenterology* 35:50–53, 1958.
15. Burnett W: An evaluation of the gastroduodenal fibrescope. *Gut* 3:361–365, 1962.
20. Takagi K, Ikeda S, Nakagawa Y, et al: Retrograde pancreatography and cholangiography by fiber duodenoscope. *Gastroenterology* 59:445–452, 1970.
21. Vennes JA, Silvis SE: Endoscopic visualization of bile and pancreatic ducts. *Gastrointest Endosc* 18:149–152, 1972.
22. Kawai K, Akasaka Y, Murakami K, et al: Endoscopic sphincterotomy of the ampulla of Vater. *Gastrointest Endosc* 20:148–151, 1974.
25. Segal HL, Watson JS: Color photography through the flexible gastroscope. *Gastroenterology* 10:575–585, 1948.
32. Wolff WI, Shinya H: Colonofiberoscopy. *JAMA* 217:1509–1512, 1971.
33. Wolff WI, Shinya H: Polypectomy via the fiberoptic colonoscope: Removal of neoplasms beyond the reach of the sigmoidoscope. *N Engl J Med* 288:329–332, 1973.
35. Lutz H, Rosch W: Transgastroscopic ultrasonography. *Endoscopy* 8:203–205, 1976.
37. DiMagno EP, Buxton JL, Regan PT, et al: Ultrasonic endoscope. *Lancet* 1:629–631, 1980.
42. Wiersema MJ, Hawes RH, Wiersema LM, et al: Endoscopic ultrasonography as an adjunct to fine needle aspiration cytology of the upper and lower gastrointestinal tract. *Gastrointest Endosc* 38:35–39, 1992.
43. Rex RK, Tarver RD, Wiersema M, et al: Endoscopic transesophageal fine needle aspiration of mediastinal masses. *Gastrointest Endosc* 37:465–468, 1991.
45. Iddan G, Meron G, Glukhovsky A, et al: Wireless capsule endoscopy. *Nature* 405:417, 2000.
47. Appleyard M, Glukhovsky A, Swain P, et al: Wireless-capsule diagnostic endoscopy for recurrent small-bowel bleeding. *N Engl J Med* 344:232–233, 2001.
53. Yamamoto H, Sekine Y, Saito Y: Total enteroscopy with a non-surgical, steerable double-balloon method. *Gastrointest Endosc* 53:216–220, 2001.
54. Inoue H, Minami H, Kobayashi Y, et al: Peroral endoscopic myotomy (POEM) for esophageal achalasia. *Endoscopy* 42:265–271, 2010.
55. ASGE Technology Committee, Pannala R, Abu Dayyeh BK, et al: Per-oral endoscopic myotomy (with video). *Gastrointest Endosc* 83(6):1051–1060, 2016.
56. Khashab MA, Stein E, Clarke JO, et al: Gastric peroral endoscopic myotomy for refractory gastroparesis: first human endoscopic pyloromyotomy (with video). *Gastrointest Endosc* 78(5):764–768, 2013.
57. Xu MD, Cai MY, Zhou PH, et al: Submucosal tunneling endoscopic resection: a new technique for treating upper GI submucosal tumors originating from the muscularis propria layer (with videos). *Gastrointest Endosc* 75(1):195–199, 2012.

A complete reference list can be found online at ExpertConsult.com

2

Setting Up an Endoscopy Facility

Klaus Mergener and Barry Tanner

INTRODUCTION

The safe and efficient performance of gastrointestinal (GI) endoscopy has the following requirements:
- A properly trained endoscopist[1] with appropriate privileges to perform specific GI endoscopic procedures[2,3]
- Properly trained nursing and ancillary personnel
- Operational, well-maintained equipment
- Adequately designed and equipped space for patient preparation, performance of procedures, and patient recovery
- Cleaning areas for reprocessing endoscopes and accessories
- Trained personnel and appropriate equipment to perform cardiopulmonary resuscitation
- A robust quality assurance/improvement program[4,5]

Many of the previously listed requirements for safe and efficient GI endoscopy depend on the careful planning and design of the endoscopy facility. This chapter describes that process, beginning with laying the groundwork, including the development of a business plan and review of regulatory issues; site selection; facility planning and design (including patient flow and space needs); equipment requirements; staffing needs; and scheduling considerations. Some additional issues, such as endoscope cleaning and storage, tissue specimen processing and handling, record keeping and documentation, and quality assurance and improvement, are discussed briefly but are covered in more detail in subsequent chapters of this book (see Chapters 4, 5, and 10).

EXPLORING POSSIBILITIES

Type of Facility

There are different types of endoscopy facilities, including hospital endoscopy units, single-specialty or multispecialty ambulatory surgery centers (ASCs), and office endoscopy suites. Each model has a unique set of advantages, disadvantages, and regulatory issues. The hospital and ASC environments are highly regulated by state and federal agencies and by third-party accreditation bodies. In the United States, these include The Joint Commission (JC), the Accreditation Association for Ambulatory Healthcare (AAAHC), and the American Association for Accreditation of Ambulatory Surgery Facilities (AAAASF). Commercial payers sometimes impose their own specific requirements. Office endoscopy suites, previously less regulated, have been subjected to more controls by state and federal agencies in recent years.

The decision regarding which type of facility to establish is affected by the practice environment (solo practitioner, small or large group, single-specialty or multispecialty group, independent or hospital-based) and local economics and politics. Regardless of the service location, high-quality care must be maintained. The American Society for Gastrointestinal Endoscopy (ASGE) has stated that the "standards for out-of-hospital endoscopic practice should be identical to those recognized guidelines followed in the hospital."[6] The hospital-based unit poses the fewest financial risks and demands for the endoscopist during the early phases of operation, and its use avoids alienating hospital administration by preserving hospital case volume. This environment, however, affords the endoscopist little control over operations, and offers him or her the lowest financial return. Office endoscopy offers control and convenience with better financial return for the physician, but it poses some safety and liability concerns.[7,8] A single-specialty endoscopic ambulatory surgery center (EASC) provides the best of control, efficiency, convenience, and reimbursement for the physician owners and is extremely popular with patients, referring physicians, and payers.[9,10] A major ASC payment reform implemented by the

Centers for Medicare and Medicaid Services (CMS) in 2008 resulted in drastic cuts of facility payments for endoscopic services.[11] Subsequently, the passage of the Affordable Care Act in 2010 led to massive hospital consolidation, which, in turn, resulted in significant increases in the prices hospitals demand for endoscopic services provided in hospital-based facilities.[12–14] How all of these changes will affect both the efforts and the ability to provide beneficial GI services to patients at a reasonable cost remains to be seen. More information about recent and ongoing health care reform efforts is available elsewhere.[15] Regardless of the type of facility being developed, formulating a business plan and understanding various regulatory issues are usually the first steps in the process.

Business Plan

The decision to set up an endoscopy facility should be made only after detailed data gathering and the formulation of a business plan (e.g., market analysis, financial pro forma, implementation time line).[16–18] For a hospital-based unit or academic medical center, facility planners and accountants often perform these functions. For an office-based suite or an EASC, the tasks fall to the physician owners, aided by numerous consultants, contractors, or corporate partners. Even with skilled help, however, development of an accurate and reliable business plan and pro forma are highly dependent on physician estimates, insights, and work habits. Physician input into the business plan makes the difference between a perfunctory exercise and an accurate predictor of future performance. Endoscopy facilities represent significant investments requiring substantial financial resources and staff. Procedure volume must be sufficient to produce adequate revenue to cover the costs of building and running the facility and to generate a profit on investment.

Many factors influence the financial performance of an endoscopy facility, including the size of the initial investment, expected volumes of service, revenue per unit of service, fixed operating costs, and variable costs per unit of service. The initial investment includes the cost of construction, equipment, and working capital for the first few months of operation. Strategic planning is important to anticipate group growth and demand for services in the next 5 to 10 years.[16,18] The impact on the GI practice of local competition and consolidation of health systems or major health plans must also be anticipated. In addition, population changes, demographics, and the possibility of new disruptive technologies might affect case volume for the practice and the endoscopy facility.

A pro forma is a calculation examining the financial feasibility of a project based on anticipated investment and operating costs and revenues. The purpose of the pro forma is to reliably predict cash flows and profitability for the project. Initial investment costs have been defined previously. Estimated total costs per case based on estimated fixed and variable costs and expected case volume are also incorporated in the pro forma. Fixed costs are costs that remain constant regardless of the number of procedures performed and include rent, interest, depreciation, taxes, insurance, amortization, and management fees. Staffing costs (salaries and benefits) are also largely fixed as most facilities operate with full-time staff for quality and efficiency reasons. Variable costs, including medical supplies, medications, equipment maintenance and repair, administrative supplies, etc., typically make up approximately 20% (i.e., a relatively minor portion) of the overall costs. Stated differently, doing one additional procedure adds a relatively small incremental cost for a significant financial benefit.

This is why optimizing efficiency as well as minimizing "no-shows" and empty slots on the schedule are critically important to the economics of an endoscopy unit.

Break-even volumes can be determined by subtracting the variable expense per procedure from the average payment per procedure to indicate the contribution available to be used for overhead and profit. Dividing fixed costs by the contribution margin per procedure indicates the number of procedures needed to pay the fixed costs, also known as the break-even point. Additional service units above that level constitute profit. Vicari and Garry[16] provided a simple example of a pro forma. The business plan and pro forma are mandatory in assessing the financial feasibility of the proposed endoscopy unit before construction. They further aid discussions in obtaining financing and help the architect design the unit for anticipated volumes.

Regulatory and Certification Issues

Before planning and designing the facility, one must understand the relevant regulatory and certification issues. As with the business plan, units developed in a hospital or academic medical center usually benefit from administrators and planners familiar with these complex issues. Physician owners of an office endoscopy suite or EASC must gain their own understanding. Various agencies provide myriad rules and regulations concerning endoscopy facilities.[19–23] Legislation can come from federal, state, or local authorities. Regulations may come from federal agencies, state departments of health, third-party accreditation organizations, and private payers. Although these rules and regulations can seem excessive and needlessly costly, their intent is to ensure safe and successful outcomes for patients. Regulations and certification issues for endoscopy facilities can be divided into six main categories, as follows:[19]

- General federal regulatory laws and rules
- Facility state licensure
- Medicare certification
- Third-party accreditation
- Physician credentialing
- Private payer requirements

General Federal Health-Related Laws

Federal regulatory laws and rules include fraud and abuse statutes (also known as antikickback laws), which are laws designed to prevent excessive or inappropriate payments. Endoscopy centers typically fall into a specific "safe harbor," a designation that protects EASC investors or shareholders from allegations of fraud or abuse. The safe harbor applies if the physician participants are surgeons or specialists engaged in the same surgical or medical practice specialty, including gastroenterology. These physicians can refer patients directly to their center and perform procedures on them as both an extension of and significant part of their practices.

Additional requirements of the safe harbor apply. Ownership of the facility, or remuneration from it, cannot be related to volume of referrals, services furnished, or the amount of business otherwise generated from that physician to the EASC. The amount of payment to physician owners from facility revenues must be directly proportional to the amount of each owner's capital investment. There must be no requirement that a passive investor make referrals to the EASC, and the EASC or any investor cannot make loans or guarantee a loan for a physician if these funds are used to purchase ownership in the EASC. Each physician must agree to treat Medicare and Medicaid patients. Finally, the physician owner must derive at least one-third of his or her medical practice income from the performance of procedures that require an EASC or hospital endoscopy unit setting.

Other general federal health-related laws and rules relevant to endoscopy facilities include the False Claims Act, copayment waivers, Stark provisions, Health Insurance Portability and Accountability Act (HIPAA) provisions, and labor and employment issues. The False Claims Act was designed to prevent false billings, claims that are medically unnecessary, and billings for inappropriately high payment. Copayment or deductible waivers may also be illegal if the government suspects such waivers are likely to induce referrals. Stark provisions stem from the Ethics in Patients Referrals Act. They are closely related to fraud and abuse statutes, but are civil rather than criminal laws. The regulatory body overseeing Medicare has ruled that a physician does not make an illegal referral for a procedure when he or she either personally performs the service or refers a patient to a partner to perform the service. HIPAA provisions are rules and regulations covering patient health information disclosed by any covered health care entity, provider, or facility. Regarding labor and employment issues, numerous rules and regulations cover discrimination, harassment, protection of the disabled, and workplace safety. The Occupational Health and Safety Act (OSHA) of 1970 seeks to protect employees from recognized work hazards that might cause death or serious harm. For endoscopy centers, OSHA requirements of major importance cover cleaning of endoscopic equipment, disinfection, and appropriate ventilation.

State Licensure

The state department of health licensing authority is interested in several features of a potential endoscopy facility. First, before any design and construction is undertaken, a careful review of the state's certificate of need (CON) requirements is needed. Some states do not allow construction of new facilities unless need is demonstrated. This process can be difficult and prospective physician owners of endoscopy facilities may encounter opposition from hospitals fearing competition and seeking to maximize use of their own facilities. Regarding specific construction guidelines, state regulators are most often interested in patient safety, the flow of the facility, cleanliness, and control of infection within the procedure areas. Many states follow guidelines from the Facility Guidelines Institute (FGI), but individual states recognize different versions of these FGI guidelines. Many states will also have their own set of regulations that must be followed and may relate to specific room sizes, acoustic regulations, door and hall size requirements, handicapped access provisions, requirements for exhaust systems, and specific fire codes.

Medicare Certification

Medicare certification is usually sought after obtaining state licensure and is required for any facility seeking reimbursement for Medicare and Medicaid work. Medicare regulations and requirements are usually more extensive than regulations of the state and address governance of the facility, transfer agreements with a nearby hospital, continuous quality improvement activities, Medicare architectural requirements, and medical records. Additional standards concern organization and staffing, administration of drugs, and procurement of laboratory and radiology services. Two other requirements warrant special attention as they relate to EASCs. First, the facility must be used exclusively for providing "surgical" services, a definition that includes GI endoscopies but not services like manometry. This requirement

also mandates a separation from other health care activities, separate staffing, and maintenance of special medical and financial records. Finally, the facility must comply with state licensure laws, which is potentially difficult in some states because of restrictive CON requirements. Medicare will survey under the ASC regulations for compliance[24] and the Medicare-adopted code set of the National Fire Protection Association (NFPA).[25]

Third-Party Accreditation

After state licensure and Medicare certification have been obtained, some states or specific payers may require a third-party accreditation before authorizing payments to an endoscopy facility. This accreditation can be provided by inspection from JC, AAAHC, or AAAASF. Although these accreditations are typically achieved after state licensure, they can sometimes be pursued simultaneously with Medicare inspection. Under certain circumstances, Medicare accepts accreditation from one of the third-party accreditation authorities in lieu of its own survey; this is known as attaining "deemed status." In a deemed-status survey, the surveyors will survey for both state regulatory compliance as well as Medicare regulatory compliance. Third-party accreditations focus on patient-related and organizational functions and, in the case of an EASC, concentrate on the "environment of care" or "facilities and environment."

Third-party inspection of a facility can be challenging and demands that the owners and operators fully understand the standards of each specific accrediting organization. A JC survey scrutinizes a variety of domains including Environment of Care, Emergency Management, Human Resources, Infection Prevention and Control, Information Management, Leadership, Life Safety, Medication Management, National Patient Safety Goals, Provision of Care, Record of Care, Rights and Responsibilities, and Waived Testing and Performance Improvement. AAAHC and AAAASF inspections assess similar functions, although these may be grouped under different organizational headings.

Physician Credentialing

Credentialing and privileging of physicians using an EASC may be mandated by federal, state, local, or third-party organizations and include a formal application process, verification of licensure and drug enforcement administration status, malpractice history, admitting privileges, advanced cardiac life support status, and documentation of training. Additional requirements may be outlined in the center's medical staff bylaws (for example, board certification of providers).

Payer Requirements

Individual health plans or insurers may have their own requirements, and these may vary significantly from payer to payer. Careful attention to local payer mix and any special requirements is necessary before designing and building an endoscopy facility to ensure qualification for payment. As outlined previously, the regulatory and certification issues for endoscopy facilities are "complex, detailed, and broad."[19] Any physician wishing to develop an endoscopy facility must understand these rules of regulation and certification. Appropriate legal counsel should be considered essential.

Choosing a Site

For hospital-based endoscopy facilities, the location of the facility is usually determined by the hospital's own planners. Although some hospitals have developed separate units for outpatient and inpatient endoscopies, most hospitals operate a single endoscopy unit. Choosing its location requires careful consideration of patient transport issues; the flow of inpatients and outpatients in and out of the unit; and the proximity to radiology, the emergency department, intensive care units, and inpatient wards. With office-based endoscopy or EASCs, physician owners choose the site. The site size and location require careful consideration because most office-based facilities or EASCs later expand to accommodate more physicians and patients. Preliminary land requirements are determined from space estimates (discussed later), parking requirements, appropriate landscaping or "green areas," and anticipated expansion. For an office endoscopy suite or EASC, proximity to a hospital is desirable to minimize travel for patients requiring hospital transfer and for physician convenience. The site should be near but perhaps not on a major street to ease patient parking. Many patients coming to an EASC or office-based facility are elderly or may be anxious about their upcoming procedures. Access should be easy. Locating the physician offices adjacent to the EASC should be strongly considered because it may be very efficient for staff and patients.

Facility Planning and Design

After forming a realistic business plan and acquiring an understanding of relevant regulatory and certification issues, attention turns to the planning and design of the facility. Although the remainder of this chapter includes some remarks about issues specifically related to hospital units, the main focus of the discussion is on the development of an outpatient endoscopy facility, details of which are equally applicable to hospital units. Objectives must be articulated to the design professionals to ensure that the facility meets the needs of patients, endoscopists, and staff. Some points to keep in mind are the following:

- Allow adequate time for planning.
- Set aside a regular block of time for discussion, review, and program development.
- Choose experienced design professionals with health care experience and knowledge of state and local health care building regulations.
- Involve staff to ensure attention to their needs and wishes.
- Prepare a statement of needs and goals to aid the architect in preparing a detailed program.
- Prepare an inventory of equipment needed and its location for the architect to be able to install the proper electrical system and plumbing.
- Visit other facilities to gather ideas worth incorporating.
- Use flow studies to evaluate placement of functional elements.
- Review preliminary drawings carefully.
- If questions arise about the size or shape of a space, lay it out with tape on the floor and simulate work practices.

Planning and design of the facility is a team project. The team mainly involves a physician representing the endoscopists who will use the facility; two staff people, including the nurse responsible for patient care activities within the unit and the appropriate administrator; the architect; engineers; and the builder. The responsible physician must be given adequate time away from clinical duties to devote to planning, design, and oversight of the construction of the facility. Designated time must be set aside because the process is ongoing and cannot be relegated to lunch hours and brief sessions whenever time can be stolen from clinical activities. The architect is the primary professional involved in overseeing the entire project. It is wise to select an architect who specializes in medical buildings, particularly one who has experience in designing endoscopy facilities. Similarly, selection of a contractor who has experience in medical construction, particularly construction of endoscopy facilities, is important. Both the architect and the contractor must thoroughly understand the requirements of regulatory and certifying bodies and local and state building codes. Sometimes the design and contracting can be provided by one company with both design and building capabilities.

Although the physician representative, designated staff persons, architect, and contractor compose the major elements of the planning and design team, additional input may be needed from engineers (mechanical, electrical, plumbing), telephone contractors, information technology experts, and attorneys. Consideration might also be given to involving a layperson or "patient" to ensure sufficient attention to issues of patient comfort, dignity, and privacy.

PLANNING

The planning stage is concerned with deciding what activities will be conducted in the facility, what equipment will be needed, and how space will be allocated.

Scope of Activities

The first consideration is which endoscopic procedures and other services will be performed in the facility. The type of facility will, to a great extent, answer this question. For a hospital unit that must provide a wide range of endoscopic services, one or more rooms must be large enough and appropriately equipped to accommodate the special equipment required for complex procedures (e.g., endoscopic retrograde cholangiopancreatography [ERCP], endoscopic ultrasound [EUS], balloon enteroscopy, laparoscopy, anesthesia cart). In some community hospitals, endoscopy units are shared with other specialties, such as cardiology or pulmonology, and have to accommodate procedures such as transesophageal echocardiography or bronchoscopy. If the hospital is part of an academic medical center, the unit may serve additional purposes, including teaching and research, requiring further modifications in space, equipment, and staffing.

For an office suite and EASC, services offered will be based on clinical considerations, safety, and logistics. In these out-of-hospital facilities, procedures are usually limited to individuals and stable patients undergoing "routine" high-volume procedures with predictable turnaround and recovery times, utilizing standard equipment and accessories. In an EASC, it is crucial that all procedures done be on the Medicare approved list to qualify for facility reimbursement. For both the office suite and the EASC, procedures are often limited to upper GI endoscopy, esophageal dilation, and colonoscopy, including polypectomy. Predictably, rapid turnaround time is crucial for an efficiently functioning EASC or office facility. Whereas EUS, ERCP, and other complex endoscopic examinations are also done in some EASCs, it is generally advisable to perform long procedures or procedures that are unpredictable in duration or clinical outcomes in the hospital. Procedures requiring prolonged recovery times, such as liver biopsy, are also best done in a hospital environment.

The question sometimes arises whether it is better to have a multispecialty or single-specialty ASC. From the standpoint of services offered and equipment, a single-specialty EASC has the advantage of being the "focus factory."[26,27] In this environment, endoscopists, skilled GI nurses, technicians, and administrative staff maximally use standardized equipment, performing predictably timed procedures with a rapid turnaround. A single-specialty EASC avoids the problem of a multispecialty facility in which highly specialized equipment lies idle much of the time while physicians from differing specialties are performing their individual procedures.

Equipment

The greatest capital expense after the basic construction is equipment. Some tabulation of the equipment needed is necessary in the early planning stages and facility design. The basic equipment needed for an endoscopy unit is listed in Box 2.1. A detailed discussion of individual items is not presented here, but a few points are useful in integrating the equipment needs into planning and design. Generally, examining or procedure tables have been replaced by height-adjustable, rolling procedural stretcher carts that allow patients, once properly gowned for endoscopy, to mount the movable cart and not leave it until ready to leave the facility. These carts allow patients to be shuttled from preparation areas to procedure rooms and back to recovery areas, and also serve as procedure tables. This capability is very important to overall system efficiency and adds to patient safety by avoiding transfer to and from a procedure table.

Another major determinant of overall system speed and efficiency is the availability of endoscopes. Adequate numbers of endoscopes, high-level disinfection systems (automatic endoscope reprocessors [AERs]), and adequate storage for extra endoscopes are required. Adequate numbers of endoscopes must be available to prevent inefficient downtime in the unit. Staff salaries, wages, and benefits make up a significant percentage of total costs of providing endoscopic services, and it is inefficient and fiscally unwise to have highly paid physicians and staff waiting for endoscopes. Regarding dilating devices and other accessories, decisions (e.g., whether to use a Savary dilator system versus dilating balloons) should first and foremost be made on clinical grounds. This decision will, however, also have economic consequences as the cost of accessory devices is bundled into the facility payment and the endoscopy center will not be able to procure additional reimbursement for higher-cost devices. Finally, with the growing use of propofol and anesthesia services for endoscopic procedures, additional medications and equipment are often required for this service.[28,29]

Physical Environment

Before beginning specific planning and design, some issues affecting space efficiency should be considered. It is the goal for physicians and staff to work as quickly and efficiently as possible while giving patients the assurance that they are receiving appropriate and safe care. System speed in the endoscopy facility usually comes from the following three delivery components:
1. Preparation and recovery of the patient.
2. Reprocessing and return of endoscopes to the procedure room.
3. Physician work habits.
If the first two components operate properly, the number of procedure rooms available is not as important as the practice habits of the physician in starting their schedule on time, performing procedures in an efficient manner, talking to patients and their families, completing medical records, and returning to the procedure room.[28] In an efficient facility, physician discipline is needed because room turnover and equipment reprocessing time can be rapid.

Flow

Architects use flow diagrams to plan movement patterns in arranging space before actual design plans. Physician and nurse input is crucial in arranging the flow relationships within the endoscopy facility to maximize efficiency, minimize travel distance, and achieve economy of movement. A basic flow diagram showing patient flow through a simple endoscopy unit is shown in Fig. 2.1. The patterns of movement may be more complicated in a hospital department. Simple flow diagrams such as these can be elaborated into a functional schematic drawing diagram as shown in Fig. 2.2. This type of functional schematic diagram shows the way that patients, staff, physicians, and equipment can move through the facility. A functional schematic diagram can be turned into a floor plan by assigning actual space requirements to the rooms that are represented. A 40% circulation allowance must be added at the end of the tabulation to account for wall thicknesses, corridors, and so forth.[30]

For hospital-based units, specific patient flow issues must be considered. Separate entrances for sick, bedridden patients and

---

BOX 2.1 Endoscopy Facility Basic Equipment List

I. Major endoscopic and electrosurgical equipment
 A. Endoscopes, light sources, video processors, and monitors
 B. Electrocautery units and accessories
 C. Hemostasis unit (e.g., heater probe, gold probe, argon plasma coagulator)
 D. Physiologic monitoring devices including pulse oximetry, blood pressure, and cardiac monitoring
II. Catheters, snares, forceps, and brushes
 A. Polypectomy snares
 B. Biopsy forceps
 C. Brushes
 1. Cleaning
 2. Cytology
 D. Graspers
 E. Retrieval baskets
III. Endoscopic report writer with photo generator and image manager
IV. Esophageal dilators
 A. Wire-guided (e.g., Savary)
 B. Balloon
V. Rolling procedural stretcher carts with adjustable heights
VI. Suction equipment
VII. Pharmaceuticals
 A. Sedation and analgesia agents
 1. Benzodiazepines
 2. Narcotic analgesics
 3. Miscellaneous preference
 B. Benzodiazepine antagonists
 C. Narcotic antagonists
 D. Glucagon
 E. Atropine
 F. Topicals
VIII. Intravenous equipment, solutions, needles, and syringes
IX. Chemicals
 A. Formalin
 B. Disinfection solutions
X. Emergency cart, resuscitation equipment, supplies, and medications
XI. High-level disinfection equipment (cleaning trays, sinks, automatic endoscope washers, and autoclave)
XII. Instrument storage cabinets
XIII. Blanket warmer
XIV. Audio/music system
XV. Eyewash station

ambulatory individuals should be considered. The monitoring and treatment requirements for sick inpatients must be taken into consideration. Separation of inpatients and outpatients in waiting or holding areas, preparation areas, and recovery areas may also be helpful. If an endoscopy facility is constructed adjacent to a clinic facility, the regulations require a firewall separation between the EASC and the clinic. Shared waiting rooms are no

longer permitted. This separation may require a 1- or 2-hour fire rated wall-door construction system depending on the state and/or the building in which the facility is located. When fire-rated walls are required, it is important that the proper rating of the wall is considered, making sure the fire-rated gypsum board on either side of the structural wall extends through the ceiling to the roof of the structure above and all penetrations through the wall are properly sealed.

Designing the Endoscopy Facility

The *Guidelines for Design and Construction of Health Care Facilities (FGI Guidelines)*, published by the American Society for Healthcare Engineering, include a section on the design and construction of GI endoscopy facilities.[31] The document is updated on a 4- to 5-year revision cycle with the latest edition published in 2014. Many states have not yet adopted this newest version and some have not officially adopted any version. A state map outlining FGI adoption is also available.[32] The *FGI Guidelines*, which are referenced by many federal and state jurisdictions, were originally conceived as minimum construction requirements for hospitals. Over time, the document has evolved to include engineering systems, infection control, and safety and architectural guidelines

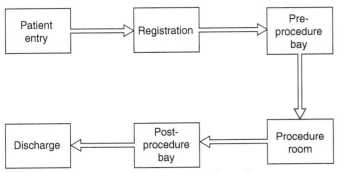

FIG 2.1 Basic endoscopy unit flow diagram.

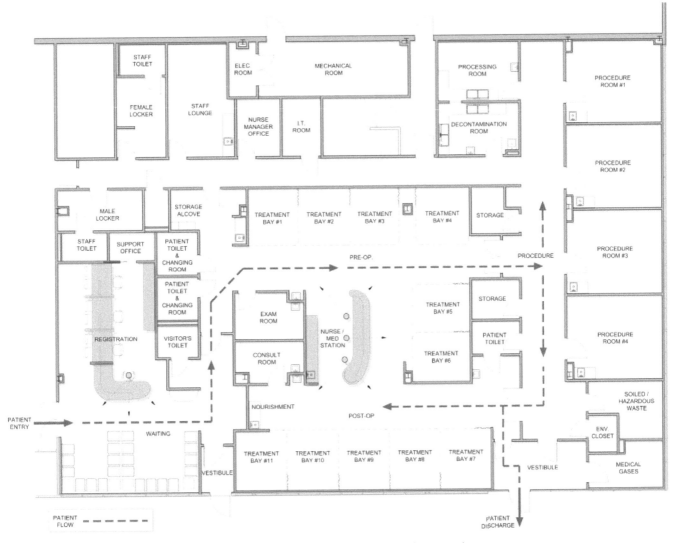

FIG 2.2 Functional relationship diagram for an ambulatory endoscopy center.

TABLE 2.1   Space Considerations

Room	Components	Considerations
Waiting	Seating Beverage counter Public restroom	Calculate the amount of seating in the waiting room based on the number of procedure rooms being constructed. Typically, 3 chairs per procedure room are needed.
Reception/business area	Registration bays needed. Billing area Medical record storage	The number of registration bays may vary depending on the number of procedure rooms. If billing functions are outsourced, less space is needed for this function. If the facility is using an EMR, medical record storage can be reduced to locking millwork.
Pre/post procedure area	Pre/post procedure bays Nurse station Nutrition area Medication area Patient belongings Handwashing sinks Restrooms/patient changing Exam/consult room	Number of procedure bays will vary with State regulations. Typically, 2–3 bays are required per procedure room. Pre- and post-op bays can be used interchangeably, provided the minimum monitoring, electrical and medical gas components are included. Nurse station must have visualization of all bays. One nurse station for all bays provides a more efficient staffing model. Medication area may be provided behind nursing station in locking millwork if State allows. Small purse lockers can be provided to secure patient belongings. Handwashing sinks typically required = 1 sink per every 4 bays.
Procedure area	Corridor Procedure rooms	The number of procedure rooms will drive the project. This calculation will be based on number of physicians and physician volume. Minimum size requirements for these rooms will vary by State. A corridor separating the pre/post area from the procedural area may be required by State. Scrub sinks – may be required in some States.
Reprocessing area	Soiled scope Reprocessing area	Separation of the soiled scope area and reprocessing area are essential. A pass-through window will allow these rooms to have two separate and distinct functions. Eyewash should be provided in the reprocessing area due to the chemicals used for reprocessing.
Staff area	Locker room(s) Shower Staff restrooms	Number and size of locker rooms will vary depending on the number of procedure rooms/staffing. Staff shower is required in some States.
Supporting functions	Storage Environmental functions Utility rooms IT room Biohazard/soiled linen/trash room	Minimum storage requirements must meet State requirements. Two environmental closets are typically required.
Mechanical	Medical gases Water heater/boiler UPS/generator Electrical room Vacuum pump room HVAC	Medical gas room is required to be rated. Depending on the number of gases, storage in this room may be required to meet certain ventilation requirements. Consider adding CO_2 to the manifold to allow for CO_2 insufflation in the procedure rooms. Work closely with the engineers to determine mechanical requirements.
Exterior	Parking Canopy	Adequate parking spaces must be provided. Number of spaces required will depend on local jurisdiction. Handicap spaces must be provided. Canopy extending to the curb may be required by some States.

EMR, electronic medical record; UPS, uninterruptible power supply.

for design and construction of hospitals and other types of health care facilities. It provides an invaluable resource for the construction of a new EASC, the construction of a hospital-based endoscopy unit, or the renovation of existing units. The *FGI Guidelines* can be purchased through the American Hospital Association.[33]

Table 2.1 provides a list of areas and components of a typical endoscopy unit as well as some key considerations for each area. The following sections highlight some of these considerations.

Arrival and Waiting Areas

The patient's experience of the endoscopy facility often begins outside the building in the parking lot. Patients arriving for endoscopy are often anxious and sometimes frightened. Maps with careful driving instructions and signs posted in the vicinity of the endoscopy facility can minimize confusion and offer reassurance. An all-weather canopy and automatic opening doors are helpful to elderly, ill, or disabled patients. The reception and waiting room area provides an early impression of the endoscopy facility and should project friendliness and efficiency. Wheelchair storage should be available in this area, with wheelchairs stored out of sight. There must be adequate room for patients' escorts because one or two people usually accompany each patient scheduled for endoscopy. If the clinic area is adjacent to the endoscopy center, there are very specific mandates in regard to separate and distinct waiting rooms. As an example, per CMS manual, the endoscopy center "must provide a waiting area for its patients within the perimeter of its 1-hour fire-rated barrier and ensure said barrier is free of penetrations."[24] Waiting areas should be well appointed and equipped with a television set and reading material. A toilet should be available near, but not directly off, the waiting room. Drinking water should be provided, either via a drinking fountain (required in some states) or bottled water (allowed in some states). The general waiting area for Northern New Jersey Endoscopy Center, Englewood Cliffs, NJ is shown in Fig. 2.3.

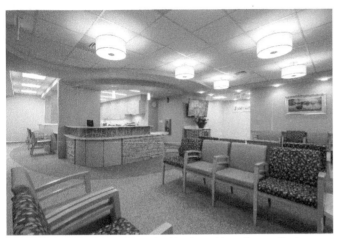

FIG 2.3 General waiting area for Northern New Jersey Endoscopy Center, Englewood Cliffs, NJ. (Photograph by Andrea Brizzi, facility designed by RSC Architects, Hackensack, NJ, http://www.rscarchitects.com.)

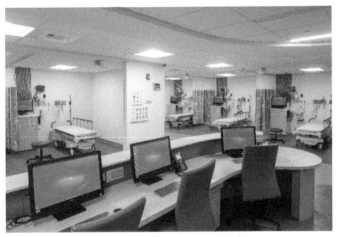

FIG 2.4 Nursing control station for preparation-recovery area, Northern New Jersey Endoscopy Center, Englewood Cliffs, NJ. (Photograph by Andrea Brizzi; facility designed by RSC Architects, Hackensack, NJ; http://www.rscarchitects.com.)

Business-Reception Area

The business-reception area includes the reception desk, registration bays, billing stations, and medical records storage. If billing functions are outsourced, square footage can be eliminated for this function. With the adoption of electronic medical records, the space needed to store paper copies of medical records can be kept at a minimum. Often this space is limited to locking cabinets located in this area.

Pre/Postprocedure Area

The preparation-recovery area of the endoscopy facility requires constant patient surveillance from the nursing staff. This area usually contains a nursing control station (Fig. 2.4), which allows unobstructed viewing of patients during the preparation and recovery stages of their visit. The most efficient arrangement for preparation and recovery is to have them occur in the same place and to set up the patient bays so they can be used interchangeably. Patient clothing can be stored in a locked cabinet

in the preparation-recovery area or can accompany the patient during transport to the procedure room and back, stored in a belonging bag underneath the rolling procedural stretcher cart. Patient valuables should be left with the patient escort or secured in a locker during the procedure. Patients can be rolled into procedure rooms on properly designed stretchers that are also used as procedure tables. In this way, patients can move from preparation to procedure and back to recovery requiring no mounting or dismounting from wheelchairs or carts. This is not only more efficient but also safer for the patient.

Per the FGI 2010 guideline, one preparation and two recovery rooms or curtained bays are required per procedure room, but state requirements may vary and need to be checked. Some patients who need additional recovery time after they are able to dismount the procedure cart can recover in recliner chairs. A few curtained recliner chair areas can provide this extra recovery space. The number and type of required recovery bays may also vary depending on the type of sedation used. Corridors between procedure areas and preparation-recovery spaces should be wide enough to provide easy patient cart movement. Toilets should be close to both preparation-recovery and procedure areas.

Procedure Room Area

The number of procedure rooms is determined by the caseload of the endoscopy facility. This number is often overestimated. More important than the number of procedure rooms is the amount of recovery space available. In an efficient facility where turnaround time is quick, the number of procedure rooms can be minimized. Turnaround between cases should be very rapid. Using procedure rooms for recovery compromises efficiency by tying up a specialized procedure room. To determine the required number of procedure rooms, consider the number of physicians and the anticipated procedural volume. An average efficient procedure room should be able to accommodate 16 to 20 endoscopy procedures per day, depending on the types of procedures being performed. Allowances should be made for anticipated growth in numbers of physicians and patients over the subsequent 5 years. By using the patient load anticipated 5 years hence, and dividing this load by the number of procedures per room per year, the number of required rooms can be calculated.

The minimum size for an endoscopy room is approximately 200 clear square feet according to the *FGI Guidelines;* however, this may vary according to state specific regulations. Clearances shall permit a minimum clearance of 3 feet 6 inches at each side, head, and foot of the stretcher/table. A hand-washing station shall be available to each procedure room. Approximately 300 square feet may be needed for higher complexity endoscopy procedures. Sometimes state licensing departments or Medicare mandates a minimum size for an "operating room" that is inappropriately large for an endoscopy room. In that instance, a variance can be requested, but it is not automatically granted.

In an endoscopy procedure room layout, placement of the light source, the video processor, video monitor(s), and electrocautery must be carefully considered. Many variations are possible to fit the preferences of the endoscopists and nursing staff. Rooms should be planned with equipment and supplies integrated into the layout and positioned strategically around the site of the patient on the procedural stretcher. An example of such a procedure room layout is provided in Fig. 2.5. The floor should be free of cables and wiring; these can be arranged along the perimeter of the room or preferably above ceiling, below the

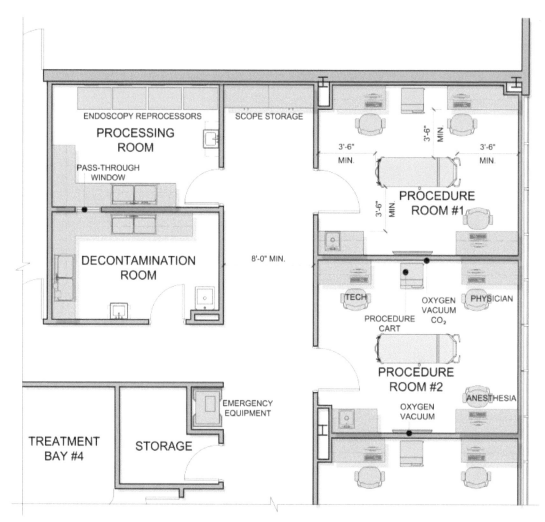

FIG 2.5 Example of procedure room and reprocessing room layout.

floor, or via conduits in the walls. This allows physicians, staff, and equipment to move unfettered by cords and cables, and it avoids damaging these sensitive components. Preplanning should include consideration of the type of endoscopes used, as this will affect the cabling needed. All endoscopic accessories, suction, oxygen, supplies, and all resuscitation equipment should be at hand. An emergency call button is required in each procedure room, and an emergency (crash) cart should be stored nearby. A typical endoscopy procedure room is shown in Fig. 2.6.

Reprocessing Areas

Efficient equipment turnover time can be achieved by having appropriate equipment for rapid cleaning and high-level disinfection. In this scenario, the speed of the endoscopy facility is determined by the efficiency of the physician between procedures rather than by the number of procedure rooms. Instrument cleaning and high-level disinfection can be accomplished by strategically placing the cleaning area between two procedure rooms or having an efficient large cleaning area within a short distance of several procedure rooms. Adequate numbers of endoscopes stored properly and reprocessed effectively and efficiently ensure that the most expensive cost elements of the endoscopy facility—the physicians and nursing staff—are not kept waiting for equipment.

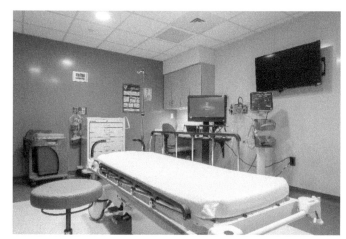

FIG 2.6 Typical endoscopy procedure room, Northern New Jersey Endoscopy Center, Englewood Cliffs, NJ. (Photograph by Andrea Brizzi; facility designed by RSC Architects, Hackensack, NJ; http://www.rscarchitects.com.)

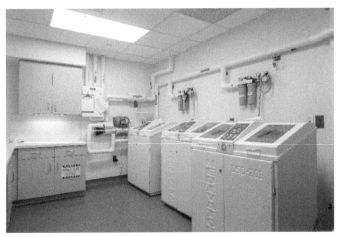

FIG 2.7 High-level disinfection processing room for multiple endoscopes. Northern New Jersey Endoscopy Center, Englewood Cliffs, NJ. (Photograph by Andrea Brizzi; facility designed by RSC Architects, Hackensack, NJ; http://www.rscarchitects.com.)

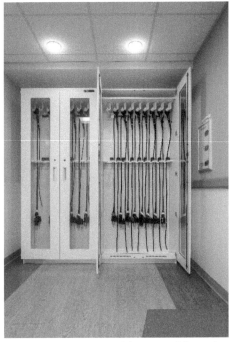

FIG 2.9 Endoscopy storage cabinet providing air circulation through endoscopy channels. Northern New Jersey Endoscopy Center, Englewood Cliffs, NJ. (Photograph by Andrea Brizzi; facility designed by RSC Architects, Hackensack, NJ; http://www.rscarchitects.com.)

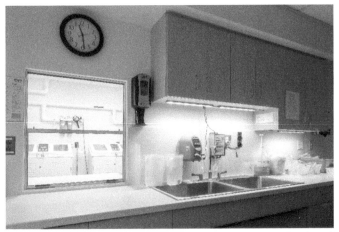

FIG 2.8 Pass-through window maintains separation of "clean" and "dirty" areas. Northern New Jersey Endoscopy Center, Englewood Cliffs, NJ. (Photograph by Andrea Brizzi; facility designed by RSC Architects, Hackensack, NJ; http://www.rscarchitects.com.)

protection against moisture and bacterial growth within channels. A storage unit with channel air circulation is shown in Fig. 2.9. It is essential that proper ventilation follow the standards to meet infection control and safety guidelines.

Support Areas

General storage for supplies must meet all temperature/humidity guidelines and be readily accessible to the preparation-recovery areas and the procedure rooms. An adequately rated room should be provided for biohazardous waste. Space should also be allocated for soiled linen and regular trash. Environmental closets are also required for this space.

Mechanical Areas

Mechanical rooms are needed to supply the medical gas manifold, vacuum pump, water heater, HVAC unit and other mechanical equipment. An alternative power source (Essential Electrical System), such as a battery backup system or generator, is necessary to ensure uninterrupted power. Providing the correct power source will be dependent on the type of anesthesia used, the type of facility, and Medicare and state regulations.

Staff Area

Requirements for dressing room spaces are different in regulated and unregulated endoscopy facilities. Rules for the EASC or hospital may be quite different from the office. It is wise to know the regulations from the state department of health and from certification agencies. Male and female locker areas are generally required, but variances can be requested to eliminate the need for unnecessary shower facilities. Fig. 2.10 shows a convenient

The soiled scope cleaning room and the reprocessing room should be large and appropriately ventilated, with ample plumbing and power provisions for future changes. Oversized sinks are required, and there should be a place for soiled endoscopes to be placed while waiting to be cleaned. Automated endoscope-reprocessing machines with multiple endoscope compartments provide an efficient way of reprocessing endoscopes (Fig. 2.7). Different instrument-reprocessing units vary in the chemicals used and their cleaning time, which has an impact on the number of endoscopes required by a busy unit. A "pass-through" window from soiled to clean processing areas, as shown in Fig. 2.8, can help maintain separation of clean and dirty areas.

A closed cabinet with proper ventilation for the storage of the clean endoscopes is essential. Endoscope storage cabinets that circulate air through the endoscope channels provide added

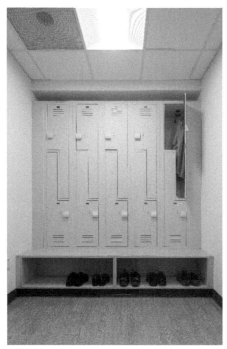

FIG 2.10 Staff changing room and lockers. Northern New Jersey Endoscopy Center, Englewood Cliffs, NJ. (Photograph by Andrea Brizzi; facility designed by RSC Architects, Hackensack, NJ; http://www.rscarchitects.com.)

locker/bench/shoe storage area in a staff locker room. An additional part of the staff area is the break room. Some state departments of health or certification bodies require a break room within the confines of the endoscopy facility. Careful attention to state and federal regulations is warranted to ensure that licensure and certification requirements are met.

Summary of Planning and Design

The design of an efficient endoscopy facility is facilitated by a functional relationship diagram showing the flow of patients through the facility. An architectural space program is developed by tabulating the areas necessary and assigning space required. This architectural space program determines the size of the facility. A procedure room utilization calculation determines the number of procedure rooms and other areas necessary to handle the patient caseload, and provisions should be made for caseload growth. Careful attention to planning and design results in the construction of a pleasant, efficient endoscopy facility that meets the needs of patients, physicians, and staff.

STAFFING AND SCHEDULING

Decisions regarding staffing and scheduling are critical to the safe and efficient operation of the endoscopy facility, have a major impact on patient outcomes, and affect the financial viability of the endoscopy unit.

Staffing

Decisions regarding staffing hinge on regulatory requirements, volumes of procedures, and case mix (disease acuity). Numerous federal and state regulations affect staffing decisions, and a thorough knowledge of these requirements is necessary to ensure compliance with state licensing requirements, Medicare certification regulations, and third-party accreditation standards.[34,35]

Medicare guidelines stipulate that a registered nurse (RN) must be available on site during all hours of operation of a hospital or ASC endoscopy facility. The nurse practice act of each individual state also affects staffing decisions. A state nurse practice act defines the scope of practice for RNs, licensed practical nurses (LPNs), and other assistants or technicians. These nurse practice acts may limit who can start intravenous (IV) lines, administer IV medications, or provide other clinical services. To determine the number of full-time equivalents (FTEs) needed for staffing, one must quantify the time needed to care for a single patient, multiply this by the number of procedures scheduled daily, and divide by the work hours per day of a full-time employee. Some factors that influence the decision to use RNs versus LPNs versus technicians include scope-of-practice regulations, salary costs, and availability. Regardless of the mix, care should always be directly supervised by an on-site RN.[36]

Scheduling

Most facilities use block scheduling to maximize efficiency and convenience.[34,35] Block scheduling also allows for time allotments based on the performance characteristics of individual endoscopists. Examples of block scheduling and tools for use in block scheduling have been published by McMillin.[34]

Time allotments for procedures vary from facility to facility. Some facilities allow 45 minutes for colonoscopy and 30 minutes for upper GI endoscopy,[34] whereas others schedule more tightly, often using 30 minute slots for all upper and lower endoscopies (Digestive Health Specialists, Tacoma, WA, unpublished data). The tighter scheduling can be accommodated by efficient endoscopists, good staffing, adequate equipment, rapid turnaround time, and ample preparation-recovery space. Careful staffing and scheduling are imperative to ensure high quality care, good patient outcomes, and optimal fiscal performance of the endoscopy facility.

DOCUMENTATION AND INFORMATION TECHNOLOGY

An accurate and complete medical record for each patient and a log of the unit's overall activities must be kept (see Chapter 10). The endoscopy report and nursing notes may include, but may not be limited to: date, patient identification data, endoscopist, specific instruments used, endoscopic procedure, indications, informed consent, extent of examination, duration of procedure, findings, notation of tissue sampling, therapeutic interventions, complications, limitations of the examination, conclusions, and recommendations. Photographs, electronic images, and biopsy reports should also be part of the record. Quality indicators and patient outcomes should be tabulated, and a method of regular peer review should be developed.[5] Information management in an endoscopy facility affects all aspects of the operation, including scheduling, billing and reimbursement, patient medical records, procedure reports, clinical laboratory and anatomic pathology reports, imaging, pharmacy, patient education, performance improvement data, financial management, materials management and inventory, budgeting and forecasting, payroll and personnel, and staffing and scheduling.[37] Modern information technology may allow more efficient and effective operations within the facility.

Information technology is changing medical practice at a rapid pace and may allow for more efficient and effective operations within the endoscopy facility.

To minimize repetitive data entry and difficulties with sharing and analyzing data across different systems, the modern endoscopy unit should plan ahead and install an information technology system that provides compatibility between the office electronic medical record (EMR), the endoscopic facility, the billing department, the endoscope manufacturer, the cardiac monitor manufacturer/model, and possibly the local hospital. The interface should allow prompt transfer of demographic data and pertinent components of the medical history and physical examination. Bidirectional transfer of information ensures that the procedure report and billing information are transmitted to the individuals who need access to it. Further increases in functionality can be envisioned. For example, the use of wireless networks and voice-recognition software for endowriters and EMRs are possible. Electronic systems can also be used to enhance service offerings to patients and families. The system can generate automatic reminder letters or offer educational material and resources for the patient and family if a new diagnosis has been made. The pathology request, endoscopy report, referral letter, discharge instructions, plans for follow-up, and billing information can be generated from the base examination and completed before the patient leaves the facility. Many of the documents can be sent electronically.

QUALITY MEASUREMENT AND IMPROVEMENT

Increasing health care costs, constrained resources, and evidence of variations in the quality of care rendered have triggered a renewed emphasis on quality measurement and improvement. Two reports by the Institute of Medicine advocate widespread changes in health care, including paying for performance as a means of achieving the delivery of high quality care.[38,39] Medicare regulations and third-party accreditors require endoscopy facilities to engage in an ongoing comprehensive self-assessment of the quality of care provided. This process includes quality improvement efforts directed toward numerous facets of the operation of the facility. Reasons for quality improvement activities include ensuring that patients receive the highest quality of care possible; providing a competitive edge when seeking contracts; and addressing the recent emphasis of legislators and regulators on quality improvement activities as part of the licensure, certification, and accreditation process. Johanson[40,41] described continuous quality improvement in the EASC. The philosophies and tools presented in this article provide a framework for quality improvement activities in all endoscopic facilities. A 2015 publication by a joint task force from the ASGE and the American College of Gastroenterology provides an excellent resource with recommendations and ranking of quality indicators that can be used as a starting point in quality measurement and improvement efforts.[5]

ACKNOWLEDGMENTS

The authors gratefully acknowledge the work of James T. Frakes, MD who authored and coauthored the previous versions of this chapter. The text of the current revision draws substantially from those previous versions. The authors are also very grateful to MaryAnn Gellenbeck for her suggestions and input related to the current revisions.

KEY REFERENCES

1. American Society for Gastrointestinal Endoscopy: Principles of training in GI endoscopy, *Gastrointest Endosc* 75:231–235, 2012.
2. American Society for Gastrointestinal Endoscopy: Methods of granting hospital privileges to perform gastrointestinal endoscopy, *Gastrointest Endosc* 55:780–783, 2002.
4. American Society for Gastrointestinal Endoscopy: Quality and outcomes assessment in gastrointestinal endoscopy, *Gastrointest Endosc* 52:827–830, 2000.
5. American Society for Gastrointestinal Endoscopy: Defining and measuring quality in endoscopy, *Gastrointest Endosc* 81(1):1–80, 2015.
6. American Society for Gastrointestinal Endoscopy: Guidelines for safety in the gastrointestinal endoscopy unit, *Gastrointest Endosc* 79:363–372, 2014.
9. Frakes JT: The ambulatory endoscopy center (AEC): what it can do for your gastroenterology practice, *Gastrointest Endosc Clin N Am* 16:687–694, 2006.
11. Vicari JJ: The future value of ambulatory endoscopy centers in the United States: challenges and opportunities, *Gastrointest Endosc* 76(2):400–405, 2012.
12. Mergener K: Impact of health care reform on the independent GI practice, *Gastrointest Endosc Clin N Am* 22:15–27, 2012.
13. Robinson JC, Miller K: Total expenditures per patient in hospital-owned and physician-owned physician organizations in California, *JAMA* 312(16):1663–1669, 2014.
14. Bai G, Anderson GF: Extreme markup: the fifty US hospitals with the highest charge-to-cost ratios, *Health Aff* 34(6):922–928, 2015.
15. Obama B: United States health care reform: progress to date and next steps, *JAMA* 316(5):525–532, 2016.
16. Vicari JJ, Garry N: Exploring possibilities: types of facilities and business plan. In Frakes JT, editor: *Ambulatory endoscopy centers: a primer*, Oak Brook, IL, 2006, American Society for Gastrointestinal Endoscopy, pp 23–27.
17. Deas TM: Assessing the financial health of the endoscopy facility, *Gastrointest Endosc Clin N Am* 12:229–244, 2002.
19. Ganz RA: Regulation and certification issues, *Gastrointest Endosc Clin N Am* 12:205–214, 2002.
24. Centers for Medicare and Medicaid Services: State Operations Manual. Appendix L: Guidance for surveyors: ambulatory surgical centers. Available at www.cms.gov/Regulations-and-Guidance/Guidance/Manuals/downloads/som107ap_l_ambulatory.pdf. (Accessed 2 December 2016).
25. National Fire Protection Association: Codes and standards. NFPA resources for CMS requirements. Available at www.nfpa.org/codes-and-standards/resources/nfpa-resources-for-cms-requirements-on-nfpa-99-and-nfpa-101. (Accessed 2 December 2016).
26. Herzlinger R: *Market-driven health care: who wins, who loses in the transformation of America's largest service industry*, Reading, MA, 1997, Addison-Wesley.
27. Deas TM, Jr, Drerup DM: Endoscopic ambulatory surgery centers: demise, service or thrive?, *J Clin Gastroenterol* 29:253–256, 1999.
29. Aisenberg J, Cohen LB: Sedation in endoscopic practice, *Gastrointest Endosc Clin N Am* 16:695–708, 2006.
31. Facility Guidelines Institute. Available at www.fgiguidelines.org. (Accessed 2 December 2016).
33. Facility Guidelines Institute: *2014 FGI guidelines for design and construction of hospitals and outpatient facilities*, Chicago, 2014, American Hospital Association.
34. McMillin DF: Staffing and scheduling in the endoscopy center, *Gastrointest Endosc Clin N Am* 12:285–296, 2002.
38. Institute of Medicine (IOM): *To Err is human: building a safer health system*, Washington, DC, 1999, National Academy Press.
39. Institute of Medicine (IOM): *Crossing the quality chasm: a new health system for the 21st century*, Washington, DC, 2001, National Academy Press.
40. Johanson JF: Continuous quality improvement in the ambulatory endoscopy center, *Gastrointest Endosc Clin N Am* 12:351–365, 2002.

A complete reference list can be found online at ExpertConsult.com

3

How Endoscopes Work

Divyanshoo R. Kohli and John Baillie

Endoscopes are flexible instruments combining fiber-optics (for illumination) and charge-coupled devices (for imaging) that are used in medicine to visualize the interior of otherwise inaccessible sites, such as the lumen of hollow organs. Endoscopes are used to examine the gastrointestinal (GI) tract, the bronchial system, the ureters and other body cavities. They have numerous uses in non-medical settings as well and are central to the modern management of many GI disorders.

ENDOSCOPE DESIGN

The endoscope consists of three basic parts: the tip, the insertion tube and the control section (Fig. 3.1).

The Control Section

The control section is the most versatile part of the endoscope. It is typically held in the left hand of the endoscopist and is used to maneuver the endoscope and introduce accessories. The tip can be maneuvered using the twin dials located on the control section. The larger dial deflects the tip up and down, whereas the smaller dial is responsible for lateral control (i.e., left or right) (Fig. 3.2). These dials can be locked into place to hold a particular position of the tip. Some ultra-thin specialized endoscopes may have only a single dial for up/down angulation and require application of torque for sideways maneuverability. Duodenoscopes used for endoscopic retrograde cholangiopancreatography (ERCP) and linear echoendoscopes have an additional dial for controlling the elevator.

There are two openings in the front of the control section that accommodate specially designed buttons. One button is used for applying suction at the tip of the endoscope. The second button has the dual functions of air insufflation and washing the camera lens. There are separate buttons that can be used to freeze and record images, selectively change the wavelength of the light (see later section on Image Processing), and alter the focus of the camera. Some buttons are also programmable for specific functions.[1]

The control section is attached to the insertion tube. It also contains an entry port ("instrument channel") that allows passage of many different endoscopic accessories, such as biopsy forceps, electrocautery probes, and snares, through the length of the endoscope. Some colonoscopes incorporate a variable-stiffness function that is controlled by a rotatable dial at the level of the control head.

Insertion Tube

The insertion tube is the part of the endoscope that enters the body. It contains a "working channel" of variable diameters, which permits passage of endoscopic accessories. It is also involved in the application of suction. Some endoscopes have a "power wash" function to direct a jet of water towards a target in the lumen. This can be very useful for cleaning debris that may coat the mucosa or obscure the lens. Angulation wires that are connected to the up-down and right-left control wheels run the length of the insertion tube. These are used to flex or even retroflex the tip of the endoscope.

The insertion tube is made from multiple layers of polymers that provide durability as well as flexibility. Spiral metal bands wound in opposite directions run through the length of the insertion tube: they transmit force and torque (twist) from the end of the tube to its tip (Fig. 3.3). Certain specialty endoscopes have devices to create variable rigidity of the insertion tube. This requires adjusting a cable that increases or decreases tension within the insertion tube (Fig. 3.4). The changes in stiffness do

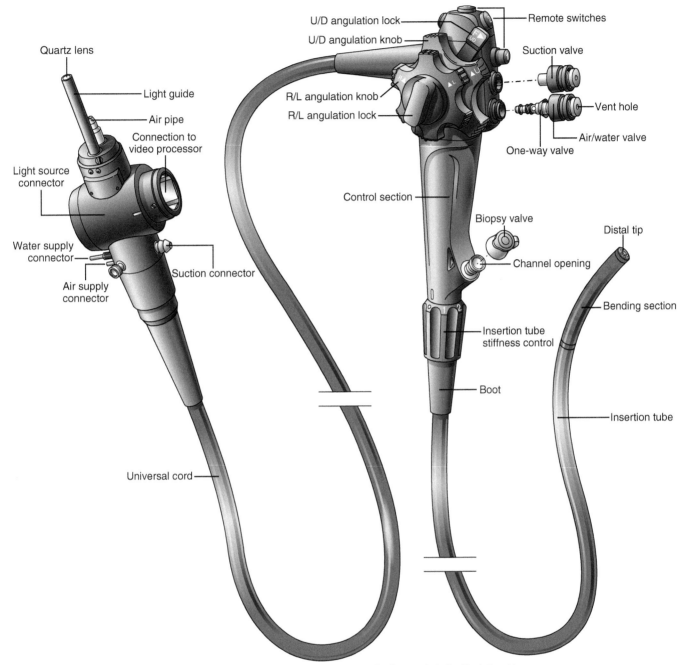

Quartz lens
Light guide
Air pipe
Connection to
video processor
Light source
connector
Water supply
connector
Air supply
connector
Suction connector
Universal cord

U/D angulation lock
U/D angulation knob
Remote switches
Suction valve
R/L angulation knob
R/L angulation lock
Vent hole
Air/water valve
One-way valve
Control section
Biopsy valve
Distal tip
Channel opening
Bending section
Insertion tube
stiffness control
Boot
Insertion tube

FIG 3.1 Components of the endoscope. *D*, down; *L*, left; *R*, right; *U*, up.

not extend to the distal 15 to 20 centimeters of the insertion tube, where separate inputs control the use of the so-called bending section.[2]

Tip of the Endoscope

The objective lens is among the many components of the endoscope mounted on the distal end or the tip of the insertion tube. This lens may be forward-facing, oblique, or side-viewing. In close proximity of the lens lies a nozzle that directs a jet of water to clean debris off the lens. A charge-coupled device (CCD) unit connected to objective lens is mounted inside the tip (Fig. 3.5A). The CCD and the objective lens form an integrated system that allows seamless transmission

of images from the tip of the endoscope through the insertion tube directly into the processing unit through an "umbilical cord" (connector).

The illumination system ("light source") transmits light into the field of view. The distal tip is also a source of air and water insufflation. The largest opening in the endoscope is a port for passage of a biopsy forceps or other endoscopic accessories. The spatial orientation of the various ports and components of the endoscopes is important (see Fig. 3.5B), especially when planning complex endoscopic interventions, such as large polypectomies.[1] Specialized endoscopes have accessories geared towards specific purposes, such as ultrasonographic (EUS) transducers in echo-endoscopes (see later).

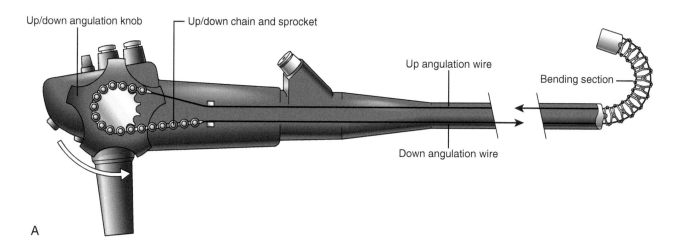

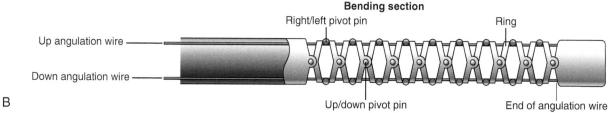

FIG 3.2 **A** and **B,** Angulation knobs in the control section cause deflection of the tip of the endoscope.

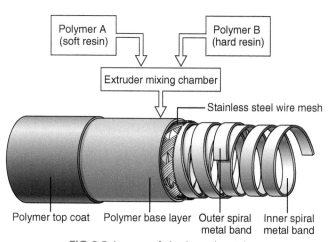

FIG 3.3 Layers of the insertion tube.

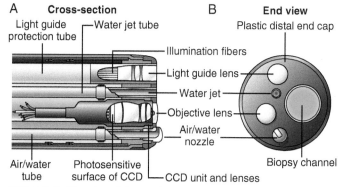

FIG 3.5 **A,** The tip of the endoscope with internal components and **B,** their spatial orientation externally. *CCD,* Charge-coupled device.

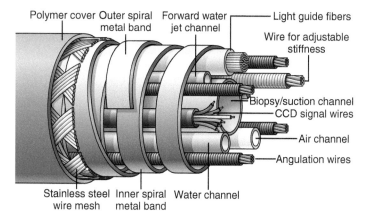

FIG 3.4 Internal components of a variable-stiffness colonoscope. *CCD,* Charge-coupled device.

The endoscope is integrated with an image processor through a connector (the umbilicus mentioned earlier). Electronic images are sent from the processor to a color monitor (TV screen). The processor also houses a powerful (usually quartz-halogen) light source, an air pump and a water bottle (Fig. 3.6). The modern endoscope is a precision tool for performing a wide range of diagnostic and therapeutic procedures.

IMAGE PROCESSING

In the earliest iteration of the endoscope, fiber-optic imaging was used to transmit the light from the illuminated end of the endoscope to the eye piece. The fiber-optics were encased in bundles that ran the length of the endoscope and used the principle of total internal reflection of light.[3] These fiber-optic

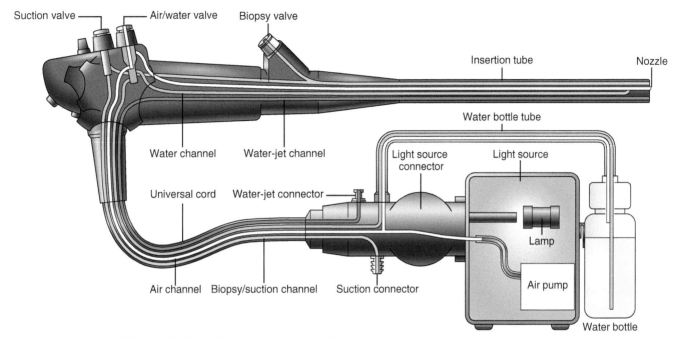

FIG 3.6 Configuration of the air, water, light, and suction systems in the endoscope.

cables were susceptible to damage and the optical arrangement required the endoscopist to hold the endoscope close to the eye.

As technology progressed, CCDs came into being and heralded the era of video endoscopy, which displays images on a screen. This freed the endoscopist from the tyranny of the eye piece, enabling an ergonomically friendly procedure with a substantially lesser risk of body fluid splashes. The CCD is an integrated circuit with photocells that generate electrical charge when hit by light (photons). The amount of charge produced is proportional to the brightness of the light. The system requires the use of a bright xenon lamp to produce white light, which is then transmitted through a filter to provide illumination. The reflected light is then processed by the CCD to an image on the monitor.[1] Using multiple filters, a mosaic of colors can be produced, resulting in a video image. Hence, the CCD essentially converts an image into a sequence of electronic signals which, after appropriate processing, are transformed into an image on the monitor screen.[4]

Before current technology allowed the etching of filters directly on to a chip, a rotating wheel with primary color filters was used to synthesize the fine-color image. This system suffered from a pronounced "flicker effect". On modern CCDs, each pixel is given one of the three primary color filters (red, blue, green) by metal oxide etching. One pixel will measure the intensity of light through a red filter; adjacent pixels do the same through blue and green filters. When the values of the colors and brightness levels from the three adjacent pixels are combined in a process repeated throughout the whole CCD, a full-color video image is the result (Fig. 3.7).[3]

Advances in CCD design and, more recently, complementary metal oxide semiconductor technology, have resulted in smaller chips with an increased number of pixels and increased resolution.[5]

Along with advances in image resolution, progress has also been made in magnifying the endoscopic images. High-magnification endoscopes are defined by the capacity to perform optical zoom by using a movable lens in the tip of the endoscope.

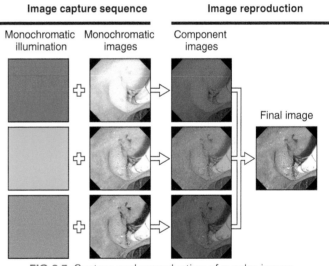

FIG 3.7 Capture and reproduction of a color image.

Optical zoom obtains a magnified image of the target while maintaining image display quality. This is distinguished from electronic or digital magnification, which simply enlarges the image on the display, with a consequent decreased pixel density and decreased image quality.[5] Certain endoscopes even employ a movable, motor-driven lens in the tip of the scope that can change the focal distance and provide a magnified view of the mucosal surface[6] (Video 3.1).

TYPES OF ENDOSCOPES

Different types of endoscopes are available to examine different areas of the human GI anatomy. The most commonly used are gastroscopes used for esophagogastroduodenoscopy (EGD) and colonoscopes for examination of the colon. Specialized endoscopes can be used to inspect the small bowel (enteroscopes), biliary and pancreatic ductal systems (duodenoscopes, choledochoscopes), as well as the extra-luminal anatomy (echoendoscopes). Therapeutic endoscopes with larger channel diameters that allow passage of complex and sophisticated accessories are also available for advanced interventional procedures.

Gastroscopes and Sigmoidoscopes

As the name suggests, gastroscopes are used for the examination of the upper GI tract, typically to the second part of duodenum. Conventional EGD endoscopes are introduced trans-orally and can be used to examine the esophagus, stomach and the first and second parts of the duodenum. These are forward-viewing endoscopes that can be used for diagnostic and therapeutic purposes. Therapeutic EGD endoscopes with enlarged or dual working channels are available to facilitate complex interventions.[7] Standard diagnostic gastroscopes are regularly used to perform flexible sigmoidoscopy.[8]

The narrow-caliber or ultra-slim endoscopes have a diameter ranging from 4.9 to 6 mm, which enables them to be introduced trans-nasally as well as trans-orally. The trans-nasal approach permits an unsedated endoscopic examination.[9] These features may provide a preferable alternative in patients who may not tolerate sedation or have narrow strictures that obstruct passage of standard-caliber endoscopes.

The narrow-caliber endoscope can examine the esophagus and stomach, but may not be long enough to reach the duodenum. Although useful for diagnostic examination, the accessory channel in these endoscopes is comparatively narrow (2 mm) and often can only allow passage of a pediatric biopsy forceps and guidewires, but not larger devices.[1] These endoscopes may also cause trauma to the nasal passages, leading to epistaxis and pain. Despite these limitations, multiple studies have shown that trans-nasal narrow-caliber endoscopes are safe and effective, and can be an alternative to standard-caliber endoscopes.[9,10] They are discussed in detail in Chapter 11.

Enteroscopes

As described previously, gastroscopes are unable to examine the GI tract distal to the duodenum due to their length. The lack of anatomic fixation of the small intestine beyond the duodenum causes standard endoscopes to "loop," which prevents deeper intubation. These limitations are overcome by enteroscopes, which are designed for deep intubation and examination of the small intestine. Enteroscopes are forward-viewing endoscopes but are substantially longer than gastroscopes and have devices designed to assist with intubation of the jejunum and ileum. These devices can be in the form of sleeves, overtubes, or inflatable balloons.

Balloon-assisted endoscopes employ an overtube with either a single- or double-balloon system mounted at the distal end. When inflated, the balloons are intended to anchor the endoscope in position during insertion to allow for pleating of the bowel over the endoscope shaft, reducing loop formation and allowing for greater insertion depth.[11] With a double-balloon enteroscope apparatus, the overtube and the enteroscope have a balloon each. Once past the major duodenal papilla, the overtube balloon is inflated to maintain a stable position and the enteroscope is advanced. Subsequently, the enteroscope balloon is inflated, the overtube balloon is deflated and the overtube is advanced to the enteroscope tip. Finally, both balloons are inflated simultaneously and the entire apparatus is carefully withdrawn to pleat the small

intestine over the apparatus. Withdrawal against the anchoring straightens the scope by reducing the loops. The preceding steps are then repeated. Double-balloon endoscopy can be done either antegrade or retrograde. Its use is limited by the often long procedure time, the need for an assistant and the need for anesthesia (usually deep sedation).

A single-balloon enteroscope does not have a balloon at the tip of the enteroscope; it only employs a balloon on the overtube. The enteroscope tip, bereft of a balloon, is anchored in place by flexing its tip in an attempt to 'hook' the mucosa at a fold. A through-the-scope system (NaviAid, Pentax Medical, Montvale, NJ) uses a disposable balloon that can be passed through the working channel of an endoscope, advanced distal to the tip of the endoscope and inflated.[12] This inflated balloon anchors the small intestine and allows distal advancement of the scope. Balloon-assisted enteroscopes may also be useful in patients with surgical altered anatomy, such as in patients with Roux-en-Y gastric bypass where access to the excluded gastric remnant is not feasible with a standard endoscope.

Enteroscopes that do not rely on balloons or overtubes are also available. A widely used technique called push enteroscopy can be used to examine the upper GI lumen as far as the proximal to mid-jejunum. Push enteroscopy can be performed using either adult or pediatric colonoscopes, or longer dedicated enteroscopes. These devices do not have any special accessories or overtubes but have a longer length and hence can go further into the small intestine when compared with a standard endoscope.[11] Spiral enteroscopes do not use balloons, but an overtube with specially designed external spirals that rotates and pleats the small intestine as the endoscope advances distally. These allow a faster advancement of the endoscope, but may have a higher complication rate.[13]

Duodenoscopes

Duodenoscopes are specialized endoscopes that are used primarily for ERCP. They are side-viewing (rather than forward-viewing) endoscopes that have the advantage of looking at the major duodenal papilla en-face. Duodenoscopes have a lever that is used to manipulate an elevator located at the tip of the endoscope. By maneuvering the elevator, the endoscopist can raise and lower accessories passed through the working channel into the field of view (Fig. 3.8). Hence, they facilitate access to the bile duct and pancreatic duct, which is helpful for cannulation of the papilla. Newer accessories, such as cholangioscopes, can be passed into the biliary duct and pancreatic duct for real-time visualization and sampling of the mucosa.[1]

Colonoscopes

Colonoscopes are designed for examining the entire colon and terminal ileum. Due to the flexibility of the colon where it is not tethered, there is a tendency for the colonoscope to form loops. The colonoscope is designed to minimize loop formation by varying the flexibility throughout the length of the insertion tube. The polymer covering the distal end of the insertion tube is relatively softer and more flexible to allow negotiating of angulations and curves, whereas the proximal end of the insertion tube is relatively firmer and less flexible to reduce loop formation. Certain instruments, called variable-stiffness colonoscopes, have a mechanism controlled by a dial on the proximal shaft that can be used to stiffen the proximal 40 to 50 cm of the insertion tube.[14] Incremental rotation of the dial adjusts the tension of a coil that runs through the insertion tube, causing the colonoscope

Cross-section through optical system

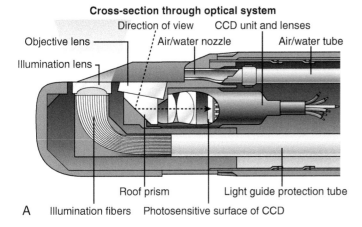

A

Cross-section through biopsy channel

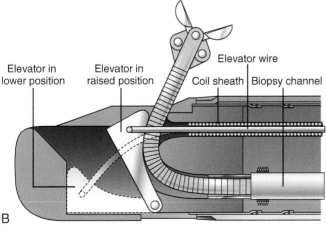

B

FIG 3.8 Cross-sectional view of the side-viewing endoscope showing **A,** the direction of view, as well as **B,** use of elevator when using endoscopic accessories. *CCD,* Charge-coupled device.

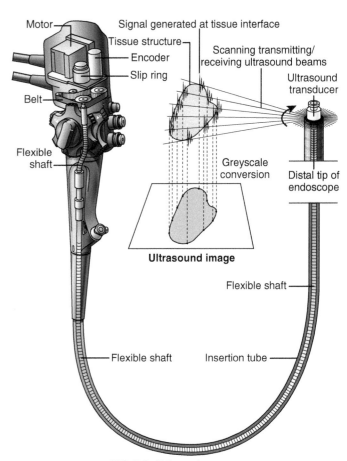

FIG 3.9 Echoendoscope.

to "stiffen."[1] Variable-stiffness colonoscopes may improve cecal intubation rates while causing less discomfort to the patient and requiring less sedation.[15] Over the years, colonoscopes have seen dramatic improvements in flexibility and image processing, and have become the principal method for diagnosis, treatment and follow-up of colorectal diseases.

Echoendoscopes

Echoendoscopes differ from the standard endoscopes as they contain an ultrasound transducer at the tip, which allows for EUS examination of the GI wall, as well as extra-luminal structures (Fig. 3.9). The EUS transducer converts electrical energy into sound waves. These travel through the wall of the GI tract and impact adjacent viscera, and are subsequently reflected back to the transducer, which reconverts them into electric energy. These electric signals are processed to create an EUS image.[16] The transducer contains piezoelectric crystals that can scan at different sound wave frequencies. Scanning at higher frequencies enhances the resolution, but reduces depth of penetration. Hence, higher frequencies are ideal for creating sharp images of structures within or adjacent to the lumen, whereas lower frequencies are needed for the imaging of more distant structures.[16] Use of Doppler signal analysis allows the endoscopist to identify (and avoid) vascular structures.[1]

Echoendoscopes may be either radial or curvilinear, which refers to the orientation of the sonographic image as it relates to the axis of the insertion tube. Thus, radial echoendoscopes produce an image that is perpendicular to the insertion tube, whereas curvilinear echoendoscopes produce an image parallel to the insertion tube. The radial echoendoscope provides a 360-degree view of the anatomy, but cannot be used for interventions such as tissue sampling via a needle or a variety of therapeutic procedures. The curvilinear echoendoscope, on the other hand, visualizes structures in the 100- to 180-degree range, but simultaneously allows real-time insertion of an EUS needle.[16] This allows the curvilinear echoendoscope to be used in diverse interventions, such as EUS-guided tissue acquisition, direct puncture of the bile duct or pancreas to relieve obstruction, trans-enteric drainage of fluid collections (e.g., endoscopic cyst-gastrostomy), fiducial marker implantation and celiac axis neurolysis.[17]

Capsule Endoscopes

Wireless capsule endoscopy is widely used in the assessment of the small bowel, especially in patients with suspected small bowel bleeding[18] or enteric Crohn's disease.[19] Recently, investigators have used this technique to evaluate more proximal pathologies, such as esophageal varices[20] and Barrett's esophagus.[21] Capsule studies have also shown encouraging results in the detection of colon polyps[22] and may have a role in patients with ulcerative colitis[23] who have had prior incomplete colonoscopies.[24]

The capsule itself is made of a clear plastic shell, a high-resolution CCD to capture images, a compact lens, a white

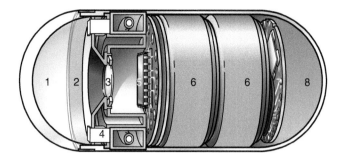

1. Optical dome
2. Lens holder
3. Lens
4. Illuminating LEDs (Light Emitting Diode)
5. CMOS (Complementary Metal Oxide Semiconductor) imager
6. Battery
7. ASIC (Application Specific Integrated Circuit) transmitter
8. Antenna

FIG 3.10 Capsule endoscope.

light-emitting diode for illumination and a battery (Fig. 3.10). The images and data are transmitted wirelessly (often via a high-frequency radio telemetry) to a sensor worn on a belt by the patient. The data from the sensor is then downloaded to a computer that has appropriate software for storage and analysis.[25] The software can be used to display the images in multiple or single frames. It can also identify and highlight pixels colored red to facilitate identification of bleeding lesions. The interpreting provider can review all the images at a variety of speeds, looking for mucosal lesions. It is also possible to calculate the time taken by the capsule to transit the small intestine.

The wireless capsule endoscopy typically requires a bowel preparation to clear the small intestine of partially digested food that may interfere with the visualization of the mucosa. Fasting or consuming only clear liquids 12 to 24 hours prior to the procedure is often recommended. The capsule is activated by removal from a magnetic holder and can be either swallowed by the patient, or endoscopically placed in the stomach or proximal small intestine. It is disposable and is designed to be excreted.[25]

Wireless capsule endoscopy may be preceded by use of a patency capsule that is made of lactose and 5% barium sulfate, and contains a radiofrequency tag. The patency capsule has the same dimensions of the capsule endoscope but can dissolve when acted upon by intestinal fluids.[26] The patency capsule is not required in all patients, but may be useful in those suspected to have tight strictures that could cause capsule retention and prevent further passage.[27]

NEWER ENDOSCOPIC MODALITIES

High-Definition Endoscopes

High-definition (HD) endoscopes may improve mucosal assessment and quality endpoints, such as adenoma detection rates (ADRs) for screening colonoscopy and dysplasia detection in Barrett's esophagus.

HD endoscopy uses a HD monitor (1080 lines of vertical resolution) and a high-resolution CCD with up to 1 million pixels, which provide much better images than standard video

endoscopy.[28] HD image displays can refresh on a line-by-line scan, which may be progressive or interlaced. Progressive scanning provides twice the temporal resolution (60 frames/sec) of interlaced scanning (30 frames/sec) and is better for video display of fast-moving objects.[5] A meta-analysis of five studies involving 4422 patients showed that HD endoscopes only marginally improved the polyp detection rate (incremental yield of 3.8%), as well as the ADR (incremental yield of 3.5%); this may hold especially true for flat or subtle lesions less than 5 mm in size.[28] Other studies have demonstrated an increase in the detection of flat and sessile polyps,[29,30] suggesting modest improvements in ADRs, especially for endoscopists with somewhat lower ADRs.[31,32]

Digital Chromoendoscopy

The primary colors–red, green and blue–form the basis of the RGB chip used in most endoscopes. A number of commercially available systems manipulate the individual components of an endoscopic image to accentuate vascular patterns and mucosal features. This can improve the visibility of surface structures and hence the identification of GI pathology (see Video 3-1).

Narrow-band imaging (NBI) available on the Olympus platform (Olympus Corporation of the Americas, Center Valley, PA) can accentuate the vascular and mucosal features using specific filters that can, for example, enhance light absorption of hemoglobin. The basic principle of NBI is that the depth of penetration of light into the mucosa depends on its wavelength.[33] Deep penetration is achieved with red light, intermediate penetration with green light and only superficial penetration with blue light.[34] The i-SCAN technology from Pentax uses different algorithms to enhance the contrast and surface structures. For example, the surface-enhancement algorithm improves the light and dark contrast, whereas the contrast-enhancement algorithm adds blue hue to dark areas. Tone enhancement breaks and then resynthesizes the individual components of an image.[34] Fujinon intelligent color enhancement (FICE; Fujifilm Medical Co., Saitama, Japan) also electronically narrows the bandwidth of conventional white light colonoscopy to improve visualization using algorithms, permitting close inspection of pit patterns and microvascular structures.[33] Thus far, multiple meta-analyses comparing NBI and white light endoscopy have failed to show a difference in polyp detection rate or ADRs.[32,35,36] There are no well-designed studies that have directly compared different commercial endoscopy systems for outcomes and image quality. A randomized tandem colonoscopy trial in South Korea compared NBI, FICE and conventional white light endoscopy in 1650 patients. The study found no increase in the detection of polyps or adenomas among the three modalities.[37] A survey of gastroenterologists, nurses and medical students who reviewed the same images had poor interobserver agreement for the quality of endoscopic images.[34]

Endoscope Modifications to Increase the Mucosal Surface Area Visualized

For endoscopists doing colonoscopies, it is of vital importance to be able to inspect the entire colonic mucosa and detect subtle lesions, such as serrated adenomas. This task is made challenging by the haustral folds in the colon. The mucosa behind colonic folds is often poorly visualized due to the inherent nature of the retrograde approach of colonic inspection. Multiple endoscopic devices are now available to increase the colonic surface area available for inspection. These devices either employ extra imaging devices or cameras with extra wide view[38] to allow visualization of mucosa behind the folds, or utilize accessories that can stretch and flatten the haustral folds for more complete inspection. An example of the former approach is the Full Spectrum Endoscopy (Fuse; EndoChoice, Inc., Alpharetta, GA) system, which adds imagers on either side of the forward-facing lens of the colonoscope. The Fuse system increases the endoscopists' view from an angle of 170 degrees to 330 degrees; it employs three large, solid-state contiguous monitors for display.[39] In an unblinded, international, randomized tandem trial, the investigators reported a significantly lower missed adenoma rate using the Fuse system compared with the standard front-viewing colonoscope.[39]

In a modification of the aforementioned system, the extra wide angle view colonoscope (Olympus Corporation) uses an extra 144- to 232-degree angle, lateral-backward viewing lens in addition to a standard 140-degree angle forward-viewing lens. The views from the two cameras are merged into a single 'panoramic' view and displayed as a single image.[40] In a small exploratory study from Japan, investigators demonstrated the safety and efficacy of the new colonoscope.[40]

Accessories That Increase the Visualized Surface Area for Examination

Multiple accessories have been developed for this purpose that can either be attached to the tip of the endoscope or passed through the working channel. Some of these accessories can be reused. These accessories can mechanically flatten or straighten the haustral folds or use imaging devices to visualize the mucosa behind the folds. The NaviAid G-EYE colonoscope (Smart Medical Systems Ltd., Ra'anana, Israel) uses a permanently integrated balloon system attached at the tip of the endoscope. In a small study on a silicone model of a colon, balloon-assisted colonoscopy had a significantly higher polyp detection rate than standard colonoscopy.[41] The interim results of a larger randomized trial indicate an improvement in the ADR, but final results are pending.[42]

A similar device is the Endocuff (Arc Medical Design Ltd., Leeds, United Kingdom), which is mounted on the distal tip of the endoscope and has multiple hinged, soft finger-like projections that can flatten the haustral folds on withdrawal.[43] This can be used to improve visualization and stabilization during complex polypectomy.[43] Randomized clinical trials have demonstrated a 14% increase in the polyp detection rate,[44] as well as a 14.7% increase in the ADR[45] using the Endocuff device. The utility of the Endocuff appears to be greater in the sigmoid colon[43,45] than other segments, which may be due to the tortuosity of this site.

Transparent caps attached to the tip of the colonoscope have been used in a similar fashion to flatten the haustral folds for inspection of the proximal mucosa. There have been conflicting data about the ability of cap-assisted colonoscopy to increase the ADR. A study in US veterans undergoing a screening or surveillance examination demonstrated that cap-assisted colonoscopy detected a higher number of adenomas per patient.[46] However, a much larger study from The Netherlands showed no difference in the ADR using cap assistance in patients undergoing a screening colonoscopy.[47] Both studies demonstrated a reduction in the cecal intubation time.[46,47] A meta-analysis of 16 randomized clinical trials of 8991 patients demonstrated that cap-assisted colonoscopy detected more polyps and reduced cecal intubation time without increasing the total colonoscopy time.[48] A Cochrane review that evaluated 14 randomized controlled trials suggested a marginally improved, but statistically insignificant, cecal intubation time.[49] A different meta-analysis concluded that use of a transparent cap increased the detection of polyps and had a higher cecal intubation rate, while having no impact on the time to cecal intubation.[50]

The Third Eye Retroscope (Avantis Medical Systems, Sunnyvale, CA) works differently from the previously mentioned accessories. Instead of mechanically flattening the haustral folds, it uses a retroflexed imaging system passed through the working channel of the endoscope. The retroflexed camera is positioned beyond the mucosal folds where it works like a rear-view mirror. It visualizes the mucosa behind the haustral folds and projects the image onto part of the TV screen. This allows the endoscopist to visualize the mucosa on either side of the haustral fold.[51] In a non-randomized study in 249 patients, Waye et al (2010) demonstrated an increase of 13.2% in the detection of polyps and an 11% increase in number of adenomas detected using the Third Eye Retroscope over standard colonoscopy.[52] In a similar study, investigators detected additional polyps and adenomas on the left and right colon using the Third Eye Retroscope and further demonstrated that the ADRs improve as endoscopists gain experience with the device.[53] Finally, in a multicenter, randomized, tandem trial comparing the Third Eye Retroscope and standard colonoscopy, the TERRACE (effect of a retrograde-viewing device on adenoma detection rate during colonoscopy) study showed 23.2% additional adenoma detection using this accessory, but with a significantly longer withdrawal and total procedure time.[54]

KEY REFERENCES

1. ASGE Technology Committee, Varadarajulu S, Banerjee S, et al: GI endoscopes, *Gastrointest Endosc* 74(1):1–6, e6, 2011.
3. Baillie J: The endoscope, *Gastrointest Endosc* 65(6):886–893, 2007.
5. ASGE Technology Committee: High-definition and high-magnification endoscopes, *Gastrointest Endosc* 80(6):919–927, 2014.
11. ASGE Technology Committee, Chauhan SS, Manfredi MA, et al: Enteroscopy, *Gastrointest Endosc* 82(6):975–990, 2015.
16. ASGE Technology Committee, Murad FM, Komanduri S, et al: Echoendoscopes, *Gastrointest Endosc* 82(2):189–202, 2015.
17. ASGE Technology Committee, Kaul V, Adler DG, et al: Interventional EUS, *Gastrointest Endosc* 72(1):1–4, 2010.
22. Rex DK, Adler SN, Aisenberg J, et al: Accuracy of capsule colonoscopy in detecting colorectal polyps in a screening population, *Gastroenterology* 148(5):948–957, e2, 2015.
25. ASGE Technology Committee, Wang A, Banerjee S, et al: Wireless capsule endoscopy, *Gastrointest Endosc* 78(6):805–815, 2013.
28. Subramanian V, Mannath J, Hawkey CJ, Ragunath K: High definition colonoscopy vs. standard video endoscopy for the detection of colonic polyps: a meta-analysis, *Endoscopy* 43(6):499–505, 2011.
30. Gross SA, Buchner AM, Crook JE, et al: A comparison of high definition-image enhanced colonoscopy and standard white-light colonoscopy for colorectal polyp detection, *Endoscopy* 43(12):1045–1051, 2011.
36. Nagorni A, Bjelakovic G, Petrovic B: Narrow band imaging versus conventional white light colonoscopy for the detection of colorectal polyps, *Cochrane Database Syst Rev* (1):CD008361, 2012.
45. Floer M, Biecker E, Fitzlaff R, et al: Higher adenoma detection rates with Endocuff-assisted colonoscopy - a randomized controlled multicenter trial, *PLoS ONE* 9(12):e114267, 2014.

A complete reference list can be found online at ExpertConsult .com

4

Cleaning and Disinfecting Gastrointestinal Endoscopy Equipment

David Lichtenstein and Michelle J. Alfa

CHAPTER OUTLINE

INTRODUCTION

The field of gastrointestinal (GI) endoscopy has expanded dramatically as new procedures, instruments, and accessories have been introduced into the medical community; more than 20 million GI endoscopies are performed annually in the United States.[1,2] Although GI endoscopes are used as a diagnostic and therapeutic tool for a broad spectrum of GI disorders, more health care–associated infectious outbreaks and patient exposures have been linked to contaminated endoscopes than to any other reusable medical device.[3–6] Failure to adhere to established reprocessing guidelines or the use of defective reprocessing equipment accounts for the majority of these cases.[7–13] In addition, complex endoscopes such as the duodenoscope and linear echoendoscope with elevator mechanisms can transmit bacterial infections even when reprocessing protocols are reportedly followed in accordance with manufacturer and societal guidelines.[14–16]

The topic of endoscope reprocessing has largely been taken for granted by many endoscopists; however, standardized cleaning and disinfection protocols have been available for some time, and, with few exceptions, changes have been gradual. This slow evolution with a high safety profile may have engendered some complacency on the part of endoscopists, to the point that many endoscopists are only vaguely aware of what goes on "behind the curtain" of the endoscope reprocessing room. Instruments are used on patients, taken away by GI nurses or other health care personnel, reprocessed, and returned ready for patient use.

As the complexity of reprocessing and recognition of its importance become a concern to the medical community and our patients, endoscopists must become more educated on these issues and thereby able to participate in informed discussions with their patients. This chapter presents a pragmatic approach to proper reprocessing of endoscopic equipment, with guidance for prevention and management of infection transmission, and includes newer sterilization and disinfection technologies.

PRINCIPLES OF REPROCESSING

Cleaning

Cleaning refers to removal of visible soiling, blood, protein substances, and other adherent foreign debris from surfaces, crevices, and lumens of instruments.[17] It is usually accomplished with mechanical action using water, detergents, and enzymatic products. Meticulous physical cleaning must always precede disinfection and sterilization procedures, because inorganic and organic materials that remain on the surfaces of instruments interfere with the effectiveness of these processes.[18] Mechanical cleaning alone reduces microbial counts by approximately 10^3 to 10^6 (three to six logs), equivalent to a 99.9% to 99.9999% reduction in microbial burden.[19–26]

Sterilization

Sterilization is defined as the destruction or inactivation of all microorganisms. The process is operationally defined as a 12-log reduction of bacterial endospores.[27] Not all sterilization processes are alike, however. Steam is the most extensively utilized process and is routinely monitored by the use of biologic indicators (e.g., spore test strips) to show that sterilization has been achieved. When liquid chemical germicides (LCGs) are used to eradicate all microorganisms, they can be called chemical sterilants; however, the US Food and Drug Administration (FDA) and other authorities have stated that these processes do not convey the same level of assurance as other sterilization methods.[28–30] Other commonly used sterilization processes include low-temperature gas such as ethylene oxide (ETO), liquid chemicals, and hydrogen peroxide gas plasma.[31]

Disinfection

Disinfection is defined broadly as the destruction of microorganisms, except bacterial spores, on inanimate objects (e.g., medical devices such as endoscopes). Three levels of disinfection are achievable depending on the amount and kind of microbial killing involved. These levels of disinfection are as follows:

1. High-level disinfection (HLD): the destruction of all viruses, vegetative bacteria, fungi, mycobacterium, and some, but not all, bacterial spores.[32,33] For LCGs, HLD is operationally defined as the ability to kill 10^6 mycobacteria (a six-log reduction). The efficacy of HLD is dependent on several factors and includes the type and level of microbial contamination; effective precleaning of the endoscope; presence of biofilm; physical properties of the object; concentration, temperature, pH, and exposure time to the germicide; and drying after rinsing to avoid diluting the disinfectant.[32]
2. Intermediate-level disinfection: the destruction of all mycobacteria, vegetative bacteria, fungal spores, and some nonlipid viruses, but not bacterial spores.
3. Low-level disinfection: a process that can kill most bacteria (except mycobacteria or bacterial spores), most viruses (except some nonlipid viruses), and some fungi.

Although this categorization for disinfection levels generally remains valid, there are examples of disinfection issues with prions, viruses, mycobacteria, and protozoa that challenge these definitions.[34]

Antiseptics are chemicals intended to reduce or destroy microorganisms on living tissue (e.g., skin), as opposed to disinfectants, which are used on inanimate objects (e.g., medical devices such as endoscopes). The difference in the way the same chemical is used to achieve different levels of disinfection and sterilization is important for endoscopy because the contact times for sterilization with any given LCG are generally much longer (hours) than for high-level disinfection (minutes) and may be detrimental to the endoscope. The relative resistance of various microorganisms to LCGs is shown in Box 4.1.

Spaulding Classification

More than 40 years ago, Earle H. Spaulding developed a rational approach to disinfection and sterilization of medical equipment based on the risk of infection involved with the use of these instruments.[35,36] The classification scheme defined these categories of medical devices and their associated level of disinfection as follows:

1. Critical: critical devices or instruments come into contact with sterile tissue or the vascular system. These devices confer a high risk for infection if they are contaminated. This category includes biopsy forceps, sphincterotomes, surgical instruments, and implants, when used in sterile anatomic locations. Reprocessing of these instruments requires sterilization.

BOX 4.1   Descending Order of Resistance of Microorganisms to Liquid Chemical Germicides

Prions (transmissible spongiform encephalopathy agents)
    Creutzfeldt-Jakob (CJD)
    Variant Creutzfeldt-Jakob (vCJD)
Bacterial spores
    Bacillus subtilis
    Clostridium sporogenes
Mycobacteria
    Mycobacterium tuberculosis
Nonlipid or small viruses
    Poliovirus
    Coxsackievirus
    Rhinovirus
Fungi
    Trichophyton spp.
    Cryptococcus spp.
    Candida spp.
Vegetative bacteria
    Pseudomonas aeruginosa
    Salmonella choleraesuis
    Enterococci
Lipid or medium-sized viruses
    Herpes simplex virus (HSV)
    Cytomegalovirus (CMV)
    Coronavirus
    Hepatitis B virus (HBV)
    Hepatitis C virus (HCV)
    Human immunodeficiency virus (HIV)
    Ebola virus

Modified from Bond WW, Ott BJ, Franke KA, et al: Effective use of liquid chemical germicides on medical devices: instrument design problems. In Block SS (ed): *Disinfection, sterilization, and preservation*, ed 4. Philadelphia, 1991, Lea & Febiger, pp 1097–1106.

---

2. Semicritical: semicritical devices contact intact mucous membranes and do not ordinarily penetrate sterile tissue. These instruments include endoscopes, bronchoscopes, transesophageal echocardiography probes, and anesthesia equipment. Reprocessing of these instruments requires a minimum of HLD.
3. Noncritical: noncritical devices contact intact skin (e.g., stethoscopes or blood pressure cuffs). These items should be cleaned by low-level disinfection.

DISINFECTION AND GI ENDOSCOPY

Endoscopes

GI endoscopes are considered semicritical devices, and the resultant minimal standard for reprocessing is HLD. This standard is endorsed by governmental agencies including the Joint Commission (JC), the Centers for Disease Control and Prevention (CDC),[37] and the FDA.[38] It is also endorsed by gastroenterology societies such as the American Society for Gastrointestinal Endoscopy (ASGE), American College of Gastroenterology (ACG), and American Gastroenterological Association (AGA), as well as medical organizations, including the Association of Perioperative Registered Nurses (AORN), Society of Gastroenterology Nurses and Associates (SGNA), Association for Professionals in Infection Control and Epidemiology (APIC), and American Society for Testing and Materials (ASTM).[39–42] HLD of endoscopes eliminates all viable microorganisms, but not necessarily all

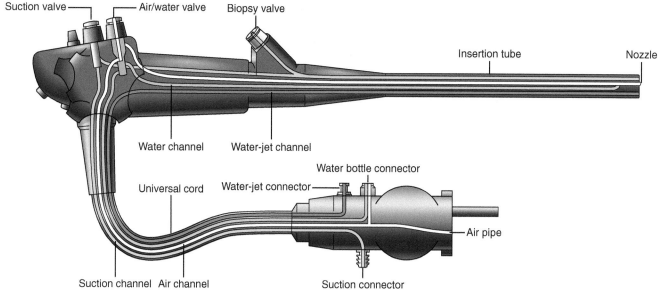

FIG 4.1 Schematic of internal channels of an endoscope. (Adapted from Olympus America. Copyright Olympus America Inc., 2003.)

bacterial spores.[43] Although spores are more resistant to HLD than other bacteria and viruses, they are likely to be killed when endoscopes undergo thorough manual cleaning. In addition, survival of small numbers of bacterial spores with HLD is considered acceptable because the intact mucosa of the GI tract is resistant to bacterial spore infection.

Endoscope sterilization, as opposed to HLD, is not required for "standard" GI endoscopy, as a reprocessing endpoint of sterilization has not been demonstrated to further reduce the risk of infectious pathogen transmission from endoscopes.[44] Sterilization of endoscopes is indicated when they are used as "critical" medical devices, such as intraoperative endoscopy when there is potential for contamination of an open surgical field.[45,46] In addition, individual institutional policies may dictate sterilization of duodenoscopes and linear endoscopic ultrasound instruments due to elevator mechanisms that have been difficult to clean and eradicate all bacterial contaminants with HLD alone (see the later section on Duodenoscope-Related Infections).

Despite the complex internal design (Fig. 4.1) of endoscopes, HLD is not difficult to achieve with rigorous adherence to currently accepted reprocessing guidelines.[47] Endoscope features that challenge the reprocessing procedures include:
- Complex endoscope design with several long, narrow internal channels and bends that make it difficult to remove all organic debris and microorganisms (e.g., elevator channel and elevator lever cavity of duodenoscopes).
- A large variety of endoscope vendors and models require different cleaning procedures and devices and materials.
- Occult damage (e.g., scratches, crevices) to the endoscope can sequester microorganisms and promote biofilm formation.

Accessories

All valves, caps, connectors, and flushing tubes need to be adequately cleaned, rinsed, and disinfected or sterilized at the same time the patient-used endoscope is being reprocessed.[48] The water bottle used to provide intraprocedural flush solution and its connecting tubing should be sterilized or receive high-level

disinfection at least once daily. The water bottle should be filled with sterile water.[49–52] Because accessory items often do not have unique identification numbers, it is critical to ensure they are dedicated to and stored with the endoscope that they are used with. This is necessary to ensure that if there is an outbreak, it is possible to identify which accessory components were used. This may require the use of disposable accessory holders or holders such as mesh bags that are also reprocessed along with the accessories.

Most accessory instruments used during endoscopy either contact the bloodstream (e.g., biopsy forceps, snares, and sphincterotomes) or enter sterile tissue spaces (e.g., biliary tract) and are classified as critical devices. As such, these devices require sterilization.[49,50] These accessories may be available as disposable "single-use" or "reusable" instruments. Reuse of devices labeled *single-use only* remains controversial but has been commonly employed in many practices, primarily for economic benefits.[44,53–56] The FDA[57] considers reprocessing a used single-use device into a ready-for-patient-use device as "manufacturing," and as a result, hospitals or third-party reprocessing[58,59] companies that reprocess these devices are required to follow the same regulations as the original equipment manufacturers (i.e., obtain 510[k] and premarket approval application; submit adverse event reports; demonstrate sterility and integrity of the reprocessed devices; and implement detailed quality assurance monitoring protocols). This includes the development of standards and policies to determine the maximum number of uses for the devices and the training of staff in the reprocessing procedures.[59–62] The regulatory burden imposed by these requirements essentially eliminated the practice of the reprocessing of single-use devices by most hospitals.

Automated Endoscope Reprocessors (AERs)

AERs were developed to replace some of the manual disinfection processes and standardize several important reprocessing steps, thereby eliminating the possibility of human error and minimizing exposure of reprocessing department personnel to chemical sterilants.[63–70] AERs continuously bathe the exterior surface of the endoscope and circulate the LCG under pressure through the endoscope channels. The AER manufacturer identifies each endoscope (brand and model) that is compatible with the AER and specifies limitations of reprocessing models of endoscopes and accessories. Variations in AERs may require customization of the facility design to accommodate requirements for ventilation; water pressure, temperature, and filtration; plumbing; power delivery; and space. All models of AERs have disinfection and rinse cycles. In addition, the AERs may also have one or more of the following automated capabilities:[32,68,71]

1. Some AERs utilize and discard small quantities of LCG per HLD cycle, whereas others have a reservoir of LCG that is reused over multiple cycles. The latter design results in gradual dilution of the LCG and requires intermittent testing to verify maintenance of the minimum effective concentration (MEC). Product-specific test strips need to be used regularly to monitor these solutions,[48] which should be discarded whenever they fall below the MEC or when the use-life expires, whichever comes first.
2. The temperature and cycle length can be altered to ensure HLD or sterilization based on the LCG and type of endoscope.
3. The AER should ensure circulation of LCGs through all endoscope channels at an equal pressure with flow sensors for automated detection of channel obstruction.
4. The AER should be self-disinfecting.
5. Vapor recovery systems are available.
6. Low intensity ultrasound waves are an option.
7. Variable number of endoscopes per cycle.
8. Some AERs flush the endoscope channels with forced air or with 70% to 80% ethyl or isopropyl alcohol followed by forced air to aid in drying the endoscope channels, thereby eliminating residual water, which reduces microbial growth during storage.
9. The AER should incorporate a self-contained or external water filtration system.

LCGs and AERs must meet specified performance levels for HLD to receive FDA clearance. This is defined as a reduction in residual organic loads and a 6-$\log_{10}$ killing of resistant indicator organisms (typically *Mycobacterium bovis*). All AERs marketed in the United States meet these criteria. The ASGE has published a summary of vendor-specific AERs and their compatible LCGs.[65] The FDA has approved labeling some AERs as washer-disinfectors due to the introduction of automated, brushless washing of endoscope channels prior to the disinfection cycle. Utilization of this AER washing cycle provides an extra margin of safety by providing redundancy of cleaning; however, the existing multisociety guideline[45] and other international standards emphasize that manual cleaning is still necessary when a washer-disinfector is used to assure the overall efficacy of HLD.[65,72]

One AER (Steris System 1E [SS1E]; Steris Corp, Mentor, OH) has received FDA approval for liquid chemical sterilization, as opposed to HLD, for heat-sensitive devices that cannot be sterilized by traditional means.[73] This system uses filtered, ultraviolet-treated water that enters the AER and mixes with a peracetic acid-based formulation that is subsequently heated to 46°C to 55°C for liquid chemical sterilization.[74] This system is designed for "point of use" sterilization, as sterile storage is not possible. For flexible endoscopes processed through the SS1E, there is still a requirement for an alcohol rinse and drying prior to placing the endoscope into a storage cabinet.

The FDA also requested that AER manufacturers conduct additional validation testing to evaluate AER reprocessing effectiveness with regard to the recess around the duodenoscope's elevator lever area.[75] An FDA communiqué released in February 2016 indicated that validation testing on three AER models (Advantage Plus [Medivators; Minneapolis, MN], DSD Edge [Medivators], and System IE [Steris Corp]) was complete and adequate.[75] In November 2015, the FDA issued a recall under consent decree for all Custom Ultrasonics (Ivyland, PA) AERs because of the company's inability to validate that their AERs were able to adequately wash and disinfect duodenoscopes to mitigate the risk of patient infection.[76] In a subsequent safety communication, the FDA recommended that health care facilities should not use Custom Ultrasonics System 83 Plus AERs for reprocessing duodenoscopes and should transition to alternative methods for duodenoscope reprocessing.[77]

Liquid Chemical Germicides and Sterilization Technologies

LCGs have inherent limitations; however, they are universally used to reprocess flexible endoscopes and accessories due to their relative convenience, safety, and rapid action. LCGs used as HLDs should ideally have the following properties: broad antimicrobial spectrum, rapid onset of action, activity in the presence of organic material, lack of toxicity for patients and endoscopy personnel, long reuse life, low cost, odorless, ability to monitor concentration, and nondamaging to the endoscope or the environment.[18,32] HLD solutions can act as sterilants if an increased exposure time is used[28,48,78]; however, the exposure time required to achieve sterilization with most LCG solutions is far longer than is practical, and therefore these formulations are only used for HLD.[48,79]

The efficacy of chemical disinfectants and sterilants is dependent on their physical properties including concentration and temperature; the length of exposure of the endoscope to the chemical solutions; the type and amount of microbial debris on the endoscope; and the mechanical components of the endoscope such as channels and crevices. Because the chemicals are toxic to humans and the environment, proper handling, thorough rinsing, and appropriate disposal are essential for human safety.[71] When selecting a HLD product, institutional requirements need to be taken into consideration with important variables including the number of endoscopes processed per day, training requirements, turnaround time, cost information, and regulatory issues regarding safe use of the HLD products. Health care workers who use HLDs need to be familiar with and have readily accessible, product/brand-specific Material Safety Data Sheets (MSDS) and keep current with regulatory changes and new product developments.[18] Users should consult with manufacturers of endoscopes and AERs for compatibility before selecting an LCG. The most commonly used FDA approved LCGs for disinfection of flexible endoscopes include glutaraldehyde, ortho-phthalaldehyde (OPA), peracetic acid, and hydrogen peroxide (Table 4.1)[71,80,81] based chemicals in varying combinations and concentrations. Some formulations contain combinations of microbicidal agents, including glutaraldehyde and phenol/phenate, peracetic acid and hydrogen peroxide, and glutaraldehyde and isopropyl alcohol. The FDA periodically updates a list of approved HLD solutions along with some of their attributes, such as contact time and temperature required for HLD.[82]

Sterilization of endoscopes is indicated on occasions when they are used as critical medical devices during open surgical procedures. The risk for contamination of the operative field exists when a nonsterile endoscope enters the abdomen through

TABLE 4.1 High-Level Disinfectants Currently Used for Endoscope Reprocessing[32,43,71,81,83]

Agent/Action	Contact Time	Advantages	Disadvantages
Glutaraldehyde Biocidal activity results from its alkylation of sulfhydryl, hydroxyl, carboxyl, and amino groups of microorganisms, which alters RNA, DNA, and protein synthesis	Minimum of 45 minutes at 25°C is indicated by the manufacturers (a minimum of 20 minutes at room temperature (20°C) is adequate according to expert opinion and published guidelines)	• Long history of use in health care settings • Excellent biocidal activity • Relatively inexpensive • Not corrosive to endoscopes • Not classified as a human carcinogen • Can be used for manual or AER systems • Some products achieve high-level disinfection with a shorter exposure time but require a higher temperature (e.g., Rapicide, Medivators, Minneapolis, MN) (US FDA, 2009)	• Fixes proteins which allows for biofilm formation; therefore, it is critical that medical devices are thoroughly cleaned prior to exposure. • Should not be used for reprocessing in patients with prion infection • Reusable for 14 to 28 days (depending on formulation) • MEC testing necessary • Vapors are sensitizing and work areas need to be properly ventilated and air quality monitored but less than glutaraldehyde. AER mitigates this issue. • Exposure may cause skin irritation or mucous membrane irritation (eye, nose, mouth), or pulmonary symptoms (epistaxis, asthma, rhinitis) • Exposure may cause colitis if the endoscope is not thoroughly rinsed • Relatively slow mycobacterial activity • Requires inactivation or special disposal protocol
Orthophthalaldehyde (OPA) Similar to glutaraldehyde interacts with amino acids, proteins, and microorganisms. However, OPA is a less potent cross-linking agent. This is compensated for by the lipophilic aromatic nature of OPA that is likely to assist its uptake through the outer layers of mycobacteria and gram-negative bacteria. OPA appears to kill spores by blocking the spore germination process.	Minimum of 10 minutes at room temperature (20°C); minimum of 5 minutes at 25°C (when used with an AER)	• Fast acting • Excellent microbiocidal activity and superior myobactericidal activity compared to glutaraldehyde • Odor not significant • No air quality monitoring required • Excellent materials compatibility • Does not coagulate blood or fix tissues to surfaces • Does not require exposure monitoring • No carcinogen classification • Stable in wide range pH 3–9 • In AERs, it lasts longer before reaching MEC limit (~80 cycles) compared to glutaraldehyde (~40 cycles). Reusable for 14 days	• An aldehyde that cross-links proteins similar to glutaraldehyde but much less active as fixative • Not used for reprocessing in patients with prion infection • Stains skin, mucous membranes, clothing and environmental surfaces • More expensive than glutaraldehyde • Slow sporicidal activity • May not be compatible with all AERs • Potential irritant of eyes, skin, nose and pulmonary tree • May require neutralization prior to disposal • Concentrate limited use to one specific AER, and contraindicated for manual reprocessing
7.5% Hydrogen Peroxide Produces destructive hydroxyl free radicals that can attack membrane lipids, DNA, and other essential cell components	15 to 30 minutes at 21°C (depending upon formulation)	• No activation required • May enhance removal of organic matter and organisms • Active against a wide range of microorganisms • No disposal issues • No odor or irritation issues • Does not coagulate blood or fix tissues to surfaces • Inactivates cryptosporidium	• Material compatibility concerns (brass, zinc, copper, and nickel/silver plating) both cosmetic and functional • Severely irritating and corrosive to eyes, skin and gastrointestinal tract if inadequately rinsed • Excessive exposure could cause irreversible tissue damage to the eyes, including blindness, inhalation of hydrogen peroxide vapors can be severely irritating to the nose, throat, and lungs
Peracetic Acid Similar to other oxidizing agents it denatures proteins, disrupts cell wall permeability, and oxidizes sulfhydryl and sulfur bonds in proteins, enzymes, and other metabolites	5 minutes as 30°C or 12 minutes at 50°C to 56°C depending on formulation	• Rapid sterilization cycle time (30–45 minutes) • Low-temperature (50°–55°C) liquid immersion sterilization • Has a significantly greater efficacy at higher temperatures (e.g., a 6-log reduction of spores at 50°C in less than 2 minutes) • Rapidly sporicidal • Environmentally friendly byproducts (acetic acid, O_2, H_2O) and leaves no residue • No adverse health effects when used under normal operating conditions • Compatible with many materials and instruments • Does not coagulate blood or fix tissues to protein • Does not allow biofilm creation and has the ability to remove glutaraldehyde hardened bioburden from biopsy channels • Has not caused resistant organisms	• Potential material incompatibility (e.g., aluminum anodized coating becomes dull) • Can corrode copper, brass, bronze, plain steel and galvanized iron • Oxidizing ability may expose the leaks in internal channels of scopes previously disinfected with glutaraldehyde • Considered unstable, particularly when diluted • More expensive (endoscope repairs, operating costs, purchase costs) • Serious eye and skin damage (concentrated solution) with contact • Concentrates are used only in specific AER

AER, automated endoscope reprocessor; FDA, Food and Drug Administration; MEC, minimum effective concentration.

TABLE 4.2 Sterilization Technologies Used for Flexible Endoscope Reprocessing[86–92]

Agent/Action	Contact Time	Advantages	Disadvantages
Steam		• Nontoxic to environment, staff, and patients • Rapid cycle time • Minimally affected by organic/inorganic soiling • Penetrates device lumens and medical packing • Rapidly microbicidal	• Deleterious for heat-sensitive instruments so only applicable for use with specially constructed flexible endoscopes as per MIFU • May leave instruments wet and susceptible to rust • Potential for burns
Ethylene oxide (ETO)	30 minutes to 1 hour exposure depending on model of ETO sterilizer (100% ETO sterilizer versus those that use a carrier gas)	• Penetrates device lumens • Compatible with most medical materials and endoscope manufacturers • Simple to operate and monitor • Sterile storage in ETO sterilization case	• Requires 8–12 hours aeration time to remove ETO residue • Only 20% of United States hospitals have ETO on-site • Long turn-around time • No microbicidal efficacy data proving SAL 10^{-6} achieved • Studies question microbicidal activity in presence of organic matter and salt • ETO is toxic, a carcinogen, flammable • May damage endoscope • Requires special exposure monitoring • Requires special exhaust "scrubbers" to remove traces of ETO prior to release in environment • Requires specific ETO case to ensure adequate ETO penetration
Vaporized hydrogen peroxide	~50 minutes	• Safe for environment and no fumes • Leaves no toxic residue • No aeration necessary • Compatible with most devices including heat sensitive (temperatures <50°C)	• Restrictions of endoscopes based on poor penetration into long and narrow lumens • Limited materials and comparative microbicidal efficacy data (not proven SAL 10^{-6} achieved)
Peracetic acid (liquid chemical sterilant)	~30–45 minutes	• Low temperature (50°–55°C) • Environmental friendly byproducts • Sterilant flows through endoscope which facilitates salt, protein and microbe removal	• Used for immersible instruments only • One scope per cycle • Potential for contact eye and skin injury • Some material incompatibility (aluminum anodized coating) • Sterile storage is not possible

MIFU; manufacturers' instructions for use; *SAL;* sterility assurance level.

an incision, as occurs with selected methods of intraoperative enteroscopy or postsurgical anatomy endoscopic retrograde cholangiopancreatography (ERCP).[84,85]

Endoscopes, when sterilized, require low-temperature methods because they are heat labile and therefore, unlike most other medical or surgical devices, they cannot undergo steam sterilization. ETO is the most commonly employed low-temperature sterilization process and a valuable method of sterilizing flexible endoscopes. However, a lengthy aeration time is required following ETO sterilization to allow desorption of all residual toxic gas from the endoscope. Additional steps must be taken, such as the application of a venting valve or the removal of the water-resistant cap to ensure proper perfusion with the gas and to prevent damage to the endoscope due to excessive pressure build-up. In addition, there are potential hazards to staff, patients, and the environment related to ETO toxicities (Table 4.2).[86] The International Agency for Research on Cancer has classified ETO as a known (group 1) human carcinogen. Within the past two decades, several new, low-temperature (< 60°C) sterilization systems have been developed, including hydrogen peroxide gas plasma, vaporized hydrogen peroxide, peracetic acid immersion, and ozone[87–92] (see Table 4.2).

GI ENDOSCOPE REPROCESSING

Over the years there has been a continuous expansion of the diagnostic and surgical techniques being performed utilizing ever more complex GI flexible endoscopes. The combination of ultrasonic capability with flexible endoscopes has opened up a new tool to use for the diagnosis and staging of cancers. However, along with these improvements that enhance diagnostic capabilities comes the increasing complexity of the endoscope channels. These complexities include double instrument channels with connector bridges, ultrasound probe channels, auxiliary channels, and elevator lever wire channels (sealed and unsealed). These complexities in endoscopes have far-reaching impacts in terms of reprocessing of reusable flexible endoscopes. This has been painfully highlighted by the recent outbreaks of antibiotic resistant bacteria associated with fully reprocessed endoscopes that remain contaminated[15,28,93–104] and act as fomites that transmit bacteria to a high percentage of subsequent patients who are exposed to the contaminated endoscope (see later section on Infection Control Issues for more detailed information on infection transmission). Such outbreaks have focused attention on the cleaning and disinfection of flexible endoscopes. There has been a paradigm change in that it is now recognized that reprocessing of GI flexible endoscopes is an extremely complex process that requires a quality systems approach, which includes specific training for reprocessing personnel, adequate monitoring of various stages in the reprocessing cycle, and ongoing documentation of staff competency.[48,95,105–114]

Human factors play a critical role in compliance with reprocessing of GI endoscopes.[115] Ofstead et al (2010) demonstrated that compliance with all the reprocessing steps occurred for only

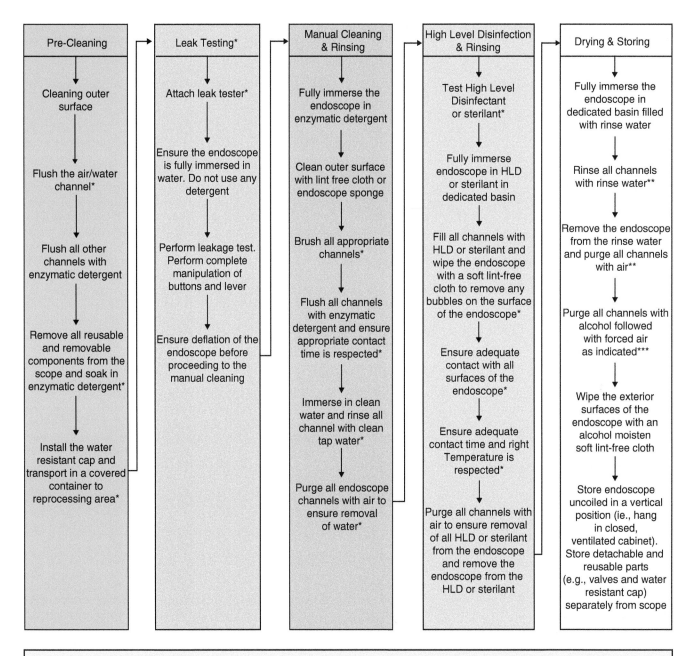

Pre-Cleaning	Leak Testing*	Manual Cleaning & Rinsing	High Level Disinfection & Rinsing	Drying & Storing
Cleaning outer surface	Attach leak tester*	Fully immerse the endoscope in enzymatic detergent	Test High Level Disinfectant or sterilant*	Fully immerse the endoscope in dedicated basin filled with rinse water
Flush the air/water channel*	Ensure the endoscope is fully immersed in water. Do not use any detergent	Clean outer surface with lint free cloth or endoscope sponge	Fully immerse endoscope in HLD or sterilant in dedicated basin	Rinse all channels with rinse water**
Flush all other channels with enzymatic detergent	Perform leakage test. Perform complete manipulation of buttons and lever	Brush all appropriate channels*	Fill all channels with HLD or sterilant and wipe the endoscope with a soft lint-free cloth to remove any bubbles on the surface of the endoscope*	Remove the endoscope from the rinse water and purge all channels with air**
Remove all reusable and removable components from the scope and soak in enzymatic detergent*	Ensure deflation of the endoscope before proceeding to the manual cleaning	Flush all channels with enzymatic detergent and ensure appropriate contact time is respected*	Ensure adequate contact with all surfaces of the endoscope*	Purge all channels with alcohol followed with forced air as indicated***
Install the water resistant cap and transport in a covered container to reprocessing area*		Immerse in clean water and rinse all channel with clean tap water*	Ensure adequate contact time and right Temperature is respected*	Wipe the exterior surfaces of the endoscope with an alcohol moisten soft lint-free cloth
		Purge all endoscope channels with air to ensure removal of water*	Purge all channels with air to ensure removal of all HLD or sterilant from the endoscope and remove the endoscope from the HLD or sterilant	Store endoscope uncoiled in a vertical position (ie., hang in closed, ventilated cabinet). Store detachable and reusable parts (e.g., valves and water resistant cap) separately from scope

* As per manufacturer of the product
** As prescribed by the manufacturer or the High Level disinfectant AND in accordance to the manufacturer of the endoscope
*** Alcohol rinse and drying is not needed if scope is used immediately on another patient, unless the final rinse was with unfiltered tap water

FIG 4.2 Overview of the reprocessing steps for GI endoscopes. (From Public Health Agency of Canada [PHAC]: Infection Prevention and Control Guideline for Flexible Gastrointestinal Endoscopy and Flexible Bronchoscopy. 2010, p 34. http://www.phac-aspc.gc.ca. [Figure 3, p 34; http://www.phac-aspc.gc.ca/nois-sinp/guide/endo/index-eng.php])

1.7% of flexible endoscopes reprocessed when cleaning steps were performed manually and disinfection was automated, compared to 75.4% compliance when both cleaning and disinfection were automated.[115] Fig. 4.2 outlines the basic steps in reprocessing of a GI flexible endoscope. Until recently, the only aspect of this process that was monitored was to test the MEC of the high-level disinfectant to ensure it contained a sufficient concentration of the active ingredient. It is easy to see from the outline provided in Fig. 4.2 how steps could be overlooked. Often staff are not aware of additional channels in new models of endoscopes and are not trained on specific cleaning requirements. The use of different sizes and types of channel brushes for the various different channel sizes, the fact that some channels cannot be brushed, and the multitude of different types of cleaning brushes available makes duodenoscope reprocessing a confusing process prone to human error.

Regulatory Changes
Major changes in GI endoscope reprocessing over the past five years have occurred and include new regulatory requirements,

device-reprocessing guidelines, and endoscope manufacturers' instructions for use. The key "domino" in this chain of changes was the 2015 FDA Guide to Manufacturers of Reusable Medical Devices (FDA, March 2015) that required manufacturers to validate that their cleaning instructions were effective and could achieve predetermined benchmarks. Cleaning validation for medical device reprocessing was not previously required; the focus was on validation of the disinfection or sterilization protocols recommended by manufacturers for their medical devices. When transmission of carbapenem-resistant *Enterobacteriaceae* (CRE) associated with contaminated duodenoscopes was recognized and first investigated and reported in the United States,[14] it was unclear why reprocessing of duodenoscopes was failing. However, it was clear that transmission rates from contaminated duodenoscopes were high (up to 45%) and that, in addition to causing infections, patients often became colonized with CRE and remained colonized long after the exposure to the CRE contaminated duodenoscope. Some health care facilities continued to report CRE transmission and suggested that the manufacturers' instructions for use (MIFUs) for endoscope reprocessing were inadequate[15,103,116] and that was why endoscope contamination was ongoing. Although there had been recent design changes by the three main duodenoscope manufacturers whereby the elevator wire channel was sealed, the transmission of CRE was reported for duodenoscopes with both sealed and unsealed elevator wire channels.[14,15,103] However, one thing was clear; it was very difficult to adequately clean the lever cavity in duodenoscopes, and visible patient debris under the elevator lever was detected in one published outbreak.[95] This has prompted new validated cleaning instructions for the lever cavity of duodenoscopes.[117] The CRE outbreaks linked to contaminated duodenoscopes prompted the FDA to convene an advisory panel meeting in May 2015, and on August 4, 2015, the FDA issued a Safety Communication[110] with the recommendations from the advisory panel meeting that included:

1. Establishing and implementing a comprehensive quality control program for endoscopy reprocessing to ensure meticulous adherence to MIFUs for duodenoscope reprocessing, adequate training of reprocessing personnel, and audits to ensure ongoing compliance.

2. Supplemental measures to be considered by sites offering ERCP procedures, including:
   - Microbiological culture with quarantine of contaminated endoscopes until culture results become available;
   - Meticulous cleaning and HLD followed by one of:
     - ETO sterilization,
     - Liquid chemical sterilization, or
     - Repeat HLD.

The FDA safety alert was followed by a CDC Health Advisory in September 2015, that indicated an immediate need for sites utilizing duodenoscopes to undertake audits of the reprocessing protocol, as well as staff training and longitudinal audits to document ongoing staff competency.

These events and actions have led to a "paradigm shift" regarding the reprocessing of flexible endoscopes,[113] whereby the need for a total quality systems approach has been recognized. It is no longer adequate to accept that endoscope cleaning is being done properly just because the MIFUs are available to staff; rather, there needs to be evidence of monitoring and ongoing audits of cleaning compliance for all staff who reprocess endoscopes. In addition, the need to ensure the endoscopes are truly dry during storage to prevent biofilm formation has been identified.[97,98,108,110,113,118–121] If biofilm forms, the ability of disinfectants to reliably kill microorganisms within biofilm is dramatically reduced.[118,122]

EFFICACY OF REPROCESSING

Overview of Quality Systems Approach

Although most published reports of infectious outbreaks related to flexible endoscopes have involved duodenoscopes, other endoscopes including colonoscopes, gastroscopes, bronchoscopes, cystoscopes, and ureteroscopes (see later sections on Reprocessing Errors and Outbreak Management and Infection Control Issues), have been shown to be contaminated and involved in infectious outbreaks. As such, every site offering flexible endoscopy procedures should ensure they have an established quality system for reprocessing these complex devices as recommended by the FDA[110] and CDC.[123] Table 4.3 provides an overview of what components are needed for such a system. As recommended by the CDC,[123] the first step that all health care facilities should undertake is to perform an audit by reviewing their current endoscopy services to ensure they meet all aspects of a quality system approach. This requires input from administration, risk management, endoscopy staff, and infection prevention and control to ensure that all components are adequately assessed and the appropriate policies and procedures documented and implemented.

Table 4.4 provides an overview of the key steps in reprocessing and outlines where mistakes are frequently made, as well as the impact of such mistakes. It is important that audits done for endoscope reprocessing are observational and based on a specific checklist of critical components, as well as data to substantiate processes (e.g., time data to show contact time with detergent during cleaning, as well as transport times to determine how frequently it exceeds 1 hour). Table 4.4 is a useful aid to review during initial training of staff, as well as during discussion of audit data on a yearly basis.

Cleaning Monitoring (Rapid Testing of Organic Residuals and Adenosine Triphosphate [ATP])

The need to monitor the adequacy of cleaning[48] is a critical step in the Total Quality System approach (see Table 4.3) to endoscope reprocessing. Appropriate benchmarks for cleaning markers have been established.[48,54,109,118,121,124–126] There are a number of rapid cleaning tests (RCT) available for monitoring organic residuals such as hemoglobin, carbohydrate, and protein, as well as those that monitor ATP residuals. There are published data for some of these rapid test methods,[112,125–132] but when selecting a rapid cleaning monitor, it is important to request that the rapid test manufacturer provide their validation data. Review of the pros and cons of the testing method based on the validation data provided by the manufacturer is an important step when selecting the RCT. Examples of the considerations for selecting the RCT are shown in Table 4.5. Once the RCT has been selected, a way to document the RCT results is needed (e.g., a record sheet that identifies the scope tested, the person doing the testing, date and time of testing, result of testing, and the result of retesting for those scopes that fail the RCT and require recleaning).

Regardless of the method selected, the site should do initial testing for ALL endoscopes to determine the current baseline status. This should be performed on the next patient use of each endoscope after completion of manual cleaning and rinsing. If the initial RCT fails for the majority of the endoscopes, this

TABLE 4.3	Overview of Quality System Requirements for Endoscopy Reprocessing Program
Area	**Specifics**
1. ***Records:*** There must be documentation of all reprocessing components to ensure there is a way to link which endoscopes (and corresponding accessories) were used on which patient.	• Document which endoscope was used in the patient's medical record • Document in the reprocessing area which personnel cleaned each endoscope, which patient the endoscope was used on, the date/time it was cleaned, and which AER (automated endoscope reprocessor) was used to disinfect the endoscope (or which sterilizer was used).
2. ***Manufacturers' instructions for use (MIFU) for all endoscopes and reprocessing equipment***	• Ensure the MIFU for reprocessing is available in the reprocessing area • Create a site-specific set of instructions that are based on the MIFU but indicate specific detergent, brushes, etc. that are used for reprocessing of each make/model of endoscope used at that site • If pump-assisted flushing is used during manual cleaning, ensure instructions for use are available • For manual cleaning, a succinct visual "aide" consisting of a summary of the process posted above the reprocessing sink, counters, etc., is useful.
3. ***Personnel*** • Qualifications • Training	• Personnel should have appropriate qualifications (e.g., certificate in medical device reprocessing and/or course in endoscope reprocessing) • Formal training MUST be provided for all reprocessing staff for each specific endoscope used in the facility. This training must include risk to reprocessing personnel, measures to reduce the risk of exposure to infectious material, appropriate use of personal protective equipment (PPE), need for meticulous attention to every step in reprocessing, risk to patients of infections if reprocessing is done improperly. Training should include review of written instructions, demonstration of proper technique, observation of trainee for a defined number of endoscopes reprocessed, and sign-off regarding competency. • Personnel files should document all qualifications and all training for each staff person. • Ongoing competency assessment should be done every year and documented for all reprocessing personnel.
4. ***Reprocessing facilities***	• Physically separate from patient service areas, treatment rooms and clean storage • Adequate sink size for flexible endoscopes • Adequate counter space for handling endoscopes • One-way work flow (dirty to clean) • Cleanable work surfaces • Adequate utilities, drains, air quality • Eye wash • Availability of appropriate PPE for staff • Appropriate equipment for automation of high-level disinfection (HLD) (e.g., AER) or sterilization process • Adequate endoscope storage facilities with restricted access
5. ***Reprocessing of endoscopes*** (see Table 4.2 for additional information)	• Traceability of each endoscope and reusable accessories used • Documentation of all monitoring performed for cleaning and minimum effective concentration (MEC) testing • Timely reprocessing • Routine cleaning and decontamination protocol for AER, flushing pump, sinks, connector tubing, endoscope storage cabinets • Policy on disposable and reusable ancillary items (e.g., water bottles, connector tubing, etc.)
6. ***Quality assurance program***	• Preventative maintenance (PM) program for endoscopes, AERs, flushing pump with repair history records • Record keeping of preventative maintenance on all equipment • Regular audits to ensure ongoing adequacy of all stages of the program
7. ***Management/oversight***	• Involvement of Infection Prevention and Control (IPAC) and workplace safety in all components of the endoscopy reprocessing is crucial • A structured management scheme with regular review of the endoscopy program that includes reprocessing considerations. • There should be regular review and reporting of monitoring data at appropriate management meetings to identify any potential issues

indicates that there may already be build-up biofilm (BBF) in the scopes being used. Remedial action would be needed for the endoscopes, which may include a longer soak time in detergent followed by extended brushing and flushing (as per scope manufacturer's input). If the endoscope fails the RCT after the remedial action, then it should be sent to the manufacturer for further remedial action (e.g., change of channels, etc.).

Surveillance Cultures

Another stage where monitoring of the endoscope can be done is post-HLD. A Rapid Post-Disinfection Test (RPDT) that could be completed just prior to the next patient use of the scope to confirm that the endoscope does not contain viable microorganisms would be ideal. However, there is little published data for

TABLE 4.4 Overview of the Issues Related to Reprocessing of Flexible Endoscopes

	Key Purpose	Reprocessing Steps	Common Errors	Impact
STEP 1: Bedside Clean	Critical to wipe exterior and flush ALL channels to dislodge patient debris while still fresh and not dried. The bedside clean reduces the load of organic material and microbes for the full manual cleaning step.	**Patient Procedure Room:** Detergent or water solution (as per endoscope manufacturer's instructions) is used to: • Wipe exterior using sponge or lint-free cloth • Suction or flush ALL channels (Note: this may require use of specific endoscope flushing adaptors as per MIFU) • Place all accessory components in detergent or water to keep moist during transport.	1. Forget to wipe exterior or forget to suction or flush some channels after patient procedure.	1. Dried patient-material is harder to remove during full cleaning. 2. Increases risk of inadequate cleaning and accumulation of organic material 3. Higher level of contamination in cleaning sink; increased risk of transmission of microbes to reprocessing personnel
TRANSPORT	An appropriate container is needed for transport of patient-used endoscopes to prevent drying of patient-material and protect endoscope from physical damage during transit Target ≤ 1 hour from time of bedside clean to commencement of full manual clean.	1. Place endoscope and all accessory components in a sealed, leak-proof rigid container for transport. Keep moist during transport. 2. Ensure patient-used endoscopes can be readily differentiated from patient-ready fully reprocessed endoscopes (e.g., specific labels on exterior of the transport container and/or the endoscope) 3. Transport endoscope to reprocessing area promptly (i.e., ≤ 1 hour)	1. Container not labeled to indicate that the endoscope inside is uncleaned and biohazardous 2. Transported in plastic bag instead of rigid container 3. Excessive time in transit (e.g., > 1 hour)	1. Contaminated endoscope is mistaken for a processed endoscope and used on another patient. 2. If transport container is not rigid there may be damage to endoscope during transport. 3. Excessive transport time leads to replication of microbes initiating biofilm formation
STEP 2: Leak Test	Ensure detection of any leaks that might allow water to enter inner scope cavity and damage light source and cause corrosion of internal components. Ensure a leaking endoscope is not used on patients as their secretions may enter damaged area and be protected from HLD and provide a reservoir for subsequent transmission to other patients.	**Reprocessing Room** **Maintain "Dirty to Clean" workflow** *Pressurize the endoscope:* **Leak test:** Manual: dry or submerged in water Automated: dry or submerged in water Observe for AT LEAST 30 seconds and manipulate the control levers to articulate the distal tip in all directions Check for bubbles if submerged in water OR: Check for a pressure drop if using the dry method of leak testing	1. Water for leak test contains detergent 2. Inadequate amount of time taken to check for bubbles 3. No articulation of the control levers 4. Failure to detect small leaks 5. Failure to decontaminate endoscope that has failed leak test before shipping for repair	1. Bubbles from leaks cannot be adequately observed when detergent bubbles are present 2. Small bubbles may go undetected and result in water damage to scope 3. Small leaks in bending section not detected without articulation to stretch the sheath. 4. Risk of patient secretions containing infectious organisms getting into the damaged area and being transmitted to subsequent patients causing infection or colonization. 5. Risk of transmitting infectious agents to biomedical technicians performing repair. Contamination of shipping container.
STEP 3: Manual Clean & Rinse	Remove as much patient-derived organic material as well as microbes. This is critical to ensure the subsequent disinfection or sterilization process works effectively and can provide an adequate margin of safety.	**Reprocessing Room** 1. Dismantle reusable components such as valves, caps, flushing connectors etc. and process along with endoscope. 2. Ensure endoscope is totally immersed in detergent solution. 3. Ideally suction detergent through all channels and discard this material (not in the cleaning basin). 4. Brush all openings including suction cylinder, air/water cylinder, instrument port, and outlets on umbilical end. 5. Adequate contact time with detergent (as per detergent manufacturer's instructions) to loosen debris. 6. Rinse away detergent using tap water.	1. Reusable components not properly cleaned. 2. Performing brushing while endoscope is not immersed. 3. No suction step before brushing so all patient material from channel brushed and flushed into the detergent solution. 4. Inadequate brushing of channels due to improper brush size or confusion regarding which brush to use. 5. Inadequate contact time with detergent. 6. Many detergents are protein solutions that need to be removed before the disinfection/sterilization step.	1. Increased risk of accumulation of organic material and biofilm forming. 2. Increased risk to personnel and environment due to aerosols of infectious debris. 3. Contamination of detergent solution with high levels of patient secretions increases the risk of high levels of organic material and microbes on exterior and in channels. 4. Inadequate brushing leads to improper cleaning and risk of excessive organic and microbial load for HLD. 5. Detergent contact inadequate results in improper cleaning and leads to accumulation of organic material and microbes. 6. If detergent is not adequately rinsed away this could lead to accumulation of protein and failure of HLD.

Continued

TABLE 4.4 Overview of the Issues Related to Reprocessing of Flexible Endoscopes—cont'd

	Key Purpose	Reprocessing Steps	Common Errors	Impact
Optional Step: Monitor manual cleaning	Monitoring of the manual cleaning ensures that the endoscope does NOT go on to HLD if it has not been properly manually cleaned. ST91 recommends that all scopes be tested for adequate cleaning at least once per week and preferably daily. This process of monitoring endoscope cleaning provides evidence of a Quality System as the cleaning adequacy is documented. It also serves as an ongoing way to monitor staff compliance with cleaning as part of annual competency assessment.	**Reprocessing Room** 1. Once manual cleaning has been completed collect a sample from the channel(s) of the endoscope. Minimally a sample from the instrument port to the distal end should be collected and tested. Follow the MIFU for the rapid cleaning monitor. If the test result is below the manufacturer's cut-off for adequate cleaning, then the scope can be transferred to the AER for HLD (or manual HLD done) or sent for sterilization. If the test result is above the MIFU cut-off, then the endoscope needs to be fully recleaned and tested after the second manual clean. NOTE: For duodenoscopes there should also be a sample from the elevator lever recess. 2. If the endoscope fails the rapid cleaning test after three rounds of cleaning it should be sent to the endoscope manufacturer for evaluation.	1. Breach of any of the manual cleaning steps shown in Fig. 4.1 can lead to patient-derived material remaining in the endoscope that is sent for HLD or sterilization. HLD or sterilization processes fix the organic residues to the channel surface leading to build-up biofilm formation (BBF).	1. Accumulation of BBF in the endoscope increases the risk of microbes in the BBF matrix surviving HLD and possibly being transmitted to subsequent patients.
STEP 4: Disinfection or Sterilization	HLD and sterilization are intended to kill any remaining microbes left after the cleaning step. HLD and sterilization can achieve 6 and 12 Log$_{10}$ microbial reductions, respectively. All reusable accessory items must also be exposed to HLD or sterilization along with the endoscope they are dedicated to.	**Reprocessing Room** 1. Ideally an automated endoscope reprocessor (AER) should be used for HLD or sterilization. Manual HLD instructions are available from manufacturers but the manual process is fraught with concerns including ensuring adequate vapor control to prevent staff exposure to toxic fumes, adequate channel perfusion when using manual syringe to inject HLD, dilution of HLD from water remaining in channels after manual cleaning, etc. 2. When using an AER, it is necessary to change the sub-micron filter inside the AER as per MIFU. 3. Fully reprocessed endoscopes and accessory components need to be handled using clean gloves to ensure skin organisms from bare hands are not transmitted to the endoscope post-HLD.	1. Inadequate HLD contact due to poor manual perfusion of channels (e.g., bubbles or inadequate immersion). 2. Breach in sub-micron filter inside AER leads to contaminated rinse water. 3. Handling of endoscope post-HLD with un-gloved hands	1. Increased risk of microbes surviving the HLD process due to inadequate contact with HLD. 2. Microbes on the endoscope when put into storage can facilitate biofilm formation. 3. Microbes on hands transferred to disinfected endoscope can survive and subsequently be transmitted to next patient that the endoscope is used for. Microbes transferred to endoscope from hands also increase the risk of biofilm formation if there is sufficient moisture.

STEP 5: Alcohol flush and forced air dry	Flush all channels with alcohol and then flush with forced air. This is intended to ensure that the channels are totally dry during storage. This step can be omitted if a channel-purge storage cabinet is used (as per cabinet manufacturer's instructions). Clean gloves should be used when handling the endoscope post-HLD during the drying process.	**Reprocessing Room** 1. Through drying of endoscope exterior and ALL channels is critical prior to storage. This can be done using appropriately filtered forced air. If a "channel-purge" storage cabinet is used the manual drying only needs to be done briefly to remove excess water prior to placing the endoscope in the cabinet (ongoing air purging once the endoscope is placed in the cabinet is preferred to ensure dryness is maintained as additional wet endoscopes are sequentially placed into the storage cabinet). There are also small air-flushing pumps that can be used to ensure channel drying prior to placing the endoscope in a regular storage cabinet. Ensure adequate time is used for air-flushing to ensure scope is totally dry before being placed in a regular storage cabinet. 2. Ensure fully reprocessed endoscopes are somehow labeled or identified so they can be easily differentiated from patient-used endoscopes that are contaminated.	1. The volume of alcohol flushed and the time for manual forced air drying is not specified in MIFU and is often sub-optimal when performed manually. 2. Contaminated endoscope may be mistaken for a fully reprocessed endoscope and accidentally used on a patient.	1. Inadequate drying during storage is one of the key factors that leads to biofilm formation. Once formed, the biofilm protects microbes from being adequately killed by HLD or sterilization and increases the risk of organisms being transmitted to patients exposed to this contaminated endoscope. 2. Use of a contaminated endoscope can lead to transmission of infectious agents that result in colonization or infection.
STEP 6: Storage	Limited access to the clean storage room ensures the endoscopes remain microorganism free and are safe to use on the next patient. Storage for 5 to 7 days is safe providing the endoscope is stored totally dry. A method of tracking the duration of individual storage time for each endoscope is recommended so that it can be reprocessed once the 5- to 7-day storage is exceeded. Reusable valves should be dedicated to and stored alongside (but not inserted into the valve cylinders of the endoscope during storage) the endoscope they are used on. This facilitates adequate tracking of the valves associated with the endoscope if an outbreak occurs.	**Clean Storage Room** 1. Place the endoscope into the storage cabinet following MIFU. If storage cabinet is not capable of purging air through the channels – the endoscope should be hung vertically during storage. For channel-purge storage cabinets the endoscope can be stored vertically or horizontally as per MIFU. Some models alarm when scope has been stored in cabinet longer than 5 to 7 days. 2. If storage exceeds 5 to 7 days the endoscope needs to be reprocessed. 3. Store the valves and other reusable accessories in a mesh bag or disposable valve holder that is hung on the endoscope to ensure these items are dedicated to a specific endoscope.	1. Endoscope storage exceeds 5 to 7 days. 2. Staff handling the endoscopes with un-gloved hands 3. Valves are inserted into the valve cylinders during storage instead of being held in a separate mesh bag/disposable holder that is hung alongside the endoscope	1. Excessively long storage may lead to fungal or other types of overgrowth or contamination. 2. Contamination of endoscope may lead to microbial replication and biofilm formation if moisture is also present. 3. Valves inserted into the valve cylinders can lead to moisture retention that facilitates microbial replication and can lead to biofilm formation.

TABLE 4.5   Overview of Rapid Cleaning Test Methods for Monitoring Manual Cleaning of Flexible Endoscopes

RCT Method	Substrate Detected	Pros	Cons	Refs
1. ATP There are many manufacturers of RCT for ATP (e.g., 3M, St. Paul, MN; Ruhof, Mineola, NY; Healthmark, Fraser, MI; etc.)	ATP from residual patient secretions and from microbes*	• Rapid (< 2 mins to do test) once sample is collected • There is a sponge device to collect channel sample (faster channel sampling method than fluid flush method) • RCT for surface and liquid testing available (i.e., can test exterior of endoscope as well as fluid used to sample channels) • Numeric measure of relative light units (RLU) provides cut-off that is less subjective.	• Cost (This is affected by the testing frequency selected by the site) • Insensitive for detection of viable bacteria (needs ~3 Log_{10}/mL of bacteria to generate 1 RLU) • Inability to link manufacturer's cut-off for acceptable cleaning to clinical outcomes (i.e., risk of infections or colonization)	125, 128–133, 135
2. Organic Residuals There are many manufacturers of RCT for organic residuals (e.g., HealthMark, Ruhoff, STERIS [Mentor, OH], etc.)	Residual patient-derived organic material such as protein, hemoglobin, carbohydrate (RCT may test one or multiples of these organic markers).	• Rapid (< 2 mins to do test) once sample is collected • Simplistic "dip & read" color change of test strip indicator pads, or test using swab for surface or channel sample, then insert swab into test reagent and assess color change.	• Inability to link manufacturer's published cut-off for acceptable cleaning to clinical outcomes (i.e., risk of infections or colonization)	124, 127, 134, 136

*Note: ATP is present in high levels in human cells and secretions whereas in microorganisms the level of ATP per cell is very low. Testing ATP post-cleaning is NOT a measure of how high the level of viable bacteria are, but rather it is an assessment as to whether manual cleaning has removed sufficient patient-derived material to be considered adequately cleaned.

ATP, adenosine triphosphate; *RCT*, rapid cleaning test.

the two RPDT tests that are currently available (Table 4.6). In the absence of validated rapid test methods, culture is the only well-studied method for detection of microbial contamination of flexible endoscopes postdisinfection/-sterilization. However, there are a number of considerations when culture is used. There have been a variety of published studies on culture results from endoscopes, but there is little data on the recovery efficiency of the various endoscope extraction methods that have been used.[137] If a patient-ready endoscope is extracted by flushing the channel with bacterial culture media or other harvesting fluids containing various proteins or buffers containing salt, then the endoscope requires recleaning and disinfection prior to being used on a patient. If sterile, high-quality water (i.e., reverse osmosis or deionized water) is used to flush endoscope channels, the endoscope can be dried and then still be safely used on the next patient.

REPROCESSING PERSONNEL

Training

Personnel who reprocess flexible endoscopes must have thorough initial training regarding the reprocessing of all makes and models of endoscopes that they will be responsible for reprocessing (see Tables 4.3 and 4.4). The training process should be documented and new staff not allowed to reprocess endoscopes on their own until they have demonstrated, under supervision, that they are competent to perform reprocessing independently. The use of rapid cleaning monitor (RCM) tests for each endoscope reprocessed during training is an excellent way to document the adequacy of the trainee's ability to perform the cleaning process. Reprocessing errors are a common underlying problem for many of the reported outbreaks.[95,97,98,123] The "human factors" study done by Ofstead et al (2010)[115] showed that inadequate cleaning of channels related to the lack of adequate channel brushing (43% of scopes) and inadequate drying (45% of scopes) prior to storage of endoscopes were the two most common breaches in

endoscope reprocessing. As outlined by recent guidelines,[48,107,108,123] initial training and ongoing competency assessment are critical to ensuring that staff can effectively reprocess flexible endoscopes.

Ongoing Competency Assessment

The compliance of reprocessing personnel with endoscope reprocessing protocols should be reviewed at least annually to document ongoing competency.[48] It is clear from some outbreaks that despite having adequate written protocols, staff may create breaches by not following some steps in the protocol.[95,98,115] As such, observational audits are a useful approach to determining if staff are fully compliant in following the site protocol. If ongoing cleaning monitoring is performed, the results of these tests can be included as part of documentation of ongoing competency.

TRANSMISSION OF PATHOGENS

Transmission of exogenous pathogens (i.e., not derived from the patient) can be categorized as "nonendoscopic," which is related to care of intravenous lines and administration of medications and anesthesia, or "endoscopic," which is related to transmission by the endoscope, water bottles, and its accessories. Outbreaks of infection have been traced to process failures, including endoscopes that are damaged or difficult to clean; AER design problems or failures such as breakdowns in AER water filtration systems; and lack of adherence to reprocessing guidelines for endoscopes and accessories. There are also data that demonstrate that all the steps associated with manual endoscope reprocessing are rarely performed and some essential steps, such as brushing all endoscope channels and adequate drying prior to storage, are frequently deficient.[115]

These deficient reprocessing practices can be summarized as follows:[32,96,115]

1. Inadequate or absent mechanical cleaning of the endoscope and channels before disinfection.

TABLE 4.6 Overview of Post-Disinfection Test Methods for Monitoring Microbial Contamination of Flexible Endoscopes

RCT Method	Substrate Detected	Pros	Cons	Refs
Rapid Endoscope Testing Methods Post-Disinfection				
1. NOW test (Commercially available; Healthmark, Fraser, MI)	Enzyme activity from any residual viable Gram negative bacteria	• Low limit of detection for Gram negative bacteria (10 CFU) • Test result available the morning after samples collected, before scope is used on patients • Targets key organisms of concern (i.e., Gram negatives)	• Test takes 18 hrs incubation so not available for scopes used multiple times the same day • Test is dependent on efficiency of sample collection; there may be false-negatives if low levels of bacteria are not extracted by fluid flushing sample collection method • Cannot detect Gram positive organisms of concern (e.g., *S. aureus*, Enterococcus, etc.) • Cannot determine if the Gram-negative bacteria are antibiotic resistant or not.	No published data
2. Polymerase chain reaction (PCR) Research PCR protocols	Residual genetic material from microbes	• Sensitive for detection of microbial genetic material • Quantitative detection is possible	• May detect genetic material from dead microbes so need to ensure the PCR test is designed to only detect genetic material in intact microbes. • Currently there are no commercial methods for rapid PCR testing. • Limit of detection not fully established • Cannot determine if the bacteria detected are antibiotic-resistant or not.	138
Traditional Culture Method				
3. Culture CDC endoscope culture protocol can be used. (Note: FDA is developing an alternative to the CDC culture protocol that is based on optimal extraction methods and optimal culture protocols.)	Detects viable microorganisms (bacteria, yeast and fungi)	• Detects viable organisms of high concern including Gram negatives and Gram positives. • Allows assessment of whether the bacteria detected are multi-antibiotic resistant • For outbreak investigation allows for genetic typing methods (e.g., PFGE) to help identify a point-source outbreak	• Requires 48 to 72 hrs before results of culture are reported. • During outbreak investigation, quarantine of the endoscope pending culture results is necessary. • For routine surveillance (i.e., not an outbreak investigation) the endoscope is often not quarantined and may be used on multiple patients before culture results are available. Sites need to have a response plan in place regarding notification if culture shows organisms of concern on an endoscope that has been used on multiple patients (i.e., notify the patient, the doctor or both?)	14, 15, 94, 97, 98–104, 107, 121, 135, 137–142

CDC, Centers for Disease Control; *CFU*, colony forming units; *FDA*, Food and Drug Administration; *PFGE*; pulsed-field gel electrophoresis.

2. Delay in reprocessing.
3. An inadequate disinfectant was used or used improperly at an incorrect concentration, temperature, or exposure period.
4. Flawed or malfunctioning AER units or use of incorrect connectors.[20,101,142]
5. Failure to disinfect or sterilize the irrigation bottle of the endoscope regularly.[143,144]
6. Endoscopic accessory instruments were not sterilized.
7. The endoscope and all channels were not dried adequately before storage.
8. Unrecognized problems with water supply.

Nonendoscopic Pathogen Transmission

Outbreaks of hepatitis B and C viruses have occurred due to failure to follow fundamental principles of aseptic technique and safe injection practices.[145,146] These included improper handling of intravenous sedation tubing, reuse of syringes and needles, and use of single-dose or single-use medical vials on multiple patients.[146–149]

The CDC guidelines for safe injection practices include the following recommendations:[150]

• Use aseptic technique when preparing and administering medications and fluids.
• A sterile, single-use, disposable needle and syringe should be used for each injection on a single patient.
• Do not administer medications from single-dose vials or use IV solutions as a common source of supply for multiple patients.
• Do not keep multidose vials in the immediate patient treatment area.
• Do not reuse a syringe to access or administer medications from a vial that may be used on multiple patients, even if the needle is changed.
• In times of critical need, medications from unopened single-dose/single-use vials can be subdivided for multiple patients. However, this should only be performed by qualified health care personnel in accordance with standards in the United States Pharmacopeia chapter on Pharmaceutical Compounding.

Endoscopic Transmission of Pathogens

More health care–associated outbreaks and patient exposures have been linked to contaminated endoscopes than to any other reusable medical device.[32,102] Nevertheless, endoscopy-related transmission of infection is very low and was originally estimated to have an incidence of approximately 1 infection per 1.8 million procedures.[3,17] This is very likely an underestimate, as many endoscopy-related infections go unrecognized because of inadequate or nonexistent surveillance programs, the absence of clinical symptoms in many patients who are colonized, a long lag time between colonization and clinical infection, and the fact that the pathogens transmitted by endoscopy are often normal enteric flora.[151] Endoscope-related transmission of bacterial infection has been rare since the adoption of the current multisociety reprocessing guidelines.[45,151] However, recent outbreaks have occurred with duodenoscopes even when the manufacturers and societal guidelines were reportedly followed correctly (see later section on Duodenoscope-Related Infections).[152]

The primary concern raised by infectious outbreaks is that current reprocessing guidelines are not adequate to ensure patient safety when undergoing endoscopic procedures. Endoscopes can harbor between 10^9 and 10^{12} enteric organisms at the completion of some patient procedures. This bioburden is reduced by cleaning (i.e., bedside precleaning followed by manual cleaning) by a factor of 2 to 6 $\log_{10}$ and the HLD step is expected to provide a 6 $\log_{10}$ reduction of any microbes remaining after cleaning.[124,153] Therefore the margin of safety associated with cleaning and HLD of GI endoscopes is low, and any deviation from proper reprocessing could lead to failure to eliminate contamination, with a possibility of subsequent patient-to-patient transmission.

Biofilms can contribute to reprocessing failure and endoscope-related infectious outbreaks.[154] Biofilms form in endoscope channels, in AERs, and within municipal and hospital water supplies as multilayered bacteria within exopolysaccharide. These biofilms protect the bacteria against physical (e.g., brushing, fluid flow) and chemical (e.g., disinfectant) forces, making the microorganisms more difficult to remove or completely kill by HLD.[151,155] There is evidence that accumulation of fixed material within endoscope channels occurs over repeated usage. Biofilms that develop in endoscopes and AERs may not be detectable by surveillance culture, as cleaning and disinfection may have destroyed bacteria within the superficial layers but not those within the deeper layers. Prompt, meticulous, manual cleaning to remove biologic material and strict adherence to reprocessing protocols is the optimal approach to reduce biofilm formation/accumulation.[155–158] Better biofilm removal protocols are needed to address this issue.

What Pathogens Are of Concern?

Pathogens of concern to the GI endoscopy community and general public include *Clostridium difficile, Helicobacter pylori, Escherichia coli,* norovirus, human immunodeficiency virus (HIV), hepatitis C virus (HCV), hepatitis B virus (HBV), and multidrug resistant organisms (MDROs) such as *M. tuberculosis,* vancomycin-resistant enterococcus (VRE), methicillin-resistant *Staphylococcus aureus* (MRSA), and CRE. All these established pathogens are susceptible to currently available chemical disinfectants and sterilants.[17,32]

Low Concern Organisms (LCO) versus High Concern Organisms (HCO)

Surveillance cultures of endoscopes are assessed for two general categories of microbial growth, LCO and HCO. HCO should not be detected after HLD as these organisms commonly result in a clinically significant infection including gram-negative bacteria (e.g., *Escherichia coli, Klebsiella spp., Shigella spp., Salmonella spp., Pseudomonas aeruginosa,* other *Enterobacteriaceae*) as well as *Staphylococcus aureus,* and *Enterococcus spp.*[159] LCO are less often associated with disease; these bacteria typically include coagulase-negative staphylococci, micrococci, diptheroids, and *Bacillus spp.* The levels of LCO on a surveillance endoscope culture can vary depending on the reprocessing, handling, and culturing practices in a facility. Typically, fewer than 10 colony forming units (CFU) of LCO does not require intervention as this most likely represents collection process contamination rather than a significant problem with the disinfection or cleaning process.[159] Interpretation of culture results with 10 or greater CFU of LCO should be considered in the context of typical culture results at the facility.[111]

Any endoscope found to be contaminated with a HCO or unacceptable CFU of LCO should cause concern and lead to repeat endoscope reprocessing followed by post-reprocessing cultures. The endoscope should be quarantined until it has been demonstrated to be free of HCO and has an acceptable level of LCO. Positive cultures should also prompt a review of the endoscopy unit reprocessing procedures to ensure adherence to the manufacturer's reprocessing instructions and to ensure proper culture methodology. If a reprocessing breach is identified, appropriate facility personnel should be notified and corrective actions should be immediately implemented. When bacteria are persistently recovered by surveillance cultures, refer to the manufacturer's instructions[111,159] for evaluating the endoscope for mechanical defects and consider having the endoscope evaluated by the manufacturer. In addition, when ineffective reprocessing is suspected based on surveillance cultures, it might be helpful to review positive cultures among affected patients to determine whether transmission of relevant pathogens could have occurred.[111,159]

Bacterial Infections

The vast majority of exogenously acquired endoscope-related infections have been caused by bacterial transmission. The bacteria involved have been true pathogens, which always have the potential to cause infection (e.g., *Salmonella spp.*), or opportunistic pathogens that cause infection if the microbial load is sufficient and/or host-factors are permissive (e.g., *Pseudomonas aeruginosa*). In the hierarchy of relative resistance to HLD, vegetative bacteria such as *Pseudomonas spp.* and *Salmonella spp.* are the most susceptible to disinfectants, whereas the mycobacteria are less susceptible and bacterial spores (e.g., *Bacillus subtilis* and *Clostridium difficile*) are the most difficult to eliminate (see Box 4.1). Nevertheless, as previously stated, all bacteria with the exception of a few bacterial spores are highly sensitive and eliminated by HLD. *Salmonella* is a serious primary pathogen, and *Pseudomonas* is ubiquitous in many water sources, and although both these pathogens have been associated most frequently with endoscopic transmission, they are both sensitive to multiple agents, including glutaraldehyde, and other HLDs. Transmission of bacterial pathogens from flexible endoscopes has been rare since the adoption of the current 2011 multisociety reprocessing guideline,[45,160] with the exception of duodenoscope-related infections (discussed later).

The most commonly reported infectious agents transmitted during GI endoscopy have been *Pseudomonas aeruginosa* (45 cases)[161–163] and *Salmonella spp.* (84 cases).[17] Isolated reports of endoscopic transmission of other enteric bacteria include *Klebsiella spp.*,[164] *Enterobacter spp.*,[165] *Serratia spp.*,[166] and *Staphylococcus aureus.*[164] The few reports of endoscopic transmission of *Helicobacter pylori* were related to inadequate reprocessing of endoscopes and biopsy forceps.[167–169] Current reprocessing guidelines are shown to inactivate *Clostridium difficile* spores,[170] and no cases of endoscopic transmission of this infection or mycobacteria have been reported. In summary, there have not been any observed GI endoscopy-related transmission of bacterial pathogens since introduction of the currently accepted reprocessing standards with the exception of duodenoscope-related outbreaks (discussed later).

Viral Infections

Much greater anxiety is associated with the possibility of transmission of viral infections. This anxiety is surprising because the viruses of greatest concern (HBV, HCV, and HIV) are among the easiest microorganisms destroyed with standard reprocessing.[171] Transmission of viral pathogens by GI endoscopy procedures is rare because these microorganisms are obligate intracellular microorganisms that cannot replicate outside living tissue. Thus, even when a flexible endoscope is contaminated with viral pathogens, the burden of virus cannot increase, as they are not capable of ex vivo replication. Enveloped viruses (e.g., HIV, HBV, HCV) die readily once dried and are more readily killed by HLD compared to nonenveloped viruses (e.g., enteroviruses, rotavirus), which can survive in dry conditions.

There has been concern about the possibility of HIV transmission by flexible GI endoscopy; however, no cases have been reported to date.[171–173] There is only one well-documented case of HBV transmission by GI endoscopy that occurred in the setting of inadequate endoscope reprocessing.[174] However, transmission of HBV is very rare or does not occur when accepted reprocessing guidelines are followed.[175]

Fungi

The presence of fungi is associated with prolonged storage of flexible endoscopes. Although transmission of *Trichosporon beigelii* and *Trichosporon asahii* occurred in the 1980s,[176,177] there are no documented cases of fungal infections by GI endoscopy when updated reprocessing guidelines are followed.

Parasites

A single publication in the 1970s reported circumstantial evidence of *Strongyloides stercoralis* transfer to four patients from a contaminated upper endoscope. No subsequent reports of parasite transmission by GI endoscopes have been identified.[178]

Prions

Creutzfeldt Jacob Disease (CJD) and variant CJD (vCJD) are degenerative neurologic disorders transmitted by proteinaceous infectious agents called prions. All prions remain infectious for years in a dried state, and resist all routine sterilization and disinfection procedures commonly used by health care facilities.[17,178–181] CJD is confined to the central nervous system (CNS) and is transmitted by exposure to infectious tissues from the brain, pituitary, or eye, whereas tissues and secretions that come into contact with the endoscope during procedures, such as saliva, gingival tissue, intestinal tissue, feces, and blood, are considered noninfectious by the World Health Organization.[17,179–182] The CDC and other infection control experts conclude that current guidelines for cleaning and disinfecting medical devices need not

be changed to protect our patients from CJD, citing no reported cases of CJD transmission by endoscopy and the lack of exposure to high-risk CNS tissue during endoscopic procedures.[17,183]

vCJD is a rare but fatal condition caused by the consumption of beef contaminated with a bovine spongiform encephalopathy agent. It differs from CJD in that the mutated prion protein can be found in lymphoid tissue throughout the body, including the gut and tonsils.[182,184] Only three cases of vCJD have been reported in the United States, and all three patients contracted the disease elsewhere.[184] As vCJD is resistant to conventional disinfectants and sterilants, endoscopy should be avoided, if at all possible, in patients known to harbor this agent.[17,184] Endoscopes used in individuals with definite, probable, or possible vCJD should be destroyed after use or quarantine to be reused exclusively on that same individual if required.[182,184]

Duodenoscope-Related Infections

Between 2012 and 2015, duodenoscopes resulted in 25 international outbreaks (at least eight in the United States) of antibiotic-resistant infections with CRE and other MDROs that sickened a reported 250 patients and resulted in 20 deaths.[16,97,103,138,185–187] In addition, transmission resulting in a long-term carrier state has been recognized as a risk of exposure to contaminated duodenoscopes. Long-term carriage has important clinical implications due to the development of a delayed infectious complication weeks to months later or patient-to-patient transmission of pathogens when these carriers are subsequently admitted to health care or chronic care facilities.

Investigative cultures identified persistent contamination of duodenoscopes as the cause for patient infections with MDROs in most of the outbreaks.[185,188] Furthermore, these duodenoscope-associated infections occurred even though the sites reported strict adherence to reprocessing procedures according to manufacturer's instructions and professional guidelines.[14,16,97,142,189] It is likely that MDROs are acting as a marker for ineffective reprocessing due to the complex design of duodenoscopes that have difficultly reaching crevices and channels involving the elevator mechanism where persistent colonization was identified.[186,190] Duodenoscopes that persistently yield positive cultures likely harbor biofilms that cannot be eradicated with standard reprocessing.[155]

In October 2015 the FDA and the CDC released an official health advisory alerting health care facilities to review their reprocessing procedures.[191–202] In response to the problems with duodenoscope reprocessing, the FDA requested all three duodenoscope manufacturers to revise and validate their reprocessing instructions with provisions for additional duodenoscope reprocessing measures.[191] This led to the modification of manufacturers' reprocessing protocols with a larger emphasis on precleaning and manual cleaning before HLD.[117,192–194] One duodenoscope manufacturer (Olympus; Center Valley, PA) subsequently modified the design of the closed elevator channel to create a tighter seal.[195,196]

In addition, the FDA has recommended that health care facilities performing ERCP consider employing supplemental measures for duodenoscope reprocessing when facilities have the resources to do so.[110] Most sites where outbreaks have occurred have chosen per procedure ETO sterilization after HLD as its primary reprocessing method, and in all reported instances, ETO has prevented further MDRO transmission.[110,185] However, one site reported failure to eliminate MDRO contamination of a duodenoscope after HLD and ETO.[116] Alternative reprocessing methods employed have included double HLD after each procedure[110,185] or HLD with duodenoscope quarantine until negative culture results are obtained.[15] Another supplemental option for reprocessing endorsed by the FDA includes the use of a liquid chemical sterilant processing system.[110,197] Surveillance microbiological culturing should be considered in addition to these supplemental reprocessing measures. This involves sampling the duodenoscope channels and the distal end of the scope to identify any bacterial contamination that may be present on the scope after reprocessing.[159,198] It must be recognized that the sensitivity of surveillance culturing of the elevator channel, the elevator lever cavity, or other scope channels is unknown. Until there are evidence-based guidelines, individual hospitals should choose from these different options based on available information and feasibility for their medical practice. However, at a minimum, there should be an audit of all facilities offering duodenoscope procedures to ensure the site has a quality system in place and is compliant with current MIFUs and guidelines.

REPROCESSING ERRORS AND OUTBREAK MANAGEMENT

Breaches of disinfection guidelines and device failures (e.g., endoscopes or AERs) are common in health care settings, resulting in potential patient injury or infection transmission.[31] The identification of such a problem may stem from the result of microbiologic surveillance cultures, an infectious outbreak within an institution or isolation of a pathogen from individuals having a recent endoscopic procedure, identification of a break in reprocessing protocol, or a visibly faulty device. Endoscopy facilities should have written policies on the roles and responsibilities within the organization to identify, report, and analyze these failures.[81]

Investigation of a Reprocessing Problem or Device Failure

The investigation of a breach in reprocessing or resultant outbreak should be undertaken using a standardized approach. It should focus on the identification of factor(s) that led to the exposure and protect patients from potential adverse events. The investigation should not be punitive and not attempt to assign blame to any particular individual. Rutala et al (2007)[199] described a process for exposure investigation, and the ASGE has published guidelines for patient assessment and notification when there is a suspected failure in the disinfection or sterilization protocol.[200] These can be summarized as follows:[199,200]

1. Confirm that the reprocessing failure occurred and assess the duration of exposure (e.g., review sterilization methods and AER records of biological parameters).
2. Quarantine any endoscopes or associated accessories that malfunctioned or are at risk for inadequate reprocessing.
3. Do not use the devices in question, such as the endoscope or AER, until proper functioning is confirmed.
4. Prepare a list of potentially exposed patients, dates of exposure, and inadequately reprocessed or malfunctioning devices used.
5. Reporting:
   • Inform facility leadership: breaches in patient safety with serious potential infection risks should be reported to facility leadership, including infection control, risk management, public relations, legal department, and selectively to local/state public health agencies, the FDA, CDC, and the manufacturers of the involved equipment.[200,203] This

will help with the investigation and lead to an expeditious correction of any deficiencies that are identified.
   • A user facility is not required to report a device malfunction, but it can voluntarily advise the FDA of such product problems using the voluntary MedWatch Form FDA 3500 under FDA's Safety Information and Adverse Event Reporting Program.[201] However, if a device failure leads to a death or serious injury, the FDA and the manufacturer must be contacted, as outlined in facility policies, by the designated individual or department at the facility.[202] The FDA encourages health care professionals, patients, caregivers, and consumers to submit voluntary reports of significant adverse events or product problems with medical products to MedWatch (https://www.accessdata.fda.-gov/scripts/medwatch/), the FDA's Safety Information and Adverse Event Reporting Program
   • Manufacturers are required to report to the FDA when they learn that any of their devices may have caused or contributed to a death or serious injury or when they become aware that their device has malfunctioned and would be likely to cause or contribute to a death or serious injury if the malfunction were to recur.[201,202]
6. Patient notification and counseling:[200,203] in instances where a breach in the reprocessing protocol or damaged equipment poses a risk to patients for adverse events, it becomes the institution's ethical obligation to notify patients in a timely manner. Notification may be accomplished by a direct meeting, telephone call, and letter sent by registered mail. The content should include an assessment of the risk, possible adverse events that may occur, symptoms and signs of the adverse event, time range for the adverse event, risk to other contacts, possible prophylactic therapy (including benefits and risks), and recommended medical follow-up. Prompt notification allows patients to take precautions to minimize the risk of transmitting infection to others and allows for early serologic testing. This may help distinguish chronic infections from those potentially acquired at the time of endoscopy and to permit earlier initiation of treatment for newly acquired infections. On the other hand, adverse publicity associated with the reporting of a reprocessing error might lead patients to avoid potentially life-saving endoscopic procedures because of an unwarranted fear of infection.
   Personal counseling should be offered to all patients. The risk of infection should be discussed and placed in context to minimize patient anxiety. Patients should be advised against donating blood and tissue products and engaging in sexual contact without barrier protection until all serologic testing is complete. A toll-free helpline should be established to provide information to all patients at risk.
7. Develop a long-term follow-up plan (e.g., long-term surveillance, changes in current policies and procedures) and prepare an after action report.

Infection Control Issues

There are risks related to infection transmission to personnel who handle patient-used endoscopes as well as to patients. Sites offering endoscopy procedures need to ensure the risk to personnel and patients is minimized.

Transporting Instruments

Flexible GI endoscopes are expensive and easily damaged. Unlike surgical instruments where the microbial load is less than 100 bacteria for 75% of instruments,[139,204] the load of microorganisms in channels of flexible endoscopes can be as high as 10^{10} bacteria[124] per instrument channel (e.g., for colonoscopes). During transport from the procedure room to the reprocessing area,[48] flexible GI endoscopes require a rigid, sealed container that is appropriately labeled as biohazardous. This protects the endoscope from accidental damage and also ensures that any patient-derived secretions and microorganisms are adequately contained and cannot drip out and contaminate the environment. All reusable accessory items (valves, flushing adaptors, cleaning valves, etc.) should be transported along with the associated endoscope. During transport, the endoscope and all accessory items should be kept moist to prevent drying of patient-derived material. If endoscopes are transported to a central reprocessing facility, evaluation of the time of transport should be conducted to determine the frequency of excessive transit times.

Personal Protection

There are risks to reprocessing personnel being exposed to patient-derived infectious materials. Endoscopes contacting the GI tract can have very high levels of infectious organisms (including bacteria, viruses, fungi, etc.) in channels or on the endoscope surface. To mitigate these risks, reprocessing personnel need to be trained regarding standard precautions, personal protective equipment (PPE), hand hygiene, disposal of sharps, and dealing with chemical and/or infectious material spills.

Standard precautions are required when reprocessing any patient-used medical device. This means that staff treat all patient-used endoscopes as potentially infectious regardless of the underlying known illnesses that patients might have (e.g. *Clostridium difficile* infection, VRE colonization, human papilloma virus infection, candidiasis, etc.). Any handling of GI endoscopes should be done with due consideration to the potential to transmit infectious microorganisms to reprocessing personnel. Staff must be trained in appropriate PPE and reprocessing considerations aimed at reducing the generation of aerosols.

It is critical that appropriate PPE be available[48,107,108] and include a gown (preferably a water-resistant gown), gloves (appropriate to the task), and a face shield/mask. Reprocessing personnel must be adequately trained in the proper donning and doffing of all PPE. Gowns, gloves, and a full-face shield (or combined face shield/mask) are required for cleaning of flexible endoscopes. The reprocessing staff needs to be trained in the appropriate use of protective gloves, as well as hand hygiene after removing gloves. Utility gloves used for cleaning of endoscopes should never be used at other stages in endoscope reprocessing (i.e., they are dedicated to the cleaning sinks). Disposable examination gloves must be available for handling cleaned endoscopes during connection to the AER. Fresh disposable gloves are needed for removing and handling fully reprocessed endoscopes from the AER and during manual channel drying and placing the endoscope into the clean storage cabinet. Fresh disposable gloves should also be used whenever an endoscope is removed from the clean storage cabinet. The use of gloves helps protect both the reprocessing personnel from contamination with patient-derived microorganisms and the fully reprocessed endoscope from contamination with skin-derived microorganisms from reprocessing personnel. Staff should always perform hand hygiene immediately after removing any type of glove. Handwashing sinks with appropriate soap, as well as waterless hand hygiene agent dispensers, must be available in the reprocessing area.

The workflow should proceed from "dirtiest to cleanest" in the reprocessing area, and there should be physical separation of "dirty" reprocessing areas and "clean" areas.[48,107,108] This requires appropriate removal of PPE and hand hygiene when leaving the dirty reprocessing area to enter any of the clean areas.

Staff should take every precaution to reduce the generation of aerosols during reprocessing of GI endoscopes. This includes total immersion of the endoscope during cleaning.[48,108] This ensures that any patient material removed from the channels during cleaning is contained within the detergent cleaning solution. Care is needed to ensure all brushing steps are done underneath the water surface to reduce aerosols. Holding the control head above water to insert the channel brush and then pulling the brush out of the channel while the control head is above the water generates significant aerosols of the contaminated detergent solution. In addition, during the air-flushing process after cleaning is completed, a piece of gauze should be placed over the distal end of the endoscope channel prior to placing it in an AER to prevent creation of aerosols when flushing out residual rinse water. A final, often overlooked step, is rinsing and decontamination of the sink after EACH endoscope is cleaned. This ensures that the sink does not accumulate microbial contamination over time and act as a reservoir within the reprocessing area to contaminate reprocessing personnel or other endoscopes. If flushing pumps are used as part of the manual cleaning step, they also require routine (usually daily) decontamination as per MIFU to ensure they do not become a reservoir of microbes that develop biofilm and subsequently contaminate endoscopes that they are used on.

Any single-use disposable sharps used in the procedure room should be disposed of in appropriate sharps containers in the procedure room. There should be **no** single-use disposable sharps transported to the reprocessing area. If there are reusable sharps (e.g., biopsy forceps) used for patient procedures, these should be appropriately transported to the reprocessing area in a labeled, rigid, sealed container that ensures separation from the endoscope. This reduces the risk that the biopsy forceps (or other sharp accessory device) could damage the endoscope during transit. Reprocessing of reusable sharps requires specific MIFU and adequate staff training to reduce the risk of sharps injuries to reprocessing personnel. Single-use, disposable accessories are preferred to eliminate the risks associated with reprocessing of reusable sharps.

KEY REFERENCES

14. Epstein L, Hunter JC, Arwady MA, et al: New Delhi metallo-beta-lactamase-producing carbapenem-resistant *Escherichia coli* associated with exposure to duodenoscopes, *JAMA* 312:1447–1455, 2014.
17. ASGE Standards of Practice Committee, Banerjee S, Chen B, et al: Infection control during GI endoscopy, *Gastrointest Endosc* 67:781–790, 2008.
32. Rutala WA, Weber DJ, Healthcare Infection Control Practices Advisory Committee (HICPAC); Centers for Disease Control and Prevention: Guideline for disinfection and sterilization in healthcare facilities. 2008. https://www.cdc.gov/infectioncontrol/pdf/guidelines/disinfection-guidelines.pdf.
45. ASGE quality Assurance in Endoscopy Committee, Petersen BT, Chennat J, et al: Multisociety guideline on reprocessing flexible gastrointestinal endoscopes: 2011, *Gastrointest Endosc* 73:1075–1084, 2011.
48. Association for the Advancement of Medical Instrumentation: *ANSI/AAMI ST91: 2015. Flexible and semi-rigid endoscope processing in health care facilities*, Arlington, VA, 2015, AAMI.

68. Ofstead CL, Wetzler HP, Snyder AK, et al: Endoscope reprocessing methods: a prospective study on the impact of human factors and automation, *Gastroenterol Nurs* 33:304–311, 2010.

69. ASGE Technology Committee, Parsi MA, Sullivan SA, et al: Automated endoscope reprocessors, *Gastrointest Endosc* 84:885–892, 2016.

71. Society of Gastroenterology Nurses and Associates: *Guideline for use of high level disinfectants & sterilants for reprocessing flexible gastrointestinal endoscopes*, Chicago, 2017, SGNA. https://www.sgna.org/Portals/0/Issues/PDF/Infection-Prevention/6_HLDGuideline_2013.pdf.

81. U.S. Food and Drug Administration: FDA-cleared sterilants and high level disinfectants with general claims for processing reusable medical and dental devices – March 2015. http://www.fda.gov/MedicalDevices/DeviceRegulationandGuidance/ReprocessingofReusableMedicalDevices/ucm437347.htm.

109. U.S. Food and Drug Administration: Reprocessing medical devices in health care settings: validation methods and labeling. Guidance for Industry and Food and Drug Administration Staff. March 15, 2015. http://www.fda.gov/downloads/medicaldevices/deviceregulationandguidance/guidancedocuments/ucm253010.pdf.

110. U.S. Food and Drug Administration: Supplemental measures to enhance reprocessing: FDA Safety Communication. August 4, 2015. www.fda.gov/MedicalDevices/Safety/AlertsandNotices/ucm454766.htm.

113. Alfa MJ: Current issues result in a paradigm shift in reprocessing medical and surgical instruments, *Am J Infect Control* 44:e41–e45, 2016.

114. Society of Gastroenterology Nurses and Associates: *Standards of infection prevention in reprocessing flexible gastrointestinal endoscopes*, Chicago, 2016, SGNA. https://www.sgna.org/Portals/0/Standards_for_reprocessing_endoscopes_FINAL.pdf?ver=2016-06-03-085449-550.

116. Naryzhny I, Silas D, Chi K: Impact of ethylene oxide gas sterilization of duodenoscopes after a carbapenem-resistant Enterobacteriaceae outbreak, *Gastrointest Endosc* 84:259–262, 2016.

120. Saliou P, Cholet F, Jézéquel J, et al: The use of channel-purge storage for gastrointestinal endoscopes reduces microbial contamination, *Infect Control Hosp Epidemiol* 36:1100–1110, 2015.

125. Alfa MJ, Olson N, Murray BL: Comparison of clinically relevant benchmarks and channel sampling methods used to assess manual cleaning compliance for flexible gastrointestinal endoscopes, *Am J Infect Control* 42(1):e1–e5, 2014.

128. Alfa MJ, Fatima I, Olson N: The ATP test is a rapid and reliable audit tool to assess manual cleaning adequacy of flexible endoscope channels, *Am J Infect Control* 41:249–253, 2013.

135. Alfa MJ, Fatima I, Olson N: The ATP test is a rapid and reliable audit tool to assess manual cleaning adequacy of flexible endoscope channels, *Am J Infect Control* 41:249–253, 2013.

137. Centers for Disease Control and Prevention: Interim sampling method for the duodenoscope – distal end and instrument channel. August 19, 2015. https://www.cdc.gov/hai/settings/lab/lab-duodenoscope-sampling.html.

159. Centers for Disease Control and Prevention: Interim protocol for healthcare facilities regarding surveillance for bacterial contamination of duodenoscopes after reprocessing. April 2015. http://www.cdc.gov/hai/organisms/cre/cre-duodenoscope-surveillance-protocol.html.

185. United States Senate; Health, Education, Labor, and Pensions Committee: Preventable tragedies: superbugs and how ineffective monitoring of medical device safety fails patients. Minority staff report. January 13, 2016. http://www.help.senate.gov/imo/media/doc/Duodenoscope%20Investigation%20FINAL%20Report.pdf.

187. Muscarella LF: Risk of transmission of carbapenem-resistant Enterobacteriaceae and related "superbugs" during gastrointestinal endoscopy, *World J Gastrointest Endosc* 6:457–474, 2014.

190. U.S. Food and Drug Administration: Design of endoscopic retrograde cholangiopancreatography (ERCP) duodenoscopes may impede effective cleaning: FDA Safety Communication. February 2015. http://www.fda.gov/MedicalDevices/Safety/AlertsandNotices/ucm434871.htm.

200. ASGE Standards of Practice Committee, Banerjee S, Nelson DB, et al: Reprocessing failure, *Gastrointest Endosc* 66:869–871, 2007.

A complete reference list can be found online at ExpertConsult.com

5

Tissue Sampling, Specimen Handling, and Laboratory Processing

Joanna A. Gibson and Robert D. Odze

CHAPTER OUTLINE

ENDOSCOPIC BIOPSY

Biopsy Techniques

Pinch Biopsy Forceps

The most common pinch biopsy forceps used worldwide fits through a 2.8-mm biopsy channel (Fig. 5.1). In general, mucosal samples vary from 4 to 8 mm in size.[1,2] A smaller-sized forcep that fits through a 2.2 mm biopsy channel is used in infants and young children. Pediatric gastroenterologists generally use narrow-bore instruments for routine diagnostic biopsies if the child weighs less than 10 kg. The primary aim of a pinch biopsy is to obtain a specimen sample that contains full-thickness mucosa, including muscularis mucosa. The tissue yield of endoscopic biopsies relies on the forceps size, amount of pressure applied on the forceps while placed against the mucosa during the biopsy procedure, and the optimal angle of the forceps when applied to the mucosal surface. In the gastric body, where mucosal folds are thick,[3] or in conditions associated with mucosal thickening, full-thickness mucosal sampling may not be achieved using a 2.8 mm channel biopsy. The inability to sample full-thickness mucosa may influence the amount of diagnostic information obtained from histologic examination.

Larger Capacity Forceps

The large-cup ("jumbo" or "max capacity") forceps requires a large channel (also termed *therapeutic*) endoscope (biopsy channel; 3.6 to 3.7 mm). Some newer designs are intended to provide larger biopsy specimens with the conventional 2.8-mm channels and intermediate-sized channels such as pediatric colonoscopes. Larger capacity forceps biopsies increase the diagnostic yield upon histologic examination. Specimens obtained with a jumbo forceps often exceed 6 mm in maximum diameter, but these are not necessarily deeper than standard biopsies.[4] Rather, a jumbo forceps typically provides more mucosa for analysis. This is particularly useful during surveillance tissue sampling, such as in patients with Barrett's esophagus (BE) or ulcerative colitis.[5] Another advantage of large capacity forceps biopsies is that larger tissue fragments enable histotechnologists to better orient the sample during tissue processing. Jumbo biopsy forceps are as safe as standard biopsy forceps, although the need to use a larger diameter channel may be less comfortable for patients.

Sampling of Submucosa

Biopsy specimens obtained with small or larger capacity pinch forceps usually contain very little submucosa, if any.[6] It is sometimes difficult to obtain specimens with sufficient submucosa, such as during a biopsy for a submucosal lesion or when the objective is to diagnose amyloid or other disorders that manifest predominantly in the submucosa. Ancillary techniques, such as fine-needle aspiration or needle core biopsy, may increase the diagnostic yield of submucosal tissue.

Hot Biopsy

Hot biopsy forceps are insulated pinch biopsy forceps through which electrical current is passed, after which the remaining tissue is ablated in situ using electrocautery.[7] Unfortunately, the result is cautery artifact in the sampled tissue, which, in small tissue samples, often makes histologic interpretation difficult (or impossible).[3,8,9] In addition, the electrocautery technique carries an excessive risk of perforation from deep tissue burn, particularly in the cecum and ascending colon.[10,11] Finally, residual dysplastic tissue on follow-up after hot forceps biopsy has been reported in 10.8% to 17% of patients post hot forceps biopsy.[12,13] For these reasons, hot biopsies have been largely abandoned by most endoscopists.

Snare Biopsy

Snare biopsy is an endoscopic technique during which a wire is placed around a polypoid lesion that protrudes into the lumen, and this allows for removal of the lesion. Snare biopsy is used primarily for colonic polyps, but polyps anywhere in the gastrointestinal (GI) tract may be removed using this technique. Snares are available in a variety of sizes and can be used in conjunction with electrocautery. Depending on their size, excised polyps are either retrieved through the suction channel of the endoscope or held by the snare after resection while the colonoscope is removed from the patient. The snare biopsy can be used to remove pedunculated or sessile polyps of various sizes.

Snare biopsy is the recommended method over pinch forceps biopsy for removal of diminutive (less than 0.5 cm) and small polyps (0.5 to 2 cm). Several randomized studies have shown a higher rate of complete resection of adenomatous polyps using cold snare biopsy compared to cold forceps biopsy.[14–16] Pedunculated polyps are generally easily removed using snare biopsy,

and the main risk of this procedure is post-polypectomy bleeding from vessels located within the stalk of the polyp.[17] In the case of larger polyps, piecemeal removal may be employed.[7,18] However, piecemeal polyp removal may limit the ability of pathologists to assess the margins of resection. Sessile polyps, or complex polyps greater than 2 cm in size, are best referred to experienced endoscopy centers for removal.

During hot snare polypectomy, the endoscopist is able to apply modulated electrosurgical current to a metal wire that cuts through pedunculated polyps at the base of the lesion. This assists tissue removal and coagulation of vessels at the base of the polyp or within the polyp stalk. Use of electrocautery versus cold snare polypectomy must be balanced against the risks of perforation and post-polypectomy bleeding. Electrocautery artifact also persists in the biopsy sample during tissue processing and is characterized by loss of nuclear and cytoplasmic detail (Fig. 5.2). Noting this effect during histologic examination can be advantageous in certain situations, such as assessment of the cauterized margin of resection. However, too much electrocautery artifact can also preclude assessment and classification of polyps, especially if the artifact is present throughout the tissue submitted for histologic examination. In general, the risk of perforation following polypectomy is minimal, and is greatest in portions of the colon covered by free serosa. Cold polypectomy, without electrical current, avoids use of cautery, thereby limiting the amount of burn artifact in the specimen and thus minimizing the risk of perforation.

Endoscopic Mucosal Resection

Endoscopic mucosal resection (EMR) is an advanced endoscopic technique used for removal of premalignant or malignant lesions that are mainly confined to the mucosa, or in some cases superficial submucosa.[19] One principle method of EMR is the use of a liquid cushion to expand the submucosa and minimize transmural cautery damage. Using this technique, the specimen usually includes mucosal and submucosal tissue. In general, EMR requires some measure of confidence that a lesion is, in fact, confined to the mucosa or submucosa. Many endoscopists rely

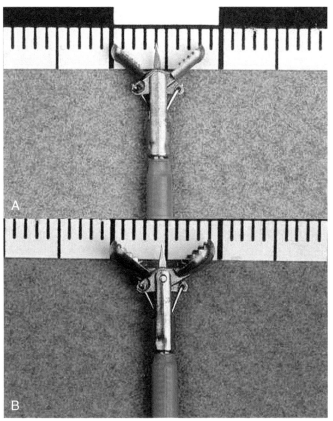

FIG 5.1 A, Standard and **B,** jumbo-sized pinch biopsy forceps.

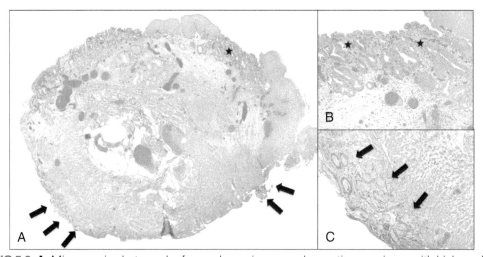

FIG 5.2 A, Microscopic photograph of an endoscopic mucosal resection specimen with high-grade dysplasia in Barrett's esophagus. Arrows point to the lateral mucosal resection margins consisting of squamous *(right)* and columnar *(left)* tissue. The *star* designates a high-grade dysplasia focus, shown at high magnification in **B. C,** Lateral resection margin showing cauterized Barrett's esophagus but without dysplasia.

on endoscopic ultrasonography (EUS) to determine the depth of a particular lesion before choosing to perform an EMR procedure. The accuracy of high-frequency EUS (15 or 20 MHz) may be as great as 95% for determining whether a lesion is limited to the mucosa.

Several variations of the EMR technique are currently used.[20] Many rely on submucosal injection of liquid, most often saline. Less commonly, diluted epinephrine is used in addition to saline, which helps constrict small blood vessels at the base of the lesion. Other techniques advocate hypertonic solutions of 3.5% saline or 50% dextrose or sodium hyaluronate. The quantity of liquid injected also varies; the idea is that the injected lesion should appear to be raised by a cushion of liquid above the mucosal surface before resection is attempted. Failure to "lift" the lesion despite generous use of submucosal saline (the so-called nonlifting sign) may be an indication that a lesion has spread deeper into the bowel wall.[21]

Two major types of EMR techniques are used: the lift and cut technique (also known as strip biopsy), without the use of suction, and aspiration mucosectomy, which employs suction as part of the method. Both methods typically also feature a snare that is used around the lifted lesion. Aspiration mucosectomy, in particular, has been widely successful for removing lesions in the GI tract.[22] A newer EMR technique is similar to aspiration mucosectomy, but after the lesion has been suctioned into the cap, a small rubber ring is released around the base of the lesion, similar to the method used during endoscopic variceal ligation. Once suction is released, the lesion appears contained within a "pseudopolyp" that may be removed by snare cautery. This is known as band-ligation EMR.[23,24]

Endoscopists and the pathologists who handle EMR specimens must recognize that these samples may contain cancer; therefore they should be handled appropriately and oriented correctly for optimal pathologic tumor staging, including assessment of depth of invasion, and the margins of resection, including assessment of the deep submucosal margin (Fig. 5.3). EMR allows the endoscopist to attempt an en bloc resection and thus, potentially, to completely resect an early malignant lesion. En bloc resection is limited, however, to lesions no more than 1.5 to 2 cm in largest diameter.[25] If deep margins are positive for neoplasia, surgical resection of the affected region is advocated.[26] Current indications for EMR include superficial carcinoma of the esophagus or stomach in patients who are not candidates for surgery; unifocal high-grade (or low-grade) dysplasia in BE; and large, flat colorectal adenomas (which might otherwise require piecemeal resection) regardless of the degree of dysplasia. EMR as a form of primary therapy for small, superficial cancer has gained increasing popularity in the United States but is even more widely used in Japan, where early gastric cancer is more common. EMR is also used as a form of primary therapy for small submucosal lesions, such as rectal carcinoid tumors or leiomyomas. In many cases, the submucosal lesion can be completely resected.[27]

Brush Cytology Samples

Brush cytology is a method used for broad sampling of the mucosal surface.[28,29] Cytology brushes share common design features: bristles, usually composed of nylon or metal fibers, branch off a thin metal shaft that runs lengthwise within a protective plastic sheath. The various brushes that are currently available do not seem to vary in terms of performance characteristics. The cytology brush is passed through an accessory channel of an endoscope. The end of the sheath is passed out of the tip of the endoscope, and the bristle portion of the brush is then extended from the sheath. The brush is rubbed back and forth several times along the surface of the mucosa, lesion, or stricture, and is then pulled back into the sheath. The sheath is withdrawn from the endoscope, and the brush is pushed out of the sheath, thus exposing the bristles. The bristle portion of the brush may be cut off, placed into fixative, and sent in its entirety to the cytopathology laboratory. Alternatively, the bristles may be rolled against a glass slide in the endoscopy suite. The slides should be immediately sprayed with fixative or submerged within it and subsequently delivered to the cytopathologist. If smears are made in the endoscopy suite, little additional benefit is derived from inclusion of the bristles for cytopathologic analysis.[30]

Brush cytology is often used in the pancreaticobiliary tree in order to sample strictures in the pancreaticobiliary tract, or in the esophagus to sample esophageal plaques or lesions suspicious of infectious esophagitis.[31,32] Of the three major potential infections of the esophagus, *Candida albicans* and herpesvirus are characterized by having organisms in surface exudate and surface epithelial slough.[33] In contrast, cytomegalovirus is typically present deeper in the tissue stroma and is not commonly detected in cytologic smears of exudate. Smears of exudates for cytologic examination for herpesvirus or *Candida* may provide a rapid diagnosis.[34] Brushings may also be used for viral culture or polymerase chain reaction (PCR) for herpesvirus, if clinically indicated.[32] For viral culture, the use of a culture medium is

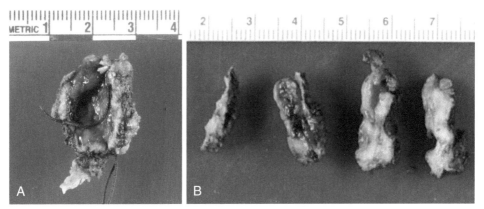

FIG 5.3 Gross photograph of endoscopic mucosal resection specimen **A,** before and **B,** after sectioning.

needed; a second brushing may be swirled around in a culture medium, or the brush tip may be cut off with wire cutters and left in the bottom of the culture medium container.

Cytologic brushings of biliary strictures are an important tool in the assessment of strictures within the pancreaticobiliary tree. Endoscopic biopsy in this location is problematic, largely due to the inability to access and visualize lesions adequately to be sampled.[35] Cancer detection rates with brush cytology sampling rates are disappointing.[36] Combining brush cytology with ancillary techniques, such as fluorescence in situ hybridization, improves accuracy and diagnostic yield.[37]

Brush cytology has been proposed as an alternative method of surveillance in patients with BE and offers the advantages of an inexpensive method and potential for sampling over a greater area of the esophagus.[38,39] In a prospective study by Kumaravel et al (2010), 530 patients were assessed using paired cytologic brushings and histologic biopsies. A concordance rate of 80% between the two methods was documented.[40] Cytology excelled at detection of high-grade dysplasia (HGD) and adenocarcinoma, but it had poor sensitivity for detection of low-grade dysplasia (LGD). Brush cytology has also previously been used in combination with fluorescence in situ hybridization for detection of DNA abnormalities in a large cohort of BE patients.[41] In another study by Timmer et al (2014), DNA gains detected in brush cytology samples of BE patients may predict a lower response rate to endoscopic therapy.[42]

Tissue Fixation

Once a biopsy has been obtained and the forceps removed from the endoscope, the tissue is retrieved or dislodged from the forceps and immediately submerged completely into a container with appropriate fixative. Avoidance of prolonged time before the tissue is placed in fixative is imperative. Care also should be taken to avoid crushing or excessively shaking the tissue sample, because this can introduce artifacts in the tissue that limit histologic assessment. For example, excessive shaking before complete fixation can lead to shearing and detaching of the surface epithelium from the mucosa and result in "denuded" mucosal sections. Excessive shaking may also shear delicate inflamed tissues, leading to tissue fragmentation that also precludes optimal histologic assessment.

Timely fixation minimizes tissue autolysis and desiccation and helps preserve mucosal architecture. The most common fixative used for GI mucosal biopsies is 10% buffered formalin. Formalin provides excellent fixation, with tissue penetration occurring at approximately 1 mm per hour.[43] The volume of formalin used for fixation should be at least 10 times greater than the amount of tissue being fixed. Importantly, formalin fixed tissue is the optimal fixative for most histochemical and immunohistochemical stains routinely performed in most laboratories. In addition, formalin fixed tissue is also suitable for use in molecular DNA or RNA based tests, including PCR and fluorescent in situ hybridization (FISH).[44-46]

On occasion, the formaldehyde in formalin may be irritating to the eyes and upper respiratory tract of personnel. In addition, formaldehyde is classified by the Environmental Protection Agency as a probable human carcinogen, at a threshold of 1.0 ppm, which is well above the level that causes sensory irritation.[47] In pathology laboratories, ventilated hoods are used to limit exposure to formalin. In the endoscopy suites, typical occupational exposure to formalin is very brief, and special ventilation is not usually required in that hospital area.

In certain circumstances, it may be required to obtain endoscopic tissue for ancillary studies other than routine histologic examination. Samples obtained for specific tests, for example, flow cytometry, tissue culture, and electron microscopy, should be handled according to the guidelines in place at the home institution. One of the more common indications for ancillary studies is flow cytometry, which can be useful when a hematologic malignancy is suspected, such as lymphoma.[48] In this example, after tissue is obtained from the lesion of interest, the tissue should be kept unfixed to send for flow cytometry; fixative should be avoided before the fresh tissue is triaged for this test. Flow cytometry cannot be performed once the tissue is fixed, and it is therefore incumbent on the endoscopist to consider the possibility of a lymphoproliferative disorder and preserve fresh tissue. Similarly, microbial culture also requires fresh tissue samples. Specimens for culture should preferably be obtained first, to minimize any extraneous contamination concerns. Ideally, fresh and unfixed tissues should be delivered to the appropriate laboratory within a few hours, but storage at 4°C overnight is acceptable.

Other diagnostic considerations may require fixing tissue in glutaraldehyde if electron microscopy is needed, or in cell culture medium for cytogenetic karyotyping. In most cases, it is customary that tissue from the same lesion, or area, should also be submitted, in a separate jar with fixative, for routine histology. This extra step confirms and ensures that tissue from the area of interest submitted for ancillary studies was, in fact, representative of the lesional tissue. Appropriate tissue triage is best achieved through collaborative discussion between the endoscopist and pathologist to understand these special procedures which frequently vary between institutions. Pathologists can also alert histotechnologists or pathology assistants in the laboratory to any special instructions to ensure timely and appropriate handling of the specimen.

Laboratory Tissue Processing

Once the specimen arrives in the pathology laboratory, the tissue is processed and glass slides are generated. Tissue processing is performed by histotechnologists, laboratory technicians who specialize in tissue handling. Histotechnologists retrieve tissues from the specimen jars and transfer the biopsy sample to a standard tissue cassette measuring $3 \times 2.5 \times 0.4$ cm. During this step, the tissue fragments in each jar are measured, counted, and recorded as part of the gross description of the pathology report. Typically, all the tissue from one jar is placed into one cassette. However, when the number of tissue fragments is high, which may in subsequent steps limit ideal tissue orientation during paraffin embedding, the tissue fragments from one jar may be divided among two or more cassettes. The cassettes are placed in an automated tissue processor, where the tissue is dehydrated and cleared in preparation for paraffin wax embedding, a process lasting several hours or overnight.

After tissue processing, histotechnologists retrieve the tissue cassettes from the processor and embed the tissue in paraffin wax to create formalin fixed paraffin embedded (FFPE) tissue blocks. During embedding, histotechnologists orient mucosal samples "on edge" to present the normal mucosal architecture at microscopy. Tiny and fragmented specimens often cannot be well oriented. Proper orientation aids in assessment of the amount of lamina propria inflammation, focal lesions such as granulomas, and intraepithelial lymphocytes (IELs) (especially small bowel). In the colon, for example, oriented sections permit accurate assessment of crypt architecture.

Orientation of intact polypectomy specimens is particularly important and requires diligent effort prior to tissue processing. The gross pathologic size and surface configuration (e.g., bosselated, villiform, or sessile) of the polyp should be noted, and the base of the polyp should be identified. Regardless of the configuration or presence of a stalk, the base of the polyp should always be inked to aid in the subsequent microscopic identification and examination of the polyp resection margins. Ink and cautery artifact on a microscopic slide are valuable landmarks for locating relevant resection margins. Small polyps (< 1 cm in diameter) should be bisected along the vertical plane of the stalk so that the surgical margin is included. Both halves of the specimen can then be submitted in one cassette for processing. For larger polyps (> 1 cm) that cannot fit easily in one cassette, the polyp is sectioned by trimming the sides away from the stalk. The stalk is submitted in a designated cassette, whereas the remainder of the polyp is submitted in separate cassettes.

To create microscopic slides, histotechnologists cut FFPE tissue blocks using a microtome, typically in a thickness of 4 microns, and place the cut tissue sections on glass slides, which are then stained with hematoxylin and eosin for routine microscopy. FFPE tissue blocks can be stored indefinitely for future use, if the clinical need arises. Tissue blocks can be recut numerous times, such as to create additional slides for various uses, including histochemical stains to detect infectious organisms or to better characterize tumors. In addition, DNA and RNA can be extracted from FFPE blocks for molecular analysis and other nuclei acid based tests.[44–46]

DISEASE SPECIFIC APPROPRIATE TISSUE SAMPLING

Esophagus

Gastroesophageal Reflux Disease

Gastroesophageal reflux disease (GERD), which occurs at an estimated prevalence rate of 20% to 40%, is a very common indication for endoscopic examination. Establishing a diagnosis of GERD includes the assessment of clinical features and endoscopic findings. Upper endoscopy (EDG) is not required in the presence of typical GERD symptoms. Endoscopy is recommended in the presence of "alarm" symptoms and for screening of patients at high risk for complications.[49,50]

Endoscopically, GERD can present with a variety of changes, ranging from normal to erosive esophagitis. Strictures and BE are common complications of GERD.[51,52] In the absence of endoscopically visible BE, there are no universally accepted biopsy protocols for the evaluation of GERD. Histologic changes in endoscopically normal appearing distal esophagus may show nonspecific features of "minimal change" esophagitis, such as papillary elongation, basal cell hyperplasia, and intercellular edema. The clinical implications of these histologic features in the absence of endoscopically visible changes are unclear. Biopsies of normal mucosa in the setting of GERD, where other diagnoses are not suspected, are not currently recommended (Table 5.1).[49,53]

Biopsies of endoscopically visible changes in GERD patients often reveal "active" esophagitis, a nonspecific injury pattern that can result from a variety of causes. GERD-associated reflux esophagitis produces a characteristic, although nonspecific, tissue injury pattern. Features of untreated active esophagitis include basal cell hyperplasia, elongation of the lamina propria papillae, epithelial cell necrosis, increased intraepithelial inflammation (including eosinophils, neutrophils, and lymphocytes), distended pale squamous "balloon" cells, intercellular edema, and, in severe cases, surface erosions or ulceration. Histologically, reflux changes are typically distributed over the distal 8 to 10 cm of the esophagus in a patchy fashion, with the most demonstrative changes typically present in the distal esophagus, and less intense change located more proximally.[54] Multiple biopsies may be necessary to consistently demonstrate histologic abnormalities. Because biopsy specimens from the lower 1 to 2 cm of the esophagus, even in asymptomatic subjects, often reveal evidence of mild basal cell hyperplasia, diagnostic biopsy specimens should also be obtained more than 2 cm above the level of the gastroesophageal junction (GEJ) to diagnose esophagitis reliably.[54–56]

TABLE 5.1	Recommendations for Optimum Location and Number of Mucosal Biopsies for
Disease	**Location and Number of Biopsy Samples**
GERD[49,53,56]	Screening endoscopy and biopsy in high risk patients and those with alarm symptoms
Eosinophilic esophagitis[101]	Multiple esophageal biopsies from several areas, and one biopsy each from duodenal and gastric mucosae Two to four biopsies from the proximal (1) and distal (1) esophagus (yield: 80%) Up to five tissue samples, including biopsies from the proximal, mid, and distal esophagus (yield: 100%)
Barrett's esophagus[59,60]	Detection of goblet cells: Four targeted biopsies that straddle the neosquamocolumnar junction, or Eight random samples obtained from the columnar-lined esophagus Surveillance for dysplasia: Four-quadrant biopsies per 2 cm of columnar-lined esophagus Additional sampling of endoscopically visible lesions Surveillance for early carcinoma in patients with high-grade dysplasia Four-quadrant biopsies per 1 cm of columnar-lined esophagus Additional sampling of endoscopically visible abnormalities
Chronic gastritis[117,143,144,145]	Five biopsies from antrum (2), corpus (2), and incisura angularis (1) Surveillance for dysplasia: Minimum of five biopsies from antrum (2), corpus (2), and incisura angularis (1) Additional sampling of endoscopically visible abnormalities If dysplasia is present: Follow up every 3 months for 1 year with topographic mapping of the stomach
Celiac disease[157]	Three biopsies of the duodenal bulb (1), proximal duodenum (1), and distal duodenum (1)

GERD, gastroesophageal reflux disease.

Pinch biopsies obtained through standard endoscopes are often not adequate for evaluation of early histologic changes resulting from reflux because they usually do not include the entire thickness of the mucosa and are difficult to orient. Endoscopes with a large-caliber biopsy channel and jumbo biopsy forceps should be used to facilitate accurate histologic diagnosis. Use of jumbo forceps does not increase the rate of complications related to endoscopy; rather, it greatly improves the quality of the histologic specimens.[5]

Barrett's Esophagus

BE is characterized by the conversion of normal squamous epithelium of the esophagus into metaplastic columnar epithelium, caused by chronic GERD in the vast majority of cases.[57,58] Patients with BE have an increased risk of developing dysplasia and adenocarcinoma. For these reasons, it is highly recommended that patients with BE undergo periodic endoscopic surveillance to detect preinvasive neoplasia (dysplasia) and prevent the development of cancer.[59,60]

The American College of Gastroenterology (ACG) and American Gastroesophageal Association (AGA) define BE as endoscopically recognizable columnar metaplasia of the esophageal mucosa that is confirmed pathologically to contain intestinal metaplasia (IM), the latter defined by the presence of goblet cells.[59,60] Based on this definition, both the endoscopic and pathologic components are required to establish a diagnosis of BE. According to this strict definition, patients who have IM (goblet cells) of the gastric cardia are not included in this disease. Columnar mucosa is visible endoscopically and is most often grossly described as *salmon-pink gastric-type* mucosa in the distal esophagus.[57,58] As much as one-third of GERD patients who lack endoscopically visible columnar mucosa within the distal esophagus show IM (goblet cells) in their otherwise anatomically normal GEJ, and these patients do not qualify as having BE based on the previously mentioned ACG and AGA guidelines.[61,62] This position is based on the assumption that the presence of a few intestinalized glands in the GEJ region of patients without endoscopically apparent columnar metaplasia of the distal esophagus does not confer the same increased risk of malignancy as endoscopically visible BE.[63] There is an absence of worldwide agreement that IM (goblet cells) should be required for a diagnosis of BE. For instance, in both the United Kingdom and Japan, IM is not required to establish a diagnosis of BE.[64–66] Studies suggest that most patients with at least 2 cm of columnar-lined esophagus are found to have IM if enough biopsy samples are obtained from the columnar-lined segment.[67] Therefore sampling error is a confounding factor. Several studies have found a similar risk of progression to dysplasia or cancer in patients with and without goblets cells in columnar-lined esophagus.[68,69]

Several anatomic landmarks are important for endoscopists to identify when evaluating patients with possible BE. The GEJ, which is the junction between the tubular esophagus and the proximal stomach, is defined in North America as the most proximal aspect of the gastric folds.[70] The squamocolumnar junction (SCJ), also known as the *Z-line*, is the junction of squamous and columnar mucosa. It does not necessarily correspond to the location of the GEJ, and is irregular in many apparently normal individuals with and without GERD symptoms. The endoscopist should provide the pathologist with knowledge about the relationship of the SCJ to the GEJ (i.e., whether it is located at or above the GEJ) and the location of the biopsy relative to these anatomic landmarks. Therefore if the SCJ is observed

to be proximally displaced relative to the GEJ, biopsies of the GEJ, the SCJ, and the intervening (salmon-pink colored) columnar mucosa should be obtained to help establish a diagnosis of BE (see Table 5.1).

An endoscopic impression of BE may be difficult if there are very short (ultrashort) segments of columnar mucosa in the esophagus.[61,71] In addition, endoscopy is challenging in patients with hiatal hernia, which makes identification of the location of the proximal gastric folds difficult. In both normal individuals and in reflux patients without BE, very short segments of endoscopically visible mucosa within the distal esophagus/GEJ region are often composed of gastric cardiac or fundic-type mucosa, but without goblet cells. In these cases, the SCJ junction is usually irregular and may project for only a few millimeters into the distal portion of the tubular esophagus. Pathologists are often asked to evaluate "GEJ" or "irregular Z-line" biopsies to "rule out BE." In the majority of cases, it is not possible for pathologists to accurately determine the true anatomic origin of the biopsy (i.e., whether it was obtained from the distal esophagus or from the proximal stomach) when evaluating biopsies from the GEJ region. Goblet cells may be present in both the distal esophagus and gastric cardia and, when present, are histologically and histochemically identical.[72,73] However, some studies have identified a variety of morphologic features that, when present, help determine whether a biopsy with columnar mucosa from the GEJ originated in the distal esophagus. For instance, in a study by Srivastava et al (2007), mucosal biopsy samples from 20 patients with BE and from 20 patients with IM of the proximal stomach were evaluated. The authors found that the presence of several features, such as buried columnar epithelium, severe crypt atrophy and disarray, multilayered epithelium, and esophageal glands and/or ducts, were indicative of esophageal origin of the columnar mucosa in the biopsy sample and thus were significantly associated with BE.[74]

Traditionally, BE has been classified into long-segment (> 3 cm), short-segment (1–3 cm), and ultrashort-segment types (< 1 cm), depending on the length of involved esophageal mucosa.[75,76] However, the biologic significance of this classification system remains unclear. Several studies have evaluated the risk of dysplasia and cancer in relation to the length of BE. A 2013 multicenter cohort study suggests an 11% increased risk of HGD and carcinoma for every 1 cm increase in BE length.[77] The increased risk associated with longer lengths of BE has been attributed to a larger surface area at risk for neoplastic progression.

Microscopically, BE is characterized by columnar epithelium composed of mucinous columnar cells with scattered goblet cells, enterocytes, and intermediate features of gastric/intestinal cells. Occasional Paneth cells and endocrine cells may be seen. Because of ongoing and recurrent inflammation, ulceration, and repair, nondysplastic BE typically shows mild architectural and cytologic changes that differ from normal intestinal epithelium. Nondysplastic BE has a relatively low nuclear-cytoplasmic (N:C) ratio and shows surface maturation. Goblet cells are irregularly distributed in BE and thus, multiple samples are usually required to detect them (Fig. 5.4). In one retrospective study of 1646 esophageal mucosal biopsies from 125 consecutive patients with BE, goblet cells were detected in 68% of cases when eight mucosal samples were taken and only in 35% when four samples were taken; no significant benefit was found in goblet cell detection with more than eight biopsies (see Table 5.1).[67] Another study found that goblet cells were more commonly detected at the

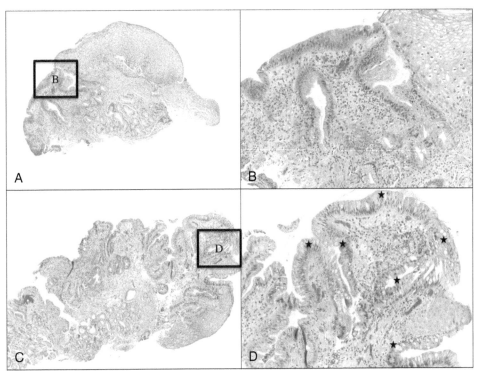

FIG 5.4 Distal esophageal biopsies from a patient with Barrett's esophagus showing fragments of squamocolumnar junctional mucosa without (**A** and **B,** low and representative high magnification, respectively) and with (**C** and **D,** low and representative high magnification, respectively) intestinal metaplasia. *Stars* highlight the scattered goblet cells.

neosquamocolumnar junction than in the distal esophagus (94% vs. 39%, respectively).[78]

Dysplasia is defined as neoplastic epithelium confined to basement membrane. Endoscopically, dysplasia may be undetectable or may appear flat, plaque-like, nodular, polypoid, or ulcerated. The histologic diagnosis and grading of dysplasia is based on evaluation of both cytologic and architectural abnormalities.[79] Intestinal type dysplasia is graded as LGD or HGD. LGD is composed of columnar cells with nuclear elongation, hyperchromasia, stratification, and retained polarity, and is often described as resembling conventional colonic tubular adenoma. In contrast, HGD exhibits architectural abnormalities and greater degree of cytologic atypia, such as marked nuclear pleomorphisms with round vesicular nuclei, prominent nucleoli, and loss of polarity. Unfortunately, there is a well-established, high degree of interobserver variability in interpretation of cytologic and architectural features among both expert GI pathologists and general pathologists.[80–82] Many pathologists, particularly those from Europe and Asia, prefer the more recently proposed Vienna classification system.[83] The Vienna system uses the terms "noninvasive neoplasia" instead of dysplasia and "suspicious for invasive carcinoma" for lesions that show equivocal cytologic or architectural features of tissue invasion. The categories in the Vienna system are as follows: negative for neoplasia, indefinite for neoplasia, noninvasive low-grade neoplasia, noninvasive high-grade neoplasia (including noninvasive carcinoma in situ and suspicion of invasive carcinoma), and invasive neoplasia (intramucosal and submucosal). The Vienna system was developed in an effort to reduce discrepancies in interpretation of dysplasia between Western and Japanese pathologists and to help reach a worldwide consensus on the nomenclature of GI neoplasia. Recent reports have also described nonintestinal forms of dysplasia, namely foveolar and serrated dysplasia, which at this time are not well characterized and the natural history of these types of dysplastic changes is poorly understood.[84–86]

Various biomarkers of progression have been studied as potential adjuncts for the diagnosis of dysplasia. For example, genomic instability as measured by copy number alteration and loss of heterozygosity were shown to be useful markers of progression.[87] Another retrospective, double-blinded validation study of eight BE methylation biomarkers proposed a methylation biomarker-based panel to predict neoplastic progression in BE with potential clinical value in improving both the efficiency of surveillance endoscopy and early detection of dysplasia.[88] More recently, p53 overexpression was associated with an increased risk of neoplastic progression in patients with BE.[89] Despite these advances, at present, there are no biomarkers, or panel of biomarkers, that have been validated in large prospective cohort studies. Morphologic assessment of dysplasia remains the gold standard for evaluating dysplasia. In their most recent position statement, the AGA does not recommend the use of molecular biomarkers to confirm a histologic diagnosis of dysplasia for patients with BE at this time.[60]

In some instances, a definite diagnosis of dysplasia cannot be established, and the term *indefinite for dysplasia* is used. This can occur when biopsies contain active inflammation, ulceration, or postulcer healing, and it may be difficult for pathologists to determine whether a biopsy with atypical changes represents true dysplasia or extreme regenerative changes. Other factors that can lead to uncertainty include technical or processing artifacts (for example, poor orientation, lack of surface epithelium, crush artifact). The rate of a diagnosis of indefinite for dysplasia varies widely between pathologists and is in part based on individual experience.[80] It is important to recognize that indefinite for dysplasia is a provisional diagnosis.

Tissue sampling in the setting of BE has been described in great detail in several other publications and various society guidelines.[59,60] Currently, recommended endoscopic surveillance consists of four-quadrant biopsies at 2-cm intervals with the use of jumbo biopsy forceps. Data that support this systematic sampling protocol include a study by Abela et al (2008), which found that systematic surveillance detected HGD, which was almost always amenable to endoscopic resection, in 2.8% of patients, compared to 0% in patients with nonsystematic sampling.[90] Furthermore, none of the patients undergoing systematic surveillance developed adenocarcinoma, whereas three patients with nonsystemic sampling died of invasive adenocarcinoma. In addition, specific endoscopic mucosal abnormalities such as ulcers, irregular lesions, nodules, and polyps should also be sampled, and these lesions should be submitted separately.

The recommended surveillance interval for dysplasia in patients with BE is determined by the presence and degree of dysplasia found. In the absence of dysplasia, the surveillance interval is every 3 to 5 years, with four-quadrant biopsies every 2 cm (see Table 5.1). If the pathology is indefinite, the biopsy should be reviewed by an expert GI pathologist. Medications for reflux treatment should be maximized to reduce the presence of inflammation, and then EGD with biopsies should be repeated. The presence of LGD should be confirmed by endoscopy within 6 months, followed by surveillance every 12 months. Studies have shown that endoscopy with magnification and narrow band imaging (NBI) allows for better localization of HGD and may also allow more targeted and fewer biopsies. For LGD, ablation therapy has also shown an advantage over surveillance alone. For instance, a 2014 multicenter randomized trial of 136 patients with LGD showed that ablation therapy reduced the risk of progression to HGD and adenocarcinoma from 26.5% to 1.5% compared with surveillance alone, over a 3-year follow-up.[91] In patients with known or suspected dysplasia, biopsies should be obtained at 1-cm intervals instead of the standard 2 cm intervals (see Table 5.1). A study of 45 BE patients with HGD reported that biopsies obtained at 2-cm intervals missed 50% of early cancers that were detected when sampling at 1-cm intervals was performed.[92]

Patients with flat HGD confirmed by an expert GI pathologist should undergo a repeat endoscopy within 3 months with four-quadrant biopsies every 1 cm if an eradication method is not used. The prevalence of cancer in resection specimens from patients who have undergone an esophagectomy for HGD ranges from 5% to 41%, and the rate of progression to cancer in patients with HGD approaches 30% at 10 years. Options for patients with flat HGD include intensive surveillance (every 3 months), esophagectomy, and ablative therapies such as BARRX radiofrequency ablation (Medtronic, Minneapolis, MN). It is recommended that patients with HGD in an area of mucosal irregularity should undergo endoscopic mucosal or surgical resection (see Fig. 5.2). EMR functions as both a diagnostic and a therapeutic procedure, and there is a growing trend toward recommending esophagectomy only for patients with either extensive HGD or invasive carcinoma.[93,94] Because EMR specimens typically consist of larger pieces of tissue than biopsies, which can also be optimally oriented during processing, EMR increases diagnostic accuracy

and allows pathologists to provide more accurate pathologic diagnostic information. For example, in a study by Mino-Kenudson et al (2007), 37% of cases of BE with dysplasia diagnosed in biopsies had a change of grade when evaluated on EMR specimens.[95] Biopsies underreported the grade of neoplasia in 21% of cases and overreported the grade in 16%. In a recent multicenter cohort study of 138 BE patients (including 15 LGD, 87 HGD, and 36 early adenocarcinoma) undergoing biopsies followed by EMR within 6 months, EMR evaluation resulted in a change in histologic diagnosis in approximately 30% of patients, irrespective of the presence or absence of visible lesions.[95a]

Eosinophilic Esophagitis

The diagnosis of eosinophilic esophagitis (EoE) is based on clinicopathologic correlation, with clinical, endoscopic and histologic findings each serving an important role in assessing a patient with dysphagia. EoE is a chronic, immune mediated disease characterized by esophageal eosinophilia and esophageal dysfunction, affecting children and adults. Endoscopically, patients with EoE can show several characteristic features, including esophageal rings, mucosal plaques or exudates, longitudinal furrows, edema, diffuse esophageal narrowing, narrow-caliber esophagus, and mucosal tears. In some cases, the esophagus appears entirely normal, but more than 90% of affected patients display one or more of these endoscopic abnormalities.[96] However, these endoscopic features have been described in other conditions and are not pathognomonic of EoE.

Histologically, many of the features of EoE overlap significantly with those of GERD, particularly in distal esophageal biopsies. EoE biopsies usually show numerous intraepithelial eosinophils, typically 15 or more per high-power field.[97] Severe GERD produces pronounced eosinophilia in this range in only a minority of cases, and in these cases, it is unclear if the patients have GERD and EoE concurrently. However, because intraepithelial eosinophils in both conditions may be patchy in distribution, sampling error can affect the ability to establish a correct diagnosis (Fig. 5.5).[98] Although not pathognomonic, additional histologic features of EoE that can aid in establishing the diagnosis include eosinophilic microabscesses, surface layering of eosinophils, surface sloughing of squamous cells mixed with abundant eosinophils, and extracellular eosinophilic granules. The distribution of disease is important, because EoE often involves long segments of the esophagus, may be patchy or focal, and typically involves the proximal or middle esophagus and the distal esophagus or GEJ equally.[99,100] In contrast, patients with GERD typically have higher eosinophil counts in the distal esophagus, an area where reflux affects the esophagus more severely, than in the proximal esophagus.

Esophageal biopsies are the only reliable diagnostic test for EoE, and therefore biopsy is required to establish the diagnosis.[101] According to experts panels and the ACG guidelines, in patients with suspected EoE, it is recommended that two to four biopsies be obtained from at least two different locations in the esophagus, most typically in the distal and proximal halves of the esophagus, regardless of endoscopic findings (see Table 5.1).[102] Biopsies targeting areas with abnormal endoscopic findings (such as rings, furrows, and plaques) are also reasonable. An interdisciplinary panel of 33 expert physicians recommends taking two to four biopsy samples from the proximal and distal esophagus, regardless of the endoscopic appearance (see Table 5.1). Biopsies should be fixed in 10% buffered formalin, which preserves eosinophils better than alternative fixatives, such as Bouin's preservative.[103]

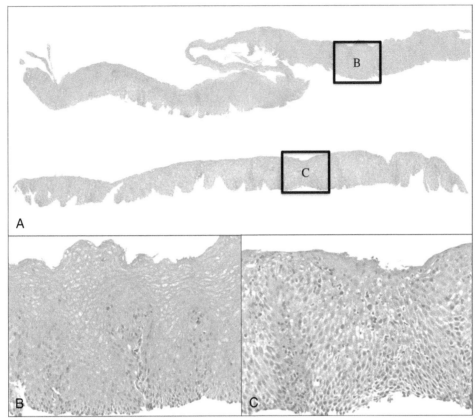

FIG 5.5 **A,** Eosinophilic esophagitis showing patchy involvement, low power view. Higher magnification shows **B,** rare scattered eosinophils in one portion of the specimen and **C,** more than 30 eosinophils per high power field in a different focus.

In addition, gastric antrum and duodenum biopsies should also be obtained if there is a clinical suspicion of more widespread eosinophilic gastroenteritis.

Infectious Esophagitis

Infectious esophagitis is an important cause of esophagitis, particularly in immunocompromised patients, but also in immunocompetent patients.[32,104] The most common causes of infectious esophagitis are viruses and fungus (Fig. 5.6). Cytomegalovirus (CMV) infects mesenchymal and columnar cells and presents macroscopically as ulcerative lesions. Biopsy for CMV detection should be concentrated at the ulcer base to optimize sampling and diagnostic accuracy.[105] In a study of HIV-infected patients with esophageal ulcers, three forceps biopsy samples from the ulcer base were diagnostic in 80% of patients with CMV esophagitis, with a maximum of 10 biopsy samples needed to confirm the diagnosis in the remaining patients.[106] The biopsy samples were examined using standard histopathologic methods, with in situ hybridization or immunohistochemical stains as needed. Qualitative CMV PCR of biopsy samples is more sensitive than standard histopathology, but likely detects latent, as well as clinical, disease. Data are inconsistent regarding the benefit of viral culture in the evaluation of CMV esophagitis. Herpes simplex virus infects squamous epithelial cells, usually present at the lateral margin of ulcers and erosions; therefore mucosal biopsy samples of the ulcer margin have the highest diagnostic yield (see Fig. 5.6C, D). Viral culture and PCR can aid in diagnosing herpes simplex virus esophagitis.[32] There are limited data on the optimal diagnostic technique for esophageal candidiasis (see Fig. 5.6A, B). White plaques are a characteristic finding and are recommended as the site of sampling, either as pinch biopsy or brush cytologic assessment.[107] Cytologic brushing may be more sensitive than histology for diagnosis.[108,109]

Stomach

Helicobacter pylori

Helicobacter pylori (HP) gastritis affects two-thirds of the world's population and is one of the most common chronic inflammatory disorders of humans.[110] Although chronic HP gastritis is asymptomatic in most infected individuals, its impact on human health is profound. HP gastritis confers a 15% to 20% lifetime risk for peptic ulcer disease, and 70% of gastric cancers and most primary gastric mucosal-associated lymphoid tissue (MALT) lymphomas are directly linked to chronic HP infection. In one British community, HP was estimated to be responsible for approximately 5% of all GI ailments.[111]

Because most patients with early HP gastritis do not undergo endoscopy, information regarding the clinical, endoscopic, and pathologic aspects of acute HP infection is limited to a few well-documented case reports, human ingestion studies, and analyses of infections acquired from inadequately disinfected endoscopic instruments.[110] Endoscopically, manifestations of acute or early HP gastritis are typically found in the antrum and characterized by hemorrhagic lesions and multiple erosions or ulcers. There are no distinct endoscopic patterns of chronic HP gastritis. Depending on the stage and type of gastritis, hyperemia,

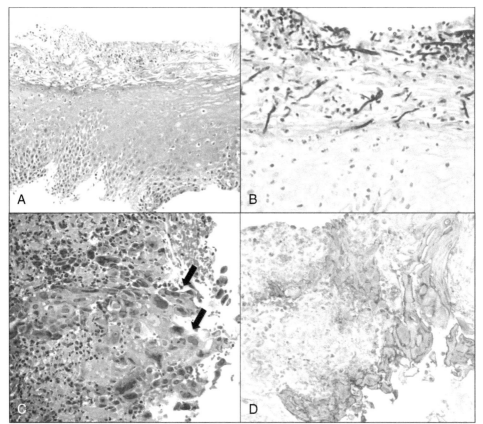

FIG 5.6 A, Candida esophagitis with superficial exudates composed of sloughed squamous epithelium and inflammatory cells. **B,** Candida organisms are highlighted by periodic acid Schiff with diastase stain. **C,** Herpes simplex virus esophagitis with superficial epithelial necrosis and sloughing, and herpetic inclusions within squamous cells *(arrow).* **D,** Immunohistochemical stain for herpes simplex virus confirms the diagnosis.

erosions, hypertrophy, and atrophy may coexist in various combinations. Unfortunately, none of these endoscopic features has proved useful for predicting the presence or absence of HP gastritis. Endoscopists should not attempt to diagnose HP gastritis based solely on the gross appearance of the gastric mucosa. The diagnosis of HP gastritis rests on pathologic evaluation of gastric mucosal biopsies or detection of urease in mucosal specimens by the Campylobacter-like organism (CLO) test or the urea breath test.[112]

Microscopically, HP chronic gastritis is characterized by a prominent lymphoplasmacytic infiltrate of the lamina propria of gastric mucosa (Fig. 5.7). In addition, mucosal neutrophils are scattered within the lamina propria or within the surface or glandular epithelium. Abundant HP organisms are usually present, characteristically attached to the surface of mucous foveolar cells.[113] After successful eradication therapy, neutrophils disappear rapidly, and their continued presence is considered a valuable indicator of therapeutic failure.[114] The intensity of the mononuclear cell infiltrate typically declines quite slowly after successful eradication of infection. As many as 30% of patients have chronic inactive gastritis that persists for several years after eradication of the organism. Other features include the presence of lymphoid follicles with germinal centers, seen in nearly all HP infected patients.[115] Occasionally, lymphoid infiltrates may be large and irregular, with destructive lymphoepithelial lesions at the periphery. In this circumstance, the possibility of gastric

lymphoma should be considered; immunohistochemical and molecular tests are often used for this purpose.

Diagnosis of HP gastritis can be made using a variety of endoscopic methods, including tissue urease activity, histologic examination, and microbial culture. The choice of test depends on the prevalence of the disease in the local population, clinical suspicion, cost considerations, and local expertise. HP normally infects antral and corpus mucosa, but in the cardia, organisms may be difficult to detect. HP organisms rarely colonize intestinal epithelium, and in patients with extensive areas of metaplastic atrophy, organisms are usually confined to the nonmetaplastic, nonatrophic areas of mucosa. The sensitivity of these endoscopic tests may be decreased by proton pump inhibitors (PPIs), bismuth compounds, antibiotics, and acute GI bleeding. Specifically, in patients who use PPIs, HP organisms tend to be rare or absent in the antrum, and they may be difficult to detect in the corpus, even in the setting of chronic active inflammation.[116] In situations of reduced sensitivity, a negative urease test result should be confirmed using a second test, and histologic exam is a convenient alternative. Similarly, patients treated with antibiotics before gastric biopsy may demonstrate a markedly reduced number of organisms and often have atypical (coccoid) forms.

There is limited data on the optimal biopsy protocol for detection of HP. Several recommendations have been published. The updated Sydney system protocol recommends five biopsies: two from the antrum, one from the angularis, two from fundus/

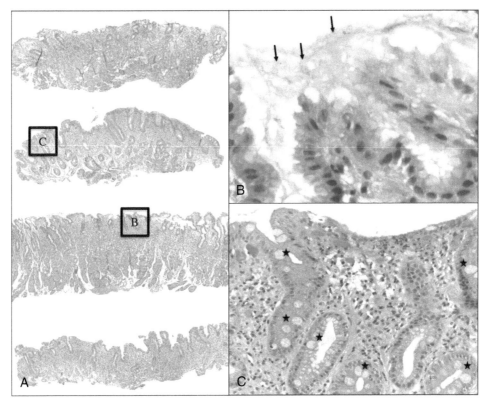

FIG 5.7 **A,** Four biopsies samples from a patient with *Helicobacter pylori* gastritis. **B,** *Helicobacter pylori* bacteria are present in the luminal aspect of the foveolar epithelium *(arrows)*. Focal intestinal metaplasia is present within a fragment of antral mucosa **C,** *Stars* highlight glands with intestinal metaplasia.

body (see Table 5.1).[117] The updated Sydney system provides pathologists with guidelines for generating systematic, uniform, and clinically relevant diagnostic reports. Another approach suggests taking three biopsies, one each from the angularis, greater curvature, and lesser curvature. El-Zimanti and Graham (1999) reported that the three biopsy protocol compared favorably with the Updated Sydney five biopsy protocol, with both methods identifying 100% of infections in a retrospective study of 46 patients.[118]

Use of ancillary stains for detection of HP, although common, is highly variable across medical centers. Commonly used and relatively inexpensive stains, such as Giemsa and Diff-Quik, are adequate for identification of most cases of HP organisms. Recently, the Rodger C. Haggitt Gastrointestinal Pathology Society recommended the use of ancillary stains when biopsies show chronic or chronic active gastritis without detectable HP on routine H&E sections, but recommended that "up front" stains on all gastric biopsies are not necessary.[119] Immunohistochemical stains for HP increase sensitivity and are particularly useful for detecting coccoid forms of the organism, rare organisms located deep within the glands, and intracytoplasmic organisms. After HP treatment, organisms may be best visualized with an immunohistochemical stain if chronic gastritis persists.

HP gastritis is associated with several possible complications. Chronic HP infection is a strong risk factor for development of gastric cancer, particularly the intestinal type, as well as lymphoma, particularly low-grade extranodal marginal zone lymphoma of mucosal-associated lymphoid tissue (MALT lymphoma). In certain regions of the world, metaplastic atrophic gastritis develops in a considerable proportion of infected persons, and this condition is a precursor to gastric carcinoma. HP gastritis with metaplasia is histologically characterized by the presence of IM and gastric gland atrophy, usually oxyntic, present in a patchy manner through the body and fundus (see Fig. 5.7C). In one study comparing HP infected patients with controls, Xia et al (2000), found that a greater proportion of HP infected individuals showed antral-type mucosa (84%) or IM (13%) at the incisura angularis, compared to uninfected patients (18% and 3%, respectively).[120] In another study, IM was found in 6% of patients at the incisura, suggesting that sampling of this area should always be included in the assessment of patients with chronic gastritis.[121] The Updated Sydney Protocol may miss the presence of IM in more than 50% of cases.[118]

Autoimmune Atrophic Metaplastic Gastritis

Autoimmune atrophic metaplastic gastritis (AMAG) preferentially affects the gastric corpus and typically spares the gastric antrum.[122,123] AMAG preferentially affects older patients and women, and is associated with other autoimmune disease.[124,125] AMAG predisposes to pernicious anemia and confers an increased risk for development of hyperplastic and dysplastic polyps, carcinoma, and endocrine tumors.[126] AMAG is associated with serum auto-antibodies, including anti-intrinsic factor and anti-parietal cell antibodies.[127] AMAG does not cause specific clinical manifestations until a critical decrease has occurred in the parietal cell mass, beyond which anemia develops.[128] Years before the onset of anemia, patients may show various degrees of hypo-chlorhydria, hypergastrinemia, and loss of pepsin and pepsinogen secretion.[129]

Endoscopically, the mucosa of the corpus in patients with autoimmune gastritis is usually thinner than normal and shows a reduction or complete absence of rugal folds. Fine submucosal vessels are usually easily recognizable on endoscopic examination in advanced cases. Hyperplastic polyps are also common in advanced-stage disease. Polyps are detected in 20% to 40% of patients with pernicious anemia; they are mostly sessile, less than 2 cm in diameter, and often multiple. Most are hyperplastic, but as many as 10% contain foci of dysplasia. Gastric cancers associated with pernicious anemia are mostly intestinal type and arise from IM, suggesting that carcinoma in autoimmune gastritis likely develops through a metaplasia-dysplasia-carcinoma pathway.[126]

Microscopically, the main pathologic features of uncomplicated autoimmune gastritis are diffuse corpus-restricted chronic atrophic gastritis with some degree of IM and enterochromaffin-like (ECL) cell hyperplasia (Fig. 5.8).[123] In the absence of comorbidities, such as concurrent HP infection or bile reflux, the antrum is typically normal. This pattern of involvement is characteristic of patients with advanced disease and is found in patients with pernicious anemia. Three pathologic phases can be identified during the course of autoimmune gastritis in corpus mucosa: early, florid, and end stage.[130,131] The early phase is characterized by diffuse or multifocal, dense lymphoplasma cell infiltration; IM and oxyntic gland destruction may be patchy in the early

stage and the possibility of sampling error limiting the diagnostic yield of biopsies exits. The florid phase of autoimmune gastritis is characterized by marked atrophy of oxyntic glands, prominent pseudopyloric and IM, diffuse lymphoplasmacytic inflammation, and normal or reduced thickness of the mucosa. At this stage of the disease, the pathologic features of autoimmune atrophic gastritis are sufficiently distinctive, particularly if the antrum is normal. However, demonstration of antibodies directed against parietal cell and intrinsic factor antigens is necessary for confirmation.[127,132] The end stage of disease is characterized by a marked reduction in oxyntic glands, foveolar hyperplasia, hyperplastic polyp formation, and increasing degrees of pseudopyloric, pancreatic, and IM. At this stage, parietal cells are difficult to detect, and inflammation is usually minimal or absent, although scattered lymphoid aggregates may persist.

During the florid and end stages, ECL cell proliferation is prominent, as a result of achlorhydria and hypergastrinemia. ECL cell carcinoids may arise during the florid phase and they are found most commonly in patients with end-stage disease.[133,134] Carcinoid tumors associated with ECL cell hyperplasia occur in 5% to 8% of patients with autoimmune gastritis and severe hypergastrinemia, and they account for 70% to 80% of all gastric carcinoid tumors.[135] ECL cell proliferation is not unique to autoimmune gastritis and may also occur in patients with Zollinger-Ellison syndrome, multiple endocrine neoplasia syndromes, and HP-associated, multifocal atrophic gastritis. Carcinoid tumors in patients with autoimmune gastritis are relatively innocuous and are associated with a more than a

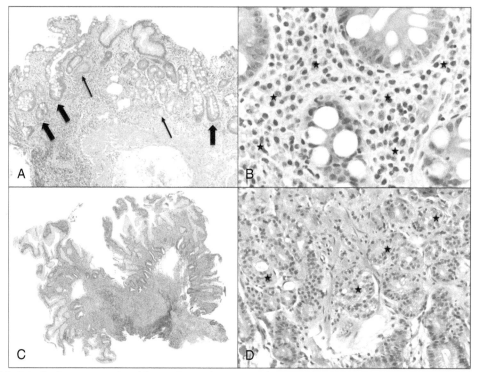

FIG 5.8 **A,** Representative biopsy from the stomach of a patient with autoimmune gastritis showing complete oxyntic gland atrophy, pseudopyloric metaplasia *(thin arrows)* and intestinal metaplasia *(thick arrows)*. Also present is a prominent lymphoplasmacytic inflammatory infiltrate in the lamina propria (**B,** lamina propria plasma cells highlighted by stars). Hyperplastic polyps (**C**) and neuroendocrine cell hyperplasia (**D,** highlighted by *stars*) are also manifestations of this disease.

95% 5-year survival rate, which sharply contrasts with the less common solitary, sporadic type of carcinoid tumors that are biologically more aggressive (< 35% 5-year survival rate).[133] It is important to convey to clinicians the clinical and pathologic context in which a gastric carcinoid is diagnosed.

Biopsy remains an important component of AMAG diagnosis and histologic exam is considered a reliable method of diagnosis. There are no standardized endoscopic mucosal biopsy protocols for AMAG.[122,130] The updated Sydney system is recommended: two biopsies from the corpus, two from the antrum, and one from the incisura angularis.[117] To establish a diagnosis of AMAG, biopsies from the antrum and body should be submitted in separate jars for independent assessment of each anatomic site, which aids in identification of the preferential gastric corpus atrophy. Biopsies should also be directed at ulcers, nodules, polyps, and masses to rule out neoplasia; these targeted biopsies should be submitted in separate jars.

Intestinal Metaplasia

IM is occasionally detected in the stomach of patients without a documented history of autoimmune gastritis or HP gastritis (see Fig. 5.7A, C). IM is defined as the replacement of gastric-type mucinous epithelial cells with intestinal type cells, including goblet cells and enterocytes.[136] IM develops in a variety of pathologic settings and usually indicates the presence of chronic atrophic gastritis, which can occur in the setting of HP gastritis. The development of extensive IM in this scenario is termed *environmental metaplastic atrophic gastritis (EMAG)*. In the absence of a complete set of biopsies from different anatomic areas of the stomach, use of a well-defined biopsy sampling protocol (such as updated Sydney system) is considered the minimum required for reliable staging of chronic gastritis. Tissue sampling in EMAG is performed to establish the diagnosis, to define the etiology and anatomic distribution of disease, and to evaluate for the presence and extent of dysplastic or neoplastic change. The stage of gastritis is determined by the combination of the extent of atrophy (scored histologically) with its topographic location (resulting from the mapping protocol). There is no standard biopsy protocol for the diagnosis and surveillance of EMAG. In a prospective, multicenter study of 112 patients with gastric IM or dysplasia, a regimen consisting of at least 12 biopsy samples had 100% sensitivity for the diagnosis of EMAG, dysplasia, and cancer, whereas one regimen consisting of seven nontargeted biopsies was able to diagnose IM in 97% of cases and all cases of dysplasia or cancer.[137] In contrast, the updated Sydney protocol detected 90% of cases of known EMAG, but also failed to identify 50% of patients with dysplasia or gastric cancer.[117]

Patients with EMAG may be at higher risk for developing dysplasia and carcinoma.[138,139] High-risk patients include those with a family history of gastric cancer, Hispanics, African-Americans, and immigrants from higher-risk geographic locations. Some studies have reported an 11% risk of adenocarcinoma for patients with atrophy or IM during a 10-year follow-up period.[140,141] No formal recommendations or data exist to support the implementation of an endoscopic surveillance program in high-risk patients who have gastric IM. Patients who have dysplasia and IM have a 100-fold increased risk of carcinoma.[142] There is no consensus regarding the appropriate time interval or biopsy surveillance protocol after a diagnosis of LGD of the stomach. Studies have suggested that in a patient with EMAG, topographic mapping of the gastric mucosa should be performed

every 3 months during the first year, followed by repeated surveillance endoscopy every 3 years if extensive metaplasia persists, along with sampling of any endoscopically visible lesions.[103,117,143–145] The American Society of Gastrointestinal Endoscopy (ASGE) recommends that patients with confirmed HGD on gastric biopsies be considered for gastrectomy or EMR.[144,146]

Gastric Polyps

Gastric epithelial polyps include fundic gland polyps, hyperplastic polyps, and adenomas. Gastric polyps are often incidentally detected on endoscopy. Polyp histology cannot be reliably distinguished by endoscopic appearance. Endoscopic forceps biopsy is inadequate to rule out dysplasia and carcinoma for polyps larger than 0.5 cm to 1 cm. Hyperplastic polyps are most common, and often occur in the setting of chronic gastritis (see Fig. 5.8C).[147,148] Fundic gland polyps that develop sporadically or in association with long-term PPI use have very low to no malignant potential.[149] It should be realized, however, that dysplasia may be found in fundic gland polyps associated with familial adenomatous polyposis.[150] Dysplastic elements may be present in as many as 20% of hyperplastic polyps.[151] Adenomatous gastric polyps also have malignant potential. Hyperplastic and adenomatous polyps may occur in the presence of HP infection and EMAG, and sampling of these entities should be performed. When hyperplastic and adenomatous polyps are identified or suspected based on endoscopic appearance, biopsy samples should also be taken from the surrounding nonpolypoid mucosa to exclude dysplasia arising in a background of metaplastic atrophic gastritis, and to determine the cause and extent of the underlying inflammatory and dysplastic condition.

Small Intestine
Celiac Disease

Celiac disease is an autoimmune-mediated disorder affecting genetically susceptible patients that results in damage to the proximal small-intestinal mucosa and of malabsorption of nutrients as a result of exposure to dietary gluten. Celiac disease may appear at any time in life, from early childhood to late adulthood. Celiac disease in adults represents a large, previously unappreciated disease population.[152–154] There has been a substantial increase in the rate of diagnosis over the last decade and celiac disease remains underdiagnosed in the United States.[155,156] It is recommended that patients suspected of having celiac disease based on clinical parameters should undergo testing.[157] Classic symptoms include abdominal discomfort, diarrhea, and steatorrhea.[158,159] However, some patients do not develop diarrhea, but instead, exhibit other signs and symptoms, including short stature, infertility, neurological disorders, recurrent aphthous stomatitis, or dermatitis herpetiformis.[158–163] In adults with occult celiac disease, fatigue and iron deficiency anemia are common, which ultimately prompt investigatory tests that uncover the correct diagnosis.[164] Some patients are entirely asymptomatic and present initially only with histologic changes on biopsy analysis ("latent celiac disease").[152,153]

No single serologic test for celiac disease has a perfect sensitivity or specificity. Immunoglobulin A (IgA) antitissue transglutaminase (TTG) antibody is the preferred initial single test for detection of celiac disease in individuals over the age of 2 years.[157,165] Serologic testing may be negative in up to 16% of patients, and if clinically indicated based on symptoms and evidence of malabsorption, additional testing should be pursued for confirmation.[166,167] Endoscopic examination and small bowel biopsy continue to play a critical role in establishing and confirming the diagnosis of celiac disease.

In patients with undiagnosed and symptomatic celiac disease, the endoscopic appearance may show classic features, characterized by a flat, scalloped appearance of the duodenum.[168] However, the endoscopic findings in patients with celiac disease can be subtle and often unreliable. One endoscopic study found that a reduction of folds, scalloping, mosaic pattern, and nodular mucosa were sensitive, but not specific, endoscopic findings in celiac disease, as they were also noted in some dyspeptic patients without celiac disease.[169] Similarly, a meta-analysis of studies testing the diagnostic sensitivity and specificity of video capsule endoscopy in celiac disease patients reports that the images seen can correctly diagnose the condition.[170] However, there is insufficient data on performance in mild histologic forms that are commonly seen.[153,154,171,172] Confocal laser microscopy shows promise as an endoscopic technique that can recognize villous irregularity and blunting, with the caveats that interobserver variability is high and the technique is not yet widely available.[173]

Histologically, the classic features of untreated celiac disease include complete villous atrophy, increased lamina propria chronic inflammation, and increased intraepithelial CD3+/CD8+ T-lymphocytes (Fig. 5.9). The histologic features of celiac disease are frequently classified according to Marsh, Marsh modified (Oberhuber), or simplified Corazza classification schema.[171,172,174]

Classic celiac disease shows greatest severity of histologic changes distally in the duodenum and proximal jejunum. The ileum may be involved in severe cases, but it is not a reliable site for biopsy diagnosis.[168,175–177] It is now widely recognized that many patients with celiac do not have diffusely abnormal duodenal histology, but instead show mild and patchy involvement in duodenal mucosal biopsies (see Fig. 5.9).[178–182] Ravelli et al (2001) prospectively evaluated 110 pediatric patients with elevated serum endomysial and/or tissue transglutaminase antibodies and clinical symptoms of celiac disease.[183] Each patient underwent mucosal biopsy of the duodenal bulb, proximal duodenum, intervening duodenum, and distal duodenum near the ligament of Treitz. Ninety-three percent of patients had changes compatible with celiac disease in at least one tissue sample, and 93% had similar findings in all samples. None of the patients had any tissue samples that were histologically normal, although complete loss of villous architecture was more commonly observed in samples from the distal small intestine. Some biopsies show preserved or minimally blunted villous architecture with a patchy increase of IELs.

Celiac disease may also be localized to the duodenal bulb. The duodenal bulb is now a recommended biopsy site because it is reliably involved in patients with patchy disease.[182,184] In a pediatric study, 16% of children had patchy villous atrophy, but all of them had involvement of the duodenal bulb, and in four patients the bulb was the only site of abnormality.[182] Similarly,

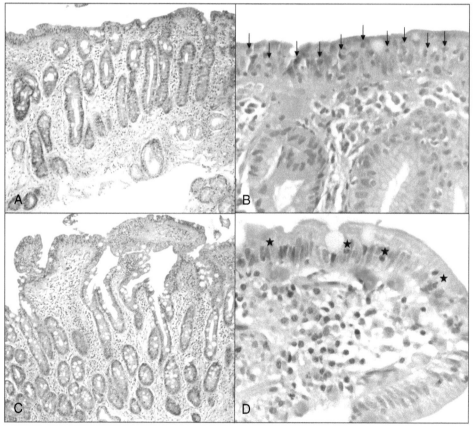

FIG 5.9 Biopsies of the duodenum from a patient with celiac disease showing variable involvement in different parts of the duodenum. In one area, complete villous atrophy along with increased intraepithelial lymphocytes is present (**A** and **B,** intraepithelial lymphocytes highlighted by *thin arrows*). A different portion of the duodenum shows preserved villi without significant increase of intraepithelial lymphocytes (**C** and **D,** occasional lymphocytes highlighted by *stars*).

Mooney et al (2016) described the features of ultrashort celiac disease limited to the duodenal bulb in a cohort of adult patients.[185] Duodenal bulb biopsies may also be more sensitive in patients following a low-gluten diet.[186] Further evidence supporting the validity of duodenal bulb biopsies as a diagnostic site is found in the study by Walker et al (2010), in which paired IEL counts were identical in the duodenal bulb and second duodenum in patients with celiac disease.[187] However, duodenal sampling had no effect on increasing detection of celiac disease in a low pretest probability cohort.[188]

Multiple samples taken from different sites of the duodenum are thought to help avoid inadequate sampling as a result of variable involvement of the disease, biopsy crush artifact, and allow for proper specimen orientation (Table 5.2). Based on studies in both adults and children, it appears that the most reliable biopsy protocol to detect all cases of celiac disease is a three- (or preferably five-) biopsy regimen that includes the duodenal bulb, the proximal duodenum, and the distal duodenum (see Table 5.2).[178,182,184,189] Although endoscopically abnormal mucosa should be preferentially targeted for sampling, it is important to realize that histologic disease may underlie normal-appearing mucosa. Historically, it was thought that well-oriented biopsy samples made it easier for pathologists to identify the cardinal features of celiac disease. Recent data, however, suggest that patients with celiac disease may only show increased intraepithelial lymphocytosis (as opposed to villous atrophy) as the key diagnostic finding.[190] Increased intraepithelial lymphocytosis is a feature that does not rely heavily on specimen orientation.

TABLE 5.2   Recommendations for Optimum Location and Number of Mucosal Biopsies for Evaluation of Common Gastrointestinal Disorders of the Lower Gastrointestinal Tract

Disease	Location and Number of Biopsy Samples
Microscopic colitis[143]	Two or more biopsies each from the transverse, descending, and sigmoid colon Additional sampling of endoscopically visible abnormalities
Inflammatory bowel disease[197,201,215-217]	Surveillance for dysplasia: Thirty-three random samples from patients with pancolitis, including five to six samples each from the right, transverse, distal, and sigmoid colon, proximal and distal colon, or Four-quadrant biopsies per 10 cm of colitic mucosa, and four-quadrant biopsies per 5 cm of colitic rectal mucosa If dysplasia is present: Complete removal of endoscopically resectable lesions, to include tissue sampling from mucosa surrounding the resection site to confirm complete excision
Graft versus host disease[143]	Optimal approach yet to be determined. Consider biopsies from upper and lower gastrointestinal tract. Avoid rectum only biopsies.

Refractory sprue is defined as a lack of or incomplete clinical response to a gluten-free diet.[191–193] Most patients with refractory sprue have histologic abnormalities similar to untreated celiac disease. However, some refractory sprue patients show loss of markers in the intraepithelial T-lymphocytes, or even monoclonality of the T cells. Collagenous sprue, characterized by a thickened subepithelial collagen layer, has since been reported in several series as a pattern of injury seen in the setting of refractory sprue, as well as associations with angiotensin receptor blockers.[191,194,195]

Colon
Inflammatory Bowel Disease
Inflammatory bowel disease (IBD), comprising ulcerative colitis (UC) and Crohn's disease, is a very common inflammatory bowel disorder affecting almost 1.5 million patients in the United States.[196] A diagnosis of IBD is established by a combination of clinical presentation and history, laboratory values, typical endoscopic features, histologic evaluation of mucosal biopsies, and radiologic findings.[197] The mucosal biopsy initial presentation is an integral component of IBD diagnosis. Microscopically, IBD mucosal biopsies, in both UC and Crohn's disease, show features of chronic colitis, including basal plasmacytosis, basal lymphoid aggregates, Paneth or pyloric metaplasia, and crypt distortion. Distinguishing between UC and Crohn's disease is based largely on the pattern and distribution of disease, rather than specific histologic features. If detected, the presence of granulomas favors Crohn's disease.[198] These histologic features are not entirely specific for IBD and might be found in other disorders, for example, IBD-like ischemia, radiation colitis or drug colitis.[199] After initiation of treatment, IBD biopsies may show mucosal healing.[200] The pathologist's role in evaluating IBD biopsies regardless of the temporal relationship to treatment, is to evaluate pathological extent of disease, degree of activity, and the presence or absence of dysplasia or cancer.

Biopsy protocols to diagnose, stage, and survey patients with IBD are based on expert consensus, case series, case-control studies, population-based cohort studies, prospective studies, and, in the case of optimal technique for surveillance colonoscopy, controlled trials (see Table 5.2).[197,201] Initial diagnosis of IBD should include confirmatory biopsy samples, to exclude the presence of other etiologies, such as infection. In patients undergoing ileocolonoscopy for suspected IBD, at least two biopsy samples should be taken from five sites, including the ileum and rectum, during the initial endoscopic evaluation. Specimens should be taken of both diseased and adjacent normal-appearing mucosa.[202] In a study of 414 consecutive patients who underwent intubation and biopsy of the terminal ileum, it was found that the diagnostic yield of ileal biopsies was highest in patients with suspected Crohn's disease, abnormal imaging studies, or endoscopic findings, but ileal sampling was not helpful when the endoscopic appearance of the ileal mucosa was normal.[203] The biopsy specimens from different locations should be separated in different jars to allow for evaluation of the extent and severity of disease. Higher detection rates for granulomas can be achieved when biopsy specimens are taken from the edge of ulcers and aphthous erosions.[204,205] If an EGD is performed for clinically suspected upper GI tract IBD, at least two biopsy samples should be taken from the esophagus, stomach, and duodenum.[205,206]

Surveillance for colorectal cancer is recommended for patients with long-standing IBD, particularly 8 to 10 years after onset of disease (see Table 5.2).[207,208] Although less common than UC, extensive colitis secondary to Crohn's disease also carries an increased risk for cancer. Data obtained from a cohort of 692 patients with IBD indicate that the standardized incidence ratio of colorectal carcinoma among Crohn's disease patients is 1.9, compared to 2.4 for patients with UC.[209] Colitis-related dysplasia may be present in endoscopically flat mucosa, or it may grow as a polyp, nodule, ulcer, or plaque. Studies indicate that most dysplasia is endoscopically visible.[210–212] Current surveillance strategies recommend extensive sampling of colonic mucosa and raised lesions, ulcers, or other suspicious areas. A study of 101 UC patients, including 81 high-risk and 20 low-risk patients, found that at least 56 jumbo-sized, nontargeted mucosal biopsies were necessary to exclude the possibility of dysplasia. This observation has led to the common practice of obtaining multiple tissue samples from every 10 to 12 cm of colon, or, alternatively, five to six samples each from the right colon, transverse colon, descending colon, sigmoid colon, proximal rectum, and distal rectum.[213] Several professional societies have proposed more recent surveillance protocols that vary slightly with respect to the time at which screening is performed following a diagnosis of colitis, the interval between surveillance examinations, and the number and location of tissue samples procured.[143,197,214,215] For instance, the ACG recommends that surveillance commence 8 to 10 years after the initial diagnosis of colitis and be repeated every 1 to 2 years with multiple biopsy samples obtained from every 10 cm of colon, regardless of the extent of colitis.[214]

The SCENIC international consensus statement, published in 2015, summarizes the evolving evidence of newer endoscopic methods for surveillance and management of dysplasia in IBD patients.[216,217] In the SCENIC statement, lesions are described according to a new nomenclature, which replaces the term *dysplasia associated lesion or mass* (DALM) and recommends using descriptive terms modified from the Paris Classification of neoplastic lesions of the gut.[218] Visible dysplasia is classified as polypoid or nonpolypoid. In addition, the term *endoscopically resectable* was defined to indicate that the lesion margins could be identified, the lesion appears to be completely removed on visual inspection, histologic examination of the specimen is consistent with complete removal, and biopsies taken from mucosa immediately adjacent to the resection site are free of dysplasia. This is a paradigm shift that has important implications for the surveillance and management of dysplasia.[219]

To optimize detection of dysplastic changes when using standard white light endoscopy, chromoendoscopy by using methylene blue or indigo carmine with targeted biopsies is recommended when expertise in this technique is available.[143,197] The SCENIC recommendations place the emphasis on chromoendoscopy for high-quality visual inspection of the mucosa.[216,217] A meta-analysis of prospective studies comparing chromoendoscopy with standard white light endoscopy found chromoendoscopy is significantly better in detecting dysplasia in patients with colonic IBD.[220] When chromoendoscopy is not available, especially if there is extensive active disease, significant pseudopolyposis, or poor preparation, random mucosal sampling with targeted biopsies of any suspicious-appearing lesions remains a reasonable alternative. In patients with documented pancolitis, biopsy specimens should be obtained in a four-quadrant fashion every 10 cm from the cecum to the rectum for a minimum of 33 total random mucosal samples in an attempt to detect dysplastic changes.[215] In patients with less extensive colitis, biopsy specimens can be limited to the greatest extent of endoscopic or histologic involvement documented by any colonoscopy. Because

of an increased risk of colorectal cancer in the rectum and sigmoid, sampling every 5 cm in the distal colon should be considered.

During colonoscopy, targeted biopsies of all visible abnormalities should be performed. Lesions should be described accordingly using the new classification and resections should be performed for endoscopically resectable lesions. According to the SCENIC recommendations, all lesions that appear endoscopically resectable should be removed in their entirety, and biopsy specimens of the flat mucosa surrounding the resection site should be obtained to ensure that the lateral margins are free of dysplasia.[214,216,217] The endoscopically removed lesion and the flat mucosa sample from the surrounding resection site should be placed in separate specimen containers and submitted for histologic confirmation of complete removal. After complete removal of endoscopically resectable dysplastic lesions, surveillance colonoscopy is recommended rather than colectomy. In patients who have endoscopically invisible dysplasia confirmed by a GI pathologist, referral to an endoscopist with IBD expertise is also recommended.

Microscopic Colitis

Microscopic colitis refers to autoimmune disorders characterized by chronic, watery, nonbloody diarrhea in patients with normal endoscopic features, but with evidence of histologic inflammation in their colonic biopsies.[221] There are two types, collagenous colitis and lymphocytic colitis. Patients are diagnosed in late adulthood, but young adults and even children may be affected.[222] Women are more commonly affected than men; the female-to-male ratio ranges from 3 : 1 to 9 : 1 in cases of collagenous colitis and slightly lower in lymphocytic colitis (F : M ratio between 2.4 : 1 and 2.7 : 1).[223] Affected patients have significant associations with other autoimmune disorders, including autoimmune thyroiditis, rheumatoid arthritis, and celiac disease, among others.

Most patients with microscopic colitis have a normal-appearing colon. Patchy erythema, edema, friability, an abnormal vascular pattern, and even frank ulcerations may occur in a small minority of patients. Some cases show pseudomembranes and linear mucosal breaks ("cat-scratch colon"). The mucosa in collagenous colitis, more so than in lymphocytic colitis, is prone to endoscope trauma and even perforation, thought to be caused by barotrauma as a result of insufflation of air into the colon at the time of endoscopy, combined with the endoscope trauma.[224–226]

Collagenous colitis and lymphocytic colitis have some overlapping histologic features. These include preservation of crypt architecture combined with an increase in inflammatory cells within the lamina propria, especially in the superficial half, and degeneration of the surface epithelium. Inflammatory cells include lymphocytes, plasma cells, and eosinophils. Eosinophils are more numerous and prominent in cases of collagenous colitis than in lymphocytic colitis. The pathognomonic finding of collagenous colitis is the presence of a thickened or irregular subepithelial collagen layer, which is usually thicker than 10 μm.[227] Collagen thickening may be continuous or patchy in distribution. Lymphocytic colitis lacks a thickened collagen layer. In lymphocytic colitis, there are increased IELs, typically greater than 20 per 100 surface epithelial cells.[228] Some cases of lymphocytic colitis show minimal histologic changes and only a slight increase in intraepithelial lymphocytosis ("atypical," "paucicellular," or "minimal change" lymphocytic colitis). In these mild cases, the disorder produces a mild increase in lamina propria inflammatory cells, usually limited to the superficial half of the mucosa. IELs are also seen in collagenous colitis; however, the degree of intraepithelial lymphocytosis is less than in lymphocytic colitis.

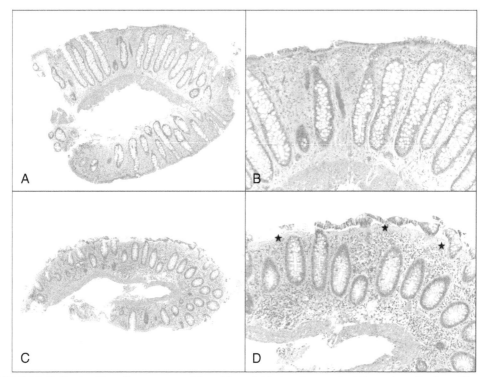

FIG 5.10 Patient with collagenous colitis with variable involvement of the colon. Rectum (**A** and **B,** low and high power respectively) showing no significant involvement compared to the right colonic biopsies (**C** and **D,** low and high power respectively) with extensive thickening of the subepithelial collagen layer (*stars* mark the thickened collagen), increased inflammation in the lamina propria and prominent surface epithelial cell detachment.

The pathologic features of microscopic colitis may be patchy and focal (Fig. 5.10).[229] Several studies have shown more severe involvement of the right versus the left colon. Rectal sparing has been observed in as many as 8% of cases.[230] No consensus exists for the optimal method of mucosal sampling in suspected microscopic colitis. Data suggest that a substantial number of patients with unexplained chronic diarrhea benefit from colonoscopy and mucosal biopsy analysis (see Table 5.2).[231–233] The potential patchy distribution of microscopic colitis sometimes requires biopsy of the right and transverse colon, in addition to the left side of the colon, for diagnosis.[229,234,235] A reasonable initial strategy may be to proceed with either flexible sigmoidoscopy or colonoscopy, with two or more biopsy samples taken from three or four areas of the colon. In situations in which flexible sigmoidoscopy is nondiagnostic, but clinical suspicion for microscopic colitis remains high, colonoscopy with additional mucosal sampling from the proximal colon should be considered. No formal comparative effectiveness analysis exists comparing and evaluating the two strategies.

Graft Versus Host Disease

Graft versus host disease (GVHD) is one of the most common complications following hematopoietic stem cell transplantation and develops in as many as 50% of patients.[236] The GI tract is commonly involved and manifests with various signs and symptoms, including nausea, vomiting, anorexia, profuse diarrhea, or ileus.[237] The diagnosis of GVHD in the GI tract is made through a combination of clinical and laboratory features, along with exclusion of other causes of GI tract dysfunction. Endoscopic biopsy and histologic examination is an important component

for assessment of patients presenting with digestive symptoms in the posthematopoietic stem cell transplant period.

The endoscopic appearance of GI GVHD is variable, ranging from mucosal edema and erythema to more severe changes of ulceration or mucosal sloughing; however, endoscopic findings do not correlate well with histologic findings.[238] Microscopically, the major histologic feature of GVHD is the presence of epithelial cell apoptosis and relatively sparse mononuclear cell inflammatory infiltrate.[239,240] In more severe examples, crypt loss and destruction are also seen. A grading scheme for GVHD has been proposed; however, correlation with clinical symptoms, endoscopic findings, and patient outcome is poor.[241,242] The histologic changes of GI GVHD are not entirely specific, and disorders such as infection, drug-related injury (in particular mycophenolate mofetil), ischemia and, rarely, IBD are part of the differential diagnosis.[243]

GVHD can affect any part of the GI tract. The optimal diagnostic approach for GI acute GVHD has yet to be determined, and studies on this topic are limited. In many centers, site of biopsy depends on clinical experience among hematooncologists and gastroenterologists in assessment of this disorder. Discordant findings between the upper and low GI tract have been reported.[244] Three small, prospective studies identified rectal or distal colon biopsy as the most sensitive test for the diagnosis of GI GVHD, even in patients presenting with primarily upper GI symptoms.[245–247] However, rectal biopsies alone can potentially miss up to 38% of GI GVHD cases.[240] One prospective study of 24 patients who had undergone stem cell transplantation identified EGD with sigmoidoscopy or ileocolonoscopy alone as equivalent strategies for the diagnosis of GVHD.[247]

KEY REFERENCES

49. Katz PO, Gerson LB, Vela MF: Guidelines for the diagnosis and management of gastroesophageal reflux disease, *Am J Gastroenterol* 108(3):308–328, quiz 329, 2013.

53. Yang YX, Brill J, Krishnan P, et al: American Gastroenterological Association Institute Guideline on the role of upper gastrointestinal biopsy to evaluate dyspepsia in the adult patient in the absence of visible mucosal lesions, *Gastroenterology* 149(4):1082–1087, 2015.

56. Kahrilas PJ, Shaheen NJ, Vaezi MF, et al: American Gastroenterological Association Medical Position Statement on the management of gastroesophageal reflux disease, *Gastroenterology* 135(4):1383–1391, 1391 e1381–1385, 2008.

59. Shaheen NJ, Falk GW, Iyer PG, et al: ACG Clinical Guideline: diagnosis and management of Barrett's Esophagus, *Am J Gastroenterol* 111(1): 30–50, quiz 51, 2016.

60. Spechler SJ, Sharma P, Souza RF, et al: American Gastroenterological Association medical position statement on the management of Barrett's esophagus, *Gastroenterology* 140(3):1084–1091, 2011.

67. Harrison R, Perry I, Haddadin W, et al: Detection of intestinal metaplasia in Barrett's esophagus: an observational comparator study suggests the need for a minimum of eight biopsies, *Am J Gastroenterol* 102(6):1154–1161, 2007.

83. Schlemper RJ, Riddell RH, Kato Y, et al: The Vienna classification of gastrointestinal epithelial neoplasia, *Gut* 47(2):251–255, 2000.

90. Abela JE, Going JJ, Mackenzie JF, et al: Systematic four-quadrant biopsy detects Barrett's dysplasia in more patients than nonsystematic biopsy, *Am J Gastroenterol* 103(4):850–855, 2008.

91. Phoa KN, van Vilsteren FG, Weusten BL, et al: Radiofrequency ablation vs endoscopic surveillance for patients with Barrett esophagus and low-grade dysplasia: a randomized clinical trial, *JAMA* 311(12): 1209–1217, 2014.

92. Reid BJ, Blount PL, Feng Z, Levine DS: Optimizing endoscopic biopsy detection of early cancers in Barrett's high-grade dysplasia, *Am J Gastroenterol* 95(11):3089–3096, 2000.

100. Saffari H, Peterson KA, Fang JC, et al: Patchy eosinophil distributions in an esophagectomy specimen from a patient with eosinophilic esophagitis: implications for endoscopic biopsy, *J Allergy Clin Immunol* 130(3):798–800, 2012.

101. Dellon ES, Gonsalves N, Hirano I, et al: ACG clinical guideline: evidenced based approach to the diagnosis and management of esophageal eosinophilia and eosinophilic esophagitis (EoE), *Am J Gastroenterol* 108(5):679–692, quiz 693, 2013.

102. Liacouras CA, Furuta GT, Hirano I, et al: Eosinophilic esophagitis: updated consensus recommendations for children and adults, *J Allergy Clin Immunol* 128(1):3–20 e26, quiz 21–22, 2011.

117. Dixon MF, Genta RM, Yardley JH, Correa P: Classification and grading of gastritis. The updated Sydney System. International Workshop on the Histopathology of Gastritis, Houston 1994, *Am J Surg Pathol* 20(10): 1161–1181, 1996.

118. El-Zimaity HM, Graham DY: Evaluation of gastric mucosal biopsy site and number for identification of Helicobacter pylori or intestinal metaplasia: role of the Sydney System, *Hum Pathol* 30(1):72–77, 1999.

143. Sharaf RN, Shergill AK, Odze RD, et al: Endoscopic mucosal tissue sampling, *Gastrointest Endosc* 78(2):216–224, 2013.

183. Ravelli AM, Tobanelli P, Minelli L, et al: Endoscopic features of celiac disease in children, *Gastrointest Endosc* 54(6):736–742, 2001.

189. Lebwohl B, Kapel RC, Neugut AI, et al: Adherence to biopsy guidelines increases celiac disease diagnosis, *Gastrointest Endosc* 74(1):103–109, 2011.

201. Kornbluth A, Sachar DB, Practice Parameters Committee of the American College of Gastroenterology: Ulcerative colitis practice guidelines in adults: American College Of Gastroenterology, Practice Parameters Committee, *Am J Gastroenterol* 105(3):501–523, quiz 524, 2010.

207. Eaden JA, Abrams KR, Mayberry JF: The risk of colorectal cancer in ulcerative colitis: a meta-analysis, *Gut* 48(4):526–535, 2001.

208. Soetikno RM, Lin OS, Heidenreich PA, et al: Increased risk of colorectal neoplasia in patients with primary sclerosing cholangitis and ulcerative colitis: a meta-analysis, *Gastrointest Endosc* 56(1):48–54, 2002.

214. Farraye FA, Odze RD, Eaden J, et al: AGA medical position statement on the diagnosis and management of colorectal neoplasia in inflammatory bowel disease, *Gastroenterology* 138(2):738–745, 2010.

215. Itzkowitz SH, Present DH, Crohn's and Colitis Foundation of America Colon Cancer in IBD Study Group: Consensus conference: colorectal cancer screening and surveillance in inflammatory bowel disease, *Inflamm Bowel Dis* 11(3):314–321, 2005.

220. Subramanian V, Mannath J, Ragunath K, Hawkey CJ: Meta-analysis: the diagnostic yield of chromoendoscopy for detecting dysplasia in patients with colonic inflammatory bowel disease, *Aliment Pharmacol Ther* 33(3):304–312, 2011.

247. Thompson B, Salzman D, Steinhauer J, et al: Prospective endoscopic evaluation for gastrointestinal graft-versus-host disease: determination of the best diagnostic approach, *Bone Marrow Transplant* 38(5): 371–376, 2006.

A complete reference list can be found online at ExpertConsult .com

6

Electrosurgery in Therapeutic Endoscopy

Marcia L. Morris and Joo Ha Hwang

CHAPTER OUTLINE

INTRODUCTION

The therapeutic basis of all electrosurgery is the use of high frequency, alternating electric current to produce heating in living cells. The heating can be manipulated to achieve a desired tissue effect such as cutting, tissue ablation, desiccation, or a combination of these. Electrical energy to produce heating and tissue effects has been a part of endoscopy since the early 1970s.[1,2] Common indications include biliary sphincterotomy, polypectomy, hemostasis, and the ablation of vascular lesions of multiple origins. Incorrect use of electrosurgery may contribute to poor patient outcomes such as post-polypectomy serositis, perforation, immediate or late hemorrhage, and sphincterotomy-associated complications.

Generator manufacturers give guidance as to suggested settings and output choices for various procedures. However, because there are many patient and physician technique variables that are outside of the manufacturer's knowledge regarding the generator's eventual impact, there can be no one "magic" setting that is guaranteed to always produce a known result. This is why physician discretion and knowledge remains important.

A clinician with no electrosurgical cognitive competence may be unable to troubleshoot, make appropriate alternate output selections, or be flexible in unusual situations. Without a good understanding of electrosurgical technology, it will be more difficult for a physician to expand his or her own clinical expertise into more advanced procedures such as endoscopic mucosal resection (EMR) or endoscopic submucosal dissection (ESD). Clinical understanding of the fundamentals of the technology is known to promote better patient outcomes.

From the clinician's point of view, this understanding and competence has been hampered by problems with nomenclature, lack of standardized training, inappropriate marketing messages, and the perpetuation of incorrect understandings and/or outdated beliefs. All these have conspired to make electrosurgery "the most commonly used, but most often misunderstood technology."[3]

There is a lack of uniformity in names for output selections used by different manufacturers (Table 6.1). Similar names may have either similar or different characteristics from one manufacturer's generator to another. The terms themselves may be intuitively misleading. For example, a waveform may be called COAG but is very capable of cutting tissue. Some terms in common usage are manufacturer trademarks. SoftCoag refers specifically to an Erbe Elektromedizin GmbH (Tübingen, Germany) generator output, whereas TouchSoft is registered to Genii, Inc. (St. Paul, MN) for a technically equivalent, very low voltage output. The constant misuse of other terms such as *electrocautery* add to the confusion and seems particularly out of step with medical practice, which relies on precise terminology in everything from reporting diagnoses (diverticulosis is not diverticulitis) to recording methodologies for others to reproduce. Recently, both the *Journal of Minimally Invasive Gynecology*[4] and the journal *Gastrointestinal Endoscopy*[5] have addressed this issue and begun to promote standardization of terms. As far as possible, this chapter conforms to these new guidelines.

This chapter outlines the basic principles of electrosurgery pertaining to flexible endoscopy and attempts to relate the fundamentals of the technology directly to common and emerging clinical procedures. The use of proprietary or brand-specific terms is minimized, and only the most reliably referenced and up-to-date information to date is included.

FUNDAMENTAL PRINCIPLES OF ELECTROSURGERY

Early pioneers of electrosurgical devices discovered that applying an electrical current to biologic tissue produces different effects.

TABLE 6.1   Output Names for Generator Units Most Commonly Marketed for Flexible Endoscopy in the USA

ConMed BiCap III	ConMed Beamer Mate	ERBE VIO300D	ERBE VIO200S	ERBE ICC200	ERBE VIO100C	Genii *gi4000*	Olympus ESG100
		Soft Coag	Soft Coag	Soft Coag	Soft Coag	TouchSoft	Soft Coag
Coag	Coag (Hot Biopsy & Pure Coag)	Forced Coag	Forced Coag	Forced Coag	Forced Coag	Coag	Forced Coag 1 & 2
		Swift Coag				Blend Coag	
Pulse Blend						Pulse Blend Cut	
Blend	Blend Cuts 1 & 2	Dry Cut			Dry Cut	Blend Cut	
Pulse Cut	Pulse Cut (Polyp and Papilla)	EndoCut I or Q	EndoCut I or Q	EndoCut		Pulse Cut	Pulse Cut Slow/Fast
Pure Cut	Pure Cut	Auto Cut	Auto Cut	Auto Cut	Auto Cut	Cut	Cut 1, 2, 3
Bipolar	BiCap & Cut	Bipolar	Bipolar	Bipolar	Bipolar	Bipolar	
	Beamer Plus: Argon Steady, Slow, Fast, Super (amplified beam) (Requires an additional unit at additional cost)	Spray Coag APC 2 Forced, Pulse 1 & 2, Precise (amplified beam) (Requires an additional unit at additional cost)	APC 2 Forced (amplified beam) (Requires an additional unit at additional cost)	APC300 Forced (standard beam) (Requires an additional unit at additional cost)		ArC Smart Beam' (linear beam) (included in unit)	

Color code: *Purple,* Monopolar contact outputs; *Blue,* Bipolar coagulation outputs; *Pink,* Non-contact coagulation modes.
Genii and TouchSoft are US Registered Trademarks of Genii, Inc., St. Paul, MN. VIO, EndoCut, Swift Coag and SoftCoag are Trademarks of Erbe Elektromedizin GmbH, Tübingen, Germany. BIcap and Beamer are Trademarks of ConMed Corporation, Utica, NY. All information taken from Operator's Manuals.
Modified from Morris ML, Bowers WJ: Math, myth and the fundamentals of electrosurgery. *J Hepatol Gastroenterol* 1(1):1–5, 2016.

The first effect is electrolytic. Charged molecules in tissue flow toward opposite electrode poles if the current applied is direct or alternates slowly. Alternating the current more rapidly eliminates the electrolytic effect and produces heating at a cellular level. However, a current alternating at less than 100 kHz results in undesired neuromuscular effects. The shocking result of applying a household current of 60 Hz is well known. Alternating at a very a high frequency (300 kHz) nearly eliminates neuromuscular effects but retains the desired cellular heating. This thermal effect is the basis of all electrosurgery.[6] Because this frequency is in the AM radio range, this energy is often referred to as *radio frequency* (RF), and a radio frequency electrosurgical generator is an acceptable term for an electrosurgical generator unit (ESU).

High-frequency alternating current is generated by an ESU and delivered to tissue via an assortment of suitable accessories. Water within cells heated very quickly vaporizes and causes the cell membranes to burst.[7] These bursting cells separate tissue. We use the accessory to guide the burst cells along a cleavage plane and say the tissue has been electrosurgically "cut."[8] Cells that heat more slowly dry out (coagulate) without bursting. The proportion of how many cells burst and how many coagulate, as well as how much tissue is involved, is referred to as the *tissue effect.* Many variables combine to make this end result (Fig. 6.1). Heating the tissue directly, producing both cutting and coagulation, sets electrosurgery apart from electrocautery. Because the intracellular water is heated directly by the RF energy and not by conduction from an already heated accessory, electrosurgery should never be referred to as *cautery.* Cautery devices produce coagulation by the passive transfer of heat from a heated accessory and can never produce electrosurgical cutting. This is why it is incorrect to use the term *electrocautery* for RF technology. True cautery devices found in gastroenterology practices include the Olympus Heat Probe (Olympus Corp., Tokyo, Japan).[9]

Variables That Impact Tissue Effect, Microprocessor Controls, and Waveforms

Current density is the defining variable in determining specific tissue effects in electrosurgery; yet it is the sum of the effects of all the other variables (see Fig. 6.1).

Current density is the measure of current concentration or, by definition, the current per unit area. The rate of heat generation, and therefore the resulting therapeutic effect, is a function of the current density. It is a measure of intensity. Mathematically, the temperature rises as a square of the current density. Current that will boil water on a square millimeter area will not even feel warm on a square-centimeter area.[10] The dramatic difference in surface area between the active electrode and the dispersive (grounding) pad is perhaps the best-known example of this principle. Current density depends on the applied voltage, current, and type of waveform, as well as the tissue impedance, the size of the electrode, and the time that current is flowing. Understanding the different characteristics of tissue heating under different circumstances is essential to understanding electrosurgery.

The physical law that relates all the electrosurgical variables is summarized by Ohm in the equation:

$$P = I^2R$$

where *P* is power, *I* is current, and *R* is resistance (for our purposes, resistance and impedance are used synonymously). The $P = V \times I$ derivation of this equation relates the type of waveform to total power (*P*). Power combines both voltage (*V*) and current (*I*). For example, if power is to remain constant as voltage

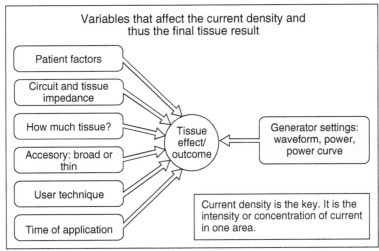

FIG 6.1 Current density variables. (Redrawn from Morris ML, Bowers WJ: Math, myth and the fundamentals of electrosurgery. *J Hepatol Gastroenterol* 1[1]:1-5, 2016.)

increases, then current must decrease. Ohm's Law defines another principle crucial to a clinical understanding of electrosurgery: as impedance in tissue rises, power (either current or voltage or both) decreases. If "nothing is done" as the therapy produces coagulation, and therefore the tissue impedance rises, the generator power must drop *(stall)*.

To address this problem, research turned in the late 1980s to using microprocessors to measure and respond to changing impedance.[11] First patented in 1986, microprocessor monitoring allows an ESU to track a resistance baseline and subsequent changes in the resistance during the electrosurgical activation. Using millions of data points, the generator's software programming (algorithm) tells the generator how to regulate the current and/or voltage (which together form power) being delivered during the activation. A graphic representation of how a particular output is designed to react to changes in impedance is called a *Power to Impedance Curve* or *Power Curve*. Sometimes marketers will use the informal term *power dosing* to explain this. Power curves associated with each output selection are so important to understanding the operation of the ESU that regulatory bodies require these graphs to be included in every user manual.

Power to impedance curves tend to be either "narrow" or "broad." By convention, power is shown on the vertical axis with increasing resistance progressing to the right on the horizontal axis (Fig. 6.2). The horizontal axis is also likely to correlate with time as tissue resistance increases when tissue becomes coagulated with increasing time of application.

The power curve dictates that the power setting displayed on an ESU is not the power that will be delivered over the entire activation. Depending on the algorithm defining the curve, the power setting displayed may be a more or less close approximation of the actual or average power delivered, or simply a target maximum power. In all cases, the average power delivered will be less than the maximum or peak power delivered.

Outputs with narrow type power curves have been long utilized in flexible endoscopy for contact coagulation using very familiar bipolar endostasis probes. Matched with low-voltage continuous outputs and a narrow power curve, this bipolar method is a frequent and effective choice for hemostasis and control of bleeding.[12]

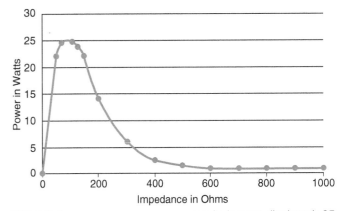

FIG 6.2 A narrow power curve example (power displayed: 25 watts).

In Fig. 6.2, 25 watts have been selected by the user and will be displayed on the ESU. To the ESU's algorithm, this selected power represents only the maximum (or target) power to be delivered.[13] The ESU is programmed to ramp up quickly in the low-resistance situation characterized by frank bleeding. The target maximum is reached, but the power drops quickly as soon as the resistance reaches approximately 100 to 300 Ohms, which correlates well with the appearance of the characteristic whitish eschar, indicating adequate coagulation. This power curve delivers exactly what is desired: rapid onset of hemostasis with self-limiting depth of injury. With the low voltage of the output and this power curve, the tissue tends not to overly dry out, which would cause the bipolar accessory to stick. This well-matched output mode, power curve, and appropriate accessory provides the desired clinical effect of reliable and quick hemostasis.

A nearly identical narrow power curve and voltage cap, matched with monopolar accessories, is usually named SoftCoag (Erbe) or TouchSoft (Genii). These soft coagulation outputs are suggested for use with monopolar hot biopsy forceps (HBF) or newer monopolar contact coagulation accessories such as the Olympus Coagrasper or the Genii TouchSoft Coagulator. One study described successful use of a snare tip with a soft coagulation

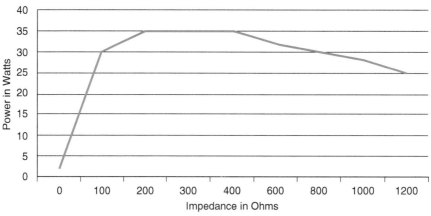

FIG 6.3 A broad power curve example.

output for touch-ups during the resection of large colonic lesions.[14] These monopolar counterparts do require the use of a return dispersive electrode (grounding pad) and require higher initial power settings to overcome the higher resistance in the monopolar circuit. TouchSoft or soft coagulation power maximums are usually set at 40, 50, or 60 watts versus the 15 to 25 watts that are very common for bipolar contact applications.

For snare polypectomy, sphincterotomy, or other procedures that depend on a smooth advance of an electrode, the narrow power curve would not be suitable, as stalling would result. Instead, a broad power curve (Fig. 6.3) where cutting with various levels of concurrent coagulation (depending upon the waveform and accessory selected) is the choice. These outputs usually ramp more slowly toward an effective power and maintain the effectiveness over a broad range of impedances. The result is a smooth and reliable transection. Again, in all cases the average power delivered over the activation will be less than the maximum or peak power. A marketing term called *constant power* is sometimes applied to broad curves but is mostly inaccurate. The power delivered is dynamically driven by the algorithm of the ESU as it responds to impedance/resistance measures. Rigid terms such as *constant*, *always*, and *never* are to be avoided in scientific and medical use for good reason. It is similarly not correct to refer to one entire ESU as a *constant power generator*. Every ESU in current use today has some outputs of both curve types included in its available selections. It is the physician's good understanding of the available outputs and their associated power curves that allow matching to suitable accessories to produce desired and optimal clinical results.

Broad power curves are ideal for most applications that require at least some cutting because the transection is done smoothly without stalling. The generator overcomes the Ohm's law directed drop in power by automatically adjusting the voltage and/or current to keep the cut progressing smoothly over a wide (broad) range of impedances. For ESUs intended for flexible endoscopy, it is now very common to also provide an additional microprocessor or software control layer over some of the broad curve output choices in order to interrupt or fractionate the cut. Named EndoCut (Erbe), Pulsed Cut (Genii), Pulsed Blend Cut (Genii), etc., these types of outputs have multiple options for adding more or less coagulation to the cutting advance. Multiple studies have shown a sole but important benefit of the pulsing or interruption of the advance: a significant reduction in uncontrolled or "zipper" cuts in sphincterotomy.[15,16]

Microprocessor control on modern generators is very precise in reading dynamic impedance and holding current and/or voltage (power) changes tightly to the algorithm design demanded by the power curve.[17] For this reason, often the "watts" shown on the generator display may be absent or only an indication of a maximum power target. In any case, and with every power curve, the average power delivered over the total activation will be less than the peak power delivered. Often the generator requires a certain lag time to reach the programmed maximum power, may on occasion even slightly overshoot it, and will ramp down from the peak depending on the impedance. It is customary for record keepers to chart only the maximum selected power shown on the generator display.

As noted, the controlling concept of the final tissue effect is the current density at the treatment site. But many variables affect the current density. Some are under the physician's control, and some are not. Only a few are functions of the ESU (see Fig. 6.1).

A defining variable that is a selection on the electrosurgery generator is the high-frequency waveform, or output mode. In solid-state generators (the only type now produced), continuous sinusoidal waveforms with fairly low voltage increasingly give way to a higher-voltage waveform that is more and more interrupted (modulated) to take the tissue effect from one of mostly cutting to one of mostly coagulation (Fig. 6.4).

A continuous high-frequency waveform with a peak voltage of at least 200Vp will produce an intensity of current sufficient to create micro electric sparks between the active electrode and the target tissue. Such high-current density along the leading edge of the electrode causes cells to literally explode, separating the tissue as if it were cut. As this cell vaporization continues, a micro steam layer is formed, which helps to propagate the cutting effect.[18]

Along the edges of the cut, there will always be a margin of cells whose distance from the active electrode allows them to heat more slowly. These cells simply coagulate. This is why it is often said, "Only a cold cut is a pure cut." It is better to use the term *cut* rather than *pure cut*, but the literature does not yet reflect this new standard. The depth of the coagulated margin along the cut is related to the height of the peak voltage in the cutting waveform, with higher voltages leaving a thicker margin of coagulation. The coagulation margin is also influenced by the thickness of the electrode. A thin wire leaves less coagulation than a flat blade or a thicker endoscopic dissection wire or knife.

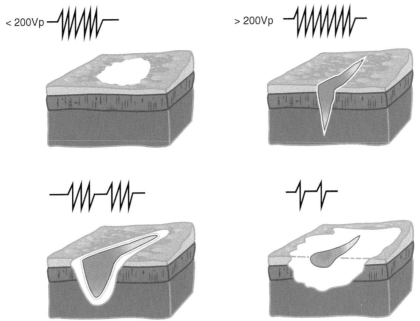

FIG 6.4 Different waveforms produce different tissue effects.

Even with a continuous waveform, if the voltage never goes above 200Vp, no cutting can occur. Such outputs lack the intensity to initiate the initial sparking necessary to produce the cutting effect. A superficial coagulation results instead. These waveforms have been described earlier in the discussion about bipolar and monopolar soft coagulation output choices with narrow power curves.

To produce deeper thermal injury with less electrosurgical cutting and an increasingly greater proportion of coagulated cells, the continuous cut waveform is interrupted or modulated. Modulating the waveform delivers the energy, even at equivalent power settings, more slowly. To increase the depth of the coagulation, the voltage spikes are increased. This is necessary because along the margins of the electrode path, the impedance is rising as the tissue is coagulated. The higher voltage spikes force the current through the desiccated layer along the cut margin, increasing the depth of the coagulation.[19]

The modulated output that for a particular generator provides the deepest coagulation (hemostasis) with only some cutting may be named either *coag* or *forced coag*. Users often erroneously call these outputs *pure coag*. The term is erroneous because as long as the voltage spikes (at least sometimes) over 200Vp, some electrosurgical cutting is expected. This common but imprecise use of terminology can promote confusion. The most common coag waveform type (which often has approximately a 6% duty cycle and crest factor of approximately six) has been a first choice for polypectomy for decades; this is because the cutting action along the snare wire allows a clean transection, whereas the coagulation remaining promotes reliable hemostasis. With the advance of ESU technology offering a greater number of output choices on many ESUs, waveforms with a bit more cutting action and comparatively less thermal spread have gained nearly equal use. These waveforms may have names such as *blend coag* or *swift coag*.[20] Robust, evidence-based data as to what waveform should be preferred is currently absent. Therefore, an optimal guideline for waveform choice is not available, leaving this to the physician's discretion, preference, and experience.[15]

Many ESUs are equipped with a varying number of modulated waveforms that fall between the extremes of nearly all cut or nearly all coag. These are typically named the *blended currents*. This is perhaps the most descriptive name, as it correctly implies that some of the cells will be vaporized, or cut, whereas some will be coagulated. Increasingly modulated waveforms with increasingly high voltages will produce tissue effects with increasing hemostasis and decreasing cutting.

Methods for Quantifying Waveforms

The qualitative descriptions of waveforms can be quantified by assigning them a duty cycle or a crest factor. The duty cycle is the numerical percentage of the time the waveform is on (spiking) and the time it is off (interrupted). A waveform with a 6% duty cycle is on 6% of the time and off 94% of the total time. The common coag or forced coag types discussed previously are those with approximately a 6% duty cycle. Any continuous waveform has a 100% duty cycle. It will be the peak voltage that will determine if a 100% duty cycle waveform produces pure (intense) electrosurgical cutting or only soft coagulation. Crest factor is similarly used to quantify the degree to which a waveform is modulated, but is more informative for modulated waves in that it includes information about the peak voltage. Modulated waveforms with low duty cycles and high crest factors produce more and deeper coagulation than waveforms with low crest factors and high duty cycles (Table 6.2). Either duty cycle or crest factor information can be found in every generator's user manual.

A physician with a good knowledge of the principles of current density, the waveform choices on the ESU at hand, and its microprocessor controlled power curves is in a very good position to control, avoid, or compensate for all the other non-ESU variables that enter into the final tissue effect (see Fig. 6.1).

One of these non-ESU variables is the operator's technique, which includes the tension applied to the accessory. Some degree of tissue tension is necessary for progression of an incision (e.g., polypectomy or sphincterotomy). However, overzealous tension

TABLE 6.2   Quantified Outputs for Several Commonly Used Generator Models

Peak Volts	Duty Cycle	Crest Factor	Conmed Beamer	BSC EndoStat	BSC EndoStat III	Erbe ICC200	Erbe VIO300	Genii gi4000	Meditron 3000B/ Pentax	Olympus ESG 100	Valleylab Force 2
< 200	100%	1.4				SoftCoag	SoftCoag	TouchSoft		Soft Coag	
> 200	100%	1.4	Pure Cut, Pulse Cut 1, 2*	Cut	Cut, Control Cut	Autocut, EndoCut	Autocut, EndoCut I, Q	Cut, Pulse Cut	Cut	Cut 1, 2, 3, Pulse Cut Slow, Fast	Cut
	70%	1.8	Blend Cut		Blend						
	50%			Blend				Blend Cut, Pulse Blend Cut	Blend 1		Blend 1 (CF 3.4)
	50%	2.5	Super Blend								
	37%										Blend 2
	30%	2.7			Coag						
		3.0	Pure Coag				Dry Cut Effect 1-4				
		3.2					Dry Cut Effect 5-6				
		3.7	Hot Bx								
		3.8					Dry Cut Effect 7-8				
	25%								Blend 2		Blend 3
	12%			Coag				Blend Coag (CF 6.3)	Blend 3		
	8%	5.0 5.4 6.0					Swift Coag Forced Coag	Coag		Forced 1,2	
	6%								Coag		
	4%					Forced Coag		Coag			
		7.4					Spray Coag				
		8.5									Coag

Increasing voltage (arrow pointing down, left side of table)

*Beamer Polyp Pulse Cut 1,2 and Papilla Pulse Cut 1,2 CF not available.
This table lists duty cycles and/or crest factors to aid endoscopists in quantifying different electrosurgery generator unit (ESU) modes. Each ESU will have additional waveform properties that contribute to tissue effect. Please refer to the operator's manual for each ESU or contact the manufacturer for further information.
Data published or provided by the manufacturers: Conmed Corp., Utica, NY; EndoStat distributed by Boston Scientific Inc., Natick, MA; Erbe USA Inc., Marietta, GA; Genii Inc., St. Paul, MN; Meditron, a division of Cooper Surgical, Trumbull, CT; Valleylab, Medtronic, Dublin, Ireland. Not all generators listed may be currently marketed.

may result in poor control of cutting, leading to a rapid incision with inadequate vessel coagulation and increased risk of hemorrhage. A slow advance can promote more coagulation. Highly skilled endoscopists performing ESD procedures are able to control small bleeding episodes simply by slowing the cut advance markedly. This holding staunches the bleeding with no change whatsoever in the accessory, the waveform output, or the power selection.

Resistance in an entire monopolar circuit or in the tissue itself varies before and during the incision. Highly fibrotic or scarred tissue is more resistant (and harder to cut) than tissue with a high water content. Tissue resistance is a dynamic variable that alters as tissue desiccates during the incision.[21] The entire resistance between an argon probe tip and the dispersive electrode plays a role in the length of the plasma arc that is generated during argon coagulation procedures. Blood flow is a variable that may help dissipate heat at the site of the tissue. Similarly, submucosal saline injection may act as a "heat sink" and help dissipate energy and prevent transmural injury during polypectomy and other procedures.[22,23]

Monopolar and Bipolar Circuits

The most common method for completing the electrical circuit in gastroenterology procedures is to use a monopolar accessory and a remotely placed dispersive (grounding) pad. The current flows from the ESU and is concentrated at the treatment site by the accessory (e.g., a snare, sphincterotome, HBF, or needle-knife). The concentrated energy at the site has high current density which promotes tissue heating. The energy then flows through the patient's tissue following a path of least resistance to the dispersive electrode on the skin and hence back to the generator, completing an electrical circuit (Fig. 6.5). Because the surface area of the pad is so much larger than the active accessory, the current density is very low at the pad site. Proper pad placement is important to evenly disperse the energy and avoid any increase in skin temperature under the pad.[24] Most modern ESUs have dispersive electrode safety alarms available when used in conjunction with "split" or "dual" pads. Patented in 1983, this technology advance is inexpensive and highly recommended, as it markedly reduces the risk of a patient skin burn under the pad.

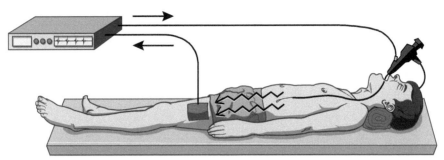

FIG 6.5 A monopolar accessory circuit.

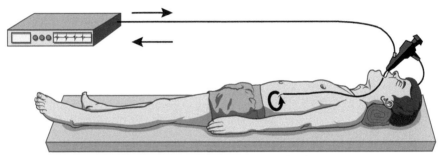

FIG 6.6 A bipolar accessory circuit.

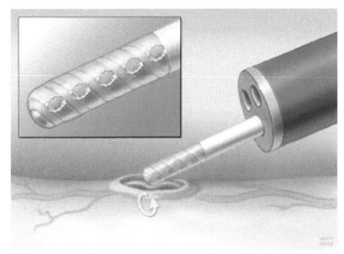

FIG 6.7 A bipolar hemostasis probe. (From Morris ML, Tucker RD, Baron TH, Song LM: Electrosurgery in in gastrointestinal endoscopy: principles to practice. *Am J Gastroenterol* 104(6); 1563–1574, 2009.)

Bipolar (multipolar) accessories are different from monopolar electrodes in that both active and return functions are included in the tip of the instrument. Current flows through a relatively small area of tissue, and there is no need for a dispersive electrode on the patient's skin (Fig. 6.6). The most common flexible endoscopic use for this technology is for contact coagulation using a flexible bipolar hemostasis probe that is supplied by many manufacturers (Fig. 6.7). Bipolar hemostasis probes have been shown to be effective devices for hemostasis for bleeding peptic ulcers, arteriovenous malformations, and other hemorrhagic lesions. Optimal results are obtained by using moderate to firm tamponade in the case of active bleeding. Power settings of 15 to 25 watts are most common. These probes are best used with generator outputs that have continuous low-voltage outputs paired with a narrow power curve in which the microprocessor control design allows the energy to ramp up quickly in the low-resistance case of frank blood, but to limit the power delivery automatically as the tissue becomes coagulated. Flexible endoscopic bipolar snares, biopsy forceps, and sphincterotomes have also been developed but have not been successfully or widely adopted.

Radio Frequency Ablation Devices

A newer, important use of bipolar current for thermal therapy is radiofrequency ablation employed to ablate Barrett's esophagus. In this situation, the current moves from one adjacent electrode on a balloon catheter to another. This energy passes via the mucosa and is sufficient to ablate the mucosa, while being superficial enough (< 1 mm depth of ablation) to prevent significant submucosal damage, and minimizing stricture formation.

Contact and Noncontact Applications

High-frequency electrosurgical energy can be applied to the tissue in either of two ways. The first and far most common method in flexible endoscopy is to have the accessory in direct contact with the surface of the tissue. A well-recognized list of common flexible endoscopic therapies and accessories employ this method: polypectomy and EMR/snares; sphincterotomy/sphincterotomes and needle-knives; contact coagulation/bipolar endostasis probes; coagraspers; and contact coagulators.

In the second way, by using especially high-voltage waveforms with or without the addition of argon (or other) gas to the treatment field, the energy can travel to the tissue surface without the accessory being in contact with the surface.

Argon-Assisted Coagulation

Argon-assisted coagulation and ablation (also called argon plasma coagulation [APC], argon beam coagulation [ABC], or simply argon coagulation [ArC]) is by far the more prominent noncontact technique in flexible endoscopy. It has many useful applications[25] including tumor debulking, ablation of vascular malformations,[26] and other hemostasis and ablation therapies.[27] Argon coagulation also has a role in "tidying up" residual adenoma after piecemeal polypectomy or EMR, although overuse in this setting may suggest suboptimal prior resection technique.[28]

In argon-assisted coagulation, argon gas flows from a special catheter tip and becomes electrically charged (ionized) by high voltage, which is concurrently delivered to an electrode in the catheter tip by a specially equipped ESU. The resulting conductive gas plasma arc provides a medium for current flow from the catheter tip to an adjacent mucosal surface. This is a monopolar application and requires the use of a dispersive pad to complete the electrical circuit. It can be used effectively by positioning the catheter tip either in a tangential or perpendicular direction to the mucosal surface. Tangential or perpendicular applications are possible because the arc will always follow the current direction to the nearest tissue without regard to the probe tip design. Although this is a noncontact method, the arc length (and therefore the distance from the tissue surface) achieved is important and variable.

This method can be controlled to promote a very superficial pliant eschar or provide deeper effects and tumor debulking by using longer activations often at higher powers.[29] Although accepted as a generally safe tool, it has been shown that argon coagulation can cause transmural injury at high power outputs,[30] and there have been reports of perforation using this device.[31] In addition, pulsed argon modes have been shown to produce a high rate of pain and patient neuromuscular responses.[32] Nonetheless, the relative ease of use, noncontact speed, ability to arc around folds, and relatively shallow depth of injury make argon coagulation a versatile and indispensable therapy.

The character of the argon beam varies with the several types of systems being marketed. In general, various manufacturers offer standard, amplified, or linear beams. Amplified beams have been termed *high power* due to their higher intensity and correspondingly greater thermal injury. These require that power settings be set lower than either standard or linear beams to compensate.[33,34]

The nature of the high-voltage waveform used to ionize the argon imparts different characteristics to each beam design. It is therefore very important not to assume that power settings or application times will be constant as a user moves from one device to another. It is important to learn and understand the power and time settings suggested by individual manufacturers. Please note that often time of application, either by a first pass of energy or repeated passes, can greatly affect the depth of thermal injury. It is possible to achieve only a few cell layers deep superficial effect or a deeper mucosal injury by varying only the time of application. See Box 6.1: Argon Clinical Pearls to aid in successful outcomes. These usage tips are appropriate no matter which ESU/argon system is in use.

It is possible to induce electrosurgical current to arc in a noncontact fashion without the aid of argon gas. To ionize mixed air in the gap between the accessory and tissue requires high voltages. (Argon gas forms a more stable plasma even in the lower range of these voltages, which is one reason argon is chosen.) The waveforms used to ionize mixed air have crest factors of at least seven or eight and may be named either *spray coag* or *fulgurate*. The ionization of mixed air is less consistent and tends to produce a variable, often charlike and less pliable eschar than when argon gas is present. Smoke may also be produced. These

---

BOX 6.1   Clinical Pearls for Best Argon Use with Any System

- Physicians should be sure to use power settings recommended for the system in use—they are NOT all the same!
- Purging the connector and argon probe with nonionized argon at least once before inserting into the endoscope is universally recommended. All systems are equipped with buttons for the automatic activation of this function.
- In addition to the initial purge, it may also be helpful to add another short purge after the probe has been inserted into the scope and is nearing the target site (be sure the tip of the probe is not touching any tissue). This helps bring the gas fully over the ignition electrode which is located at the end of the probe and makes sure an adequate non-ionized argon cloud is surrounding the target site.
- Sometimes approaching the tissue with the probe in a tangential position will help get close to the target treatment site without touching.
- It is OK to gently "lay down" the probe tip and then pull back without delivering energy to gauge distance from the tissue.
- Don't extend the probe too far out of the scope; working closely gives better control. Be sure you see the tip of the probe extending beyond the tip of the endoscope.
- Keep your foot on the energy delivery pedal long enough to get ignition started.
- There are three popular application techniques: "spot welding," "painting," and "ignite and drag." Each has different uses and slightly different techniques. It helps to practice on ex vivo or animal models.
- For the painting technique, move the scope not the probe.
- Increasing the time increases the penetration depth.
- Putting the dispersive (grounding pad) on the flank can shorten the impedance path and help make the beam longer.
- Don't turn up the gas flow trying to make the beam longer. This will only dilute the ions already activated.
- 1 liter per minute flow rate is sufficient for most applications. Increasing the gas flow will lead to more distension of the patient's gut.
- Monitor the patient for distension during the procedure, and use suction frequently, especially for lengthy or pediatric applications. Recall that argon gas is flowing when the foot pedal is depressed even if the beam has not ignited.
- It is not true that having a side or circumferential tip on the argon probe will make it safe to touch the tissue.
- Do not use argon coagulation to treat varices, hemorrhoids, or other lesions requiring tamponade or coaption.

---

drawbacks, along with historic concerns about capacitive coupling when high voltages are used with endoscopes, have made the use of these nonargon-assisted methods rare in flexible endoscopy, although the method is fairly common in open surgery.

Recently, however, the use of spray coag/fulgurate waveforms have been introduced by some Japanese physicians as an optional output choice for the dissection stage of ESD and peroral endoscopic myotomy (POEM) procedures. No studies of tissue effect and safety of this waveform in these settings are known to have been published to date.

Electrical Hazards

Being mindful of the monopolar circuit can help prevent some of the most common types of electrosurgical injuries. Once a monopolar snare, for example, is attached to an active cord inserted into the generator socket and the generator is on, it is a potential "active electrode." If the dispersive pad has also been placed on the patient, it is imperative not to place that active electrode (snare) on the bed next to the patient while turning your attention elsewhere. If someone were to activate the footswitch, the patient could be burned wherever they were in contact with the snare lying on the bed. The best-practice rule is to carefully manage all active electrodes. Disconnect the accessory from the active cord, or place the generator in "standby" mode, if available, until everyone is actually ready for the electrosurgical procedure. Carefully managing active cords and accessories can also prevent shocks and burns to staff. Handle active electrodes by their plastic insulated areas only, and never attempt to connect or disconnect accessories while current is flowing.[35,36]

Although a published report of an electrosurgical pad burn during a flexible endoscopic procedure is unknown, it is still wise to take advantage of the inexpensive, well-studied safety advantages of using split/dual/sensing dispersive pads. When using any of the many generators that include pad safety and tissue sensing technology in their design, these pads are able to communicate with the generator's computer and alarm system and produce both a visual and audible warning to the operator that the pad is sensing an unbalanced impedance situation that, if not corrected, could result in a temperature rise on the patient's skin under the pad and might increase the risk of a burn. Support staff should be well trained in best practices for the placement of dispersive electrodes.

Electrosurgery With Implanted Devices

Implanted cardiac pacemakers and cardioverter defibrillators (ICDs) are designed to sense and react to electric signals from the heart. This makes them vulnerable to interference from electrical signals that are not cardiac in origin, and it has long been known that extra care must be taken when using electrosurgery for treating these patients. Patients with these implanted devices can safely undergo electrosurgery as long as certain precautions are taken.[37,38] Newer pacemakers have been engineered to be resistant to electric interference, and alteration in function from electrosurgery is extremely rare in gastroenterology. However, the risk exists, and if interference with the implanted device occurs, the effects could be highly variable and dependent not only on the source and character of the interfering signal, but on the design of the device itself.

Pacemakers can be temporarily inhibited from outputting a signal, or the interference might be interpreted by the device as noise, which can cause the device to revert to an asynchronous pacing mode (a mode in which the device paces but does not sense) at a rate preset by the manufacturer. The interference might be interpreted by the device as a programming signal leading to inappropriate programming of the device. Sometimes the battery life might be affected, or, in the case of ICDs, they may trigger an inappropriate therapy shock to the patient. Most ventricular assist devices have sensitive components contained in external controllers and are not usually affected by electrosurgery, but checking the manufacturer's recommendation is advisable for these devices as well.[24]

Current recommendations for the management of patients with these cardiac devices are based on consensus statements published by individual societies such as the American College of Cardiology Foundation/American Heart Association (ACCF/AHA), the Heart Rhythm Society/American Society of Anesthesiologists (HRS/ASA), and the American Society of Gastrointestinal Endoscopy (ASGE). Whereas agreement between societies is not completely consistent, there is universal agreement that it is recommended that each endoscopy practice have a protocol in place that will be followed when a patient with an implanted device is scheduled. These protocols should be initiated and reviewed by qualified personnel trained in the operation of implanted cardiac devices. All societies agree that it is imperative to identify the approximately 20% of cardiac pacemaker implant patients who are dependent on their pacemakers for moment-to-moment maintenance of adequate rhythm and hemodynamics.

Bowel Explosion Risk

It is possible to ignite a fire in the colon in the presence of naturally occurring gases such as hydrogen and methane in the presence of oxygen. Thorough colon preparation using approved preparation techniques with solutions that do not contain mannitol or sorbitol is necessary even if the electrosurgery, including argon coagulation, is used only in the sigmoid colon or rectum.[39,40] Explosion has been reported with the use of ArC in the rectum after enema preparation.[41,42] If electrosurgery must be performed on an unprepared colon, efforts to exchange the gas in the colon with repeated insufflation and suction should be undertaken. Carbon dioxide (CO_2) insufflation, mainly used for patient comfort, may reduce the risk of gas ignition further.

Fundamentals in Practice

The following are a summary of key principles of ESU use in flexible endoscopy:
- The final tissue effect seen is the result of both non-ESU and ESU variables
- The ESU variables are the power selection, the waveform selection, and the power curve built into the generator for that waveform selection.
- Non-ESU variables that include the accessory chosen, the time of application, operator technique, and the tissue character can have a defining impact on the final result.
- Current density is the arbiter of the tissue effect. For example, sphincterotomy progresses much better when a small amount of wire is in contact with the tissue. Smaller amounts of tissue have higher current density when everything else is equal.
- Polypectomy cutting may be difficult to initiate if the polyp has a very thick stalk and a large circumference of tissue is in contact with the snare, or if the snare is squeezed too tightly so that more of it is surrounded by tissue. These factors lower the current density. The lower current density tends to slow the heating, producing a greater proportion of coagulation to cutting. A "loosely-snug-and-smooth" snare closing technique is recommended to promote smooth polypectomies.
- Thin accessories focus the energy and raise the current density, thus promoting cutting, whereas broader accessories spread the energy over a wider area and lower the current density, which promotes more coagulation effect.

Biliary and Pancreatic Sphincterotomy

Transpapillary division of the biliary sphincter has become a routine part of endoscopic retrograde cholangiopancreatography (ERCP) to facilitate biliary access, remove calculi, improve drainage in biliary dyskinesia, prevent biliary stenosis after ampullectomy, and aid in stent placement. Sphincterotomies are done using monopolar current. Most sphincterotomies are performed using a "pull" type of sphinctertome. The tip of the instrument has an exposed wire (20 to 30 mm) that forms a bow with the catheter when a handle is tightened; this puts tension between the cutting wire and the roof of the papilla. Only the tip of the exposed wire is used for cutting (to increase current density and improve operator control of the incision). Most procedures are wire guided with a shielded guidewire in the bile duct to ensure that the pancreatic duct is not inadvertently incised. Cutting may be performed with either pure cut (100% duty cycle with peak voltage > 200 V; see Table 6.2) or blended (37% to 70% duty cycle; see Table 6.2) current. The use of a cut current results in a more rapid incision with less edema of surrounding tissues, but less hemostasis. Elta[43] et al (1998) first demonstrated that the use of a cut current in lieu of a blended coag waveform (25% duty cycle) resulted in a lower rate of pancreatitis.

As would be expected with less coagulation, increased mild hemorrhage is seen, but this does not translate into clinically significant bleeding.[44] However, because of the potential for less control of a rapid incision with a nonfractionated cut current, great care must be taken with this current output. As mentioned earlier, most new generators have waveform selections that automatically fractionate or interrupt (pulse) the cut current during the course of the incision. As with colonic polypectomy, excessive tissue desiccation should be avoided because this may lead to stalling of the incision.

Needle-Knife Sphincterotomy

Needle-knife sphincterotomy employs a fine, stiff wire projecting approximately 5 mm beyond the tip of a catheter. This type of sphincterotomy is used to cut a pathway into the bile duct and is usually reserved for cases of failed cannulation in which biliary access is of particular importance.

Complications of Sphincterotomy—Link With Electrosurgery

Common complications of endoscopic sphincterotomy include pancreatitis, hemorrhage, and perforation. Each complication may be influenced by the type of current used.

Pancreatitis. Acute pancreatitis is the most common complication of endoscopic sphincterotomy, occurring in at least 5% of cases.[45,46] Development of pancreatitis may be partly a function of iatrogenic trauma to the periampullary region (this trauma results in edema and obstruction to pancreatic flow) or to patient factors such as the presence of Sphincter of Oddi dysfunction. Most current research indicates that generator waveform choice has little effect on post-ERCP pancreatitis as long as a coagulation or blended coagulation waveform with a 25% duty cycle or lower is avoided (see Table 6.2).[15]

Hemorrhage. Hemorrhage during endoscopic sphincterotomy is due in part to inadequate coagulation effect of tissue during the incision. Mild oozing at the sphincterotomy site at the time of endoscopic sphincterotomy is common, settles spontaneously, and is of no clinical significance. Minor bleeding at the time of sphincterotomy may be more common with pure cut technique. Significant hemorrhage occurs in 1% to 3% of patients[47] with an associated mortality of less than 1%.[48] This hemorrhage is due to incision of a significant vessel, which is partly "bad luck" and sometimes due to poor orientation of the incision, cutting into a diverticulum or overcutting the incision. Arterial bleeding is not prevented by one electrosurgical output versus another. It is believed, however, that a half-incised vessel (the ends of which cannot retract) bleeds much more than a fully cut one, implying that cutting a little more may be useful in this situation.

Perforation. Duodenal perforation during endoscopic sphincterotomy is usually the result of a poorly aligned or too-long incision beyond the boundaries of the intramural common bile duct. Clinically significant perforation occurs in less than 1% of sphincterotomies.[49,50] The risk of perforation may be 8% in patients with a small papilla and patients with papillary stenosis.[51]

Asymptomatic perforation may be more common, possibly occurring in 15% of sphincterotomies.[52] Duodenal perforation may occur during a rapid, uncontrolled cut of the sphincter *(zipper cut)*. The occurrence of this type of rapid incision is a function of current delivery to the tissue and operator experience. The use of a pulsed or interrupted advance type of waveform has been shown to reduce this risk.[53]

Polypectomy

Polypectomy is most commonly used to remove colonic polyps, either in one piece or piecemeal. Polypectomy and other thermal ablative techniques such as hot biopsy and ablation have the potential to cause transmural damage, resulting in either serosal inflammation (post-polypectomy syndrome) or perforation. The risk of perforation with all colonoscopies has been estimated to be one perforation in a range between 1000 to 2000 colonoscopies.[54] Serositis without perforation occurs in 1% of polypectomies[55] and manifests 6 hours to 5 days after the procedure with pain, fever, and leukocytosis. The right side of the colon is particularly at risk because of its thinner wall.

Immediate hemorrhage occurs in approximately 1% of polypectomies, and delayed bleeding may occur in 2% of polypectomies.[56] Significant hemorrhage is much more likely when cutting through a thick stalk. Delayed bleeding may occur anytime up to 2 weeks after the procedure. From the preceding discussion, it can be seen that sphincterotomy and polypectomy complications may be related partly to either an overrapid, poorly controlled incision or an overdesiccated, poorly progressed incision.

Modern generators use microprocessor-controlled feedback to help produce predictable tissue results in spite of changes in tissue resistance. However, there are patient factors and operator technique that cannot be accounted for by the generator's algorithm (see Fig. 6.1). Bleeding risk, for example, is greatly influenced by patient factors such as anticoagulant use. Dobrowolski et al (2006)[57] reported variance in bleeding rates with polyp size, morphology, and malignant state, whereas Watabe et al (2006)[58] also noted that hypertension puts patients at risk for a delayed post-polypectomy hemorrhage. It is at this intersection of electrosurgery fundamentals and the characteristics of the particular patient presenting for treatment that the physician well schooled in both will consistently experience the best outcomes.

Hot Biopsy Forceps

HBF have been a popular means of removing diminutive polyps for many years.[59] HBF employs monopolar circuitry. Blended or coagulation current should be used at a relatively low setting and applied only until blanching of the tissue occurs (1 to 2 seconds). The bowel should be deflated before power application, and care must be taken not to touch other parts of the bowel wall with the cups while coagulating. Post-polypectomy syndrome, perforation, and significant bleeding have all been reported after removal of diminutive polyps using HBF.[19,58] This technique is also relatively poor at removing all polyp tissue.[60]

Endoscopic Mucosal Resection

EMR is a method of removing sessile or flat neoplasms involving the mucosal layer of the GI tract. Several methods of EMR exist including injection, cap, and ligation-assisted techniques.[61] All forms of EMR utilize snares to perform the resection. The resection is typically performed using either some form of a blended-cut current (crest factors of approximately 2.5 to 5.5 [see Table 6.2]) or a coagulation mode similar to that used to perform polypectomy (i.e., broad power curve with a crest factor of approximately 6 [see Table 6.2]). Potential complications associated with EMR include hemorrhage (immediate and delayed) and perforation/full thickness resection.

Endoscopic Submucosal Dissection

ESD is a method for resecting neoplastic lesions en bloc. In performing ESD, the perimeter of the margin is typically marked using a needle-knife or snare tip using a low-voltage contact coagulation current (100% duty cycle, < 200 V; see Table 6.2). The submucosa is then injected with a solution (typically saline-based) followed by incision of the mucosa around the perimeter of the initial markings. The incision is made using an electrosurgical knife with an ESU setting that delivers a blended current capable of both cutting and coagulation. Following the mucosal incision of the perimeter of the lesion, dissection of the submucosa can be performed with various electrosurgical knives (discussed in detail in Chapters 32 and 37). Various ESU settings will allow the endoscopist to perform the dissection. In selecting the appropriate ESU setting for performing the dissection, factors such as the vascularity and extent of fibrosis need to be considered and often need to be modified during the procedure depending on what is encountered during the resection. If a large vessel or active bleeding is encountered during the resection, the vessel should be coagulated using coagulation graspers with a soft coagulation current (100% duty cycle, < 200 V; see Table 6.2). As previously mentioned in this chapter, the specific ESU settings used for the various aspects of ESD depend on the technique used by the endoscopist, with the tissue effect being largely impacted by the technique and accessory used (see Fig. 6.1). Therefore, a physician performing ESD should have a thorough understanding of electrosurgical principles and the specific operating characteristics of their ESU.

Peroral Endoscopic Myotomy

POEM is a method to treat achalasia and other esophageal motility disorders by performing a myotomy endoscopically.[62] The procedure and indications are discussed in detail in Chapters 19 and 45. In regard to electrosurgical principles for performing POEM, the procedure utilizes similar devices and techniques to ESD. A submucosal injection is performed proximal to where the myotomy is performed. This is followed by a longitudinal mucosal incision (approximately 2 cm in length) using an electrosurgical knife with ESU setting similar to that for performing the mucosal incision in ESD. The submucosal space is then entered through the mucosal incision. A submucosal tunnel is then created by performing a series of injections into the submucosal space followed by dissection of the submucosa. Various electrosurgical knives and ESU settings can be used for performing the dissection of the submucosal space. The use of "spray coag" (high voltage, high crest factor, short duty cycle current; see Table 6.2) has been reported to be used successfully for dissecting the submucosal space.[62] However, other ESU settings (e.g., blended cut currents or coagulation current with a crest factor of approximately 6; see Table 6.2) can also be utilized to perform the submucosal dissection. Following the creation of the submucosal tunnel past the gastroesophageal junction, the myotomy is then performed using an electrosurgical knife. Again, the choice of ESU setting is dependent on the accessory used, tissue factors, and the operator technique. The setting should

produce a cutting effect along with coagulation. Large vessels and active bleeding can be managed using coagulation graspers using a continuous coagulation current less than 200 V (see Table 6.2).

SUMMARY

There are a variety of indications for electrosurgery throughout the gastrointestinal tract for cutting or ablating tissue. All these techniques involve manageable risks of perforation or hemorrhage. New accessory devices, techniques, and generators intended to reduce these risks do not replace the responsibility of the clinician to have a working knowledge of the principles underlying the tools in use.

KEY REFERENCES

5. Wong Kee Song LM, Gostout CJ, Tucker RD, et al: Electrosurgery in gastrointestinal endoscopy: terminology matters. Letters to the Editor, *Gastrointest Endosc* 83:271–273, 2016.

11. Tucker RD, Hudrlik TR, Silvis SE, et al: Automated impedance: a case study in microprocessor programming, *Comput Biol Med* 11(3):153–160, 1981.

13. Laine L, Long GL, Bakos GJ, et al: Optimizing bipolar electrocoagulation for endoscopic hemostasis: assessment of factors influencing energy delivery and coagulation, *Gastrointest Endosc* 67:502–508, 2008.

14. Fahrtash-Bahin F, Holt B, Jayasekeran V, et al: Snare tip soft coagulation achieves effective and safe endoscopic hemostasis during wide-field endoscopic resection of large colonic lesions, *Gastrointest Endosc* 78(1):158–163, 2013.

15. ASGE Technology Committee, Tokar JL, Barth BA, et al: Electrosurgical generators, *Gastrointest Endosc* 78(2):197–208, 2013.

16. Norton ID, Petersen BT, Bosco J, et al: A randomized trial of endoscopic biliary sphincterotomy using pure cut versus combined cut and coagulation waveforms, *Clin Gastroenterol Hepatol* 3(10):1029–1033, 2005.

17. Morris ML, Bowers WJ: Math, myth and the fundamentals of electrosurgery, *J Hepatol Gastroenterol* 1(1):1–5, 2016.

18. Munro MG: Fundamentals of electrosurgery part I: principles of radiofrequency energy for surgery. In Feldman LS, Fuchshuber P, Jones DB, editors: *The SAGES manual on the fundamental use of surgical energy (FUSE)*, New York, 2012, Springer.

19. Morris ML, Tucker RD, Baron TH, et al: Electrosurgery in in gastrointestinal endoscopy: principles to practice, *Am J Gastroenterol* 104(6):1563–1574, 2009.

20. Singh N, Harrison M, Rex DK: A survey of colonoscopic polypectomy practices among clinical gastroenterologists, *Gastrointest Endosc* 60(3):414–418, 2004.

21. Rey JF, Bellenhoff U, Dumonceau JM: ESGE Guideline: the use of electrosurgical units, *Endoscopy* 42:764–771, 2010.

24. Nelson G, Morris ML: Electrosurgery in the gastroenterology suite, *Gastroenterol Nurs* 38:430–439, 2015.

27. Ginsberg G, Barkun AN, Bosco J, et al: Technology status evaluation report: the argon plasma coagulator, *Gastrointest Endosc* 55(7):807–810, 2002.

29. Eickhoff A, Jakobs R, Schilling D, et al: Prospective nonrandomized comparison of two modes of argon beamer (APC) tumor desobstruction: effectiveness of the new pulsed APC versus forced APC, *Endoscopy* 39(7):637–642, 2007.

32. Eickhoff A, Hartmann D, Eickhoff JC, et al: Pain sensation and neuromuscular stimulation during argon plasma coagulation in gastrointestinal endoscopy, *Surg Endosc* 22(7):1701–1707, 2008.

33. Manner E, May A, Faerber M, et al: Safety and efficacy of a new high power argon plasma coagulation system (hp-APC) in lesions of the upper gastrointestinal tract, *Dig Liver Dis* 38(7):471–478, 2006.

35. Association of periOperative Registered Nurses (AORN): Recommended practices for electrosurgery. In *Perioperative standards and recommended practices*, Denver, 2010, AORN, pp 105–125.

41. Manner H, Plum N, Pech O, et al: Colon explosion during argon plasma coagulation, *Gastrointest Endosc* 67:1123–1127, 2008.

43. Elta GH, Barnett JL, Wille RT, et al: Pure cut electrocautery current for sphincterotomy causes less post procedure pancreatitis than blended current, *Gastrointest Endosc* 47:149–153, 1998.

50. Freeman ML: Adverse outcomes in ERCP, *Gastrointest Endosc* 56:S273–S282, 2002.

54. Fyock CJ, Draganov PV: Colonoscopic polypectomy and associated techniques, *World J Gastroenterol* 16(29):3630–3637, 2010.

58. Watabe H, Yamaji Y, Okamoto M, et al: Risk assessment for delayed hemorrhagic complication of colonic polypectomy: polyp related factors and patient related factors, *Gastrointest Endosc* 64:73–78, 2006.

61. ASGE Technology Committee, Hwang JH, Konda V, et al: Endoscopic mucosal resection, *Gastrointest Endosc* 82(2):215–226, 2015.

62. Inoue H, Minami H, Kobayashi Y, et al: Peroral endoscopic myotomy (POEM) for esophageal achalasia, *Endoscopy* 42(4):265–271, 2010.

A complete reference list can be found online at ExpertConsult .com

7

Sedation and Monitoring in Endoscopy

Vaibhav Wadhwa and John Joseph Vargo II

INTRODUCTION

Sedation is regularly used to facilitate the performance of endoscopic procedures. Sedation practices have noticeably changed over the past decade, with a shift from no or moderate sedation to monitored anesthesia care (MAC) for gastrointestinal (GI) endoscopy.[1]

Sedation during an endoscopic procedure helps in two ways; first, by decreasing procedural pain, thereby making the patient more comfortable, and second, by decreasing any untimely patient movements, thereby reducing complications.[2] Both these factors affect the overall quality and safety of endoscopic procedures.

Sedation is associated with its own potential problems. Sedation-related complications, such as aspiration, oversedation, hypoventilation, and airway obstruction, make up more than half of all reported endoscopic complications.[3,4]

Sedation use requires additional monitoring and recovery, and therefore has implications in the form of time, cost, and staffing. Due to these issues, some prior studies have advocated for the use of unsedated endoscopy[5-7]; however, the rate of use of unsedated endoscopy remains very low in the United States.[8] The main reason for that is unpredictable patient tolerability during the endoscopic procedures. Several studies have shown that even though patients agree to undergo the procedure without sedation initially, the need for sedation later in the procedure causes significant delays in procedure completion when compared to patients who are sedated throughout the procedure.[9,10]

The length and complexity of procedures and the comorbidities of the patient are the most important factors for sedation use. These factors may influence the choice of sedative, the level of sedation, and the need for an anesthesiologist during the procedure. Patients also vary in their sensitivity to sedation and their tolerance of endoscopy. The American Society of Anesthesiologists (ASA) defines the level of sedation on a spectrum of four recognizable levels, from minimal sedation to general anesthesia[11] (Table 7.1). The most commonly used level in endoscopic procedures is moderate sedation, wherein the patient demonstrates purposeful response to visual or tactile stimuli. This level of sedation can be achieved with a benzodiazepine alone or combined with an opiate. Due to the increased use of MAC, propofol use to target balanced propofol sedation (concurrent use with midazolam and/or fentanyl) is being increasingly used for mild to moderate sedation and is associated with improved patient outcomes.[12,13]

This chapter focuses on all aspects of sedation and patient safety. Patient evaluation and risk assessment, presedation preparation, patient monitoring during sedation, sedation providers, sedation in high-risk populations, and issues of consent are discussed. The attributes of commonly used sedative drugs are discussed in the context of level of sedation and monitoring required.

TABLE 7.1	**Levels of Sedation**
Level 1: Minimal sedation	Drug-induced state, during which patient responds normally to verbal commands. Cognitive function and coordination may be impaired. Ventilatory and cardiovascular function are unaffected
Level 2: Conscious sedation	Drug-induced depression of consciousness, during which patient responds purposefully to verbal commands, either alone or accompanied by light tactile stimulation. Patent airway is maintained without help. Spontaneous ventilation is adequate, and cardiovascular function is usually maintained
Level 3: Deep sedation	Drug-induced depression of consciousness, during which patient cannot be easily aroused but responds purposefully to repeated or painful stimulation. Patient may require assistance maintaining an airway. Spontaneous ventilation may be inadequate, and cardiovascular function is maintained
Level 4: General anesthesia	Patient is not able to be aroused even by painful stimuli. Patient often requires assistance in maintaining patent airway. Positive-pressure ventilation may be required owing to respiratory depression or neuromuscular blockade. Cardiovascular function may be impaired

From Bryson HM, Fulton BR, Faulds D: Propofol: an update of its use in anesthesia and conscious sedation. *Drugs* 50(3):513–559, 1995.

TABLE 7.2	**Definition of American Society of Anesthesiologists Status**
Class 1	Patient has no organic, physiologic, biochemical, or psychiatric disturbance. Pathologic process for which operation is to be performed is localized and does not entail systemic disturbance
Class 2	Mild to moderate systemic disturbance caused either by the condition to be treated surgically or by other pathophysiologic processes
Class 3	Severe systemic disturbance or disease from whatever cause; it may be impossible to define degree of disability with finality
Class 4	Severe systemic disorders that are already life-threatening, not always correctable by operation
Class 5	Moribund patient who has little chance of survival but is submitted to operation in desperation

PATIENT EVALUATION, PREPARATION, AND RISK STRATIFICATION

The risk of adverse outcomes can be reduced by appropriate preprocedural evaluation of the patient's history and physical findings. The clinicians responsible for sedation should familiarize themselves with specific and relevant aspects of the medical history, including abnormalities of major organ systems, previous adverse experience with sedation and analgesia, current medications and drug allergies, time of the last oral intake, and history of alcohol or recreational drug use. A thorough physical examination should be done, particularly to assess the heart and lungs, in addition to assessing the airway anatomy. It may be useful to consider the patient in terms of the ASA status classification (Table 7.2), as increasing number and severity of comorbidities are associated with an increased incidence of cardiopulmonary unplanned events. Patients undergoing sedation should be informed of the benefits, risks, and limitations associated with sedation and possible alternatives. This should be completed as part of the patient consent.

Patients undergoing sedation should be stratified according to the risk for sedation-related complications to receive either moderate sedation or MAC. The Stratifying Clinical Outcomes Prior to Endoscopy score (the SCOPE score) is a validated score that can be used to predict difficult moderate sedation for endoscopy based on several factors.[14] The purpose of the risk stratification is to reduce the incidence of sedation-related adverse events.

PROCEDURAL MONITORING

Patients should have continuous monitoring while undergoing endoscopic procedures and also before, during, and after the administration of sedative agents. Standard monitoring procedures include electrocardiography, pulse oximetry, blood pressure measurement, and capnography. Monitoring should be discontinued only when the patient is fully awake. According to the ASA guidelines, it is recommended that continuous recording of the patient's level of consciousness, respiratory function, and hemodynamics reduces the risk of sedation-related adverse outcomes.[11] Close monitoring helps in early detection of adverse events induced by sedatives, such as apnea, hypoxemia, hypotension, and arrhythmias, which allows for early intervention to prevent any life-threatening complications. Each of the monitored parameters is addressed in the following sections.

Level of Consciousness

Alteration in the level of consciousness while under sedation serves as a guide to the depth of sedation the patients. With a decrease in level of consciousness being associated with a loss of reflexes that normally protect the airway and prevent hypoventilation, it is important to assess patient response to commands during sedation (see Table 7.1). Verbal responses also provide information indicating that the patient is breathing. In procedures where verbal responses are impossible, such as upper GI endoscopy, nonverbal responses such as hand movements, finger squeezing, toe wiggling, etc., should be sought. A lack of response to verbal or tactile stimuli suggests a higher depth of sedation and should be managed accordingly.

Pulse Oximetry

A common noninvasive method of measuring oxygen saturation is pulse oximetry, which uses a light signal transmitted through tissue and takes into account the pulsatile volume changes that occur. The pulse oximeter measures the pulsatile signals across perfused tissue at two distinct wavelengths: the infrared band, which corresponds to oxyhemoglobin, and the red band, which corresponds to reduced hemoglobin.

However, the sole use of pulse oximetry is inadequate for detecting alveolar hypoventilation in patients undergoing endoscopy.[15] This is demonstrated by the oxyhemoglobin dissociation curve. A high oxyhemoglobin concentration is preserved despite a decrease in partial pressure of oxygen in the blood (Pao_2) until the Pao_2 falls below 60 mm Hg, at which point the pulse oximeter reading reflects the decreasing Pao_2 with a rapid decrease in oxygen saturation. Therefore, alveolar hypoventilation is detected earlier with the use of capnography (described later) than pulse oximetry.[16]

Pulmonary Ventilation

Respiratory depression in the form of transient hypoxemia is not uncommon with sedation use and is usually trivial. It is also encountered in unsedated procedures. Extended periods of hypoxemia, however, can cause tachycardia and coronary ischemia. Therefore, respiratory monitoring is very important to reduce the risk of adverse outcomes.

Direct observation of respiratory movement or direct pulmonary auscultation is the simplest way to monitor ventilator function. A noninvasive method for measuring arterial carbon dioxide is transcutaneous carbon dioxide monitoring ($PtCO_2$), which entails placing a heated electrode on the skin, causing the microcirculation to "arterialize." The eventual production of carbonic acid due to diffusion of carbon dioxide into an electrolyte solution provides a pH reading by using the Henderson-Hasselbalch equation, which allows for calculation of the arterial carbon dioxide level. The use of this technique was validated by Nelson et al (2000), who demonstrated significantly more CO_2 retention in patients with standard monitoring than those with standard monitoring coupled with $PtCO_2$ monitoring in patients undergoing endoscopic retrograde cholangiopancreatography (ERCP).[17]

Capnography is the gold standard for respiratory monitoring. It works by measuring the CO_2 indirectly by virtue of light absorption in the infrared region of the electromagnetic spectrum. CO_2 retention is identified as an early event on capnography and is a sign of ventilation compromise. It serves as a qualitative method for detection of CO_2 levels in nonintubated patients undergoing endoscopy, as the exact measurement of CO_2 is inaccurate unless the breathing system is a closed circuit, such as in intubated patients. There have been several studies that have demonstrated that use of capnography detects significantly more hypoxemia in patients undergoing GI endoscopy than standard monitoring.[16,18] However, a 2016 trial did not demonstrate any reduction in the incidence of hypoxemia events in healthy individuals undergoing routine endoscopy targeting moderate sedation.[19]

Bispectral index (BIS) monitors are often used in the operating room to assess the adequacy of the depth of anesthesia while under a general anesthetic in patients undergoing surgical procedures. However, the BIS monitor has significant overlap of scores across sedation levels when it is used to detect deep sedation, resulting in an overall lower accuracy rate.[20]

Hemodynamic Measurements

Hemodynamic complications, such as hypotension, arrhythmias, and cardiovascular response to stress, are some of the mild direct effects of sedative agents and analgesics that may happen during sedation. Regular measurements of pulse and blood pressure can help detect these changes, which may represent responses to hypoxemia, oversedation, or possibly patient distress to procedure-induced pain. Although no evidence shows that blood pressure monitoring during endoscopy influences morbidity and mortality, it has been recommended that both regular blood pressure measurements and pulse be monitored throughout procedures performed under sedation.[1] Continuous electrocardiogram (ECG) monitoring should be considered in high-risk patients, such as patients with known disturbances in cardiac rhythm, cardiomyopathies, or ischemic heart disease. The requirement for ECG monitoring has not been evaluated in clinical trials.

Supplemental Oxygen

Supplemental oxygen administered via nasal cannulas or a mask has been shown to reduce the incidence of desaturation during endoscopy performed under sedation[21,22] and hence it should be given to all patients receiving sedation. However, as supplemental oxygen may delay the onset of hypoxemia in sedated patients with decreased pulmonary ventilation, it is essential not to rely solely on pulse oximetry to monitor ventilation but to employ additional techniques, such as capnography or a BIS monitor.

INTRAVENOUS ACCESS

Intravenous access should be maintained throughout the procedure until the patient is no longer at risk from cardiopulmonary or respiratory depression. It facilitates the immediate availability of vascular access in the event of oversedation for administration of reversal agents or for using emergency drugs in the event of cardiopulmonary compromise. In patients who are receiving sedatives via nonintravascular routes (e.g., pediatric patients undergoing endoscopic procedures), intravenous access should also be obtained if the likelihood of any cardiopulmonary depression is high.

SEDATION AND CONSENT

There are a couple of important things to keep in mind when it comes to consent and sedation. First and foremost, the patient should be fully informed of the indications, risks, and alternatives to sedation before he or she consents to the procedure. The second important issue is whether a patient, while under sedation, can withdraw consent for the procedure. If a sedated patient indicates during endoscopy that he or she wishes to have the procedure stopped, should the endoscopist stop or complete the procedure, bearing in mind that it would be in the patient's best interests to complete it? A study from the United Kingdom researched this issue and found that 88% of gastroenterologists stated that they would only stop after repeated requests by the sedated patient, and only 45% of gastroenterologists thought patients were capable of making rational decisions while under sedation.[23] When looked at from the patient's perspective, the study found that opinion was evenly divided into terminating the procedure immediately or completing it.[23]

STAFFING LEVELS AND TRAINING

Adequate patient monitoring during sedation is difficult for a clinician performing the procedure. There should be additional individuals available to monitor the patient's status in terms of level of consciousness, ventilatory function, and hemodynamic parameters. The presence of another individual is likely to improve patient comfort and satisfaction. Several areas of expertise are required while managing sedated patients, including knowledge of administered drugs and management of adverse events. All staff members administering sedative drugs should be made familiar with the pharmacology of all drugs used prior to their involvement. Particularly, staff members should be aware of the basics such as the time to onset of action, elimination half-life,

---

BOX 7.1   Appropriate Emergency Equipment to Have Available When Using Sedative or Analgesic Drugs Capable of Causing Cardiorespiratory Depression

Appropriate emergency equipment should be available whenever sedative or analgesic drugs capable of causing cardiorespiratory depression are administered. The following lists should be used as a guide, which should be modified depending on the individual practice circumstances. Items in brackets are recommended when infants or children are sedated.

Intravenous Equipment
- Gloves
- Tourniquets
- Alcohol wipes
- Sterile gauze pads
- Intravenous catheters [24–22-gauge]
- Intravenous tubing [pediatric "microdrip" (60 drops/mL)]
- Intravenous fluid
- Assorted needles for drug aspiration, intramuscular injection (intraosseous bone marrow needle)
- Appropriately sized syringes [1-mL syringes]
- Tape

Basic Airway Management Equipment
- Source of compressed oxygen (tank with regulator or pipeline supply with flowmeter)
- Source of suction
- Suction catheters [pediatric suction catheters]
- Yankauer-type suction
- Face masks [infant/child]
- Self-inflating breathing bag-valve set [pediatric]
- Oral and nasal airways [infant/child-sized]
- Lubricant

Advanced Airway Management Equipment (for practitioners with intubation skills)
- Laryngeal mask airways [pediatric]
- Laryngoscope handles (tested)
- Laryngoscope blades [pediatric]
- Endotracheal tubes
  - Cuffed 6.0, 7.0, 8.0 mm ID
  - [Uncuffed 2.5, 3.0, 3.5, 4.0, 4.5, 5.0, 5.5, 6.0 mm ID]
- Stylet (appropriately sized for endotracheal tubes)

Pharmacologic Antagonists
- Naloxone
- Flumazenil

Emergency Medications
- Epinephrine
- Ephedrine
- Vasopressin
- Atropine
- Nitroglycerin (tablets or spray)
- Amiodarone
- Lidocaine
- Glucose, 50% [10% or 25%]
- Diphenhydramine
- Hydrocortisone, methylprednisolone, or dexamethasone
- Diazepam or midazolam

ID, internal diameter.
From American Society of Anesthesiologists Task Force on Sedation and Analgesia by Non-Anesthesiologists: Practice guidelines for sedation and analgesia by non-anesthesiologists. *Anesthesiology* 96(4):1004–1017, 2002.

---

interactions, adverse reactions, contraindications, and pharmacology of appropriate antagonists.

Individuals monitoring sedated patients should be able to recognize complications associated with the sedative drugs. Since most of the complications associated with sedatives are cardiopulmonary in nature, at least one individual should be familiar with advanced airway and ventilation management. Guidelines recommend an advanced resuscitation provider be immediately available in the event of an emergency.[11] Resuscitation equipment should be readily available and must include a cardiac defibrillator, advanced airway and positive-pressure ventilation equipment, and all the appropriate drugs, including sedative antagonists (Box 7.1).

POSTPROCEDURAL MONITORING

The patients remain at risk of sedative-related complications even after completion of the procedure. The risk of upper airway obstruction and hypoxemia after significant moderate sedation for ERCP seems to be greatest immediately after removal of the endoscope. Monitoring of the patient should be continued until the patient has reached an acceptable level of consciousness, with normal ventilation, oxygenation, and hemodynamic parameters. Before discharging the patient, it should be recognized that there may be a prolonged period of amnesia with impairment of cognition and judgment, even though the patient's conscious level may appear normal. Patients may also be mildly dehydrated, especially after colonoscopy, and fluid replacement should be addressed before discharge planning.

After an outpatient procedure, the following instructions should apply for at least 24 hours after discharge:
- Patients should not drive.
- Patients should not operate heavy or dangerous machinery.
- Patients should not sign any legally binding documents.
- Patients should be given written instructions regarding "warning signs and symptoms" of any adverse outcomes of the procedure and contact numbers for 24-hour advice.

In addition to the previous points, patients should arrange for a ride home beforehand, and that should be confirmed with the patient before starting the procedure.

In a placebo-controlled study, flumazenil use was shown to augment recovery from sedation and amnesia without any apparent risk for resedation.[24] Although use of flumazenil adds to the costs of the procedure, it still may be preferable for some patients. Use of flumazenil does not preclude the need for postprocedural monitoring, and there is currently not enough evidence to support its routine use.

DRUGS FOR SEDATION

An ideal sedative agent should have the following characteristics:
- Rapid onset of action
- Practical means of delivery
- Short half-life with rapid recovery

- Safe with predictable sedative response (pharmacodynamics)
- Minimal or no cardiovascular or respiratory effects
- Effective in producing a calm, pain-free, cooperative patient

The most commonly used class of drugs are benzodiazepines, which are used alone or in combination with an opiate. It is vital that clinicians are familiar with a few specific sedatives (e.g., midazolam or fentanyl). Most recently, propofol has become the agent of choice to induce deep sedation. Midazolam and diazepam are also frequently used and have been shown to have similar efficacy when compared to each other.[25,26] Midazolam is an attractive agent for endoscopy owing to its rapid onset of action, short half-life, and amnestic properties.

Fentanyl and meperidine are the most frequently used opiates, with fentanyl being preferred and commonly used because of its rapid action and absence of nausea.

The use of a benzodiazepine and an opiate is the most frequently utilized combination in endoscopic procedures, although this concurrent use may lead to an increased incidence of sedation-related complications.[27] Combination therapy in colonoscopy and upper GI endoscopy, however, does not seem to improve pain and tolerance when compared with individual agents.[27–29]

The safest method of administration is by giving small incremental doses until the desired level of sedation is attained, rather than giving a single bolus dose based on patient weight.

Droperidol used to be used in the sedation of agitated patients; however, due to its numerous side effects, it is not widely utilized anymore. Nitrous oxide has also been infrequently used as a form of patient-controlled analgesia in several studies involving colonoscopy.[30,31] Potential benefits of its use include an absence of sedation-related risks and a rapid recovery. However, studies utilizing nitrous oxide were inconsistent and showed minimal to no benefit compared with traditional sedation.

PROPOFOL AND DEEP SEDATION

In certain circumstances, standard moderate sedation is not sufficient, and patients may require a higher level of sedation. These circumstances include patients who are not tolerant of endoscopy under moderate sedation and in procedures that are painful, longer, or complex, such as ERCP, endoscopic ultrasound (EUS), balloon enteroscopy, and endoscopic submucosal dissection (ESD). Deep sedation can be achieved with benzodiazepine and narcotic combinations. Fentanyl, remifentanil, and meperidine all have been combined with benzodiazepines and narcotics to accentuate sedative effects to achieve deep sedation.

Propofol is a popular drug that is frequently used for GI endoscopy because of its highly favorable pharmacokinetics. Its short half-life, rapid onset of action, rapid recovery times, and attainable depth of sedation make an attractive agent for endoscopic procedures. It has no analgesic properties. Patients who regularly use sedatives and narcotics are often insensitive to standard benzodiazepine sedation and may benefit from propofol sedation. There are several disadvantages associated with propofol use. Propofol has to be continuously titrated to maintain sedation due to its short half-life. The narrow therapeutic window between moderate sedation, deep sedation, and anesthesia necessitates close monitoring. As a result of peripheral vasodilation and impairment of cardiac contractility, propofol may cause profound hypotension. Propofol causes apnea more readily than midazolam, so managing the airway and pulmonary ventilation is more critical if propofol is used.

NEWER AGENTS

Remimazolam is the latest drug innovation in anesthesia. It is an ester-based benzodiazepine designed to be used for short-duration sedation. It has an organ independent metabolism and is rapidly hydrolyzed by tissue esterases without producing any active metabolites. The sedation effect is shorter than midazolam, and frequent dosing may be required for procedure completion. Preliminary studies have suggested that the recovery time is similar to midazolam, although remimazolam recovery times lack the long outliers seen with midazolam sedation.[32]

Fospropofol is a prodrug that is enzymatically converted to propofol in the liver with a delayed onset of action (4–8 min) and extended duration of action (20–30 min).[33] It may decrease the need for frequent administration, which is often seen with propofol; however, because it needs to be converted to propofol, it has a decreased clinical effect compared to propofol. Fospropofol failed to gain popularity due to several inaccuracies that were reported in the published fospropofol pharmacokinetic-pharmacodynamic data. This led to the retraction of six studies, and correct data is yet to be made available.[34]

Dexmedetomidine is an α_2-adrenoreceptor agonist with sedative, anxiolytic, and analgesic effects. Its effects on respiratory system are minimal, and it does not cause clinically significant respiratory depression.[35,36] It can be administered either intranasally or intravenously, although the latter is preferred.[37] Dexmedetomidine is delivered as an initial bolus infusion of 1 µg/kg over 10 min followed by continuous infusion of 0.6 µg/kg per hr that may be titrated between 0.2 to 1.0 µg/kg per hr. Dose modification is often necessary in elderly or critically ill patients. Side effects include bradycardia and a biphasic change in blood pressure (high then low) with administration of increasing concentrations.[38] Dexmedetomidine alone or dexmedetomidine with meperidine and midazolam has shown to have less respiratory depression and higher patient satisfaction scores for routine endoscopy and more advanced procedures (e.g., ERCP) than midazolam alone or midazolam with meperidine.[39,40] Dexmedetomidine causes less respiratory depression even when administered with propofol as compared to propofol administered with sufentanil, meperidine, or midazolam.[41]

SEDATION PROVIDERS

In the United States, moderate sedation is usually administered by an endoscopist, whereas anesthesiologists are the ones managing sedation for MAC or general anesthesia. There are several alternative methods of sedation for endoscopy, which include patient-controlled sedation (PCS), automated delivery using methods such as the SEDASYS system (Ethicon Endosurgery, Inc., Somerville, NJ), and nonanesthesiologist-administered sedation using centrally acting agents such as propofol.

Nearly all endoscopic procedures in the United States are completed with some form of sedation, whereas nearly three-fourths of all endoscopies performed in Europe and Asia are completed without sedation.[42] The percentage of patients undergoing endoscopic procedures (simple or advanced) with MAC or deep sedation in the United States continues to rise. A national survey in 2006 concluded that roughly 75% of patients undergoing endoscopic procedures in the United States received moderate sedation and 25% received deep sedation. Presently, the regions with the highest anesthesiologist-administered sedation rates are the South and Mid-Atlantic states.[43] Cooper et al

(2013) showed that from 2000 to 2009, anesthesia services were used in 40% of the total endoscopies performed in the northeastern United States.[44]

SEDASYS

In 2013, the US Food and Drug Administration (FDA) approved the SEDASYS system (Ethicon) for minimal to moderate sedation in ASA class 1–2 patients who are at least 18 years old and have a body mass index (BMI) less than 35 for elective esophagogastroduodenoscopy (EGD) and colonoscopy with a requirement that an anesthesiologist be "immediately available" in case of any complications. It was designed to be used with an initial fentanyl dose, followed by a propofol bolus delivered over 3 to 5 minutes, and then an adaptable propofol infusion. It had shown promise when compared with moderate sedation for endoscopy in low-risk patients, with better recovery times and greater satisfaction with SEDASYS among patients and clinicians.[45] There is no direct comparison between SEDASYS and anesthesiologist-delivered sedation in the current literature. A very limited number of hospitals in the United States adopted SEDASYS. As a result, in May 2016, the manufacturer (Johnson & Johnson, New Brunswick, NJ) decided to remove it from the market due to a lack of popularity.

Patient-Controlled Sedation (PCS)

PCS uses the same hardware as patient-controlled analgesia with drugs (propofol, opioid, and/or benzodiazepines) chosen by the endoscopist. PCS has been shown to be successful in several small studies of both simple and advanced endoscopic procedures.[46,47] Anesthesiologist-administered propofol and PCS have equal satisfaction for ERCP but with shorter recovery times and less frequent use of minor airway interventions, such as chin lifts, in the PCS group. In one study, anesthesiologist intervention was required to complete ERCP in 7% of PCS cases.[46]

Gastroenterologist-Directed Propofol Sedation

Worldwide, gastroenterologists favor using propofol as a sedative for endoscopic procedures over traditional sedatives. In Switzerland, gastroenterologists administer propofol in both hospital and private practice settings, reflecting successful implementation of nonanesthesiologist-administered propofol-based sedation in other countries.[48] A 2014 large German study of 24,441 endoscopic procedures with gastroenterologist-directed propofol sedation in ASA class 1–3 patients with BMI less than 40 and without obstructive sleep apnea (OSA) (ASA class 3 patients with cardiac issues were also excluded) concluded that the incidence rate for major adverse events (such as apnea or laryngospasm requiring mask ventilation or intubation) was only 0.016%, with the incidence of minor adverse events being just 0.46%. All affected patients made a full recovery.[49] Anesthesia was titrated between moderate to deep sedation.

The latest guidelines of the European Society of Gastrointestinal Endoscopy for the administration of propofol for GI endoscopy by nonanesthesiologists consist of involving an anesthesiologist in high-risk patients, such as those with an ASA classification of 3 or higher, with a Mallampati score of 3 or higher, with conditions that put them at risk for airway obstruction, chronically receiving significant amounts of narcotics, or for whom a lengthy or a complicated procedure is anticipated.[50]

The FDA regulations on propofol state, "For general anesthesia or MAC sedation, Diprivan Injectable Emulsion (Fresenius Kabi USA LLC, Lake Zurich, IL) should be administered only by persons trained in the administration of general anesthesia and not involved in the conduct of the surgical/diagnostic procedure."[51] This statement has grossly limited the use of propofol by nonanesthesia providers in the United States.

A fairly large 2017 meta-analysis found no difference in rates of overall complications between endoscopist-directed propofol administration and nonendoscopist-directed propofol administration.[52]

SEDATION IN DIFFERENT PATIENT POPULATIONS

Endoscopy in Patients With Cirrhosis

Chronic liver disease is one of the most common indications for emergent endoscopy. Liver dysfunction reduces both the clearance of the drugs eliminated by hepatic metabolism and plasma protein binding. It is also associated with a reduction in drug-metabolizing enzyme activities such as the Cytochrome P450 (CYP450) enzymes. Therefore, in patients with advanced liver disease, it is imperative to adjust the dose of those drugs eliminated by renal excretion.[53]

A 2015 meta-analysis concluded that propofol provided more prompt sedation and recovery from EGD than midazolam in cirrhotic patients, with no difference in incidence of side effects.[54]

Endoscopy Without Sedation

Unsedated endoscopy is facilitated by use of ultraslim endoscopes (<5.9 mm in diameter). The transnasal route of EGD has a higher patient acceptance rate and is preferred by more patients as compared to conventional EGD with or without sedation.[55] However, the disadvantages of the transnasal EGD are the inferior image and the smaller biopsy samples.[56]

Endoscopy and Pregnancy

Endoscopic procedures in pregnant patients are rarely required and should only be done for the most convincing indications, such as significant GI bleeding, severe nausea and vomiting, dysphagia, and severe diarrhea (all of which may impact maternal and fetal nutrition), as well as biliary pancreatitis or cholangitis.[57] The procedures should be deferred to the second trimester whenever possible to decrease the impact of anesthesia drugs on fetal development.

Both the mother and fetus are at risk for adverse events with endoscopy and, more significantly, anesthesia. A comprehensive discussion of the risks to the fetus and mother with a preoperative obstetrician consultation should be compulsory during the informed consent process for endoscopy. Monitoring of fetal heart rate may be performed during the endoscopy or before and after the procedure.

The left lateral position is recommended for the procedure to avoid compression of inferior vena cava or aorta and prevent compromise of the fetal circulation. Any exposure to radiation should absolutely be avoided. If an ERCP is required, patient position should be appropriate with a lead apron shielding the uterus. An expert should perform the procedure and preferably use a nonfluoroscopy technique.[57]

Anesthesiology services are recommended to be involved during endoscopic procedures involving pregnant patients. There is an increased risk for aspiration in pregnant patients due to elevated intraabdominal pressure and decreased lower esophageal sphincter tone. Maternal hypoxia and/or hypotension may result in reduced uterine blood flow and affect fetal viability.[58]

To summarize, endoscopic procedure time should be minimized, special attention must be paid to the indication for the procedure and patient positioning, fetal monitoring should be made a priority and, if possible, all procedures should be deferred to at least the second trimester.

Endoscopy in Obese Patients

Obese patients are at risk for OSA and adverse cardiovascular events during endoscopic procedures.[59] These patients can be stratified into groups at high and low risk for OSA using the STOP-BANG (Snoring, Tiredness, Observed apnea, blood Pressure, Body mass index, Age, Neck circumference, and Gender) screening tool.[60] The STOP-BANG score may help in predicting sedation-related adverse events in obese patients undergoing advanced, but not routine, endoscopic procedures.[61,62]

EGD can be safely performed with moderate sedation in most patients with a Roux-en-Y gastric bypass unless the coexisting medical conditions necessitate anesthesia monitoring.[63] In a comparison with those without a bypass, patients with Roux-en-Y gastric bypass required higher doses of fentanyl and midazolam during EGD. The dose of drugs required for sedation increased after gastric bypass despite the resulting weight loss.[64]

SEDATION FOR DIFFERENT ENDOSCOPIC PROCEDURES

Standard Endoscopic Procedures

Propofol has been compared with traditional sedative agents such as midazolam, meperidine, and fentanyl in several trials during standard endoscopic procedures.[65–68]

Propofol was shown to be safer and more effective than traditional sedative agents for maintaining an adequate level of sedation during endoscopy, resulting in better titration of the level of sedation and a shorter recovery time.[69] A 2017 meta-analysis of 27 studies did not find any difference in cardiopulmonary complications between propofol and traditional sedative agents for GI endoscopy.[52]

Balanced propofol sedation targeted to induce moderate sedation in patients undergoing upper GI endoscopy was also shown to result in better patient satisfaction and a shorter recovery time than standard sedation alone.[12]

Propofol Use in Complex Endoscopic Procedures

The use of propofol in complex and prolonged procedures has also been investigated extensively.[70–72] Patients undergoing ERCP are increasingly using MAC instead of moderate sedation. Most of these procedures are performed today without any need for endotracheal intubation.[73] Studies have evaluated the use of balanced propofol sedation in patients undergoing ERCP, with recovery times being longer than in patients undergoing sedation only with propofol.[74] In addition, deep biliary cannulation rates for moderate and deep sedation have shown to be similar.[75]

In Europe, gastroenterologists have transitioned to using propofol sedation in patients undergoing EUS. Recently, a study from Spain (2012) concluded that nonanesthesiologist-administered propofol-based sedation for upper EUS in high-risk and average-risk patients had a low rate of minor complications and no major complications.[76] General anesthesia use assists in EUS-guided fine-needle aspiration of pancreatic masses by decreasing patient movement and resulting in an increased diagnostic yield.[77]

ESD is an emerging procedure in the United States. Unlike standard endoscopy, ESD is associated with pain throughout the procedure, such as during the incision and dissection phases, as well as the distension and endoscope movement required to perform the procedure. Therefore, deep sedation is a prerequisite for these patients. MAC without endotracheal intubation in patients undergoing esophageal or gastric ESD reduces body movement and provides a safer treatment environment in these difficult and prolonged cases.[78] A 2015 comparison of two sedation protocols, moderate sedation with analgesic supplementation (MSAS) and analgesia-targeted light sedation (ATLS), showed that ATLS did not affect the ESD performance while producing a lower incidence of desaturation events and decreased incidence of aspiration pneumonia.[79] Propofol-remifentanil infusion regimens were used in this study to achieve the desired level of sedation.[79]

PHARYNGEAL ANESTHESIA IN SEDATION

Topical anesthetic agents are frequently used to suppress the gag reflex in upper endoscopy in addition to sedation. The most commonly used agents are lidocaine, benzocaine, and tetracaine, administered as an aerosol spray to the pharynx. Pharyngeal anesthesia in conjunction with intravenous or intramuscular sedation during upper endoscopy was shown to improve ease of endoscopy and patient tolerance in a meta-analysis.[80] Topical anesthetics have been associated with severe adverse effects such as aspiration, anaphylaxis, or methemoglobinemia and hence should be used cautiously.

MANAGEMENT OF OVERSEDATION

Sedative agents have been associated with more than 50% of all endoscopy-related complications, the most common being oversedation, hypotension, and respiratory depression. Studies have shown that the expected mean desaturation during all endoscopic procedures is approximately 3% from baseline during sedation.[81] The availability of reversal agents for sedative drugs (i.e., benzodiazepines and opioids) are associated with a reduced risk of sedation-related adverse events. The specific antagonists that are available are flumazenil for benzodiazepines and naloxone for opioids.

However, no such antagonists exist for propofol and that is the biggest disadvantage of using this drug. Even though its short half-life may lead to a rapid reversal of sedation, cardiopulmonary compromise in the interim may prove to be disastrous in the absence of an anesthesiologist.

In patients who have received both a benzodiazepine and an opioid, flumazenil reverses sedation but not respiratory depression. Similarly, naloxone monotherapy has not been shown to reverse respiratory depression induced by opioid and benzodiazepine combinations. In the setting of combination therapy-induced respiratory depression, it is recommended that naloxone is given in addition to flumazenil. At the time of reversal or before reversal, the following should be done:
- Perform basic airway management
  - Clear airway including suction (if appropriate)
  - Jaw thrust maneuver
  - Guedel airway if necessary
- Administer supplemental oxygen or increased oxygen
- Encourage or stimulate deep breaths
- Administer positive-pressure ventilation if spontaneous ventilation is inadequate

Flumazenil and naloxone were previously reserved only for treatment of oversedation and respiratory depression. However, the long recovery times experienced with benzodiazepine use have prompted some research into the feasibility of routine use of flumazenil with potential cost savings.[24,82] The cost-effectiveness of this routine use is still under investigation.

REVIEW OF SPECIFIC DRUGS

Benzodiazepines

Benzodiazepines are central nervous system (CNS) depressants that induce sedation, hypnosis, amnesia, and anesthesia. The mechanism of action seems to intensify the physiologic inhibitory mechanisms mediated by γ-aminobutyric acid (GABA).

Midazolam

Pharmacology. Midazolam is a short-acting benzodiazepine with an intravenous peak onset of action of 2 to 5 minutes depending on the dose given and level of consciousness attained. If given with an opioid, the onset of action is more rapid (1.5 minutes), sedation is deeper, and a dose reduction of 30% is recommended. At doses sufficient to induce sedation, midazolam decreases the ventilatory response to increased CO_2 in normal patients and in specific patients with chronic airway limitation. The pharmacokinetic profile of midazolam is linear, over 0.05 to 0.4 mg/kg, lending predictable dosage titration. The elimination half-life is 1 to 2.8 hours with a large volume of distribution. The drug is metabolized rapidly to 1-hydroxymethyl midazolam in the liver, conjugated, and secreted in the urine. The elimination half-life is increased in elderly patients and patients with renal failure.

Administration. Midazolam should be titrated in doses of 0.5 to 2 mg at intervals of 2 to 3 minutes to a total dose of 5 mg. Higher doses may be required but should be used with caution.

Precautions and adverse reactions. When given with an opioid analgesic, there is an increased sedative effect necessitating administration in small incremental steps and a usual requirement of a 30% reduction in dose. Sensitivity increases with age. Caution is required when using midazolam in elderly patients, patients with hepatic or renal impairment, and patients with airflow limitation. Owing to a reduced rate of plasma clearance, patients with heart failure eliminate midazolam more slowly. Paradoxic reactions may occur with restlessness, agitation, and disinhibition. Hypotension is a recognized association of midazolam, particularly if given with an opioid.

Contraindications. Midazolam should not be given to patients with myasthenia gravis, alcohol intoxication, or narrow-angle glaucoma.

Interactions. The sedative effects of midazolam are enhanced by other CNS depressants, including neuroleptics, alcohol, tranquilizers, antidepressants, analgesics, antiepileptics, and anxiolytics. The effects of midazolam are attenuated by drugs that induce cytochrome P450 (rifampicin, carbamazepine, and phenytoin) and enhanced by inhibitors (erythromycin, diltiazem, antiviral agents, and fluconazole). In particular, midazolam should be given with care in patients receiving combination antiretroviral therapy.

Diazepam

Pharmacology. Diazepam is metabolized in the liver to the active metabolites temazepam, nordiazepam, and oxazepam, all of which are renally excreted. Plasma concentrations of diazepam and its active metabolites exhibit considerable interpatient variation. The intravenous plasma time curve is biphasic, with an initial rapid increase with a half-life of up to 3 hours and a second elimination phase with a half-life of 20 to 70 hours. The elimination half-life is increased in elderly patients and in patients with renal and hepatic impairment.

Administration. Diazepam should be titrated in doses of 2 to 4 mg to a total of 10 to 20 mg in some circumstances.

Precautions and adverse reactions. Caution is required in patients with renal, hepatic, and cardiopulmonary impairment. Hypotension occurs rarely. Other precautions, contraindications, and drug interactions are similar to midazolam.

Opioid Analgesics

Fentanyl

Pharmacology. Fentanyl is a synthetic opioid with an estimated 80-fold greater potency than morphine. In contrast to other opioids, fentanyl does not induce histamine release. After intravenous injection, fentanyl reaches peak analgesic effects within 1 to 2 minutes, with a duration of 30 to 60 minutes. Serum concentrations decrease rapidly within 5 minutes to 20% of peak concentrations, followed by a slow decrease over 30 minutes. The drug is metabolized in the liver to active metabolites, all of which are excreted in the urine.

Administration. A dose of 50 to 100 μg should be given before administering a benzodiazepine to enable accurate sedative dose titration.

Precautions and adverse reactions. Fentanyl causes respiratory depression for periods extending beyond the analgesic effect. In light of the route of elimination, a reduced dose should be used in hepatic and renal impairment. In view of the marked respiratory depression that can occur with its use, caution is required in patients with pulmonary disease.

Contraindications. Fentanyl may cause severe bronchospasm and is contraindicated in patients with asthma. Fentanyl may cause severe muscle rigidity and is contraindicated in patients with myasthenia gravis.

Interactions. The sedative effect of fentanyl is enhanced by other CNS depressants, such as other opioids, benzodiazepines, alcohol, neuroleptics, and tranquilizers. In particular, fentanyl has been associated with hypotensive adverse events with monoamine oxidase inhibitors and neuroleptics.

Meperidine

Pharmacology. Meperidine is a synthetic opioid with sedative and analgesic properties. Similar to other narcotics, meperidine causes respiratory depression and suppresses the cough reflex. The sedative and analgesic effects of meperidine after intravenous dosing occur within 2 to 4 minutes, and the analgesic effects can last 4 hours. The elimination half-life is 3.2 hours, and metabolism is predominantly hepatic conjugation. Meperidine elimination is prolonged in patients with hepatic impairment.

Precautions and adverse reactions. Care should be taken when giving meperidine concurrently with other neurodepressants. The most common adverse reaction is respiratory depression. Meperidine may also result in profound hypotension. One active meperidine metabolite, normeperidine, has convulsant properties, and elimination is prolonged in patients with renal impairment and elderly patients. In these patients, high doses of meperidine may lead to convulsions, agitation, irritability, and tremors.

Administration. Meperidine should be given at an intravenous dose of 25 to 50 mg. Higher doses are more likely to result in adverse events.

Drug interactions. The sedative effects of neurodepressants all are potentiated by meperidine. In addition, when given with phenothiazines, CNS toxicity and hypotension may occur. Interactions with monoamine oxidase inhibitors may be fatal and result in excitation, sweating, rigidity, hypertension or hypotension, and coma.

Propofol
Pharmacology
Propofol is distributed rapidly and induces sedation within 30 to 60 seconds. The context-sensitive half-life is only 2 to 8 minutes. Metabolism is by hepatic conjugation with renal excretion of inactive metabolites. Propofol is a centrally acting neural depressant without any analgesic properties and rapidly crosses the blood-brain barrier to potentiate GABA activity.

Contraindications
Propofol is contraindicated in patients with known allergy to propofol.

Precautions and Adverse Reactions
The most important effects to be monitored with propofol are respiratory depression and apnea, occurring frequently with deep sedation. Hypotension is also common. Patients with ASA class 3 or higher, elderly patients, and patients using sedatives or opioid agents are at particular high risk for developing these cardiorespiratory complications. Apnea and hypotension can occur in 75% of patients. In endoscopic trials using propofol, ventilatory support was necessary in 10% of patients, although incidence of respiratory depression necessitating support was far greater in complex procedures requiring a cooperative patient.[34] Excitatory phenomena such as tremors, twitches, hypertonus, and hiccups can occur in 14% of patients. Rarely, pulmonary edema, hypertension, cardiac arrhythmias, bronchospasm, and laryngospasm have occurred. Pain at the injection site is the most frequent local complication and occurs in 5% to 50% of patients.[52]

Administration
Propofol has been given in endoscopic studies by repeated bolus injections or as an infusion. Propofol is usually administered as an initial bolus dose of 20 to 40 mg followed by maintenance doses of 10 to 20 mg to attain the required level of sedation. Alternatively, propofol can be infused at a dose of 0.5 to 1.0 mg/kg over 1 to 5 minutes to induce deep sedation, followed by maintenance infusion at a dose of 1.5 to 3 mg/kg per hr. For anything other than very short procedures, administration of propofol as an infusion is preferable because this produces better steady-state levels and more stable operating conditions.

Interactions
The sedative effect of propofol is enhanced by other sedative agents and analgesics.

Flumazenil
Pharmacology
Flumazenil is an imidazobenzodiazepine and antagonizes benzodiazepines through competitively inhibiting central receptors. Its effects are rapid, within 30 to 60 seconds, and it has an elimination half-life of 53 minutes. Clearance is entirely hepatic, where it is conjugated to form inactive metabolites.

Contraindications
Flumazenil should not be given to patients with known sensitivity to flumazenil.

Precautions and Adverse Reactions
Care should be taken when administering flumazenil to patients with known benzodiazepine dependence because this may precipitate withdrawal or convulsions. Consideration should be given to the possibility of resedation and respiratory depression following the use of flumazenil. Patients should be monitored for an appropriate period based on the dose and duration of effect of the benzodiazepine used. Despite the use of reversal agents, patients should still be given postprocedural warnings, as previously described. Flumazenil is not recommended in epileptic patients taking benzodiazepines because this may give rise to convulsions. Seizures have been reported in patients with epilepsy and hepatic impairment.

Interactions
Flumazenil also blocks the effects of nonbenzodiazepines acting on benzodiazepine receptors such as zopiclone.

Administration
The recommended initial dose is 0.2 mg administered intravenously over 15 seconds. This dose can be repeated using 0.1-mg doses every 60 seconds to achieve reversal to a total dose of 2 mg.

Naloxone
Pharmacology
Naloxone is a competitive antagonist at opiate receptor sites and can reverse the sedative and respiratory effects of opiates. The effects of intravenous naloxone are apparent within 2 minutes, and a single dose from an ampule of 0.2 mg lasts 20 to 30 minutes. The effects of meperidine and other opioids last longer than this, therefore repeated doses of naloxone may need to be given. Naloxone is conjugated in the liver with renal excretion of the metabolites. Elimination half-life is 60 to 90 minutes.

Contraindications
Naloxone should not be administered to patients with known hypersensitivity to this medication.

Precautions and Adverse Reactions
Care is required in patients who are dependent on opiates because naloxone can precipitate withdrawal syndrome. A rapid reversal of opioids can induce catecholamine release and cause excitation, ventricular arrhythmias, hypotension, pulmonary edema, convulsions, and death. Care should be used in patients with preexisting cardiac abnormalities.

Administration
Naloxone can be given intravenously or intramuscularly at an initial dose of 0.4 to 2 mg. Doses can be repeated at 2- to 3-minute intervals until a total dose of 10 mg is reached.

ACKNOWLEDGEMENT

We would like to thank Drs. Matthew R. Banks, George J.M. Webster, and Liang H. Wee for their valuable book chapter on the same topic in the previous edition of *Clinical Gastrointestinal Endoscopy.* The framework from their excellent chapter was used to write the current version of this book chapter.

KEY REFERENCES

1. Vargo JJ, DeLegge MH, Feld AD, et al: Multisociety sedation curriculum for gastrointestinal endoscopy, *Am J Gastroenterol* 76(1):e1–e25, 2012.
2. Igea F, Casellas JA, Gonzalez-Huix F, et al: Sedation for gastrointestinal endoscopy, *Endoscopy* 46(8):720–731, 2014.
3. Freeman ML: Sedation and monitoring for gastrointestinal endoscopy, *Gastrointest Endosc Clin N Am* 4(3):475–499, 1994.
8. Arrowsmith JB, Burt Gerstman B, Fleischer DE, et al: Results from the American Society for Gastrointestinal Endoscopy/U.S. Food and Drug Administration collaborative study on complication rates and drug use during gastrointestinal endoscopy, *Gastrointest Endosc* 37(4):421–427, 1991.
9. Petrini JL, Egan JV, Hahn WV: Unsedated colonoscopy: patient characteristics and satisfaction in a community-based endoscopy unit, *Gastrointest Endosc* 69(3 Pt 1):567–572, 2009.
11. American Society of Anesthesiologists Task Force on Sedation and Analgesia by Non-Anesthesiologists: Practice guidelines for sedation and analgesia by non-anesthesiologists, *Anesthesiology* 96(4):1004–1017, 2002.
13. Cohen LB, Hightower CD, Wood DA, et al: Moderate level sedation during endoscopy: a prospective study using low-dose propofol, meperidine/fentanyl, and midazolam, *Gastrointest Endosc* 59(7):795–803, 2004.
17. Nelson DB, Freeman ML, Silvis SE, et al: A randomized, controlled trial of transcutaneous carbon dioxide monitoring during ERCP, *Gastrointest Endosc* 51(3):288–295, 2000.
18. Vargo JJ, Zuccaro G, Jr, Dumot JA, et al: Automated graphic assessment of respiratory activity is superior to pulse oximetry and visual assessment for the detection of early respiratory depression during therapeutic upper endoscopy, *Gastrointest Endosc* 55(7):826–831, 2002.
19. Mehta PP, Kochhar G, Albeldawi M, et al: Capnographic monitoring in routine EGD and colonoscopy with moderate sedation: a prospective, randomized, controlled trial, *Am J Gastroenterol* 111(3):395–404, 2016.
20. Qadeer MA, Vargo JJ, Patel S, et al: Bispectral index monitoring of conscious sedation with the combination of meperidine and midazolam during endoscopy, *Clin Gastroenterol Hepatol* 6(1):102–108, 2008.
32. Borkett KM, Riff DS, Schwartz HI, et al: A phase IIa, randomized, double-blind study of remimazolam (CNS 7056) versus midazolam for sedation in upper gastrointestinal endoscopy, *Anesth Analg* 120(4):771–780, 2015.
44. Cooper GS, Kou TD, Rex DK: Complications following colonoscopy with anesthesia assistance, *JAMA Intern Med* 173(7):551–556, 2013.
48. Heuss L, Froehlich F, Beglinger C: Nonanesthesiologist-administered propofol sedation: from the exception to standard practice. Sedation and monitoring trends over 20 years, *Endoscopy* 44(05):504–511, 2012.
49. Sieg A, Beck S, Scholl SG, et al: Safety analysis of endoscopist-directed propofol sedation: a prospective, national multicenter study of 24 441 patients in German outpatient practices, *J Gastroenterol Hepatol* 29(3):517–523, 2014.
50. Dumonceau J-M, Riphaus A, Schreiber F, et al: Non-anesthesiologist administration of propofol for gastrointestinal endoscopy: European Society of Gastrointestinal Endoscopy, European Society of Gastroenterology and Endoscopy Nurses and Associates Guideline – Updated June 2015, *Endoscopy* 47(12):1175–1189, 2015.
52. Wadhwa V, Issa D, Garg S, et al: Similar risk of cardiopulmonary adverse events between propofol and traditional anesthesia for gastrointestinal endoscopy: a systematic review and meta-analysis, *Clin Gastroenterol Hepatol* 15(2):194–206, 2017.
57. Shergill AK, Ben-Menachem T, Chandrasekhara V, et al: Guidelines for endoscopy in pregnant and lactating women, *Gastrointest Endosc* 76(1):18–24, 2012.
60. Chung F, Abdullah HR, Liao P: STOP-Bang Questionnaire, *Chest* 149(3):631–638, 2016.
61. Coté GA, Hovis CE, Hovis RM, et al: A screening instrument for sleep apnea predicts airway maneuvers in patients undergoing advanced endoscopic procedures, *Clin Gastroenterol Hepatol* 8(8):660–665.e1, 2010.
62. Mehta PP, Kochhar G, Kalra S, et al: Can a validated sleep apnea scoring system predict cardiopulmonary events using propofol sedation for routine EGD or colonoscopy? A prospective cohort study, *Gastrointest Endosc* 79(3):436–444, 2014.
75. Mehta PP, Vargo JJ, Dumot JA, et al: Does anesthesiologist-directed sedation for ERCP improve deep cannulation and complication rates? *Dig Dis Sci* 56(7):2185–2190, 2011.
79. Yoo YC, Park CH, Shin S, et al: A comparison of sedation protocols for gastric endoscopic submucosal dissection: moderate sedation with analgesic supplementation vs analgesia targeted light sedation, *Br J Anaesth* 115(1):84–88, 2015.
80. Evans LT, Saberi S, Kim HM, et al: Pharyngeal anesthesia during sedated EGDs: is "the spray" beneficial? A meta-analysis and systematic review, *Gastrointest Endosc* 63(6):761–766, 2006.

A complete reference list can be found online at ExpertConsult .com

8

Patient Preparation and Pharmacotherapeutic Considerations

Mark Schoeman and Nam Q. Nguyen

INTRODUCTION

Correct patient preparation is essential for all endoscopic procedures because it contributes significantly to the safety and success of the procedure. Many requirements must be considered during the preparatory phase; patient preparation is not limited to statements regarding fasting or how to complete a bowel preparation. The clinician must consider issues such as timing and patient-specific factors that must be taken into account when preparing for an endoscopic procedure. If the patient has had this type of information explained, he or she is more likely to comply with preparation instructions in a safe manner. As part of this phase and as part of the explanation about what the procedure involves, it is also necessary to explain potential risks and complications. All this communication with the patient contributes to the process of obtaining informed consent, which is a crucial part of the preparation process.

INFORMED CONSENT

The process of informed consent varies from country to country. In many parts of Europe, a formal consent is not required before endoscopic examinations. If the patient comes to have the procedure performed, these systems assume an implied consent. In other parts of the world, such as the United States and Australia, the consent process is a very detailed and potentially complex process that requires considerable attention by the endoscopist (see Chapter 10).

GENERAL INFORMATION ABOUT PATIENT PREPARATION

Numerous aspects must be considered when preparing patients for endoscopic examinations, including the following:
- Understanding of the patient's particular clinical problem
- Awareness of the patient's clinical history
- Knowledge of the patient's recent (and past) medication history
- Requirements of procedure-specific preparation
- Requirements of patient-specific preparation
- Informed consent
- Postprocedure observation and discharge planning

The endoscopist must have knowledge of the indication for the procedure because this determines not only what procedure is performed but also what interventions or treatment might be required during the procedure. Implicit also is an understanding of the patient's clinical history and the results of any recent investigations. The preprocedure assessment must extend to the patient's past medical and surgical history, previous endoscopy results, current medical therapy (including over-the-counter and intermittent medications), and drug allergies. Specific clinical history such as diabetes, a personal or family history of bleeding disorder, anesthetic reactions, or previous adverse reactions to other medical interventions (including reactions to radiologic contrast agents) should also be considered. Armed with this information, the endoscopist is able to determine the proper preparation and any specific modifications regarding sedation that might be required for the individual patient (see Chapter 7).

After the procedure preparation, risks, and potential complications have been discussed, the next phase of the explanatory process is to discuss discharge guidelines. Most endoscopic examinations are performed as day procedures, and frequently patient sedation is administered. Most institutions require that sedated patients are discharged in the care of a responsible person who not only can supervise transportation of the patient home but who also is able to respond to any delayed complications or difficulties. The level of postprocedure supervision depends on the type of intervention and sedation, specific patient factors such as mobility and age, and other factors such as geographic isolation. These issues must be brought to the patient's attention before the procedure so that proper planning can occur. Difficulties with discharge arrangements should always be resolved before the endoscopic procedure and never left to be discussed after the procedure has been performed. Although the previous process may seem cumbersome, there are significant advantages for the patient and the endoscopist, such as the following:

- Ability to obtain informed consent
- Proper patient preparation
- Greater patient confidence with preparation
- Decreased failure of patient to attend endoscopic examination
- Correct procedure being performed
- Improved diagnostic yield
- Decreased patient anxiety and potentially improved patient tolerance of the procedure
- Improved discharge outcome

ROUTINE LABORATORY TESTING BEFORE ENDOSCOPIC PROCEDURES

Routine preprocedure laboratory testing is the practice of ordering a set panel of tests for all patients undergoing a given procedure, irrespective of specific information obtained from the history and physical examination. There are insufficient data to determine the benefit of routine laboratory testing before endoscopic procedures.[1] Most studies indicate that physicians overuse laboratory testing and that routine preoperative screening tests are usually unnecessary. In one large study, only 40% of preoperative tests were done for a recognizable indication, and less than 1% of the tests revealed abnormalities that would have potentially influenced perioperative management.[2] Moreover, no adverse events were attributable to the identified laboratory abnormalities. An evaluation of routine laboratory testing in the periendoscopic period should consider the frequency of abnormal test results within a given population, the accuracy of the tests, the risks of the planned procedure, the use of moderate sedation versus anesthesia, and whether an abnormal result will affect the decision

to perform endoscopy or alter periprocedural management or outcome. Individual patient and procedure risks should be factored into the decision to perform periendoscopic laboratory tests. The cost of screening and the expense of follow-up testing to evaluate often minor abnormalities that seldom improve patient care must also be considered. Furthermore, falsely abnormal test results may unnecessarily delay endoscopy and subject the patient to additional risks, with untoward health and economic consequences.

PREPARATION FOR ENDOSCOPY AND ENTEROSCOPY

Patients should not eat solid food for 6 to 8 hours or drink clear fluids for at 2 to 4 hours before an elective endoscopy.[3] If a delay in gastric emptying is known or suspected, longer fasting or a period of a fluid-only diet should be considered. Many centers use prokinetic agents to speed gastric emptying in patients when fasting time is inadequate (see subsequent section on special circumstances). In situations in which there is a delay in gastric emptying or in which there is inadequate fasting time, there is a significant risk of pulmonary aspiration, and airway protection with airway intubation should be considered. Normally, it is acceptable for patients to take their usual medicines with a sip of water before endoscopy. Special consideration must be given to patients taking anticoagulant medication or medication to treat diabetes (see subsequent section on Special Circumstances).

If a bleeding disorder is suspected or known, tests to evaluate this and direct therapy are indicated. Similarly, if the patient's clinical condition is unstable or indicates that an abnormality in the blood tests is likely to be present, appropriate testing and correction of relevant abnormalities is indicated. Preparation for antegrade enteroscopy is the same as described earlier. If retrograde enteroscopy is to be performed, preparation requirements are the same as for colonoscopy.

PREPARATION FOR ENDOSCOPIC RETROGRADE CHOLANGIOPANCREATOGRAPHY

The preparation of patients for endoscopic retrograde cholangiopancreatography (ERCP) is similar to the preparation for endoscopy.[3] Generally, patients undergoing ERCP almost always require sedation and the duration of the procedure is longer; this should be taken into account for purposes of discharge planning. Patients with suspected or proven biliary or pancreatic duct obstruction are generally given prophylactic intravenous antibiotics if there is a clinical suspicion of inadequate duct drainage (Table 8.1). Antibiotics may also be given in patients with sclerosing cholangitis and in patients after liver transplantation. Before ERCP, it is important to determine if the patient has a known history of reaction to iodinated contrast agents. Although reaction to the contrast agent in allergic patients during ERCP is rare, it is generally considered appropriate to administer prophylactic steroids, often in combination with an intravenous antihistamine agent. In severe cases, enlisting support of an anesthetist in case of a reaction is a prudent precaution. The use of a noniodinated contrast agent is an additional strategy.

Because ERCP is performed with radiologic imaging of the abdomen, patients who have had recent barium studies or other oral contrast agents should be checked to ensure that the field of view is clear for the ERCP to be successfully completed. If there is residual contrast material in the gut, a formal bowel

TABLE 8.1   Antibiotic Prophylaxis and/or Treatment to Prevent Local Infections

Patient Condition	Procedure	Need for Antibiotic Prophylaxis	Goal of Antibiotic Prophylaxis
Biliary obstruction without cholangitis	ERCP with complete drainage ERCP with incomplete drainage	Not recommended Recommended, continue antibiotics after procedure	Not applicable (NA) Prevention of cholangitis
Solid lesion in the upper and lower GI tract	EUS-fine-needle biopsy	Not recommended	NA
Cystic lesion in mediastinum or pancreas	EUS-fine-needle aspiration	Suggested	Prevention of cyst infection
All patients	PEG or PEJ insertion	Recommended	Prevention of peri-stomal infection
Cirrhosis with acute GI bleeding	All patients, regardless of the nature of endoscopic procedure	Recommended on admission	Prevention of infectious events and reduction of mortality
Synthetic vascular graft and other nonvalvular cardiovascular devices	Any endoscopic procedures	Not recommended	NA
Prosthetic joints	Any endoscopic procedures	Not recommended	NA
Peritoneal dialysis	Lower GI endoscopy	Suggested	Prevention of peritonitis
Solid malignancy of upper GI tract	EUS guided fiducial insertion	Suggested	Prevent seeding infection at insertion site

ERCP, endoscopic retrograde cholangiopancreatography; *EUS,* endoscopic ultrasound; *GI,* gastrointestinal; *PEG,* percutaneous endoscopic gastrostomy; *PEJ,* percutaneous endoscopic jejunostomy.
Adapted from ASGE Standards of Practice Committee, Khashab MA, Chithadi KV, et al: Antibiotic prophylaxis for GI endoscopy. *Gastrointest Endosc* 81(1):81–89, 2015.

preparation may be required. Women of childbearing age must be asked if they are pregnant. If there is uncertainty, the ERCP may need to be deferred until a pregnancy test can be done. If ERCP is considered necessary in a pregnant woman, appropriate lead shielding of the lower abdomen is recommended to protect the fetus. Similarly, pelvic shielding is appropriate for any premenopausal woman.

No data support routine blood tests before diagnostic ERCP, and screening tests are generally not required. If a bleeding disorder is suspected or known, tests to evaluate this and direct therapy are indicated. Similarly, if the patient's clinical condition is unstable or indicates that an abnormality in the blood tests is likely to be present, appropriate testing and correction of relevant abnormalities is indicated. In patients presenting for ERCP with a history or signs of biliary obstruction, the possibility of disordered coagulation exists. Correction of this type of abnormality before the procedure is appropriate.

The European Society of Gastrointestinal Endoscopy now recommends routine rectal administration of 100 mg of diclofenac or indomethacin immediately before (or after) in all patients without contraindication to the medication.[4]

PREPARATION FOR COLONOSCOPY

Of all endoscopic procedures, the quality of the preparation before colonoscopy has the greatest effect on the outcome of the procedure.[3] The preparation is often regarded as the most unpleasant part of colonoscopy, and many patients are more concerned about this aspect than having the procedure performed. It is vital that the patient be given detailed verbal and written instructions to complete the preparation safely. If the correct preparation is not followed, the procedure usually has to be deferred. Good bowel preparation is essential to provide an optimal view for colonic examination and to minimize the risk of colonic trauma during the procedure resulting from a poor view. The method of administration and types of bowel preparation are discussed in detail in the next chapter (Chapter 9).

To achieve an optimal preparation, a careful patient assessment is needed to determine which bowel cleansing agent should be used and what modifications to the patient's diet and regular medications are required. The addition of simethicone to the bowel preparation does not improve cleansing but does reduce bubbles, which may improve the endoscopic view.[5] As part of the preparation, most patients are advised to have only a clear liquid diet for 24 hours before the examination.[3] Routine blood testing before colonoscopy is not required. Management of patients taking antiplatelet and anticoagulation medications should be carefully considered before the examination to minimize the risk of procedure-related bleeding (see later guidelines). In addition, any medication that might be associated with constipation should be temporarily stopped to facilitate the bowel cleansing process. In particular, oral iron can make the stool black and viscous, and iron should be stopped at least 5 days before the colonoscopy.[3] Last, specific instructions should be given to diabetic patients who are taking oral hypoglycemic medications or insulin to avoid periprocedural hypoglycemia.

Intravenous sedation is administered to most patients who undergo colonoscopy. It is necessary for the patient to fast before the procedure to reduce the potential for aspiration. The duration of fasting can be comparatively brief because the patient will have been on clear fluids only for 24 hours before the procedure while undergoing bowel preparation. A fasting time of 2 to 4 hours is generally considered adequate.

There are many independent predictors for a potential inadequate bowel preparation, such as a late colonoscopy start time; failure to follow preparation instructions; inpatient status; procedural indication of constipation; use of drugs that impair gut motility (e.g., tricyclic antidepressants, calcium channel blockers, iron); male gender; and a history of cirrhosis, stroke, dementia, obesity, or diabetes mellitus.[6-9] A prior history of failed colonoscopy preparation is also highly predictive of a failed second or subsequent attempt at preparation.[10] In these various patient groups, a more prolonged bowel preparation may be required. Other options to improve the quality of the preparation include abstinence from dietary fat for 1 week and a morning procedure time. In patients who develop nausea, vomiting, or excessive bloating and patients who do not tolerate the preparation, one of the following measures can be used:

- Stop the preparation early if a clear fecal fluid output is achieved
- Interrupt the preparation temporarily for 1 to 2 hours and then resume
- Use a trial dose of metoclopramide or another prokinetic agent
- Chill the bowel preparation solution (very cold solution is not recommended)
- Add clear, sugar-free flavor enhancers or lemon juice (avoid red colors)
- Slow the rate of consumption of the solution

PREPARATION FOR FLEXIBLE SIGMOIDOSCOPY

Preparation before flexible sigmoidoscopy generally requires cleansing of only the left colon.[3] In most cases, this cleansing can be achieved by administering one or two enemas 1 hour before the procedure. Several types of enemas are available:

- Microlax enema (sodium citrate 450 mg, sodium lauryl sulfoacetate 45 mg, and sorbitol 3.125 g)
- Fleet enema (sodium phosphate)
- Tap water enema
- G&O enema (three parts glycerin, three parts olive oil, and three parts water)

A more extensive bowel preparation may be required in severely constipated patients or in patients in whom a therapeutic procedure is required, such as polypectomy or argon plasma coagulation therapy. In these cases, 2 L of polyethylene glycol (PEG)-based bowel preparation with 24 hours of clear fluid may be adequate. In contrast, bowel preparation may be unnecessary in patients with active colitis or watery diarrhea. Generally, patients undergoing flexible sigmoidoscopy do not require intravenous sedation. If sedation is required, the patient should be advised to follow a protocol similar to other endoscopic procedures requiring sedation.

PREPARATION FOR ENDOSCOPIC ULTRASOUND

Patient preparation for endoscopic ultrasound (EUS), including the dietary guidelines, is similar to preparation for upper gastrointestinal (GI) endoscopy.[3] In patients in whom a biopsy or therapeutic intervention is considered necessary, a platelet count and coagulation studies may be appropriate before the procedure if a bleeding disorder is suspected. In addition, antiplatelet and anticoagulation therapies must be reviewed, and if EUS-guided biopsy is likely to be performed, appropriate modification or cessation of these agents is necessary given that EUS-fine-needle aspiration (FNA) is a high-risk procedure for bleeding (see later discussion). Diagnostic EUS is considered a low-risk procedure and thus antiplatelet and anticoagulation therapies can be continued. For those who are on double-antiplatelet therapy for coronary stent(s), EUS-FNA can be performed with cessation of clopidogrel but continuation of aspirin. A 2017 retrospective study indicated that the risk of bleeding in patients who underwent EUS-FNA while on aspirin was not significantly higher than those without aspirin use (1.6% vs. 1.0%).[11]

Antibiotic prophylaxis is not generally required unless FNA of a cystic lesion or fiducial insertion is being performed (see Table 8.1). FNA of cystic lesions is considered high risk for

infection, and antibiotics are recommended. Available limited data indicated that the risk of infection after fiducial placement varies between 0.6% and 1.6%.[12,13] Given the inability to remove these markers after implantation, antibiotic prophylaxis is generally recommended and adopted by most centers.[14] In contrast, FNA of solid lesions in the upper GI tract[15,16] or in the lower GI tract[17] has been shown to be a low-risk procedure and does not warrant antibiotic prophylaxis. The use of antibiotic prophylaxis in EUS-guided celiac plexus block or neurolysis has not been established, as infectious complications after this procedure are rare.[18]

PREPARATION FOR CAPSULE ENDOSCOPY

Optimizing conditions for capsule endoscopy continues to be an area of interest. Most centers prefer a slightly longer fasting time than for routine endoscopy. Generally, clear fluids are given after lunch on the day before the examination, and the patient fasts for 12 hours before the examination is scheduled to begin. No medication should be taken within 2 hours of ingestion of the capsule. In some centers, 2 L of a PEG-based bowel preparation regimen is given before the patient begins the 12-hour fast.[19,20] This additional step might be particularly important if the patient has had a recent barium study or has had some other form of oral radiologic contrast agent. Some units ask the patient to ingest a small amount of simethicone preparation before the procedure to improve visual quality, as well as a prokinetic such as metoclopramide.[21] The use of a purgative preparation may improve the quality of the small bowel images obtained during the capsule endoscopy study and increase the diagnostic yield.[22] This benefit has not been confirmed in other studies. The purgative preparation does not seem to influence completion rate of the study, however. The optimal preparation regimen is not yet established, so instructions may be individualized for the patient. It is prudent to review the patient's medications and consider withholding any medication that might slow GI motility. Iron supplements should be stopped at least 3 days before the examination.

PREPARATION FOR ENDOSCOPIC PROCEDURES IN PATIENTS WITH DIABETES

There are no controlled trials to guide preparation for endoscopic procedures in diabetic patients.[3] The approach to these patients must be individualized, and factors such as usual glycemic control and the patient's ability to manage his or her diabetes are important considerations. There are no specific requirements in diabetic patients who are controlled on diet alone. In patients taking oral hypoglycemic agents, medications are generally withheld during preparation for the procedure. During this time, the patient must monitor his or her serum glucose and be able to manage or get assistance if there is evidence of progressive hyperglycemia. Hypoglycemia is managed with sugar-containing clear fluids or candy. In patients taking insulin, dose reduction while undergoing the preparation is normal. For upper GI procedures, the usual dose may be given the evening before the procedure, but only half the dose is given on the morning of the examination. The remaining dose can be given, if appropriate, after the procedure has been completed.

Insulin-dependent diabetics undergoing preparation for colonoscopy should have their diabetic treatment individually modified with clear instructions provided as to how hypoglycemia and hyperglycemia should be managed. Diabetic patients should preferentially be scheduled for a morning procedure and ideally be the first case for the day. During the preparation, the patient must be advised to monitor serum glucose regularly. Patients with brittle diabetic control, patients unable to manage hypoglycemia or hyperglycemia, and patients with significant other comorbidity may need medical or nursing supervision during bowel preparation.

SPECIAL CIRCUMSTANCES

Preparation for Endoscopy in Case of Ingestion of a Foreign Body or for Food Bolus Obstruction

Ingestion of foreign bodies occurs mainly in children and mentally disabled patients. Food bolus obstruction is relatively common in adults, particularly with the increasing incidence of eosinophilic esophagitis.[23,24] Endoscopic assessment and removal is the main modality of treatment for objects below the level of the cricopharyngeal muscle. The nature of the patient's symptoms and what has been ingested determines the urgency of the procedure. Emergency procedures should be performed for patients who are unable to swallow their saliva, patients with sharp objects (e.g., fish bones, pins, dentures, razor blades), and patients with impacted disk batteries.[24,25] The procedure is probably technically easier if performed early. Plain x-rays of the chest and neck may be advisable before the endoscopic procedure if the nature of the object or the site of obstruction is unclear from the history. The x-ray film may also show ectopic gas patterns to indicate a silent perforation. Oral radiologic contrast material is generally best avoided because of the risk of aspiration and because it may obscure the endoscopic field.[26,27]

With regard to food bolus impaction, glucagon or another prokinetic can be given while the patient is waiting for endoscopy, but this is usually unsuccessful and should not delay endoscopy.[28,29] Special attention should be given to airway protection to avoid the risk of airway obstruction during the procedure. Continuous oral suction and the availability of a laryngoscope are also important. General anesthesia with endotracheal intubation is usually required if airway protection is needed. Whereas the literature suggests that airway intubation is required in less than 25% of cases,[30] it is probably performed more frequently than not in modern endoscopic units and is probably a prudent precaution. An alternative strategy to protect the airway is the use of an esophageal overtube, but this should be used with caution due to the risk of perforation. General anesthesia with muscle relaxation often facilitates removal of difficult or large items, particularly as they pass through the upper esophageal sphincter; this is particularly true for swallowed dentures (see Chapter 22).

Preparation for Endoscopy in Patients With Upper Gastrointestinal Bleeding

Preparation of an acutely bleeding patient for endoscopy requires additional precautions and care. The first step is to ensure that the patient is adequately resuscitated because any subsequent endoscopy is best performed when the patient is hemodynamically stable. Volume replacement and correction of any coagulation or platelet function disturbance are important. If there is evidence of ongoing bleeding, urgent endoscopy with airway protection, even in an unstable patient, may be the best way of getting better clinical control of the situation. If time permits, a 6-hour fast is desirable because this would improve the endoscopic view.

However, a fast is often not practical, particularly if there is evidence of active bleeding. Sometimes gastric lavage can be used to empty the stomach of blood before endoscopy is performed. Care must be taken not to suck too aggressively with the gastric lavage tube because significant mucosal trauma can occur, and this can make interpretation of the subsequent endoscopic findings difficult. Available data, including from a randomized, placebo-controlled study, have demonstrated the benefit of an intravenous dose of erythromycin given 2 hours before endoscopy to improve endoscopic view in patients with upper gastrointestinal bleeding.[31] Three meta-analyses have also concluded that the administration of intravenous erythromycin is beneficial in this situation.[32-34]

Endoscopy in patients with upper GI bleeding is usually performed after the patient has received intravenous sedation.[35] General anesthesia and endotracheal intubation should be considered in patients with active hematemesis or if there is a perceived increased risk of aspiration. If the patient is suspected of having a bleeding peptic ulcer, an intravenous proton pump inhibitor (PPI) should be given before the endoscopy. Studies have suggested that a PPI can significantly improve outcome in these patients.[36-39] Similarly, patients suspected of having variceal bleeding may benefit from an octreotide or terlipressin infusion[40-42] (see Chapter 15). Patients who present with suspected variceal bleeding due to known chronic liver disease should receive preprocedure intravenous antibiotics (see subsequent section on antibiotic prophylaxis).

Preparation for Colonoscopy in Patients With Lower Gastrointestinal Bleeding

In patients with lower GI bleeding, colonoscopy is the procedure of choice to identify the site of bleeding and, in some circumstances, allows therapeutic intervention (see Chapter 16).[43] Before the procedure, patients should be resuscitated, and their general condition should be stabilized. Routine blood tests and coagulation profiles are generally performed in patients with upper GI bleeding, and these should be corrected if abnormal. Generally, colonoscopies in patients with lower GI bleeding are performed on a semi-urgent basis, and when the patient is hemodynamically stable to allow time for some form of bowel preparation. The view at colonoscopy if the patient is actively bleeding is often a problem in procedures performed urgently, although some studies suggest that urgent colonoscopy is not only technically possible and safe but also effective in controlling bleeding.[44,45] Blood itself is a cathartic; some clinicians perform the procedure in an unprepared bowel.[46] Other clinicians preferring a bowel preparation generally give 4 L of PEG over 4 hours before the procedure.[3,44,47,48] This solution can be given orally or via a nasogastric tube. In elective procedures, the colon can be prepared in a standard fashion. Because these patients are at higher risk of a disturbance of intravascular volume, it is generally advisable to avoid sodium phosphate–based preparations. A prokinetic agent may facilitate the bowel preparation. In general, patients should not have barium studies before colonoscopy because it would interfere with the view and may obscure flat mucosal lesions such as angiodysplasia. If an obstructive lesion is suspected, a clear water-soluble contrast agent such as Gastrografin should be used.

Antiplatelet and Anticoagulation Therapy

Endoscopic procedures are being performed more frequently in patients who are receiving antiplatelet and/or anticoagulant

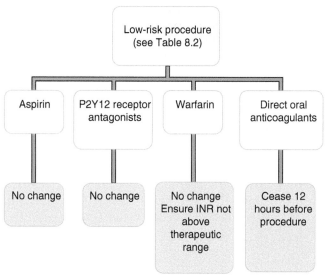

FIG 8.1 Low-Risk Endoscopic Procedure. *INR*, international normalized ratio.

TABLE 8.2 Endoscopic Procedures Considered to Be at Low- and High-Risk of Bleeding	
Low Risk	**High Risk**
Diagnostic procedures ± biopsy	Polypectomy
ERCP without sphincterotomy	ERCP with sphincterotomy/ ampullectomy
Biliary or pancreatic stenting	Dilation of strictures
Diagnostic EUS	Therapy of varices
Enteroscopy	PEG or PEJ insertion
Argon plasma coagulation	EMR/ESD
Barrett's ablation therapy	EUS with FNA
	Esophageal/enteral/colonic stent (controversial)
	Cystogastrostomy

EMR, endoscopic mucosal resection; *ERCP*, endoscopic retrograde cholangiopancreatography; *ESD*, endoscopic submucosal dissection; *EUS*, endoscopic ultrasound; *FNA*, fine needle aspiration; *PEG*, percutaneous endoscopic gastrostomy; *PEJ*, Percutaneous endoscopic jejunostomy (direct).

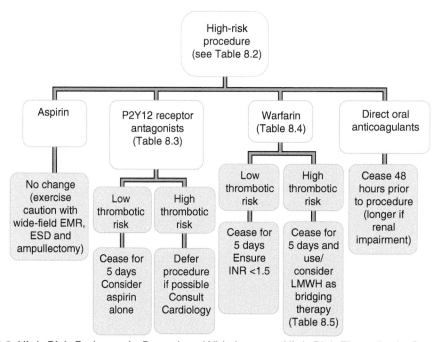

FIG 8.2 High-Risk Endoscopic Procedure With Low- or High-Risk Thrombotic Condition. *EMR*, endoscopic mucosal resection; *ESD*, endoscopic submucosal dissection; *INR*, international normalized ratio; *LMWH*, low molecular weight heparin.

therapy. Management of these patients and their medications in the periprocedural period requires clinical judgement and an understanding of risks involved; the latter includes both the risks of hemorrhage when performing endoscopic procedures on antiplatelet or anticoagulant therapy and the risks of thromboembolism and other adverse events when ceasing these medications (Figs. 8.1 and 8.2). Patients will need an individualized assessment, and it is not possible to give guidance to cover all situations.

All endoscopic procedures have an inherent risk of bleeding. Minor bleeding is common; however, clinically relevant bleeding, defined as bleeding requiring specific intervention, unplanned

admission to hospital, or blood transfusion, should be rare. Traditionally, procedures have been divided into those at low and high risk for hemorrhage (Table 8.2).[49,50] The risk of thromboembolism from conditions treated by antiplatelet agents is summarized in Table 8.3 and from conditions treated by warfarin are summarized in Table 8.4. Both these aspects need to be considered before a decision is made to cease antiplatelet or anticoagulant medication. In some high-risk situations, these medications cannot be ceased without very significant consequences. The recommendations made in this chapter are in keeping with the 2016 guidelines from the American Society for Gastrointestinal Endoscopy (ASGE),[49] the British Society of

TABLE 8.3 Low- and High-Risk Conditions for Ceasing Clopidogrel

Low Risk	High Risk
Ischemic heart disease without stent	Bare metal stent (within 1 month)
Cerebrovascular disease	Drug-eluting stent (within 12 months)
Peripheral vascular disease	

TABLE 8.4 Low- and High-Risk Conditions for Ceasing Warfarin

Low Risk	High Risk
Prosthetic (metal) aortic valve	Prosthetic (metal) mitral valve
Prosthetic (xenograft) valve	Prosthetic (metal) valve and AF or prior thromboembolic event
AF without valvular heart disease	AF and valvular heart disease (especially mitral stenosis)
Over 3 months since VTE	Under three months since VTE
Thrombophilia syndromes	

AF, atrial fibrillation; *VTE,* venous thromboembolic event.

Gastroenterology, and the European Society of Gastrointestinal Endoscopy.[50]

RISK STRATIFICATION

For all endoscopic procedures there is a risk of intraprocedure or postprocedure bleeding. Many patients who present for elective endoscopic procedures are taking antithrombotic therapy to reduce the risk of thromboembolic events associated with conditions such as atrial fibrillation, acute coronary syndromes, deep vein thrombosis (DVT), hypercoagulable states, endoprostheses, etc. Recent guidelines summarized in this document consider the risk of bleeding from an endoscopic intervention versus the risks of antithrombotic drug cessation. The recommendations are mostly supported by clinical evidence, but in some cases only expert opinion is available to provide a best guess on the risk analysis of bleeding versus thrombosis. Many experts also recognize that bleeding is rarely fatal whereas the consequences of a major thromboembolic event can have very serious and lifelong effects on the patient. When considering discontinuing antithrombotic therapy, it is crucial to consider patient preference in addition to clinical opinion. A postpolypectomy hemorrhage might be considered a better outcome than a major CVA with permanent disability from the patient's perspective.

Bleeding: Low-Risk Procedures

These are generally diagnostic procedures with or without biopsy (see Table 8.2). ERCP without sphincterotomy but with stent insertion, argon plasma coagulation, and Barrett's ablation therapy are also categorized as low-risk procedures. Aspirin does not increase the risk of clinically significant bleeding following low-risk endoscopic procedures, and thus can be continued (see Fig. 8.1). Data regarding the bleeding risk during low-risk endoscopic procedures when patients are on P2Y12 receptor antagonists (clopidogrel, prasugrel, ticagrelor, ticlopidine) are limited. The

previous recommendations of stopping P2Y12 receptor antagonists for low-risk procedures were based indirectly on data derived from surgical procedures (see Fig. 8.1). It remains common practice in patients taking dual antiplatelet agents to consider continuing aspirin and ceasing the P2Y12 receptor antagonist in the periprocedural period. In a systematic review of 161 reported cases of late drug-eluting stent thrombosis (> 30 days but < 1 year after stent placement) and very late drug-eluting stent thrombosis (> 1 year after stent placement), patients who discontinued both aspirin and a P2Y12 receptor antagonist had a median time to event of 7 days. In those who discontinued P2Y12 receptor antagonist but remained on aspirin, the median time to an event was 122 days. There were a total of six cases (6%) of stent thrombosis within 10 days of P2Y12 receptor antagonist cessation, suggesting that short-term discontinuation between 30 days and 1 year from drug-eluting coronary stent placement (late stent thrombosis) might be relatively safe but still carry some risk. The British and European guidelines more definitively state that P2Y12 receptor antagonists can be continued for low-risk procedures.

There are no data regarding bleeding risk in patients on low molecular weight heparin (LMWH) undergoing low-risk procedures. Decision making should therefore be individualized. For low-risk procedures, it can probably be continued (see Fig. 8.1).[51] Similarly, patients taking warfarin can continue their medication for low-risk procedures, providing the international normalized ratio (INR) is in the therapeutic range. The data to support this recommendation are, however, weak.

Advice on the use of direct oral anticoagulants (DOACs), such as dabigatran, rivaroxaban, and apixaban during low-risk procedures is difficult. Given these new anticoagulants do not need blood monitoring for their therapeutic range, they are increasingly used for prevention of: (1) venous thromboembolic events after major orthopedic surgery (hip and knee replacement); (2) stroke and systemic embolus in nonvalvular atrial fibrillation; and (3) DVT/pulmonary embolism recurrence. Clinicians should be cautious, as the degree of anticoagulation cannot be assessed, and the availability of reversal agent(s) are currently limited. In general, the peak anticoagulant effect of DOACs is between 2 and 6 hours after oral ingestion; this is prolonged in patients with renal impairment.[49] This is because DOACs, especially dabigatran, are cleared predominantly by the kidneys. Dabigatran also has limited bioavailability, and high concentrations of the drug may be found in the stool. This may cause a local bowel wall effect and account for reports of increased risk of lower GI bleeding in some studies. Given these factors, the general advice is to omit DOACs on the morning of a low-risk procedure[49] (see Fig. 8.1).

Bleeding: High-Risk Procedures

Aspirin does not increase the risk of clinically significant bleeding following high-risk endoscopic procedures, including procedures like colonic polypectomy and biliary sphincterotomy (see Fig. 8.2). Cold snare polypectomy is associated with less delayed bleeding than diathermy-assisted polypectomy and may be a preferred resection technique where possible in patients taking aspirin. Advice regarding aspirin and wide-field endoscopic mucosal resection (EMR) or endoscopic submucosal dissection (ESD) is still not clear, and data are not conclusive. Similarly, the use of aspirin in patients undergoing ampullectomy should be cautious, as the risk of bleeding is significant, and informed consent is important.

P2Y12 receptor antagonists should be stopped for 5 days in patients undergoing a high-risk procedure who are considered at low thrombotic risk (see Fig. 8.2). As for low-risk procedures, it is recommended for patients taking dual antiplatelet agents to consider continuing aspirin and stopping the P2Y12 receptor antagonist 5 days prior to the procedure. There are recent data in a small number of patients showing an excessive bleeding risk when transbronchial lung biopsies are taken while patients are on clopidogrel (3.4% vs. 89%).[49–51] The risk of bleeding after transbronchial biopsy is not increased in patients taking aspirin. The latter finding is similar to the endoscopic data and, by extrapolation, clopidogrel should be used with great caution in patients undergoing high-risk procedures. If the thrombotic risk is high, then the procedure should be deferred, or, if not possible, bridging therapy with LMWH should be considered.

A significant risk of hemorrhage exists when high-risk endoscopic procedures are performed on patients taking warfarin. Published data in this area are limited given that anticoagulation is generally avoided when high-risk procedures are performed; however, one study did show a high rate of bleeding when colonic polypectomy was performed with patients on warfarin (0.8% vs. 10.8%; odds ratio [OR] 13.37).[49,50] There are also data showing a high risk (10% to 15%) of significant bleeding when performing an ERCP with sphincterotomy in patients where warfarin is restarted within 72 hours.[49] Guidelines suggest cessation of warfarin 5 days prior to a high-risk procedure allowing the INR to drift back to normal during this time (see Fig. 8.2). The INR preprocedure should be less than 1.5.[49,50] If the procedure is uneventful and the risk of postprocedure bleeding is considered low, the warfarin can be restarted immediately after the procedure. In patients with a high thrombotic risk, warfarin should be ceased and bridging therapy be given using a LMWH, which should be stopped 12 hours prior to the procedure. All patients should be advised that there is an increased risk of postprocedure hemorrhage compared to nonanticoagulated patients.

In patients who are taking DOACs and undergoing high-risk procedures, the DOACs should be ceased 48 hours prior to the endoscopic procedure[49,50] (see Fig. 8.2). For patients with impaired renal function, the drug should be stopped 72 hours prior to the procedure. In those who are still on the DOACs and require an emergency procedure, urgent consultation with a hematologist is essential.

Postprocedure Therapy Resumption

If antithrombotic therapy is stopped prior to a procedure, then it is recommended the therapy be resumed within 24 to 48 hours after the procedure depending on the perceived bleeding and thrombotic risks.

Risk of Thromboembolism

Extreme care must be taken in discontinuation of antiplatelet therapy for endoscopy in patients who have a cardiac stent, as the risk of coronary stent thrombosis can be as high as 29%, leading to myocardial infarction with a significant risk of death.[49,50] The risks apply to both bare metal and drug-eluting stents, but the period for which most risk is present differs. Clopidogrel should preferably not be stopped for at least 1 month after insertion of a bare metal stent. When clopidogrel is prescribed following placement of a drug-eluting stent, cessation of therapy should be discussed with the patient's cardiologist. In general, antiplatelet therapy (usually dual therapy) should not be stopped within 12 months. If clopidogrel is to be ceased, the duration

should be less than 7 days, and, in most cases, aspirin should be continued.

Cessation of warfarin results in varying risks of thromboembolism, depending on the underlying condition (see Table 8.4). The highest risk exists for conditions such as prosthetic heart valves and atrial fibrillation (AF) with high risk features; there is a risk of thromboembolism (3.6%) in these situations despite bridging therapy with LMWH. The risk of thromboembolism in patients undergoing endoscopy who have their anticoagulation adjusted for the procedure, ranges from 0.31% to 2.93%. The risk of thromboembolism in AF without anticoagulation ranges from 1.9% to 18.2% depending on concomitant risk factors.[49,50] The risk of discontinuing warfarin in the setting of treatment for venous thromboembolism is probably low, particularly if more than 3 months have passed since the event.

Given that DOACs are frequently used for low-risk thrombotic conditions, they can be safely stopped prior to high-risk endoscopic procedures without bridging therapy. If these drugs are prescribed for conditions outside these indications, individual consideration is needed in consultation with the prescriber of the relevant agent.

Bridging Therapy (Table 8.5)

In patients with nonvalvular AF, bridging with LMWH is not required. In a 2015 large randomized controlled trial that examined the role of bridging therapy with heparin for endoscopic procedure in AF patients, bridging therapy was associated with an increased risk of major bleeding events (3.2% vs. 1.3% [placebo]) and a similar rate of thrombotic events (0.3% vs. 0.4%).[52] Thus, in uncomplicated AF, bridging therapy is not necessary. The proportion of high-risk AF patients, such as those with concomitant mitral stenosis or high CHADS2 (congestive heart failure, hypertension, age ≥ 75 years, diabetes mellitus, stroke [double weight]) score was small; therefore, a firm recommendation on no bridging therapy in these patients cannot be made and consultation with a cardiologist is recommended. In contrast, bridging therapy is usually required for patients with

TABLE 8.5 Approach to Bridge Therapy for Warfarin		
Condition	**Associated Diagnosis**	**Management**
Atrial fibrillation	None CHA2DS2-VASc score < 2	No bridge recommended
	Mechanical valves/mitral stenosis History of CVA CHA2DS2-VASc score ≥ 2	Consider bridge therapy
Valvular heart disease	Bileaflet mechanical AVR	No bridge recommended
	Mechanical AVR and any thromboembolic risk factor Older generation mechanical AVR Mechanical mitral valve	Bridge therapy recommended

CHA2DS2-VASc = congestive heart failure, hypertension, age > 75 years [2 points], diabetes mellitus, stroke [2 points], vascular disease, age 65–74 years, sex category [i.e., female sex].
AF, atrial fibrillation; *AVR,* aortic valve replacement; *CVA,* cerebral vascular accident.
Adapted from ASGE Standards of Practice Committee, Acosta RD, Abraham NS, et al: The management of antithrombotic agents for patients undergoing GI endoscopy. *Gastrointest Endosc* 83(1):3–16, 2016.

metal heart valves and appears safe and effective for this indication. Some patients with newer metal aortic valves may not require bridging therapy. In patients with a thrombophilia, the risk of thrombotic events after temporary cessation of anticoagulation therapy is minimal and bridging is therefore not required. Thrombophilia syndromes have been recently reclassified as low-risk conditions, especially factor V Leiden and F2G20210A thrombotic mutation. Even in patients with deficiencies of antithrombin and protein C or S, who are at a higher risk of thrombosis, bridging is not required in most cases.

Endoscopy Procedures in a Bleeding Patient on Antithrombotic Therapy

In general, performing endoscopic procedures in an acutely bleeding patient taking antithrombotic therapy is reasonable and safe. Patients taking antiplatelet agents who bleed can be given a platelet transfusion. Once bleeding is controlled, then the antiplatelet therapy can resume. Data suggests that for patients who develop bleeding from aspirin-related peptic ulcer disease, resumption of aspirin with concurrent PPI therapy is better than switching to clopidogrel alone for prevention of recurrent bleeding. Prompt resumption of antiplatelet therapy after cessation of bleeding is crucial, as the risk of rebleeding is not significantly increased, but there is a clear increase in 30-day mortality in patients where antiplatelet therapy was not restarted.

In patients taking warfarin, reversal of the INR to a range of 2.5 or less allows successful intervention and outcomes comparable to nonanticoagulated patients. Preprocedure INR does not appear to correlate with procedure outcome in various studies. The Rockall and Glasgow-Blatchford scores assessing rebleeding risk or outcome do not include INR in their calculations. The predominant clinical concern is how best to correct the thrombotic defect and how to balance this reversal against the preexisting thrombotic risks. In general, plasma products, platelet transfusions, clotting factors, and vitamin K have all been used to reverse antithrombotic agent effects. Which product to use and how aggressive therapy is given will depend on the severity of bleeding and the thrombotic risk, as well as consideration of how best to resume antithrombotic therapy once bleeding has been controlled.

In the event of massive bleeding in patients taking the DOACs, hemodialysis can be used. In clinical practice, however, such an unstable patient is unlikely to be able to tolerate hemodialysis. Urgent hematology review is recommended, and often clotting factors are used but their effectiveness is uncertain. Specific monoclonal antibodies have been developed as antidotes for the DOAC agents and can reverse the anticoagulant effects within minutes. At present, idarucizumab, a monoclonal antibody against dabigatran, is available for use in the United States and Europe, but not currently in Asia-Pacific regions. Antidotes to other DOAC agents are under development and the results of clinical trials are eagerly awaited.

Management of Disorders of Hemostasis Before Endoscopic Examinations

Management of patients with hemostasis disorders should be individualized and when possible should be in close collaboration with an experienced hematologist in a specialized center with a specialist coagulation laboratory. The endoscopist must assess the risk of bleeding based on the procedural risk and the severity of the underlying disorder of hemostasis and plan the endoscopic procedure accordingly.[52]

Von Willebrand's Disease

von Willebrand's disease (vWD) is the most common inherited disorder of hemostasis; therapy before endoscopic procedures depends on the type of vWD. For less severe type I disease, treatment with desmopressin (DDAVP) starting 1 hour before the procedure and once daily thereafter for 2 to 3 days is adequate for patients undergoing diagnostic procedures and mucosal biopsies. However, for therapeutic procedures, infusion of factor VIII 1 hour before the procedure to achieve a factor VIII activity of 0.80 to 1.20 U/mL is required. After the procedure, factor VIII activity of at least 0.30 to 0.50 U/mL must be maintained for up to 2 weeks to minimize the risk of rebleeding.[41] For more severe type II and type III disease, the same factor VIII replacement regimen is required for diagnostic (maintenance duration of 2 to 3 days) and therapeutic procedures (up to 2 weeks).[53]

Hemophilia A and B

Preprocedural assay of factor VIII or IX activity is essential to determine the dosage of replacement therapy in patients with hemophilia. Before the procedure, factor VIII infusion is required to achieve an activity of 0.80 to 1.20 U/mL. Postinfusion factor assay should be obtained to determine the patient's response to the infusion. For purely diagnostic procedures, no further infusion is required. If mucosal biopsies are performed, 75% of the initial dose should be given every 24 hours for an additional 2 to 3 days. If therapeutic procedures are performed, twice-daily factor VIII infusion is required to achieve a maintenance activity of 0.30 to 0.50 U/mL for up to 2 weeks. Adequate factor VIII maintenance activity must be confirmed by at least daily factor VIII assay. Indications for factor IX replacement are identical to the indications for factor VIII infusion except that the maintenance dose is administered at intervals of 24 hours because the half-life of factor IX is longer.[53]

Liver Disease

The possible hemostatic defects in patients with liver disease are coagulopathy and thrombocytopenia. Correction is usually not required for diagnostic endoscopic procedures, but most centers would consider correction if the INR is greater than 2.5. Correction is necessary if therapeutic maneuvers are needed. These recommendations are based on limited data. If high-risk procedures are done, correction of an INR to less than 1.5 is advisable[53]; this can be accomplished by a combination of fresh frozen plasma and vitamin K replacement. Correction of significant thrombocytopenia is discussed later under "Thrombocytopenia" subsection.

Renal Failure

The main hemostatic defect in patients with renal failure is an acquired qualitative platelet defect secondary to uremia. Bleeding complications in these patients undergoing renal biopsy, abdominal surgery, liver and bone biopsies, or tooth extraction are rare.[54] In addition, measurement of preprocedural bleeding time is not helpful because it does not predict outcome.[54] Platelet infusion is not routinely recommended, unless concurrent significant thrombocytopenia exists.[53] Because uremia is thought to be the cause of platelet dysfunction, dialysis with limited heparin shortly before high-risk procedures is recommended to reduce serum urea nitrogen to less than 50 to 75 mg/dL.[53,55]

Thrombocytopenia

There are no prospective data on the need for prophylactic platelet transfusion, and the following guidelines have been based on decision analysis.[53,56,57] Platelet transfusion to increase the platelet count to greater than 20×10^9 platelets/L is required for low-risk procedures, and a count greater than 50×10^9 platelets/L is required for high-risk therapeutic procedures. For patients with immune thrombocytopenia, elective procedures should be postponed until an appropriate improvement in platelet count (20 to 30×10^9 platelets/L) is observed with standard therapy. If endoscopic procedures cannot be postponed and immediate intervention is necessary, a platelet transfusion should be given just before the procedure.[53] If bleeding occurs after the procedure, further platelet transfusion should be given. Input from a hematologist is recommended if response to platelet transfusion is poor.[53]

ANTIBIOTIC PROPHYLAXIS

Although endoscopic procedures within the GI tract can be associated with bacteremia, clinically significant complications from the bacteremia are rare. There are, however, specific high-risk procedures and high-risk patient conditions for which it is considered appropriate to use prophylactic antibiotics (see Table 8.1; adapted from the 2015 ASGE guideline). The major high-risk procedures are esophageal dilation, sclerotherapy of varices, percutaneous endoscopic gastrostomy insertion, ERCP in patients who have an obstructed pancreaticobiliary tract, or those with inadequate duct drainage on completion of the procedure. High-risk patient factors that warrant specific consideration for antibiotic prophylaxis include patients with cirrhosis and ascites, patients with primary sclerosing cholangitis, and those with a preexisting immune-deficiency condition. The choice of antibiotic to be used in the previously listed circumstances is beyond the scope of this chapter. Local guidelines should be followed, and microbiologic advice should be sought if necessary. Recent positive cultures, if available, should be taken into account when deciding on antibiotic regimens. In addition, many institutions modify recommendations depending on whether the patient is an existing inpatient or presents to the hospital from the community. If local guidelines are not available, international guidelines from the British Society of Gastroenterology (2009)[58] or the American Society of Gastrointestinal Endoscopy (2015)[59] can be used.

Antibiotic Prophylaxis for Prevention of Infective Endocarditis

The practice of antibiotic prophylaxis in GI endoscopy to prevent infective endocarditis has previously been common. Antibiotic guidelines no longer recommend routine antibiotic prophylaxis for the prevention of infective endocarditis as has previously been suggested.[59] A consensus document has been published looking at the role of antibiotic prophylaxis for the prevention of infective endocarditis.[60] These guidelines were prepared in collaboration with many learned societies and advisory groups and have been broadly adopted internationally. The guidelines conclude that:

- Only an extremely small number of cases of infective endocarditis might be prevented by antibiotic prophylaxis.
- Antibiotic prophylaxis is not recommended based solely on an increased lifetime risk of acquisition of infective endocarditis.

- Administration of antibiotics solely to prevent endocarditis is not recommended for patients who undergo GI tract procedures.
- Antibiotic prophylaxis is reasonable only for patients with an underlying cardiac condition associated with the highest risk of an adverse outcome from infective endocarditis.

Antibiotic prophylaxis may be considered in very high-risk cardiac conditions. The cardiac conditions that are considered the highest risk for adverse outcome from endocarditis include the following:

- Prosthetic cardiac valve or prosthetic material used for cardiac valve repair
- Previous history of infective endocarditis
- Congenital heart disease
- Unrepaired cyanotic congenital heart disease, including palliative shunts and conduits
- Completely repaired congenital heart defect with prosthetic material or device during 6 months after the procedure
- Repaired congenital heart disease with residual defects at the site or adjacent to the site of a prosthetic patch or prosthetic device
- Cardiac transplant recipients who develop cardiac valvulopathy

The major ongoing challenge that exists with the introduction of these new guidelines is patient education, but, with time, patient acceptance is definitely increasing. Many patients remain anxious and require reassurance that their expected administration of antibiotics is no longer required.

If antibiotics are required, it is recommended that a single dose be given before the procedure. If the antibiotic inadvertently is not administered before the procedure, it may be given up to 2 hours after the procedure. The gut contains a wide variety of bacteria, but of these, Enterococci are the most likely to cause infective endocarditis. If an antibiotic is required for a high-risk patient, amoxicillin and ampicillin are the preferred agents for enterococcal coverage. Vancomycin (1 gm IV) may be used in patients who are allergic to penicillin. Vancomycin administration should be slow (maximum rate 10 mg/min) to avoid complications. If patients are already receiving antibiotics, a different class of agent should be chosen rather than increasing the dose of the existing treatment. Antibiotic prophylaxis is generally given intravenously. Intramuscular injections should be avoided in patients who are anticoagulated.

Antibiotic Prophylaxis for Patients With Vascular Grafts and Other Implanted Devices

It has been suggested that some delayed infections of orthopedic, neurosurgical, and other prostheses may be due to bacteremia associated with endoscopic procedures.[58] However, the risk from endoscopic procedures is negligible compared with other daily activities associated with bacteremia, such as chewing, or oral hygiene measures such as toothbrushing. Any benefit of antibiotics to cover these activities would be outweighed by the adverse effects. The British Society of Gastroenterology, the ASGE, and the American Society of Colon and Rectal Surgeons do not recommend the use of antibiotics before endoscopy in patients with orthopedic prostheses, central nervous system vascular shunts, vascular grafts or stents, penile prostheses, intraocular lenses, pacemakers, or local tissue augmentation materials.

Antibiotic Prophylaxis for Percutaneous Endoscopic Gastrostomy or Percutaneous Endoscopic Jejunostomy

A single dose of an appropriate antibiotic given 30 minutes before percutaneous endoscopic gastrostomy or jejunostomy insertion is routinely recommended for all patients who are not already receiving antibiotics because the risk of peristomal wound infection is significantly reduced.[58] However, for patients who are already receiving appropriate antibiotics, no additional prophylaxis may be required. Patients known to be colonized with multiple resistant organisms or patients who have been hospitalized for some time before percutaneous endoscopic gastrostomy or jejunostomy insertion and who are likely to be colonized with resistant organisms should receive antibiotic prophylaxis appropriate to cover multiple resistant organisms. Local guidelines should be followed when choosing the antibiotic before percutaneous endoscopic gastrostomy or jejunostomy insertion. The choice of drug should be carefully considered in patients who are allergic to penicillin.

Antibiotic Prophylaxis for Patients With Variceal Bleeding or Patients With Decompensated Liver Disease Who Develop Acute Gastrointestinal Bleeding

Prophylactic antibiotics in patients with variceal bleeding or in patients with decompensated liver disease who develop acute GI bleeding improves short-term survival and may be associated with a reduced risk of rebleeding.[58] It is recommended that patients receive antibiotics before endoscopy. The choice of antibiotics is determined by local guidelines, but ceftriaxone is frequently used.

Antibiotic Prophylaxis for Patients With Neutropenia or Who Are Immunocompromised

Neutropenia ($< 0.5 \times 10^9$/L) predisposes patients to sepsis after procedures such as endoscopy, but the level of risk is unclear.[57] Patients who are febrile should already be treated with empiric antibiotics according to local hematology guidelines. In afebrile patients, antibiotic prophylaxis should be offered for high-risk procedures such as sclerotherapy, esophageal dilation, or ERCP with duct obstruction. Gram-negative aerobic and, less frequently, anaerobic organisms are likely pathogens, and the choice of antibiotic should reflect local sensitivities. No data support the use of prophylactic antibiotics in patients who have a normal neutrophil count but who are nonetheless immunocompromised (e.g., organ transplants). Routine antibiotic prophylaxis is not recommended in patients with human immunodeficiency virus (HIV) infection.

KEY REFERENCES

1. ASGE Standards of Practice Committee, Pasha SF, Acosta R, et al: Routine laboratory testing before endoscopic procedures, *Gastrointest Endosc* 80:28–33, 2014.
4. Dumonceau JM, Andriulli A, Elmunzer BJ, et al: Prophylaxis of post-ERCP pancreatitis: European Society of Gastrointestinal Endoscopy (ESGE) Guideline – updated June 2014, *Endoscopy* 46:799–815, 2014.
11. Inoue T, Okumura F, Sano H, et al: Bleeding risk of endoscopic ultrasound-guided fine-needle aspiration in patients undergoing antithrombotic therapy, *Dig Endosc* 29(1):91–96, 2017.
12. Dhadham GC, Hoffe S, Harris CL, et al: Endoscopic ultrasound-guided fiducial marker placement for image-guided radiation therapy without fluoroscopy: safety and technical feasibility, *Endosc Int Open* 4(3): E378–E382, 2016.
13. Chavalitdhamrong D, DiMaio CJ, Siersema PD, et al: Technical advances in endoscopic ultrasound-guided fiducial placement for the treatment of pancreatic cancer, *Endosc Int Open* 3(4):E373–E377, 2015.
14. Alkhatib AA, Mahayni AA, Yoder LJ: A single dose of prophylactic antibiotic may be sufficient to prevent postprocedural infection in upper endosonography guided fiducial marker placement, *Minerva Gastroenterol Dietol* 61(3):121–124, 2015.
18. Chantarojanasiri T, Aswakul P, Prachayakul V: Uncommon complications of therapeutic endoscopic ultrasonography: what, why, and how to prevent, *World J Gastrointest Endosc* 7(10):960–968, 2015.
49. ASGE Standards of Practice Committee, Acosta RD, Abraham NS, et al: The management of antithrombotic agents for patients undergoing GI endoscopy, *Gastrointest Endosc* 836:3–16, 2016.
50. Veitch AM, Vanbiervliet G, Gershlick AH, et al: Endoscopy in patients on antiplatelet or anticoagulant therapy including direct oral anticoagulants: British Society of Gastroenterology (BSG) and European Society of Gastrointestinal Endoscopy (ESGE) guidelines, *Gut* 65:374–389, 2016.
52. Douketis JD, Spyropoulos AC, Kaatz S, et al: Perioperative bridging anti-coagulation in patients with atrial fibrillation, *N Engl J Med* 373: 823–833, 2015.
59. ASGE Standards of Practice Committee, Khashab MA, Chithadi KV, et al: Antibiotic prophylaxis for GI endoscopy, *Gastrointest Endosc* 81:81–89, 2015.

A complete reference list can be found online at ExpertConsult .com

9

Bowel Preparation for Colonoscopy

Parth J. Parekh, Edward C. Oldfield IV, and David A. Johnson

CHAPTER OUTLINE

INTRODUCTION

Colorectal cancer (CRC) is the third leading cancer diagnosis and the third leading cause of cancer-related death in both men and women in the United States.[1] Colonoscopy is currently the gold standard in CRC prevention by allowing clinicians to detect and remove precancerous lesions. In addition, colonoscopy can be used for CRC surveillance and diagnostic evaluation of other positive CRC screening tests (e.g., fecal occult blood tests, fecal immunochemical tests, virtual colonography, etc.), as well other symptomatic complaints (e.g., diarrhea, hematochezia, etc.). The diagnostic accuracy and therapeutic safety of colonoscopy hinges on the quality of the colonic cleansing or preparation.

Unfortunately, current estimates suggest that up to 25% of bowel preparations are inadequate,[2] defined as the inability to achieve cecal intubation and effectively visualize the colonic mucosa.[3] Inadequate preparations can result in failed detection of precancerous or neoplastic lesions,[4] longer procedural times,[5] lower cecal intubation rates,[6] increased electrocautery risk,[7] and subjecting patients to multiple procedures due to the need for shorter intervals between endoscopic evaluations.[2,6]

There are several bowel-preparation formulations currently available on the market. Available formulations are assessed on their safety profile, efficacy, and patient tolerability. Studies have identified several independent patient-related predictors that increase the likelihood of an inadequate preparation: a previous inadequate colonoscopy, being non-English speaking, having Medicaid insurance, evidence of polypharmacy (particularly using medications that alter colon motility, i.e., tricyclic agents and opiates), obesity, advanced age, male sex, and comorbidities including diabetes mellitus, prior stroke, dementia, cirrhosis, prior gastrointestinal surgery, and Parkinson's disease.[8–10] Several physician- and procedure-related predictors that increase the likelihood of an inadequate preparation have also been identified: longer appointment wait times for colonoscopy, a procedural indication of constipation, a later colonoscopy time, and inpatient status.[8–10] The ideal colonic preparation should be effective in evacuating the colon of all fecal material without resulting in any patient discomfort, fluid shifts, or electrolyte imbalances. Here we review the available colonoscopy preparations and discuss the optimal timing for taking the preparations. In addition, this review will provide up-to-date literature for clinicians to ensure patient safety and to potentially modify patient-, physician-, and procedure-related factors to optimize bowel preparation quality.

AVAILABLE REGIMENS FOR COLONIC LAVAGE PRIOR TO COLONOSCOPY

Clinicians should be cognizant of cost, patient tolerability, and comorbid conditions when prescribing colon preparations. The available colon preparations are summarized later and in Table 9.1.

Isosmotic Agents

Isosmotic agents are polyethylene glycol (PEG)-containing preparations that are osmotically balanced with non-fermentable electrolyte solutions, thus theoretically minimizing significant fluid and electrolyte shifts. These preparations cleanse the intestinal lumen through the cathartic effect that results from large-volume lavage.

PEG-electrolyte solutions (PEG-ELS) (GoLytely, Braintree Laboratories, Braintree, MA) is one of the most commonly prescribed colon preparations. There were no significant physiologic changes (e.g., weight, vital signs, serum electrolytes, blood chemistries, or blood counts) seen in clinical trials.[11–13] Thus, PEG-ELS is considered generally safe in patients with preexisting electrolyte disorders or those who cannot otherwise tolerate a significant sodium load (e.g., patients with advanced renal or hepatic impairment, or congestive heart failure).[14] Finally, PEG-ELS does not alter histologic features of colonic

TABLE 9.1 Summary of Available Bowel Preparations

Brand (Company)	Formulation	Volume (L)	FDA Approved?	Dosing Regimen	Caution	Hyper/Hypo/ Iso Osmotic
GoLytely (Braintree Laboratories)	PEG Sodium sulfate Sodium bicarbonate Sodium chloride Potassium chloride	4	Yes	Split dose (2 L day before and 2 L day of procedure) Single dose (4 L day before)	Least palatable	Iso
NuLYTELY Trilyte (Braintree Laboratories)	PEG Sodium bicarbonate Sodium chloride Potassium chloride	4	Yes	Split dose (2 L day before and 2 L day of procedure) Single dose (4 L day before)	More palatable (Sodium sulfate removed from formulation)	Iso
Moviprep (Salix Pharmaceutical)	PEG-3350 Sodium sulfate Sodium chloride Ascorbic acid	2	Yes	Split dose (1 L day before and 1 L day of procedure) Single dose (2 L day before)	Potential to precipitate hemolysis in patients with G6PD	Iso
Miralax (Merck)	PEG-3350	238 g mixed with 64 oz of Gatorade to create a 2-L PEG-SD	No	Split dose (1 L day before and 1 L day of procedure) Single dose (2 L day before)	Fluid shifts and electrolyte derangements may occur Caution in patients with hepatic/renal impairment or CHF	Hypo
Suprep (Braintree Laboratories)	PEG-3350 Sodium sulfate Potassium sulfate Magnesium sulfate	12 oz in 2.5 L of water	Yes	Split dose (6 oz OSS with 10 oz of water + 32 oz of water the day before and 6 oz OSS + 10 oz of water + 32 oz of water day of procedure)		Hyper
Suclear (Braintree Laboratories)	PEG-3550 Sodium sulfate Potassium sulfate Magnesium sulfate	6 oz OSS and 2 L PEG-ELS in 1.25 L of water	Yes	Split dose (6 oz OSS with 10 oz of water + 32 oz of water the day before and 2 L PEG-ELS day of procedure) Single dose (6 oz OSS with 10 oz of water + 16 oz of water followed by 2 L PEG-ELS + 16 oz of water 2 hours after OSS)		Hyper
Prepopik (Ferring Pharmaceutical)	Sodium picosulfate Magnesium sulfate Anhydric citric acid	10 oz in 2 L of water	Yes	Split dose (5 oz Prepopik day before + 40 oz of clear liquid and 5 oz Prepopkik + 24 oz of clear liquids day of procedure) Single dose (5 oz Prepopkik + 24 oz clear liquids the afternoon or early evening day before procedure and 5 oz Prepopkik + 24 oz of clear liquids 6 hours later	Risk of magnesium toxicity Avoid in patients with nephrotic impairment	Hyper
Magnesium citrate (OTC)	Magnesium citrate	20–30 oz in 2 L of water	No	Split dose (1–1.5 10-oz bottles the day before and 1–1.5 10 oz bottles day of procedure)	Risk of magnesium toxicity Avoid in patients with nephrotic impairment	Hyper
Osmoprep (Salix Pharmaceuticals)	NaP	32 tablets in 2 L of water	Yes	Split dose (20 tablets day before and 12 tablets day of procedure)	Risk of calcium and phosphate nephropathy, particularly in those highly susceptible	Hyper

CHF, Congestive heart failure; *FDA,* Food and Drug Administration; *PEG,* polyethylene glycol; *PEG-ELS,* PEG-electrolyte solutions; *PEG-SD,* PEF + sports drink; *OSS,* oral sodium sulfate; *OTC,* over the counter.

mucosa and as a result can be used in patients suspected of having inflammatory bowel disease without affecting the diagnostic yield.[15]

One major pitfall of large-volume PEG-ELS is that nearly 15% of patients are unable to complete the preparation due to the large volume (resulting in abdominal fullness and cramping) and/or palatability (due to sulfate-associated taste).[16] To overcome these shortcomings, Food and Drug Administration (FDA)-approved reduced-volume PEG-ELS and sulfate-free PEG-ELS formulations were developed.

Low-volume PEG-ELS (Moviprep, Merck, Kenilworth, NJ), containing supplemental ascorbate and sodium sulfate, were formulated to provide a more tolerable preparation. Several studies have demonstrated similar efficacy with low-volume PEG-ELS compared with the standard 4-L PEG-ELS preparation.[17–20] The safety profile of low-volume PEG-ELS is comparable to that of standard large-volume PEG-ELS, with the exception of patients with glucose-6-phosphate dehydrogenase deficiency, as ascorbate may precipitate hemolysis in these patients.[21]

Sulfate-free PEG-ELS (SF-PEG-ELS) (NuLYTELY or Trilyte, Braintree Laboratories, Braintree, MA) was formulated to overcome the palatability issues of standard large-volume PEG-ELS by completely removing sodium sulfate, decreasing potassium concentration, and increasing chloride concentration.[13] This results in lower luminal sodium concentrations, thus SF-PEG-ELS formulations are solely dependent on its osmotic effects. Clinical data have demonstrated SF-PEG-ELS to be as efficacious and safe when compared with standard PEG-ELS.[22]

Hyperosmotic Agents

Hyperosmotic agents draw water and electrolytes into the bowel lumen, resulting in fluid loss, peristalsis, and ultimately evacuation of the bowel. As a result, these small-volume preparations cause fluid shifts and can result in electrolyte derangements.

Magnesium Citrate

Magnesium citrate is a commonly used agent that has an osmotic effect (as described earlier) and additionally stimulates the release of cholecystokinin, which results in intraluminal accumulation of fluid and electrolytes thought to promote colonic transit.[23] To date, there have been four randomized controlled trials evaluating the use of magnesium citrate for colonoscopy preparation, which included two trials that combined it with either PEG-ELS or sodium phosphate (NaP) solution.[24–27] Park et al (2010) evaluated the efficacy and tolerance of split-dose magnesium citrate and low-volume PEG for morning colonoscopy.[24] A total of 232 patients were randomized to receive 4-L PEG (group 1; day prior to procedure; n = 79), split-dose PEG (group 2; 2-L PEG day before the procedure followed by another 2-L PEG day of the procedure; n = 80), or magnesium citrate and PEG (group 3; 250 mL of magnesium citrate day before procedure followed by 2-L PEG day of the procedure; n = 73). They found that satisfactory bowel preparations were more frequently reported in group 3 when compared with group 1, and similar to that of group 2. In addition, they found that patients in group 3 were more willing to repeat the same preparation, if necessary, than those in group 1 (93% vs. 38%, $p < 0.001$) or group 2 (93% vs. 62%, $p < 0.001$), which led the authors to conclude that split-dose magnesium citrate low-volume PEG regimen was more efficient than the convention 4-L PEG regimen, and equally efficient but preferable to the split-dose regimen for morning colonoscopy. Magnesium citrate does result in transient elevations in serum magnesium levels; however, this has not been linked to any adverse outcomes in healthy persons.[28] It does undergo renal excretion, however, and thus should be avoided in patients with chronic kidney disease because of possible magnesium toxicity (resulting in bradycardia, hypotension, nausea, drowsiness, and even death).[29,30]

Sodium Phosphate and Oral Sodium Sulfate

NaP (Osmoprep, Salix pharmaceuticals, Raleigh, NC) is a hyperosmotic solution that has recently lost favor due to the rare occurrence of calcium[31] and phostphate[32] nephropathy. Patient characteristics associated with a higher predilection toward phosphate nephropathy include compromised renal function, female gender, inadequate hydration during bowel preparation, hypertension treated with angiotensin-converting enzyme inhibitors or angiotensin receptor blockers, older age, or concomitant use of certain medications (diuretics or nonsteroidal antiinflammatory drugs).[33] Additionally, NaP can cause significant fluid shifts and electrolyte derangements, particularly in elderly patients or those with impaired gut motility, renal or hepatic impairment, or congestive heart failure.[34] Thus, the FDA has recently issued a black box warning for the tablet form of NaP.[23] It is not currently recommended for use in bowel preparation.[24,28]

Oral sodium sulfate (OSS) (Suprep or Suclear, Braintree Laboratories, Braintree, MA) is a hyperosmotic prep that is not associated with significant fluid shifts and electrolyte derangements, owning to the fact that sulfate is a poorly absorbed anion. Di Palma et al (2009) evaluated the efficacy of OSS as a bowel preparation for colonoscopy in adult patients.[35] This multicenter, single-blind, randomized, non-inferiority study compared the efficacy of OSS with PEG-ELS. The study, totaling 364 patients, randomized each patient to split-dose administration, in which the first portion was taken the evening before the colonoscopy and the second the morning of. They found that there was no difference between OSS and PEG-ELS, with successful preparations seen in 97.2% and 95.6%, respectively. Patients who received OSS did report slightly more gastrointestinal events (i.e., cramping, bloating, nausea and vomiting) than those that received PEG-ELS ($p = 0.009$). The investigators concluded that OSS is an effective alternative to PEG-ELS with a comparable safety profile. Another multicenter, single-blind, randomized, non-inferiority study by Rex et al (2010) randomized 136 adult patients undergoing outpatient colonoscopy to 4-L SF-PEG-ELS (given the night prior to colonoscopy) or OSS given in equally divided doses the evening prior to and morning of colonoscopy.[36] They found that a successful bowel preparation (98.4% vs. 89.6%; $p = 0.04$), in particular preparations rated as excellent (71.4% vs. 34.3%; $p < 0.001$), was achieved more frequently with OSS than SF-PEG-ELS. Given similar side effect profiles, the authors concluded that OSS was a safe alternative as a low-volume preparation for colonoscopy. A limitation of the study is the fact that SF-PEG-ELS was entirely administered the evening prior and not as a split dose.

Sodium Picosulfate-Magnesium Citrate

The combination of sodium picosulfate-magnesium citrate (P/MC) (Prepopik, Ferring Pharmaceutical, Parsippany, NJ) was introduced to the United States market in 2012. P/MC has a dual mechanism as it combines the stimulant laxative properties of sodium picosulfate (which increases the frequency and force of peristalsis) and the hyperosmotic properties of magnesium citrate.[37] Rex et al (2013) evaluated the efficacy of P/MC in a multicenter, assessor-blinded, randomized, non-inferiority study.[38] This phase 3 study randomized 601 patients to P/MC (n = 304) or to day-before 2-L PEG-3350 and bisacodyl tablets (n = 297). P/MC was superior to 2-L PEG-3350 in overall colon cleaning (84.2% vs. 74.4%) and in cleaning of the ascending (89.5% vs. 78.8%), transverse and descending colon (92.4% vs. 85.9%), and rectosigmoid (92.4% vs. 87.2%). Patients also reported higher tolerability (ease of consumption and taste) for P/MC than PEG-3350, leading the authors to conclude that the bowel-cleansing effects and tolerability of split-dose P/MC were superior to day-before preparation with 2-L PEG-3350 and bisacodyl tablets.

Hyposmotic Agents

PEG-3350 powder (Miralax, Merck, Kenilworth, NJ) is an over-the-counter laxative (marketed for constipation) available as an 8.3-ounce bottle. It is often mixed with 64 ounces of Gatorade (PepsiCo, Chicago, IL) to formulate a 2-L PEG formulation (PEG-SD). In the clinical setting it is often combined with adjunctive medications such as bisacodyl.[39] Given conflicting data at present, the routine use of PEG-SD is not currently recommended.[23] Hjelkrem et al (2011) compared split-dose PEG-ELS to split-dose PEG-SD alone and in combination with pretreatment medications (bisacodyl or lubiprostone) to determine the efficacy and tolerability of PEG-SD for bowel preparation.[40] This prospective, blinded, randomized controlled trial totaling 403 patients randomly assigned patients to receive GoLytely (Braintree Laboratories, Braintree, MA), MiraLAX (Merck, Kenilworth, NJ), Miralax with bisacodyl (10 mg), or Miralax with lubiprostone (24 μg). They found GoLytely was more effective at bowel cleansing than Miralax alone or in combination with lubiprostone or bisacodyl (average Ottowa bowel preparation scores for each group were 5.1, 6.9, 6.8 and 6.3, respectively; $p < 0.001$). One study suggested that the use of PEG-SD results in lower adenoma detection rates (ADRs) compared with standard PEG-ELS due to differences in preparation quality.[41] However, several studies have demonstrated PEG-SD to be as efficacious as PEG-ELS with a comparable side effect profile.[42–45]

Adjunctive Therapy

There have been a multitude of adjunctive agents that have been investigated with the hopes to enhance bowel preparation and/or visualization of the mucosa. Agents have included simethicone, flavored electrolyte solutions, prokinetics, spasmolytics, bisacodyl, senna, olive oil, and probiotics. None of these agents have consistently shown improved efficacy, safety, or increased patient tolerability of the bowel preparation; accordingly, they are not currently recommended for routine use as adjunct therapy.[28] However, prescribing physicians may find these agents useful in select circumstances. A summary of key studies evaluating adjunctive therapies for bowel preparation is presented here.

Wu et al (2011) conducted a meta-analysis evaluating the supplemental use of simethicone.[45] This review, totaling seven studies that compared the efficacy of simethicone with a purgative to a purgative alone, found that the overall efficacy of colon preparation was comparable (odds ratio [OR], 2.06; 95% confidence interval [CI], 0.56–7.53; $p = 0.27$), despite a notable reduction in the presence of intraluminal bubbles (OR, 39.3; 95% CI, 11.4–135.9; $p < 0.01$) in the simethicone cohort.

The use of prokinetic agents in combination use with purgative laxatives has not demonstrated adjunctive benefit. Metoclopramide is a prokinetic agent that increases the amplitude of gastric contraction and peristalsis of the duodenum and jejunum without affecting colonic motility. The data indicate that prokinetic agents such as metoclopramide do not improve colonic cleaning but are conflicting as to their effect on patient tolerability,[12] thus it is not currently recommended as an adjunct to bowel preparation.[23,28] Senna and bisacodyl have been used as adjuncts to PEG-ELS, and although they have been demonstrated to improve tolerability,[47] they have not been as effective as standard colon preparation.[48,49]

A randomized trial by Repici et al (2012) comparing two low-volume PEG-ELS preparations (PEG-ELS citrate-simethicone with bisacodyl and PEG-ascorbate) did not demonstrate any difference in tolerability, safety, acceptability, and compliance.[50] Another study, which involved 107 patients, demonstrated that colon cleansing with 2-L PEG-ELS ascorbate was superior when compared to PEG-ELS with bisacodyl.[19] Pretreatment with olive oil has been shown to enhance both patient satisfaction and tolerability in addition to quality of right-side colonic cleansing; however, it did not impact the left colon when compared with 4-L PEG-ELS.[51] Finally, Lee et al (2010) evaluated the efficacy of a 2-week probiotic treatment (containing a mixture of *Bacillus subtilis* and *Streptococcus faecium*) or placebo with oral NaP in patients with and without constipation with the primary outcome measure being the quality of bowel cleansing.[52] They found that patients suffering from constipation were more likely to benefit from probiotic pretreatment compared with placebo (54.9% vs. 20.8%, respectively; $p < 0.001$). However, patients with normal defecation did not benefit from probiotic pretreatment. Thus, they concluded that probiotic pretreatment may be considered in patients suffering from constipation, but did not appear to be of value in patients with normal defecation.

SPLIT DOSING

A split-dose preparation is currently strongly recommended by the most recent multi-society guidelines on bowel preparation.[23,28,53] Since the publication of these guidelines, even more evidence supporting split-dose preparation has been made available, including two recent meta-analyses that reviewed all available randomized trials utilizing split-dose versus non-split-dose preparations.[54,55] The meta-analysis by Bucci et al (2014), which included 29 studies, evaluated the efficacy of split dose versus non-split dosing.[54] The overall results demonstrated that split-dose preparations were superior to non-split dosing. An adequate preparation was achieved in 85% and 63% of patients, respectively. Of note, this was independent of the laxative used. A secondary analysis, however, highlights an important consideration that likely explains the derived benefit of using split prep over a non-split prep: the concept of runway time. Runway time refers to the time elapsed between the last dose of purge and the beginning of the colonoscopy. The quality of colon preparation is inversely related to the duration of runway time owing to the arrival of liquid stool from the ileum, which produces a film in the proximal colon and impairs the detection of polyps, particularly flat lesions.[28,56] As such, the authors established that the optimal runway time after completion of the oral preparation is 3 hours. It is important to note that prep quality decreases after 4 to 5 hours and is negated after 5 hours, independent of the laxative used.[54]

A meta-analysis by Martel et al (2015), which included 47 trials (13,487 patients), also compared split-dose preparation to day-before preparation.[55] Overall, split-dose preparations had a significantly better quality of colon cleansing when compared with day-before preparation, irrespective of the type of preparation used (OR, 2.51; 95% CI, 1.86–3.29). In addition, patients were more willing to repeat split-dose compared with day-before preparation (OR, 1.90; 95% CI, 1.05–3.46). Other studies have also found that patients were more willing to comply with a split-dose regimen.[54,57] Altawil et al (2014) surveyed 149 patients, scheduled for morning procedures, regarding their opinion about a split-dose regimen.[57] Among the 149 survey participants, 64% (95/149) of patients were willing to wake up early to complete the split prep; of these patients, the majority (68%) preferred an early-morning appointment, with 29% preferring late morning and only 3% preferring an afternoon appointment. In comparison, only 56% of primary care providers who were also surveyed on their opinion about the willingness of their patients to undergo morning bowel preparation thought their patients would be willing to undergo split dosing. Overall, these studies suggest that a split-dose preparation does not significantly impair patient compliance, despite the fact it often requires patients to wake early in the morning to complete the preparation. The only exception for performing non-split dosing is for same-day preparation on the day of colonoscopy, which has also demonstrated a similar efficacy.[28]

A 2017 randomized controlled trial totaling 690 patients undergoing colonoscopy for positive fecal immunochemical testing compared ADRs with use of split-dose preparation and day-before preparation.[58] Patients were randomized to receive either low-volume split-dose or day-before regimens. The proportion of patients with at least one adenoma detected was significantly higher in the split-dose group compared with the day-before group (53% [183/345] vs. 40.9% [141/345], respectively; relative risk [RR], 1.22; 95% CI, 1.03–1.46). Furthermore, the split-dose prep was associated with a significantly higher rate of detecting advanced adenomas compared with the day-before group (26.4% [91/345] vs. 20% [69/345], respectively [RR, 1.35; 95% CI, 1.06–1.73]). Per-polyp analysis found that the total number of adenomas and advanced adenomas per patient were significantly higher in the split-dose group compared with the day-before group (1.15 vs. 0.8, $p < 0.001$; 0.36 vs. 0.22, $p < 0.001$). Subgroup analysis evaluating the detection of sessile serrate lesions (7.8% vs. 4.1%, $p = 0.053$) and right-sided adenomas (0.96% vs. 0.85%, $p = 0.29$) favored the use of split-dose prep but failed to achieve statistical significance.

Overall, these studies support the current multi-society guidelines on bowel preparation that endorse the use of split dosing over day-before preparation for patients undergoing morning procedures.[24,28] For patients undergoing an afternoon procedure, same-day preparation is considered an acceptable alternative due to runway time. When using split dosing, patients and providers should time the second dose of the split preparation such that it begins 4 to 6 hours before procedure and is completed at least 2 hours before the scheduled time. As described earlier, split-dose preparation is associated with improved colon cleansing, increased patient compliance, and, most importantly, increased ADRs.

DOCUMENTATION OF THE QUALITY OF BOWEL PREPARATION

There are several scoring systems available for evaluating the adequacy of bowel preparation. This section will outline and discuss the Aronchick Scale, Ottawa Scale, and Boston Bowel Preparation Scale (BBPS). Table 9.2 summarizes the different scoring systems.

Aronchick Scale

The Aronchick Scale rates the quality of preparation based on percentage of residual stool during initial inspection before any attempted washing or suctioning of the mucosa.[59] The scale ranges from 1 to 5 and assigns a whole, rather than segmental, score. Grading scores are: (1) excellent: small volume of clear liquid or greater than 95% mucosa seen; (2) good: large volume of clear liquid covering 5% to 25% of surface but greater than 90% of mucosa seen; (3) fair: some semisolid stool that could not be suctioned or washed away, but greater than 90% of mucosa seen; (4) poor: semisolid stool could not be suctioned or washed away and less than 90% of mucosa seen; (5) inadequate: repeat preparation needed. The Aronchick Scale has often been used as the gold standard for comparison of other bowel preparation scales because it assesses preparation quality on initial inspection, despite the fact that it has not been fully validated.[23,60]

Ottawa Scale

The Ottawa Scale differs from the Aronchick Scale in that it assesses the quality of preparation in different segments (i.e., right colon, mid colon, and rectosigmoid). In addition, it provides an overall global score for colonic fluid. Total scores range from 0 (excellent) to 14 (very poor/inadequate). Segment scores range from 0 to 4: (0) excellent: mucosal detail clearly visible; (1) good: minimal turbid fluid in segment; (2) fair: necessary to suction liquid stool to adequately visualize colonic wall; (3) poor: necessary to wash and suction to obtain view; (4) inadequate: solid stool not cleared with washing and suctioning.[60,61] Global colonic fluid is rated as being either a 0, 1, or 2, which indicates a small, moderate, or large volume of fluid, respectively. The Ottawa Scale has demonstrated high global inter-rater reliability, as well as high reliability when applied to the individual colon segments.[61]

Boston Bowel Preparation Scale

The BBPS assesses bowel preparation after the mucosa has been cleaned to the best of the endoscopist's ability. The scoring system is applied to each of the three areas of the colon: right side (including cecum and ascending colon), transverse section (including hepatic and splenic flexures), and left side of the colon (including the descending colon, sigmoid colon, and rectum). Point assignments are 0 to 3 for each segment, with total scores ranging from 0 to 9. The scoring system for each segment is as follows: (0) unprepared colon segment with mucosa not seen because of solid stool that cannot be cleared; (1) portion of mucosa of the colon segment seen, but other areas of the colon segment are not well seen because of straining, residual stool and/or opaque liquid; (2) minor amount of residual staining, small fragments of stool and/or opaque liquid, but mucosa of colon segment is seen well; (3) entire mucosa of colon segment seen well, with no residual staining, small fragments of stool, or opaque liquid. If the procedure is aborted due to inadequate preparation, any non-visualized segments are assigned a score of 0.

In a comprehensive validation study, the BBPS demonstrated near-perfect inter-rater reliability and substantial intra-rater reliability.[62] BBPS scores also correlated with polyp detection rates, as scores of 5 or over had a higher polyp detection rate than scores lower than 5 (40% vs. 24%, respectively; $p < 0.02$).[63]

TABLE 9.2 Summary of Bowel-Preparation Scoring Scales

Aronchick Scale

Score	Rating	Description
1	Excellent	Small volume of clear liquid or > 95% mucosa seen
2	Good	Large volume of clear liquid covering 5%–25% of surface but > 90% of mucosa seen
3	Fair	Some semisolid stool that could not be suctioned or washed away, but > 90% of mucosa seen
4	Poor	Semisolid stool could not be suctioned or washed away and < 90% of mucosa seen
5	Inadequate	Inadequate; repeat preparation needed

Ottawa Scale

Segment Score[a]

0	Excellent	Mucosal detail clearly visible
1	Good	Minimal turbid fluid in segment
2	Fair	Necessary to suction liquid stool to adequately visualize colonic wall
3	Poor	Necessary to wash and suction to obtain view
4	Inadequate	Solid stool not cleared with washing and suctioning

Global Score for Retained Fluid

0	Small
1	Moderate
2	Large volume

[a]Segment scores are applied to each of the three colonic segments: right colon, mid colon, and rectosigmoid.
Total scores include the sum of the three segments scores plus the global fluid score. Total scores range from 0 (excellent) to 14 (very poor/inadequate). Scores for the Ottawa and Aronchick Scale are based on assessments performed prior to colonoscopic suction and lavage.

Boston Bowel Preparation Scale

Score	Description
0	Unprepared colon segment with mucosa not seen because of solid stool that cannot be cleared
1	Portion of mucosa of the colon segment seen, but other areas of the colon segment are not well seen because of straining, residual stool, and/or opaque liquid
2	Minor amount of residual staining, small fragments of stool, and/or opaque liquid, but mucosa of colon segment is seen well
3	Entire mucosa of colon segment seen well, with no residual staining, small fragments of stool, or opaque liquid

Score applied to three segments:
1. Right side (including cecum and ascending colon)
2. Transverse section (including hepatic and splenic flexures)
3. Left side of the colon (including the descending colon, sigmoid colon, and rectum)
Point assignments are 0–3 for each segment, with total scores ranging from 0–9.
If the procedure is aborted due to inadequate preparation, any non-visualized segments are assigned a score of 0.
Scores are based on assessments performed after completion of colonoscopic suction and lavage.

Additionally, a segment score of 2 or 3 was associated with improved polyp detection for both right- (OR, 1.60; 95% CI, 1.01–2.55) and left-sided polyps (OR, 2.58; 95% CI, 1.34–4.98) compared with a segment score of 0 or 1.[6]

Comparison and Recommendations

According to the United States Multi-Society Task Force (USMSTF), quality indicators for colonoscopy include a primary goal to achieve a bowel preparation adequate to detect a lesion of greater than 5 mm.[28] In addition, the USMSTF also recommends that endoscopists achieve a minimum of 85% adequate bowel preparation rate in their practice.[28] If the threshold is not met, the process of preparation, patient education, navigation tools, and medication selection all warrant closer review in order to better optimize outcome.[28] The European Society of Gastrointestinal Endoscopy guidelines on adequate bowel preparation propose that at least 90% of screening examinations be rated as having an "adequate" or better bowel cleansing.[53]

A systematic review and meta-analysis totaling 11 studies by Clark et al (2014) investigated the impact of bowel preparation quality on the ADRs using the Aronchick Scale, comparing high-quality (excellent/good), intermediate-quality (fair), and low-quality (poor/insufficient) bowel preparation.[64] Overall, ADRs were significantly higher for both the high- and intermediate-quality preparation groups compared with the poor-quality group (OR, 1.41; 95% CI, 1.21–1.64 and OR, 1.39; 95% CI, 1.08–1.79, respectively). However, there was no significant difference in ADR between the high- and intermediate-quality groups (OR, 0.94; 95% CI, 0.80–1.10). A 2016 meta-analysis by Sulz et al investigated the effects of bowel preparation on ADR, advanced adenomas, and CRC.[65] They found that detection of early adenomas was significantly reduced with inadequate (poor or insufficient) preparations compared with adequate (excellent, good, or fair) preparations (OR, 0.53; 95% CI, 0.46–0.62). This was also true for advanced adenomas (OR, 0.74; 95% CI, 0.62–0.87). Thus, it appears that an inadequate bowel preparation affects the detection of early colonic lesions more so than for advanced lesions, but both are reduced.

A 2016 prospective observational study by Clark et al sought to provide an objective definition of an adequate preparation using the BBPS.[66] Data were collected from 438 male patients undergoing screening and surveillance colonoscopies who then underwent a repeat colonoscopy within 60 days by a different blinded endoscopist. BBPS was used to quantify adequacy of bowel preparation. They found that a BBPS segment score of 2 or 3 for all colon segments was sufficient for detection of adenomas of 5 mm or greater and that patients meeting these criteria should return for screening or surveillance colonoscopy at standard guideline-recommended intervals, and these colonic preparations were thus considered adequate. Conversely, segments with a BBPS score of 1 had a significantly higher rate of missed adenomas of 5 mm or greater, when compared with segments with scores of 2 or 3.

Despite an adequate ADR for both intermediate- and high-quality bowel preparation, evidence from 2016 suggests that only high-quality bowel preparation is adequate for the detection of sessile serrated adenomas/polyps (SSPs).[67] A prospective trial comparing the SSP detection rate among 749 patients undergoing screening and surveillance colonoscopies in which the endoscopists graded the quality of bowel preparation using both the Aronchick Scale and the BBPS was performed.[67] When using the Aronchick Scale, detection of SSPs was significantly lower in patients with intermediate-quality preparation (4.6%) compared with high-quality preparation (12.0%; OR, 0.37; 95% CI, 0.15–0.87). This finding also held true for the BBPS, where significantly fewer SSPs were detected in patients with a BPPS of less than 7 compared with a score of 7 to 9 (4.7% vs. 12.6%; OR, 0.36; 95% CI, 0.19–0.67).

Currently, the multi-society guidelines on bowel preparation for CRC screening strongly recommend documentation of the adequacy of the bowel preparation, ideally assessed after all appropriate efforts to clear residual debris have been completed.[23,28] As a result, the guidelines do not recommend the use of the Aronchick Scale or Ottawa Scale because these scales score retained fluid.[28] Based on the currently available evidence, if employing the BBPS to assess colon cleansing, any score less than 5 warrants a repeat colonoscopy in less than 1 year, whereas those with totals scores of 7 or higher, or if all segment scores are 2 or greater, can follow appropriate guideline-recommended screening intervals.

DIET DURING BOWEL CLEANSING

Traditionally, patients are instructed to ingest only a clear liquid diet (e.g., transparent liquids) the day prior to colonoscopy to decrease the likelihood of residual food contents. A 2016 meta-analysis, however, evaluating nine studies totaling 1686 patients evaluated the outcomes of patients undergoing colonoscopy who consumed a clear liquid diet versus a low-residue diet the day prior to colonoscopy.[68] They found that patients consuming a low-residue diet demonstrated significantly higher odds of tolerability (OR, 1.92; 95% CI, 1.36–2.70; $p < 0.01$) and willingness to repeat preparation (OR, 1.86; 95% CI, 1.34–2.59; $p < 0.01$) when compared with those who underwent a clear liquid diet. In addition, they found no difference in adequate bowel preparations (OR, 1.21; 95% CI, 0.64–2.28; $p = 0.58$) or adverse effects (OR, 0.88; 95% CI, 0.58–1.35; $p = 0.57$). It should be noted, however, that the diet regimens in these trials were variable

(heterogeneity: $p = 0.008$, I = 62%). Regimens included a regular diet until 6 PM, regular breakfast, low-residue breakfast, lunch and snack, a soft diet, and a semi-liquid diet. Thus, consensus guidelines include full liquids until the evening on the day prior to colonoscopy and consideration of a low-residue diet for part or all of the day prior to colonoscopy, particularly in patients without identifiable pre-procedural risks for inadequate bowel preparation (e.g., constipation).[28]

FUTURE DIRECTION OF BOWEL PREPARATION

Colon Hydrotherapy

The Angel of Water device (Lifestream, Austin, TX), referred to as the Prep System, was initially developed by institutes promoting "well-being" via a method of comfortable colonic hydrotherapy to achieve colon cleansing. A 2016 prospective, non-inferiority study compared a standard PEG protocol with bowel cleansing by low-pressure water infusion into the colon (Prep System, Lifestream, Austin, TX). Patients were randomly assigned to either a split-dose 2 L + 2 L PEG or the Prep System, after 5 days on a low-residue diet.[69] Prep System cleansing consisted of infusion of 35-L water ($\times 2$) at 37°C into the rectum over a 1-hour period. The quality of bowel cleansing was assessed using the BBPS by a colonoscopist blinded to the preparation. Groups were comparable for age, sex, and colonoscopy indication.

The total median BBPS (7 in both groups) and segmental scores did not differ between groups. Mean duration of colonoscopy, blood electrolytes after bowel cleansing, and patient satisfaction (89% in the patients who underwent prep using the Prep System vs. 76% in the PEG cohort) did not differ between the two groups. Adverse events, mainly nausea, were more frequent in the PEG group ($p = 0.03$). In the setting of this study, the Prep System appeared as effective as the split-dose prep using PEG for bowel cleansing before colonoscopy with similar, if not better, patient tolerance.

The system is currently licensed by HyGIeaCare (Austin, TX), with over 4600 patients successfully having undergone this procedure to date with excellent success and acceptability by patients.[70] HyGIeaCare Prep provides a FDA-cleared colon lavage system to replace the traditional oral prep. The patient sits comfortable on a padded recliner while a colon purge with low-pressure warm water is delivered comfortably via a small soft rectal tube (Fig. 9.1). The colonic effluent washes out the

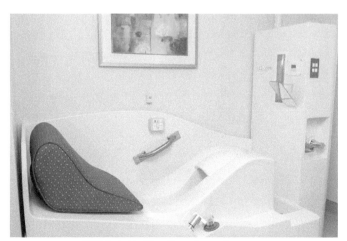

FIG 9.1 HyGleaCare Prep System.

rectum, and colonic cleansing is achieved typically within 45 minutes. The HyGIeaCare Prep is private, uses low-pressure flow of warm water, is odorless, and effective. The patient undergoes their scheduled colonoscopy immediately after undergoing their prep, which offers a novel alternative to the traditional preparation by overcoming several barriers to effective colonoscopy preparation (e.g., intolerance of large-volume oral purgatives).

CONCLUSION

Colonoscopy is the mainstay in CRC diagnosis and prevention; however, the effectiveness of colonoscopy hinges on an adequate colon preparation. Ineffective bowel cleaning results in missed lesions, increased cost, and repeated procedures. National guidelines in the United States have emphasized the hurdles faced with bowel preparation for colonoscopy and the consequences of inadequate colon preparation. These challenges include intolerance of the preparation and inadequate preparation quality, which then impacts important benchmarks for quality, including ADRs, compliance with appropriate surveillance intervals, and in achieving the new threshold benchmark for adequate preparation (now set at 85%). There are several scoring systems available that can be used to calculate whether a prep is adequate or inadequate. The quality of the bowel preparation should be determined after the endoscopist has thoroughly attempted to cleanse the bowel. The choice of bowel preparation for colonoscopy should be individualized to the patient based on a number of factors including cost, tolerability, and patient comorbidities. Any method that improves the acceptability and effectiveness of the colon preparation prior to colonoscopy is a key and critical step toward the ultimate goal: achieving a quality colonoscopy!

KEY REFERENCES

2. Harewood GC, Sharma VK, De Garmo P: Impact of colonoscopy preparation quality on detection of suspected colonic neoplasia, *Gastrointest Endosc* 58(1):76–79, 2003.
3. Shah HA, Paszat LF, Saskin R, et al: Factors associated with incomplete colonoscopy: a population-based study, *Gastroenterology* 132(7): 2297–2303, 2007.
4. Chokshi RV, Hovis CE, Hollander T, et al: Prevalence of missed adenomas in patients with inadequate bowel preparation on screening colonoscopy, *Gastrointest Endosc* 75(6):1197–1203, 2012.
5. Rex DK, Imperiale TF, Latinovich DR, Bratcher LL: Impact of bowel preparation on efficiency and cost of colonoscopy, *Am J Gastroenterol* 97(7):1696–1700, 2002.
8. Hassan C, Fuccio L, Bruno M, et al: A predictive model identifies patients most likely to have inadequate bowel preparation for colonoscopy, *Clin Gastroenterol Hepatol* 10(5):501–506, 2012.
10. Ness RM, Manam R, Hoen H, Chalasani N: Predictors of inadequate bowel preparation for colonoscopy, *Am J Gastroenterol* 96(6):1797–1802, 2001.
12. Brady CE, Dipalma JA, Pierson WP: Golytely lavage–is metoclopramide necessary?, *Am J Gastroenterol* 80(3):180–184, 1985.
23. Saltzman JR, Cash BD, Pasha SF, et al: Bowel preparation before colonoscopy, *Gastrointest Endosc* 81(4):781–794, 2015.
24. Park SS, Sinn DH, Kim YH, et al: Efficacy and tolerability of split-dose magnesium citrate: low-volume (2 liters) polyethylene glycol vs.

28. single- or split-dose polyethylene glycol bowel preparation for morning colonoscopy, *Am J Gastroenterol* 105(6):1319–1326, 2010.
28. Johnson DA, Barkun AN, Cohen LB, et al: Optimizing adequacy of bowel cleansing for colonoscopy: recommendations from the US multi-society task force on colorectal cancer, *Gastroenterology* 147(4):903–924, 2014.
32. Heher EC, Thier SO, Rennke H, Humphreys BD: Adverse renal and metabolic effects associated with oral sodium phosphate bowel preparation, *Clin J Am Soc Nephrol* 3(5):1494–1503, 2008.
35. Di Palma JA, Rodriguez R, Mcgowan J, Cleveland Mv: A randomized clinical study evaluating the safety and efficacy of a new, reduced-volume, oral sulfate colon-cleansing preparation for colonoscopy, *Am J Gastroenterol* 104(9):2275–2284, 2009.
36. Rex DK, Di Palma JA, Rodriguez R, et al: A randomized clinical study comparing reduced-volume oral sulfate solution with standard 4-liter sulfate-free electrolyte lavage solution as preparation for colonoscopy, *Gastrointest Endosc* 72(2):328–336, 2010.
38. Rex DK, Katz PO, Bertiger G, et al: Split-dose administration of a dual-action, low-volume bowel cleanser for colonoscopy: the SEE CLEAR I study, *Gastrointest Endosc* 78(1):132–141, 2013.
40. Hjelkrem M, Stengel J, Liu M, et al: MiraLAX is not as effective as GoLytely in bowel cleansing before screening colonoscopies, *Clin Gastroenterol Hepatol* 9(4):326–332, e1, 2011.
42. Samarasena JB, Muthusamy VR, Jamal MM: Split-dosed MiraLAX/Gatorade is an effective, safe, and tolerable option for bowel preparation in low-risk patients: a randomized controlled study, *Am J Gastroenterol* 107(7):1036–1042, 2012.
43. Shieh FK, Gunaratnam N, Mohamud SO, Schoenfeld P: MiraLAX-Gatorade bowel prep versus GoLytely before screening colonoscopy: an endoscopic database study in a community hospital, *J Clin Gastroenterol* 46(10):e96–e100, 2012.
47. Dipalma JA, Wolff BG, Meagher A, Cleveland Mv: Comparison of reduced volume versus four liters sulfate-free electrolyte lavage solutions for colonoscopy colon cleansing, *Am J Gastroenterol* 98(10):2187–2191, 2003.
53. Hassan C, Bretthauer M, Kaminski MF, et al: Bowel preparation for colonoscopy: European Society of Gastrointestinal Endoscopy (ESGE) guideline, *Endoscopy* 45(2):142–150, 2013.
54. Bucci C, Rotondano G, Hassan C, et al: Optimal bowel cleansing for colonoscopy: split the dose! A series of meta-analyses of controlled studies, *Gastrointest Endosc* 80(4):566–576, e2, 2014.
55. Martel M, Barkun AN, Menard C, et al: Split-dose preparations are superior to day-before bowel cleansing regimens: a meta-analysis, *Gastroenterology* 149(1):79–88, 2015.
57. Altawil J, Miller LA, Antaki F: Acceptance of split-dose bowel preparation regimen for colonoscopy by patients and providers, *J Clin Gastroenterol* 48(6):e47–e49, 2014.
58. Radaelli F, Paggi S, Hassan C, et al: Split-dose preparation for colonoscopy increases adenoma detection rate: a randomised controlled trial in an organised screening programme, *Gut* 66(2):270–277, 2017.
64. Clark BT, Rustagi T, Laine L: What level of bowel prep quality requires early repeat colonoscopy: systematic review and meta-analysis of the impact of preparation quality on adenoma detection rate, *Am J Gastroenterol* 109(11):1714–1723, 2014.
66. Clark BT, Protiva P, Nagar A, et al: Quantification of adequate bowel preparation for screening or surveillance colonoscopy in men, *Gastroenterology* 150(2):396–405, 2016.
67. Clark BT, Laine L: High-quality bowel preparation is required for detection of sessile serrated polyps, *Clin Gastroenterol Hepatol* 14(8): 1155–1162, 2016.

A complete reference list can be found online at ExpertConsult .com

10

Legal Concepts for Gastroenterologists

Kayla Feld, Sarah Blankstein, and Andrew Feld

CHAPTER OUTLINE

Endoscopic evaluation has become an indispensable and powerful tool for prevention, diagnosis, and therapy for digestive disorders. Performance of endoscopic procedures is not without risk, however. In the event of a bad outcome, physicians may face legal liability. It is therefore important that gastroenterologists understand the types of legal risk they may face and best practices for managing those risks.

This chapter briefly addresses legal aspects of gastrointestinal endoscopy. Part I of this chapter describes the types of malpractice lawsuits faced by gastroenterologists. Part II describes the anatomy of a malpractice suit, including the role of adherence to the applicable standard of care. Part III describes the basic elements and importance of obtaining and documenting informed consent. Part IV briefly summarizes legal obligations regarding protected health information. Finally, part V concludes with a discussion of risk management approaches, including good documentation practices, use of clinical practice guidelines (CPGs), and best practices for managing complications and errors once they have occurred.

TYPES OF LAWSUITS FACED BY GASTROENTEROLOGISTS

Malpractice lawsuits are a fact of practice for physicians in the United States. Beginning in the 1990s, several large studies, including the landmark Harvard Medical Malpractice Study, revealed surprising levels of medical errors and malpractice suits and provided an important impetus for the safety movement.[1–3]

More recently, a published study of claims data from 1991 through 2005 for all physicians covered by a large, national professional liability insurer revealed that each year 7.4% of physicians had a malpractice claim, with 1.6% having a claim

leading to payment.[4] The study identified a large degree of variation by specialty in physicians' risk of facing a malpractice lawsuit. Gastroenterologists during the study period faced a higher degree of malpractice risk than US physicians overall, with over 10% of gastroenterologists facing a malpractice claim annually.[4] Because gastroenterology involves the performance of invasive procedures, such as colonoscopies, this slightly elevated malpractice risk is not surprising.

To avoid potential lawsuits, it is important for gastroenterologists practicing in the United States to be familiar with the types of malpractice claims gastroenterologists most often face. One common type of malpractice claim gastroenterologists face is a claim of missed or delayed diagnosis. These claims often stem from a delayed diagnosis of colorectal cancer (CRC) due to missteps such as failure to conduct an initial CRC screening with the appropriate level of care, failure to notify patients of abnormal test results, and failure to ensure that patients complete follow-up appointments.[5] Other types of malpractice claims gastroenterologists face include claims related to improper performance of a procedure (e.g., a perforated bowel resulting from poor colonoscopy technique) or failure to monitor a patient's case. In addition to claims arising from medical error, malpractice liability may also result from "nonmedical" conduct, such as failure to obtain informed consent or breach of patient confidentiality and privacy protections.

Data on the relative frequency of different types of malpractice claims against gastroenterologists is limited. However, a review of gastroenterology claims data compiled by the Physician Insurers Association of America (PIAA) from 1985 through 2005 revealed that the most common reasons gastroenterologists face malpractice lawsuits are "error in diagnosis" (28% of claims), "improper performance" of a procedure (25% of claims), "failure to supervise or monitor case" (9% of claims), and performance of a procedure "when not indicated or contraindicated" (2.3% of claims).[6] There was no "medical misadventure" identified in 19% of claims.[6]

LEGAL PRINCIPLES IN MEDICAL PRACTICE

Medical malpractice actions are typically based on the legal theory of negligence. A claim of negligence requires the plaintiff's attorney to prove four elements:

1. Duty: The physician owed an obligation of care to the plaintiff;
2. Breach of Duty: The physician violated that duty by practice below the applicable standard of care;
3. Causation: The physician's substandard practice caused harm to that individual; and
4. Damages: The plaintiff suffered cognizable and compensable harm.

Duty

To prove the element of duty, it generally suffices to establish the existence of a physician-patient relationship. Although a physician has no legal duty to accept a person as a patient or to provide care to a person with whom the physician does not have a physician-patient relationship, once the physician establishes a physician-patient relationship with an individual, the physician has a duty to provide competent care to that person and could be held liable for failure to do so.

It is generally evident when such duty has been established. For example, a physician-patient relationship may be established by the patient entering the hospital or clinic and the physician accepting to or beginning to treat the patient. The duty of care may also be established in less obvious situations, however, such as when advising an emergency room physician about a patient while on call or providing a "curbside consult" to a patient while not on call.

As less formal methods of medical communication, such as medical web platforms or emails that allow patients to interact with physicians, become more prevalent, it is important for physicians to remain cognizant of the potential for such venues to lead to the establishment of a physician-patient relationship and the corresponding duty of care.

Breach of Duty

To prove the element of breach, the plaintiff must show that the physician did not provide the level of care that a reasonable and prudent member of the medical profession would undertake under the same or similar circumstances.[7,8] Breach may be established by showing that the treatment itself was substandard or that the physician failed to obtain informed consent to the procedure from the patient. With respect to substandard treatment, whether a physician has breached his or her duty to the patient and provided inadequate care is determined in reference to the standard of care that the physician was expected to provide. The standard of care is based on prevailing practice and may be established by the testimony of an expert in the field as to whether the physician's care was adequate or, with increasing frequency, reference to CPGs or quality measures. Importantly, it is not the negative result that determines whether the physician breached his or her duty to the patient, but whether the physician acted with the degree of skill and care of a reasonable physician in the circumstances. One must distinguish a "bad outcome" from negligence.

The current standard of care and whether the physician's conduct fell short of this standard has traditionally been established through expert witness testimony, but courts are increasingly relying on respected national guidelines as well. CPGs are treatment standards developed by practitioners (typically medical associations) and are informed by a systematic review of evidence and assessment of the benefits and harms of alternative care options.[9] While a court will regard such guidelines as relevant evidence, it generally will not allow them, standing alone, to establish the standard of care in any given situation.[10] Nevertheless, CPGs and quality measures may be cited by experts and become important determinants of the standard of care.

While in many cases breach must be established by reference to expert testimony or medical guidelines, in certain cases the breach falls within the "common knowledge"[11] or "obvious occurrence"[12] exception, wherein the wrong committed is within the realm of a layperson's comprehension (e.g., a sponge retained in the abdomen at surgery, or amputation of the wrong limb). Expert witnesses are also unnecessary under a similar but technically separate doctrine called *res ipsa loquitur* (the thing speaks for itself), a legal term applying to a narrow category of malpractice cases in which the jury may infer negligence from the mere fact of an accident's occurrence.[13] Whereas some jurisdictions openly disfavor application of *res ipsa loquitur* in medical malpractice cases,[14] other jurisdictions apply it in common knowledge or obvious occurrence cases.

Causation

The third element, causation, may be established by showing that the physician's substandard medical care directly led to the harm experienced by the plaintiff. Causation is frequently the most complicated and difficult element for plaintiffs to prove in medical malpractice cases. Because patients commonly have preexisting conditions, it is often difficult to determine whether the physician's substandard practice "caused" the patient's bad outcome or whether the patient's harm would have happened anyway.

Although the causation analysis varies from state to state, a 2014 case involving a gastroenterologist in Pennsylvania provides a good illustration of how courts have handled complex causation analysis in malpractice cases.[15] The plaintiff in this case suffered from chronic constipation for which her gastroenterologist prescribed Visicol. Visicol is approved for cleansing the colon for a colonoscopy; use of Visicol for long-term treatment of chronic constipation was an off-label use. The plaintiff was on Visicol for five years before her nephrologist took her off the medication after diagnosing her with permanent, progressive kidney disease. At trial, the plaintiff presented evidence that her kidney failure was caused by long-term ingestion of Visicol as prescribed by her gastroenterologist. The defendant gastroenterologist responded by raising the patient's history of bulimia, hypertension, and nonsteroidal antiinflammatory drug (NSAID) use as alternative explanations for the kidney disease.

Following the trial, a jury determined that the gastroenterologist was negligent, but denied recovery to the plaintiff, finding that she had failed to prove causation. As interpreted by the lower court, causation required a showing that *but for* the Visicol prescription, the plaintiff would not have experienced the injury of progressive kidney disease. Given the plaintiff's preexisting conditions, this could not be established. The case did not end there, however. The patient appealed the case, and the appellate court remanded the case for a new trial with an instruction to apply an alternative theory of causation, the increased risk theory. Under the increased risk theory, a plaintiff may prove causation based on a showing that the defendant's conduct increased the risk that the harm sustained by the plaintiff would occur. Thus, even though Visicol may not have caused the plaintiff's kidney disease, the plaintiff could recover by demonstrating that chronic use of Visicol caused an increased risk of developing kidney disease.

Damages

Finally, plaintiffs must prove the fourth element, damages, by showing that they experienced some form of compensable harm. Once the plaintiff has established each of the elements of the malpractice suit, the defendant physician or medical practice is required to pay all damages suffered by the plaintiff, even if surprisingly great in scope.

The amount of damages a plaintiff can recover explains why some types of malpractice cases are brought with significantly greater frequency than others. For example, missed or delayed diagnosis of CRC is the most frequent and serious lawsuit against gastroenterologists.[6,16] CRC is a serious illness and may therefore result in a large damages award. Similarly, a young patient with inflammatory bowel disease who becomes disabled after a negligent event may have a large claim for medical expenses and future lost income. The potential for a large settlement or judgment is enough to justify to the plaintiff's attorney the expense of bringing a malpractice suit.

Apportioning Damages Among Multiple Defendants

In many malpractice cases, the patient sues multiple providers who were involved in his or her care. This creates complex questions about how damages in the case will be apportioned among the defendants. One question that arises is how responsibility for payment of damages is handled where one of the defendants is either unable to or does not pay. There are two main ways states handle this issue, though many states have modified these models in some respects. Under a "joint and several liability" system, each defendant is individually liable for all the damages in the case. If all defendants are able to pay, the plaintiff recovers the damages from all the defendants. If one or more of the defendants is unable to pay, the other defendants are responsible for paying all the damages. Conversely, under a "several liability" system, defendants are responsible for their proportionate share of the damages, and if one of the defendants does not pay, the other defendants are not responsible for covering that share of the damages.

As of 2014, the National Conference of State Legislatures reports that about half of the states allow for joint and several liability and half have a several liability system.[17] This is an oversimplification of the landscape, however, as most states have modified these systems to some extent. For example, some states have hybrid liability rules, where joint and several liability applies to some portion of damages (e.g., joint and several liability for economic damages and several liability for noneconomic damages). In some states, whether joint and several liability or several liability applies depends on some aspect of the case, such as the defendant's percentage fault in the case.

Vicarious Liability

Another critical issue that arises in many malpractice cases is the question of "vicarious liability." Vicarious liability is a legal concept that extends liability for a wrongdoing beyond the original wrongdoer to persons who have not directly committed a wrong, but on whose behalf the wrongdoers acted. The primary practical importance of this concept is that it provides the plaintiff with additional financially responsible defendants who likely have

greater resources than the original defendant. For example, in the context of medical malpractice lawsuits, a hospital could be held directly liable for its own negligence (e.g., due to poorly maintained equipment) and could also be held vicariously liable for the negligence of its employees (e.g., if a nurse administered the wrong medication).

For the practicing physician, the implication of vicarious liability is that physicians can be held legally liable not only for their own actions but also for the actions of others whom they are responsible for supervising. This holds even if the gastroenterologist had neither personally committed nor even was aware of the wrongful act. Thus, if a nurse involved in an endoscopy procedure failed to use sterile technique or appropriately monitor the patient, causing the patient harm, the gastroenterologist performing the procedure could be vicariously liable for the injuries caused by the nurse. In another example, if the physician's medical assistant fails to provide notification of an urgent postprocedure call regarding a developing complication, or gives incorrect postprocedure advice, the supervising gastroenterologist could be held liable, despite being unaware of the call or advice.

Defenses

When faced with a medical malpractice claim, there are certain "affirmative defenses" available to physicians. One defense that may be raised is a statute of limitations defense. If the plaintiff does not bring a malpractice claim until after the time period specified in the relevant state's statute of limitations has lapsed, then the case is barred. The statute of limitation varies by state, but typically is in the realm of two to three years.

Another affirmative defense that may be raised in a malpractice case is "contributory negligence" of the patient. This is an important defense in the medical malpractice context, because plaintiffs are often at least partially responsible for their own injuries (e.g., if the patient skipped follow-up appointments or failed to take medications as recommended). In the past, contributory negligence was a complete defense, and plaintiffs could not recover anything if they were partially responsible for their own injury. This is not the current state of the law, however, and contributory negligence will typically only serve as a partial defense that may reduce damages. Different states take different approaches to handling contributory negligence. In states that have a "pure" comparative negligence system, the plaintiff is entitled to the percentage of the damages for which the defendant is liable. Other states have modified this comparative negligence system by, for example, only allowing the plaintiff to recover damages if the defendant was at least 50% responsible for the damages.

INFORMED CONSENT

Failure to obtain effective informed consent may provide a basis for establishing breach of duty in a medical malpractice case. A physician violates his or her duty to obtain a patient's informed consent if he or she fails to disclose facts necessary for the patient to form intelligent consent to the proposed treatment.[18]

It is critical to recognize that the duty to obtain informed consent requires more than the patient's pro forma consent to treatment. For consent to be valid, the patient must voluntarily consent to treatment after receiving information on, and understanding, the material risks and benefits of the proposed treatment and available alternative treatments.[19] Thus, while some malpractice suits may involve a complete failure to obtain a patient's consent to treatment, most malpractice suits with an informed consent element involve allegations that the physician did not disclose sufficient information to allow the patient to make a truly informed decision when giving consent.[20]

In determining whether the physician satisfied his duty to inform the patient of material risks and alternative treatments, courts apply one of two standards. In some states, courts apply a "reasonable person" standard, under which physicians are required to disclose that information which a reasonable person would find important in deciding about a treatment. Other states have adopted a "prudent physician" standard. Under this approach, physicians must disclose that information which a reasonable physician in similar circumstances would disclose.

It is also important to keep in mind that informed consent may be withdrawn, potentially subjecting the physician to liability for any treatment administered after consent was withdrawn.[21–24] The question of liability based on withdrawal of consent is handled differently from state to state. In some states, for example, providers are liable only if the patient's withdrawal of consent satisfies a two-part test. First, the patient's withdrawal must have been done in a manner as to "leave no room for doubt in the minds of reasonable men that in view of all the circumstances consent was actually withdrawn."[25] Second, at the time the patient withdrew consent, it must have been medically feasible to desist in the treatment without the cessation being detrimental to the patient's health.[25]

There are a number of steps gastroenterologists may take to reduce the risk of liability for failure to obtain informed consent. These steps are particularly relevant for open access or direct access procedures. As an initial step, gastroenterologists should adopt an intake process where the patient is mailed or verbally given information about the relevant procedure (e.g., CRC screening). This mailing or discussion should include a description of the procedure, the purpose of the procedure, the risks and benefits of the procedure, and alternative treatments or diagnostic options. The office should document the patient's receipt of this information and whether the patient had any questions or concerns about the procedure. For any patients who appear uncertain or have many questions, the office should schedule a preprocedure consultation appointment with the physician. Finally, on the day of the procedure, the physician should obtain the patient's documented consent to the procedure. Where thorough information is provided to the patient through a process similar to that described here, the physician can fulfill his or her legal obligation to obtain informed consent by summarizing the information at the time he or she obtains the patient's consent.

DISCLOSURE OF PROTECTED HEALTH INFORMATION

As the practice of medicine shifts to incorporate information technology, there have been many improvements in physicians' ability to document, store, and exchange patient data, communicate between physicians and with patients, monitor patients more effectively, and reduce administrative inefficiencies. Alongside these improvements, a host of legal risks for physicians have emerged, such as new standards of care arising from increased access to patient records, liability for failure to respond adequately and rapidly to questions sent over email, and issues relating to the focus of this section, the disclosure of protected health information.

Patients have a legal right to, and in many cases are dependent on, the confidentiality of their medical records. Disclosure of such protected health information can lead to liability for the physician, hospital, or storing facility for the data. The United States has a network of laws and standards relating to the protection of patient health information.

Two important rules to keep in mind are the Health Insurance Portability and Accountability Act of 1996 (HIPAA) Privacy Rule and the HIPAA Security Rule. The former establishes national standards to protect the privacy and limit use and disclosure of all individually identifiable health information relating to the individual's past, present, or future physical or mental health condition, the provision of health care to that individual, or the payment for such care where the individual is identified. The HIPAA Security Rule deals with electronic protected health information and requires the implementation of administrative, physical, and technical safeguards to protect the information covered in the HIPAA Privacy Rule. The penalty for breaching the rights of patients under these rules was increased in 2010 with the introduction of the Health Information Technology for Economic and Clinical Health (HITECH) Act from a maximum of $250,000 to over $1.5 million.

Unless a statutory exception applies, physicians should ensure that they do not disclose, intentionally or through a failure to include sufficient safety mechanisms, identifying patient information, unless they have consent for such disclosure. When communicating with patients over email, physicians should ensure that all email communication with patients is compliant with HIPAA, transferred over secure networks, and with sufficient disclaimers or precautions about the timeliness of email communication and potential outsider access.

RISK MANAGEMENT APPROACHES

While there is no way to entirely insulate a medical practice from malpractice risk, there are a number of steps that can be taken to reduce risk. Many gastroenterology practices have implemented risk management programs designed to reduce legal risk through implementation of proactive strategies.

Elements of a risk management program in gastroenterology may include[26–29]:

1. A codified peer review process, which may include reviews of complications and sentinel events;
2. Unit reviews, which should include, among other things, monitoring of infection control steps for colonoscopy and other procedures, and assessment of the adequacy of appointment reminder systems and results notification;
3. Use of CPGs and documented practice plans (e.g., a written policy for responding to postprocedure patient concerns or complications);
4. Training of office staff on malpractice risks, risk mitigation techniques, and effective communication with patients[30,31];
5. Documentation of all aspects of a patient's care (such as informed consent, patient experience during procedures, and instructions given to patients)[26,32]; and
6. Coverage by adequate malpractice insurance.

Good Documentation Practices

As described previously, one aspect of an effective risk management program is the implementation of good documentation practices. Documentation demonstrating that proper procedures were followed at each step establishes a record of appropriate care in the event that a patient brings a malpractice suit after treatment. To ensure that the documented record is credible and available as a defense, it is therefore critical that all entries be dated and that notations never be altered. To the extent that there is an error in the record, the correction should be made, signed, and dated. The error should be struck through or otherwise denoted as an error, but should remain legible.

Documentation must be thorough to best protect the physician in the event that malpractice litigation arises. At a minimum, the record should include a description of the informed consent process and the patient's consent, any findings, interventions performed, complications, recommendations and patient instructions, and recommended follow-up. Documentation is particularly important when a gastroenterologist is performing an invasive procedure because patients are at an increased risk of experiencing harm. Generally acceptable components of complete documentation for a colonoscopy, for example, include the following:

1. Photographic recording of the cecum and landmarks;
2. Description of the colon preparation, including a recommendation for early repeat of colonoscopy when the preparation is inadequate;
3. Notation of slow and careful withdrawal with adequate clearing of residual pools of liquid;
4. Record of compliance with the informed consent process, including that the physician mentioned the possibility of missed diagnosis;
5. An established process for managing patients' postprocedure questions or complications;
6. A secure method to notify patients and referring physicians of procedure results, including pathology and recommendations for further examinations; and
7. A system to monitor procedure quality and results.[33]

Clinical Practice Guidelines

Another effective risk management tool in gastroenterology is the use of CPGs. As described earlier, CPGs are evidence-based treatment guidelines developed to assist practitioners determine preferable approaches to treat specific clinical problems.[34,35] CPGs are developed by practitioners (primarily medical societies) based on a variety of sources, such as clinical trials, other peer-reviewed studies, and expert consensus. Because CPGs are developed based on scientific evidence and reflect the practice recommendations of well-respected physicians in the field, adhering to CPGs is one way to improve patient care and reduce the malpractice risk. Nevertheless, it is important to keep in mind that CPGs have limitations. In particular, CPGs may become outdated and no longer represent the standard of care.[36] Physicians are still required to follow and apply advancements in medicine, regardless of the outdated status of the CPG. The quality movement, with quality assessment measures, has a similar impact on standard of care and risk management.

Best Practice for Managing Complications and Error

The most cautious and meticulous approach to the practice of medicine cannot guarantee that no complications or errors will occur. A significant determinant of the ultimate outcome of such issues is how the physician responds. Although traditional medical training curriculums do not allocate much time to addressing the optimal response,[37] proper management of these issues is important to the patient's health, perception of the physician and likelihood to sue, as well as the avoidance of similar complications or errors in the future. While a normal response

may be to attempt to hide the issue and avoid informing the patient, particularly if the complication arose as a result of error on the part of the physician, this can have dangerous consequences for the patient's health and will likely erode the patient's trust in the physician if he or she ultimately does find out about the error. A more positive and productive response, for example, would be for the physician to promptly inform the patient and their family of the issue, express empathy, and recommend follow-up care. One study of a program instituted at the University of Michigan Health System in 2001, whereby physicians were encouraged to disclose errors to patients and offer compensation, determined that in the 9 years after the program was instituted, claims dropped 36% and lawsuits dropped 65%.[38] Approximately 15 years after the institution of the program, a second study found a 58% drop in claims per patient encounters, despite a 72% increase in clinical activity.[38]

When a complication or error arises, the appropriate response for the physician is to engage in frank discussion and open dialogue with the patient and/or family, provide empathy, and suggest next steps.[39] An empathetic response is always appropriate in the face of an adverse outcome. Physicians should be careful to distinguish offering empathy (i.e., "I am sorry this happened to you") from an apology or admission of error. Engaging with the hospital's risk management team to determine the best course of action can also assist physicians in determining the appropriate response. When a lawsuit is brought, it is important to communicate properly with the risk management department and/ or defense attorney and to understand the timeline and proceedings involved in a lawsuit.[40]

KEY REFERENCES

1. Harvard Medical Malpractice Study: A Report of the Harvard Medical Practice Study to the State of New York. Cambridge, MA, The President & Fellows of Harvard College, 1990.
2. Brennan TA, Leape LL, Laird NM, et al: Incidence of adverse events and negligence in hospitalized patients. Results of the Harvard Medical Practice Study I, *N Engl J Med* 324(6):370–376, 1991.
3. Thomas EJ, Studdert DM, Burstin HR, et al: Incidence and types of adverse events and negligent care in Utah and Colorado, *Med Care* 38(3):261–271, 2000.
4. Jena AB, Seabury S, Lakdawalla D, Chandra A: Malpractice risk according to physician specialty, *N Engl J Med* 365(7):629–636, 2011.
5. Wahls TL, Peleg I: Patient and system-related barriers for the earlier diagnosis of colorectal cancer, *BMC Fam Pract* 10:65, 2009.
7. Hood v. Phillips, 554 S.W.2d 160, 165 (Texas 1977).
8. Moses RE, Feld AD: Legal risks of clinical practice guidelines, *Am J Gastroenterol* 103:7–11, 2008.
9. Institute of Medicine (IOM): *Clinical practice guidelines we can trust.* Washington, DC, The National Academies Press, 2011.
10. Halls v. Kiyici, 104 A.D.3d 502, 504-05, 960 N.Y.S.2d 423, 425 (2013).
16. Gerstnberger PD, Plumeri PL: Malpractice claims in gastrointestinal endoscopy: analysis of an insurance industry database, *Gastrointest Endosc* 39:132–138, 1993.
19. Berg JW, Appelbaum PS, Lidz CW, et al: *Informed consent: legal theory and clinical practice*, ed 2, Oxford, Oxford University Press, 2001.
23. Vargo JJ, Delegge MH, Feld AD, et al: Multi-society sedation curriculum for gastrointestinal endoscopy, *Am J Gastroenterol* 143(1):e18–e41, 2012.
26. Feld KA, Feld AD: Risk management and legal issues for colonoscopy, *Gastrointest Endosc Clin N Am* 20(4):599–600, 2010.
27. Feld KA, Blankstein SF, Feld AD: Medical legal aspects of quality improvement, *Colorectal Cancer Screen* 173–192, 2015.
28. Cotton PB: Analysis of 59 ERCP lawsuits: mainly about indications, *Gastrointest Endosc* 63(3):378–382, 2006.

29. Rex DK: Avoiding and defending malpractice suits for post-colonoscopy cancer: advice from an expert witness, *Clin Gastroenterol Hepatol* 11(7): 768–773, 2013.

30. Levenson W, Roter DL, Mullooly JP, et al: Physician-patient communication. The relationship with malpractice claims among primary care physicians and surgeons, *JAMA* 277:553–559, 1997.

31. Gallagher TH, Studdert D, Levinson W: Disclosing harmful medical errors to patients, *N Engl J Med* 356:2713–2719, 2007.

32. Petrini DA, Petrini JL: Risk assessment and management for endoscopists in an ambulatory surgery center, *Gastrointest Endosc Clin N Am* 16: 801–815, 2006.

33. Rex DK, Bond JH, Feld AD: Medical legal risks of incident cancers after clearing colonoscopy, *Am J Gastroenterol* 96(4):952–957, 2001.

37. Feld KA, Feld AD: Time to put managing endoscopic complications into the curriculum, *Am J Gastroenterol* 111(3):353–354, 2016.

38. Adams MA, Elmunzer BJ, Scheiman JM: Effect of a health system's medical error disclosure program on gastroenterology-related claims rates and costs, *Am J Gastroenterol* 109:460–464, 2014.

39. Richter JM, Kelsey PB, Campbell EJ: Adverse event and complication management in gastrointestinal endoscopy, *Am J Gastroenterol* 111(3): 348–352, 2016.

40. Feld AD, Moses RM: Most doctors win: what to do if sued for medical malpractice, *Am J Gastroenterol* 104:1346–1351, 2009.

A complete reference list can be found online at ExpertConsult .com

11

Small-Caliber Endoscopy

Mathieu Pioche, Jérôme Rivory, Jérôme Dumortier, and Thierry Ponchon

RATIONALE

Upper endoscopy is an important diagnostic tool in the care of patients with gastrointestinal (GI) diseases. Unfortunately, there is a certain amount of discomfort and patient intolerance associated with unsedated procedures. For this reason, physicians are hesitant to use unsedated endoscopy as a first-line of investigation in patients with various GI problems, including gastroesophageal reflux disease (GERD). Thus, proton pump inhibitors are often used as a diagnostic test or for prolonged periods before proceeding to endoscopy. Different approaches have been proposed to improve patient tolerance during upper GI endoscopy. The most common and most widely used approach is intravenous sedation.[1–5] Most patients wish to be sedated for upper endoscopy to avoid discomfort, but sedation introduces the need for numerous guidelines not otherwise required during endoscopy. Pre-, intra-, and postprocedure monitoring and assessment are required. Sedation related issues are responsible for up to 40% of the total endoscopic cost (cost of medication, cost of specialized nursing care, work loss) and one-half of the risk.[2,4] Most patients would prefer to return quickly to normal activities as afforded by unsedated endoscopy.[6] In some countries, general anesthesia is used broadly, which seems extreme for routine upper endoscopy. Less intensive approaches to sedation include premedication, topical anesthesia, and more anecdotal methods (such as ambient music), but they are less effective than intravenous sedation. The goal of all these methods is to reduce the patient's level of sensation, but they fail to modify the nature of the examination itself.

Transnasal introduction has been widely employed for bronchoscopy and laryngoscopy. With the advent of thinner endoscopes, transnasal esophagogastroduodenoscopy (EGD, or upper endoscopy) was originally considered an alternate option when transoral intubation was not possible for anatomical reasons.[7,8] With time, transnasal intubation appeared to be a logical alternative to standard peroral EGD on a routine basis, as oral intubation of the esophagus is a major source of discomfort for patients.[9] The transoral route induces protective glottal reflexes as the endoscope passes the base of the tongue and is swallowed. With the transnasal route, the patient does not swallow and does not have protective reflexes; patients can control their laryngeal motility and do not feel any sensation of asphyxia, as illustrated by the fact that they are able to talk during the procedure, further decreasing symptoms associated with anxiety.

In this chapter, we will discuss two major topics: tolerance and performance. This association is essential to allow transnasal endoscopy to expand and potentially replace conventional oral endoscopy in certain situations.

TRANSNASAL ENDOSCOPY

History

Since the first publications in the 1990s, studies concerning patient tolerance of unsedated transnasal endoscopy have shown conflicting results.[8–12] The authors of one study[13] observed that the overall assessment of patients regarding transnasal endoscopy is worse than with standard endoscopy, whereas another study[14] concluded exactly the opposite. Patient tolerance of transnasal endoscopy is a major issue. The majority of published studies to date are in favor of the transnasal approach. One study of 20 volunteers noted significantly less risk of gagging and vomiting during transnasal insertion.[15] Another evaluated 24 patients who underwent sequential transnasal EGD (5.3-mm diameter scope) followed by standard EGD.[16] The transnasal group had less choking, sore throat, discomfort, and a higher rate of acceptability than the peroral group. A randomized study with 181 patients found tolerance was better with transnasal EGD (5.3-mm diameter) compared to conventional, peroral EGD.[17] This study found that only 3% of patients undergoing transnasal endoscopy desired sedation on a future exam versus 15% in the peroral group. Another study that enrolled 60 patients observed that patients undergoing transnasal endoscopy (5.3-mm diameter) rated the procedure only slightly less comfortable than those undergoing sedated conventional endoscopy. Unsedated transnasal endoscopy was associated with significantly less procedure and recovery room time.[18] One researcher placed 150 patients into three groups to elucidate the respective effect of the nasal route versus the small endoscope diameter on the patient's level of tolerance.[10] One group had an oral route with a 9.8-mm diameter endoscope, the second group had an oral route with a 5.9-mm diameter endoscope, and the third group had a transnasal route (5.9 mm). They found less choking and nausea in the transnasal route group and therefore concluded that the tolerance was dependent on the route and not the endoscope diameter. A similar study was conducted on 150 patients.[14] The authors observed that an ultrathin instrument was better tolerated and required less sedation than conventional endoscopes. Whereas the transnasal route caused less gagging than the peroral route, the tolerance was more dependent on the diameter of the endoscope than on the route of passage. This was demonstrated by the improvement noted with transnasal scopes with only two-way tip deflection, which have a reduction in diameter from 5.5 mm (four-way tip deflection) to 4.9 mm. Finally, a comparative prospective study demonstrated that improved tolerance and less nasal pain was associated with the use of smaller diameter endoscopes when transnasal access was utilized.[19] An example of a transnasal procedure is presented in Video 11.1.

Is the Nasal Route or the Smaller Endoscope Easier to Tolerate?

Four randomized studies have compared the nasal route and the oral route using ultrathin endoscopes. One study used 5.3-mm and 5.9-mm diameter endoscopes in 170 unsedated patients.[20] The authors found the tolerance similar in the two groups. In contrast, another author demonstrated better tolerance with a 4.9-mm two-way tip deflection scope versus a 5.5-mm nasal scope.[19] One researcher enrolled 60 patients in a study comparing the unsedated transnasal and peroral routes using a 6-mm endoscope for both routes.[11] Overall, tolerance was similar in both groups. The main difference found was that the transnasal group had significantly more nasal pain on insertion and thus 85% of the patients in the transoral group versus only 69% in the transnasal group were willing to undergo unsedated endoscopy in the future ($p = 0.07$). In the fourth study, researchers randomized 260 patients undergoing EGD to have it performed with an ultrathin transnasal (6-mm videoendoscope), an ultrathin oral (6-mm videoendoscope), or standard endoscope (9.6-mm videoendoscope).[13] The study results were not in favor of the transnasal route; the overall assessment was better for standard EGD. However, gagging was reduced in transnasal endoscopy. Of note, it is often gagging that makes oral intubation difficult, thus necessitating increased sedation. It is therefore important to note that all these studies have noted less gagging with the transnasal approach.

How Can We Explain Tolerance Discrepancies Between Different Studies?

Optimal preparation of the patient is a key factor in achieving improved tolerance. First, a topical anesthetic (lidocaine) has to be administered with pledgets or by spraying deeply within the nostrils at least 5 minutes prior to endoscope insertion.[21,22] Second, a topical vasoconstricting agent (naphazoline) should be administered as an adjunct to the anesthetic drug to enlarge the nasal passages. Finally, a pharyngeal local anesthetic should be administered at the same time. However, these preparation factors likely do not explain the differences observed. In fact, it is likely that the endoscopists themselves have a large influence on patient preferences. The method of presentation and explanation of the study, as well as the way the questionnaire is obtained, are probably decisive factors (e.g., in one study, patients were questioned by an assistant nurse who did not attend the endoscopy procedure), and the opinions of the patients could reflect the opinions of the endoscopists.[10,12,19] Additionally, if patients are questioned after some time has elapsed since the procedure, their responses may change. The manner in which the patients are recruited may also explain the mixed results, and education is also an important factor. At some institutions, transnasal endoscopy has become the initial approach to EGD, and all patients receive transnasal endoscopy as the initial method of upper endoscopy. Patient age does not seem to affect tolerance of transnasal endoscopy, as demonstrated in a comparative study between young and older patients.[23,25] In a recent meta-analysis including 6659 patients, the technical success of transnasal endoscopy was slightly reduced compared to transoral (−2% lower) but tolerance was significantly improved, with 63% of patients preferring transnasal endoscopy to oral endoscopy.

Results
Technical Success
Several studies highlight the trade-off between the potential improved tolerance of transnasal endoscopy and the concomitant loss of diagnostic accuracy. One issue is the higher rate of failure to pass the endoscope into the second portion of the duodenum via a transnasal approach. These technical problems are related to the smaller scope diameter and increased flexibility. In one study, the failure rate was 18% with transnasal endoscopy versus 3% for peroral endoscopy. A higher transnasal failure rate was also found in a second study.[20] The failure to intubate the duodenum via the transnasal route is due to a combination of factors. First, endoscopists are less familiar with this approach, as they are traditionally taught the peroral method. However, the technical success of transnasal endoscopy can be quickly improved with a rapid self-learning curve for experienced endoscopists.[24] Second, due to its more flexible nature, looping occurs frequently in transnasal endoscopy, often making it impossible to reach the second duodenum. The final and likely most important factor is the size of the nasal passage compared to the oral passage. It is the diameter of the endoscope (5.3 mm vs. 5.9 mm) that accounts for the significantly higher proportion of failures (8 of 41 vs. 2 of 43 for the 5.9- vs. 5.3-mm scope, respectively).[20] The larger diameter also accounted for the significantly higher proportion of epistaxis (12 of 33 vs. 4 of 41). The difference in diameter of the 5.3-mm fiberscope versus the 5.9-mm videoscope may account for the differing results seen in published studies. Similar results were demonstrated using a 4.9-mm endoscope compared to a 5.9-mm two-way tip deflection transnasal scope (Olympus, Tokyo, Japan), with a 97.6% success rate for the 4.9-mm scope versus an 88.8% success rate for the 5.9-mm scope ($p < 0.05$). A meta-analysis has demonstrated the effectiveness of transnasal endoscopy, with a 95% technical success rate versus a 97.8% rate with the transoral route (difference:

−2%, confidence interval [CI] −4% to −1%); however, this difference was not significant if a smaller endoscope (< 5.9 mm) was used (difference: −1%, CI −3% to 0.9%).[25]

Procedure Length

In two studies comparing the transnasal and transoral technique,[17,20] the examination time was 2 minutes longer in the transnasal group than in the transoral group, but this was not observed in a third study.[14] The reason for these differing results is ambiguous and the previously discussed meta-analysis did not analyze procedure time. On one hand, the transnasal approach could be longer, as suctioning of the gastric juice is more difficult and analysis of the mucosa is more challenging. Improved endoscope maneuverability using four-way 5.5-mm diameter endoscopes reduces procedure duration compared to two-way angulation 4.9-mm endoscopes in gastric cancer screening.[26] This difference may also be explained, however, by improved patient tolerance via the transnasal route that permits a more comfortable and thus longer analysis of the mucosa, especially within the stomach, whereas with the transoral

route, the operator may perform an expedited exam to reduce discomfort.

Optical Diagnostic Quality

Despite the improved patient tolerance with the unsedated transnasal approach, decreased optical quality has been observed with the thin, 5.3-mm fiberoptic scope (Fig. 11.1).[27] This may lead to missed lesions. The authors of one study noted a sensitivity of 89% for the transnasal approach,[16] and in another study using the ultrathin endoscope, 5 out of 59 endoscopic findings that were identified on standard endoscopy were missed.[11] Due to the smaller channels, the air/water and suction were suboptimal when compared to present conventional upper endoscopes. Sacrificing optimal visualization for a small diameter is a challenging trade-off. Recently, image quality has been dramatically improved in transnasal video endoscopes with virtual chromo-endoscopy (such as narrow band imaging [NBI; Olympus] and FUJI Intelligent Chromo Endoscopy [FICE; Fujinon, Fujifilm Medical Co., Saitama, Japan]).[28,29] Nevertheless, transnasal endoscopy is typically used for evaluating upper GI symptoms,

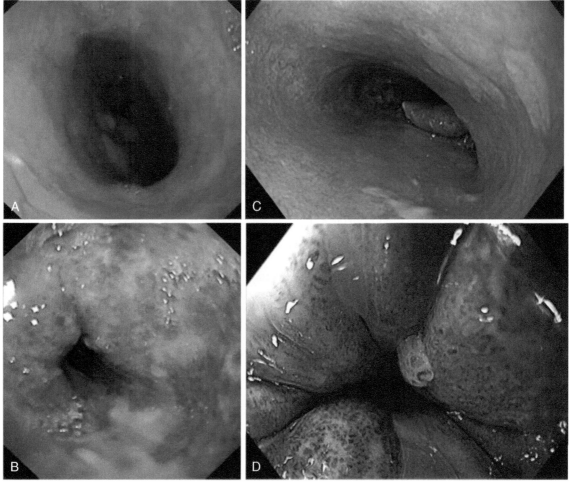

FIG 11.1 Example of an esophageal carcinoma viewed with a transnasal endoscope (Olympus N180, Tokyo, Japan) and a conventional gastroscope (Olympus HQ 190, Tokyo, Japan). **A,** Transnasal endoscopy picture with white light imaging. **B,** Transnasal endoscopy picture with narrow band imaging. **C,** Conventional endoscopy picture with white light imaging. **D,** Conventional endoscopy picture with narrow band imaging and dual focus magnification.

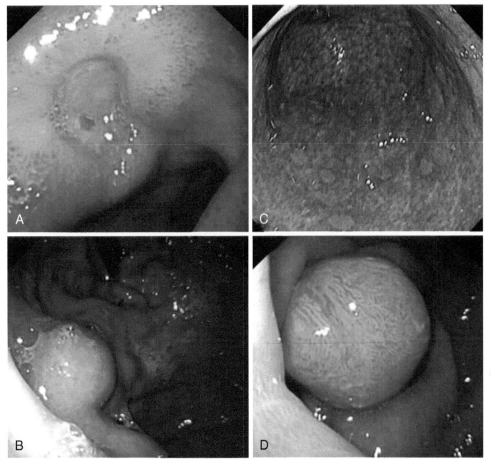

FIG 11.2 Example of upper GI pathology viewed with a transnasal endoscopy. **A,** Ulcer in the antrum. **B,** Gastroesophageal varices. **C,** Intestinal metaplasia in the antrum using NBI. **D,** Antral hyperplastic polyp.

suspected portal hypertension, and screening for Barrett's esophagus (Fig. 11.2), but not for the precise examination of preneoplastic lesions, for which upper GI scopes with zoom capability are preferred (see Fig. 11.1).[30,31]

Adverse Events

Epistaxis is the major side effect of transnasal gastroscopy. For some authors, use of the 5.9-mm videoendoscope resulted in epistaxis in 36% of patients, whereas the 5.3-mm endoscope was associated with epistaxis in 10% of cases. In a large study with 450 transnasal endoscopy procedures, the rate of epistaxis was 5.8%, all of which resulted in limited bleeding.[32] In one series, the epistaxis rate was only 2%.[14] In addition to epistaxis, vertigo may occur after administration of nasal topical anesthesia, probably due to the passage of lidocaine into the inner ear through the eustachian tube.

Biopsy Sampling

Several studies have demonstrated that biopsy sampling can be performed successfully using the small diameter endoscope with a pediatric biopsy forceps (1.8 mm).[10,14,20] The quality of sampling was found to be satisfactory by a histopathologist. In a 2010 prospective comparative study, 1355 biopsy samples were examined, and their quality was analyzed by expert pathologists. The mean size of samples was inferior when the 1.8-mm diameter

pediatric forceps was compared to a 2.2-mm diameter forceps ($p < 0.01$), but the mucosal depth and specimen quality needed to achieve a definitive histologic diagnosis were similar.[33]

Specific Diagnostic Indications

As previously discussed, despite recent improvements in imaging with newer devices, transnasal endoscopy does not provide imaging comparable to standard upper endoscopes because standard endoscopes have a 9-mm diameter and are equipped with zoom lenses, a powerful light source, and better charge-coupled device or complementary metal-oxide semiconductor technology.[34] Thus, when high-resolution picture quality is needed, such as for detection of gastric neoplasia, lesion characterization, and margin delineation, most experts use sedated transoral endoscopy with standard endoscopes to reduce discomfort from longer procedures (as inspection is often done using white light, virtual chromoendoscopy, and dye) and maximize visualization. On the other hand, some lesions are not endoscopically challenging and can easily be detected by transnasal endoscopy, such as ulcers, esophagitis, varices, and Barrett's esophagus.[30,35] Furthermore, some of these easy to diagnose lesions occur in patients with severe comorbidities, making sedated procedures challenging and dangerous. In these cases, unsedated procedures aid in reducing patient risks and allow for repeated procedures during follow-up with good patient acceptance.

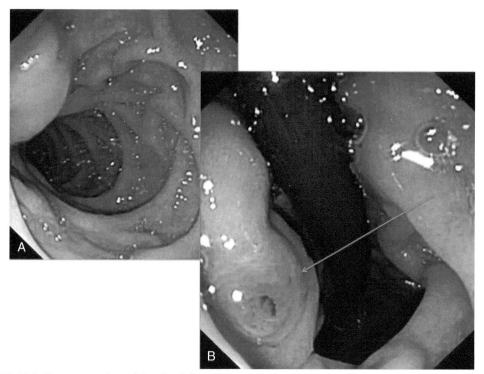

FIG 11.3 Demonstration of the flexibility of transnasal endoscope. **A,** Anterograde view of the second duodenum and the ampulla. **B,** Duodenal retroflexion with retrograde imaging of the major papilla.

Anatomical Reasons

Transnasal endoscopy is sometimes the only viable option when the oral route is not accessible. This is true for patients with trismus or after tongue surgery.[36] Due to its excellent flexibility, transnasal scopes allow for retroflexion almost everywhere in the digestive tract. For example, retroflexion is possible in the second duodenum to optimize visualization of the papilla when an ampullary adenoma is suspected (Fig. 11.3).

Esophageal and Pharyngeal Cancer Screening

High-risk patients, including those with a history of head and neck cancers, have an increased risk of esophageal and pharyngeal cancers. In addition, they may have consequences of tobacco or alcohol use such as respiratory or chronic liver disease. Thus, unsedated procedures are beneficial by avoiding sedation and intubation, particularly for patients with a history of ear, nose and throat (ENT) surgery.[37]

Transnasal unsedated endoscopy is significantly more effective than oral endoscopy (98.9% vs. 73.2%, $p < 0.01$) to examine the pharyngeal area; this is due to the better endoscope axis and to a reduction in the gag reflex.[38] Nevertheless, as discussed previously, virtual chromoendoscopy or iodine staining are needed to improve the sensitivity of endoscopic detection.[39–41] The superiority of chromoendoscopy versus white light endoscopy was also demonstrated in transnasal endoscopy with NBI, Lugol staining, and FICE.[42–44] The Valsalva maneuver is a helpful aid to fix the esophagogastric junction and to improve visualization in the lower esophagus.[45] Transnasal endoscopy with chromoendoscopy is an option to detect esophageal cancer in high-risk patients, although prospective comparative studies are needed to demonstrate its noninferiority compared to standard peroral endoscopy.

Portal Hypertension

Esophageal and gastric varices are easy to diagnose, and patients with cirrhosis typically undergo several endoscopy procedures to detect signs of portal hypertension in the esophagus and stomach. These patients are fragile with severe comorbidities; sedation in these patients can carry significant risk. Transnasal unsedated endoscopy has been studied for this specific indication in several prospective studies, demonstrating superior tolerability compared to transoral endoscopy and with similar effectiveness in diagnosing esophageal and gastric varices, as well as stigmata of recent bleeding.[30,35,46] Virtual chromoendoscopy with FICE may aid in diagnosing esophageal varices.[47] In cirrhotic patients, capsule endoscopy has also been evaluated to assess patients via a less invasive technique. One study demonstrated improved tolerance with capsule endoscopy with the same diagnostic effectiveness when compared to transnasal endoscopy.[48] All patients in this study preferred capsule endoscopy for their follow-up, but the cost effectiveness of this strategy was not evaluated. Due to its cost, capsule endoscopy is not currently recommended to assess portal hypertension in cirrhotic patients and endoscopy is still the initial option.

Preoperative Endoscopy Before Bariatric Surgery in Obese Patients

EGD is an important facet of the preoperative evaluation for bariatric surgery. Morbidly obese patients are at high risk for airway complications during sedated procedures, and transnasal EGD is thus an attractive option. This technique is effective in identifying pathology that requires preoperative treatment or long-term follow-up and offers a complete examination with biopsy capabilities to detect *Helicobacter pylori* or preneoplastic conditions.[33,49]

First Look Endoscopy for Upper GI Bleeding

Upper GI bleeding (UGIB) can be classified into two types a priori according to severity scores: severe bleeding needing resuscitation in intensive care units, and bleeding without hemodynamic consequences that can be medically managed. Patients with severe bleeding usually need intubation and urgent endoscopy to stop the bleeding effectively. In patients with bleeding without hemodynamic compromise, the bleeding source is usually uncertain or due to lesions that can be effectively treated with antisecretory medications such as proton pump inhibitors (esophagitis, ulcer, gastritis). For those patients, transnasal endoscopy is an option to reduce the morbidity of sedated endoscopy. In a prospective study, 145 patients with suspected UGIB were evaluated, and 89 without severe bleeding were considered for transnasal endoscopy.[31] This was effectively performed in 52 cases with five failures; the remainder of the exams were contraindicated for reasons such as patients being on anticoagulant medications. Only two patients had actively bleeding lesions requiring conversion to a sedated endoscopy with intubation.

Assessing and Traversing Esophageal Strictures

Esophageal strictures are sometimes difficult to evaluate due to the narrowed luminal diameter. Patients with a history of esophageal cancer treated with radiation therapy may develop a stenosis but also have a risk of metachronous esophageal cancer above and below the stricture. Using a small-caliber endoscope via a transnasal or transoral technique is useful to traverse the stricture and to examine the distal esophagus.[50] Furthermore, once the stricture is passed, a guidewire can be safely placed to allow subsequent dilation or stent placement.[51]

Therapeutic Transnasal Endoscopy

Guidewire Placement

Transnasal endoscopy is well suited to certain situations involving guidewire placement.[51] This includes traversing strictures to allow for guidewire placement prior to dilation or stenting as mentioned previously. In addition, transnasal endoscopy has been used for placement of feeding tubes for quite some time, especially for patients with severe comorbidities.[7,8,50,52]

Transnasal Endoscopic Gastrostomy

Initially used in cases of oral obstruction, transnasal unsedated endoscopic gastrostomy tube placement was subsequently described and evaluated in several studies involving medically fragile patients.[51,53–57] This technique appears less invasive and is effective and safe when compared to conventional transoral gastrostomy tube placement.[58] It represents a good option in cases of oral obstruction by head and neck cancer.[59] However, the recent description of ostomy metastases in cases utilizing the "pull" technique have changed the approach to this situation.[60–62] Push gastrostomy is now recommended (radiologically or endoscopically) in these situations to avoid metastasis of tumor cells into the gastrostomy tract.[63]

Argon Plasma Coagulation

The endoscopic diagnosis of gastric vascular ectasia and varices can be improved using virtual chromoendoscopy during transnasal endoscopy, as discussed previously.[47,64] Furthermore, a small-size argon plasma probe has been developed (Erbe, Tübingen, Germany) that can pass through the operating channel of 5.5-mm transnasal scopes to treat lesions. Thus, it is possible to treat lesions such as gastric antral vascular ectasia and telangiectasia without sedation by argon plasma coagulation in patients with significant sedative risks.[64,65] This technique has also been used in Peutz-Jeghers syndrome to allow for the destruction/ablation of residual hamartomas after resection.[66]

Endoscopic Resection

Commonly, endoscopic resection requires conventional upper or lower GI endoscopes that have a large operating channel and a water-jet channel to use the relatively large tools needed for resection and to provide adequate lavage in case of bleeding. Nevertheless, there are reports of endoscopic resection using transnasal scopes. The first involved the treatment of Peutz-Jeghers polyps using a combination of snare polypectomy and argon plasma coagulation.[66] Subsequently, a transnasal endoscope was placed in parallel with a conventional endoscope to retract a lesion during a gastric endoscopic submucosal dissection (ESD) procedure.[67–69] More recently (2013), a Japanese team developed a dedicated cap for a transnasal endoscope to perform ESD.[70] This group subsequently described ESD cases in the esophagus and in the duodenal bulb using a transnasal endoscope because of the difficult location in the esophagus and the inability to perform retroflexion with a conventional endoscope in the duodenal bulb.[71,72]

BILIARY TRACT DIAGNOSIS AND TREATMENT

Small-caliber endoscopes have been increasingly used to access the common bile duct to explore strictures or to perform intracorporeal lithotripsy of bile stones.[73] Three types of cholangioscopy are possible: percutaneously after a period of drainage (to make a mature fistula track), using a mother-baby endoscope system through the operating channel of a duodenoscope, and direct peroral cholangioscopy with or without a guidewire. Whatever the technique used, cholangioscopy allows for the examination and targeted biopsy of strictures, as well as the destruction and removal of stones or polyps. Those techniques have become the first-line option, especially when surgery is not suitable or difficult, such as after liver transplantation or a complex biliopancreatic surgery.[74,75]

Percutaneous Anterograde Approach

After percutaneous drainage has been performed and an appropriate period of time has elapsed to create a fistula, a small-caliber endoscope (cholangioscope, transnasal scope) can be introduced into the bile duct to evaluate, biopsy, and dilate strictures and to treat (lithotripsy) and remove bile duct stones.[76,77] Although mother-baby endoscopy has been dramatically improved, the percutaneous approach is still used in certain situations.[78] One example is for biliary diseases occurring in patients with a history of digestive surgery and a hepaticojejunal anastomosis (gastric bypass, Roux en Y).[79] In these cases, a jejunal loop is connected to the biliary tree and endoscopic access to the anastomosis is difficult or impossible, even when using single- or double-balloon enteroscopy.[80] In this situation, percutaneous access may be the only option when a repeat surgery is not feasible. A benefit of the percutaneous approach is the maneuverability of the scope, as the distance between the skin and the papilla is short. Furthermore, as the scope is introduced from the liver to the papilla, examination of the distal bile duct just above the papilla is likely easier.[81] This approach allows shorter scopes with better maneuverability to be used.[82] Commonly, percutaneous cholangioscopy needs two operators and a percutaneous drain that has been present for several weeks or even months to allow for maturation of the fistula track. This long period of drainage may not be well tolerated for many patients, and different strategies avoiding percutaneous drainage have been developed to achieve direct access to the bile duct via the digestive tract.

Mother-Baby Endoscope System

This technique consists of introducing a small-caliber endoscope into the operating channel of a duodenoscope (4.2 mm) over a guidewire and advancing it over the guidewire across the papilla.[83] The main advantage of this approach is the lack of need for a percutaneous fistula, but serious limitations were initially described. The first types of cholangioscopes appeared in 1985 and were ultrathin fiberscopes.[81] From the beginning, the benefits of the mother-baby system in exploring the middle portions of the bile duct were apparent, although the distal bile duct was easier to visualize and examine by the percutaneous approach. These systems were extremely fragile because they were passed into the duodenoscope and across the elevator and progressively the need for disposable systems appeared. The SpyGlass system (Boston Scientific, Marlborough, MA) was developed to allow examination of the bile duct though a duodenoscope with a reusable optic fiber within a disposable scope.[84,85] The concept was well received, but the maneuverability of the scope and the optical quality of the fiber posed serious limitations.[86] The second-generation SpyGlass device (SpyGlass DS, Boston Scientific) with integrated digital imaging and improved scope mobility has dramatically improved the quality of the system, as demonstrated by several publications.[75,87] This new system allows for high-quality exploration of the bile duct to aid in performing targeted biopsies and lithotripsy through a small operating channel; however, the device is currently quite expensive. Several new disposable cholangioscopes are being developed.

Direct Retrograde Cholangioscopy

The final solution to access the bile or pancreatic duct is direct cholangiopancreatoscopy using a small-caliber endoscope (transnasal scope, cholangioscope, or pediatric/standard upper endoscope) on a guidewire directly from the mouth to the papilla. If a pediatric/standard upper endoscope is used, a guidewire may not be needed if balloon papilloplasty has been performed on the biliary orifice. This strategy typically involves first performing an endoscopic retrograde cholangiopancreatography (ERCP) to put the guidewire into the duct and then exchanging the duodenoscope over the wire and subsequently inserting the transnasal endoscope or cholangioscope onto this guidewire. Compared to mother-baby systems, the size of the scopes passed over the wire can reach 5.5 mm, and image quality is improved, as is the maneuverability and the mechanical strength of the scope.[88] In addition, even larger pediatric/standard endoscopes can be advanced over stiffer wires or directly inserted into the biliary tree after balloon papilloplasty. The main limitation is that the technical success rate of this option is between 72% and 89% even when using an intraductal balloon to stabilize the guidewire.[88–90]

DISPOSABLE TRANSNASAL ENDOSCOPES

Finally, a general trend in endoscopy and gastroenterology is to reduce the constraints and costs associated with endoscopy while improving our ability to detect digestive lesions at an early stage,

which is the best approach to improve patient prognosis. For the general population to accept and be compliant with endoscopic screening and follow-up, the examinations must be easy to perform, well tolerated, and inexpensive. Unsedated transnasal endoscopy could be a possible solution, but it is certainly not the only one. Endoscope reprocessing is another constraint related to the practice of endoscopy. It is time consuming, costly, and represents an occupational hazard to the reprocessing staff who have contact with disinfectants. Furthermore, there is still a risk of residual contamination of the endoscope resulting from inadequate reprocessing and, albeit rare, there are no acceptable and effective methods of disinfection for preventing the transmission of prion diseases. One solution for reducing the risk of contamination and the need for disinfection is the so-called disposable-sheathed endoscope. Mayinger et al (1998, 1999) demonstrated the feasibility of disposable-sheathed gastroscopy in 50 patients.[91,92] The performance of endoscopy outside of traditional endoscopy units with reprocessing facilities might be an important advance in achieving a more widespread use of endoscopy. Such a device might be useful should a gastroenterologist feel endoscopy is appropriate immediately after examining a patient in the office and would allow for performance of the procedure within the exam room. The combination of a transnasal route and a disposable sheath may prove to be an attractive alternative for patients by not only resulting in a reduction in health care expenses, but also allowing for earlier detection of digestive tract lesions. Potential applications of this approach could be used in screening for esophageal varices and Barrett's esophagus.

In conclusion, transnasal EGD using small-caliber endoscopes is an important technique in GI endoscopy. It is well tolerated by patients and offers the possibility of performing endoscopy without sedation. Thus, it could significantly bring down the costs and associated risks of EGD. Ongoing improvements and continued development are warranted in the areas of optics and air/water channels before this promising method will replace conventional upper endoscopy. At present, select patients intolerant of peroral endoscopy may benefit from the transnasal approach.

CONTROVERSIES: COMPETITION WITH CAPSULE ENDOSCOPY

Capsule endoscopy, whose role in the management of obscure GI bleeding is well established, has been utilized since 2004 to examine the esophagus.[48] The three primary applications of esophageal capsule endoscopy involve the detection and follow-up of Barrett's esophagus, the detection of squamous cell carcinoma, and the detection and follow-up of esophageal varices in cirrhotic patients. Capsule endoscopy is a direct competitor to transnasal endoscopy, with its main advantage being the same as that for transnasal endoscopy (i.e., improved patient tolerance). Furthermore, capsule endoscopy also has a major advantage in that it is a single-use device and therefore does not require equipment reprocessing. Capsule endoscopy does not permit complete gastric evaluation, despite the recent ability of a prototype capsule to achieve percutaneous magnetic control, and does not currently provide the ability to sample tissue.[93,94] For these reasons, the potential role of capsule endoscopy for the identification and surveillance of preneoplastic or neoplastic tissue such as Barrett's esophagus or squamous cell carcinoma of the esophagus is limited. For these indications, transnasal endoscopy provides a better option and is also currently less expensive than the disposable capsule.

KEY REFERENCES

12. Dumortier J, Napoleon B, Hedelius F, et al: Unsedated transnasal EGD in daily practice: results with 1100 consecutive patients, *Gastrointest Endosc* 57(2):198–204, 2003.

13. Birkner B, Fritz N, Schatke W, Hasford J: A prospective randomized comparison of unsedated ultrathin versus standard esophagogastroduodenoscopy in routine outpatient gastroenterology practice: does it work better through the nose?, *Endoscopy* 35(8):647–651, 2003.

19. Dumortier J, Josso C, Roman S, et al: Prospective evaluation of a new ultrathin one-plane bending videoendoscope for transnasal EGD: a comparative study on performance and tolerance, *Gastrointest Endosc* 66(1):13–19, 2007.

25. Sami SS, Subramanian V, Ortiz-Fernández-Sordo J, et al: Performance characteristics of unsedated ultrathin video endoscopy in the assessment of the upper GI tract: systematic review and meta-analysis, *Gastrointest Endosc* 82(5):782–792, 2015.

35. Saeian K, Staff D, Knox J, et al: Unsedated transnasal endoscopy: a new technique for accurately detecting and grading esophageal varices in cirrhotic patients, *Am J Gastroenterol* 97(9):2246–2249, 2002.

36. Johnson DA, Cattau EL, Khan A, et al: Fiberoptic esophagogastroscopy via nasal intubation, *Gastrointest Endosc* 33(1):32–33, 1987.

54. Lustberg A, Fleisher AS, Darwin PE: Transnasal placement of percutaneous endoscopic gastrostomy with a pediatric endoscope in oropharyngeal obstruction, *Am J Gastroenterol* 96(3):936–937, 2001.

55. Lustberg AM, Darwin PE: A pilot study of transnasal percutaneous endoscopic gastrostomy, *Am J Gastroenterol* 97(5):1273–1274, 2002.

83. Bogardus ST, Hanan I, Ruchim M, Goldberg MJ: "Mother-baby" biliary endoscopy: the University of Chicago experience, *Am J Gastroenterol* 91(1):105–110, 1996.

A complete reference list can be found online at ExpertConsult .com

12

Postsurgical Endoscopic Anatomy

Sreeni Jonnalagadda and Alisa Likhitsup

INTRODUCTION

Patients who have undergone surgical procedures that altered the upper gastrointestinal (GI) anatomy are often referred for endoscopic evaluation.[1] It is essential for gastroenterologists to understand the postoperative anatomical alterations to select the appropriate endoscope and accessories and obtain meaningful and accurate diagnostic information.[2–5]

This chapter discusses the most common surgical procedures involving the upper GI tract. Technical details and common variations are described for each surgical procedure. The endoscopic correlates to anatomical alterations are described. Available surgical reports should always be reviewed before the endoscopic examination.

ANTIREFLUX PROCEDURES

Nissen Fundoplication

Fundoplication is an effective antireflux operation, performed by creating a gastric plication over the distal esophagus just proximal to the cardioesophageal junction to restore the competency of lower esophageal sphincter. This is a standard operative treatment in select patients with gastroesophageal reflux disease (GERD) (Fig. 12.1).[6]

Fundoplication was first described by Dr. Rudolph Nissen in 1955.[7] This procedure is frequently performed along with hiatal hernia surgery.[8,9] A modified technique called a *floppy Nissen fundoplication* can be accomplished by shortening the wrap from 5 cm to 2 cm. Despite being more lax than a conventional Nissen fundoplication, it is equally effective for GERD management, with the additional benefit of a lower incidence of postoperative gas-bloat syndrome or dysphagia. A laparoscopic approach to this procedure has proved to be safe and reliable. Laparoscopic floppy Nissen fundoplication has become the surgical gold standard treatment for GERD.[10–12]

To perform Nissen surgery, the distal esophagus, the cardioesophageal junction, the gastric fundus, and the right and left crura are dissected. Careful dissection is required to avoid transection of the nerve of Latarjet, a branch of anterior vagal trunk supplying the pylorus. Damage to this branch can result in delayed gastric emptying.[13,14] After hernia reduction, the right and left crura are approximated with sutures (see Fig. 12.1A). Division of the short gastric vessels may be required to mobilize the fundus.[15,16] The gastric fundus is mobilized posterior to the cardioesophageal junction, creating a 360-degree wrap by the placement of two or three sutures involving stomach-esophagus-stomach in the anterior portion of the wrap (see Fig. 12.1B1). The anterior and posterior vagus nerves are usually contained in the wrap and attached to the esophagus. At the end of the procedure, the wrap must lie below the diaphragm without tension.[17,18]

During endoscopy, an intact Nissen fundoplication is easily identifiable. During antegrade endoscope passage, the gastroesophageal junction appears tight on visualization, but offers mild resistance to passage of the endoscope. The retroflexed view reveals an encircling redundant mucosa with several parallel rugal folds overlying the gastric cardia, as well as less capacious stomach fundus (see Figs. 12.1B2). Although this is a 360-degreee wrap, the redundant fold appears as a 270-degree free cuff margin because the border continuous with the lesser curvature is not evident.[19] The crural closure should maintain the cardia below the diaphragm with the stomach completely insufflated with air. Occasionally, sutures in the distal esophagus may be observed, indicating migration through the wall or inappropriate penetration depth of the stitches during the procedure; this may or may not be associated with symptoms.[20]

Findings associated with failure of the fundoplication include esophagitis, lack of the encircling fold on a retroflexed view, patulous gastroesophageal junction, migration of the wrap through an enlarged esophageal hiatus, or hourglass appearance

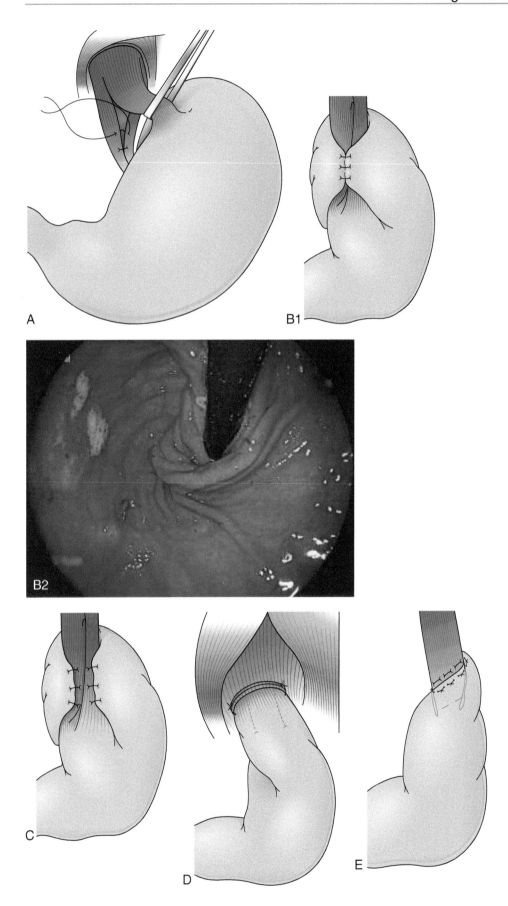

A

B1

B2

C

D

E

FIG 12.1 Antireflux procedures. **A,** Esophageal hiatus is narrowed by sutures that approximate the crura of the diaphragm. **B1,** Nissen fundoplication: a short and loose 360-degree wrap is created around the distal esophagus; **B2,** Parallel rugal folds encircle the cardia and the insertion tube of the endoscope. The cardia is below the diaphragm, and there is no hiatal enlargement. **C,** Toupet fundoplication: a posterior partial wrap is created by suturing the edges of the stomach to the anterior esophagus, leaving a space in between. **D,** Dor procedure: a partial anterior fundoplication usually performed following a Heller myotomy. **E,** Belsey-Mark IV procedure: a partial wrap is created through a thoracotomy by progressive invagination of the esophagus into the stomach.

of the proximal stomach (indicating slippage and irregularity in the dome shape of the fundus, which in turn indicates parahiatal hernia). A squamocolumnar junction located more than 1 cm proximal to the margin of the wrap has been reported to be a major endoscopic clue in diagnosis of postfundoplication problems.[21] An upper GI contrast study can delineate the precise relationship between the wrap and diaphragmatic hiatus when endoscopic examination is unable to clarify if the wrap is intact. Gastric food retention secondary to gastroparesis may be related to damage to the vagus nerves during the procedure.[21] Some patients with persistent dysphagia have a tight wrap that causes resistance to the advancement of the endoscope and these patients may benefit from endoscopic dilation.[22]

Partial Fundoplications (Dor and Toupet)

A partial fundoplication is created with the fundus partially enveloping the distal esophagus, enabling a reduction in postoperative dysphagia and gas-related side effects.[23] A Dor fundoplication is performed anteriorly, and is usually performed in patients who also require a Heller myotomy (see Fig. 12.1C). Toupet fundoplication is performed posteriorly and is best indicated in patients with impaired esophageal body motility (see Fig. 12.1D).[24–26] Partial fundoplications also have a prominent fold overlying the cardia, which is less evident than 360-degree wraps when observed endoscopically.[27]

Belsey Mark IV

The Belsey Mark IV fundoplication requires a thoracotomy. A partial 240-degree anterior wrap is created by the placement of three sutures involving stomach fundus and distal esophagus, resulting in a progressive invagination of the esophagus into the proximal stomach. The crura are also sutured to narrow the esophageal hiatus (see Fig. 12.1E).[28] Endoscopically, the Belsey Mark IV and Nissen fundoplications appear similar, with folds encircling the endoscope at the level of the cardia. However, coils of gastric rugae as seen after Nissen repair are not evident, and there is an anterior compression that corresponds to the attachment of the esophagus to the diaphragm.[19]

Collis Gastroplasty

A short esophagus, usually caused by chronic scarring resulting from GERD, can be repaired surgically through a Collis gastroplasty. This gastroplasty creates a tubular segment of stomach in continuity to the esophagus, long enough to be encircled by a 360-degree fundoplication placed below the diaphragm. The fundoplication around this tubular segment within the positive pressure of the abdomen prevents the gastroesophageal reflux.[29] Short esophagus is identified less often presently, because GERD is diagnosed and treated earlier, reducing the incidence of esophageal scarring and shortening.[30] Endoscopically, the squamocolumnar junction is observed above a short tubular segment of stomach, which may not distend properly because of the wrap. The Collis gastroplasty resembles the Nissen fundoplication on a retroflexed view, except with a less capacious fundus.

OPERATIONS WITHOUT ALTERATION OF THE PANCREATICOBILIARY ANATOMY

Billroth I

The Billroth I operation is a type of reconstruction after a partial gastrectomy in which the stomach is anastomosed to the duodenum (Fig. 12.2A).[31] The gastric resection is usually limited to the antrum, and a truncal vagotomy is often performed in conjunction with the resection. The gastroduodenostomy anastomosis is found toward the greater curvature. A prominent gastric fold representing the closed part of the stomach is often observed along the lesser curvature ending at the gastroduodenostomy. A mucosal pattern change from gastric folds to flat duodenal surface indicates the anastomosis site. The duodenal bulb is partially resected, and the circular folds of the second portion are visualized endoscopically immediately distal to the anastomosis. Major and minor papillae appear to be more proximal in the duodenum than in a patient with intact anatomy. Following the loss of the pylorus, bile reflux is very commonly seen.

Billroth II

In a Billroth II reconstruction after a partial gastrectomy, the duodenal stump is closed and a gastrojejunostomy is created (see Fig. 12.2B). This type of reconstruction is commonly used for complicated peptic ulcer disease or localized gastric antral carcinoma wherein extensive resection is required. The remaining stomach is variable in length and may allow retroflexion maneuver if an adequate residual stomach remains. The gastric remnant usually contains frothy bile and mucosal erythema from the alkaline reflux.[32] The gastrojejunostomy is located at the distal end of the stomach where two stomal openings corresponding to an end-to-side anastomosis can be identified (see Fig. 12.2C).

There are several variations in surgical technique to perform the gastrojejunostomy, each with a distinct endoscopic appearance. The technique selected depends on surgeon preference, and there is no uniform approach. The gastrojejunostomy can vary with regard to the size of the anastomosis, orientation of the jejunal loop to the stomach, and position of the anastomosis relative to the transverse colon. If the whole length of the transected stomach is anastomosed to the jejunum (oralis totalis or Polya), several rows of jejunal folds are observed between the two stomal openings (Fig. 12.3A). Conversely, if only a segment of the transected stomach is anastomosed to the jejunum (oralis partialis or Hoffmeister), few or no folds are evident. In this case, the stomach is partially closed from the lesser curvature to reduce the diameter of the anastomosis, which is located toward the greater curvature. A prominent fold may be seen emanating from the lesser curvature to the anastomosis. Some surgeons attach the jejunal limb to the suture line that is closing the stomach to prevent dehiscence when performing an oralis partialis anastomosis (see Fig. 12.3B).[33] In this case, a sharp angulation might be negotiated to enter the corresponding jejunal limb. The small anastomosis diameter in association with the sharp angulation of this type of reconstruction may make the anatomy difficult to define endoscopically.

In some cases, the stomach is completely closed at the distal end, and the gastrojejunal anastomosis is performed with a linear or a circular stapler in a side-to-side fashion at the posterior wall, 2 cm proximal to the end of the stomach.[34] When observed endoscopically, however, this side-to-side anastomosis is almost indistinguishable from a short end-to-side anastomosis. The jejunum can be anastomosed to the stomach with the afferent limb attached to the greater curvature (isoperistaltic) or to the lesser curvature (antiperistaltic). The afferent limb refers to the jejunal limb that is in continuity with the duodenum, whereas the efferent limb refers to the one that leaves the stomach toward the distal jejunum. The two stomal openings observed

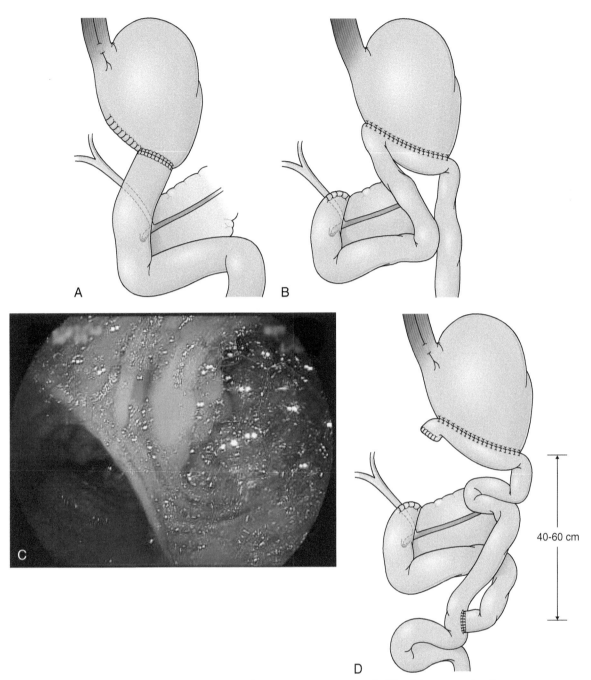

FIG 12.2 Three types of reconstruction after partial gastrectomy. **A,** Billroth I: a gastroduodenostomy is performed toward the greater curvature. **B,** Billroth II: a gastrojejunostomy is created to reestablish the alimentary transit. Several variations may be observed in this type of reconstruction. **C,** Bile coming from the anastomotic opening linked to the lesser curvature indicates the afferent limb (anisoperistaltic anastomosis). **D,** Roux-en-Y: a gastrojejunostomy only is created with the efferent limb to prevent biliopancreatic reflux into the stomach. A 40-cm to 60-cm efferent limb leads to the jejunojejunostomy and afferent limb.

endoscopically may represent the afferent or efferent limb depending on how the reconstruction was performed (see Fig. 12.3C and D). If the reconstruction is isoperistaltic, the opening linked to the greater curvature corresponds to the afferent limb. If the reconstruction is antiperistaltic, the opening linked to the greater curvature corresponds to the efferent limb. Usually the stomal opening linked to the lesser curvature is more difficult

to access with the endoscope because of the relative tangential approach of the endoscope to the anastomosis (see Fig. 12.3E).[35]

Gastrectomies usually include the lesser curvature more than the greater curvature in the resection. In addition, the information from surgical notes about the type of reconstruction, peristalsis, and bile flow might help define the limbs endoscopically. On careful observation of the anastomosis, bile may be seen coming

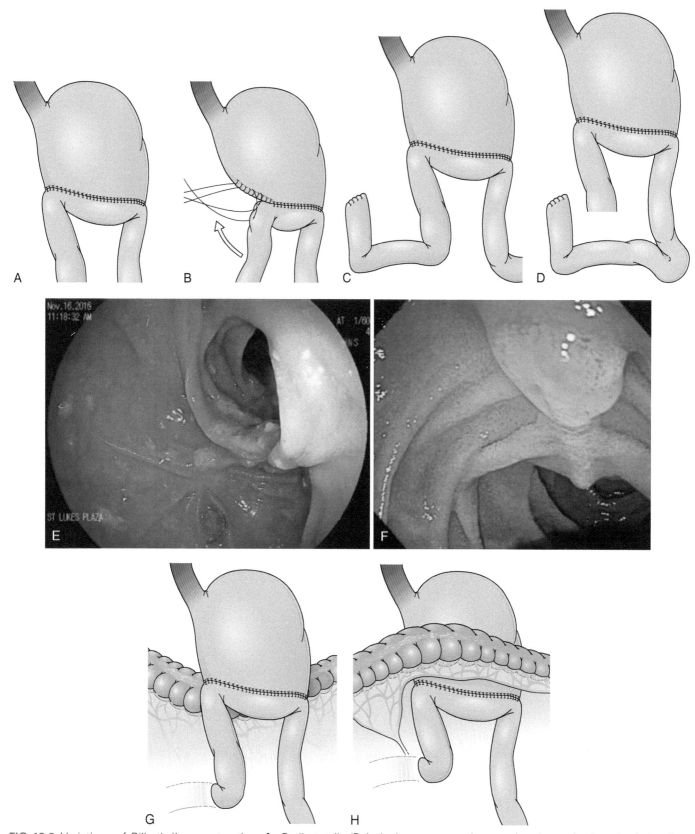

FIG 12.3 Variations of Billroth II reconstruction. **A,** Oralis totalis (Polya): the anastomosis occupies the entire length of the distal stomach. **B,** Oralis partialis (Hoffmeister): the anastomosis occupies only part of the distal stomach. In some cases, the jejunal limb is sutured to the lesser curvature to protect the suture line of the stomach from disruption. In this scenario, a sharp angulation must be negotiated to advance the endoscope through the stomal opening linked to the lesser curvature. **C,** Antiperistaltic anastomosis: the afferent limb is attached to the lesser curvature. **D,** Isoperistaltic anastomosis: the afferent limb is attached to greater curvature. **E,** Sharp verticalization of the gastroenteroanastomosis impairs advance of the endoscope to this afferent limb. **F,** Retrograde view of the major papilla through the afferent limb. **G,** Antecolic reconstruction: the anastomosis is anterior to the transverse colon leading to a longer afferent limb. **H,** Retrocolic reconstruction: the anastomosis passes through the mesocolon creating a shorter afferent limb.

predominantly from the afferent limb. Introducing the endoscope through this opening should reveal an increasing volume of bile as the endoscope advances toward the bulb, although bile may also be observed in the efferent limb. Visible peristaltic waves advancing away from the endoscope suggest that the instrument is in the efferent limb. When the duodenal stump is reached, the flat mucosa of the residual bulb with a scar-like deformity in a cul-de-sac can be identified. A careful withdrawal of the endoscope exposes the major papilla, usually located at the right upper quadrant at radiography (see Fig. 12.3F).

In patients with Billroth II anatomy, the papilla is rotated 180 degrees in the endoscopic visual field. This "upside down" position requires distinct techniques to perform endoscopic retrograde cholangiopancreatography (ERCP), including dedicated sphincterotomes, needle-knife cut technique over the stent, or balloon dilation of the papilla.[36–40] If the duodenal stump cannot be identified, the endoscope should be withdrawn, and the other limb should be intubated as far as possible. Fluoroscopic visualization may indicate that the efferent limb has been entered when the instrument is seen to pass deep into the pelvis. Conversely, passage of the endoscope into the right upper quadrant toward the liver or previous cholecystectomy clips suggests entry into the afferent limb.[41]

The length of the afferent limb also varies depending on the surgical technique. The afferent limb, naturally fixed at the ligament of Treitz and surgically fixed to the stomach, should be tensionless but not redundant. There are two ways to position the afferent limb in relation to the transverse colon during a Billroth II reconstruction. If an antecolic anastomosis is performed, the gastrojejunostomy is placed anterior to the transverse colon (see Fig. 12.3G). Antecolic reconstructions frequently have long afferent limbs because of the distance between the ligament of Treitz and the remaining stomach, over the mesocolon, omentum, and transverse colon. Conversely, retrocolic reconstructions are performed through an opening in the transverse mesocolon, shortening the distance between the ligament of Treitz and the remaining stomach (see Fig. 12.3H).[42,43] Antecolic and retrocolic anastomoses are similar endoscopically except for the the length of the limbs. Caution should be taken if a percutaneous endoscopic gastrostomy is indicated for a patient with a previous partial gastrectomy and retrocolic reconstruction.

Billroth II reconstruction can be created as a side-to-side jejunojejunostomy, referred to as the Braun procedure (Fig. 12.4A).[44] This variant results in an anastomosis between the afferent and the efferent limb to divert bile from the gastric remnant and to release the pressure of the afferent limb, supposedly preventing duodenal stump fistula.[45] The Braun anastomosis is performed 10 to 15 cm distal to the gastrojejunostomy and requires a longer afferent limb to accommodate the jejunojejunostomy.[46] Endoscopically, the gastrojejunostomy is similar to a standard Billroth II. Frothy bile is present in the stomach because the Braun procedure only partially diverts biliopancreatic fluids from the gastrojejunostomy. After advancing the endoscope through either opening of the gastrojejunostomy, the side-to-side Braun anastomosis can be found in the afferent and efferent limb, and three openings can be identified (see Fig. 12.4B). One leads to the distal jejunum, another leads to the afferent limb, and the third one leads back to the stomach. A complete reverse intubation of the stomach may be carried out through the loop created with the Braun anastomosis. The same anatomic landmarks described for other Billroth II procedures are helpful in directing the endoscope through the limbs. However, a

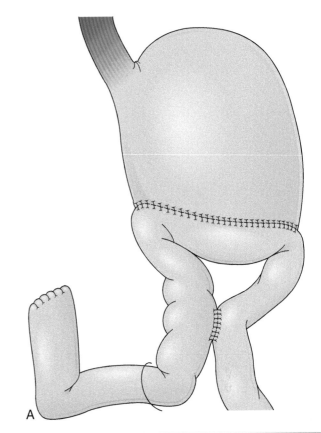

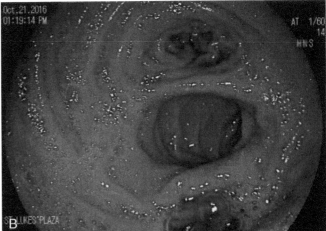

FIG 12.4 **A,** Braun procedure after a Billroth II gastrectomy: an anastomosis between the afferent and efferent limb is created to prevent biliopancreatic reflux to the stomach or alleviate pressure in the afferent limb. **B,** Braun jejunojejunostomy: three openings resulting from a side-to-side enteroanastomosis.

trial-and-error approach may be ultimately necessary to reach the duodenal stump.

A higher rate of perforation has been reported during ERCP while traversing the afferent limb compared with standard ERCP, particularly when a stiff therapeutic duodenoscope is used.[47,48] The Braun procedure has also been associated with perforations during ERCP. The use of a forward-viewing endoscope in these patients can reduce the risk of jejunal perforations.[49] The ability to use a duodenoscope elevator may increase the success of the procedure, and a flexible diagnostic duodenoscope may be safer than a stiff therapeutic instrument. If the papilla cannot be located with a side-viewing endoscope, the forward-viewing endoscope used should be either a pediatric colonoscope or one of the deep small bowel intubation technologies such as single or double balloon endoscopes to maximize the chances of reaching the papilla.

Roux-en-Y Gastrectomy

In a Roux-en-Y reconstruction, the jejunum is transected close to the ligament of Treitz, creating two distinct segments. The distal segment is sutured to the gastric remnant (gastrojejunostomy), becoming the efferent limb. The proximal segment is sutured to this efferent limb (jejunojejunostomy) approximately 40 cm below the gastrojejunal anastomosis (see Fig. 12.2D). The proximal segment is called the afferent limb, which connects the duodenum to the efferent limb instead of the stomach as in Billroth II reconstructions. The Roux-en-Y reconstruction prevents biliopancreatic fluids from refluxing into the stomach in patients who have undergone gastric resection. It can be performed as the initial reconstruction after a gastrectomy or as the treatment for postgastrectomy syndrome resulting from a previous Billroth II reconstruction.[50–53] Truncal vagotomy is commonly performed in association with Roux-en-Y to prevent peptic ulcers in the efferent limb, which is no longer washed by the alkaline contents of the biliopancreatic fluid.[54]

The gastrojejunal anastomosis is end-to-side, and two stomal openings are seen. The reconstruction can be oralis totalis or partialis, isoperistaltic or antiperistaltic, and antecolic or retrocolic, as described for Billroth II. In contrast to the Billroth II, one of the two limbs is extremely short and ends blindly almost immediately. On entering a long limb with a patent lumen, it is almost certain that the endoscope is within the efferent limb. If the Roux-en-Y was performed after an initial Billroth II reconstruction, the endoscopist should be aware that the blind limb might be patent for several centimeters before ending in a cul-de-sac. This short segment of patent limb occurs because conversion from a Billroth II to a Roux-en-Y sometimes has to be performed farther from the gastrojejunostomy to avoid adhesions from the initial surgery.

In effective Roux-en-Y reconstructions, the remnant stomach is completely clean of bile (Fig. 12.5A and B). The absence of bile in an operated stomach should always alert the endoscopist for a Roux-en-Y reconstruction, and the presence of residual food in this case should not lead to an erroneous conclusion of efferent limb obstruction. Total obstruction of the afferent limb in a Billroth II reconstruction could also prevent bile to reflux to the stomach, mimicking a Roux-en-Y, but this is uncommon.[55] Conversely, presence of bile does not exclude a Roux-en-Y reconstruction. In this case, a short-length efferent limb may be responsible for the reflux. To be effective, the efferent limb has to measure at least 40 cm from the gastrojejunal anastomosis to the jejunojejunal anastomosis.[56] Longer limbs (up to 60 cm) may also be encountered.[57]

Intubation through the efferent limb usually follows a straight route with variable looping. The enteroenteric anastomosis is usually end-to-side, but it may be side-to-side with a blind end. In either case, the endoscope has to leave the efferent limb and enter the afferent limb to reach the major papilla in the duodenum (see Fig. 12.5C). If a side-to-side anastomosis is present, three openings can be observed. The opening in continuity with the efferent limb leads to the distal jejunum, the second opening leads to a blind distal end of the afferent limb, and the third one

leads to the duodenum through the afferent limb (see Fig. 12.5D). An end-to-side anastomosis has two openings. One is a continuation of the efferent limb and leads to the distal jejunum; the other opening leads to the afferent limb. Different degrees of angulation have to be negotiated to enter the afferent limb depending on the anastomosis configuration. Once the afferent limb is entered, progressively more bile should be seen until the duodenal stump is reached.

A complete visualization of the Roux-en-Y gastrojejunostomy during a routine upper endoscopy can be performed with a forward-viewing gastroscope, including the jejunojejunostomy. In contrast, if patients require ERCP, a longer insertion tube is usually needed (pediatric and adult colonoscopies, dedicated enteroscopes, single or double balloon enteroscopes).[58] Overtube-assisted enteroscopy (OAE) techniques, single or double balloon enteroscopes, have increased the ability to perform ERCP in patients with altered upper GI anatomy. ERCP success rates are 90% in patients with Billroth II anatomy, 76% in patients who had undergone either a Roux-en-Y or a pancreaticoduodenectomy, pylorus-preserving pancreaticoduodenectomy, or hepaticojejunostomy, and 70% in patients who underwent Roux-en-Y with gastric bypass surgery. Cannulation success rates appeared to be equivalent in patients with both native papilla and biliary-enteric or pancreaticoenteric anastomoses (90%–92%).[59–61]

Gastrojejunostomy Without Gastric Resection

Gastrojejunostomy without gastric resection is performed to bypass the distal stomach or the duodenum, mostly in cases of malignant obstruction that cannot be resected. In major duodenopancreatic trauma with a high risk for fistulas, a gastrojejunostomy may also be performed in association with a temporary closure of the pylorus as part of the duodenal exclusion.[62] Occasionally, the gastrojejunostomy is created prophylactically during the surgical exploration of a patient with unresectable adenocarcinoma of the head of the pancreas to prevent subsequent gastric outlet obstruction.[63] The gastrojejunostomy is usually performed along the greater curvature of the distal body or the proximal antrum of the stomach (Fig. 12.6A). It may involve the anterior or the posterior wall at the surgeon's discretion. In all cases, a side-to-side anastomosis is performed with the first jejunal loop that can be sutured without tension to the stomach. The anastomosis can be isoperistaltic or antiperistaltic, antecolic or retrocolic, as described for a Billroth II gastroenteroanastomosis. The definition for the length of the anastomosis does not apply (oralis totalis or oralis partialis) because this is a side-to-side anastomosis. However, this anastomosis usually resembles an oralis partialis in length.

The gastrojejunostomy appears endoscopically as a vertical anastomosis with two stomal openings that correspond to the afferent and efferent limbs. Either one of the limbs may be in a superior (upper) or inferior (lower) position, depending on the technique used during the surgery. If an isoperistaltic gastrojejunostomy has been created, the opening of the afferent limb should be expected in the upper position. The endoscopist should look carefully for a gastrojejunostomy in a patient with an upper tract obstruction who had undergone surgery. This anastomosis may become easily overlooked because it is typically not large, usually located among edematous gastric folds, and associated with gastric contents resulting from outlet obstruction (see Fig. 12.6B). Ulcerations are also common and may impair intubation of the jejunal openings resulting from tissue retraction.[64] Access to the papilla can be achieved by passing the endoscope retrograde

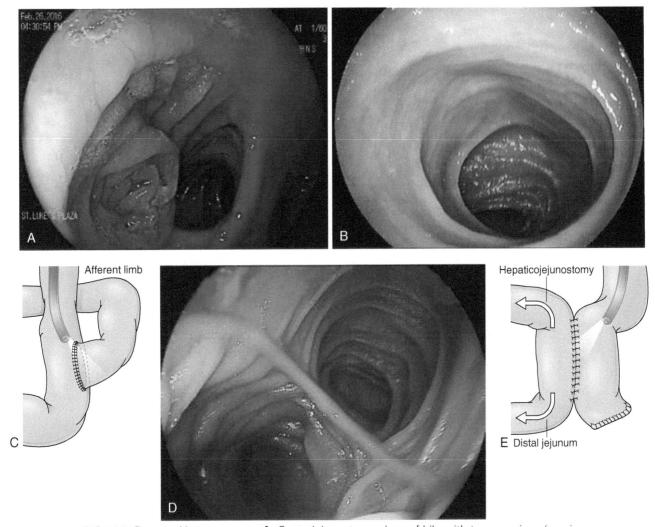

FIG 12.5 Roux-en-Y gastrectomy. **A,** Gastrojejunostomy clean of bile with two openings (one is short and ends blindly). **B,** Lack of bile in typical Roux-en-Y efferent limb. **C,** Terminolateral anastomosis in a Roux-en-Y gastrectomy: two openings are observed at this level; one leads to the distal jejunum, and the other leads to the ampulla via the afferent limb. **D,** Two openings are at the level of a side-to-side jejunojejunostomy. The third opening is located proximally and out of the field. Bile is usual at this level where the efferent limb connects to the afferent limb. **E,** Laterolateral anastomosis in a hepaticojejunostomy: the endoscope has passed through the stomach, duodenum, and proximal jejunum reaching the jejunojejunal anastomosis. Three openings are noted, including a blind one. In contrast to a Roux-en-Y gastrectomy **(A),** the loop in which the endoscope is located ends blindly.

through the afferent limb when a gastric outlet obstruction has been established. The Braun procedure may be added to the gastrojejunostomy as previously described for Billroth II reconstruction (see Fig. 12.6C).

Bariatric Surgery

Obesity is associated with serious health consequences including hypertension, type 2 diabetes, hyperlipidemia, coronary artery disease, peripheral vascular disease, cerebral vascular accidents, thromboembolic conditions, obstructive sleep apnea, obesity-hypoventilation syndrome, weight-bearing osteoarthritis, nonalcoholic fatty liver disease, hepatic cirrhosis, and an increased risk of developing colorectal and pancreatic cancer.[65–67] Indications for bariatric procedures are increasing because of the increase in

prevalence of obesity, including childhood obesity, and the lack of effective nonsurgical treatments. The National Institutes of Health (NIH) Consensus Conference in 2004 recognized bariatric surgery as the most effective therapy available for morbid obesity and that it can result in improvement or complete resolution of obesity-related comorbidities.[67] Bariatric surgical procedures include laparoscopic or open Roux-en-Y gastric bypass, sleeve gastrectomy (SG), vertical banded gastroplasty (VBG), laparoscopic adjustable gastric band (LAGB), biliopancreatic diversion with duodenal switch (BPD/DS), and laparoscopic mini gastric bypass.[5,67] A growing number of patients with altered anatomy should be expected in endoscopy units because GI complaints are frequent after bariatric surgery. The same complaints in uncomplicated postoperative courses can be present in patients

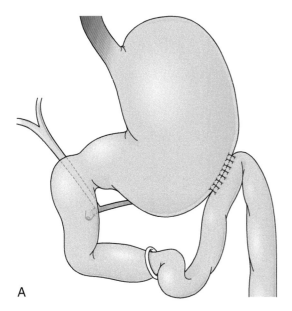

A

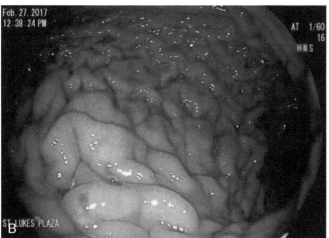

B

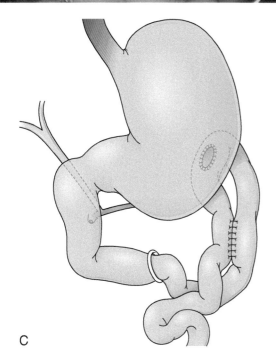

C

FIG 12.6 Gastroenteroanastomosis. **A,** Antiperistaltic gastroenteroanastomosis is created along greater curvature. **B,** Gastrojejunostomy without gastric resection: residual contents, enlarged gastric folds, and suboptimal air insufflation may obscure this anastomosis. **C,** Isoperistaltic gastroenteroanastomosis is created on the posterior wall of the stomach in association with Braun procedure.

with important surgical complications, which may require surgical revision.[68–70] Early post–bariatric surgery complications include early postoperative hemorrhage, anastomotic leak, and fistula. Late complications include anastomotic stricture, marginal ulcer, obscure GI bleeding, and gastric band slippage.[5]

Some endoscopic findings may represent either a normal postsurgical appearance or a complication depending on the surgery that was performed.[71] An example is the endoscopic finding of a communication between a short proximal gastric pouch and a normal-size remnant stomach. This communication is normally expected in a VBG, but it represents a failure (gastrogastric fistula) if the surgical procedure was a gastric bypass (GB). Familiarity with the most common bariatric procedures is essential for optimal endoscopic assistance to bariatric patients and surgeons. Surgical procedures to treat obesity have evolved during the last 6 decades. They can be simplified into two types, restrictive and malabsortive.[72] Selection of a procedure is based on individual patient characteristics and surgeon preference.[73–75]

Jejunoileal Bypass

Jejunoileal bypass (JIB) was the first procedure proposed to induce malabsorption in 1954.[76] It is technically simple and safe because it involves only enteroanastomosis, and the surgical steps are performed in the middle abdomen. In JIB, the proximal jejunum and the distal ileum are transected. The long jejunoileal segment in between these two transections is excluded from the intestinal transit by closing the proximal margin and connecting the distal margin to the sigmoid colon. An enteroanastomosis is performed between the proximal jejunum and the distal ileum, leaving a short segment of small bowel for absorption (Fig. 12.7). This procedure does not alter the endoscopic anatomy of the upper GI tract. JIB is no longer performed because of severe hepatic complications.[77] Patients with an intact JIB should consider reversion of the operation.

Gastric Bypass

GB is a restrictive and malabsorptive procedure.[78] It is the most popular bariatric procedure performed worldwide along with sleeve gastrectomy.[79,80] The operation includes partition of the stomach, creating a small-volume pouch (15 to 50 mL) in the proximal stomach.[79,81] With the distal stomach completely disconnected, the proximal gastric pouch is anastomosed with a Roux-en-Y limb that ranges from 75 to 150 cm in length to reestablish the alimentary transit. The extent of the bypass of the intestinal tract determines the degree of macronutrient malabsorption (Fig. 12.8A).[67,82]

Gastric bypass can be performed by both open and laparoscopic techniques. The laparoscopic approach has a higher rate of intraabdominal complications but a shorter duration of hospitalization, fewer wound complications, and improved postoperative patient comfort.[67] Surgical technical variations can

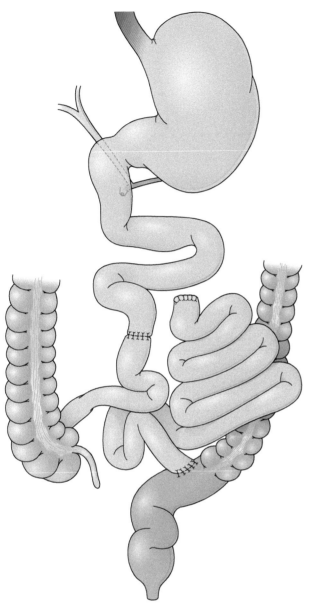

FIG 12.7 Jejunoileal bypass. This operation reduces the small bowel absorptive surface and leaves a long, nonfunctional segment of small bowel. Endoscopically, there is no change in the anatomy for upper endoscopy and endoscopic retrograde cholangiopancreatography (ERCP).

be observed in GB in regard to the orientation of the pouch (horizontal vs. vertical), partition of the stomach (transection vs. no transection), use of a Silastic ring around the gastrojejunal stoma, and the length of the Roux-en-Y limbs.[83–85]

The procedure proposed by Capella et al (2002)[86] incorporates a Silastic ring in the upper gastric pouch to prevent late stretching and the suturing of the Roux-en-Y limb to the staple line of the pouch to prevent late gastrogastric fistulas (see Fig. 12.8B–D).

For the endoscopist, GB may be compared with a Roux-en-Y gastrectomy. The differences are the size of the proximal gastric pouch, the length of the Roux-en-Y limb, and the fact that the distal stomach is not resected. Upper endoscopy in a patient with GB shows a small proximal pouch immediately after the esophagogastric junction with a narrow stoma leading to the

small bowel and a long limb before reaching the jejunojejunal anastomosis, which may be inaccessible depending on the length of the limb (see Fig. 12.8E). The gastric partition may include only the staple line, without division of the stomach (undivided bypass), or a complete transection of the stomach (divided bypass) (see Fig. 12.8F). Undivided bypass presents a higher rate of fistulas between the pouch and the distal stomach compared with divided bypass. A gastrogastric fistula leads to a failure in weight loss and to a higher incidence of peptic ulcers beyond the gastrojejunal anastomosis.

The gastrojejunostomy may be to the side or to the end of the jejunum or stomach. The small gastric pouch makes lateral and terminal gastric anastomoses indistinguishable. However, lateral and terminal anastomoses are different on the jejunal side. A lateral jejunal anastomosis has two openings. One ends blindly shortly after the anastomosis; the other leads to the distal jejunum (efferent limb) (see Fig. 12.8G). A terminal anastomosis has one opening that should be readily accessible endoscopically. The blind end of a lateral anastomosis should not be confused with stenosis of the efferent limb, particularly when scarring alters the anatomy. Abnormal endoscopic findings include esophagitis, pouch or esophagus dilation, stomal stenosis, stomal ulceration, prosthesis erosion at the stoma, and breakdown of the partition staple line. Stomal ulceration has been related to staple line dehiscence in which a gastrogastric fistula occurs, although other factors may be involved.[87,88]

Access to the major papilla and to the disconnected part of the stomach is often impossible transorally in patients with GB using regular endoscopes.[89–91] A percutaneous gastrostomy tract created in the distal stomach is used as an alternative to access these areas with the endoscope.[92,93] Double-balloon and single-balloon enteroscopy has emerged as an alternative to access the biliopancreatic ducts and the disconnected part of the stomach in these patients.[94–97]

Sleeve Gastrectomy

SG is a restrictive laparoscopic procedure in which the greater curvature is removed and a small gastric tube is left. Over the past decade, SG has emerged as a popular bariatric surgical approach. It was first introduced as the two-staged approach to duodenal switch (DS) or GB for the super obese patient.[98] The stand-alone SG has provided comparable results with the GB operation in regards to weight reduction and amelioration of obesity-related comorbidities.[99–101] Although GB is still the most common bariatric operation performed worldwide (45%), SG is now the most common bariatric operation performed in the United States/Canada (43%) and Asian/Pacific regions (49%) and the second most common worldwide (37%).[80]

The endoscopic view after sleeve gastrectomy reveals a long, tubular stomach limited in expansion by a staple line that parallels the lesser curvature (Fig. 12.9). The DS procedure is often performed in conjunction with a SG, but also includes a duodenojejunal anastomosis visible just distal to an intact gastric pylorus. In the latter, the ampulla is thus not available for visualization or ERCP in a standard fashion.

Vertical Banded Gastroplasty

The initial gastroplasty procedure was inadequate in terms of weight loss and was refined by Mason into VBG. VBG is a purely restrictive procedure resulting from a search for a simpler operation compared with GB.[102] VBG involves the creation of a small pouch in the proximal stomach and the encirclement of the

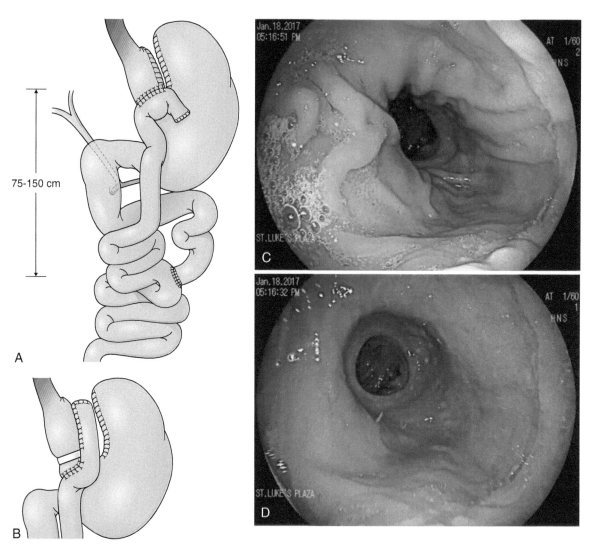

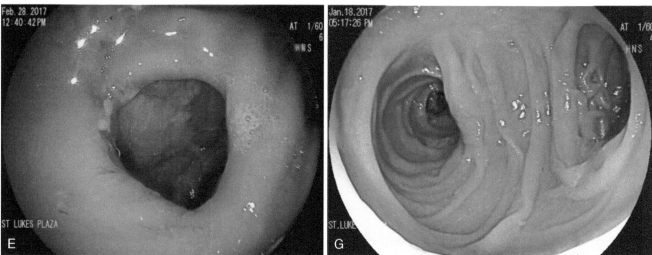

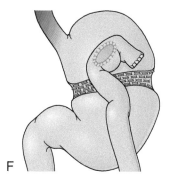

FIG 12.8 Gastric bypass. **A,** Small-volume pouch (15 to 50 mL) is created just beyond the gastroesophageal junction and is anastomosed to a jejunal loop in a Roux-en-Y fashion. The efferent limb ranges from 75 to 150 cm. The distal stomach is not resected and may be used to create a gastrostomy through which the endoscope can be advanced to perform endoscopic retrograde cholangiopancreatography (ERCP) or gastroduodenoscopy. **B,** A technical variation includes the attachment of the jejunal limb to the gastric partitioning to prevent gastrogastric fistulas and the placement of a Silastic ring in the distal portion of the pouch to prevent dilation. **C,** Small gastric pouch with a subtle circumferential compression proximal to the anastomosis indicating an external ring. **D,** Intact stapler line at the gastric pouch. **E,** Small-diameter gastro-jejunostomy. **F,** Undivided gastric bypass: The staple line is not transected, and the pouch is horizontal. This type of gastric bypass has been associated with failures in weight loss because of dilation of the pouch and disruption of the staple line. **G,** End-to-side gastrojejunostomy with two openings. The right one is the efferent limb. The left one ends blindly.

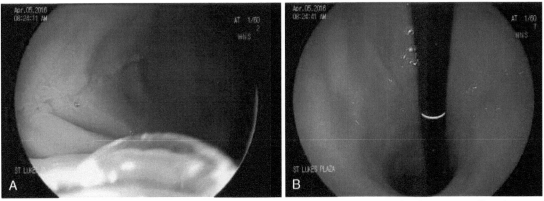

FIG 12.9 Sleeve gastrectomy. **A,** Long tubular stomach limited in expansion by a suture line that parallels the lesser curvature. **B,** Retroflex view.

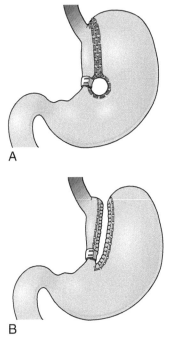

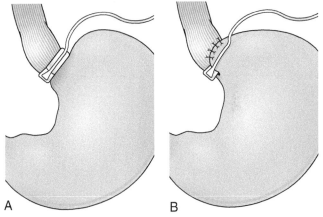

FIG 12.11 Laparoscopic adjustable gastric banding. **A,** A 15-mL pouch is created in the proximal stomach with a banding device. The device can be adjusted to narrow the opening to the distal stomach by percutaneous injection of fluids. **B,** A gastrogastric suture is placed anteriorly over the band to prevent gastric herniation.

FIG 12.10 Vertical banded gastroplasty. A 15-mL pouch is created at the angle of His, and the outlet channel is encircled by a circumferential band. **A,** Circular and linear staplers are used to create this uncut gastroplasty. **B,** The staple line may be divided, separating the two gastric parts to prevent gastrogastric fistula.

outlet channel to prevent dilation. The pouch is created along the lesser curvature with a stapled partition precisely at the angle of His to accommodate a volume of 15 mL or less. The outlet channel of the pouch is stabilized by the encirclement of a 5-cm circumference band or a Silastic ring (Fig. 12.10A). A technical variation includes dividing the stapled partition (see Fig. 12.10B).

Upper endoscopy in patients with intact VBG shows a small tubular pouch immediately after the esophagogastric junction with a narrow outlet channel that, once traversed, leads to the remaining distal stomach. Abnormal endoscopic findings include esophagitis, staple line dehiscence, food impaction, stenosis of the pouch outlet, and erosion of the gastric wall by the material used to encircle the outlet channel.[103,104] The remaining stomach,

duodenal bulb, and biliopancreatic ducts are readily accessible for endoscopy if the outlet channel permits passage of the endoscope. The outlet channel is ideally 11 mm wide and 15 mm long, and is amenable to endoscopic dilation in case of stenosis.

Laparoscopic Adjustable Gastric Banding

LAGB is the least invasive of the purely restrictive bariatric surgery procedure. LAGB was commonly performed in European countries and Australia, but now GB and SG account for almost 75% of bariatric surgery outside of the United States.[80,105,106] LAGB involves placing a band around the proximal stomach to create a 15-mL pouch without the need of resecting or stapling the stomach (Fig. 12.11A).

LAGB is now performed using a silicone material device that can be inflated with saline solution to adjust the gastric-pouch outflow. The inflatable part of the band device is connected by tubing to a reservoir, then implanted and secured to the abdominal fascia, which can be accessed via a needle.[107] There are unique long-term complications of LAGB, which include gastric prolapse, stomal obstruction, esophageal and gastric pouch dilation, gastric erosion and necrosis, and access port problems. Use of a prosthetic device introduces additional potential problems of malfunction and infection.

Upper endoscopy in a patient with LAGB shows a small gastric pouch at the level of the cardia with a narrow outlet channel that leads to the distal normal stomach. Esophageal dilation, esophagitis, gastric pouch dilation, gastric slippage, outlet channel stenosis, and gastric wall erosion by the band device are the most common abnormal findings observed after LAGB.[108,109] Occasionally, a marked gastric fold surrounding the pouch outlet channel can be observed in a retroflexed view within the distal stomach. This fold corresponds to the gastrogastric sutures placed anteriorly over the band device to decrease the risks of gastric herniation (see Fig. 12.11B). Similar to VBG, once the endoscope is advanced through the pouch-outlet channel, examination of the distal stomach, duodenum, and biliopancreatic ducts can be performed as in a regular endoscopy.

Biliopancreatic Diversion

Biliopancreatic diversion (BPD) is a malabsorptive procedure to delay contact between ingested food material, bile, and pancreatic juice.[110] BPD was first reported in 1979 by Scopinaro

et al and is also known as the Scopinaro procedure.[111] In BPD, the small bowel is divided, creating two limbs. The distal limb is anastomosed to the stomach, and the proximal limb is anastomosed to the ileum. After completion, the small bowel has a new anatomic configuration with three distinct channels: common, alimentary, and biliopancreatic (Fig. 12.12A). BPD requires no small bowel resection and does not leave a nonfunctional small bowel segment. The results of the procedure depend on the length of the channels, which are variable because of the individual patient characteristics and surgeon preferences. Typically, a 50-cm to 100-cm common channel and a 150-cm to 200-cm alimentary channel are created. The remaining small bowel constitutes the biliopancreatic channel.

The common channel length is the determinant for long-term weight maintenance and steatorrhea, and the total common alimentary channel is for the temporary mild short-gut syndrome. In addition, the stomach is altered via a partial resection or a GB to prevent peptic ulcer and to limit food intake. The gastric component of the BPD is easily accessible endoscopically, and the findings vary according to the procedure performed. Nevertheless, bile should never be observed, and peptic ulceration at the gastroenteroanastomosis and small bowel always should be

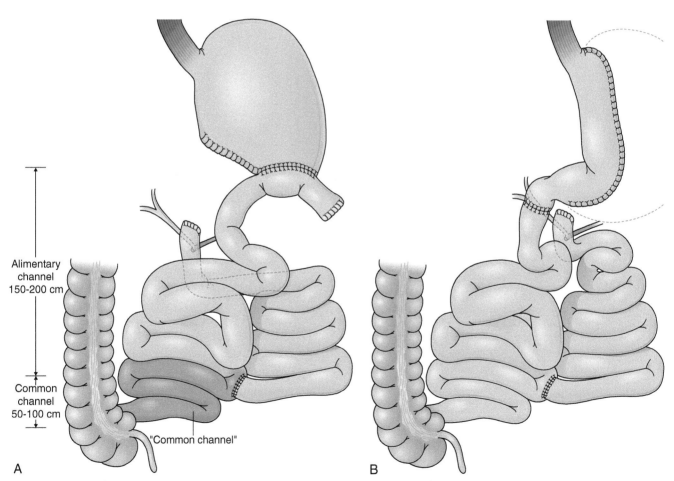

FIG 12.12 Malabsorptive bariatric surgeries. **A,** Biliopancreatic diversion: a partial gastrectomy is reconstructed in a Roux-en-Y fashion with long afferent and efferent limbs (biliopancreatic and alimentary channels). Shadowed area represents the short length common channel (50 to 100 cm). **B,** Duodenal switch: a sleeve gastrectomy with preservation of the pylorus leads to a duodeno-jejunostomy rather than a gastrojejunostomy. Jejunal limbs are reconstructed as in a biliopancreatic diversion.

carefully investigated. If a partial gastrectomy was chosen, the stomach resembles a Roux-en-Y gastrectomy with a short proximal gastric pouch. A GB may appear as a vertical small gastric pouch or a horizontal pouch that includes the fundus. In a horizontal pouch, the anastomosis with the jejunum should be observed toward the greater curvature. A GB does not include stomach resection, leaving a nonfunctional distal gastric segment, and it can be divided or undivided.

Performing ERCP in a patient with BPD is nearly impossible per os because the endoscope has to be advanced all the way through the small bowel, except for the common channel, to reach the major papilla. Alternatives to access the major papilla are through a gastrostomy (surgical or radiologic) or through a disrupted staple line between the pouch and the stomach. These alternatives apply only for patients who had a GB because gastric resection precludes both options. Double-balloon enteroscopy has the potential to advance through the altered BPD anatomy and reach the major papilla.

Duodenal Switch

The DS procedure is a variation of BPD. This procedure includes an SG preserving the pylorus and anastomosis of the enteric limb end-to-end with the postpyloric duodenum (see Fig. 12.12B).[110] A lower prevalence of side effects has been reported for DS compared with BPD. The same principles described in regard to BPD apply to DS during the endoscopic evaluation, except that a duodenojejunostomy rather than a gastrojejunostomy is present.

OPERATIONS WITH ALTERATION OF THE PANCREATICOBILIARY ANATOMY

Pancreaticoduodenectomy (Whipple Procedure)

The Whipple procedure is performed to resect malignant or benign lesions in the head of the pancreas, distal bile duct, or in the second portion of the duodenum.[112] The extent of the resection classifies this procedure as classic or pylorus-preserving.

Classic Whipple Procedure

In the classic Whipple procedure, the gastric antrum, duodenum, head of the pancreas, and distal bile duct are resected. There are over 68 variations for reconstruction of the alimentary and pancreaticobiliary tract.[113] Currently, one well-accepted technique is to create all necessary anastomoses with a single limb of small bowel (Fig. 12.13A).[114,115] In this case, a side-to-side gastroenteroanastomosis is encountered endoscopically, usually oralis partialis and with the resection limited to the antrum. All the variations regarding orientation, position to the transverse colon, and stoma size described for the Billroth II gastroenteroanastomosis apply here. On entering the afferent limb, which may range from 40 to 60 cm and include a Braun procedure, the anastomosis with the biliary and pancreatic ducts can be identified. Sharp angulations resulting from fixation to adjacent organs may be encountered before reaching the blind end of the most proximal portion of the afferent limb, where the pancreaticojejunostomy is found.

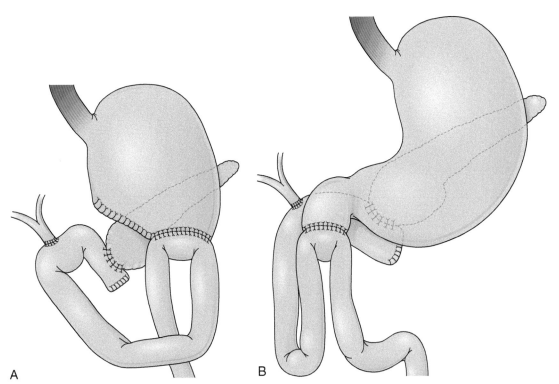

FIG 12.13 Whipple operations. **A,** Classic Whipple: the distal stomach, head of the pancreas, distal biliary duct, and duodenum are resected. A single loop of jejunum is used to the anastomoses with the stomach and biliary and pancreatic ducts. A partial isoperistaltic gastroenteroanastomosis is shown. **B,** Pylorus-preserving Whipple: a duodenojejunostomy rather than a gastrojejunostomy is created in this procedure.

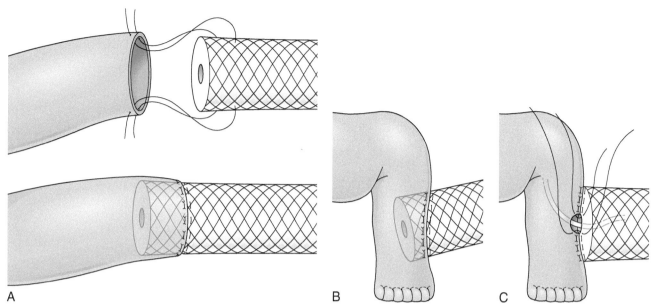

FIG 12.14 Pancreaticojejunostomies. **A,** Terminoterminal dunking anastomosis in which the pancreas is invaginated into the jejunum. **B,** Terminolateral dunking anastomosis. **C,** Mucosa-to-mucosa pancreaticojejunostomy.

The pancreaticojejunostomy may be end-to-end or end-to-side. In either case, the pancreaticojejunostomy may also be a mucosa-to-mucosa or a "dunking" anastomosis.[116] A mucosa-to-mucosa anastomosis creates a small opening by suturing the pancreatic duct to the jejunal mucosa. The dunking anastomosis differs from the mucosa-to-mucosa anastomosis in that the pancreas is invaginated into the jejunum (Fig. 12.14). The opening of the pancreatic duct varies from a flat, small-diameter anastomosis (mucosa-to-mucosa) to a protuberant, sometimes downward-oriented anastomosis (lateral dunking), making the identification and cannulation of this duct technically challenging. The hepaticojejunostomy is located approximately 10 cm proximal to the pancreaticojejunostomy. It is always an end-to-side anastomosis located in the antimesenteric border of the limb, occasionally subtle or hidden by a fold.

Pylorus-Preserving Whipple Procedure

The pylorus-preserving Whipple procedure differs from the classic Whipple operation in that the stomach is not resected and a short segment of the proximal bulb remains to be anastomosed with the jejunum (see Fig. 12.13B).[117] This modification has proved to decrease the morbidity of pancreaticoduodenectomies, such as malnutrition due to the reduced volume of the stomach, without compromising the oncologic principles of the resection.[118] A duodenojejunostomy rather than a gastrojejunostomy is observed in patients with a pylorus-preserving Whipple procedure. After traversing a normal stomach and the pylorus, a two-opening, small-diameter anastomosis is identified in a short segment of bulb. Depending on the orientation of the reconstruction, the afferent limb is to the right (antiperistaltic) or to the left (iso-peristaltic). Antecolic or retrocolic anastomosis can also be observed, creating variations on the length of the jejunal limb. Usually, a trial-and-error approach is necessary to define the afferent limb, in which the pancreatic and biliary anastomosis are performed as described for the classic Whipple procedure. In patients who have undergone either Whipple operation, the biliary and pancreatic anastomosis may be reached with a side-viewing or a forward-viewing endoscope, owing to the relatively short afferent limb.

Roux-en-Y Hepaticojejunostomy

Anastomosis of the hepatic duct to a loop of jejunum without disturbing the gastroduodenal anatomy is usually performed for biliary disease or during liver transplantation when the native bile duct cannot be used to create a duct-to-duct anastomosis (e.g., in the setting of sclerosing cholangitis).[119] The hepaticojejunostomy is usually end-to-side, but side-to-side anastomosis can also be encountered (Fig. 12.15A). The anatomy of the stomach, duodenum, and pancreas is not altered, and endoscopic evaluation of these organs is similar to a nonoperated stomach. If the bile duct must be accessed, the endoscope has to be advanced through a normal stomach and duodenum before reaching the jejunojejunal anastomosis that leads to a Roux-en-Y limb with the hepaticojejunostomy. Long-length endoscopes are usually necessary, and in most cases balloon enteroscopy systems employing an overtube are now used.[120–122]

In contrast to the anatomy after a Roux-en-Y gastrectomy, the duodenojejunal limb merges into the small bowel rather than merging with a loop of small bowel. At the level of the jejunojejunostomy, three lumens (side-to-side) or two lumens (end-to-side) can be observed, depending on the reconstruction (see Fig. 12.5E). One lumen leads to the distal jejunum, and the other leads to the limb that contains the hepaticojejunostomy. The third lumen (only if side-to-side) observed along the initial limb occupied by the endoscope ends blindly just beyond the anastomosis. A trial-and-error approach to the first two limbs reveals the one with the hepaticojejunostomy. The end-to-side hepaticojejunostomy is similar to the one described in the Whipple procedure except that here the location is closer to the blind end of the limb. In contrast to the end-to-side hepaticojejunostomy, the side-to-side hepaticojejunostomy preserves the access to the biliary ducts through the major papilla if the distal common

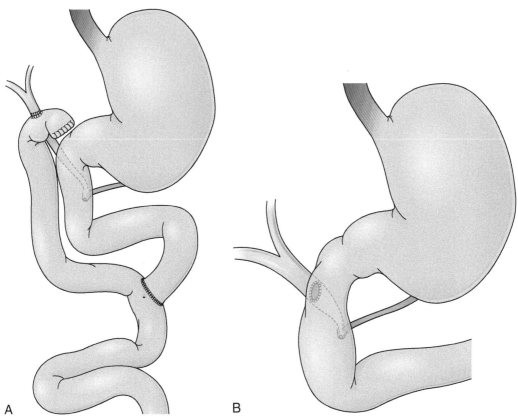

A   B

FIG 12.15 Bilioenteric anastomoses. **A,** Roux-en-Y hepaticojejunostomy: the bile duct is anastomosed to a limb of jejunum in a lateral or terminal fashion. A side-to-side anastomosis preserves cannulation of the intrahepatic ducts through the papilla if no obstruction is present. The pancreatic duct remains accessible through the second portion of the duodenum. **B,** Choledochoduodenostomy: usually a side-to-side anastomosis is accessible on the second portion of the duodenum. The distal bile duct may be filled with residual enteric contents leading to the sump syndrome.

bile duct is not obstructed. In this case, a cholangiogram can be obtained with the aid of an occlusion balloon inflated proximal to the hepaticojejunostomy, avoiding the demanding insertion of the endoscope through the Roux-en-Y limb. Air within the intrahepatic ducts is common in bilioenteric anastomosis and may be useful to evaluate patients in whom the hepaticojejunostomy is not reachable with the endoscope (air cholangiogram).[4,123]

Choledochoduodenostomy

Choledochoduodenostomy is the anastomosis of the bile duct to the second portion of the duodenum, usually performed in a side-to-side fashion (see Fig. 12.15B). Endoscopically, after traversing the pylorus, the choledochoduodenostomy is found proximal to the major papilla. The anastomosis may be sufficiently wide to allow visualization and partial intubation of the extrahepatic ducts. A side-to-side anastomosis has two lumens. One lumen leads to the proximal biliary tree, and the other leads to the distal common bile duct. Because there is no alimentary diversion from the anastomosis, food impaction may occur in the distal common bile duct causing the sump syndrome, which may require an ERCP.[124] Because the biliary duct can be accessed both through the major papilla and through the choledochoduodenostomy, a combination of accesses can be used to manipulate the different portions of the ducts, including anterograde cannulation of the papilla. The approach to the pancreatic duct is the same as for standard ERCP.

KEY REFERENCES

1. Max MH, West B, Knutson CO: Evaluation of postoperative gastroduodenal symptoms: endoscopy or upper gastrointestinal roentgenography? *Surgery* 86:578–582, 1979. 483167.
2. Donahue PE, Nyhus LM: Surgeon-endoscopists and the assessment of postoperative patients, *South Med J* 75:1570–1575, 1982. 7146998.
3. Feitoza AB, Baron TH: Endoscopy and ERCP in the setting of previous upper GI tract surgery. Part I. Reconstruction without alteration of pancreaticobiliary anatomy, *Gastrointest Endosc* 54:743–749, 2001. 11726851.
4. Feitoza AB, Baron TH: Endoscopy and ERCP in the setting of previous upper GI tract surgery. Part II. Postsurgical anatomy with alteration of the pancreaticobiliary tree, *Gastrointest Endosc* 55:75–79, 2002. 11756919.
5. Malli CP, Sioulas AD, Emmanouil T, et al: Endoscopy after bariatric surgery, *Ann Gastroenterol* 29:249–257, 2016.
17. Horgan S, Pellegrini CA: Surgical treatment of gastroesophageal reflux disease, *Surg Clin North Am* 77:1063–1082, 1997. 9347831.
19. Johnson DA, Younes Z, Hogan WJ: Endoscopic assessment of hiatal hernia repair, *Gastrointest Endosc* 52:650–659, 2000. 11060191.
21. Jailwala J, Massey B, Staff D, et al: Post-fundoplication symptoms: the role for endoscopic assessment of fundoplication integrity, *Gastrointest Endosc* 54:351–356, 2001. 11522977.
25. Hunter JG, Richardson WS: Surgical management of achalasia, *Surg Clin North Am* 77:993–1015, 1997. 9347828.
27. Mellinger JD, Ponsky JL: Endoscopic evaluation of the postoperative stomach, *Gastrointest Endosc Clin N Am* 6:621–639, 1996. 8803571.

43. Lin LF, Siauw CP, Ho KS, et al: ERCP in post-Billroth II gastrectomy patients: emphasis on technique, *Am J Gastroenterol* 94:144–148, 1999. 9934745.

44. Hintze RE, Adler A, Veltzke W, et al: Endoscopic access to the papilla of Vater for endoscopic retrograde cholangiopancreatography in patients with Billroth II or Roux-en-Y gastrojejunostomy, *Endoscopy* 29:69–73, 1997. 9101141.

53. Xiong JJ, Altaf K, Javed MA, et al: Roux-en-Y versus Billroth I reconstruction after distal gastrectomy for gastric cancer: a meta-analysis, *World J Gastroenterol* 19(7):1124–1134, 2013.

58. Testoni PA, Mariani A, Aabakken L, et al: Papillary cannulation and sphincterotomy techniques at ERCP: European Society of Gastrointestinal Endoscopy (ESGE) Clinical Guideline, *Endoscopy* 48:657–683, 2016.

59. Skinner M, Popa D, Neumann H, et al: ERCP with overtube-assisted enteroscopy technique: a systematic review, *Endoscopy* 46:560–572, 2014.

67. Buchwald H: Consensus Conference Statement Bariatric surgery for morbid obesity: health implications for patients, health professionals, and third-party payers, *J Am Coll Surg* 200:593–604, 2005.

68. Stellato TA, Crouse C, Hallowell PT: Bariatric surgery: creating new challenges for the endoscopist, *Gastrointest Endosc* 57:86–94, 2003. 12518137.

71. Papavramidis ST, Theocharidis AJ, Zaraboukas TG, et al: Upper gastrointestinal endoscopic and histologic findings before and after vertical banded gastroplasty, *Surg Endosc* 10:825–830, 1996. 8694947.

75. Needleman BJ, Happel LC: Bariatric surgery: choosing the optimal procedure, *Surg Clin North Am* 88:991–1007, 2008. 18790150.

80. Angrisani L, Santonicola A, Iovino P, et al: Bariatric surgery worldwide 2013, *Obes Surg* 25:1822–1832, 2015.

91. Wright BE, Cass OW, Freeman ML: ERCP in patients with long-limb Roux-en-Y gastrojejunostomy and intact papilla, *Gastrointest Endosc* 56:225–232, 2002. 12145601.

96. Chu YC, Yang CC, Yeh YH, et al: Double-balloon enteroscopy application in biliary tract disease-its therapeutic and diagnostic functions, *Gastrointest Endosc* 68:585–591, 2008. 18561917.

106. Abd Ellatif ME, Alfalah H, Asker WA, et al: Place of upper endoscopy before and after bariatric surgery: a multicenter experience with 3219 patients, *World J Gastrointest Endosc* 8(10):409–417, 2016.

113. Trede M: Technique of Whipple pancreatoduodenectomy. In Trede M, Carter DC, Longmire WP, editors: *Surgery of the pancreas*, New York, 1997, Churchill Livingstone, pp 487–498.

114. Farnell MB, Nagorney DM, Sarr MG: The Mayo Clinic approach to the surgical treatment of adenocarcinoma of the pancreas, *Surg Clin North Am* 81:611–623, 2001. 11459275.

A complete reference list can be found online at ExpertConsult .com

13

Endoscopic Simulators

Catharine M. Walsh and Jonathan Cohen

CHAPTER OUTLINE

INTRODUCTION

Safe performance of gastrointestinal endoscopic procedures requires extensive and high-quality training. Endoscopy skills have traditionally been taught within the clinical setting, in the form of a mentor-apprenticeship model in which novice endoscopists learn skills under the supervision of experienced preceptors. Concerns with regard to patient safety and training efficiency have prompted the endoscopy community to reconsider this training model. It is becoming increasingly less acceptable that endoscopic techniques are learned entirely in the clinical setting before trainees have shown some proficiency in their skills in a safe, controlled, simulated training environment.

Several factors have contributed to the shift toward incorporation of simulation into gastrointestinal endoscopy training. First, recent guidelines from endoscopy focused organizations such as the American Society for Gastrointestinal Endoscopy (ASGE)[1] have encouraged the use of simulation-based training, and it is now mandated by accreditation organizations in certain jurisdictions such as the United States.[2,3] Secondly, whereas the "ideal" training platform has traditionally been considered the patient, gastrointestinal endoscopy is uniquely challenging to teach in the clinical environment, as preceptors are required to relinquish complete control of the endoscope to allow trainees to learn the technique.[4] Clinical training also adds time to each procedure, which has implications with regard to capacity and economics.[5] Additionally, clinical demands and time restrictions often limit a preceptors' capacity to provide detailed instruction and feedback. Furthermore, training on patients occurs through chance encounters, which may limit exposure to particular pathologies. Finally, concern for patient comfort and safety can often impact the learning experience and act to limit case availability and training exposure, especially for certain higher risk procedures such as endoscopic retrograde cholangiopancreatography (ERCP).

There are also a number of recognized benefits of endoscopic simulators that have helped drive their integration into training. Simulators provide learners with the opportunity to practice cognitive, technical, and integrative competencies related to endoscopy in a controlled environment.[6,7] Learners can build a framework of basic techniques through sustained deliberate practice in a setting where errors can be allowed to progress so trainees can learn from their mistakes without adverse consequences.[8] For novice learners, mastery of basic skills in a low-risk controlled environment, prior to performance on real patients, enables trainees to then focus on more complex skills once they progress to clinically-based training. Simulation also permits individualized learning, as cases can be adapted to a learner's unique needs and the nature and difficulty of the simulation tasks can be systematically varied over time to adapt to the skill level of the learner. Additionally, trainers do not have to juggle teaching and clinical demands and can instead focus solely on learners to provide a learner-centered educational experience and take full advantage of learning opportunities without distraction. Simulation can also be used to expose learners to patient pathophysiology or techniques (e.g., variceal banding) that might be rarely encountered in the clinical setting. In addition, the hands-on lab affords trainees with an optimal opportunity to develop critical communication skills needed to perform procedures that require coordination with one or more assistants. Finally, simulators can play a potential role in maintaining skills for practicing physicians who perform fewer endoscopic procedures or have taken a break in their training and/or practice.

Despite the shift towards simulation-based training and the potential benefits of simulation, a 2014 survey revealed that less than half of adult gastroenterology programs in the United States utilize simulation and it is mandated in only 15% of programs.[9] Across programs, simulation is being employed in a markedly heterogeneous fashion with regard to the manner in which it is integrated into training, the time spent on simulators, and the training tasks and types of simulators employed. Additionally, whereas program directors widely recognize the role that simulation can play with regard to assessment, no programs directors reported using simulation to assess endoscopic competence.[9]

As outlined in the ASGE's 2012 Preservation and Incorporation of Valuable Endoscopic Innovations (PIVI) report, the decision about whether to incorporate simulation technologies into endoscopy training must rely on data regarding the magnitude of training benefits, any cost savings resulting from accelerated learning, associated expenses, and training needs.[1] The use of simulation within a training curricula needs to be justified and outweigh the associated costs. The rationale for using simulation should be based on evidence with regard to the potential benefits for patients, trainees, preceptors, and training programs.[1]

With regard to upper endoscopy and colonoscopy, extensive systematic reviews on the topic have shown endoscopy simulation-based training to be beneficial for novice endoscopists in developing knowledge and technical skills in a safe and controlled environment, prior to clinical practice.[10–12] Existing randomized control trials (RCTs) have primarily shown benefit during the early phase of clinical work and potential benefit in shortening the learning curve to competency; however, a reduction in the learning curve of more than 25%, as proposed in the ASGE's PIVI report as a threshold for widespread adoption to their use, has yet to be demonstrated.[1,10–14] Additionally, diagnostic and therapeutic gastrointestinal endoscopy skills learned within the simulated setting have been shown to transfer to patient care.[10–12,15] To date, there is little evidence that patients benefit materially with regard to factors such as adverse events or satisfaction when a procedure is performed by a trainee with previous simulator experience. Potential cost and manpower reductions resulting from simulation training have also not been examined in depth.[1] Additionally, validated models for training more advanced therapeutic procedures such as polypectomy and stenting are lacking or sparse.

Whereas evidence to date suggests that simulation-based endoscopy training is effective and learning outcomes transfer to the clinical setting, simulation must be integrated into training and assessment in a thoughtful and purposeful manner to maximize its benefit. This chapter will outline factors to consider in choosing an appropriate simulator for training, elaborate on the use of simulation to train endoscopic nontechnical skills, discuss instructional design features that can be used to enhance endoscopic training using simulators, and outline the potential use of simulation for assessment of endoscopic competence. The value of simulation for basic endoscopy training[10–12,16] and details of available simulator models for specific procedures[17–20] have been reviewed extensively elsewhere and will not be discussed in depth.

CHOICE OF SIMULATORS IN THE TRAINING ENVIRONMENT

Traditionally educators have favored high-fidelity computerized simulators for teaching technical skills based on the assumption that they provide the optimal context to prepare learners for the clinical environment.[8,21] However, this assumption is not based on empirical data. Over the past decade, the capabilities of endoscopic simulators have steadily expanded. Currently, there are a wide variety of simulators available to teach endoscopy and one's choice of simulator should be based on the educational and/or assessment goals, as well as cost, as opposed to technology. Effective use of simulation is highly dependent on a close match of educational goals with simulation tools.

The use of simulation to teach gastrointestinal endoscopy dates back to the 1960s.[4] In general, there are five types of endoscopic simulators: (1) inanimate static models or mechanical simulators, (2) virtual reality computer generated models, (3) ex vivo (explanted organ) animal models, (4) live animal models, and (4) hybrid simulations. Every training model has its advantages and disadvantages and is best suited to training specific tasks and levels of learners (Table 13.1). Inanimate static models or mechanical simulators are part-task trainers that generally involve performance of characteristic motor tasks with a real endoscope within an inanimate closed environment with realistic visual and motor requirements and haptic feedback.[22–24] They generally do not provide summative feedback like some computerized endoscopy simulators do; therefore, a mentor must be present to guide training. However, they are inexpensive, portable, and allow for deconstruction of specific tasks such as retroflexion, torque steering, and tip control. Virtual reality computerized simulators, which became commercially available in the 1990s, are advantageous in that many are capable of providing real-time feedback and a library of clinical cases with varying degrees of difficulty of anatomy and complexity of tasks.[4] Whereas the virtual reality computer simulators incorporate pathology recognition, the relative value of simulator training in this core component of competency, as compared to didactic resources (e.g., web-based atlases, lectures) in combination with mentored clinical endoscopy experience, has not yet been determined. Additionally, virtual reality simulators are costly and not easily portable. Ex vivo (explanted) models are fabricated from a combination of plastic parts and explanted animal organs which can be used to train specific tasks such as endoscopic mucosal resection (EMR), ERCP, or hemostasis techniques.[15,19,25,26] Live animal models (e.g., anesthetized porcine model) are the most realistic endoscopy simulators. Although the haptic feedback closely resembles human tissue, there are distinct differences with regard to wall thickness and organ orientation, resulting in a slightly different "feel."[18,19] Animal models in general are difficult to prepare and use. They require procurement of animals and/or animal organs, extensive preparation and disposal processes, use of animal-use endoscopes, and they cannot be used indefinitely.[18,19] Ex vivo models have the advantage of being easier to assemble, more affordable, and raising less ethical issues when compared to use of live animals; however, they have unfavorable tissue characteristics compared with vital tissue.[19] Due to the aforementioned limitations, many endoscopy training programs do not use these simulator models locally and they are most often employed at specially equipped regional or national training courses or meetings. Finally, hybrid simulation links a simulated patient (i.e., an actor) with a computer-driven virtual reality simulator or inanimate model in a simulated clinical environment. It is advantageous in that it allows learners to perform endoscopic procedures in a holistic clinical context without risk of causing harm. Additionally, multidisciplinary team members, such as an endoscopic nurse and/or anesthesiologist, can participate in scenarios to facilitate

TABLE 13.1   The Role of Various Endoscopic Simulation Models for Training

Simulator	Learner Level for a Given Task	Whole and/ or Part-Task Training	Procedure(s)	Cost	Advantages	Disadvantages
Inanimate Static Models (Mechanical Simulators)	• Novice	• Part-task	Basic skills related to EGD, FS colonoscopy and ERCP	• Low	• Inexpensive • Portable • Minimal set-up • Task-specific • Allows for task-deconstruction • Real endoscope • +/– Variety of cases	• Cost • Feedback metrics not generated automatically
Virtual Reality Computer Generated Models	• Novice • Intermediate	• Part-task • Whole task	EGD, FS, colonoscopy, EUS, ERCP, sedation, hemostasis techniques, polypectomy, working with an endoscopic assistant	• High	• Automated feedback (although expert feedback superior[35]) • Variety of cases • Minimal set-up • Permits team training with assistant	• Expensive • Bulky / not portable • Real endoscope not used
Ex vivo Animal Models	• Novice • Intermediate • Advanced	• Part-task • Whole task	Hemostasis techniques, polypectomy, EMR, ESD, PEG tube insertion, ERCP, foreign body removal, stent placement, ablation techniques, suturing and defect closure, EUS/FNA, double balloon enteroscopy, working with an endoscopic assistant	• Medium	• Realistic • Allows for task-deconstruction • Real endoscope • Permits team training with assistant	• Requires specially equipped facilities • Cannot be used indefinitely • Somewhat resource intensive to set up • Feedback metrics not generated automatically
Live Animal Models	• Intermediate • Advanced	• Part-task • Whole task	ERCP, Hemostasis, EUS, ESD, manometry, working with an endoscopic assistant	• High	• Very realistic (including peristalsis and breathing movements) • Real endoscope • Permits team training with assistant • Ideal when bleeding control is a key skill (e.g., ESD)	• Expensive • Requires specially equipped facilities • Can't be used indefinitely • Resource intensive to set up • Ethical concerns • Feedback metrics not generated automatically
Hybrid Simulation	• Intermediate • Advanced • Endoscopic assistants • Anesthesia	• Whole task • Higher level integrative competencies (ENTS)	ENTS, working with an endoscopy team	• Medium	• Realistic • Ability to train higher-level integrative competencies[6,7] such as teamwork and communication	• Resource intensive to set up • Logistically can be hard to schedule multiple endoscopy team members for a single session

EGD, esophagogastroduodenoscopy; *EMR*, endoscopic mucosal resection; *ENTS*, endoscopic non-technical skills; *ERCP*, endoscopic retrograde cholangiopancreatography; *ESD*, endoscopic submucosal dissection; *EUS*, endoscopic ultrasound; *FNA*, fine needle aspirate; *FS*, flexible sigmoidoscopy; *PEG*, percutaneous endoscopic gastrostomy.

training of integrative competencies related to endoscopy, such as situational awareness, professionalism, and communication. Integrative competencies are higher-level competencies required to perform an endoscopic procedure that complement an individual's technical skills and clinical knowledge to facilitate effective delivery of high-quality endoscopic care in varied contexts.[6] Integrative competencies include core skills, such as communication and clinical judgment, that allow individuals to integrate their knowledge and technical expertise to function effectively within a health care team, adapt to varied contexts, tolerate uncertainty, and ultimately provide safe and effective patient care.

As mentioned previously, educational goals, and not technology, should guide decisions about which simulator to use for

training and assessment. Certain simulators, such as virtual reality computer generated models and live animal models, are useful to teach performance of the procedure as a whole, whereas education in basic endoscopic procedural elements, such as video image interpretation, endoscope handling, and torque steering, can be delivered using simple and less expensive inanimate part-task trainers.[22,23] Becoming familiar with the endoscope and learning a procedure at the same time creates increased cognitive work load and slows skills acquisition.[27] Pretraining on a mechanical simulator until a certain level of proficiency is reached may help shorten the learning curve and better protect patients. Part-task simulators (including mechanical and ex vivo models) are useful to teach and/or reinforce particular skill sets or components of the procedure, such as polypectomy or bleeding

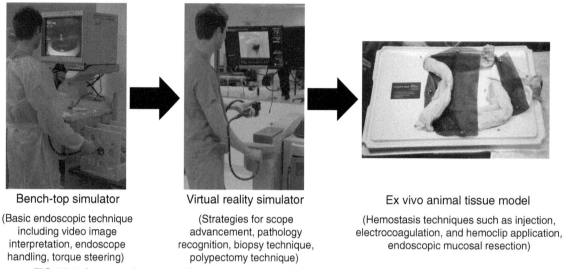

Bench-top simulator

(Basic endoscopic technique including video image interpretation, endoscope handling, torque steering)

Virtual reality simulator

(Strategies for scope advancement, pathology recognition, biopsy technique, polypectomy technique)

Ex vivo animal tissue model

(Hemostasis techniques such as injection, electrocoagulation, and hemoclip application, endoscopic mucosal resection)

FIG 13.1 An example progressive endoscopic simulation-based curriculum where learners proceed to training at progressively increasing levels of difficulty over time and simulator models are matched to the task.

control, as they deconstruct the skill set, allowing the learner to focus on the task at hand. Finally, more complex clinical events and behaviors, such as team training, benefit from use of more sophisticated hybrid simulations which involve use of inanimate or computerized simulators in conjunction with simulated patients (see the section entitled, Simulation to Train Endoscopic Nontechnical Skills).

In deciding which simulator one should use for a given training goal or stage of training, one should consider both the capabilities of the simulator itself and the training program that will be used to support the model. Simulators can be used to teach and/ or reinforce multiple training tasks depending on how they are integrated within a curriculum. Ultimately, the choice of simulator(s) must reflect the desired educational goals. We propose a three-stage framework for endoscopy simulation-based training that can be applied to help select simulators for a comprehensive endoscopy curriculum. The framework encompasses (1) task deconstruction using part-task trainers, followed by (2) use of simulators suited to whole procedural training and finally, (3) use of hybrid simulation to train higher-level integrative competencies related to endoscopic nontechnical skills.[6,7] This framework is theoretically in line with a progressive model of simulation-based training which is outlined in the following section. As mentioned previously, the utility of various simulators for specific training tasks is detailed in Table 13.1.

Progressive Model of Simulation-Based Training

Progressive learning, which involves planned and gradual increases in the difficulty or complexity of simulation-based tasks as learners' abilities improve, can be used by educators to guide selection of simulators for educational programs.[28,29] In this way instruction is matched to the learner's developmental level and simulators are chosen based on their ability to train a specific task. Range of task difficulty can be varied longitudinally across a curriculum or within a single session. An example curriculum for endoscopy that is based on the progressive model of simulation-based training could start trainees on a low-fidelity, bench-top colonoscopy simulator[22] which is ideal to teach basic endoscopic skills with regard to interpretation of the video image,

endoscope handling, and torque steering (Fig. 13.1). A virtual reality simulator could then be used to teach leaners various strategies for endoscope advancement (e.g., loop reduction, patient position change), pathology recognition, and basic biopsy and polypectomy technique. Subsequently, ex vivo animal tissue models could be used to train more advanced techniques such as EMR, or hemostasis skills including injection, electrocoagulation, and hemoclip application. This model of progressive simulation-based training has been used within the field of aviation with success.[30] In aviation training, as the situations grow more complex, trainees are increasingly required to troubleshoot difficult and unexpected situations. By analogy, particularly with the ex vivo models and hybrid simulation, and to an extent with difficult anatomy cases on the virtual reality simulator, progressive challenges can be created and trainees may be tasked to manage an unplanned adverse event in the controlled environment of the hands-on lab.

A recent RCT by Grover et al (2017)[31] within the field of gastrointestinal endoscopy has shown that a progressive simulation-based training curriculum that involves a deliberate transition from low to high task complexity and task difficulty improves colonoscopy skill acquisition and transfer to the clinical setting, compared to a curriculum utilizing high-fidelity simulation in isolation. It is thought that progressive simulation-based training is effective as task difficulty is adapted to align with the current skill of the learner, thus allowing learners to be optimally challenged as their skills improve; this is a factor known to enhance learning and promote task engagement.[28] As learners progress through training they can build upon previously attained competencies by engaging in activities of increasing difficulty without being cognitively overloaded. The aim is to train learners on progressively more challenging and difficult tasks that do not result in overwhelming the trainee in terms of cognitive load.

SIMULATION TO TRAIN ENDOSCOPIC NONTECHNICAL SKILLS

Use of simulation enables learners to practice and receive feedback in a safe, learner-centered environment. Simulation can be used to improve not only competence of endoscopic technical skills but also cognitive and integrative skills such as teamwork and decision-making.[6,7] Over the past decade there has been increasing recognition of the importance of endoscopic nontechnical skills (ENTS). In addition to the knowledge and technical skills required to perform endoscopy safely and proficiently, nontechnical skills play a central role in high-quality endoscopic practice. The vast majority of recommendations stemming from a report by the National Confidential Enquiry into Patient Outcomes and Death,[32] which investigated deaths occurring within 30 days of adult therapeutic gastrointestinal endoscopy procedures in the United Kingdom, highlight failings in nontechnical skills and behaviors such as communication, situational awareness, decision making, and teamwork, as opposed to technical skills. Nontechnical skills are an integral facet of competent endoscopic practice and an important contributor to patient safety and clinical outcomes.

Currently there is limited recognition, training or assessment of ENTS within endoscopy training programs. Training with regard to appropriate communication with an endoscopic assistant to coordinate techniques such as wire passage, injection, or polypectomy is often taught using ex vivo or virtual reality endoscopy simulator models. However, such training does not address the full breadth of nontechnical skills related to endoscopy, such as situation awareness. Hybrid simulation is a potential means of effectively training ENTS. Hybrid simulation is a term coined by Kneebone (2003)[33] to describe the process of attaching a simulator to a simulated patient. With regard to endoscopy, hybrid simulation involves a learner performing a procedure on an endoscopy simulator in a naturalistic setting (i.e., endoscopy suite), while interacting with an actor portraying a patient (i.e., a simulated or standardized patient) (Fig. 13.2). Multidisciplinary team members, such as an endoscopic nurse or anesthesiologist, can also be introduced into the scenarios. In this way, aspects of ENTS such as communication, decision making, leadership, teamwork, role clarity, coordination, shared goals, mutual respect, crisis management, and empathy can be taught during the simulations. Incorporation of debriefing that focuses on ENTS into team training allows team members to develop a shared mental model of the team's performance, reflect on their performance, and identify positive and negative aspects of performance to develop a plan for improvement and identify and mitigate causes of errors or near misses.[34] Recently published

studies by Grover et al (2015 and 2017)[35,35a] support the use of a curriculum integrating hybrid simulation as a means to improve nontechnical skill acquisition in novice endoscopists and transfer of skills to the clinical environment. Salas et al (2008)[36] have identified evidenced-based principles for effective team training that can be integrated when designing endoscopy simulation-based team training sessions, including: (1) focusing team training on identified critical teamwork competencies; (2) emphasizing teamwork over task work; (3) ensuring training is relevant to the clinical environment; and (4) providing timely, descriptive and relative feedback, which is essential to correct and reinforce desired teamwork behaviors.

INTEGRATING SIMULATORS INTO TRAINING

Health professions education has placed increased reliance on simulation in recent decades to enhance learner knowledge, skills, and attitudes, as well as to provide opportunities for practice in a safe and controlled environment. Development of any simulation-based training program should be evidence based, much like the practice of medicine. Integration of instructional design features known to enhance simulation-based instruction are required to optimize transfer of learner skills and behavior to the clinical workplace. Incorporation of these principles would advance the current state of endoscopic simulation-based training and enhance the effectiveness of endoscopy training. The following sections outline several educational principles that may be applied to develop well-designed endoscopy simulation-based training curricula to enhance learning.

Curricular Integration

Thoughtful integration of simulation into an overarching curriculum is known to be an essential feature of its effective use.[8] Simulation is one of several teaching strategies available to educators to achieve learning outcomes. It is important to determine where simulation can be used most effectively within the context of a broader endoscopic curriculum by matching learning objectives to the educational method(s) best suited to teach those objectives. Maximal learning benefit is achieved by having an organized and systematic approach to the incorporation of simulation.[37] Simulation should ideally be a required component of standard adult and pediatric endoscopy training curricula and built into learner's regular training schedule to help facilitate learner engagement in deliberate practice. Additionally, core skills that are taught within the simulation-based environment should reflect the ways in which learner performance is assessed, as assessment is known to drive learning.[38] Currently, endoscopy curricula are lacking across many training programs.[39] There remains a need to develop a standardized endoscopy curriculum that integrates simulation in a thoughtful and purposeful manner to augment and reinforce clinical learning of technical, cognitive, and integrative (nontechnical) competencies related to endoscopy. The American Board of Surgery has recently developed the Flexible Endoscopy Curriculum as part of the Fundamentals of Endoscopic Surgery (FES) Program which focuses on equipping surgical residents with the knowledge and technical skill to be a surgical endoscopist.[3,40] This effort, which was sparked by limited numbers of clinical cases available for surgical residents to complete under direct expert supervision, is a first step in the generation of a milestone-based curriculum that includes both didactic and hands-on simulator training. However, the curriculum only focuses on cognitive and technical

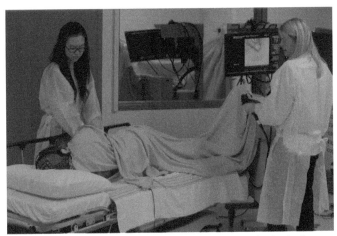

FIG 13.2 Colonoscopy hybrid simulation scenario, including an endoscopy nurse and the combination of a virtual reality simulator with a standardized patient.

milestones and fails to include training with regard to higher-level integrative (nontechnical) competencies required to perform endoscopic procedures safely and effectively, such as teamwork, decision making, and communication.[6,7,41] To date, validity evidence in support of the curriculum is lacking. Most important to the development of this and any future innovative curricula that integrate the use of simulators into training and assessment is the need to validate the results with evidence from objective performance data on real, unassisted procedures. For this purpose, the ASGE's PIVI report criteria serve as a useful guide.[1]

Deliberate Practice

Deliberate practice, a term initially used by Ericsson (2004) in instructional science,[42] involves focused repetitive performance of intended skills, coupled with informative feedback that promotes monitoring and error correction to improve performance in a specific domain. Deliberate practice is more predictive of expert performance than experience or natural aptitude.[43] Simulation is important as it affords trainees opportunities for deliberate practice of rarer or higher risk endoscopic procedures, such as management of gastrointestinal bleeding, in a controlled, low-risk environment. For deliberate practice to be effective, there have to be multiple different simulation experiences which increase in levels of challenge. Additionally, it is reliant on keen observers who are skilled feedback providers.

Mastery Learning

Reflective of the movement towards outcomes-based medical education, mastery learning is an instructional approach that requires learners to achieve a defined proficiency before proceeding to the next instructional objective.[44] The time needed to achieve a mastery standard will vary between learners. Simulation-based training in other domains, such as surgery, that incorporates mastery learning has been shown to significantly improve skills acquisition and improve patient outcomes.[44] Three small feasibility studies have examined use of mastery learning for colonoscopy on a virtual reality simulator, the results of which indicate potential benefit, although none have directly compared mastery-based learning with other simulation-based learning strategies.[45–47] Key features of simulation-based mastery training include a baseline assessment, clear learning objectives, defined minimal mastery standards that must be sequentially met, and educational activities focused on achievement of mastery objectives with concurrent formative assessment to enhance learning and gauge progress.[48] Challenges to implementing mastery learning principles include the development of clearly defined goals, defensible mastery standards, and complementary assessment instruments with strong validity and reliability evidence.[37,48] To date, this has not been done within the field of endoscopy. Additionally, instruction using a mastery model takes more time.

Task Variability

Real endoscopy provides marked variation in terms of anatomy, pathology, and procedural difficulty. Therefore, it is important to introduce task variability during practice to ensure learners have opportunities to engage in practice of endoscopic skills that capture or represent a wide range of patients.[8] Additionally, research from the motor learning literature has shown that skill acquisition and long-term retention of skills is enhanced when task parameters (e.g., difficulty, pathology encountered) are variable during practice. Simulation-based training that incorporates task variability can also help promote adaptive expertise.

Experts are flexible in their thinking and performance and are able to adapt to change and create new approaches to adapt to unexpected and complex problems. Research from the laparoscopic surgery literature has shown that learners who are exposed to variability during simulation-based training have improved flexibility of trained skills as compared to those who did not encounter task variability.[49]

Distributed Practice

Although distributed and massed practice schedules have not been directly compared for endoscopy, studies from the surgical domain indicate that best training results are obtained when training is scheduled as multiple short training sessions distributed over time, as opposed to one long block of training.[50,51] With distributed practice learners tend to have less mental fatigue and thus are able to devote more cognitive resources to learning.[51] Distributed practice also allows more time for memory consolidation and mental rehearsal; both are considered key factors in enhancing the performance of procedures.[52] Before each spaced practice session, learners have to retrieve key aspects of the skill being learned from their memory, resulting in deeper encoding. Additionally, learners forget information over time; therefore, they have to invest more cognitive effort into learning, with a resultant positive effect on long-term retention.[51] Distributed practice is especially important for complex skills that take a number of practice attempts to achieve a plateau in skill acquisition. A distributed practice schedule, however, is often logistically more complicated to implement and thus most skills courses are predominantly conducted using massed practice schedules. Varying the task load during a session can potentially help reduce the detrimental effects of mental fatigue.

Performance Enhancing Feedback

Provision of constructive feedback is a cornerstone of effective training and is recognized as the most important feature of simulation-based training.[37] The power of feedback depends largely on the properties of the information given, the manner in which it is delivered, and the way it is interpreted. Instructional feedback is a key motivator for trainees and has been shown to provide a distinct advantage in the acquisition of endoscopy skills.[31,53] Mahmood et al (2004)[54] showed that there is no improvement in endoscopy skills acquisition in the simulated setting in the absence of feedback, and studies comparing instructor-derived feedback with simulator-generator feedback have shown a distinct advantage with regard to instructor-derived feedback.[53] Additionally, the results of Grover et al's (2015)[35] recent randomized controlled study support integration of endoscopy simulation into a structured curriculum incorporating instructional feedback as a means to augment technical, cognitive, and integrative skills acquisition, as compared with self-regulated learning on virtual reality simulators.

Feedback that is tied to prespecified objectives and is followed by correction of performance forms the basis for deliberate practice, an essential component of attainment of expertise.[42,55] Feedback should focus on simple, well-defined, and achievable points to avoid overburdening the trainee. Feedback should ideally be a two-way process between the trainer and learner that is delivered in a nonjudgmental manner and is based on observable actions and linked to specific suggestions for improvement.[56,57] Additionally, it should be constructive, focused on improvement, and should strive to foster the trainee's conscious understanding of the steps required for performance. Incorporation of problem solving and active decision making, especially with more advanced trainees, serves to improve self-reflection and ultimately conscious competence.[56] This is achieved by focusing feedback discussions on critical challenges during the procedure, having the learner diagnose the problem, review potential options and decide, in consultation with the instructor, which option to try. Questioning on the part of the trainer encourages active engagement and reflection and encourages learners to think independently and weigh potential solutions rather than simply being informed of the best option.[56]

The simulated setting provides an ideal environment for feedback provision as learners can work through errors independently and feedback delivery can be structured to enhance learning without compromising patient safety. For example, Walsh et al (2009)[58] found that the timing of feedback provision is an important factor influencing skill acquisition in novice endoscopists in the simulated setting. Terminal feedback that is given at the end of completion of a simulated task is more effective in promoting endoscopy skills acquisition and retention of skills as compared with feedback that is given during task performance.[58] Constant feedback may lead learners to depend on the feedback for guidance such that a learners' performance declines when the feedback is withheld. Additionally, constant feedback may cognitively overload learners as they are required to focus their attention on listening to the feedback, rather than engaging in the cognitive processing essential for learning (schema acquisition and rule automation).[27] Provision of continuous feedback may also disrupt the concentration of trainers and ultimately impair feedback provision as the simultaneous tasks of observation and feedback provision may place excessive cognitive demands on the instructor. Terminal feedback permits time for learners to focus their cognitive efforts on problem solving around difficulties; this is a factor known to enhance learning. Concerns for patient safety do not permit the use of terminal feedback within the clinical setting, pointing to the idea that simulation technology allows educators to use strategies known to enhance learning, such as terminal feedback, which are not possible to use when teaching in the clinical setting due to concerns for patient safety.

With regard to feedback interpretation, the perceived credibility of the feedback provider influences feedback effectiveness,[59–61] thus supporting the use of instructors with expertise in endoscopy and an awareness of principles of adult education. Additionally, feedback incorporating some objective indicators of performance increases the perceived credibility of the content of the feedback and likelihood that it is accepted. This supports the use of video to demonstrate errors or incorporation of simulator-generated metrics or validated assessment tools into feedback provision. Additionally, formative endoscopy assessment tools, such as the Gastrointestinal Endoscopy Competency Assessment Tool (GiECAT),[6,62] the Mayo Colonoscopy Skills Assessment Tool (MCSAT),[63] or the Assessment of Competency in Endoscopy (ACE) tool[64] can be used by endoscopy trainers to help guide feedback delivery as they help trainers identify areas the trainee needs to focus on to improve.

Debriefing after a simulation-based session allows learners the opportunity to engage in self-assessment, reflect on their performance, identify errors and successes, identify areas for development, and mitigate any lack of insight with the trainee. Debriefing discussions should be tied to the prespecified objectives for the training session. A useful guide for debriefing that is based on empirical evidence and educational theory is Rudolph et al's (2008)[65] four-step model which includes (1) noting pertinent performance gaps related to predetermined objectives; (2) providing feedback that describes the gap(s); (3) investigating the basis for the gap(s) by exploring the frames (assumptions, goals, knowledge base) and emotions contributing to the current performance level; and (4) helping close the performance gap through discussion or targeted instruction about principles and skills relevant to performance. Every simulation-based training session should conclude with the generation of mutually agreed upon learning goals for future training episodes to continually reinforce and build upon existing competencies.

Instructor Training

With regard to the effectiveness of simulation-based training, there is increasing recognition that the role of the instructor[57] is a vital component to effective education and both endoscopy trainees and trainers believe more formal instruction on how to teach endoscopy to be benficial.[39,48] The ability to teach endoscopy is an important skillset that can likely be enhanced with instruction.[65a] Although research evaluating instructor training is lacking, it is increasingly recognized that endoscopy training should be ideally provided by individuals with the requisite skills and behaviors to teach endoscopy effectively and efficiently, including an awareness of adult education principles and best practices in procedural skills education. Observation and experience have shown that effective instruction is not easy or intuitive and that clinical experience is not a proxy for instructor effectiveness.[48] Endoscopy instructor courses aimed at teaching trainers essential components of an effective technical skills training session are increasingly being implemented across jurisdictions such as Canada[66] and the United States[67] and are now mandatory for adult gastroenterology endoscopy trainers in the United Kingdom.[68,69] These courses teach instructors evidence-based educational principles, such as use of performance enhancing feedback and standardized language, that can be applied by trainers to enhance learning in the clinical setting.[70] Although anecdotally very effective, with some evidence to show improvement in trainer confidence and skill,[71] the short- and long-term value and utility of these educational opportunities and their application to teaching in the simulated setting are currently unknown.

SIMULATION-BASED ASSESSMENTS

An increased emphasis on quality, patient safety, learner-centeredness and social accountability has resulted in a paradigm shift across medical education from a process-based system that specifies the amount of time required to learn specified content to a competency-based system that is focused on describing and assessing outcomes that can be demonstrated in practice.[72] Competency-based medical education signifies a training process that results in documented achievement of the requisite knowledge, skills, attitudes, and behaviors for competent independent practice.[73] Reflective of this, endoscopy training programs are required to ensure that trainees are competent to perform endoscopic procedures safely, independently and competently upon the completion of training. Key to this need for quality assurance is the requirement for reliable, accurate and objective assessments of a trainee's skill.

High quality assessment is reliant on the existence of tools and measures that are both reliable and valid. Within the clinical setting, direct observation of procedural skills is the preferred method to support ongoing skills assessment.[7] Direct observational assessment tools can be used during clinical training to monitor the learner's progress, guide performance-enhancing feedback, augment learning, identify learners who require more focused training, and ultimately to determine when a trainee has demonstrated sufficient competence to enter unsupervised practice.[7] With regard to colonoscopy, there are four direct observational assessment tools that have been developed and validated in a more systematic manner when compared with other published tools[7]: The GiECAT,[6,62,74] the MCSAT,[63,75] the ACE[64,76] Colonoscopy Skills Assessment Tool, and the Joint Advisory Committee on GI Endoscopy's Direct Observation of Procedure (JAG-DOPS) Assessment Tool.[77] With regard to upper endoscopy, the ACE EGD Skills Assessment Tool[76] has been published, but studies evaluating its evidence of reliability and validity are lacking. An assessment tool with strong evidence of reliability and validity also exists for polypectomy, the Direct Observation of Polypectomy Skills (DOPyS) tool.[78–80] Rigorously developed direct observational clinical assessment tools, such as the aforementioned examples, are also useful with regard to simulation-based training, as they can help trainers pinpoint specific deficiencies that may be amenable to training on simulators. Additionally, psychometrically sound clinical assessment tools play an important role in the effort to develop and validate alternative assessment methods using simulators, as simulator-based assessment tools should be predictive of independently defined minimal competence parameters such as those generated by high-quality, direct, observational assessment tools.[1]

Simulation-based assessments are appealing to educators as they offer a proxy for clinical observations, thus enabling assessment at the "shows how" level of Miller's (1990)[81] pyramid. They are advantageous in that they are capable of providing assessments in a controlled environment that are less subject to assessor bias. Additionally, they are capable of delivering standardized, highly reproducible assessment scenarios across trainees (i.e., simulation is capable of eliminating variability due to pathology and/or anatomy) and learners at all stages of training can carry out assessment tasks independently on simulators in a risk-free environment, thus mitigating concerns for patient safety. Furthermore, simulation can be used to assess integrative competencies such as communication within immersive team-based scenarios.[6,7] For example, through use of an Integrated Procedural Performance Instrument (IPPI) format assessment scenario, initially described by Kneebone (2003),[33] during which participants are assessed performing a procedure on a endoscopy simulator in a naturalistic setting while interacting with team members (e.g., endoscopic nurse, anesthesiologist) and a standardized patient (i.e., a hybrid simulation as described previously).

Whereas simulation-based assessment has many potential advantages, what remains a challenge for the field of simulation is the development of models capable of providing accurate and reliable skills assessment. Prior to implementation of simulation-based assessment, tools for measuring endoscopy skills within the simulated environment must demonstrate acceptable evidence of reliability and validity. Currently, performance during an endoscopy simulation-based assessment is generally assessed by one of three means: virtual reality simulator metrics, motion analysis, and direct observational assessment tools.[82]

Simulator Generated Performance Metrics

Virtual reality endoscopy simulators typically provide immediate and automatic assessment by generating computer measured metrics of "performance" such as percentage of mucosa visualized, time to reach the cecum, and patient discomfort during the simulated procedure.[83] Simulator-derived metrics are advantageous in that they are objective and assessments can potentially be completed in the absence of an experienced endoscopist. A number of studies have been carried out to validate these metrics for various commercially available virtual reality colonoscopy simulators.[14,84–94] However, research assessing the validity of such metrics has yet to demonstrate that they are capable of meaningfully discriminating between endoscopists across varying levels of skill.[14,76,84–95] A reason for this limitation in some cases has been the observation that many of the modules are not difficult enough to perform to allow for such graded skill differentiation. Additionally, two studies of moderate quality which compared simulated and live performance ratings using poor quality direct observational assessment tools revealed that these metrics do not correlate with performance scores assigned by blinded expert endoscopists.[96,97] Furthermore, the use of computerized simulators for assessment purposes is often cost-prohibitive.

Virtual reality endoscopic simulation has recently been integrated into the board certification process for general surgery in the United States through the FES program. Modeled after the validated Fundamentals of Laparoscopic Surgery,[98–100] the FES program consists of web-based didactic material, a written examination to assess cognitive aspects of endoscopy, and a hands-on skill test on a virtual reality simulator. The FES performance-based manual skills assessment consists of five simulation-based tasks designed to assess fundamental endoscopy-related technical skills.[101] Although the assessment has good test-retest reliability (intraclass correlation coefficient [ICC] = 0.85), scores correlated only modestly with real-life colonoscopy performance ($r = 0.78$) as assessed using the Global Assessment of Gastrointestinal Endoscopic Skills–Colonoscopy (GAGES-C)[102,103]; the GAGES-C is a direct observational assessment tool with moderate quality validity evidence that only assesses the technical aspects of endoscopic competence.[7] Proper validation of the FES or any other simulator-based assessment will require use of a clinical assessment tool with strong evidence of validity and reliability that incorporates cognitive and integrative components of endoscopic competence, as well as technical competencies, such as the previously mentioned GiECAT,[66,62,74] MCSAT,[63,75] ACE,[64] or JAG-DOPS[77] assessment tools, or from actual objective clinical outcome data. Additionally, assessors were not blinded with regard to the endoscopist's skill level.[104] Whereas this is a promising first step in the application of endoscopic simulation-based assessment, further research is required to determine whether a passing FES score is a reliable and valid marker of competence in performing clinical endoscopic procedures. In line with ASGE's PIVI report, it is recommended that simulator-based assessment tools must be procedure-specific and predictive of independently defined minimal competence parameters from real procedures with a kappa value of at least 0.70 for high-stakes assessment.[1]

Performance metrics derived from tasks performed on low-fidelity, part-task endoscopy simulators (e.g., precision, speed) are also being studied as a means to assess technical skills.[23,105] In particular, the Thompson Endoscopic Skills Trainer (TEST), which was developed to emphasize fundamental endoscopic technical skills for basic maneuvers including retroflexion, tip deflection, torque, polypectomy, navigation, and loop reduction, has been shown to differentiate technical skill accurately among all training levels (construct validity).[23,105] Whereas low-cost simulators, such as the TEST, potentially enable assessment of particular tasks (e.g., retroflexion, torque) that could be used to help track achievement of specific technical milestones during training, further validity evidence is required before they are adopted broadly, including studies to establish learning curves and to correlate use to the simulator with improved clinical aptitude.

For simulator-derived metrics to be useful for formative assessment, they must be able to discriminate between endoscopists with small differences in experience (discriminative validity) in a manner that allows educators to identify discrete areas of deficiency and provide specific feedback and remediation. This might also allow program directors to implement mastery learning principles, requiring trainees to reach sufficient proficiency on simulators prior to advancing to further training with regard to more complex and higher risk procedures such as ERCP or EMR. For summative high-stakes assessment such as credentialing, not only would simulator metrics be required to demonstrate excellent discriminative validity, they would also need to correlate closely with competency in performing live endoscopy procedures in a reproducible, accurate, and reliable manner, preferably with a kappa of 0.7 of better.[1,83]

Motion Analysis

Motion analysis can also be used to assess endoscopic performance within the simulated setting. Assessments based on motion analysis aim to quantify procedural dexterity using parameters generated by motion tracking hardware and/or software that are extracted from movements of the hands and/or procedural instrument(s) (e.g., force applied, path length, instrument trajectory).[106] The advantage of assessments based on motion analysis is that they are objective. However, they only permit quantification of technical skills and they are reliant on hardware and/or software resources which can potentially interfere with procedural performance (e.g., motion tracking sensors on an endoscopist's hands), thus limiting their feasibility. Additionally, whereas motion analysis can objectively assess procedural dexterity, it does not assess the full range of competencies required to perform a colonoscopy. Furthermore, motion-analysis research to date has been limited[107–111] and further validity evidence of the technology and appropriate metrics is required prior to widespread implementation.

Direct Observational Simulator Assessment Tools

Direct observational assessment tools rely on an external rater to observe and assess learners using predefined criteria that are based on an assessment framework. Such tools are advantageous, as compared with simulator-generated metrics and motion analysis, as they are capable of providing trainees with more specific feedback with regard to performance quality and areas requiring improvement. Additionally, they allow for assessment of cognitive and integrative aspects of endoscopic competence such as knowledge of accessories, clinical judgment, and communication. Furthermore, they potentially enable one to measure direct transfer of skills between the simulated and clinical environment. To date, however, there are limited data examining reliability and validity evidence of a direct observational tool for simulated endoscopy.[12,96,97,112,113] Direct observation tools that have been assessed to date in the simulated setting lack the discriminative power to assess performance and determine competence in actual clinical performance. Further work is required to assess the psychometric properties of a comprehensive observational assessment tool within both the simulated and clinical setting to enable measurement of transfer of skills between the two environments.

There are a number of compelling reasons to implement endoscopic simulation-based assessments; however, as mentioned previously, prior to widespread adoption further research is required to ensure these assessments can reliably distinguish between endoscopists with a range of endoscopic experience and predict competence in patient-based endoscopy.[17] Challenges remain with regard to the use of simulation for assessment, including the limited realism of simulators, lack of assessments with strong validity and reliability evidence, and the inability to control for potential simulator related behaviors, such as a "cavalier" attitude given trainees are aware that no real patients are at risk. Additional effort is needed to address these concerns, including improved assessment metrics and the development of assessments that utilize an adequate number of scenarios and raters to demonstrate acceptable reliability and validity. Further work is also needed to help determine where simulation is best placed within an overarching program of assessment and whether simulation-based skills assessment can be used to guide decisions with regard to progression of training (i.e., when to advance trainees' clinical responsibilities with regard to endoscopy) within a competency-based training model.

LOOKING TO THE FUTURE

The past three decades have been characterized by a rapid expansion of simulation modalities designed to train individuals learning endoscopic procedures and a general acceptance of their use. However, there remains a need for integration of evidence-based principles to facilitate effectiveness of endoscopy simulation-based training, including curricular integration, deliberate practice, mastery learning, task variability, and performance enhancing feedback. Expert benchmarks of performance need to be established for various training tasks on simulators to create clearly defined metrics that can form the basis of proficiency-based training goals. And although goals are ideally determined in terms of mastery standards, training should ideally focus on provision of performance-enhancing feedback to augment learning. More efforts to develop and evaluate courses designed to train endoscopic instructors with regard to best practices for teaching in the simulated setting are also required to ensure widespread application of evidence-based educational principles known to enhance learning.

Much work also remains to clarify the optimal use of simulation-based training to supplement conventional endoscopy training. There is a paucity of comparative effectiveness studies (studies comparing one simulation modality with another active simulation-based intervention[11]) examining the effectiveness of instructional design features and best practice for selection of simulation modalities to train specific tasks. Furthermore, more work is needed to help elucidate how to best integrate simulation within a broader endoscopy curriculum to optimize safety, cost-effectiveness, learning, and skill transfer to the clinical setting. The timing, frequency, and duration of endoscopy simulation-based training required to optimize skill transfer to the clinical setting has yet to be fully elucidated. It also remains unknown whether ongoing work on simulators during patient-based clinical training has any complementary benefit, and if so, how much and for what specific techniques is the extra training worthwhile.

The major limiters with regard to implementation of endoscopic simulation into training remain cost and accessibility.[9] Advances in cloud-based technology and reductions in the cost of computing have yet to translate into far less expensive virtual reality simulators with processing centralized in the cloud via local dummy terminals. This obstacle continues to incentivize programs to try to do more with less costly static and ex vivo models. For broader adoption of simulation across training programs, affordable, validated, and easily accessible endoscopic simulators are required. Additionally, studies comparing the cost effectiveness of simulation as compared to other forms of training are needed, including examination of potential cost savings resulting from accelerated learning and the initial and ongoing expenses associated with simulation training.[1]

Based on current evidence, endoscopy simulation-based training has been shown to be useful in the early training phase in helping speed up the initial phase of the endoscopy learning curve and reduce patient burden.[10,11] To date, simulation has primarily been studied as a means to train novice endoscopists. Simulators have untapped potential to improve nontechnical aspects of endoscopic performance that has yet to be examined fully. Specifically, further studies are needed to assess simulation as a means to train broader integrative competencies related to the skill of endoscopy, such as teamwork and communication, and higher level competencies, such as crisis management, that require the integration of both technical and nontechnical skills for successful management.[6,7] Other potential expanded methods of using simulators that have yet to be explored can be drawn from the aviation industry, such as the use of simulation to help individuals learn how to troubleshoot difficult situations (e.g., perforation) that occur infrequently but must be mastered.[30]

The potential role of simulators as a means to train cognitive skills, in particular pathology recognition, also remains underemphasized. Future work is required to determine how best to train in pathology recognition using simulators and how to optimally integrate other learning modalities, such as web-based pathology recognition e-learning modules, into an overarching simulation curriculum to maximize learning.

The role simulators can potentially play in maintaining skills related to endoscopy also remains unexplored, especially with regard to procedures where there may be insufficient clinical volume for adequate maintenance of skill. An evidence base also needs to be further established with respect to best practices in the use of simulation for training of more advanced endoscopic skills. It is important to continue to improve upon simulator models to allow for the deliberate practice of therapeutic interventions, such as polypectomy, injection techniques, hemostasis techniques, stent deployment, and closure of defects with clips.

In addition to training, simulation is increasingly being used as a tool for credentialing, licensing, and certification across disciplines.[114] With regard to gastrointestinal endoscopy, the field is still a long way from achieving such a goal. An important challenge for the endoscopy simulation field will be the development of models capable of providing accurate skills assessments that can reliably predict clinical performance at preestablished benchmarks of competency. Such assessments could be used during the course of training to help guide when trainees might advance to subsequent levels of clinical responsibilities, allowing them to perform more technically demanding procedures. Additionally, reliable and valid simulator-based assessments would be of enormous value as they would provide unbiased and reproducible measures for credentialing purposes and help ensure

patients that the individuals performing their endoscopy have been trained to sufficient minimum standards of quality.[1]

There remains a need to develop further high-quality procedure specific clinical assessment tools, such as the GiECAT,[6] MCSAT,[63] ACE,[64] and JAG-DOPS,[77] that possess strong validity and reliability evidence to establish learning curves and performance benchmarks for all endoscopic procedures against which simulator-based metrics can be validated. Once key, clinically relevant, metrics for a technique are identified, assessment tools based on these metrics need to be developed that are accurate, reliable, and capable of distinguishing individuals with a range of endoscopic experience. These tools should also accurately predict actual clinical performance and correlate with clinical performance benchmarks in prospective validation studies.[1] To achieve this goal, better tracking of longitudinal outcomes, such as cecal intubation and adenoma detection rates, is needed across procedures as a means to validate simulation-based assessments and help examine the long-term impact of simulator enhanced training. Finally, additional research is required to determine where simulation-based assessments are best placed within an overall program of assessment to maximally augment learning. Ultimately, improving the use of simulation for assessment purposes will greatly broaden the appeal and value of simulators to hospitals who are responsible for credentialing individuals to perform endoscopic procedures and aid in improving learner access to simulators and integration across training programs.

KEY REFERENCES

1. Cohen J, Bosworth BP, Chak A, et al: Preservation and Incorporation of Valuable Endoscopic Innovations (PIVI) on the use of endoscopy simulators for training and assessing skill, *Gastrointest Endosc* 76:471–475, 2012.
4. Dunkin BJ: Flexible endoscopy simulators, *Semin Laparosc Surg* 10:29–35, 2003.
6. Walsh CM, Ling SC, Khanna N, et al: Gastrointestinal endoscopy competency assessment tool: reliability and validity evidence, *Gastrointest Endosc* 81:1417–1424, 2015.
7. Walsh CM: In-training gastrointestinal endoscopy competency assessment tools: types of tools, validation and impact, *Best Pract Res Clin Gastroenterol* 30:357–374, 2016.
8. Issenberg SB, McGaghie WC, Petrusa ER, et al: Features and uses of high-fidelity medical simulations that lead to effective learning: a BEME systematic review, *Med Teach* 27:10–28, 2005.
9. Jirapinyo P, Thompson CC: Current status of endoscopic simulation in gastroenterology fellowship training programs, *Surg Endosc* 29:1913–1919, 2015.
10. Walsh C, Sherlock M, Ling S, Carnahan H: Virtual reality simulation training for health professions trainees in gastrointestinal endoscopy, *Cochrane Database Syst Rev* CD008237, 2012.
11. Singh S, Sedlack RE, Cook DA: Effects of simulation-based training in gastrointestinal endoscopy: a systematic review and meta-analysis, *Clin Gastroenterol Hepatol* 12:1611–1623, 2014.
12. Ekkelenkamp VE, Koch AD, de Man RA, Kuipers EJ: Training and competence assessment in GI endoscopy: a systematic review, *Gut* 65:607–615, 2016.
13. Cohen J, Cohen SA, Vora KC, et al: Multicenter, randomized, controlled trial of virtual-reality simulator training in acquisition of competency in colonoscopy, *Gastrointest Endosc* 64:361–368, 2006.
17. Cohen J, Thompson CC: The next generation of endoscopic simulation, *Am J Gastroenterol* 108:1036–1039, 2013.
18. van der Wiel SE, Magalhães RK, Dinis-Ribeiro M, et al: Simulator training in gastrointestinal endoscopy From basic training to advanced endoscopic procedures, *Best Pract Res Clin Gastroenterol* 30:375–387, 2016.

22. Walsh CM, Cooper MA, Rabeneck L, Carnahan H: High versus low fidelity simulation training in gastroenterology: expertise discrimination, *Can J Gastroenterol* 22:Abstract 164, 2008.

23. Jirapinyo P, Kumar N, Thompson CC: Validation of an endoscopic part-task training box as a skill assessment tool, *Gastrointest Endosc* 81:967–973, 2015.

26. Matthes K, Cohen J: The Neo-Papilla: a new modification of porcine ex vivo simulators for ERCP training (with videos), *Gastrointest Endosc* 64:570–576, 2006.

27. van Merriënboer JJG, Sweller J: Cognitive load theory in health professional education: design principles and strategies, *Med Educ* 44:85–93, 2010.

28. Guadagnoli M, Morin M-P, Dubrowski A: The application of the challenge point framework in medical education, *Med Educ* 46:447–453, 2012.

30. Cohen J, Nuckolls L, Mourant RR: Endoscopy simulators: lessons from the aviation and automobile industries, *Gastrointest Endosc Clin N Am* 16:407–423, 2006.

31. Grover SC, Scaffidi MA, Khan R, et al: Progressive learning in endoscopy simulation training improves clinical performance: a blinded randomized trial, *Gastrointest Endosc* 86(5):881–889, 2017.

33. Kneebone RL, Nestel D, Moorthy K, et al: Learning the skills of flexible sigmoidoscopy—the wider perspective, *Med Educ* 37:50–58, 2003.

35. Grover SC, Garg A, Scaffidi MA, et al: Impact of a simulation training curriculum on technical and nontechnical skills in colonoscopy: a randomized trial, *Gastrointest Endosc* 82:1072–1079, 2015.

35a. Grover SC, Scaffidi MA, Khan R: A virtual reality curriculum in non-technical skills improves colonoscopic performance: A randomized trial, *Gastrointest Endosc* 85:AB181, 2017, (Abstract Sa1075).

36. Salas E, DiazGranados D, Weaver SJ, King H: Does team training work? Principles for health care, *Acad Emerg Med* 15:1002–1009, 2008.

41. Vassiliou MC, Dunkin BJ, Marks JM, Fried GM: FLS and FES: comprehensive models of training and assessment, *Surg Clin North Am* 90:535–558, 2010.

42. Ericsson KA: Deliberate practice and the acquisition and maintenance of expert performance in medicine and related domains, *Acad Med* 79:S70–S81, 2004.

44. Cook DA, Brydges R, Zendejas B, et al: Mastery learning for health professionals using technology-enhanced simulation: a systematic review and meta-analysis, *Acad Med* 88:1178–1186, 2013.

51. Spruit EN, Band GPH, Hamming JF, Ridderinkhof KR: Optimal training design for procedural motor skills: a review and application to laparoscopic surgery, *Psychol Res* 78:878–891, 2014.

54. Mahmood T, Darzi A: The learning curve for a colonoscopy simulator in the absence of any feedback: no feedback, no learning, *Surg Endosc* 18:1224–1230, 2004.

55. Fried GM, Waschke KA: How endoscopy is learned: deconstructing skill sets. In Cohen J, editor: *Successful training in gastrointestinal endoscopy*, Oxford, 2011, Wiley-Blackwell, pp 16–21.

58. Walsh CM, Ling SC, Wang CS, Carnahan H: Concurrent versus terminal feedback: it may be better to wait, *Acad Med* 84:S54–S57, 2009.

59. Watling C, Driessen E, van der Vleuten CPM, Lingard L: Learning from clinical work: the roles of learning cues and credibility judgements, *Med Educ* 46:192–200, 2012.

62. Walsh CM, Ling SC, Mamula P, et al: The gastrointestinal endoscopy competency assessment tool for pediatric colonoscopy, *J Pediatr Gastroenterol Nutr* 60:474–480, 2015.

63. Sedlack RE: The Mayo Colonoscopy Skills Assessment Tool: validation of a unique instrument to assess colonoscopy skills in trainees, *Gastrointest Endosc* 72:1125–1133, 2010.

64. Sedlack RE, Coyle WJ: Assessment of competency in endoscopy: establishing and validating generalizable competency benchmarks for colonoscopy, *Gastrointest Endosc* 83:516–523, 2016.

65. Rudolph JW, Simon R, Raemer DB, Eppich WJ: Debriefing as formative assessment: closing performance gaps in medical education, *Acad Emerg Med* 15:1010–1016, 2008.

65a. Walsh CM, Anderson JT, Fishman DS: Evidence-based approach to training pediatric gastrointestinal endoscopy trainers, *J Pediatr Gastroenterol Nutr* 64(4):501–504, 2017.

68. Anderson JT: Assessments and skills improvement for endoscopists, *Best Pract Res Clin Gastroenterol* 30:453–471, 2016.

71. Matthes K, Cohen J, Kochman ML, et al: Efficacy and costs of a one-day hands-on EASIE endoscopy simulator train-the-trainer workshop, *Gastrointest Endosc* 62:921–927, 2005.

74. Walsh CM, Ling SC, Walters TD, et al: Development of the gastrointestinal endoscopy competency assessment tool for pediatric colonoscopy (GiECATKIDS), *J Pediatr Gastroenterol Nutr* 59:480–486, 2014.

75. Sedlack RE: Training to competency in colonoscopy: assessing and defining competency standards, *Gastrointest Endosc* 74:355–366, 2011.

76. Sedlack RE, Coyle WJ, Obstein KL, et al: ASGE's assessment of competency in endoscopy evaluation tools for colonoscopy and EGD, *Gastrointest Endosc* 79:1–7, 2014.

77. Barton JR, Corbett S, van der Vleuten CP: The validity and reliability of a Direct Observation of Procedural Skills assessment tool: assessing colonoscopic skills of senior endoscopists, *Gastrointest Endosc* 75:591–597, 2012.

79. Gupta S, Anderson J, Bhandari P, et al: Development and validation of a novel method for assessing competency in polypectomy: direct observation of polypectomy skills, *Gastrointest Endosc* 73:1232–1239, e2, 2011.

81. Miller GE: The assessment of clinical skills/competence/performance, *Acad Med* 65:S63–S67, 1990.

96. Moorthy K, Munz Y, Orchard TR, et al: An innovative method for the assessment of skills in lower gastrointestinal endoscopy, *Surg Endosc* 18:1613–1619, 2004.

97. Sarker SK, Albrani T, Zaman A, Kumar I: Procedural performance in gastrointestinal endoscopy: live and simulated, *World J Surg* 34:1764–1770, 2010.

101. Vassiliou MC, Dunkin BJ, Fried GM, et al: Fundamentals of endoscopic surgery: creation and validation of the hands-on test, *Surg Endosc* 28:704–711, 2014.

102. Vassiliou MC, Kaneva PA, Poulose BK, et al: Global Assessment of Gastrointestinal Endoscopic Skills (GAGES): a valid measurement tool for technical skills in flexible endoscopy, *Surg Endosc* 24:1834–1841, 2010.

104. Mueller CL, Kaneva P, Fried GM, et al: Colonoscopy performance correlates with scores on the FES™ manual skills test, *Surg Endosc* 28:3081–3085, 2014.

105. Thompson CC, Jirapinyo P, Kumar N, et al: Development and initial validation of an endoscopic part-task training box, *Endoscopy* 46:735–744, 2014.

107. Mohankumar D, Garner H, Ruff K, et al: Characterization of right wrist posture during simulated colonoscopy: an application of kinematic analysis to the study of endoscopic maneuvers, *Gastrointest Endosc* 79:480–489, 2014.

112. Haycock A, Koch AD, Familiari P, et al: Training and transfer of colonoscopy skills: a multinational, randomized, blinded, controlled trial of simulator versus bedside training, *Gastrointest Endosc* 71:298–307, 2010.

A complete reference list can be found online at ExpertConsult.com

Luminal Gastrointestinal Disorders

14

Nonvariceal Upper Gastrointestinal Bleeding

Kyle J. Fortinsky and Alan N. Barkun

CHAPTER OUTLINE

INTRODUCTION

The annual incidence of upper gastrointestinal bleeding (UGIB) is 48 to 160 events per 100,000 adults in the United States, where it is the cause of approximately 300,000 hospital admissions per year.[1,2] In Europe, the annual incidence of UGIB in the general population ranges from 19.4[3,4] to 57.0[3,5] events per 100,000 individuals. There is no formal explanation for the breadth of the range between countries, although differences in health care systems and case recording capacities may be substantial.[4,5] Additional contributing factors may include alcohol intake and *H. pylori* prevalence.

In both North America and Europe, in a general practice setting, approximately 80%–90% of acute UGIB episodes have a nonvariceal etiology with peptic ulcers and gastroduodenal erosions accounting for the majority of lesions.[6,7] UGIB-related mortality rates have decreased in the past two decades, but still range from 2% to 15%.[8–10] Two studies conducted in the United Kingdom highlighted that, despite a notable decrease in mortality in patients with UGIB from 1993 to 2007, mortality from peptic ulcer bleeding is still 10%–13%.[7,9]

This chapter discusses the various management principles of medical therapy in nonvariceal UGIB (NVUGIB) put forth by guidelines from the multidisciplinary international consensus group in 2010, the American College of Gastroenterology in 2012, and the European Society of Gastrointestinal Endoscopy in 2015.[2,11,12] When applicable, more recent evidence is included with a focus on randomized controlled trials (RCTs) and metaanalyses.

Each section of this chapter presents the most current evidence and provides recommendations for practice. This chapter focuses on providing an evidence-based approach to initial resuscitation, the role of blood transfusion, preendoscopic, endoscopic, and postendoscopic management for patients presenting with NVUGIB.

CLINICAL PRESENTATION

The presentation of GI bleeding is dependent on the site, volume, and rate of bleeding. The most common clinical presentation of UGIB, defined as a source proximal to the ligament of Treitz, includes either hematemesis or melena. Occasionally, the emesis can appear to resemble coffee-grounds, which can occur when older blood in the stomach is reduced by stomach acid. The appearance of melena (black, tarry, and foul-smelling stool) is caused by the degradation of blood as it passes through the small bowel and colon. Bleeding that originates from the small bowel or proximal colon can also present with melena. Importantly, a massive UGIB can manifest as hematochezia (bright red blood per rectum) since the rapid passage of blood through the GI tract does not have time to be degraded. Presentation with hematochezia accounts for approximately 10% of patients with NVUGIB and is more common in patients presenting with hemodynamic instability.[6,13]

INITIAL EVALUATION

The immediate priority in management is to secure the patient's airway, and tend to breathing and circulation.[14] The patient should be placed in a monitored setting, at which point large-bore venous access should be established. Resuscitation should be initiated for patients with NVUGIB prior to any other procedure, and should include stabilization of the blood pressure with appropriate infusion of sufficient fluid volumes.[15,16] In the intensive care unit (ICU), saline or Ringer acetate is preferred to hydroxyethyl starch (HES), as HES has been shown to increase the need for renal-replacement therapy in ICU patients, and may increase severe bleeding.[17]

The primary objectives of resuscitation are to restore blood volume and to maintain adequate tissue perfusion, in the hope of preventing hypovolemic shock and ultimately death. No data suggest that any particular type of colloid solution is safer or more effective in patients needing volume replacement.[18] Certain patients will require resuscitation with blood products including red blood cells, platelets, and, rarely, clotting factors (e.g., fresh frozen plasma).

LABORATORY DATA

Certain laboratory tests are required at initial presentation to guide resuscitation and to risk-stratify patients based on established scoring systems.[19] Initial blood work should include: hemoglobin level, platelet count, blood urea nitrogen, creatinine, prothrombin time, and partial thromboplastin time.[20] A type and screen or cross-match is indicated if transfusion is being considered. Other investigations including liver enzymes and liver function testing, cardiac enzyme testing, and an electrocardiogram are often performed to exclude potential confounding diagnoses or complicating conditions. Additional investigations can be guided by individual patient characteristics noted on history or physical examination.

ROLE OF NASOGASTRIC ASPIRATE

The routine placement of a nasogastric tube (NGT) in patients presenting with NVUGIB remains controversial and is not recommended by current guidelines.[2,12] One 2013 retrospective study of 166 patients was able to predict active bleeding at endoscopy by combining NGT aspirate results with blood pressure and heart rate parameters.[21] Opinions vary as high-quality evidence is lacking to decide whether certain patients benefit from NGT aspiration and lavage to help aid in both diagnosing UGIB, as well as improving visualization during endoscopy.[22–25] Studies have failed to show any improvement in clinical outcomes attributable to the insertion of an NGT.[26–29] One study identified 520 patients with UGIB who had a documented nasogastric aspirate prior to endoscopy and found that a bloody aspirate was associated with high-risk lesions (odds ratio [OR] 4.82) although the negative predictive value was only 77.9%.[22] Importantly, a clear nasogastric aspirate reduced the likelihood to 0.15. There are, however, certain patients in whom the source of GI bleeding is unclear and who may benefit from placement of an NGT to confirm an upper GI source.[30] Current guidelines do not suggest routine use of NGT placement prior to endoscopy.[11]

RISK STRATIFICATION

Several scoring systems have been created to risk-stratify patients presenting with NVUGIB.[31–33] Patients who are deemed high-risk may benefit from earlier and more aggressive treatments, including admission to the ICU and more rapid endoscopic evaluation.[34–36] Moreover, low-risk patients may be appropriate for outpatient management, which could be safe and more cost-effective.[37–40] Each scoring system has strengths and limitations that we will briefly outline hereafter. For detailed descriptions of the components of the most studied scores, see Table 14.1.

The Rockall score has been shown to accurately predict rebleeding and mortality rates for patients presenting with NVUGIB.[41,42] This scoring system incorporates clinical and endoscopic information to provide a total score for each patient. Multiple studies have validated the Rockall score and suggest that patients with a low score have a lower likelihood of rebleeding and mortality.[43–45] Specifically, a score of less than 3 predicts a rebleeding rate of approximately 5% and a mortality rate of 0%. The major limitation of the Rockall score is that endoscopy must be performed to calculate the total score, thus limiting its usefulness in preendoscopic risk stratification.

The Glasgow-Blatchford score (GBS) uses clinical data on presentation to determine whether a patient with NVUGIB will require a blood transfusion, endoscopic intervention, or surgery.[46] Several prospective studies have evaluated whether certain patients with low GBS scores can be discharged safely from the emergency department without immediate endoscopic evaluation.[37,47,48] One prospective, multicenter study found that patients presenting to the emergency department with a GBS score of 0 could be safely managed as outpatients because none of these patients returned to their index hospital with recurrent UGIB or death within 6 months.[45] More recently (2012), a metaanalysis found that a GBS score of 2 or more was 98% sensitive at identifying patients who require urgent evaluation.[49]

The AIMS65 score represents one of the most recently developed tools for risk-stratifying patients and may be superior to previous scoring systems with regards to predicting inpatient mortality.[50] Using only 5 clinical variables available at presentation,

TABLE 14.1 Components of the AIMS65, Glasgow-Blatchford, and Rockall Scores

AIMS65		GLASGOW-BLATCHFORD		ROCKALL	
Variable	**Score**	**Variable**	**Score**	**Variable**	**Score**
Albumin < 3.0 g/dL	1	**Blood urea nitrogen (mg/dL)**		**Age**	
INR > 1.5	1	≥ 6.5 to < 8.0	2	< 60	0
Altered **M**ental Status	1	≥ 8.0 to < 10.0	3	60 to 79	1
SBP ≤ 90 mm Hg	1	≥ 10.0 to < 25	4	> 80	2
Age > **65**	1	≥ 25	6		
				Shock	
		Hemoglobin (g/dL): Men		No shock	0
		≥ 12.0 to < 13.0	1	Heart rate > 100	1
		≥ 10.0 to < 12.0	3	HR > 100, SBP < 100	2
		<10.0	6		
				Comorbidity	
		Hemoglobin (g/dL): Women		Heart failure or IHD	2
		≥ 10.0 to < 12.0	1	Renal or liver failure or	3
		<10.0	6	Metastatic cancer	
		Systolic BP (mm Hg)		**Endoscopic Diagnosis**	
		100 to 109	1	No lesion or MWT	0
		90 to 99	2	All other diagnoses	1
		< 90	3	Malignancy	2
		Other Variables		**High-Risk Stigmata**	
		Heart rate >100	1	None or dark spot	0
		Melena at presentation	1	Active bleeding or clot or visible vessel	2
		Syncope	2		
		Hepatic disease	2		
		Heart failure	2		
Maximum Score	5	**Maximum Score**	23	**Maximum Score**	11

HR, heart rate; *INR,* international normalized ratio; *MWT,* Mallory-Weiss tear; *SBP,* systolic blood pressure; *IHD,* ischemic heart disease.
Data from Saltzman JR, Tabak YP, Hyett BH, et al: A simple risk score accurately predicts in-hospital mortality, length of stay, and cost in acute upper GI bleeding. *Gastrointest Endosc* 74(6):1215–1224, 2011.

it is more accurate at predicting mortality than the GBS score.[51] The AIMS65 score, however, was less accurate at predicting the need for blood transfusion than GBS score, and similar in predicting in-hospital rebleeding.[52]

Limitations of all three scores include disparate comparative study results, variations in performance based on study populations and (surprisingly) geographic regions, and the absence of true interventional trials assessing patient outcomes following the introduction of a score early on in patient management.[53,54]

RED BLOOD CELL TRANSFUSION

The decision whether to transfuse red blood cells is based on the presenting hemoglobin level, hemodynamic status, patient comorbidities such as cardiac disease, and symptoms of anemia. A large Cochrane review put into question the usefulness of red blood cell transfusions in UGIB, demonstrating no overall survival benefit.[55]

A 2013 single-center RCT of 921 patients with acute UGIB found a restrictive transfusion strategy (transfusion threshold < 7 g/dL with target hemoglobin of 7–9 g/dL) significantly decreased 6-week mortality, length of stay, and transfusion-related adverse events compared with a liberal transfusion strategy (transfusion threshold < 9 g/dL with target hemoglobin of 9–11 g/dL).[56] The overall mortality benefit conferred by the restrictive transfusion strategy appears to have been driven by results obtained in patients with Child-Pugh class A and B cirrhosis. The subgroup of patients with NVUGIB did not exhibit a significant decrease in their overall mortality with a restrictive

transfusion policy, although there was a trend towards benefit with no suggestion of harm. Importantly, this study excluded all patients presenting with severe hemorrhagic shock, acute coronary syndrome, symptomatic peripheral vasculopathy, stroke, or transient ischemic attack in keeping with consensus guidelines, suggesting higher hemoglobin targets for some of these patients.

Current guidelines suggest that patients with hemoglobin levels of 7 g/dL or less should receive blood transfusions to reach a target hemoglobin level of 7–9 g/dL, provided that the individual has no coronary artery disease, evidence of tissue hypoperfusion or acute hemorrhage.[2] In patients with acute coronary syndrome, UGIB is associated with a markedly increased mortality, and a higher hemoglobin target level, above 10 g/dL, may be required.[2,57,58]

As part of a recent UK audit, despite 73% of patients with UGIB presenting with a hemoglobin level greater than 8 g/dL, approximately 43% received red blood cell transfusions.[59] A recently published metaanalysis (2014) not restricted to NVUGIB suggests that a restrictive transfusion approach reduces health care associated infections.[60] Additional randomized trials are needed to address the issue of hemoglobin transfusion thresholds in patients with NVUGIB, including patients with significant cardiac disease. One large multicenter randomized trial is currently being completed in the United Kingdom, which may help answer such uncertainties.[61]

Platelet Transfusion

A 2012 systematic review of 18 studies examining platelet transfusion thresholds in patients with NVUGIB found insufficient evidence supporting an optimal platelet count.[62] However, based primarily on expert opinion, the authors proposed a platelet transfusion threshold of 50×10^9/L (or 100×10^9/L if altered platelet function is suspected). Additional high-quality data are needed to confirm these recommendations.

REVERSAL OF ANTICOAGULATION

Many patients who present with NVUGIB will be on anticoagulation for a variety of reasons, most commonly due to atrial fibrillation. Of these patients, many are on warfarin, which can be monitored using the international normalized ratio (INR). Several retrospective studies have shown no difference in rebleeding, mortality, length of stay, or transfusion requirements between patients with an INR between 1.3 and 2.7.[63] One cohort study compared patients with UGIB not on anticoagulation to patients on warfarin that had their INR corrected to 2.5 or under using fresh frozen plasma.[64] They found no differences in rebleeding, surgery, mortality, or complication rates between the two groups. As such, upper endoscopy (EGD) in patients with therapeutic INR levels on warfarin appears to be safe to allow for early endoscopy. Current guidelines suggest that endoscopy should not be delayed to correct anticoagulation in patients on warfarin who have a therapeutic INR.[2] For patients with an INR above 3, rapid reversal can be considered with either prothrombin complex concentrate or fresh frozen plasma in addition to vitamin K.[65]

Several new direct-acting oral anticoagulants are commonly prescribed to patients given their higher efficacy at preventing stroke and systemic thromboembolism in patients with atrial fibrillation.[66] These direct-acting anticoagulants now account for approximately 62% of all prescriptions for nonvalvular atrial fibrillation within the United States.[67] Some of these drugs may increase GI bleeding when compared to warfarin.[68,69] One major concern with these direct-acting oral anticoagulants is that there is no reliable way to monitor their efficacy on routine blood work.[70] Furthermore, only dabigatran (Pradaxa) currently has an approved reversal agent, known as idarucizumab (Praxbind), whereas reversal for the other agents await commercialization in most countries.[71] At this time, there are no clear guidelines as to the precise management of NVUGIB patients taking these newer anticoagulants.[72] There have been some reports of clotting factors such as fresh frozen plasma, activated factor VII, or prothrombin complex concentrate being used for partial reversal of anticoagulation.[73] Experts have suggested that early consultation with a hematologist and/or cardiologist should be considered in all patients with suspected GI bleeding on any of the direct acting oral anticoagulants.[74]

TIMING OF ENDOSCOPY

The timing of endoscopic evaluation depends on patient factors (hemodynamic stability, airway protection) and hospital factors (monitored setting, availability of endoscopic expertise, dedicated nurses and equipment). Several studies have confirmed that emergency endoscopy (within 6–12 hours) for UGIB has no advantage in terms of rebleeding, surgical rates, or mortality when compared to routine endoscopy within 24 hours.[75,76] In one large retrospective study of 934 patients, Lim et al (2011) found that early endoscopy (defined as endoscopy within 13 hours of presentation) was associated with a lower mortality rate for high-risk patients with GBS scores of 12or higher.[77] Interestingly, there was no difference in rebleeding rate, transfusion requirements, or surgery. Moreover, for low-risk patients with GBS scores less than 12 there were no differences in any outcomes when comparing early endoscopy to endoscopy within 24 hours of presentation. There is ongoing controversy as to the existence of a "weekend effect" whereby mortality from UGIB may be higher after regular working hours compared with patients treated at other times. Some authors postulate this effect may be due to a patient selection bias (sickest presenting at any time, including after hours) or decreased resources including delays to endoscopy and other treatments.[78–81]

Current guidelines suggest that endoscopy should be performed within 24 hours in all patients presenting with UGIB who are admitted to hospital because this practice has been shown to decrease length of stay, rebleeding rates, and need for surgery.[2] Some experts believe that, based on the limited evidence, endoscopy should be considered within 12 hours in selected high-risk patients.[12,82]

Prokinetics

The use of prokinetic agents (such as erythromycin) before GI endoscopy has been shown to significantly shorten the duration of endoscopy, reduce the need for repeat endoscopy, and decrease the need for blood transfusions.[83–87] In a large, multicenter RCT involving 253 patients presenting with either melena of hematemesis, erythromycin alone was equally efficacious at improving endoscopic visualization as NGT aspirate alone or in combination with erythromycin.[29] One metaanalysis which included 313 patients found that either intravenous erythromycin or metoclopramide immediately before EGD in patients with UGIB decreased the need for repeat endoscopy, but did not improve other clinically relevant measurable outcomes.[85]

More recently, another small-sized, low-quality randomized trial (2013) compared NGT aspirate alone versus NGT aspirate with erythromycin and found the combination provided superior visualization, reduced hospital admissions, and decreased blood transfusions.[83] No data suggest that the administration of prokinetic agents can decrease mortality, the risk of rebleeding, or the need for surgery.[84–86,88] Nonetheless, given improved visibility at endoscopy and other potential benefits discussed previously, especially in light of the favorable benefit-harm profile of erythromycin, current guidelines suggest that after ruling out contraindications to these agents (such as hypokalemia or a prolonged QT interval) a 250 mg bolus of erythromycin should be administered approximately 30 to 45 minutes prior to endoscopy. This recommendation is for patients with clinical evidence of active hemorrhage (hematemesis or melena) or acute anemia requiring resuscitation, or in those who have recently eaten, but should not be used routinely in all patients presenting with UGIB.[2,29]

Preendoscopic Proton Pump Inhibitors

Despite theoretical pharmacological differences between the different proton pump inhibitors (PPIs), no data support the use of a particular intravenous PPI over another when treating patients with UGIB. In the rest of this chapter, PPI will be used as a generic term for all such agents.

Starting PPI treatment before endoscopy for UGIB remains a controversial practice. A metaanalysis that included 2,223 participants from six randomized, clinical trials found that preendoscopic PPI treatment reduces the proportion of patients identified as having high-risk lesions (active bleeding, non-bleeding visible vessel, and adherent clot) thus reducing the need

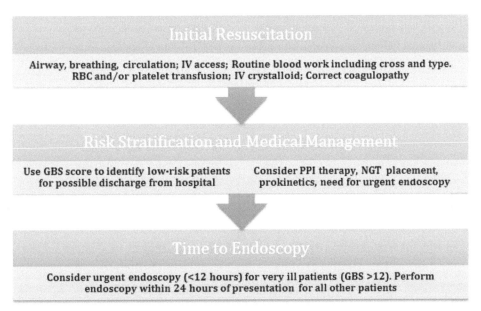

FIG 14.1 Steps for Initial Management of Upper Gastrointestinal Bleeding. *GBS,* Glasgow-Blatchford score; *IV,* intravenous; *NGT,* nasogastric tube; *PPI,* proton pump inhibitor; *RBC,* red blood cell.

for endoscopic therapy (i.e., down-staging of high-risk endoscopic lesions).[89] Despite these advantages, there is no evidence that preendoscopic PPI treatment affects mortality, risk of rebleeding, or need for surgery. For this reason, current guidelines recommend initiating PPI therapy on presentation to hospital, although it should never delay optimal resuscitation.[2] PPI therapy pre-endoscopy is especially cost-effective in certain scenarios: when endoscopy is delayed for more than 16 hours after admission, or if patients have a high likelihood of nonvariceal bleeding, especially in those with high-risk symptoms, such as hematemesis.[90,91] Current guidelines advise against the use of histamine-2 receptor antagonists in acute ulcer bleeding.[2]

No recommendations can be made regarding the optimal dose or optimal route of administration of PPIs administered preendoscopy. A reasonable strategy may be to adopt a high-dose intravenous bolus (e.g., 80 mg) followed by a continuous infusion (e.g., 8 mg/hour) regimen.[92] This infusion can be continued until endoscopy, at which point reassessment is required depending on the appearance of the bleeding lesion and the need for therapeutic intervention (see section on postendoscopic PPI therapy). A recent budget impact analysis assessing PPI institutional costs both pre- and postendoscopy suggest minimal incremental costs when opting for high-dose PPI infusion[93] (Fig. 14.1).

ETIOLOGY OF NONVARICEAL UPPER GASTROINTESTINAL BLEEDING

The most common causes of NVUGIB include: gastroduodenal ulcers, angiodysplastic lesions, Dieulafoy lesions, Mallory-Weiss tears (MWT), malignancy, esophagitis, and erosive gastritis among other causes.[94–96] Endoscopy allows for both the diagnosis and treatment of these lesions. The relative frequency of the causes of UGIB from a recent audit of 5004 patients presenting with UGIB can be seen in Table 14.2.[97]

TABLE 14.2   Frequency of Endoscopic Diagnoses for Patients Presenting With Upper Gastrointestinal Bleeding

Endoscopic Diagnosis	Frequency
Peptic ulcer disease	36%
Esophagitis	24%
Gastritis or gastric erosions	22%
Erosive duodenitis	13%
Esophageal or gastric varices	11%
Portal hypertensive gastropathy	5.5%
Mallory-Weiss tear	4.3%
Upper GI malignancy	3.7%
Angiodysplasia or vascular lesion	2.7%

Summary of Findings	Frequency
One diagnosis found	50%
Two or more diagnoses found	31%
No abnormality seen	19%

Modified from Hearnshaw SA, Logan RF, Lowe D, et al: Use of endoscopy for management of acute upper gastrointestinal bleeding in the UK: results of a nationwide audit. *Gut* 59(8):1022–1029, 2010.

Indications for Endoscopic Therapy for Gastroduodenal Ulcers

The role of endoscopic therapy for the management of gastroduodenal ulcers is based on the Forrest classification, which categorizes ulcer into high and low risk in terms of rebleeding risk (Table 14.3).[98–101] Several studies have since validated the Forrest classification in terms of predicting risk of rebleeding and the need for endoscopic intervention.[100,101] Overall, endoscopic

TABLE 14.3   Risk of Rebleeding Peptic Ulcer Disease Despite Medical Management Alone Based on Forrest Classification on Initial Endoscopic Evaluation

Endoscopic Stigmata (Forrest)	Frequency	Rebleeding on Medical Management
Spurting vessel (IA)	10%	90%
Oozing vessel (IB)	10%	10–20%
Nonbleeding visible vessel (IIA)	25%	50%
Adherent clot (IIB)	10%	25–30%
Flat pigmented ulcer base (IIC)	10%	7–10%
Clean-based ulcer (III)	35%	3–5%

TABLE 14.4   Forrest Classification for Endoscopic Appearance of Gastroduodenal Ulcers

Forrest Classification	Endoscopic Appearance	Endoscopic Therapy
IA	Spurting vessel	Therapy required
IB	Oozing vessel	Therapy required
IIA	Nonbleeding visible vessel	Therapy required
IIB	Adherent clot	Consider therapy
IIC	Flat pigmented ulcer base	No therapy required
III	Clean-based ulcer	No therapy required

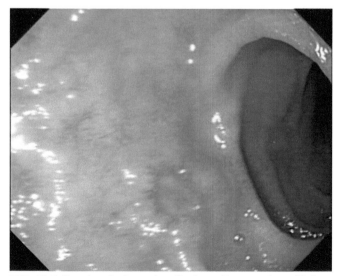

FIG 14.2 Duodenal ulcer classified as Forrest class III (i.e., clean-based).

therapy is required for patients with ulcers classified as IA, IB, or IIA, and is controversial for patients with an adherent clot (see section titled Nonbleeding Adherent Clot).[102–104] For ulcers with IIC and III classification (Fig. 14.2), endoscopic therapy is not warranted, as rebleeding risks are low (Table 14.4; Fig. 14.3).[98]

Nonbleeding Adherent Clot

The endoscopic management of an adherent clot overlying an ulcer base remains controversial in the literature (Fig. 14.4). Consideration must be given to endoscopic removal of the clot and treatment of the underlying lesion if it satisfies criteria for high-risk stigmata (e.g., Forrest classification IA, IB, or IIA). Vigorous irrigation of the clot using a water pump has been shown to expose the underlying stigmata in 26%–43% of cases, of which 70% were high risk stigmata requiring endoscopic therapy.[105,106] The rebleeding risk for clots that remain despite irrigation has been estimated between 0%–35% in several studies.[104,105,107,108] One metaanalysis of 6 RCTs comprising 240 patients with adherent clots found that although endoscopic therapy was associated with a lower rebleeding risk than medical therapy alone (8.2% vs. 24.7%, $p = 0.01$), other endpoints, including length of hospital stay (6.8 vs. 5.6 days; $p = 0.27$), transfusion requirements (3.0 vs. 2.8 units; $p = 0.75$), and mortality (9.8% vs. 7%, $p = 0.54$), were no different between the two groups.[103] This metaanalysis did have several limitations including the vastly different patient populations, and statistical tests used to assess the impact of heterogeneity.[109]

Endoscopic therapy for adherent clots consists of preinjection with epinephrine followed by removing the adherent clot using a cold snare. Once the clot is removed, combination therapy can be applied to the underlying stigmata as indicated.[104,108] One 2015 observational study suggested that endoscopic therapy was preferred over conservative therapy alone for adherent clots in terms of mortality but did not demonstrate lower rebleeding rates.[102] Future multicenter randomized controlled studies are required to better identify patients who may benefit from endoscopic intervention compared to PPI therapy alone.

MODALITIES FOR ENDOSCOPIC THERAPY

The most commonly used endoscopic techniques for management of a bleeding ulcer include: injection therapy, thermal coaptive therapy, endoscopic clipping, and hemostatic powders.[110] Each method has its strengths and weaknesses and often more than one technique can be used for a given case.[111] Each modality will be discussed separately, including the role of combination therapy.

Injection Therapy

Epinephrine is the most established injection agent used for peptic ulcer injection therapy, although studies have been done using normal saline along with a sclerosant agent.[112] The mechanism of action is thought to be local tamponade and vasoconstriction (Fig. 14.5). Epinephrine diluted to 1 : 10,000 in normal saline is found to be most effective and safest. A large RCT of 165 patients with actively bleeding ulcers or visible vessels was performed to determine the ideal amount of epinephrine injection (1 : 10,000). This RCT, which was largely representative of the existing literature, found that large volume injection (13–20 mL) compared to small volume injection (5–10 mL) was associated with less rebleeding (15.4% vs. 30.8%, $p = 0.037$).[113] A large metaanalysis of 1673 patients revealed that epinephrine injection alone is inferior to either clips or thermal therapy.[114] An additional metaanalysis confirmed these findings.[115] One of the roles of epinephrine injection is to temporize and control bleeding to achieve better visualization and so apply more definitive therapy (e.g., thermal therapy or clipping) to the lesion. Overall, injection

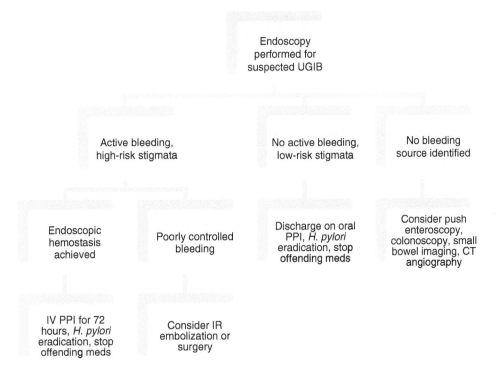

FIG 14.3 Approach to Endoscopic Management of Upper Gastrointestinal Bleeding (UGIB). *CT*, computed tomography; *IR*, interventional radiology; *IV*, intravenous; *PPI*, proton pump inhibitor.

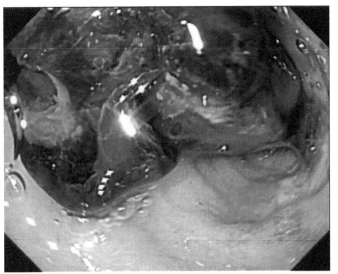

FIG 14.4 Duodenal ulcer with adherent clot.

therapy is a useful technique to incorporate into the management of ulcer bleeding but should not be used as monotherapy.

Technique for Injection

A disposable injection needle with a retractable tip is used. The most commonly used needles are the 23- or 25-gauge needles, with a needle length of approximately 3 to 5 mm.[116] Injection is undertaken in 0.5- to 2.0-mL increments in all four quadrants around the target lesion because the path of the underlying artery is often unknown.[117] Randomized studies found that a total volume of 20 to 45 mL may be injected to achieve the desired results, although the studies were performed using

monotherapy.[113,118] In the setting of active bleeding, if the initial injection results in noticeable slowing and, more so, cessation of bleeding, a single injection site may suffice. Additional volume may be injected via a single site as long as any lifting effect does not impair access to the bleeding vessel for second-line therapy with coaptive coagulation or hemoclips.

Thermal Coaptive Therapy

The most widely used modalities to provide contact thermal therapy include the bipolar probes (delivers electrical current) and the heater probe (aluminum garnet that provides heat). The advantages of these devices are their excellent efficacy, safety, portability, cost, and for some, the ability to combine irrigation, and coagulation.[119-122] The probes are used to place manual compression over the lesion to tamponade the bleeding vessel and obliterate the lumen of the offending arteriole in the base of the bleeding lesion through so-called coaptive electrocoagulation (Fig. 14.6). Regardless of the probe being used, the endpoint for successful hemostasis for contact thermal hemostasis, especially when treating large arteries, is firm pressure on the bleeding lesion until a "footprint" is obtained.[116]

Coagulation can be achieved by using either the tip or side of the probe depending on the location, but *en-face* treatment is favored. Specific details about the two most commonly used probes are given in the following sections. Other forms of thermal therapy have recently been assessed, such as using soft coagulation delivered with hemostatic forceps, as is done for endoscopic mucosal resection and endoscopic submucosal dissection. Comparative trials amongst treatment modalities are few, but a recent RCT compared the effectiveness of soft coagulation using hemostatic forceps with a heater probe in 111 patients presenting with ulcer bleeding. Overall, patients randomized to hemostatic forceps had lower rebleeding rates, fewer perforations, and fewer surgeries.[123]

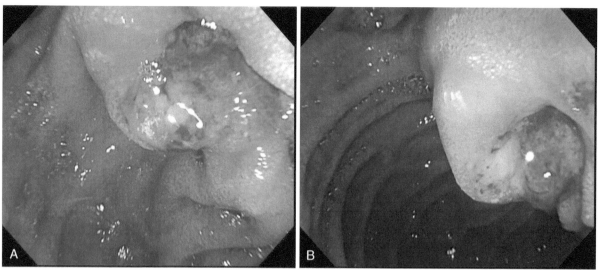

FIG 14.5 A, Duodenal ulcer with visible vessel injected with epinephrine causing vasoconstriction evidenced by **B,** blanching of the mucosa.

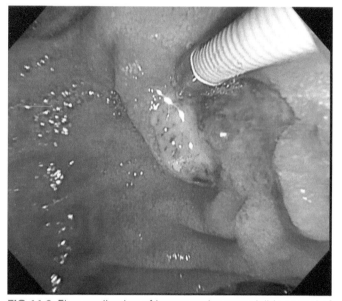

FIG 14.6 Firm application of heater probe onto visible vessel of duodenal ulcer to obtain a "footprint."

In one metaanalysis, the use of thermal coaptive therapy for patients with high-risk lesions was shown to reduce rebleeding (OR 0.44), need for surgery (OR 0.39), and mortality rates (OR 0.58) when compared with no endoscopic treatment.[115] In a separate metaanalysis the impact on mortality was not reproduced (OR 0.64).[124] Although pooled metaanalytical data comparing thermal monotherapy with the combination of injection and thermal therapy did not reveal any significant differences in rebleeding, subgroup analysis favored combination therapy after two less generalizable trials were removed, resulting in decreased risks of rebleeding (OR 0.37).[124]

Bipolar Probe Technique

The technique for applying bipolar electrocoagulating energy has not been standardized and varies among reported clinical trials. One expert recommends forcefully applying a large (3.2-mm) bipolar circumactive probe (BICAP) on a power setting of 3 to 5 for a prolonged duration, such as 14 seconds, or seven pulses of 2 seconds each.[125] Another expert used a setting of 3 or 4 with 10-second pulses on a BICAP II generator.[126]

Heater Probe Technique

The present technique for bleeding peptic ulcers involves using the larger heater probe and placing firm tamponade directly on the bleeding point or visible vessel, and coagulation with at least 120 J (four pulses of 30 J each) before moving the probe.[127,128] An additional application of energy when using the heater probe or bipolar probes as the probe is removed from the treatment site can reduce unwanted tissue adhesion and the inadvertent tearing of the coagulated sealant with resultant rebleeding.[129,130]

Argon Plasma Coagulator

Argon plasma coagulation (APC) is a noncontact method that allows for controlled electrocoagulation via high-frequency monopolar energy to be delivered to the tissue through an ionized gas (argon plasma). In a large retrospective study of 194 patients presenting with a visible vessel overlying an ulcer, APC was equally effective as hemoclips in controlling bleeding in terms of rebleeding rate, need for transfusion, and mortality.[131] In a prospective trial of 41 patients, Cipolletta et al (1998) compared APC with heater probe therapy; rates of initial hemostasis, recurrent bleeding, emergency surgery, and 30-day mortality were comparable in both groups.[132] Chau et al (2003) reported similar results in a large (185 cases) randomized trial comparing epinephrine plus heater probe with epinephrine plus APC.[133]

APC has proven to be an effective therapy for managing angiodysplastic lesions as evidenced by a reduction in need for transfusion and surgery.[134] Importantly, however, recurrence of these lesions, in spite of any therapy, is evident in approximately one-third of patients. One 2016 cohort study of 53 patients found that APC treatment as opposed to no endoscopic treatment did not improve 30-day rebleeding rates or mortality rates in patients presenting with UGIB secondary to a malignancy.[135] Overall, APC appears to be an effective, safe, and relatively low cost alternative that can be used for many different causes of UGIB including peptic ulcers, angiodysplastic lesions (including

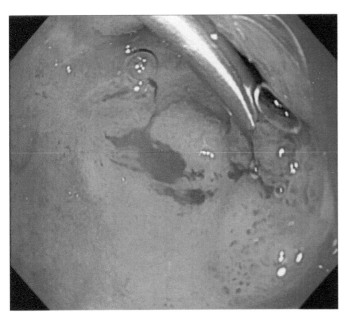

FIG 14.7 Duodenal ulcer treated with endoscopic clip.

gastric antral vascular ectasia), and perhaps malignancy related bleeding.[136–138]

Endoscopic Clipping

The underlying mechanism of clips is the mechanical ligation of the bleeding vessel (Fig. 14.7). Most studies have been performed on first-generation clips. Clips are easier to apply with the scope in the straight position. An example of an endoscopic clip being applied to an actively bleeding peptic ulcer can be seen in Video 14.1. Tangential access makes application a challenge because of the simple mechanics allowing the clip to be extruded from the catheter, opened, and finally closed.[139] Other regions shown to be difficult to clip include the posterior wall of the antrum and the superior duodenal recess.[140] The advantages of using clips include that no additional equipment is required, there is no thermal injury or special setup, and they are easily applied. The one drawback is the cost associated with disposable clips and that some clips may not deploy properly and must then be discarded. The proposed method of deploying the clip is to visualize the ulcer or visible vessel and to capture the lesion within the clip. When applying the clip, it should be maximally opened and gentle pressure applied with the clip over the lesion. Using suction to help approximate the edges helps capture tissue and then the clip is deployed. Sometimes additional clips are required to adequately achieve hemostasis.

One metaanalysis of 4261 patients found that any form of endoscopic treatment was superior to pharmacotherapy alone.[124] Optimal endoscopic therapies include thermal therapy or clips, either alone or in combination with other methods. Interestingly, injection followed by thermal therapy did not decrease rebleeding compared with clips (OR 0.82) or thermal therapy alone (OR 0.79) Overall, clips were superior to thermal therapy (OR 0.24) but, when followed by injection, were not superior to clips alone (OR 1.30).

Several RCTs investigating the use of endoscopic clips alone or in combination with other endoscopic modalities have reported variable success. The most important factor seems to be the location of the lesion, such as high on the lesser curvature and posterior duodenal wall, which are challenging locations for clip deployment.[141] Improvements in endoscopic clip devices have included single-use, rotatable, and reopening features.[142] Lastly, in certain cases endoscopic therapy may be unsuccessful at controlling acute bleeding; for these situations, placing clips near the site of the bleeding can help interventional radiologists localize the site for embolization.[143]

Combination Therapy

There is a theoretical advantage of combining therapies because hemostasis is achieved by different mechanisms. Combination therapy with injection and coaptive therapy has consistently shown superiority over medical therapy.[144] In a prospective study by Bianco et al (2004), combined therapy with epinephrine injection with bipolar probe showed better results than epinephrine alone.[145] Most of the RCTs looking at combination therapy with clips and injection therapy utilize clips prior to injection to avoid possible displacement of the clip as the tissue edema resorbs.

Calvet et al (2004) performed a metaanalysis of trials comparing epinephrine injection alone with epinephrine plus a second method (thermal, mechanical, sclerosant) for patients with UGIB.[114] The analysis included 16 studies of 1673 patients who had high-risk stigmata of bleeding defined by Forrest criteria IA, IIA, and IIB. Addition of a second endoscopic method reduced rate of rebleeding (18.4% vs. 10.6%), need for surgery (11.3% vs. 7.6%), and mortality (5.1% vs. 2.6%) compared with epinephrine injection alone. Risk of further bleeding decreased regardless of the type of second method used. Risk of significant complications, including massive bleeding, gastric wall necrosis, and perforation, was the same in both groups (1.1%).

A recent Cochrane review metaanalysis from 2014 compared combination therapy versus monotherapy with epinephrine injection alone in patients with high-risk peptic ulcer bleeding. This review included 2033 patients and found that combination therapy (i.e., epinephrine injection with either injection of another substance, coaptive therapy, or mechanical clipping) was more effective than monotherapy with epinephrine injection alone. Specifically, combination therapy had a significantly lower risk of rebleeding (relative risk [RR] 0.53), the need for surgery (RR 0.68), and mortality (RR 0.50). Overall, combination therapy was associated with a reduced risk of rebleeding (RR 0.57), a reduced need for emergency surgery (RR 0.68) and a lower mortality (RR 0.50).[146] Sub-analysis was unable to determine which combination therapy was most effective.

Hemostatic Powders

Various hemostatic powders are a new and emerging modality being used for the management of patients with UGIB. The advantage of these powders is their noncontact and nontraumatic application whereby a bleeding lesion is sprayed with the powder. This treatment modality also allows for treatment of large surface areas and does not require the same precision as other interventions like coaptive therapy or clipping. Some powders require direct application to an actively bleeding lesion.[147,148] Available products for endoscopic application include Tc-325 (Hemospray, Cook Medical, Bloomington, IN), Endoclot TM (EndoClot Plus, Inc., Santa Clara, CA), and Ankaferd (Ankaferd Health Products Ltd., Turkey). Data and availability of some of these products are limited and thus we will concentrate on the discussion on Tc-325 (Hemospray). For a more complete description of other available powders, readers can refer to a 2015 review article.[149]

Systematic reviews of case series suggest Tc-325 is extremely effective in achieving immediate hemostasis.[149] Additional roles may exist for Tc-325 as rescue therapy, arresting bleeding for transfer to a site with more expertise in endoscopic hemostasis and malignant bleeding. There has only been one reported RCT to date (in patients exhibiting high-risk ulcer lesions) suggesting worsened efficacy if used in peptic ulcer disease bleeding owing to the limited 12–24-hour residency time of the powder that is exceeded by the 72-hour delayed rebleeding period following endoscopic hemostasis.[147–149]

The largest multicenter study to date included 63 patients with NVUGIB of which 55 (87%) patients had Tc-325 used as initial monotherapy to control bleeding.[150] Hemospray was effective as monotherapy at controlling bleeding in 85% (47/55) of patients and the rebleeding rate was 15% at 1-week. Of the 8 patients who were managed with traditional endoscopic therapy at initial presentation, Tc-325 effectively managed all episodes of rebleeding and prevented the need for interventional radiology or surgery. Several additional studies, including one metaanalysis, have shown similar results in terms of initial management and recurrent bleeding with the use of Tc-325, including use in patients with thrombocytopenia and those on anticoagulation.[151–154]

Other indications that seem to have derived benefit from the use of hemostatic powders include anastomotic ulcer bleeding, ischemic colitis, and postpolypectomy bleeding.[155–157] Importantly, Tc-325 is a temporary treatment and is not recommended as monotherapy for lesions with a high risk of rebleeding such as peptic ulcers with high-risk stigmata.[152] Tc-325 may still be used is these situations, but only in combination with more definitive ulcer therapy as discussed previously.[151] Future studies will delineate the precise use of Tc-325 in various patients and compare its use to traditional endoscopic therapies. Given its ease of use and apparent safety, Tc-325 appears to be at the very least a cost-effective option for temporizing bleeding while more definitive therapeutic options are being considered.[158]

POSTENDOSCOPIC PROTON PUMP INHIBITORS

The goal of PPI therapy is to raise the gastric pH sufficiently to promote clot stability and to reduce the effect of pepsin and gastric acid.[159] In a study that aimed to identify the lowest effective dose of PPI, rather than using a high (or low) dose, continuous infusion was the key to maintain an intragastric pH above 6.[160] Two metaanalyses have confirmed that an intravenous PPI bolus followed by continuous PPI infusion over 72 hours reduces the rates of mortality (RR = 0.40, 0.28–0.59; number needed to treat [NNT] = 12), rebleeding (RR = 0.40, 0.28–0.59; NNT = 12), and surgery (RR = 0.43, 0.24–0.76; NNT = 28). Mortality was only reduced in patients who had previously undergone successful endoscopic hemostasis.[115,161] Cost-effectiveness analyses have demonstrated the economic dominance of high-dose intravenous PPI over no treatment strategies, principally due to the high incremental cost of an additional hospitalization for rebleeding in light of the modest NNT.[162]

More recently, a systematic review and metaanalysis (2014) compared intermittent versus continuous PPI therapy for the treatment of high-risk bleeding ulcers after endoscopic therapy.[163] This study revealed that intermittent PPI therapy may be as effective as continuous infusion high-dose therapy in these high-risk patients, which may have benefits in terms of cost-savings, and the authors firmly conclude that guidelines should be revised to recommend intermittent PPI therapy. Current guidelines remain ambivalent towards optimal postendoscopy PPI dosing due to an overall lower quality of evidence secondary to a high risk of bias and imprecision in the aforementioned systematic review.[12]

High-dose oral PPI treatment after endoscopy was efficacious in early trials conducted in India and Iran, but differences in the physiological and pharmacokinetic characteristics of the patients, as well as local high *Helicobacter pylori* carriage rate and limited comorbidities make the results of these studies difficult to apply to other populations. The endoscopic treatment administered was also not the current recommended standard.[164] A further study published in 2009 assessed gastric pH in patients receiving a 90-mg oral dose of lansoprazole followed by 30 mg every 3 hours (total dose 300 mg in 24 hours) after successful endoscopic treatment for peptic ulcer bleeding.[165] The primary endpoint was the proportion of the 24-hour period that the patients had a gastric pH greater than 6 (median 55%). However, large differences in this value were evident between individuals (range 6%–99%), and only 1 of 14 patients (7%) reached a pH above 6 in at least 80% of this time.[165] Accordingly, the evidence is insufficient to support the use of oral PPI therapy immediately after endoscopy in high-risk patients. Current recommendations are for oral PPI therapy in patients with lower-risk stigmata on endoscopy, such as a clean-based ulcer or a flat-pigmented spot.[166]

A recent RCT of 293 patients investigated the efficacy of double-dose oral PPI (esomeprazole 40 mg PO twice daily for 11 days, followed by once daily dosing for another 14 days) compared to single-dose oral PPI (esomeprazole 40 mg PO once daily for 25 days) after 3 days of intravenous PPI infusion for patients with high Rockall scores of 6 or higher at increased risk for rebleeding.[167] Cheng et al (2014) found less rebleeding rates with the twice-daily PPI regimen (10.8% vs. 28.7%, $p = 0.002$). We recommend routinely prescribing double-dose PPI for at least 14 days following intravenous PPI infusion in these high-risk patients and single dose thereafter.

The decision to continue oral PPI past 28 days must be judged on an individualized basis as there is insufficient evidence to guide practice and it is determined by the nature of the bleeding lesion. For example, longer courses of PPI therapy may be warranted for patients with bleeding erosive esophagitis compared to a patient with a duodenal ulcer.[2] The optimal duration of treatment with oral PPI is unknown and also depends on patient ongoing risk factors, and sometimes the severity of the presentation. For example, a patient treated for peptic ulcer disease related to either *H. pylori* or nonsteroidal antiinflammatory drug (NSAID) use, may only require a short course of PPI so long as the *H. pylori* is eradicated or the NSAID discontinued.[2,12] The benefits and risks of ongoing PPI therapy should be discussed with individual patients.[168]

SECOND-LOOK ENDOSCOPY

Prior to the widespread use of PPI therapy for peptic ulcer disease, several studies suggested that routine second-look endoscopy could be utilized for the purpose of preventing rebleeding.[169–172] More recently, Chiu et al (2016) randomized 305 patients with a high-risk peptic ulcer (either actively bleeding or a visible vessel) to either an intravenous PPI infusion or intravenous PPI bolus along with a second-look endoscopy within 24 hours after the initial endoscopy.[173] Based on the results of this RCT, there was no significant difference in rebleeding, transfusion requirements, need for surgery, or mortality between the two groups. A metaanalysis by El Ouali et al (2012) that included this trial in abstract form, suggested that the only compelling evidence for second look endoscopy is in patients with peptic ulcers exhibiting high-risk stigmata who did not undergo modern recommended endoscopic therapy or who were not provided PPI therapy.[169] Current guidelines do not recommend routine second-look endoscopy but rather only to be considered in patients who are at high risk for rebleeding.[2,11]

PREVENTION OF RECURRENT BLEEDING

To prevent recurrent bleeding, underlying risk factors for recurrent bleeding must be identified and addressed. Patients undergoing endoscopic therapy for high-risk stigmata should be kept *nil per os* (NPO) for 24 hours, and hospitalized for 72 hours to provide intravenous PPI therapy.[2] Risk factors for peptic ulcer disease recurrence include presence of *H. pylori*, NSAID use, and the need for prolonged antiplatelet medications and/or anticoagulants.[168,174] Each risk factor will be addressed separately (Fig. 14.8). If there is no identifiable cause of the peptic ulcer (e.g., *H. pylori* negative, no aspirin or NSAID use), guidelines suggest indefinite long-term PPI therapy because the incidence of recurrent ulcer bleeding in this population has been reported at 42%.[12,175,176]

NSAID Therapy

Any patient who develops peptic ulcer disease while on NSAID should be considered for either NSAID discontinuation or PPI prophylaxis.[177] If the NSAID can be discontinued, PPI therapy is only required for 4 to 8 weeks to allow for ulcer healing.[178] Often, however, NSAIDs must be continued either for either their pain management or antiinflammatory properties. Should NSAID treatment be necessary, guidelines recommend considering a COX-2-selective NSAID at the lowest possible dose along with daily PPI therapy.[2,12,179] Studies have shown a synergistic effect of *H. pylori* and NSAIDs with regard to UGIB so all patients who require ongoing NSAID therapy should be tested for *H. pylori* and treated as necessary.

Antiplatelet Therapy

The indication for antiplatelet therapy must be considered and weighed against the risk of ongoing or recurrent bleeding. For patients on aspirin for primary prevention, withholding the aspirin during acute bleeding and restarting it within 3–5 days is recommended by current guidelines based on RCT data suggesting increased overall mortality in the group in whom acetylsalicylic acid (ASA) was withheld for up to 2 months.[11,180,181] Certainly if there is no indication for aspirin therapy, then consultation with a cardiologist or neurologist may allow for discontinuation.

If aspirin is required for secondary prevention, long-term PPI therapy should be continued indefinitely to prevent rebleeding.[12,181,182] Pooled results of two RCTs[183,184] showed a significant reduction in rebleeding with ASA combined with PPI compared with clopidogrel alone (OR 0.06). There was no difference in cardiovascular events, cerebrovascular events, or mortality between the two groups.[2] *H. pylori* testing and eradication should be performed in all patients with peptic ulcer disease to reduce the risk of recurrent bleeding.[2]

Current guidelines suggest primary, let alone secondary PPI prophylaxis in all patients who are on dual antiplatelet therapy after coronary artery stenting because the risk of bleeding on dual antiplatelet therapy is significantly higher than being on aspirin alone.[185–187] Although there was controversy regarding the effect of PPI on the efficacy of clopidogrel, one 2016 RCT of 1970 patients showed no detrimental effect of PPI when added to dual antiplatelet therapy.[188] There are no high-quality studies that address the important question of withholding or resuming dual antiplatelet therapy during a UGIB; however, due to the high risk of stent thrombosis, most guidelines suggest continuing aspirin and withholding clopidogrel in severe bleeding and considering resuming as soon as bleeding is adequately controlled.[189] Certainly, the endoscopist must weigh the risk of stent thrombosis with the perceived risk of rebleeding and often consultation with cardiology is helpful (Fig. 14.9).

Restarting Anticoagulation

Many patients who present with UGIB are on anticoagulants on admission to hospital, and depending on the severity of bleeding, may have their anticoagulation interrupted during their hospitalization.[190] The ideal time to restart anticoagulation once the bleeding source has been controlled is unknown.[72] The

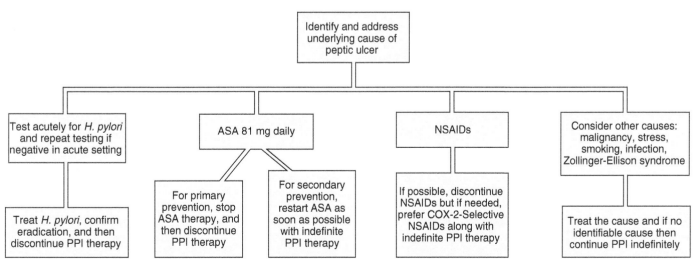

FIG 14.8 Diagnosis and Management of Peptic Ulcers After Endoscopy. *ASA,* acetylsalicylic acid; *NSAIDs,* nonsteroidal antiinflammatory drugs; *PPI,* proton pump inhibitor.

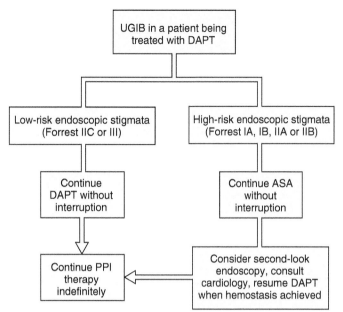

FIG 14.9 Approach to Management of Dual Anti-Platelet Therapy (Dapt) in Patients Presenting With Upper Gastrointestinal Bleeding (UGIB). *ASA,* acetylsalicylic acid; *PPI,* proton pump inhibitor. (Modified from Gralnek IM, Dumonceau JM, Kuipers EJ, et al: Diagnosis and management of nonvariceal upper gastrointestinal hemorrhage: European Society of Gastrointestinal Endoscopy (ESGE) Guideline. *Endoscopy* 47[10]:a1–a46, 2015.)

BOX 14.1   Considerations for Early Reintroduction of Anticoagulation After UGIB

Factors That Favor Early Reintroduction of Anticoagulation

Patient has a high CHADS2 or CHADS-VASC score

Ulcer or lesion with low-risk of rebleeding (e.g., Forrest IIC or III)

Successful hemostasis on initial endoscopy with low likelihood of rebleeding

Patient has normal platelet number and function

No additional risk factors for bleeding (i.e., no anti-platelets or NSAIDs)

Patient is clinically stable with no evidence of ongoing bleeding after endoscopy

Close observation and follow-up is possible after restarting anticoagulation

Patient has sufficient hemoglobin reserve in case of rebleeding

Patient has adequate clearance of the anticoagulant (i.e., no renal/liver failure)

There are no concomitant medications that could interfere with anticoagulant drug levels

Data from Desai J, Kolb JM, Weitz JI, Aisenberg J: Gastrointestinal bleeding with the new oral anticoagulants–defining the issues and the management strategies. *Thromb Haemost* 110(2):205–212, 2013.

---

decision about restarting anticoagulation often depends on the perceived risk of rebleeding, as well as the indication for anticoagulation and the risks of its interruption. One retrospective study examined 1329 patients who were on warfarin at the time of major GI bleeding to see whether restarting anticoagulation afterwards was associated with increased bleeding or mortality.[191] They found that restarting warfarin after 7 days was associated with a lower risk of thromboembolism and mortality without an increased risk of rebleeding.

More recently, Sengupta et al (2015) conducted a prospective observational study of 197 patients on anticoagulation presenting with GI bleeding.[192] At 90 days of follow-up, anticoagulation continuation at hospital discharge was associated with a significantly lower risk of thrombotic episodes (hazard ratio [HR]=0.121, $p = 0.03$) which was most pronounced in patients with underlying malignancy. There was a nonsignificant trend towards increased rebleeding (HR=2.17, $p = 0.10$), as well as a trend toward decreased mortality (HR 0.63, $p = 0.40$) in patients who were restarted on anticoagulation upon discharge.

Based on limited evidence, current European Society of Gastrointestinal Endoscopy guidelines suggest that resumption of anticoagulation be considered in patients between 7 to 14 days after an episode of GI bleeding. Earlier resumption of anticoagulation may be considered in patients with a low risk of rebleeding and in those in whom the interruption of anticoagulation for over 1 week could be hazardous, such as those with mechanical heart valves, high CHADS2 scores, known thrombotic disorders, or recent thromboembolism.[193,194] Individual patient factors must be considered and consultation with a cardiologist, hematologist, and/or neurologist is often warranted.[195]

Reintroduction of direct-acting oral anticoagulants is a particular issue because of the rapid onset of systemic anticoagulation (often within hours of the first dose), as well as the current paucity of reversal agents in cases of rebleeding.[189,196] A 2013 review article provided practical algorithms for management of anticoagulation in patients with GI bleeding and outlined various factors that can contribute to the decision of restarting anticoagulation (Box 14.1).[197]

HELICOBACTER PYLORI

All patients with NVUGIB due to erosions or ulcers should be tested for infection with *H. pylori*, which is one of the principal causes of bleeding ulcers. Without eradication, ulcer relapse and subsequent rebleeding is especially high in these patients.[198,199] Several different testing methods are available including urea-breath testing, histological tests, and serology.[200,201] Testing for *H. pylori* should be performed during the acute UGIB episode and treatment should immediately follow a positive test result.[202] A second test should be performed if an initial one during the acute UGIB episode is negative because false negative rates are high in the acute setting (up to 55%).[2] Real-time polymerase chain reaction (PCR) might improve *H. pylori* detection in patients with peptic ulcer bleeding. Real-time PCR testing for a combination of *H. pylori* 16S rRNA and urease A had a sensitivity of 64% and a specificity of 80% in tissue samples that had previously been considered negative by histological testing alone.[203]

After the completion of antibiotic and PPI treatment, a urea-breath test might be the most convenient approach to assess the effectiveness of *H. pylori* eradication treatment, unless repeat endoscopy is indicated, at which time gastric biopsies can be performed. Regardless of the method being used, checking for eradication is mandatory because of the risk of ulcer recurrence with bleeding as mentioned earlier, and because *H. pylori* infection is a major cause of gastric cancer, specifically noncardia gastric cancer.[204,205] In patients with *H. pylori*-associated bleeding ulcers, continuing PPI therapy after *H. pylori* eradication is not required, unless there persist other ongoing risk factors, including aspirin or NSAID use.

IRON REPLACEMENT THERAPY

Patients who present with UGIB should have iron studies performed after the acute bleeding episode. Anemic patients and even nonanemic patients with evidence of iron deficiency should be offered iron replacement therapy upon discharge from hospital as it may improve their quality of life and cognitive function.[206,207] In one study, only 16% of anemic patients post UGIB were prescribed oral supplementation upon discharge from hospital.[208] Correcting anemia rapidly after discharge may be crucial in minimizing both mortality risk and the possible need for a transfusion during a rebleeding episode. In a large prospective study, patients discharged after UGIB with hemoglobin values less than 100 g/L had twice the mortality rates when compared to patients with hemoglobin levels greater than 100 g/L.[209]

Intriguingly, current international consensus and American College of Gastroenterology (ACG) guidelines do not discuss the role of iron replacement post UGIB.[2,12] A 2014 RCT of 97 patients highlighted the importance of iron replacement by comparing intravenous iron, oral iron, and placebo in patients with anemia secondary to NVUGIB.[210] Patients receiving iron therapy had significantly lower rates of anemia (hemoglobin level < 12 g/dL for women and hemoglobin level < 13 g/dL for men) compared to patients receiving placebo at 3 months post UGIB (17% on iron therapy vs. 70% on placebo, $p < 0.01$). Importantly, there was no difference in efficacy between one dose of intravenous iron and 3 months of oral iron replacement, although compliance in patients taking oral iron was only 56%.

The primary limitation to oral iron supplementation seems to be GI tolerability likely attributable to nonabsorbed iron.[211] All iron salts (ferrous sulfate, ferrous fumarate, and ferrous gluconate) demonstrated similar efficacy and side effect profiles in a randomized trial.[212] A certain controlled-release iron preparation (extended-release ferrous sulfate with mucoproteose) has fewer GI side effects than the iron salts according to a large metaanalysis.[213] There are currently no studies evaluating the tolerability of the newer polysaccharide–iron complexes, although previous studies evaluating similar formulations (e.g., ferric-dextrin complex) have not shown any clear benefit.[214]

VASCULAR LESIONS

Dieulafoy Lesion

A Dieulafoy lesion is a dilated aberrant submucosal blood vessel that erodes through the overlying epithelium without an associated mucosal ulcer. The caliber of the artery is much larger than usual mucosal capillaries and measures approximately 1 to 3 mm.[215] One study of 109 patients with Dieulafoy lesions found that most lesions were found in the stomach (53%), followed by the duodenum or jejunum (33%) and lastly colon or rectum (13%).[215–217] There have been rare reports of lesions within the esophagus.[218] Dieulafoy lesions cause approximately 1%–2% of NVUGIB.[7] The 90-day mortality rate has been described between 10%–17%.[215,219] There are no clearly defined risk factors for these lesions: however, NSAIDs and cardiovascular risk factors such as hypertension, chronic kidney disease, and diabetes have been implicated.[215,220]

The natural history of Dieulafoy lesions is that of profuse bleeding; recurrent bleeding occurs in approximately 10% of

patients.[219] Initial evaluation with endoscopy can sometimes reveal the culprit vessel during active bleeding episodes. However, the lesion may be missed in up to 70% of patients in between bleeding episodes and, as such, Dieulafoy lesions remain in the differential for recurrent UGIB without a clear source identifiable on endoscopy.[221] Occasionally, a raised nipple or visible vessel can be visualized and treated.[222] More recently, endoscopic ultrasound has been used to confirm the diagnosis. Once a lesion is found and treated, consideration can be given to tattooing to easily relocate the lesion on follow-up endoscopic evaluation. Capsule endoscopy has been found to be useful at detecting small bowel Dieulafoy lesions and can be considered in patients when esophagogastroduodenoscopy and colonoscopy are unrevealing.[223]

Various endoscopic therapies have been studied in the management of patients with Dieulafoy lesions, including epinephrine injections with bipolar probe coagulation, hemoclip, APC, endoscopic band ligation (EBL), and cyanoacrylate injections.[215,217,224–228] The choice of specific therapy may be guided by local expertise, endoscopist preference, and the location of the lesion. Endoscopic banding ligation has been associated with ulcer bleeding once the band has fallen off, as well as perforation, especially in the gastric fundus, small bowel and right colon.[229] One small study of 9 patients found no difference in outcomes using either hemoclips or EBL in the management of patients with bleeding duodenal Dieulafoy lesions.[224] An older observational study suggested that band ligation may be superior to injection therapy.[230]

Some studies have shown that Doppler ultrasound can be considered to confirm ablation of the culprit vessel as a method to prevent rebleeding.[231] Newer therapeutic techniques using endoscopic-ultrasound guidance report more targeted therapy.[222,232,233] For recurrent bleeding refractory to endoscopic therapy, embolization or surgery may be required.[234,235]

Angiodysplasia

Angiodysplastic lesions appear as flat, cherry-red lesions with a fern-like pattern of ectatic blood vessels radiating from a central vessel (Fig. 14.10). These lesions in the stomach and small bowel may be the source of bleeding in 3%–5% of patients presenting

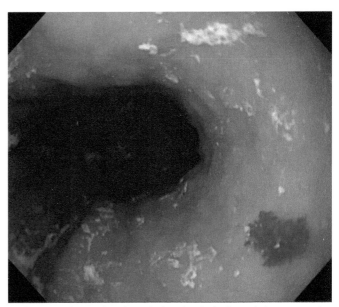

FIG 14.10 Example of angiodysplastic lesion of the stomach.

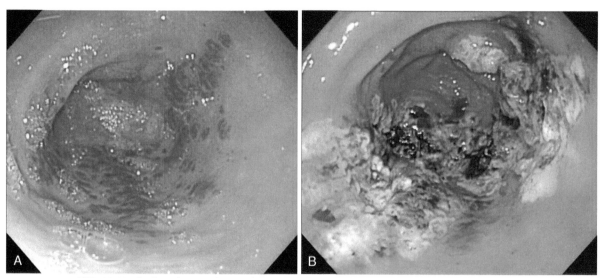

FIG 14.11 **A,** Gastric antral vascular ectasia **B,** treated with argon plasma coagulation.

with UGIB.[236] More commonly, however, these patients will often present with occult GI bleeding and iron deficiency anemia.[237] The diagnosis is usually made on endoscopy, but can also be made using capsule enterography, computed tomography (CT) enterography, or conventional angiography. There are several risk factors that have been implicated in developing angiodysplastic lesions including chronic kidney disease, von Willebrand disease, aortic stenosis, and left-ventricular assist devices.[238–241]

Several endoscopic modalities have proven effective at controlling bleeding angiodysplastic lesions, including APC, bipolar electrocautery, and hemoclips.[134,242] The most widely used method seems to be APC due to its ease-of-use and presumed safety profile. One study found that submucosal injection of normal saline prior to treatment with APC significantly reduced the risk of tissue injury. Although initial therapy is effective, rebleeding rates are reported at 36% at 22 months.[243]

Gastric Antral Vascular Ectasia (GAVE)

GAVE, also known as "watermelon stomach," has a characteristic appearance of longitudinal rows of flat and reddish spots.[244] These lesions tend to present more often with occult GI bleeding and iron deficiency anemia. GAVE has been associated with female gender, older age (> 70 years old), systemic sclerosis, and cirrhosis.[245,246] The diagnosis is made endoscopically and can be confirmed with biopsy, endoscopic ultrasound, or CT scan.[247]

Endoscopic management options are identical to other vascular lesions and include: APC, bipolar probe, heater probe, cryotherapy, radiofrequency ablation, and EBL (Fig. 14.11).[242,248–251] A systematic review found that patients with GAVE treated with EBL have fewer episodes of rebleeding (8%) compared to those treated with APC (68%, $p = 0.01$) Importantly, there is no evidence that portal decompression with a transjugular intrahepatic portosystemic shunt (TIPS) procedure provides any reduction in bleeding.[252] For bleeding refractory to endoscopic management, antrectomy has been shown to prevent rebleeding.[253]

MALLORY-WEISS TEARS

Epidemiology and Risk Factors

MWT account for approximately 3%–10% of NVUGIB.[254–256] MWT was first described in 1929 as a linear mucosal laceration of the distal esophagus often including the gastroesophageal junction and upper part of the stomach.[257] The mechanism responsible for the tear is thought to be rapid propulsion of the gastric cardia into the thoracic cavity through the hiatus, most commonly due to vomiting or retching.[258] The most cited risk factors for a MWT include male gender, age 30 to 50, hiatal hernia, and alcohol use. Alcohol intake has been found to be a contributing factor in 44% of patients presenting with a tear and hiatal hernia is present in 40% to 100% of patients.[259,260] Other factors that may be associated with tears include: severe coughing, pregnancy, heavy lifting or straining, hiccupping, and colonic lavage with polyethylene glycol.[254,260–262] MWT has been described as a rare complication of esophagogastroduodenoscopy and transesophageal echocardiography.[261,263,264] One prospective study of 281 patients found that 30-day mortality was equivalent between MWT and peptic ulcer disease (5.3% vs. 4.6%, $p = 0.578$).[265]

Risk Stratification

As the diagnosis of MWT is made endoscopically, initial management is identical to that of all NVUGIB (described in Fig. 14.1). Aspects on clinical history, including retching prior to hematemesis, or other risk factors as mentioned earlier, may increase the likelihood of a tear. Physical examination should be performed to look for signs of crepitus over the chest suggestive of subcutaneous emphysema as a result of an associated (Boerhaave's syndrome) esophageal perforation.[266] A chest x-ray should be performed in all patients to exclude free air under the diaphragm (suggesting a perforation), a pneumomediastinum, or a pneumothorax.[267–270] If there is any concern of possible esophageal rupture, urgent surgical consultation is needed and additional imaging may be required. One retrospective study of 38 patients found that the GBS could be used to predict outcome in patients with MWT.[271] Specifically, they noted that patients with a GBS score less than 6 did not require endoscopic intervention or blood transfusion. Of the patients with a GBS score of 6 or higher, 39% required endoscopic intervention and 74% required a blood transfusion. Recent reports (2016, 2015) describe successful closure of a full thickness tear using an over-the-scope clip and an uncovered metal stent.[272,273] Rebleeding rates from MWT have been reported as 5%–10% depending on various clinical factors including any bleeding diathesis.[262]

Endoscopic Stigmata

Endoscopic stigmata that predict a high risk of rebleeding in peptic ulcer disease (i.e., Forrest classification) do not apply to MWT. Kim et al (2005) reviewed 159 patients with a MWT with a rebleeding rate of 10.7% of patients; the greatest predictor of rebleeding was active bleeding at time of endoscopy (OR 9.89),[274] whereas another study of 76 patients with MWT suggested that neither a visible vessel nor an adherent clot are associated with rebleeding.[275] As a result, current guidelines suggest that endoscopic therapy be reserved for an actively bleeding MWT and not performed for nonbleeding lesions, including those with visible vessels or adherent clots.[11] In all patients, high-dose PPI therapy is recommended after endoscopic evaluation, although the timing and route of delivery have not been well studied. Extra caution should be taken in patients with coagulopathy, liver disease, and those with hemodynamic instability or transfusion requirements while in hospital.

Endoscopic Therapy

There are several effective options for endoscopic management of bleeding secondary to a MWT including: injection therapy, hemoclip, electrocoagulation, APC, and EBL.[276] Epinephrine injection by itself may be effective at controlling initial bleeding but has been associated with higher rebleeding rates when compared to combination therapy.[277,278] EBL and hemoclip placement have both proven to be highly effective therapies for MWT.[279] Hemoclip placement can be challenging within the esophagus, especially at the gastroesophageal (GE) junction. EBL, on the other hand, may be somewhat easier to deploy.

One RCT of 41 patients found no significant difference between EBL and hemoclip plus injection in terms of rebleeding rates, need for transfusion, or duration of hospital stay.[280] Another RCT of 56 patients compared EBL and hemoclip plus epinephrine for a bleeding MWT and found that recurrent bleeding was significantly higher in the hemoclip plus injection group compared to the EBL group (18% vs. 0%, $p = 0.02$).[281] It was suspected that injecting with epinephrine prior to deploying the clips led to issue edema, which perhaps increased the likelihood of clip

detachment. It is therefore suggested that epinephrine injection be administered after the clip has been put in place. Endoscopic electrocoagulaton and APC have also been shown to be effective treatments, although both therapies can cause tissue injury, possibly leading to perforation of the esophageal wall.[276]

Overall, clinicians should tailor their choice of endoscopic therapy to their patient, as well as their experience and skillset. If endoscopic therapy fails to control the bleeding, urgent referral should be made for either angiography-guided embolization or surgery.[276] Certainly, urgent surgical referral must be made if esophageal perforation is suspected at any time.

MALIGNANT BLEEDING

Roughly 1%–5% of all UGIB is caused by either primary GI malignancy or metastatic disease.[282–284] Moreover, UGIB is often the initial presentation in patients with various GI malignancies. Similar to patients with nonmalignancy related bleeding, endoscopy is usually performed within 24 hours in these patients and various modalities including epinephrine or alcohol injections, endoscopic clipping, APC, and bipolar electrocoagulation are often used to control bleeding.[285–287] Compared to peptic ulcer bleeding, however, rates of rebleeding, surgery, and mortality are much higher in patients with malignant bleeding.[282] Indeed, patients with malignancy related bleeding will often require chemotherapy, radiation, interventional radiologic procedures, or surgery to control bleeding.[285] One retrospective study noted rebleeding rates of 49% in patients with UGIB related to malignancy.[282,288]

Studies have found some success at initial endoscopic management with Tc-325 hemostatic powder as it is a noncontact approach that will not traumatize the friable malignant tissue and can be applied to a broad surface area with multiple bleeding points, as is often the case (Fig. 14.12).[148] Although this hemostatic powder can be effective at managing acute malignant bleeding, the powder washes off after approximately 24 hours.[147] Based on uncontrolled studies[148] the powder may be effective at temporarily managing UGIB while other modalities such as radiation, interventional radiologic procedures, or surgery are

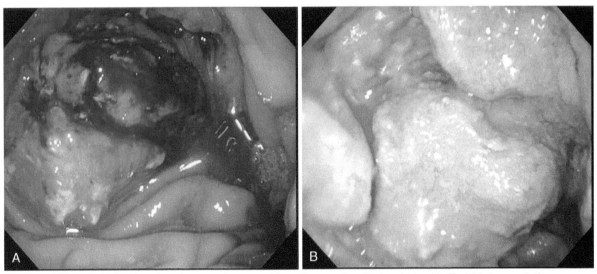

FIG 14.12 **A,** Gastric adenocarcinoma with active oozing **B,** treated with Tc-325 hemostatic powder.

being considered; some patients have experienced prolonged bleed-free episodes. Considering how difficult initial endoscopic management of malignant UGIB can be, and the high rate of recurrent bleeding, gastroenterologists must consider using all options within their armamentarium when faced with a patient with malignant UGIB. The exact role of Tc-325 and other hemostatic powders in malignant bleeding is unknown and awaits results from controlled trials.

COMPLICATIONS OF ENDOSCOPIC THERAPY

There are several potential complications with all endoscopic therapies and the benefits of each procedure should be carefully weighed against its associated risks.[289] Informed consent must be obtained from the patient or substitute decision maker prior to any procedure.[290–292] Procedural sedation and cardiopulmonary complications including cardiac or respiratory arrest, angina or myocardial infarction, hypotension, hypoxia, and aspiration pneumonia are a few of the many potential complications related to sedation.[293–295] Consideration must always be given to the use of anesthesia and airway protection prior to any procedure, especially in patients with comorbidities such as obstructive sleep apnea or known cardiovascular disease.[293]

One 2016 metaanalysis found that endoscopy performed shortly after an acute coronary syndrome (in most cases, an EGD for bleeding indications) was associated with a higher complication rate and mortality rate; thus, extra care should be taken in deciding the optimal time for endoscopy in this subgroup of patients.[57] Ongoing monitoring and assessment is required before, during, and after the procedure.[296,297] Reversal agents and resuscitation equipment should also be readily available in case of complications.[298]

FAILURE OF ENDOSCOPIC THERAPY

Despite initial resuscitation, medical management, and endoscopic therapy a subset of patients will have recurrent bleeding requiring additional interventions. A management algorithm was recently proposed and is shown in slightly modified version in Fig. 14.13.

TRANSCATHETER ARTERIAL EMBOLIZATION

Embolization is a safe and effective alternative to surgery when endoscopic therapy has failed to control the source of UGIB.[299] By itself, angiography can be used to locate the site of bleeding in the context of massive UGIB whereby endoscopic visualization is limited.[300] If active extravasation of blood is noted, which occurs in approximately 40% of cases, directed embolization can be performed to treat the underlying bleeding vessel.[301,302] If no culprit vessel is identified on angiography, empiric embolization towards a suspected location can be performed as well.[303–305] One study showed that endoscopic clips placed at the time of the failed therapeutic endoscopy near the bleeding site can be helpful in localizing the target location for empiric embolization.[143]

The technical success of embolization ranges between 60% and 100% and the clinical success ranges between 69% and 99%.[301,306,307] The most common reason for ongoing bleeding after embolization is a lesion being fed by the gastroduodenal artery, which often has several collaterals that can continue bleeding despite initial embolization. One study of 60 patients found that 15 of the 16 patients who had rebleeding after initial

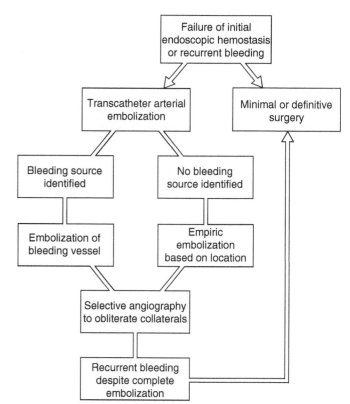

FIG 14.13 Algorithm for failure of initial endoscopic hemostasis or recurrent bleeding. (Modified from Lu Y, Loffroy R, Lau JY, Barkun A: Multidisciplinary management strategies for acute nonvariceal upper gastrointestinal bleeding. *Br J Surg* 101[1]:e34–e50, 2014.)

embolization had so due to ongoing bleeding from the collaterals of the gastroduodenal artery.[301]

Immediate complications of angiography include infection or bleeding from the vascular access site, as well as dissection of the target vessel.[300] Other worrisome complications include bowel ischemia and perforation, which have now been minimized by more precise embolization and newer imaging techniques.[308] In a large case series, approximately 9% of patients had minor or major complications including intestinal ischemia, perforation, and duodenal stenosis.[300,309]

Current guidelines suggest that embolization be considered after two endoscopic attempts have been made to control the bleeding.[2,11] RCTs have shown that percutaneous embolization is efficacious and has a lower mortality rate than surgery.[310,311] Occasionally, for patients found to have large ulcers or those with unfavorable locations for endoscopic therapy, embolization may be used as second-line therapy instead of a repeat endoscopy. Some studies have even suggested a role for prophylactic embolization to prevent recurrent bleeding in certain patients with high-risk endoscopic features.[312–314] In general, embolization is preferred over surgery due to its equivalent efficacy and favorable safety profile.[312] The precise role of technique of embolization will continue to be defined as studies address important clinical dilemmas.

EMERGENCY SURGERY

The need for emergency surgery for bleeding peptic ulcers has decreased significantly over the past 2 decades.[315] In the United

Kingdom, the rate of surgery for peptic ulcer disease decreased from 8% in 1993 to 2% in 2006.[7,316] In the United States, the rate of emergency ulcer surgery has decreased by over 21%.[317] The reasons for the decreased need for surgery include the routine use of PPI therapy, as well as the improvements in endoscopic management.[318,319] Surgical intervention, however, is still needed in certain cases of refractory UGIB whereby endoscopic and radiologic procedures are either not possible or unsuccessful.[320] As the risks of surgical intervention are greater than the risks of either endoscopic or radiologic intervention, surgery is only reserved for those who have failed other less-invasive alternatives.

Surgical options include simple intraluminal ligature or plication alone, which is less invasive, or the more conventional surgery, which includes ulcer excision with either vagotomy and pyloroplasty or a partial or total gastrectomy.[321] Although several randomized trials have suggested a lower rebleeding risk with a partial or complete gastrectomy, mortality rates are no different than with the less invasive surgical options.[322,323]

Overall, surgery remains a valuable option for certain patients but should not be considered unless there is ongoing bleeding after failing both endoscopic and radiologic therapies. In certain patients with massive hemorrhage or endoscopic findings suggestive of high-risk lesions that may not be amenable to endoscopic therapy, early surgical referral may be considered.

FUTURE DIRECTIONS FOR ENDOSCOPIC THERAPY

Over-the-Scope Clip

Novel endoscopic techniques continue to be developed to better manage patients with NVUGIB.[324] One case series of 9 patients used an over-the-scope clip to manage patients with refractory UGIB after initial endoscopic therapies were used.[325] Chan et al (2014) found that over-the-scope clip could be deployed successfully in all patients and clinical bleeding was stopped in 77% (7/9) of patients. Another retrospective review of 14 patients with recurrent UGIB despite endoscopic therapy found that an over-the-scope clip was successful in 86% (12/14) of patients at preventing further bleeding with no adverse events.[326] Future studies will evaluate this technique as initial therapy for larger, high-risk ulcers, as well as those with recurrent bleeding despite routine endoscopic management.

Doppler Endoscopic Probe

Newer endoscopic modalities such as a Doppler endoscopic probe have been used to better characterize peptic ulcer rebleeding risk when compared to traditional measures, such as the Forrest classification. Some studies have shown no added benefit of the Doppler probe in the management of patients with UGIB.[327,328] One prospective study of 163 patients with bleeding peptic ulcers found that the Doppler probe was useful in correlating arterial blood flow at the base of the ulcer with subsequent rebleeding rates.[329] They also showed that the Doppler flow seen after endoscopic treatment correlates with rebleeding risk as well. This study suggests that using Doppler in addition to the Forrest classification may have a beneficial effect in identifying patients who are at the highest risk of rebleeding and also as a method of determining whether patients may benefit from additional endoscopic interventions to achieve definitive hemostasis. Future multicenter randomized controlled studies are needed to confirm these findings.

CONCLUSIONS

The management of NVUGIB begins with resuscitation, risk stratification, and preendoscopic medical management, including prokinetics and PPI therapy. Endoscopy should be performed in all patients within 24 hours, although certain high-risk patients may benefit from earlier endoscopy, whereas other patients who are low-risk may be discharged home with close follow-up. Endoscopic findings and technical expertise will determine which endoscopic modality, if any, will be used for hemostasis, although injection of epinephrine alone is less effective than other approaches. Postendoscopic management is based on the etiology and endoscopic appearance of the lesion, and patients with high-risk lesions should receive intravenous PPI therapy for 3 days before being discharged on an oral regimen. Any reversible risk factors should be addressed, including anti-platelets, NSAIDs, anticoagulation, and *H. pylori*. Patients with recurrent bleeding episodes should undergo repeat endoscopy followed by percutaneous embolization and surgery, if needed. Future research will continue to identify the role of emerging therapies, including hemostatic powders, in view of their continuing to improve the outcomes of patients presenting with NVUGIB.

KEY REFERENCES

2. Barkun AN, Bardou M, Kuipers EJ, et al: International consensus recommendations on the management of patients with nonvariceal upper gastrointestinal bleeding, *Ann Intern Med* 152(2):101–113, 2010.
11. Gralnek IM, Dumonceau JM, Kuipers EJ, et al: Diagnosis and management of nonvariceal upper gastrointestinal hemorrhage: European Society of Gastrointestinal Endoscopy (ESGE) Guideline, *Endoscopy* 47(10):a1–a46, 2015.
12. Laine L, Jensen DM: Management of patients with ulcer bleeding, *Am J Gastroenterol* 107(3):345–360, quiz 361, 2012.
19. Saltzman JR: Advances and improvements in the management of upper gastrointestinal bleeding, *Gastrointest Endosc Clin N Am* 25(3):xv–xvi, 2015.
48. Aquarius M, Smeets FG, Konijn HW, et al: Prospective multicenter validation of the Glasgow Blatchford bleeding score in the management of patients with upper gastrointestinal hemorrhage presenting at an emergency department, *Eur J Gastroenterol Hepatol* 27(9):1011–1016, 2015.
51. Abougergi MS, Charpentier JP, Bethea E, et al: A Prospective, Multicenter study of the AIMS65 score compared with the glasgow-blatchford score in predicting upper gastrointestinal hemorrhage outcomes, *J Clin Gastroenterol* 50(6):464–469, 2016.
56. Villanueva C, Colomo A, Bosch A: Transfusion for acute upper gastrointestinal bleeding, *N Engl J Med* 368(14):1362–1363, 2013.
69. Abraham NS, Singh S, Alexander GC, et al: Comparative risk of gastrointestinal bleeding with dabigatran, rivaroxaban, and warfarin: population based cohort study, *BMJ* 350:h1857, 2015.
72. Radaelli F, Dentali F, Repici A, et al: Management of anticoagulation in patients with acute gastrointestinal bleeding, *Dig Liver Dis* 47(8): 621–627, 2015.
77. Lim LG, Ho KY, Chan YH, et al: Urgent endoscopy is associated with lower mortality in high-risk but not low-risk nonvariceal upper gastrointestinal bleeding, *Endoscopy* 43(4):300–306, 2011.
92. Lau JY, Leung WK, Wu JC, et al: Omeprazole before endoscopy in patients with gastrointestinal bleeding, *N Engl J Med* 356(16): 1631–1640, 2007.
98. Forrest JA, Finlayson ND, Shearman DJ: Endoscopy in gastrointestinal bleeding, *Lancet* 2(7877):394–397, 1974.
103. Kahi CJ, Jensen DM, Sung JJ, et al: Endoscopic therapy versus medical therapy for bleeding peptic ulcer with adherent clot: a meta-analysis, *Gastroenterology* 129(3):855–862, 2005.

116. Muguruma N, Kitamura S, Kimura T, et al: Endoscopic management of nonvariceal upper gastrointestinal bleeding: state of the art, *Clin Endosc* 48(2):96–101, 2015.

124. Barkun AN, Martel M, Toubouti Y, et al: Endoscopic hemostasis in peptic ulcer bleeding for patients with high-risk lesions: a series of meta-analyses, *Gastrointest Endosc* 69(4):786–799, 2009.

146. Vergara M, Calvet X, Gisbert JP: Epinephrine injection versus epinephrine injection and a second endoscopic method in high risk bleeding ulcers, *Cochrane Database Syst Rev* (2):CD005584, 2007.

149. Chen YI, Barkun AN: Hemostatic powders in gastrointestinal bleeding: a systematic review, *Gastrointest Endosc Clin N Am* 25(3):535–552, 2015.

161. Leontiadis GI, Sharma VK, Howden CW: Proton pump inhibitor therapy for peptic ulcer bleeding: cochrane collaboration meta-analysis of randomized controlled trials, *Mayo Clin Proc* 82(3):286–296, 2007.

163. Sachar H, Vaidya K, Laine L: Intermittent vs continuous proton pump inhibitor therapy for high-risk bleeding ulcers: a systematic review and meta-analysis, *JAMA Intern Med* 174(11):1755–1762, 2014.

184. Chan FK, Ching JY, Hung LC, et al: Clopidogrel versus aspirin and esomeprazole to prevent recurrent ulcer bleeding, *N Engl J Med* 352(3):238–244, 2005.

192. Sengupta N, Feuerstein JD, Patwardhan VR, et al: The risks of thromboembolism vs. recurrent gastrointestinal bleeding after interruption of systemic anticoagulation in hospitalized inpatients with gastrointestinal bleeding: a prospective study, *Am J Gastroenterol* 110(2):328–335, 2015.

210. Bager P, Dahlerup JF: Randomised clinical trial: oral vs. intravenous iron after upper gastrointestinal haemorrhage–a placebo-controlled study, *Aliment Pharmacol Ther* 39(2):176–187, 2014.

299. Lu Y, Loffroy R, Lau JY, Barkun A: Multidisciplinary management strategies for acute non-variceal upper gastrointestinal bleeding, *Br J Surg* 101(1):e34–e50, 2014.

315. Lau JY, Barkun A, Fan DM, et al: Challenges in the management of acute peptic ulcer bleeding, *Lancet* 381(9882):2033–2043, 2013.

329. Jensen DM, Ohning GV, Kovacs TO, et al: Doppler endoscopic probe as a guide to risk stratification and definitive hemostasis of peptic ulcer bleeding, *Gastrointest Endosc* 83(1):129–136, 2016.

A complete reference list can be found online at ExpertConsult .com

15

Portal Hypertensive Bleeding

*Anna Baiges, Virginia Hernández-Gea, Andrés Cárdenas,
and Juan Carlos García-Pagán*

CHAPTER OUTLINE

INTRODUCTION

Portal hypertension is defined by a pathologic increase in portal pressure in which the pressure gradient between the portal vein and inferior vena cava (the portal pressure gradient, PPG) is increased above the upper normal limit of 5 mm Hg.[1] Portal hypertension becomes clinically significant when the PPG increases above the threshold of 10 mm Hg (formation of varices) or 12 mm Hg (variceal bleeding, ascites).[2,3]

Acute variceal bleeding (AVB) is the most dreaded complication of portal hypertension because, even though mortality rates have decreased due to improvement in general management, medical treatment, and endoscopic therapy, mortality is still approximately 15%. Moreover, variceal bleeding leads to deterioration in liver function and can trigger other complications of cirrhosis such as bacterial infections, hepatic encephalopathy (HE), or hepatorenal syndrome. Therapy to prevent rebleeding (secondary prophylaxis) is mandatory given that patients surviving a variceal bleeding episode have a very high risk of rebleeding, which is associated with mortality as high as that of the first bleed.

NATURAL HISTORY OF VARICES IN CIRRHOSIS

The natural history of cirrhosis is considered to be a progression from compensated cirrhosis to decompensated cirrhosis. Compensated cirrhosis is defined as the absence of jaundice, variceal hemorrhage (VH), ascites, and HE. On the other hand, decompensated cirrhosis is defined as the presence of one of these features. The transition from compensated to decompensated cirrhosis occurs at a rate of 5% to 7% per year.[4,5] The development

of portal hypertension directly leads to the formation of portal-systemic collaterals such as esophageal and gastric varices and represents a key stage in this natural history of cirrhosis.

When cirrhosis is diagnosed, varices are present in approximately 30% to 40% of compensated patients and in 60% of those with decompensated cirrhosis.[6] The annual incidence of new varices is approximately 5% to 10%[7]; these initially develop as small varices and gradually dilate at a rate of 5% per year. The factor that has been most consistently associated with variceal progression is baseline Child-Pugh or its worsening during follow-up.[8] Variceal bleeding usually occurs late in the natural history of portal hypertension and in order for varices to bleed the hepatic venous pressure gradient (HVPG) must rise above 12 mm Hg.[7,9] Certain characteristics, such as the severity of liver disease, the size of the varix, and the presence of red wale marks (specially on thin areas of the variceal wall), place the varices at higher risk of bleeding, which can occur with an incidence of 4% to 15% per year.[6,10,11] The risk of bleeding is very low (between 1% and 2%) in patients without varices at the first examination, and increases to approximately 5% per year in those with small varices and to 15% per year if medium or large varices are present at diagnosis.[12]

PREVENTION OF FIRST BLEEDING FROM ESOPHAGEAL VARICES

Screening for Esophageal Varices

Until recently, the current consensus was that every cirrhotic patient should be endoscopically screened for varices at the time of diagnosis[13] to detect those requiring prophylactic treatment.

However, the introduction of transient elastography (Fibroscan) of the liver has changed this scenario in some patients. Fibroscan is used to estimate the degree of liver fibrosis but also to determine if patients are at risk of having varices and portal hypertension. This has been extensively studied and validated in patients with cirrhosis due to hepatitis C (HCV); current guidelines suggest that patients with HCV and elastography values of stiffness less than 20 kPa and a platelet count over 150,000 could avoid screening endoscopy because the risk of having varices is extremely low.[14]

In patients without varices on initial endoscopy, follow-up evaluation should be performed after 2 to 3 years (2 if there is a deterioration in liver function).[14] In patients with small varices, a follow-up endoscopy should be performed every 1 to 2 years to check for a possible increase in size, based on an expected 10% to 15% per year rate of progression of small to large varices. This time interval should be shortened in cases of clinical decompensation. Primary prophylaxis with nonselective β-blockers (NSBBs, propranolol, nadolol, carvedilol) or endoscopic band ligation (EBL) must be initiated when the patient develops medium to large varices or small varices with red wale signs in those with Child-Pugh class C cirrhosis.[14] No follow-up endoscopy is needed once NSBBs are started, but once initiated, NSBBs should be maintained through the patient's life. Although still not discussed in guidelines, there is recent evidence (2016) suggesting that carvedilol might delay the progression of small to large esophageal varices (EVs).[15]

Nonselective β-Blockers Versus Endoscopic Banding Ligation for Primary Prophylaxis

NSBBs are effective in the prevention of variceal bleeding. These drugs reduce portal pressure by decreasing portal venous inflow through vasoconstriction of the splanchnic circulation and by decreasing cardiac output.[16] A reduction in HVPG to 12 mm Hg or less, or 20% or less from baseline, protects from VH[17,18] and also decreases the incidence of clinical decompensation.[19] NSBB side effects (hypotension, fatigue, weakness) can be managed by adjusting the dose. However, up to 20% of patients may have absolute or relative contraindications.

Propranolol is typically started at 20 mg twice daily and nadolol at 40 mg once a day. These drugs are given in a stepwise fashion, increasing the dose until it is maximally tolerated or the resting heart rate is between 50 and 60 beats/min. Carvedilol is more effective than propranolol in reducing HVPG[19–21] through an anti α-adrenergic activity and a mildly vasodilating effect. Carvedilol is started with 6.25 mg once a day and afterwards the dose is increased to 6.5 mg twice a day (higher doses may not further decrease portal pressure, yet may increase the risk of arterial hypotension). Indirect data suggests that carvedilol is more effective than propranolol/nadolol in primary prophylaxis, although this has not been adequately studied in head-to-head clinical trials.

Variceal ligation is performed every 3 to 4 weeks until variceal eradication is achieved, which typically occurs after 2 to 4 sessions. Eradication is defined by either the disappearance of the varices or the impossibility of grasping and banding them with the ligator. Meta-analyses of randomized controlled trials (RCTs) of β-blockers versus band ligation indicate that ligation is associated with a lower incidence of first VH without differences in mortality.[23,24] Nonetheless, endoscopic ligation requires several sessions and may be associated with important side effects, such as bleeding from postligation ulcers. Although the choice of

β-blockers or endoscopic therapy should be made depending on the local resources, availability of experienced endoscopists, patient preference, side effects, and contraindications, a reasonable approach is to begin with β-blockers if there are no contraindications because they are inexpensive, easy to use, and relatively safe.[25] Those patients who develop side effects or have contraindications to β-blockers should then be offered endoscopic variceal band ligation. If the patient tolerates NSBBs, no follow-up endoscopy is needed. In those that undergo EBL and for whom varices are eradicated, follow-up endoscopies approximately 3 months after the complete eradication should be performed and varices should be reeradicated upon recurrence.

All randomized studies and meta-analyses comparing the combination of NSBB plus EBL versus EBL alone in primary prophylaxis had failed to demonstrate a clear benefit from combination therapy, with a predicted higher number of adverse events in the combination therapy group[26] not supporting the use of combination therapy for primary prophylaxis. However, a 2017 study has challenged this recommendation, suggesting that the combination therapy of NSBB and EBL may be more effective in primary prophylaxis than NSBB alone or EBL alone for the prevention of acute variceal bleeding, although with similar mortality rates at 2 years. Until more data is available, it is wise to follow the current guidelines of using either NSBB or EBL, but not in combination.[27]

GENERAL MANAGEMENT OF ACUTE VARICEAL BLEEDING (AVB)

Ruptured EV cause 80% of all upper gastrointestinal bleeding episodes in patients with portal hypertension.[28] Diagnosis is established at emergency endoscopy based on observing one of the following: (1) active bleeding from a varix (observation of blood spurting or oozing from the varix); (2) white nipple or clot adherent to a varix; or (3) presence of varices without other potential sources of bleeding (Fig. 15.1). Endoscopy should be performed within the first 12 hours of admission, especially in patients with hematemesis or hemodynamic instability.

AVB should be managed in an intensive care setting. The initial ABCs (airway, breathing, circulation) of resuscitation should be applied with the aim of maintaining aerobic metabolism and restoring an appropriate oxygen transport to the tissues. At least two large bore venous accesses should be placed on admission, as they can be necessary for rapid administration of volume during initial resuscitation. An airway should be immediately secured, and endotracheal intubation is mandatory before endoscopy if there is any concern about the safety of the airway, especially in encephalopathic or actively bleeding patients, as they are at risk of bronchoaspiration of gastric content and blood; this risk is further exacerbated by endoscopic procedures.[29,30]

Avoiding prolonged hypotension is particularly important to prevent further complications such as renal failure and ischemic hepatitis, which are associated with increased risk of rebleeding and death,[31] and therefore blood volume replacement with plasma expanders must be used, aiming at maintaining a mean arterial pressure of at least 65 mm Hg. However, overexpansion must also be avoided as it may induce rebound increases in portal pressure and facilitate rebleeding. Therefore, a delicate fluid balance is needed. In fact, an RCT showed that a restrictive transfusion strategy in which patients were only transfused if hemoglobin levels dropped below 7 g/dL improved survival in

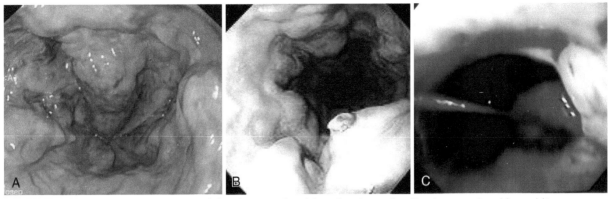

FIG 15.1 Endoscopic view of **A,** a large varix with red wale marks, **B,** a large varix with a white nipple sign, **C,** and an actively bleeding (spurting) esophageal varix in a patient with cirrhosis.

Child-Pugh A and B patients, except in patients with shock, ongoing bleeding, or ischemic heart disease.[32]

As mentioned earlier, the main associated complications of AVB are bacterial infections, HE, and impaired renal function. Infections may be both a consequence and a precipitating event leading to AVB. Antibiotic treatment significantly decreases the risk of rebleeding and improves survival.[33] In most cases, either norfloxacin 400 mg by mouth twice daily for 7 days or IV ceftriaxone 1 to 2 g/day can be given, although intravenous antibiotics are preferred in those patients with hypovolemic shock and advanced cirrhosis,[34] in hospital settings of high prevalence of quinolone-resistant bacterial infections, and in patients on previous quinolone prophylaxis.[14] Variceal bleeding can trigger HE, mainly because of the intestinal absorption of toxic substances generated from blood proteins. Even though there is no strong data supporting the need of prophylactic treatment, both lactulose and rifaximin should be used to prevent HE.

The rapid implementation of vasoconstrictors and performance of endoscopy should be instituted within the first 12 hours of admission; however this interval can be shortened to 6 hours in those with hematemesis once they are stabilized in a monitored unit.[35]

Finally, it is important to consider if the patient is at high risk for treatment failure, which is known to occur in approximately 15% of patients. Critically, this is the population where mortality-related bleeding concentrates.[36] A multicenter European randomized clinical trial[37] showed that high-risk patients (defined as Child-Pugh C up to 13 points, or Child B plus active bleeding at endoscopy) benefit from a preemptive transjugular intrahepatic portosystemic shunt (TIPS) within 72 hours of admission. This approach markedly decreased rebleeding and mortality without increasing the incidence of HE. Beneficial effects of the use of preemptive TIPS in high-risk patients were confirmed in an observational retrospective study.[38]

HEMOSTATIC THERAPIES

Initial therapy for acute variceal bleeding is based on the combination of vasoactive drugs with endoscopic therapies.[39] The early use of vasoconstrictors in most cases can initially arrest bleeding, which translates to better visualization at endoscopy. These drugs also reduce rebleeding and improve survival among patients with cirrhosis and AVB.[40–44]

TABLE 15.1 **Vasoconstrictors Used in Acute Variceal Bleeding**	
Drug	**Dose**
Terlipressin	Intravenous bolus 2 mg/4 hr for 24–48 hr then 1 mg/4 hr
Somatostatin	Intravenous bolus 250 mcg followed by infusion of 250–500 µg/hr
Octreotide	Intravenous bolus of 50–100 µg followed by infusion of 50 µg/hr

All drugs are administered for a minimum of 2 days and may be extended for up to 5 days.

Pharmacological Treatment

The drug selection will depend mainly on local resources as different studies and meta-analysis have not found significant differences in efficacy when comparing the different vasoactive agents.[44] The most commonly used vasoactive drugs are terlipressin, somatostatin, and its analogue (octreotide) (Table 15.1).

Terlipressin is a long-acting derivative of vasopressin that has been shown to effectively control AVB, decrease transfusion requirements, and decrease bleeding-related mortality.[45,46] As soon as variceal bleeding is suspected, terlipressin should be initiated at a dose of 2 mg every 4 hours during the first 24 hours, and it may be maintained for up to 5 days at a dose of 1 mg every 4 hours to prevent rebleeding.[42] As it is a potent vasoconstrictor, terlipressin may be associated with mild adverse events such as abdominal pain, diarrhea, or bradycardia[47]; it can also induce cardiac ischemia and it is therefore contraindicated in patients with known ischemic heart disease.[46] Hyponatremia in varying degrees has been described in patients treated with terlipressin, especially those with preserved liver function, and therefore sodium levels must be monitored.[47]

Somatostatin reduces portal pressure by inducing selective splanchnic vasoconstriction without systemic effects.[48] It is commonly used as an initial bolus of 250 µg followed by a 250 µg/hr or 500 µg/hr infusion that is maintained for 5 days or until the achievement of a 24 hours bleed-free period.[49] The 500 µg/hr dose causes a greater fall in HVPG (13% vs. 6% compared to 250 µg/hr) and seems to have greater clinical efficacy in the subset of patients with active variceal bleeding at emergent endoscopy.[50]

Octreotide is a somatostatin analogue with a longer half-life[51] but similar safety profile than somatostatin. The optimal doses are not well determined, but it is usually given as an initial bolus of 50 to 100 μg, followed by an infusion of 25 or 50 μg/hr.[52] As with somatostatin, therapy can be maintained for 5 days to prevent early rebleeding. Octreotide may improve the results of endoscopic therapy but has uncertain effects if used alone.[16,43]

Endoscopic Therapy

Endoscopy is one of the cornerstones of the management of AVB because it confirms the diagnosis and allows specific therapy during the same session. An important consideration before considering endoscopy is choosing the type of sedation for the procedure, as patients need to be fully sedated for the procedure to be successful. Intravenous sedation with propofol is a safe and better tolerated option than benzodiazepines (midazolam) plus an opiate (meperidine or fentanyl), which can potentially trigger episodes of minimal HE.[53–55] Endoscopic therapies for varices are effective because they cause obliteration of the varix. The two endoscopic methods available for AVB are endoscopic sclerotherapy (ES) and EBL (Figs. 15.2 and 15.3).

ES consists of the injection of a sclerosing agent (sodium morrhuate [5%], ethanolamine oleate [5%] or polidocanol [1%–2%]) into the variceal lumen or adjacent to it. This causes inflammation and thrombosis, creating a scar over the site of the varix. Although it is easy to perform (only an injection catheter

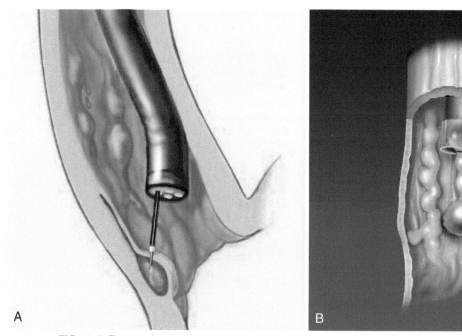

FIG 15.2 Two endoscopic methods used for the management of varices: **A,** sclerotherapy and **B,** band ligation.

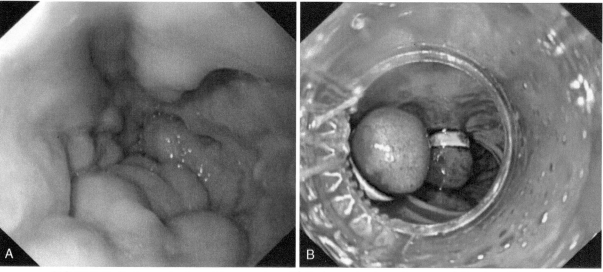

FIG 15.3 A, Endoscopic view of large varices. **B,** Endoscopic view of successfully placed bands in the distal esophagus.

and the sclerosant are needed) there are a significant number of local and systemic complications, which include esophageal ulcers, strictures, substernal chest pain, fever, dysphagia, and even the development of pleural effusions.[56,57] ES also increases the risk of bacteremia and can predispose one to spontaneous bacterial peritonitis or distal abscesses.[58,59] Other rare complications include perforation, mediastinitis, pericarditis, chylothorax, and esophageal motility disorders.[56,57,60,61]

EBL consists in the placement of several elastic bands (range between 4 to 10) on the varices to occlude the varix and cause thrombosis. Ligation of the varix and the surrounding mucosa eventually leads to necrosis of the mucosa. The bands fall off within 5 to 7 days, leaving a shallow ulcer that heals and subsequently scars. After the index treatment of an episode of AVB, scheduled repeated sessions need to be performed at 3- to 4-week intervals to completely obliterate the varices and reduce the risk of rebleeding.[62]

There are several commercially available multiband devices. They have between 4 and 10 preloaded bands (Fig. 15.4). Beginning the procedure with a 6- or 7-band device will allow for enough bands to be placed in a single session without having to repeatedly intubate the patient with the gastroscope. After the index diagnostic endoscopy is performed in a patient with AVB and the suspected varix is identified, the endoscope is withdrawn and the ligation device is loaded. After the varix is identified, the tip of the scope is pushed toward it and continuous suction applied so the mucosa of the varix fills the cap and causes a "red out" sign; at this point the band can be fired and a click is felt. The red out sign is always required; otherwise the band will inevitably be misfired. Afterwards, the scope should not be advanced distally. Band ligation should always commence in the most distal portion of the esophagus near the gastro-esophageal (GE) junction (Video 15.1). Bands are applied in a spiral pattern progressing up the esophagus until all major columns of varices of the lower third of the esophagus (no more than 8 to 10 cm above the GE junction) are banded. If there is a limited view because of ongoing bleeding, an option is to aggressively flush with water, perform suction, and start placing bands at the GE junction. This reduces the heavy bleeding and further bands can be fired afterwards.

The procedure can be associated with adverse events such as transient dysphagia and chest pain, which respond well to analgesics (i.e., liquid acetaminophen), as well as an oral suspension of antacids. A liquid diet should be started the same day and soft foods the next day. Shallow ulcers at the site of bands are frequent and can bleed in up to 4% of cases.[63] The use of a proton pump inhibitor (i.e., pantoprazole 40 mg/day for 10 days) decreases the size of ulcers but does not prevent them from bleeding.[64] Severe and rare complications such as massive bleeding from ulcers or rarely from variceal rupture, esophageal perforation, esophageal strictures, or altered esophageal motility, may occur with EBL.[65] If a patient bleeds due to an ulcer after EBL, ES may be performed if there is active bleeding or oozing, but this approach is often ineffective. Where available, an option is applying Hemospray (Cook Medical, Winston-Salem, NC) (a hemostatic powder) to the bleeding site. This powder, which is used for nonvariceal gastrointestinal bleeding, seems to be promising as a hemostatic technique for patients with portal gastropathy, variceal bleeding, and bleeding post-EBL ulcers.[66–68]

EBL is highly effective in the control of AVB, with an immediate efficacy in 90% of cases.[69] Several clinical trials and a meta-analysis indicate that EBL is better than ES for all major outcomes, including initial control of bleeding, recurrent bleeding, time to variceal eradication, and survival[70,71]; in addition, it is associated with less adverse events.[72] Therefore, EBL is considered the endoscopic therapy of choice in AVB. Although EBL is preferred over ES for an episode of AVB, in the setting of active hemorrhage or torrential bleeding, EBL may sometimes be difficult to perform due to lack of visibility. Therefore, both techniques are reasonable options in the setting of AVB.

Prevention of Recurrent Bleeding From Esophageal Varices

The combination of drug therapy with EBL is the recommended strategy for preventing variceal rebleeding.[73,74,75] Recent data suggest that NSBBs are the main drug responsible for the benefit of the combination.[76]

FAILURE TO CONTROL BLEEDING

During an acute episode of variceal bleeding, approximately 10% to 15% of patients do not respond to the previously mentioned therapies and controlled bleeding is not achieved. In such cases, if the patient is stable, a second therapeutic endoscopy may be performed. However, if this is unsuccessful or there is massive bleeding, the patient should be offered alternate treatment, before the clinical status further deteriorates. Both TIPS and surgical shunts are extremely effective at controlling

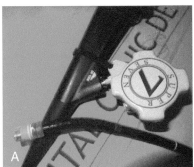 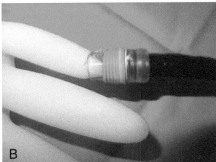 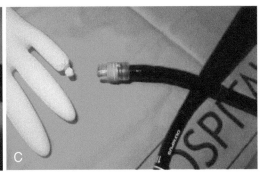

FIG 15.4 **A,** Band ligator placed on the shaft of the endoscope, the knob is attached to the working channel. **B,** The proximal end of the endoscope has a cap with premounted bands that allows for suction of the varix (in this case a glove is used). **C,** Once the varix is suctioned into the cap, the band is fired and the varix is ligated.

variceal bleeding, although TIPS is the first-choice treatment because most patients requiring rescue treatment have advanced liver disease.[14,77,78] However, until definitive treatments such as TIPS can be instituted, patients may require temporary placement of balloon tamponade or esophageal stents.

Current guidelines recommend using balloon tamponade only in massive bleeding, as a temporary "bridge" until definitive treatment can be instituted (for a maximum of 24 hours) in an intensive care unit.[79,80] Esophageal balloon tamponade, which is typically performed with a Sengstaken-Blakemore tube, causes hemostasis by direct compression of the bleeding varices. If placed properly, tamponade may provide initial control of bleeding in up to 85% of cases, but rebleeding is observed in 50% of the patients after deflation of the balloon.[81] The most common complications include aspiration pneumonia and esophageal perforation, which may occur in 30% of patients, with a mortality rate of 5% mainly due to perforation.[60] The incidence of complications increases with the duration of tamponade and when tubes are inserted by inexperienced staff. Therefore, tamponade should only be performed by skilled and experienced personnel in intensive care facilities and with special caution in patients with respiratory failure or cardiac arrhythmias. Because of the high risk of aspiration pneumonia, tamponade should be preceded by prophylactic orotracheal intubation.

A safer alternative to balloon tamponade is placing fully covered self-expandable metal stents which act as tamponade mechanism on the esophagus.[82] The main advantages include fewer side effects, ability to maintain enteral feeding, and the possibility to leave the stent in place for 1 week, which allows for stabilization of the patient in order to plan bridge therapies such as TIPS. The SX-Ella Danis stent (135 mm × 25 mm; ELLA-CS, Hradec Kralove, Czech Republic) is a removable, fully covered, self-expanding nitinol metal stent with atraumatic edges specifically designed for AVB (Fig. 15.5). It comes in a ready to use procedure pack that contains all items necessary for its placement. In addition, it has radiopaque markers at both ends

and at the midportion for monitoring with plain chest x-rays. The stent can be deployed in the lower esophagus without radiological or endoscopic assistance; however in some cases a prior endoscopy is useful as a means of leaving a rigid guidewire in the stomach, which later aids in placing the premounted stent. The procedure is relatively easy to perform but basic training is needed. The stent can be removed 7 days later endoscopically using an overtube system (Extractor for SX-ELLA Danis stent) without causing trauma to the esophagus.

A 2016 RCT comparing esophageal metal stent versus tamponade by using the Sengstaken-Blakemore balloon in patients with esophageal variceal bleeding refractory to medical and endoscopic treatment showed that success of therapy, defined as survival at day 15 with control of bleeding and without serious adverse events, was more frequent in the stent than in the tamponade group, with similar survival but less serious adverse events. Therefore, these findings favor the use of esophageal stent for refractory variceal bleeding.[83]

GASTRIC VARICEAL BLEEDING

Gastric varices (GV) are present in approximately 20% of patients with portal hypertension and are the source of 5% to 10% of all upper digestive bleeding episodes in patients with cirrhosis. The classification of GV by Sarin et al (1992) is the most commonly used for risk stratification and management[84] (Fig. 15.6). The most common are gastroesophageal varices type 1 (GOV1): EV extending below the cardia into the lesser curvature (75% of GV). These are usually managed as the EV. GOV type 2 (GOV2)

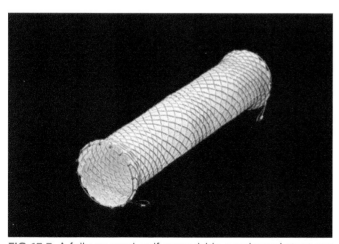

FIG 15.5 A fully covered, self-expandable esophageal stent can be placed in the esophagus as a rescue therapy in patients in whom variceal bleeding cannot be controlled by endoscopic therapy plus vasoactive drugs. The stent (SX-Ella Danis) is 135 mm long × 25 mm wide and has two threads in the distal and proximal end that allows the stent to be pulled endoscopically. (Courtesy ELLA-CS, Hradec Kralove, Czech Republic.)

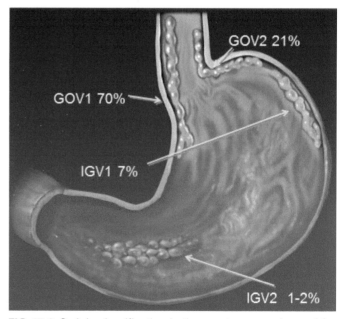

FIG 15.6 Sarin's classification is the most commonly used for risk stratification and management of gastric varices. GOV1: EV extend below the cardia into the lesser curvature. GOV type 2 (GOV2) are EV extending into the fundus, isolated GV type 1 (IGV1) are located in the fundus, whereas isolated GV type 2 (IGV2) are located elsewhere in the stomach. *EV*, esophageal varices; *GV*, gastric varices; *GOV*, gastroesophageal varices; *IGV*, isolated GV.

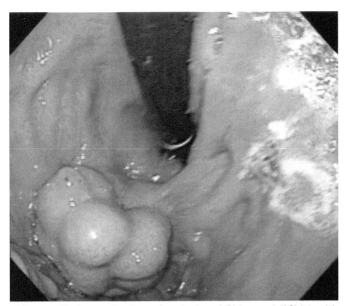

FIG 15.7 Endoscopic view of an isolated GV type 1 (IGV1) with stigmata of recent bleeding.

are EV extending into the fundus and account for 21% of GV. Isolated GV type 1 (IGV1) are located in the fundus (7%) (Fig. 15.7), whereas isolated GV type 2 (IGV2) are located elsewhere in the stomach (1%–2%).

The evidence to support management recommendations of GV bleeding is less robust than that for EV, as most data come from retrospective series. Few RCTs are available, and those that are have a small sample size and, in many occasions, no adequate stratification according to the type of GV or presence/severity of liver disease.

Prevention of First Hemorrhage From Gastric Varices

There is only one RCT on the primary prevention of gastric VH, including 89 patients with large (≥ 1 cm) GOV2 and IGV1 that were randomized to endoscopic obturation by cyanoacrylate (CYA) (glue) injection, NSBBs, and observation.[85] The number of patients with IGV1 was small (15%). Glue injection was associated with lower bleeding rates (10%) than NSBBs (38%) and observation (53%). Survival was better in the glue-treated group (93%) compared to observation (74%), but no different from NSBBs (83%). Although firm recommendations cannot be derived from this trial, the least invasive treatment is NSBBs and has the advantage that it may prevent other complications of cirrhosis.

Management of Gastric Variceal Bleeding

The current recommendations are to treat GOV1 (75% of all GV) as EV. By contrast, endoscopic therapy with tissue adhesives, mainly CYA,[86] is the recommended therapy for acute bleeding from GOV2 and IGV, including IGV1 (located in the fundus) and IGV2 (located anywhere in the stomach).[87–89] Lately, delivery of CYA under endoscopic ultrasound (EUS) guidance has been suggested to enable precise delivery of glue into the varix lumen and may improve the achieved obliteration rate and diminish adverse events.[90,91] Follow-up EUS may also be important to evaluate obliteration of larger varices and to retreat if necessary. Band ligation may be used in small GOV2 varices if obliteration

with tissue adhesives is not available. Balloon tamponade with the Linton-Nachlas tube may serve as a bridge to derivative treatments in massive bleedings.[92]

Prevention of Rebleeding From Gastric Varices
Endoscopic Variceal Obturation (CYA Glue Injection)
In one RCT, repeated CYA injection was superior to NSBBs preventing rebleeding and mortality in patients with cardiofundal varices.[93] In another trial, addition of NSBBs to CYA injection did not improve rebleeding or mortality compared to CYA injection alone.[94]

Transjugular Intrahepatic Portosystemic Shunt
AN RCT including patients with GOV1 and GOV2 varices showed TIPS to be more effective than glue injection in preventing rebleeding,[95] with more than a 90% success rate for initial hemostasis and a very low rebleeding rate, although survival was similar.

Balloon Occluded Retrograde Transvenous Obliteration (BRTO)
This procedure for treatment of fundal varices associated with a large gastro/splenorenal collateral involves retrograde catheterization of the left renal vein, followed by balloon occlusion and slow infusion of sclerosant to obliterate the gastro/splenorenal collateral and fundal varices.[96–98] BRTO could be an alternative treatment when TIPS cannot be performed, especially in patients with extrahepatic portal vein obstruction. BRTO presents the potential advantage over TIPS that it does not shunt portal blood flow away from the liver and therefore can be performed on patients with poor hepatic reserve.

PORTAL HYPERTENSIVE GASTROPATHY

Portal hypertensive gastropathy, and other gastric vascular lesions observed in patients with cirrhosis, is discussed in Chapter 18.

SUMMARY (FIG. 15.8)

Portal hypertensive bleeding is a dreaded complication of patients with cirrhosis and portal hypertension. Primary prophylaxis to avoid bleeding from varices should be done in patients with a high risk of bleeding (i.e., Child B or C cirrhosis or presence of red wale marks). Patients should receive therapy with nonselective β-blockers if there are no contraindications. Those patients who develop side effects or have contraindications to β-blockers should be offered endoscopic variceal band ligation. Initial management of acute variceal bleeding should focus on resuscitation with adequate volume replacement, careful blood transfusions of blood to keep hemoglobin levels at 7 g/L, antibiotic prophylaxis, and endotracheal intubation in selected cases. Standard of care mandates for early administration of vasoactive drugs and EBL within the first 12 hours of the index bleed. In addition, patients should be evaluated to decide if they are candidates for a preemptive TIPS. Patients that fail combined pharmacological and endoscopic therapy may require temporary placement of balloon tamponade or esophageal stents until definitive treatment (preferably TIPS) can be instituted. Given the available data, esophageal stents in this setting are preferred. Patients that fail the previously mentioned therapies should undergo an evaluation for TIPS. Patients that recover from an episode of variceal bleeding should undergo combination therapy with endoscopic

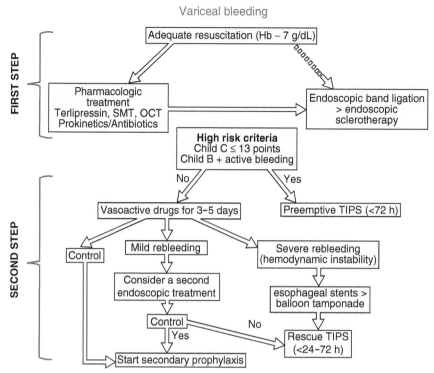

FIG 15.8 Recommended algorithm for the treatment of an episode of acute variceal bleeding (AVB). Placement of transjugular intrahepatic portosystemic shunts (TIPS) (within 72 hrs) for patients AVB with Child B actively bleeding or C cirrhosis (< 13 points) is associated with a significant reduction in rebleeding and mortality and can be considered in such cases. Temporary measures include placement of an esophageal stent or balloon tamponade. Esophageal stents are preferred, as they are safer and more effective. The use of the balloon is associated with potentially lethal complications such as aspiration and perforation of the esophagus. *Hb*, haemoglobin; *OCT*, octreotide; *SMT*, somatostatin.

variceal ligation plus nonselective β-blockers for the prevention of recurrent VH. Bleeding episodes from gastric varices GOV2 + IGV1 are usually severe and sometimes difficult to control. Endoscopic injection of *N*-butyl-2-cyanoacrylate glue is one of the cornerstones of therapy as this measure is effective in over 90% to 95% of patients presenting with acute bleeding from gastric varices. Patients that cannot be controlled by this measure require TIPS.

KEY REFERENCES

1. de Franchis R, Baveno V Faculty: Revising consensus in portal hypertension: report of the Baveno V consensus workshop on methodology of diagnosis and therapy in portal hypertension, *J Hepatol* 54:1082–1083, 2011.
7. Merli M, Nicolini G, Angeloni S, et al: Incidence and natural history of small esophageal varices in cirrhotic patients, *J Hepatol* 38:266–272, 2003.
11. Groszmann RJ, Bosch J, Grace ND, et al: Hemodynamic events in a prospective randomized trial of propranolol versus placebo in the prevention of a first variceal hemorrhage, *Gastroenterology* 99:1401–1407, 1990.
13. Merkel C, Marin R, Angeli P, et al: A placebo-controlled clinical trial of nadolol in the prophylaxis of growth of small esophageal varices in cirrhosis, *Gastroenterology* 127:476–484, 2004.
14. de Franchis R: Baveno VI Faculty: Expanding consensus in portal hypertension. Report of the Baveno VI Consensus Workshop: stratifying

risk and individualizing care for portal hypertension, *J Hepatol* 63:743–752, 2015.
16. D'Amico G, Pagliaro L, Bosch J: Pharmacological treatment of portal hypertension: an evidence-based approach, *Semin Liver Dis* 19:475–505, 1999.
19. Reiberger T, Ulbrich G, Ferlitsch A, et al: Carvedilol for primary prophylaxis of variceal bleeding in cirrhotic patients with haemodynamic non-response to propranolol, *Gut* 62:1634–1641, 2013.
24. Gluud LL, Krag A: Banding ligation versus beta-blockers for primary prevention in oesophageal varices in adults, *Cochrane Database Syst Rev* (8):CD004544, 2012.
25. Garcia-Tsao G, Sanyal A, Grace N, et al: Prevention and management of gastroesophageal varices and variceal hemorrhage in cirrhosis, *Am J Gastroenterol* 102:2086–2102, 2007.
26. Sarin SK, Wadhawan M, Agarwal SR, et al: Endoscopic variceal ligation plus propranolol versus endoscopic variceal ligation alone in primary prophylaxis of variceal bleeding, *Am J Gastroenterol* 100:797–804, 2005.
31. Cárdenas A, Ginès P, Uriz J, et al: Renal failure after upper gastrointestinal bleeding in cirrhosis: incidence, clinical course, predictive factors, and short-term prognosis, *Hepatology* 34:671–676, 2001.
37. García-Pagán JC, Caca K, Bureau C, et al: Early use of TIPS in patients with cirrhosis and variceal bleeding, *N Engl J Med* 362:2370–2379, 2010.
38. Garcia-Pagán JC, Di Pascoli M, Caca K, et al: Use of early-TIPS for high-risk variceal bleeding: results of a post-RCT surveillance study, *J Hepatol* 58:45–50, 2013.

49. Escorsell À, Bordas J, del Arbol L, et al: Randomized controlled trial of sclerotherapy versus somatostatin infusion in the prevention of early rebleeding following acute variceal hemorrhage in patients with cirrhosis, *J Hepatol* 29:779–788, 1998.

73. Villanueva C, Minana J, Ortiz J, et al: Endoscopic ligation compared with combined treatment with nadolol and isosorbide mononitrate to prevent recurrent variceal bleeding, *N Engl J Med* 345:647–655, 2001.

83. Escorsell A, Pavel O, Cardenas A, et al: Esophageal balloon tamponade versus esophageal stent in controlling acute refractory variceal bleeding: a multicenter randomized, controlled trial, *Hepatology* 63:1957–1967, 2016.

84. Sarin SK, Lahoti D, Saxena SP, et al: Prevalence, classification and natural history of gastric varices: a long-term follow-up study in 568 portal hypertension patients, *Hepatology* 16:1343–1349, 1992.

A complete reference list can be found online at ExpertConsult .com

16

Lower Gastrointestinal Bleeding

Wilson T. Kwong and Thomas J. Savides

INTRODUCTION

Acute severe lower gastrointestinal (GI) bleeding is a common problem and frequent reason for hospitalization. Colonoscopy is often performed for diagnosis and potential therapeutic intervention. This chapter focuses on moderate to severe acute lower GI bleeding, defined as hematochezia, from a bleeding source distal to the ileocecal valve with an onset of less than 3 days of duration. This presentation usually prompts presentation to the emergency room and subsequent hospitalization.

EPIDEMIOLOGY

Lower GI bleeding occurs at a rate of 36.5 per 100,000 in the adult population, based on a national inpatient database.[1] Assuming that an average, full-time clinical gastroenterologist is responsible for 50,000 adult lives, he or she would see approximately 20 cases per year. Most cases occur in elderly patients, given the increased frequency and risk for diverticulosis, vascular disease, and colonic malignancy.[2] Risk of lower GI bleeding is also associated with the use of aspirin and nonsteroidal antiinflammatory drugs (NSAIDs).[3,4]

A large US database study comprising 227,000 patients with discharge diagnoses of lower GI bleeds in 2002 reported an overall mortality rate of 3.9%.[5] A more recent (2012) study examining a national inpatient database revealed a lower mortality rate of 1.5% in 2009.[1]

INITIAL APPROACH TO A PATIENT WITH HEMATOCHEZIA

The initial approach to a patient with lower GI bleeding is directed towards determining the severity of bleeding, the etiology, and volume resuscitation. This includes obtaining a thorough history, orthostatic vital signs, laboratory testing, and physical and rectal examinations. Patients should be asked about whether they saw red blood or dark maroon blood, duration of symptoms, previous episodes of GI bleeding, a history of peptic ulcer disease, symptoms of abdominal pain or fever, travel history, prior colonoscopy or endoscopy results, prior pelvic radiation, surgical history, history of diverticulosis, and prior abdominal imaging studies. Patients should also be asked about use of medications associated with GI bleeding (e.g., aspirin, NSAIDs, and anticoagulants). Accompanying symptoms of weight loss or a change in bowel habits suggests possible colon cancer. Abdominal pain usually suggests ischemic colitis, although abdominal pain can be present in other colitides and malignancy. The presence of fever and leukocytosis is also suggestive of a colitis.

The most important parts of the physical examination are the vital signs and the stool/rectal examination. The presence of bright red blood on rectal examination strongly suggests the possibility of colonic bleeding. Bright red blood per rectum is generally from a colonic source, unless it is accompanied by hypotension, which can either occur during a severe upper GI bleed or a small bowel bleed with rapid transit of blood.[6] An elevated blood urea nitrogen/creatinine (BUN/Cr) ratio of greater than 30 is suggestive of an upper GI source of bleeding.[7] In the setting of hematochezia without hypotension, placement of a diagnostic nasogastric (NG) tube is usually unnecessary because it is unlikely that there is a severe upper GI bleed without hypotension. If there is hypotension and hematochezia, a severe upper GI bleed is possible, and an NG tube should be placed. A clear NG tube lavage does not always imply a lower GI source because 16% of patients with duodenal ulcer bleeds have negative NG lavage.[8] If bile is seen in the NG tube lavage, it is unlikely to be an upper GI bleed. Physical examination should also focus on abdominal tenderness, surgical scars, and stigmata of liver disease. At least one large bore intravenous catheter should be placed, with two placed in the setting of ongoing bleeding to allow for adequate resuscitation and transfusion as needed.

Blood should be sent for complete blood count, international normalized ratio (INR), chemistry panel, and type and crossmatch for packed red blood cells. Resuscitation should be initiated simultaneously with assessment. Intravenous fluids should be infused as fast as needed to keep systolic blood pressure greater than 100 mm Hg and pulse lower than 100 beats/min. Patients are transfused with packed red blood cells with a goal of 7 g/dL or a higher goal of 9 g/dL in the setting of massive bleeding or cardiac ischemia.[9]

Most patients with lower GI bleeding can be admitted to a medical ward. Patients with active bleeding should be admitted to a monitored intermediate care unit or intensive care unit (ICU), especially if there is persistent tachycardia or hypotension despite initial resuscitation. Hemoglobin levels should be obtained every 4 to 6 hours until the patient has a stable level. Patients older than age 60 or with risk factors for coronary artery disease should be evaluated for potential cardiac ischemia induced by anemia, hypotension, and blood loss.

Endoscopy of any sort should be done only when it can be performed safely and when the information may influence patient care. Patients should be resuscitated with fluids and transfusions before endoscopy. Ideally, patients should be hemodynamically stable, with a heart rate of less than 100 beats/min and systolic blood pressure greater than 100 mm Hg. Hemoglobin should be at least 7 g/dL. Severe thrombocytopenia (platelet count < 50,000/mm³) should be corrected with transfusions before emergency endoscopy, and elevated INR above 2.5 should be considered for correction with intravenous vitamin K or fresh frozen plasma. However, decisions to reverse anticoagulation should be made on an individual basis based on risk of thrombosis and severity of bleeding. Patients taking direct oral anticoagulants including rivaroxaban, apixaban, edoxaban, and dabigatran appear to have a similar risk of GI bleeding compared to patients taking warfarin.[10–12]

Early Predictors of Severity in Acute Lower Gastrointestinal Bleeding

Early predictors (within 4 hours of admission) of severity for continued or recurrent bleeding after 24 hours of hospitalization include a heart rate greater than 100 beats/min, systolic blood pressure less than 115 mm Hg, syncope, nontender abdominal examination, observed rectal bleeding during the first 4 hours of hospital evaluation, aspirin ingestion, and the presence of more than two comorbid conditions (Box 16.1).[13,14] This prediction model has been prospectively validated; the low-risk group (no risk factors) had a 0% risk of rebleeding, the moderate-risk group (1–3 risk factors) had a 45% risk of rebleeding, and the high-risk group (> 3 risk factors) had a 77% risk of rebleeding.[14] It is possible that factors such as these can be used to help triage patients to the appropriate level of care, such as ICU, hospital ward, or outpatient evaluation, as well as urgent versus elective endoscopic evaluation.

Multivariate analysis found that independent predictors of in-hospital mortality were age (> 70 years), intestinal ischemia, presence of two or more comorbid illnesses, bleeding while hospitalized for a separate condition, coagulopathies, hypovolemia, transfusion of packed red blood cells, and male gender. Colorectal polyps and hemorrhoids were associated with a lower mortality

---

> **BOX 16.1   Early Predictors of Severity of Continued or Recurrent Lower Gastrointestinal**
>
> **Bleeding**
> Heart rate >100 beats/min
> Systolic blood pressure < 115 mm Hg
> Syncope
> Nontender abdominal examination
> Observed rectal bleeding during first 4 hours of hospital evaluation
> Aspirin
> More than two comorbid conditions

From Strate LL, Orav EJ, Syngal S: Early predictors of severity in acute lower intestinal tract bleeding. *Arch Intern Med* 163:838–843, 2003; and Strate LL, Saltzman JR, Ookubo R, et al: Validation of a clinical prediction rule for severe acute lower intestinal bleeding. *Am J Gastroenterol* 100:1821–1827, 2005.

---

risk. Patients who develop severe lower GI bleeding while hospitalized for other lesions have a much higher mortality rate than patients admitted with lower GI bleeding. In a large retrospective study, the in-hospital mortality rate for patients with lower GI bleeding who began as outpatients was 2.4% compared with 23% for patients with in-hospital lower GI bleeding ($P < .001$).[2]

DIAGNOSTIC OPTIONS

Most patients should undergo initial evaluation with colonoscopy after adequate bowel preparation. However, in selected cases, flexible sigmoidoscopy with enema or oral bowel preparation can be considered. Other diagnostic tests such as angiography, computed tomography (CT) scans (including CT colonography and CT angiography), and tagged red blood cell nuclear scans, can be considered.

Anoscopy

Anoscopy can be useful if actively bleeding hemorrhoids are suspected. However, nearly every patient requires additional visualization of the more proximal colon using colonoscopy or possibly sigmoidoscopy. Therefore anoscopy is of limited utility in the setting of moderate to severe lower GI bleeding and is rarely performed for this purpose.

Flexible Sigmoidoscopy

Occasionally, flexible sigmoidoscopy may be performed to quickly evaluate the left side of the colon for any bleeding site stigmata, rather than waiting for a full colonoscopy bowel preparation, and this results in a diagnosis in approximately 9% of cases.[15] Flexible sigmoidoscopy can be considered in those with imaging studies such as CT scan or prior colonoscopy, suggesting a distal source of bleeding or postpolypectomy bleeding where the location of blood loss is strongly suspected to be distal. This may also be appropriate for patients with a suspected left-sided colitis or obstructing mass.

Nuclear Medicine Scintigraphy

Nuclear medicine scintigraphy involves injecting a radiolabeled substance in the patient's bloodstream and then performing serial scintigraphy to detect focal collections of radiolabeled material. It has been reported to detect bleeding at a rate of 0.1 mL/min.[16] The overall positive diagnostic rate is approximately 45%, with a 78% accuracy in the localization of the true bleeding site.[17] The most common false-positive result occurs when there is rapid transit of luminal blood such that labeled blood is detected in the colon, although it originated in the upper GI tract. The main drawback to nuclear medicine scintigraphy is that it results in a delay to therapeutic intervention in those with active bleeding. Scintigraphy may be better suited for intermittent, obscure, overt GI bleeding despite evaluation with endoscopy and colonoscopy.[9]

Angiography

In patients with severe hematochezia from a lower GI source felt to be too unstable for colonoscopy, angiography with the intention of embolization should be considered. NG tube placement or upper endoscopy (EGD) should be considered first to rule out a brisk upper GI bleed. Angiography is positive when the arterial bleeding rate is at least 0.5 mL/min.[18] The diagnostic yield depends on patient selection, timing of the procedure, and the skill of the angiographer, with positive yields in 12% to 69% of cases. Advantages of angiography are the ability to perform the procedure immediately without the need for bowel preparation, the opportunity for therapeutic embolization at the same time, and the ability to manage upper GI or small bowel bleeds that were incorrectly presumed to be a lower GI bleed. Disadvantages include a 3% rate of major complications, including hematoma formation, femoral artery thrombosis, contrast dye reactions, renal failure, and transient ischemic attacks.[19] Another disadvantage is the requirement for active bleeding at the time of angiography, otherwise a target is not visible for embolization.

Computed Tomography

Urgent contrast enhanced multidetector CT has been studied in the evaluation of lower GI bleeding. A large retrospective series of 1604 patients with a lower GI bleed who underwent urgent CT scan performed within the first 24 hours reported higher rates of bleeding source identification during colonoscopy (68% vs. 20%) in diverticular bleeding when contrast extravasation was detected on CT scan.[20] The same study also suggested that CT scan also helps determine optimal timing of colonoscopy as elective colonoscopy can be done in patients with colonic thickening on CT, suggesting colitis or malignancy, and urgent colonoscopy should be done in the absence of these findings. CT scan should be considered early in the course of evaluation in patients with significant abdominal pain, fevers, leukocytosis, and risk factors for vascular disease to evaluate for colitis, which may preclude the need for urgent colonoscopy in patients with self-limited lower GI bleeding. Colonoscopy can be performed on an elective basis in these patients, especially at centers where colonoscopy is not readily available.

Colonoscopy

Urgent colonoscopy using a rapid purge has been shown to be safe, to provide important diagnostic information, and sometimes to allow therapeutic intervention.[21] Patients usually ingest 4 to 8 L of polyethylene glycol either orally or via NG tube over 3 to 5 hours until the rectal effluent is clear of stool, blood, and clots. Metoclopramide may be given intravenously before the purge and repeated after 3 to 4 hours to facilitate gastric emptying and reduce nausea.

Most "urgent" colonoscopies for lower GI bleeds are performed 6 to 36 hours after the patient is admitted to the hospital. Because most bleeding stops spontaneously, cases are often performed electively the day after hospitalization to allow the patient to receive blood transfusions and to finish the bowel preparation.

The overall diagnostic yield of a presumed or definite etiology using colonoscopy in lower GI bleeding ranges from 48% to 90%, with an average of 68%, based on a review of 13 studies.[17] The problem with interpreting these data is that it is often impossible to determine a definite diagnosis of the cause of the bleeding, unless bleeding stigmata are identified, such as active bleeding, a visible vessel, an adherent clot, mucosal friability or ulceration, or the presence of fresh blood limited to a specific part of the colon. A presumptive diagnosis is often made, especially in the case of diverticular bleeding, in which no blood is seen but there is a potential bleeding site present.

The optimal time for performing urgent bowel preparation and colonoscopy is unknown. Theoretically, the sooner the colonoscopy is performed, the higher the likelihood of finding a lesion that might be amenable to hemostasis, such as a bleeding diverticulum or polyp stalk. However, a retrospective study from the Mayo Clinic suggested that there was no significant association between the time of endoscopy (0 to 12 hours, 12 to 24 hours, > 24 hours) and the findings of active bleeding or other stigmata that would prompt colonoscopic hemostasis in patients with diverticular bleeding.[22] A randomized trial comparing urgent colonoscopy within 12 hours to colonoscopy performed within 36 to 60 hours reported similar outcomes with regards to further bleeding, blood transfusions, hospital days, subsequent therapeutic interventions for bleeding, and hospital charges.[1] Therefore, the benefit of urgent over elective colonoscopy has not been clearly established.

Surgery

Surgical management is rarely needed for lower GI bleeding because most bleeding is either self-limited or managed with endoscopic therapy or angiography. The main indications for surgery are malignant lesions and recurrent bleeding from diverticula.

ETIOLOGY AND PATHOGENESIS OF SEVERE LOWER GASTROINTESTINAL BLEEDING

It is not always possible to visualize active bleeding during colonoscopy. A definite diagnosis of a bleeding lesion can usually be made if active bleeding is seen or if there are obvious stigmata, such as an adherent clot or visible vessel. A presumptive diagnosis can be made if there is a suspicious lesion and no other possible sources. Table 16.1 lists the frequency of various presumed or definite sites of acute colonic bleeding.[23] Potential colonic lesions amenable to endoscopic hemostasis include diverticula, postpolypectomy bleeding, angiodysplasia, hemorrhoids, Dieulafoy's lesions, tumors, ulcers, varices, and radiation proctitis.

Diverticular Bleeding

Colonic diverticula are herniations of colonic mucosa and submucosa through the muscular layers of the colon. Diverticula in the colon are actually pathologic pseudodiverticula because true diverticula contain all layers of the intestinal wall. Colonic diverticula seem to form when colonic tissue is pushed out by intraluminal pressure. Diverticula occur at the point of entry of the small arteries that supply the colon, the vasa recta, as they penetrate the circular muscle layer of the colonic wall (Fig. 16.1). The entry points of the vasa recta are areas of relative weakness

TABLE 16.1   Etiology of Severe Lower Gastrointestinal Bleeding*

Cause	Cases (%)
Diverticulosis	33
Cancer/polyps	19
Colitis	18
Unknown	16
Angiodysplasia	8
Other	8
Postpolypectomy	6
Anorectal	4

*Summary of 1333 patients in seven published studies.
From Zuckerman GR, Prakash C: Acute lower intestinal bleeding. Part II. Etiology, therapy, and outcomes. *Gastrointest Endosc* 49:228–238, 1999.

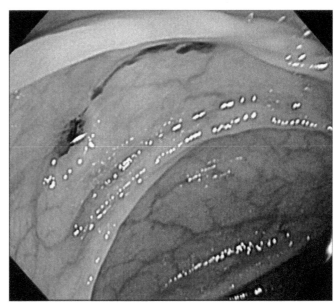

FIG 16.2 Stigmata of recent bleeding from a diverticulum.

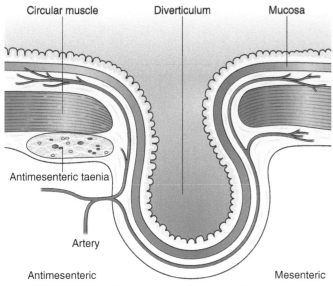

FIG 16.1 Vascular anatomy of colonic diverticulum.

through which the mucosa and submucosa can herniate when under increased intraluminal pressure. They vary in diameter from a few milliliters to several centimeters. The most common location is the left colon.

Most colonic diverticula are asymptomatic and remain uncomplicated. Bleeding may occur from vessels at the neck or base of the diverticulum.[24] Diverticula are common in Western countries, with a prevalence of 50% in older adults.[25] In contrast, less than 1% of people living in continental Africa and Asia have diverticula.[26] This finding has led to the hypothesis that regional differences in prevalence can be explained by the low amounts of dietary fiber in Western diets. Presumably, a low-fiber diet results in less stool content, longer fecal transit time, increased colonic muscle contraction, and, ultimately, increased intraluminal pressure that results in the formation of pulsion diverticula. In addition, diverticula occur with increasing frequency with advanced age, which could be a result of weakening of the colonic wall and muscle tone.

It has been estimated that 3% to 5% of patients with diverticulosis develop diverticular bleeding.[27] Although most diverticula are in the left colon, several series suggest that bleeding diverticula

occur more often in the right colon.[24,27-29] Patients with diverticular bleeding are typically elderly and present with painless hematochezia. They have often been taking aspirin or NSAIDs. In at least 75% of patients with diverticular bleeding, the bleeding stops spontaneously.[28] Patients in whom bleeding stops usually require less than 4 units of blood transfusion. Patients with successful resection of a bleeding diverticulum had a rebleeding rate of 4%.[28] Among patients in whom bleeding stopped spontaneously, the rebleeding rate from colonic diverticulosis was 25% to 38% over the next 4 years.[2,28] Urgent colonoscopy after rapid bowel preparation often reveals that bleeding has stopped by the time of colonoscopy, and only nonbleeding diverticula are detected. These patients are given the diagnosis of "presumptive diverticular bleed" because the diverticula are the only likely source of bleeding, although no stigmata were identified.

Occasionally, urgent colonoscopy reveals stigmata of recent bleeding, such as active bleeding, a visible vessel, clot, or blood limited to one segment of the colon (Fig. 16.2). It seems possible that earlier colonoscopy in lower GI bleeding would result in a greater frequency of finding stigmata of recent diverticular bleeding. However, a small case series did not find any differences in the detection rate of active bleeding or bleeding stigmata if colonoscopy was performed between 0 and 12 hours, 12 and 24 hours, or more than 24 hours from the time of hospital admission.[22] There have been attempts to stratify patients with diverticular bleeding at increased risk for rebleeding, employing the same endoscopic stigmata used in high-risk peptic ulcer bleeding (active bleeding, visible vessel, and clot), although the natural history for each of these untreated stigmata is unknown. The "pigmented protuberance" found on the edge of some diverticula at histopathology is usually clot at the edge of a ruptured blood vessel.[30]

The UCLA/CURE group found that among patients with stigmata of recent diverticular hemorrhage (six active bleeding, four visible vessels, and seven adherent clots), there was a very high rebleed rate of 53% and an emergency surgery rate of 35%.[31] Colonoscopic hemostasis of actively bleeding diverticula has been reported using bipolar probe coagulation, epinephrine injection, metallic clips, rubber band ligation, and fibrin glue.[30–37] If fresh red blood is seen in a focal segment of colon, we try to examine this segment of bowel carefully to detect the exact bleeding site. If the bleeding is coming from the edge of the diverticulum or there is a pigmented protuberance on the edge, we initially inject 1:10,000 epinephrine in 1-mL aliquots using a sclerotherapy needle into four quadrants around the bleeding site. Then we use either an endoscopic clip or a bipolar probe at a low power setting (10 to 15 W) and light pressure for a 1-second pulse duration to cauterize the diverticular edge and stop bleeding or flatten the visible vessel. If there is a nonbleeding adherent clot, we inject around the clot with 1:10,000 epinephrine in four quadrants with 1 mL per quadrant and remove the clot in piecemeal fashion using a cold snare. The clot is shaved down until it is 3 mm above the diverticulum, and then the underlying stigma is treated with either endoscopic clip or bipolar probe coagulation as discussed previously. After performing endoscopic hemostasis of a bleeding diverticulum, a permanent submucosal tattoo and a metal clip (if not previously placed) should be placed in the adjacent mucosa to identify the site in case colonoscopy, angiographic embolization, or surgery is required for recurrent bleeding. For long-term management after colonoscopic hemostasis, patients are told to avoid NSAIDs.

In 2000, Jensen and colleagues in the UCLA/CURE group[31] published their results on urgent colonoscopy for diagnosis and treatment of severe diverticular hemorrhage. The investigators found that 20% of patients with severe hematochezia had endoscopic stigmata suggesting a definite diverticular bleed. Compared with a historical control group with high-risk stigmata but no colonoscopic hemostasis, the group receiving colonoscopic hemostasis had a rebleed rate of 0% versus 53% and an emergency hemicolectomy rate of 0% versus 35%. After 3 years of follow-up, there were no rebleeding episodes in the patients who underwent colonoscopic hemostasis. In contrast to the UCLA experience, a smaller, retrospective review of the Duke University reported 13 patients with active bleeding or stigmata who received endoscopic treatment with epinephrine or bipolar coagulation or both.[38] The 30-day rebleed rate was 38%; four of these patients underwent surgery. The long-term rebleed rate was 23% with a mean follow-up of 3 years.

Angiographic embolization can also be performed in selected cases of diverticular bleeding, but there is a risk of bowel infarction and renal failure. Surgical resection for diverticular bleeding is usually reserved for recurrent bleeding episodes. Resection should be guided by colonoscopic, angiographic, or nuclear medicine studies showing the likely bleeding site. The need for surgery is often guided by certainty regarding the bleeding site and medical comorbidity because diverticular bleeding is often mild, and the risks of surgical complications are increased in elderly patients.

Colon Cancer

Most patients with colon cancer present with occult GI blood loss rather than hematochezia. For adult patients with hematochezia, determining the presence or absence of a colon cancer is imperative because early diagnosis improves survival. Because a cancer must ulcerate for overt bleeding to occur, most bleeding cancers are at a relatively advanced tumor stage (Fig. 16.3A) but can be seen with nonmalignant polyps (see Fig. 16.3B). Bleeding is usually mild and self-limited. Active bleeding from a malignant colonic lesion is often challenging given the large size of lesions, abnormal nature of the tissue, and often diffuse nature. For instances of bleeding from a focal area of a malignant lesion, endoscopic clipping either with traditional or over the scope clips, bipolar cauterization, or epinephrine injection can be considered. There are reports of successful hemostasis on bleeding colonic malignancies with hemostatic powders that have the benefit of ease of use and ability to treat larger areas.[39]

Colitis

The term *colitis* refers to any form of inflammation of the colon. With regard to severe lower GI bleeding, this is usually ischemic colitis, inflammatory bowel disease, or possibly infectious colitis. Ischemic colitis generally manifests as hematochezia with left-sided abdominal discomfort. It results from mucosal hypoxia and is thought to be caused by hypoperfusion of the intramural vessels of the intestinal wall rather than by large vessel occlusion. Most cases do not have a recognizable cause, but associated conditions include recent aortic or cardiac surgery, vasculitis, and medications.[40,41] Because of collateral circulation, ischemic involvement is usually segmental and primarily affects the mucosal aspect of

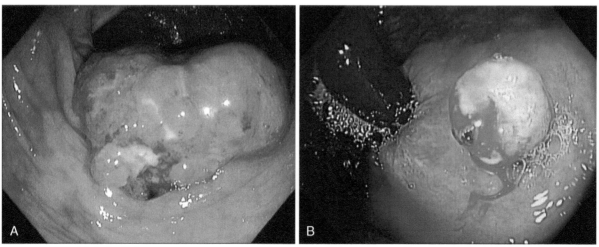

FIG 16.3 A, Colon cancer as source of hematochezia. **B,** Nonmalignant polyp as source of hematochezia.

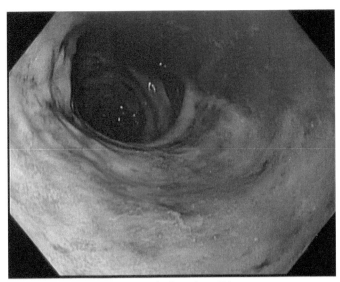

FIG 16.4 Ischemic colitis.

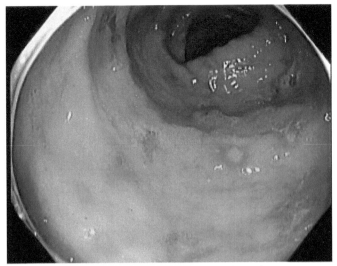

FIG 16.6 Infectious colitis with ulceration.

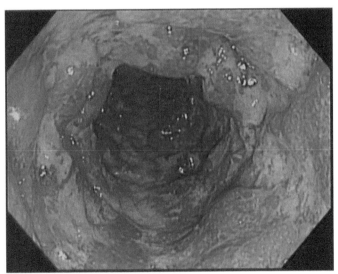

FIG 16.5 Crohn's colitis with ulceration.

the intestine. The colon is mostly affected in the watershed areas, such as the splenic flexure or rectosigmoid junction in which there is reduced collateral circulation, although ischemia can occur anywhere.

The diagnosis of ischemic colitis is usually confirmed by colonoscopy but can be suspected by "thumbprinting" on plain film radiographs or, more commonly, colonic wall thickening on CT scan. The colonoscopic appearance includes erythema, friability, and exudate (Fig. 16.4). Biopsy specimens may be suggestive of ischemic changes but, more importantly, are used to exclude Crohn's disease and infection. Ischemic colitis generally resolves in a few days and does not require colonoscopic hemostasis. In a large retrospective series from Kaiser Permanente San Diego, there were no episodes of rebleeding from ischemic colitis over a 4-year period.[2] Inflammatory bowel disease affecting the colon can cause friability and ulceration of the colon (Fig. 16.5) though rarely cause severe acute lower GI bleeding. In a case series from the Mayo Clinic, most patients had Crohn's disease[42] and were successfully treated medically. Three of the 31 patients in the

series received endoscopic therapy with epinephrine injection alone or with bipolar coagulation for adherent clots or oozing ulcers in Crohn's disease. Of the patients with Crohn's disease with severe bleeding, 39% required surgical management.

Infectious colitis should be excluded in any patient with severe lower GI bleeding and colitis. Lower GI bleeding can occur with infection by *Campylobacter jejuni*, *Salmonella*, *Shigella*, invasive *Escherichia coli*, *E. coli* 0157, *Clostridium difficile*, or *cytomegalovirus*. Significant blood loss is rare. Diagnosis is made by stool testing and flexible sigmoidoscopy which can reveal a nonspecific colitis or ulcers (Fig. 16.6).

Angiodysplasia

Colonic angiomas are also referred to as angiodysplasia, arteriovenous malformations, or vascular ectasias. These appear as flat or slightly raised, red, ectatic vessels that have been described to have a spider-like appearance (Fig. 16.7A, B). They are generally uncommon; less than 1% of asymptomatic patients undergoing screening colonoscopy were found to have angiodysplasia.[43] The lesions seem to increase with age and may represent degeneration of previously normal blood vessels in the cecum and proximal ascending colon. Histopathology reveals a large, dilated, submucosal vein and, in advanced cases, dilated mucosal veins with small arteriovenous communications. Proposed explanations for angioma formation include the partial obstruction of submucosal veins passing through the colonic muscle layers, with eventual dilation of the submucosal and mucosal veins, and local mucosal ischemia.

Medical conditions associated with angiomas include chronic renal failure and hereditary hemorrhagic telangiectasia (Osler-Weber-Rendu syndrome). There have been reports suggesting that aortic stenosis is associated with lower GI bleeding, presumably from colonic angiomas.[44] The potential biologic explanation is that aortic stenosis causes defects in von Willebrand factor, which causes the patient to have decreased platelet adhesion and increased bleeding tendency, especially if there were preexisting mucosal GI lesions such as angiomas.[45,46] Clinical studies do not support the association between aortic stenosis and the presence of angiomas, however.[47,48] Bleeding from angiodysplasia is usually painless and usually occurs from the right colon.

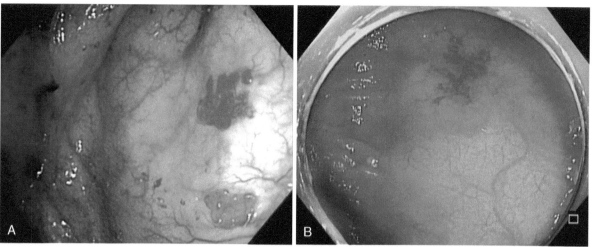

FIG 16.7 **A** and **B,** Arteriovenous malformations.

In recent decades, it seems that the reported frequency of angiomas as the source of lower GI bleeding has decreased.[21,31] This may be because of better recognition of angiomas with improved endoscope technology and increased attribution to presumed diverticular bleeding as the cause of hematochezia. Endoscopic hemostasis with argon plasma coagulation is reported to be successful in 85% of cases though endoscopic clipping can be considered in patients on antiplatelet agents or anticoagulation (Video 16.1). In patients with persistent bleeding from angiodysplasia, treatment with thalidomide or octreotide can lead to a clinical response in 71% and 77% of patients, respectively.[49]

Postpolypectomy Bleeding

Postpolypectomy bleeding occurs after between 1% and 6% of polypectomies, usually within the first 7 days.[50] It is generally mild and self-limited. Reported risk factors for postpolypectomy bleeding include large polyps (> 2 cm), thick stalks, sessile polyps, and right colon polyps.[50] The endoscopic appearance of delayed postpolypectomy bleeding can be variable depending on the timing of colonoscopy. The appearance can range from a well-defined, clean-based ulceration (Fig. 16.8A, B) to active bleeding from a poorly defined ulcerated region (see Fig. 16.8C). Endoscopic management techniques include hemoclips, epinephrine injection, thermal coagulation, and endoloops (Fig. 16.9, Videos 16.2 and 16.3).[50–53] In a case series from the Mayo Clinic, the median time to bleeding after polypectomy was 5 days (range 0 to 17 days).[52] Of patients, 65% received aspirin, NSAIDs, warfarin, heparin, or steroids after polypectomy; 76% required transfusions; and 96% were managed endoscopically with coagulation or epinephrine injection or both. A randomized trial of 413 patients demonstrated no reduction in the risk of postpolypectomy with routine clipping in polyps with a mean size of 8 mm.[54] A 2013 series on polypectomy of sessile or flat polyps greater than 2 cm in size demonstrated a significant reduction in postpolypectomy bleeding from 10% to 2% when the defect is completely closed.[55]

Radiation Proctitis

Radiation proctitis usually causes mild, chronic hematochezia but occasionally can cause acute severe lower GI bleeding. Ionizing radiation can cause acute and chronic damage to the normal colon and rectum after radiation treatment for gynecologic, prostatic, bladder, or rectal tumors. Approximately 75% of patients who receive 4000 rad develop acute, self-limited diarrhea, tenesmus, abdominal cramping, and, rarely, bleeding during the first few weeks. Chronic radiation effects occur 6 to 18 months after completion of treatment. Bowel injury resulting from chronic radiation is related to vascular damage, with subsequent mucosal ischemia, thickening, and ulceration. Much of this damage is believed to be due to chronic hypoxic ischemia and oxidative stress. Flexible sigmoidoscopy reveals telangiectasia, friability, and ulceration in the rectum (Fig. 16.10).

Patients should be instructed to avoid all aspirin and NSAIDs and should be put on a high-fiber diet. Medical therapies with topical or oral 5-aminosalicylic acid, sucralfate, or formalin can be tried with variable success.[56–60] Thermal therapy with argon plasma coagulation (APC), bipolar probe coagulation, radiofrequency ablation, and cryotherapy can be quite successful.[57–59] However, thermal therapy has the potential to result in ulceration which can result in further bleeding, especially in those on antiplatelet agents or anticoagulants (Fig. 16.11). Patients with refractory radiation proctitis may experience improvement with hyperbaric oxygen therapy.[61]

Hemorrhoids

Hemorrhoids are a plexus of veins just above the rectal squamocolumnar junction. Internal hemorrhoids are located above the dentate line, and external hemorrhoids are located below the dentate line. Symptomatic hemorrhoids are common in adults, mostly associated with prolonged straining during bowel movements, chronic constipation, pregnancy, obesity, and low-fiber diet. Bleeding is characterized by bright red blood per rectum that can coat the outside of the stool, may drip into the toilet bowel, and is present when wiping with tissue. Usually this is mild bleeding, but occasionally severe bleeding may occur from hemorrhoids. Treatment of hemorrhoids usually starts with medical therapy consisting of fiber supplementation to soften stool, lubricant rectal suppositories (with or without steroids), and warm sitz baths. Anoscopic therapy can also be used, including rubber band ligation, injection sclerotherapy, cryosurgery, infrared photocoagulation, and bipolar and direct current electrocoagulation. The use of a flexible endoscope and band ligation devices have also been described.[62] A disposable bander has been shown

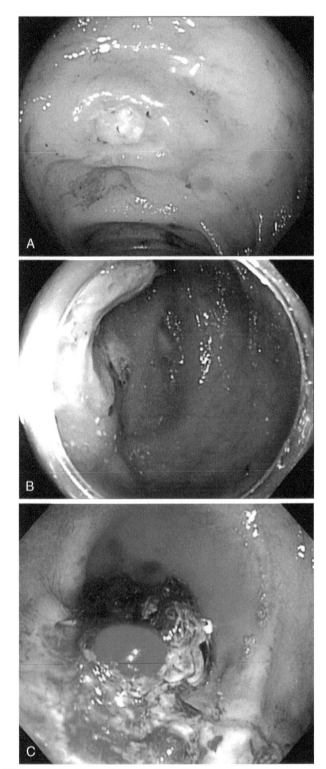

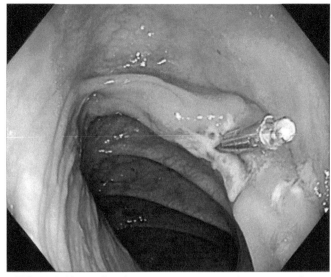

FIG 16.9 Hemoclip placement over postpolypectomy ulcer.

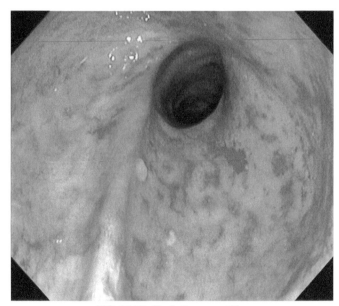

FIG 16.10 Radiation proctitis.

FIG 16.8 **A,** Clean based ulcer from postpolypectomy site. **B,** Large ulceration from postpolypectomy site. **C,** Active bleeding from postpolypectomy site.

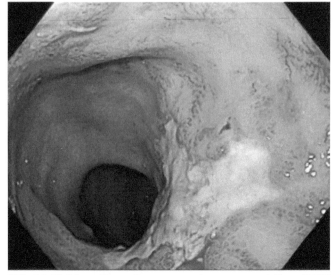

FIG 16.11 Ulceration after argon plasma coagulation (APC) treatment of radiation proctitis.

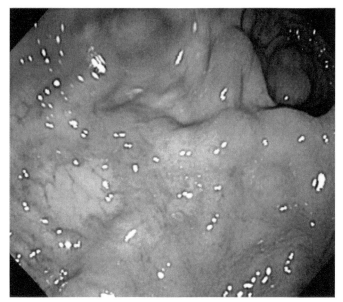

FIG 16.12 Rectal varices.

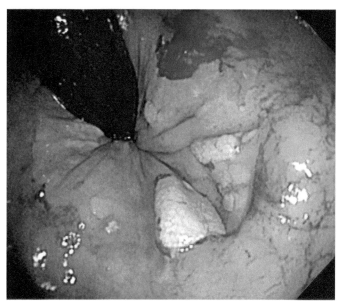

FIG 16.13 Active bleeding from a rectal Dieulafoy's lesion.

to be a technically simple method of hemorrhoid treatment with good results with a low rate of complications.[63] Surgery is reserved for refractory bleeding not controlled with other mechanisms. Most patients respond to medical management.

Rectal Varices

In response to portal hypertension, varices can develop in the rectal mucosa between the superior hemorrhoidal veins (portal circulation) and the middle and inferior hemorrhoidal veins (systemic circulation). On endoscopic examination, rectal varices are seen as vascular structures located several centimeters above the dentate line (Fig. 16.12). The incidence of rectal varices increases with the degree of portal hypertension. Approximately 60% of patients with a history of bleeding esophageal varices have rectal varices. Rectal varices can be treated similarly to esophageal varices, with sclerotherapy, rubber band ligation, or portosystemic shunts.[64,65] Endoscopic ultrasound-guided coil and/or glue treatment of rectal varices can be considered in refractory cases or where visualization is impaired due to brisk bleeding.[66]

Dieulafoy's Lesion

Dieulafoy's lesions are large submucosal arteries without overlying mucosal ulceration, which can cause massive bleeding from the colon and rectum (Fig. 16.13). There have been reports of bleeding Dieulafoy's lesions in the rectum that were treated successfully with endoscopic hemostasis, including cauterization and hemoclip placement.[67,68]

SUMMARY

The source of severe lower GI bleeding can usually be diagnosed by urgent colonoscopy. The differential diagnosis of lower GI bleeding includes diverticulosis, cancer, colitis, angiomas, postpolypectomy sites, radiation proctitis, internal hemorrhoids, and rectal varices. Patients should be stabilized with medical resuscitation and transfusion before urgent colonoscopy. Urgent colonic purge allows for earlier colonoscopy and the increased possibility for colonoscopic hemostasis. Bleeding diverticula and postpol-

ypectomy bleeding can be treated with epinephrine injection, bipolar coagulation, or clipping. Radiation proctitis and angiomas can be treated with thermal coagulation. Most patients who have successful colonoscopic hemostasis do not experience rebleeding. After endoscopic hemostasis, medical management can often help reduce the chances of rebleeding. Urgent colonoscopy should be performed in all patients with severe hematochezia who are suspected of having a lower GI bleed.

KEY REFERENCES

1. Laine L, Yang H, Chang SC, et al: Trends for incidence of hospitalization and death due to GI complications in the United States from 2001 to 2009, *Am J Gastroenterol* 107(8):1190–1195, 2012.
2. Longstreth GF: Epidemiology and outcome of patients hospitalized with acute lower gastrointestinal hemorrhage: a population-based study, *Am J Gastroenterol* 92:419–424, 1997.
3. Fouch PG: Diverticular bleeding: are nonsteroidal anti-inflammatory drugs risk factors for hemorrhage and can colonoscopy predict outcome for patients? *Am J Gastroenterol* 90:1779–1784, 1995.
4. Laine L, Connors LG, Reicin A, et al: Serious lower gastrointestinal clinical events with nonselective NSAID or coxib use, *Gastroenterology* 124:288–292, 2003.
5. Strate LL, Ayanian JZ, Kotler G, et al: Risk factors for mortality in lower intestinal bleeding, *Clin Gastroenterol Hepatol* 6:1004–1010, 2008.
7. Srygley FD, Gerardo CJ, Tran T, et al: Does this patient have a severe upper gastrointestinal bleed? *JAMA* 307(10):1072–1079, 2012.
9. Strate LL, Gralnek IM: ACG clinical guideline: management of patients with acute lower gastrointestinal bleeding, *Am J Gastroenterol* 111(4):459–474, 2016.
10. Abraham NS, Singh S, Alexander GC, et al: Comparative risk of gastrointestinal bleeding with dabigatran, rivaroxaban, and warfarin: population based cohort study, *BMJ* 350:h1857, 2015.
11. Larsen TB, Rasmussen LH, Skjøth F, et al: Efficacy and safety of dabigatran etexilate and warfarin in "real-world" patients with atrial fibrillation: a prospective nationwide cohort study, *J Am Coll Cardiol* 61(22):2264–2273, 2013.
12. Sherwood MW, Nessel CC, Hellkamp AS, et al: Gastrointestinal bleeding in patients with atrial fibrillation treated with rivaroxaban or warfarin: ROCKET AF trial, *J Am Coll Cardiol* 66(21):2271–2281, 2015.

13. Strate LL, Orav EJ, Syngal S: Early predictors of severity in acute lower intestinal tract bleeding, *Arch Intern Med* 163:838–843, 2003.

14. Strate LL, Saltzman JR, Ookubo R, et al: Validation of a clinical prediction rule for severe acute lower intestinal bleeding, *Am J Gastroenterol* 100:1821–1827, 2005.

20. Nakatsu S, Yasuda H, Maehata T, et al: Urgent computed tomography for determining the optimal timing of colonoscopy in patients with acute lower gastrointestinal bleeding, *Intern Med* 54(6):553–558, 2015.

21. Jensen DM, Machicado GA: Diagnosis and treatment of severe hematochezia: the role of urgent colonoscopy after purge, *Gastroenterology* 95:1569–1574, 1988.

22. Smoot R, Gostout CJ, Rajan E, et al: Is early colonoscopy after admission for acute diverticular bleeding needed? *Am J Gastroenterol* 98:1996–1999, 2003.

31. Jensen DM, Machicado GA, Jutabha R, et al: Urgent colonoscopy for the diagnosis and treatment of severe diverticular hemorrhage, *N Engl J Med* 342:78–82, 2000.

38. Bloomfeld RS, Rockey DC, Shetzline MA: Endoscopic therapy of acute diverticular hemorrhage, *Am J Gastroenterol* 96:2367–2372, 2001.

43. Foutch PG, Rex DK, Lieberman DA: Prevalence and natural history of colonic angiodysplasia among healthy asymptomatic people, *Am J Gastroenterol* 90:564–567, 1995.

44. Heyde EC: Gastrointestinal bleeding in aortic stenosis, *N Engl J Med* 259:196, 1958.

45. Vincentelli A, Susen S, Le Tourneau T, et al: Acquired von Willebrand syndrome in aortic stenosis, *N Engl J Med* 349:343–349, 2003.

46. Sadler JE: Aortic stenosis, von Willebrand factor, and bleeding, *N Engl J Med* 349:323–325, 2003.

48. Bhutani MS, Gupta SC, Markert RJ, et al: A prospective controlled evaluation of endoscopic detection of angiodysplasia and its association with aortic valve disease, *Gastrointest Endosc* 42:398–402, 1995.

53. Parra-Blanco A, Kaminaga N, Kojima T, et al: Hemoclipping for postpolypectomy and postbiopsy colonic bleeding, *Gastrointest Endosc* 51:37–41, 2000.

54. Shioji K, Suzuki Y, Kobayashi M, et al: Prophylactic clip application does not decrease delayed bleeding after colonoscopic polypectomy, *Gastrointest Endosc* 57:691–694, 2003.

55. Liaquat H, Rohn E, Rex DK: Prophylactic clip closure reduced the risk of delayed postpolypectomy hemorrhage: experience in 277 clipped large sessile or flat colorectal lesions and 247 control lesions, *Gastrointest Endosc* 77(3):401–407, 2013.

A complete reference list can be found online at ExpertConsult .com

17

Middle Gastrointestinal Bleeding

Stas Bezobchuk and Ian M. Gralnek

INTRODUCTION

Traditionally, obscure gastrointestinal bleeding (OGIB) is reported to account for approximately 5% of all gastrointestinal (GI) bleeding and is defined as bleeding from an unknown source that persists or recurs after negative bidirectional endoscopic diagnostic evaluations.[1,2] A negative bidirectional endoscopic diagnostic evaluation is defined as a negative upper endoscopy (esophagogastroduodenoscopy [EGD]) and negative colonoscopy with careful evaluation of the terminal ileum.[1,2] However, with the introduction of video capsule endoscopy (VCE) in 2001 and device-assisted deep enteroscopy in 2004 (e.g., double-balloon enteroscopy), and the ability to endoscopically visualize the entire length of the small bowel, the majority of patients who were previously classified as having "OGIB" were found to have a small bowel source of bleeding. Small bowel bleeding is now referred to as *middle GI bleeding* if the source of bleeding is located between the ligament of Treitz and the ileocecal valve. Thus today, following negative upper and lower endoscopic examinations and before performance of VCE, patients should be classified as having "suspected middle GI bleeding" with the diagnosis of true OGIB reserved only for patients who have also undergone a negative VCE examination.[1,2]

Overt middle GI bleeding refers to patients presenting with either melena or hematochezia with a source of bleeding identified in the small bowel. Furthermore, the term *occult middle GI bleeding* can be reserved for patients presenting with iron-deficiency anemia, with or without guaiac-positive stools, who are found to have a small bowel source of bleeding.[1,2]

INVESTIGATING SUSPECTED MIDDLE GASTROINTESTINAL BLEEDING

Push Enteroscopy

Push enteroscopy permits evaluation of the proximal small intestine to a distance that is approximately 50 to 100 cm beyond the ligament of Treitz. Dedicated video-enteroscopes (250 cm in length) are commercially available, but if these instruments are not available at the endoscopy site, a pediatric or standard adult colonoscope can be used with distance of insertion 40 to 50 cm beyond the ligament of Treitz. The use of an overtube, back-loaded onto the endoscope insertion tube, may help limit looping of the enteroscope within the stomach and facilitate deeper small bowel intubation.[4] Although the use of an overtube may allow for deeper small bowel intubation, it does not appear to increase the diagnostic yield of the test.[4] The diagnostic yield of push enteroscopy is reported to range from 3% to 70%, with most small bowel findings being vascular lesions (e.g., arteriovenous malformations). Interestingly, most of the lesions diagnosed during push enteroscopy have been found in locations accessible to standard EGD.[9]

With the development of endoscopic tools/devices for dedicated video-enteroscopes, such as biopsy forceps, snares, thermal probes (contact and noncontact), and injection needles, push enteroscopy is preferred over radiologic diagnostic modalities because of the ability to obtain tissue, perform polypectomy or hemostasis if necessary, and mark lesion sites with an India ink tattoo or an endoscopic clip. However, push enteroscopy does not allow for the visualization of the entire small bowel, and

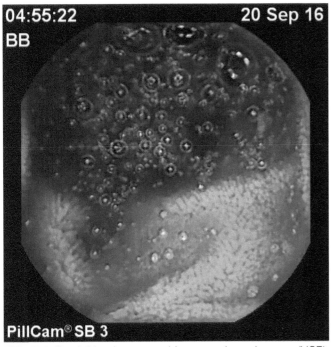

FIG 17.1 Fresh blood seen at video capsule endoscopy (VCE).

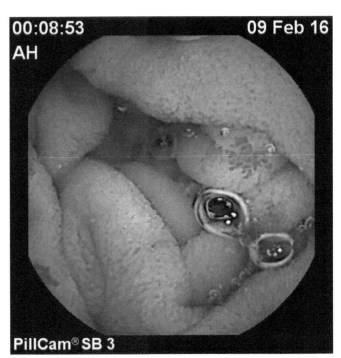

FIG 17.2 Angioectasia seen at video capsule endoscopy (VCE).

adverse events, including perforation and mucosal laceration, have been reported with the use of an overtube. With the advent of small bowel VCE and device-assisted "deep" enteroscopy, diagnostic push enteroscopy is less commonly used today.

Video Capsule Endoscopy

VCE is an endoscopic technology that is readily available worldwide and capable of obtaining endoscopic images from the entire small bowel.[1,2] VCE is easy, minimally invasive, safe, patient-friendly, and is the first-line diagnostic tool in imaging the small bowel for pathologies. With this realization, there has been rapid uptake and wide acceptance of this endoscopic technology for detecting small bowel abnormalities.

VCE allows complete evaluation of the small bowel (from the duodenum to the ileocecal valve) in 79% to 90% of patients, with a reported diagnostic yield of 38% to 83% in patients with suspected small bowel bleeding (Figs. 17.1 and 17.2; Video 17.1).[1,2] The main utility of VCE lies in its high positive (94%-97%) and negative (83%-100%) predictive values in the evaluation of GI bleeding.[10–12] Findings at VCE leading to endoscopic or surgical intervention or a change in medical management have been reported in 37% to 87% of patients (Figs. 17.3 to 17.10; Videos 17.2 to 17.10).[13] In addition, 50% to 66% of patients have been reported to remain transfusion free without recurrent bleeding at follow-up after VCE-directed interventions.[14] In patients who have had a negative VCE study, rebleeding occurs in 6% to 27%.[15,16]

The diagnostic yield of VCE may be influenced by multiple factors, with a higher likelihood of positive findings in patients with a hemoglobin less than 10 g/dL, longer duration of bleeding (> 6 months), more than one episode of bleeding, overt as compared with occult bleeding (60% vs. 46%), and performance of VCE within 14 days of a bleeding episode (91% vs. 34%).[17–19] It has also been shown that detecting a source of bleeding depends on the timing of VCE investigation. In a study by Pennazio et al (2004), evaluating 100 consecutive patients undergoing VCE,

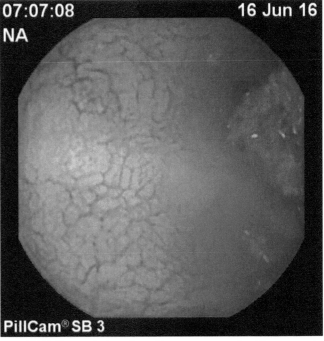

FIG 17.3 Suspected celiac disease seen at video capsule endoscopy (VCE).

the diagnostic yield of VCE was 92% for patients with overt bleeding, 44% for occult bleeders, 67% for patients with prior overt bleeding who were studied within 10 to 14 days of their bleeding episode, and only 33% for those studied by VCE at 3 to 4 weeks after the bleeding episode.[20]

Limitations of VCE include lack of biopsy or therapeutic capabilities, inability to perform endoscopic marking, inability

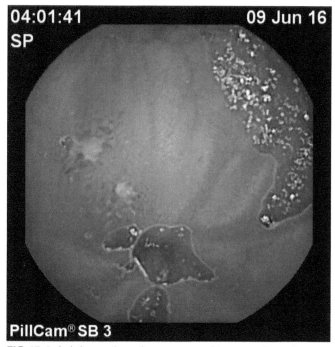

FIG 17.4 Aphthous ulcerations seen at video capsule endoscopy (VCE).

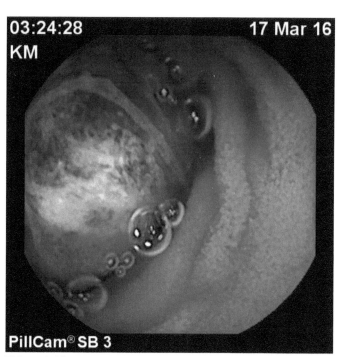

FIG 17.6 Ulcerated mass lesion seen at video capsule endoscopy (VCE).

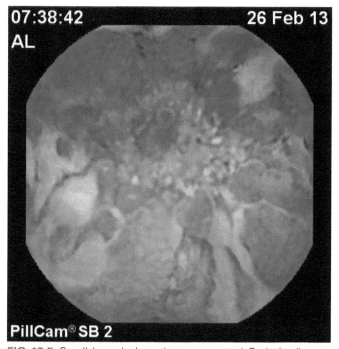

FIG 17.5 Small bowel ulcerations suspected Crohn's disease seen at video capsule endoscopy (VCE).

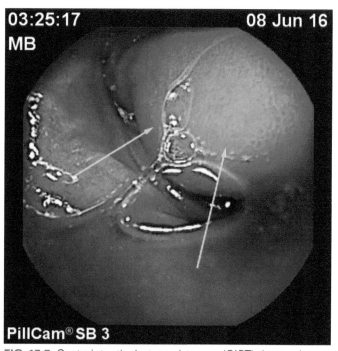

FIG 17.7 Gastrointestinal stromal tumor (GIST) *(arrows)* seen at video capsule endoscopy (VCE).

to control movement of the capsule through the GI tract, and difficulty in localizing lesions. Other limitations of VCE include a lack of specificity, with 14% incidental findings in healthy volunteers[21] and a 10% to 36% false-negative rate.[22] Finally, VCE fails to identify the major papilla in a majority of cases[23,24] and therefore may miss important duodenal lesions because of rapid

transit through the duodenal loop. This deficiency may be improved to 60% if a dual camera capsule is used. There are studies to suggest that repeat VCE may be of benefit and increase the diagnostic yield, even when the first VCE study is negative. Diagnostic yield of a repeated VCE was reported to be between 35% and 75% with subsequent management change reported

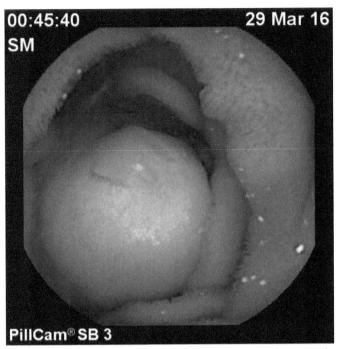

FIG 17.8 Large submucosal mass lesion seen at video capsule endoscopy (VCE).

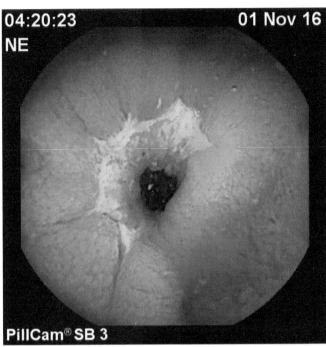

FIG 17.10 Nonsteroidal antiinflammatory drug (NSAID) enteropathy seen at video capsule endoscopy (VCE).

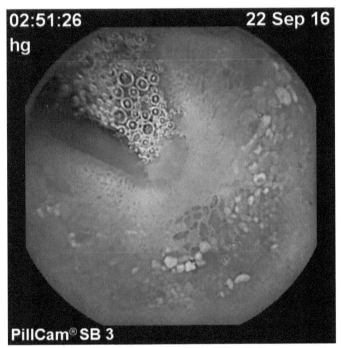

FIG 17.9 Nonsteroidal antiinflammatory drug (NSAID) enteropathy seen at video capsule endoscopy (VCE).

in 39% to 62.5% of the patients, particularly when the type of bleeding changes from occult to overt or there is a hemoglobin drop greater than 4 g/dL.[25–27] In some patients, luminal debris and bubbles interfere with endoscopic viewing. Some physicians use polyethylene glycol-based preparations, prokinetic agents, simethicone, or a combination of these products before capsule

ingestion; however there is no consensus as to the necessity of a pre-VCE bowel preparation.[1,2]

Some patients may be considered unsuitable candidates for VCE, including patients with cardiac pacemakers, implanted defibrillators, left ventricular assist devices, and patients with suspected small bowel obstruction. Yet, multiple case series suggest that VCE, when performed with careful patient monitoring, is safe in patients with pacemakers and implanted cardiac defibrillators.[28–31] Patients with swallowing disorders or an unwillingness to voluntarily swallow the capsule may have the capsule endoscopically placed into the duodenum. Historically, overtubes have been used to deliver the capsule into the stomach, whereas standard polypectomy snares and nets have been used for capsule delivery directly into the duodenum.[32–34] The AdvanCE (US Endoscopy, Mentor, OH) allows endoscopic delivery of the video capsule. The system is a disposable catheter with a sheath diameter of 2.5 mm that is preloaded through the accessory channel of an endoscope. A specialized capsule cup is screwed onto its distal end, and the activated video capsule is loaded into the cup. The upper endoscope and the device are then advanced to the desired anatomical area, and the capsule is released via a deployment apparatus located at the proximal catheter. Additionally, a capsule paired with a magnetic wand (Navi Capsule, IntroMedic, Seoul, Korea) has been created to assist with mobilizing the device through the esophagus, stomach, and into the duodenum to facilitate delivery in patients with delayed gastric emptying.

Capsule retention is a potential adverse event of VCE.[35] The reported incidence of capsule retention ranges from 0% in healthy volunteers, to 1.4% in patients with obscure GI hemorrhage, to 2.1% in patients with suspected small bowel obstruction due to neoplastic lesions, and up to 2.6% in small bowel Crohn's disease, which limits its use in patients with suspected bowel obstruction or strictures until luminal patency is documented.[36–38] Pre-VCE screening small bowel radiographs have not been able to eliminate capsule retention. To address the problem of capsule retention, the Agile Patency Capsule (PC) was developed (by Given Imaging, now Medtronic, Minneapolis, MN). The PC, being the same size as a video capsule, serves as dummy to assess the patency of the small bowel prior to VCE examination. As one of the major contraindications for VCE is suspicion of small bowel stenosis, routine administration of PCs could enable safe VCE use in a larger patient population by ruling out possible stenosis.[39] The PC system consists of two main parts: the capsule itself, with a radio frequency identification tag (RFID tag), and an external detector system to capture radio frequency signals. The PC is made of lactose and 10% barium, which dissolves when coming into contact with intestinal fluids through the window located at the edge of the capsule, also known as the timer plug. To ensure that the timer plug is not blocked by capsule impaction in a stricture, the second-generation PCs consist of two timer plugs. If PC excretion does not occur, dissolution starts at 30 hours. After 35 hours, 38% of the capsule is dissolved and is 100% dissolved within 72 hours.[40] After dissolution, the remains of the PC encounter no difficulties in passing a small bowel stricture. One drawback of the RFID tag system is the possibility of impaction in a stricture and resultant small bowel ileus or obstruction. Recently however, the use of a "tag-less" Agile PC was reported by Nakamura et al (2014)[41]

The PillCam SB video capsule endoscope (Medtronic) is a wireless capsule (11 mm × 26 mm) composed of a light source, lens, complementary metal oxide semiconductor imager, battery, and wireless transmitter. The PillCam SB has a battery life of approximately 7 to 8 hours, in which time the capsule captures two images per second (approximately 60,000 total images per examination) in a 140-degree field of view and 8:1 magnification. The smooth outer coating of the capsule allows easy ingestion and prevents adhesion of intestinal contents as the capsule moves via natural peristalsis from the mouth to the anus. Endoscopic images are transmitted via sensor arrays to a recording device worn as a belt by the patient. The recorded images are downloaded into a Reporting and Processing of Images and Data (RAPID) computer workstation and reviewed as a continuous video by the physician. The PillCam SB VCE offers advanced optics and a wider field of view for imaging the small bowel and also provides

Automatic Light Control for optimal illumination of each image. The third generation of PillCam SB (Pillcam SB 3) is now available. CapsoCam by Capsovision (Saratoga, CA) renewed the concept of VCE by offering a capsule with a 360-degree view and on-board image storage, which enables the retrieval of images wire-free after interception of the capsule in the feces. The capsule contains four cameras, which offer high-resolution images and a frame rate up to 20 fps max. Furthermore, two new technologies were developed, Smart Motion Sense Technology and Auto Illumination Technology. Smart Motion Sense Technology enables the capsule to activate its cameras only during capsule motion. When the capsule is stationary, a sensor is used to compare the current frame with the previous frame to control reactivation. Auto Illumination Technology controls the 16 white LEDs to provide the optimal level of illumination. When the capsule is located near the bowel wall, a low light intensity is optimal to capture the best images. A position further away from the wall necessitates a higher light intensity. By adding these software features, battery life is extended up to 15 hours. The first clinical trial that used the CapsoCam reported its safety and efficacy in small bowel evaluation.[42] In a French study by Pioche et al (2014), the concordance between the PillCam SB2 and CapsoCam was evaluated in terms of diagnostic yield and image quality. A kappa value of 0.63 was reported, confirming good concordance between the two capsules. Although the reading time of the CapsoCam was longer, the CapsoCam detected significantly more lesions in a per-lesion analysis.[43] Olympus (Center Valley, PA) has also introduced a next-generation video capsule: ENDOCAPSULE EC-10. With the ENDOCAPSULE EC-10 System, there is improvement in the angle of view, 160 degrees as opposed to 145 degrees in the previous model, battery life has been extended from 8 hours to 12 hours, and there has been an improvement in image quality. Other small bowel capsules with technical features are listed in Table 17.1.

Device-Assisted Enteroscopy

Deep evaluation of the small bowel can be accomplished with balloon-assisted or non–balloon-assisted enteroscopes coupled with a specialized overtube apparatus. The procedure can be performed via an antegrade approach (via the mouth) or via a retrograde approach (via the anus). In the United States, current

TABLE 17.1	Available Video Capsule Endoscopy (VCE) Devices			
Capsule	**PillCam SB 3** Given Imaging	**EndoCapsule** Olympus America	**MiroCam** Intromedic Company	**OMOM** Jianshan Science and Technology
Size	Length: 26.2 mm Diameter: 11.4 mm	Length: 26 mm Diameter: 11 mm	Length: 24.5 mm Diameter: 10.8 mm	Length: 27.9 mm Diameter: 13 mm
Weight	3.00 g	3.50 g	3.25–4.70 g	6.00 g
Battery life	8 hr or longer	8 hr or longer	11 hr or longer	6–8 hr or longer
Resolution	340 × 340 30% better than SB2	512 × 512	320 × 320	640 × 480
Frames per second	2 fps or 2–6 fps	2 fps	3 fps	2 fps
Field of view	156 degrees	145 degrees	170 degrees	140 degrees
Communication	Radio frequency communication	Radio frequency communication	Human body communication	Radio frequency communication
FDA approval	Yes	Yes	Yes	No
Price per capsule	$500	$500	$500	$250

options for device-assisted enteroscopes include double-balloon enteroscopy (DBE), single-balloon enteroscopy (SBE), and spiral enteroscopy. A newer, through-the-scope balloon-assisted device that allows "on-demand" enteroscopy is also available.

DBE, initially described and reported by Yamamoto et al (2004), is a novel endoscopic insertion technique that attempts to improve on currently available endoscopic insertion methods to evaluate the entire length of the small bowel.[44] The DBE system (Fujinon Inc, Saitama, Japan), uses a high-resolution, dedicated video enteroscope that has a working length of 200 cm and two soft, latex balloons; one balloon is attached to the tip of the enteroscope, and the other is attached to the distal end of a soft, flexible overt-tube (Fig. 17.11). The balloons can be inflated and deflated using an air pump that is controlled by the endoscopist while monitoring air pressure.[45] The balloons grip the wall of the bowel, allowing the endoscope to be advanced without looping.

The procedure can be performed via an oral or anal approach with or without fluoroscopic guidance. Choice of peroral or transanal approach is usually dictated by suspicion of the location of a possible lesion as determined by preceding small bowel VCE or other small bowel imaging technique.[46,47] In a peroral approach, when the two balloons reach the duodenum, the overtube balloon is inflated to fix the overtube to the small bowel wall. The overtube is held in place as the endoscope is further inserted. Once the tip of the endoscope is maximally inserted, the balloon on the tip of the endoscope is inflated, the balloon on the overtube is deflated, and the overtube is advanced over the shaft of the endoscope. When the distal end of the overtube reaches the tip of the endoscope, the overtube balloon is reinflated, again fixing

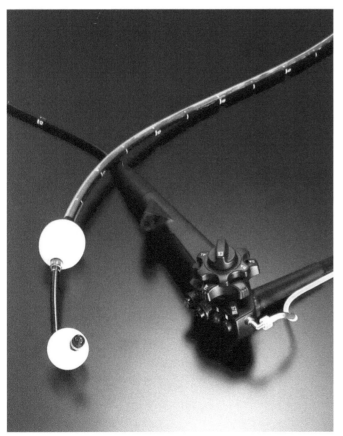

FIG 17.11 Double-balloon enteroscope.

the overtube to a second point on the small bowel wall. This sequence is repeated until the entire small bowel is evaluated or further advancement of the endoscope is unable to be performed.

The mean reported procedure times for DBE range from 73 to 123 minutes. The estimated depth of insertion for the peroral antegrade approach is reported to be between 220 and 360 cm and for the transanal retrograde approach between 120 and 180 cm. Reported rates of complete enteroscopy widely vary. Whereas Japanese studies have reported complete enteroscopy rates in the 70% to 86% range, Western series have generally reported much lower completion rates. Reported DBE diagnostic yields have ranged from 40% to 80%, with therapeutic yields of 15% to 55%.[48–52] In a 2010 study of 200 patients with OGIB bleeding undergoing DBE, the diagnostic yield was 77% for overt bleeding, 67% for patients with occult hemorrhage, and 59% for patients with prior overt bleeding.[53] Moreover, as compared with VCE, DBE has been shown to have similar diagnostic yields in evaluating small bowel disease.[54] Successful performance of endoscopic therapeutic interventions has been reported in 40% to 73% of patients undergoing DBE. Urgent DBE may be better than nonurgent DBE and is associated with a lower recurrent bleeding rate.[55] In addition, one study suggests higher diagnostic yields of DBE for patients with overt bleeding, yet higher recurrence rates in patients presenting with obscure overt bleeding.[56] Moreover, repeat DBE from the same direction may be beneficial, particularly if the patient had a prior positive DBE.[57]

DBE has technical nuances that require specialized training. Furthermore, two operators are needed for the procedure. The procedures are lengthy and potentially uncomfortable for the patient and may be fatiguing for the operators. It is not recommended that both antegrade and retrograde approach procedures be performed on the same day.[58] Antegrade examinations are thought to be easier than retrograde examinations because of difficulty in intubating the terminal ileum via the retrograde approach, with reported failure rates of ileal intubation with retrograde examination ranging from 7% to 30%. Previous abdominal surgery and resultant adhesions can also make the procedure more difficult. The most commonly reported adverse events with DBE include pancreatitis, bleeding, and perforation with an overall rate ranging between 1.2% and 1.6%. Specifically, the rate of pancreatitis is reported to be 0.3% and that of perforation to be between 0.3% and 0.4%. Of note, the perforation risk seems to be higher in patients with surgically altered anatomy, and thus caution is advised in such cases (Videos 17.11 to 17.16).

Single-Balloon Enteroscopy

SBE was introduced in 2007, and uses a dedicated enteroscope with an overtube (SIF-Q180; Olympus America Inc., Center Valley, PA) and a balloon inflation control device that allows automatic balloon pressure control. In contrast to DBE, only the disposable overtube has a nonlatex balloon at its distal end. The enteroscope has a working length of 200 cm, an outer diameter of 9.2 mm, and a 2.8-mm diameter working channel. The overtube (ST-SB1; Olympus) is 140 cm long with a 13.2-mm outer diameter, and its distal end has an inflatable silicone balloon (Fig. 17.12). The balloon is controlled by pressing buttons on the front panel of the Olympus balloon control unit or on a remote control. The internal surface of the overtube is hydrophilic, and lubrication between the outer surface of the enteroscope and the inner surface of the overtube is facilitated by flushing the internal surface of the overtube with water.[59,60]

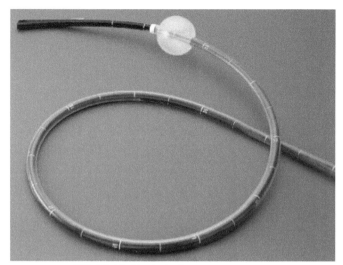

FIG 17.12 Single-balloon enteroscope.

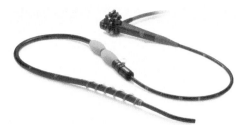

FIG 17.13 Spiral enteroscope.

The technique for SBE is similar to DBE. The overtube is backloaded onto the enteroscope, and the enteroscope is advanced as far as possible into the small bowel, then anchored by using its flexible tip (as opposed to enteroscope tip balloon-assisted anchoring used in DBE). Subsequently, the overtube is advanced with its balloon deflated to the tip of the enteroscope. The overtube balloon is then inflated while keeping the enteroscope tip flexed. Subsequently, the entire apparatus is withdrawn to allow pleating of the small bowel over the enteroscope and overtube. The efficacy of SBE is generally similar to DBE. Reported diagnostic yields have ranged from 41% to 65% and therapeutic yields from 7% to 50%.[61–63] The reported range for depth of insertion is 130 to 270 cm for antegrade examinations and 70 to 200 cm for retrograde examinations. Studies suggest that the rate of total enteroscopy with SBE may be lower than that with DBE by up to 24%. SBE is associated with challenges similar to DBE, but overall, SBE is technically less complicated given that only a single balloon must be inflated and deflated by the endoscopist. However, it has been suggested that, due to a lack of an anchoring mechanism on the enteroscope, there can be difficulty in maintaining the enteroscope position in the small bowel as the overtube is advanced. Similar to DBE, transanal retrograde ileal intubation during SBE can be challenging. The procedure times for antegrade and retrograde approaches are similar, and the overall procedure times are comparable to those of DBE. Adverse events reported with SBE are rare and include abdominal pain, fever, mucosal tears, pancreatitis, and perforation.

Spiral Enteroscopy

Spiral enteroscopy was also introduced in 2007, with the potential to provide a simpler and faster deep enteroscopy technique compared with balloon-assisted enteroscopy (Video 17.17). Spiral enteroscopy uses a disposable overtube with a soft, raised spiral ridge that is designed to pleat the small bowel. The overtube is 118 cm long with a soft, raised, spiral helix at its distal end that is either 4.5 mm (low profile) or 5.5 mm (standard profile) in height. The overtube is compatible with enteroscopes that are 200 cm in length and between 9.1 mm and 9.5 mm in diameter (Fig. 17.13). Two different overtubes are available for antegrade (Endo-Ease Discovery SB, Spirus Medical LLC., West Bridgewater,

MA) or retrograde (Endo-Ease Vista, Spirus Medical) examinations. The overtube has a coupling device on its proximal end that affixes itself to the enteroscope. This allows for free rotation of the overtube independent of the enteroscope but prevents independent movement of the enteroscope (advancement or withdrawal) relative to the overtube. When the overtube is uncoupled, the enteroscope can then be advanced or withdrawn independent of the overtube.[64,65] A motorized spiral enteroscopy system has been developed by Olympus and early pilot data in a small group of patients was recently reported in abstract form.[66] Spiral enteroscopy is rather simple to perform, and forward progress through the small bowel can be completed in approximately 18 minutes.[64] Based on the prior literature, the mean procedure times for the anterograde approach have been estimated to be 79 ± 15 min for DBE (10 studies), 65 ± 16 min for SBE (5 studies), and 35 + 6 min for spiral enteroscopy (4 studies). Two operators are required to perform spiral enteroscopy: an endoscopist and an assistant to operate the overtube. Before insertion, the inner lining of the overtube is generously lubricated with the proprietary lubricant supplied with the device. The overtube is then backloaded onto the enteroscope so that approximately 20 cm of the enteroscope protrudes past the distal tip of the overtube. When the overtube and enteroscope are coupled, the overtube should be rotated clockwise for advancement and counterclockwise for withdrawal. For antegrade examination, the overtube and enteroscope are advanced slowly with clockwise rotation of the overtube until the enteroscope tip ideally reaches the ligament of Treitz.

The diagnostic yield of the initial cases of spiral enteroscopy has been reported to be only 33%.[65] More recent prospective data (2011) suggest that the diagnostic yield in patients with a positive VCE study was 57%.[67] Questions have been raised regarding safety concerns with bowel trauma and difficulty in rapid device removal during an emergency. However, there were no major adverse events reported in the early published literature.[68] In a series of 75 patients, 12% reported a sore throat, 27% had superficial mucosal trauma, and 7% had moderate esophageal trauma that did not require intervention. In a retrospective registry study involving 1750 patients, the rate of severe adverse events was reported to be 0.3%, with a small bowel perforation rate of 0.3%.[69]

On-Demand Enteroscopy

The NaviAid (SMART Medical Systems Ltd, Ra'anana, Israel) is a newer device that consists of a disposable balloon component that is advanced through the working channel of an upper endoscope or colonoscope (NaviAid AB and NaviAid ABC).[70] The NaviAid AB has a working length of 350 cm with a balloon diameter of 40 mm. The minimum endoscope working channel diameter needed for passage of the device is 3.8 mm. The inflation/

deflation of the balloon is controlled by an air supply unit, and balloon pressure is regulated. The balloon device can be advanced through the channel of the endoscope if deep enteroscopy is required "on demand." The NaviAid device requires no specific premounting or preprocedural preparation. The procedure technique is conceptually similar to balloon-assisted enteroscopy. The balloon is advanced beyond the tip of the endoscope through the working channel and inflated to anchor itself to the bowel wall. Subsequently, repetitive push-pull maneuverers are performed with the endoscope sliding over the catheter as a rail until it reaches the inflated balloon distally. The balloon catheter can be withdrawn to allow for therapeutic interventions as needed and reinserted for further advancement of the endoscope. The NaviAid enteroscopy platform is balloon-guided, whereas DBE and SBE are scope-guided and balloon-assisted techniques. Achieving deeper insertion is often better achieved with a scope-guided enteroscopy platform. Preliminary studies of the NaviAid on-demand enteroscopy system report mean antegrade insertion depths of 120 to 190 cm with mean procedure times of 16 to 52 minutes. Data on retrograde examinations have reported a mean depth of insertion of 89 to 110 cm. Diagnostic and therapeutic yields for antegrade examinations are 45% and 36%, respectively, and for retrograde examinations, 59% and 47%, respectively.[70]

Few studies have directly compared DBE, SBE, and spiral enteroscopy. Parameters evaluated have included depths of insertion, rates of complete enteroscopy, procedure times, clinical outcomes, learning curves, and safety.[71–76] Currently, there are no comparative data for the NaviAid on-demand enteroscopy system.

A few studies, with limited numbers of patients, have evaluated the role of emergency DBE in actively bleeding patients.[77–79] Diagnostic yields and short-term outcomes appear to be promising. Deep enteroscopy as an initial diagnostic and therapeutic step in actively bleeding patients is an included consideration in the European Society of Gastrointestinal Endoscopy (ESGE) and American College of Gastroenterology (ACG) guidelines on management of small bowel bleeding.[1,2]

Intraoperative Enteroscopy

Exploratory laparotomy with intraoperative enteroscopy (IOE) has been used since the 1980s and is a diagnostic and potentially therapeutic endoscopic modality in suspected small bowel disease; it is also considered the ultimate endoscopic evaluation of the small bowel.[80–83] In addition to being able to diagnose small bowel sources of bleeding, IOE allows for identification of lesions for definitive surgical resection. A colonoscope (pediatric or adult size) or, more optimally, a dedicated small bowel video enteroscope, can be advanced beyond the ligament of Treitz into the proximal jejunum by peroral route or by way of a small bowel enterotomy. The latter technique expedites the examination, especially of the distal small bowel, and minimizes the potential for iatrogenic trauma to the small bowel arising from excessive manipulation of the endoscope that can arise from peroral passage. Once inserted, the surgeon gently telescopes the small bowel over the shaft of the endoscope, allowing for the careful inspection of the mucosa.

Inspection of the small bowel mucosa should be performed in an anterograde manner. When using a small bowel enterotomy, the endoscope is first advanced to the terminal ileum/cecum and then withdrawn with careful inspection. Dimming the operating room lights facilitates endoscopic visualization by the

endoscopist and external inspection of the bowel by the surgeons. Lesions identified endoscopically can be marked for resection by the surgeon with a suture placed on the serosal aspect of the bowel. After completion of the enteroscopy and withdrawal of the endoscope, the marked sites can then be surgically resected. An alternative approach to IOE involves insertion of a sterilized (or sterile-covered) endoscope through multiple, surgically created enterotomies, rectal insertion, or laparoscopy-assisted enteroscopy. Reported adverse events associated with IOE include mucosal lacerations, perforations, prolonged ileus, abdominal abscess, and bowel ischemia.[80–83] Due to its invasive nature and potential for adverse events, the decision to perform IOE must not be taken lightly. All risks and benefits need to be fully considered and explained to the patient; only experienced endoscopists and surgeons should perform this procedure. Currently, this technique is reserved as a last option if deep enteroscopy using DBE, SBE, or spiral enteroscopy cannot be performed successfully because of the presence of abdominal adhesions, obesity, or other technical factors.

RADIOGRAPHIC IMAGING STUDIES

Small Bowel Contrast Radiography

A small bowel series (upper GI series with small bowel follow-through) involves the oral ingestion of a dilute barium solution with serial abdominal images obtained of the small bowel. Enteroclysis is a double-contrast study performed by passing a tube into the proximal small bowel and injecting barium, methylcellulose, and air, and is considered superior to standard small bowel follow-through. An upper GI series with small bowel follow-through is sometimes used to evaluate obscure GI bleeding either before performing push enteroscopy or after a negative push enteroscopy examination. The role of small bowel series and enteroclysis in the evaluation of obscure GI bleeding has declined substantially because of its very low diagnostic yield (0% to 6% for small bowel follow-through and 10% to 25% for enteroclysis) and the advent of improved endoscopic diagnostic techniques for the small bowel.[1,2] In addition to limited diagnostic sensitivity in middle GI bleeding, enteroclysis can be uncomfortable for the patient and involves more radiation exposure than small bowel follow-through. Generally, the role of enteroclysis in the evaluation of middle GI bleeding is limited to settings in which VCE and enteroscopy are unavailable or contraindicated, such as clinical situations that suggest small bowel obstruction secondary to malignancy, Crohn's disease, or prior significant nonsteroidal antiinflammatory drug use. Otherwise, there is little or no role today for either small bowel series or enteroclysis in the evaluation of suspected middle GI bleeding.

Cross-Sectional Imaging

Novel cross-sectional imaging techniques for evaluation of the small bowel include helical computed tomography enteroclysis (CTE), helical CT angiography, and magnetic resonance (MR) and CT enteroclysis/enterography. In a meta-analysis of 18 studies, CTE had a pooled yield of 40% compared with 53% for VCE.[84] Several studies have shown that VCE has higher yields for detecting vascular and inflammatory lesions compared with CTE.[85,86] However, some studies have shown that CTE can detect vascular and inflammatory abnormalities, which may be missed on VCE.[87] The detection of subtle vascular abnormalities at CTE may be influenced by technique and experience. An advantage of CTE over VCE is the improved detection of small bowel masses, especially those that are mural-based. In a study by Huprich et al (2011), CTE detected 9/9 (100%) small bowel tumors, whereas VCE only detected 3/9 (33%) of the lesions.[87] Therefore CTE and VCE are complementary examinations. For example, in a study of 30 patients with negative CTE, subsequent VCE was positive in 57%.[86] In another study of 52 patients with nondiagnostic VCE, subsequent CTE had a 50% positive yield in those patients with overt small bowel bleeding.[88] Because of the limited number of studies using MR enterography (MRE), this exam is not routinely recommended in lieu of CTE, but can be considered in patients less than 40 years of age because of absence of radiation exposure.[89,90]

An advantage of cross-sectional small bowel imaging techniques is the ability to screen for contraindications to VCE. In one study, 11% of patients being evaluated for suspected small bowel bleeding were excluded from VCE secondary to high-grade strictures identified on MRE.[90]

Nuclear Medicine Studies

Tagged red blood cell (RBC) scans are noninvasive, safe, and readily available. Most commonly performed with technetium-labeled RBCs, a radionuclide bleeding scan detects bleeding that is occurring at a rate of 0.1 to 0.5 mL/min. It is of little or no value in patients with suspected, occult, middle GI bleeding who appear to have a low rate of blood loss because the rate of bleeding is too slow to be detected. Bleeding scans may be more sensitive than angiography, but less specific than either a positive endoscopic or angiographic examination.[91,92] Early scans (up to 4 hours after initial injection) may be helpful in gross localization of bleeding when the rate of blood loss exceeds 0.1 to 0.5 mL/min. However, tagged RBC scans can identify only a general area of bleeding, and assessment with other diagnostic modalities, such as angiography, is usually necessary after nuclear scans. The role of nuclear medicine scans is very limited, if at all relevant today in patients with suspected middle GI bleeding, because the ability to accurately localize the source of bleeding is poor at best and better, more readily available technologies exist (e.g., multidetector CT angiography).[93]

CT Angiography

Most studies using CT to evaluate GI bleeding are performed during multiphase contrast enhancement with one of the phases occurring during the arterial phase of enhancement. When performed with oral contrast, this is referred to as multiphasic CTE. When no oral contrast is administered, the technique has been termed multiphasic CT or CT angiography (CTA). Multiphasic CT or CTA is usually performed to detect the site of active bleeding in cases of acute overt bleeding, which can occur sporadically or in the setting of small bowel bleeding. CTA has been shown to be able to detect bleeding rates as slow as 0.3 mL/min compared with 0.5 to 1.0 mL/min for conventional angiography and 0.2 mL/min for ^{99m}Tc tagged RBC scintigraphy. A meta-analysis of nine studies including 198 patients showed CTA had a pooled sensitivity of 89% and specificity of 85% in diagnosing acute GI bleeding throughout the GI tract.[94] Several of these studies demonstrated detection by CTA when other techniques were negative. CTA is widely available and can be performed rapidly during the time of bleeding, which may aid in detection compared with other techniques. CTA has also been shown to accurately localize the site of bleeding.[95] Other studies have shown sensitivities of 79% to 94% and specificity of 95% to 100% for detecting active bleeding throughout the GI tract.[96–98] In a study

of 113 consecutive patients with active GI bleeding, CTA was positive in 80/113 (70.8%), all of which were confirmed. Negative studies were seen in 33 patients (29.2%). Out of the 33 patients, 27 required no further intervention.[95] In a retrospective analysis of 31 patients with suspected overt small bowel bleeding, CTA had a yield of 45% (86% tumor yield and 33% nontumor yield) compared with 94% for DBE. CTA detected one of seven ulcers, six of seven tumors, and both angioectasias seen at DBE. In addition, CTA provided correct guidance for DBE in 100% of cases.[99] CTA can also be used to help triage patients for further management. In one study, 64/86 CTA was negative and 92% of these patients required no further intervention. There were no cases with a negative CTA that had a subsequent positive conventional angiogram within 24 hours.[97] Therefore some have recommended watchful waiting in cases with a negative CTA as the bleeding rate may be low or intermittent and conventional angiography rarely shows an additional site of bleeding. Factors predictive of a positive conventional angiogram following a positive CTA include nondiverticular etiologies and lower hemoglobin levels and should be performed soon after the CTA to enhance detection.[100] To detect contrast extravasation, the patient must be actively bleeding at the time of the scan. The findings of blood within the lumen or sentinel clot may help localize the source if the bleeding is subtle or absent. If no active bleeding or source is identified at the time of the CTA, additional workup may be necessary. In elderly patients with decreased renal function, the administration of intravenous contrast for CT may increase the risk of renal adverse events if subsequent conventional angiography is required.

Angiography

The data on the clinical utility of angiography in the setting of suspected middle GI bleeding are very limited.[101] Compared with tagged RBC scans, mesenteric angiography is more likely to document the specific site of bleeding, yet the rate of bleeding must be greater than 0.5 mL/min. Angiography can also identify lesions that are not actively bleeding because of demonstration of typical vascular features seen in vascular ectasias (e.g., slow-emptying veins, a vascular tuft, and early-filling veins) and neoplasms. It is possible to administer embolization therapy if an amenable lesion is detected. Provocative angiography using anticoagulants, vasodilators, or thrombolytic agents may increase the likelihood that a source of bleeding can be identified and has been advocated by some investigators.[102,103] However, the risk of inducing uncontrolled bleeding limits the use of this technique and should only be performed at centers with appropriate experience. Throughout the years, catheter-based intervention has shown significant advances with transition from vasopressin infusion to superselective transarterial embolization, resulting in improved results and decreased adverse events. In 15 studies from 1992 to 2006, consisting of 309 patients and using superselective transarterial embolization, there was an 82% technical success rate, 95% overall clinical success rate, 76% 30-day success rate, and a rebleed rate of 12%.[104] However, most cases were for bleeding sources located outside of the small bowel. In a 2014 retrospective study of 70 patients, investigators reported a 99% technical success rate, 71% primary clinical success rate, and 79% secondary clinical success rate after repeat embolization and bowel infarction in 4%.[105] Predictors of failure to achieve 30-day hemostasis included a hemoglobin level of less than 8 g/dL, coagulopathy and upper GI bleeding, contrast extravasation, and more than one vessel needing to be embolized.

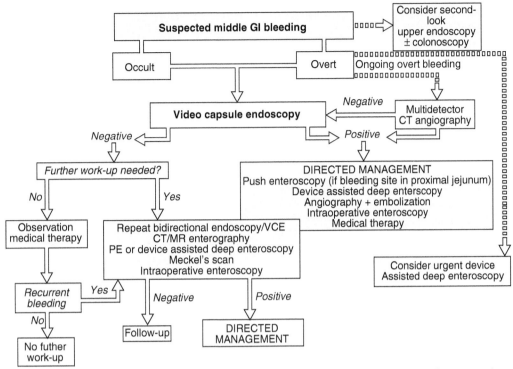

FIG 17.14 Diagnostic algorithm for middle gastrointestinal bleeding. *CT,* computed tomography; *MR,* magnetic resonance; *PE,* push enteroscopy; *VEC,* video capsule endoscopy.

Proposed Diagnostic Strategy

According to the recent ACG and ESGE evidence-based guidelines, we propose similar recommendations for diagnosing a cause of suspected middle GI bleeding (Fig. 17.14).

1. Second-look upper endoscopy should be considered in cases of recurrent hematemesis, melena, or a previous incomplete upper endoscopy exam. Push enteroscopy can be performed as this second-look examination.
2. Second-look colonoscopy should be considered in the setting of recurrent hematochezia, a previous incomplete ileocolonoscopy, or documentation of an inadequate colon preparation at previous colonoscopy.
3. If second-look examinations do not diagnose a bleeding source, the next step should be small bowel evaluation for suspected middle GI bleeding. Unless contraindicated, VCE should be the first-line procedure for small bowel evaluation and before deep enteroscopy to increase diagnostic yield.
4. Device-assisted deep enteroscopy should be attempted if there is a strong suspicion of a small bowel lesion based on clinical presentation or an abnormal VCE study. Any method of device-assisted deep enteroscopy can be used when small bowel endoscopic evaluation and therapy is required.
5. IOE should be limited to clinical situations where deep enteroscopy cannot be performed, such as in patients with prior intraabdominal surgeries and/or intestinal adhesions.
6. Initial "emergency" deep enteroscopy can be considered in cases of massive hemorrhage or when VCE is contraindicated.

Suspected Overt Middle GI Bleeding

1. In acute, overt, massive GI bleeding suspected to be from the middle GI tract, conventional angiography should be performed emergently for hemodynamically unstable patients.

2. In hemodynamically stable patients with evidence of active bleeding, multiphasic CT (CTA) can be performed to identify the site of bleeding and guide further management.
3. In patients with acute overt GI bleeding and slower rates of bleeding (0.1–0.2 mL/min), or uncertainty of active bleeding, tagged RBC scintigraphy can be performed if deep enteroscopy or VCE are not available to guide timing of angiography.
4. In brisk, active, overt bleeding, CTA is preferred over CTE.
5. Conventional angiography should not be performed as a diagnostic test in patients without overt bleeding. Provocative angiography can be considered in the setting of ongoing overt bleeding and negative VCE, deep enteroscopy, and/or CT, but should only be performed at centers with appropriate experience.
6. In younger patients with ongoing overt bleeding and unremarkable evaluation with VCE and MR/CT enterography examinations, a Meckel's scan should be performed.

TREATMENT OF SMALL BOWEL VASCULAR LESIONS

Endoscopic Therapy

Due to its ease of use, availability, and safety, argon plasma coagulation has been the endoscopic treatment of choice for small bowel vascular lesions. To date, there have been no published trials comparing endoscopic therapy of angioectasias compared with sham therapy or trials where only actively bleeding vascular lesions or lesions of a certain size are treated compared with therapy for all visualized lesions. Given these limitations, recurrence of bleeding has been used as a surrogate for the effectiveness of treatment. Two randomized controlled studies demonstrated a lack of benefit for either intervention, VCE versus radiology, or with hormonal therapy compared with placebo.[106,107] A 2014 meta-analysis of 14 studies including 623 subjects with small bowel angioectasia treated with endoscopic therapy demonstrated a pooled rebleeding rate of 34% (95% confidence interval [CI]: 27%-42%) after a mean follow up of 22 ± 13 months.[108] Risk factors for recurrent bleeding from small bowel angioectasia include the overall burden of vascular lesions, age greater than 65 years, jejunal location, presence of concomitant cardiac valvular disease, chronic renal disease, use of anticoagulant medications, and need for blood transfusion. Heyde syndrome is a controversial association between the presence of aortic stenosis and angioectasia and is thought to be secondary to an acquired type 2 von Willebrand's deficiency.[109,110] In support of this association is the fact that some patients with aortic stenosis have demonstrated resolution of GI bleeding after aortic valve replacement.[108] Patients with left ventricular assist devices are also at risk for angioectasias and recurrent bleeding again thought secondary to an acquired von Willebrand's deficiency syndrome.[111]

Medical Therapy of Middle GI Bleeding

Supportive care with iron, given orally or intravenously, is the mainstay of treatment for mild small intestinal bleeding.[112] This not only helps maintain an adequate hemoglobin level but in more severe cases reduces the frequency of transfusion. In more severe bleeding, transfusion of packed RBCs is an essential element of treatment, particularly when mechanistic and medical methods fail. There are no prospective data showing that withdrawal of anticoagulation therapy is beneficial. In a retrospective study assessing 162 patients with small bowel bleeding, risk factors for recurrent bleeding following DBE included the presence of small bowel vascular disorders and comorbid conditions, but not the usage of anticoagulants or antiplatelet agents.[113]

Hormonal Therapy

There have been several trials of hormonal therapy, all done in the pre-VCE era. Thus, the precise nature of what was treated was largely unknown with respect to the small intestine. At the present time, hormonal therapy does not have a role in the treatment of small bowel bleeding.

Somatostatin Analogs

There has been long time interest in the use of somatostatin analogs for treating angioectasias.[114] The proposed mechanism of action for these agents has included reduction of bleeding by the inhibition of angiogenesis, decrease in splanchnic blood flow, increase in vascular resistance, and improved platelet aggregation. Most recently, Nardone et al (2014) performed a retrospective analysis on the use of octreotide in 98 patients with bleeding from angiodysplasia.[115] Over a mean follow-up period of 78 months, the investigators demonstrated a reduction of transfusion requirements. Forty percent of subjects were categorized as complete responders, 32% as partial responders, and 26% as nonresponders. The treatment protocol used was subcutaneous octreotide 100 µg (three times/day) for 1 month; then at 2 weeks, patients received a depot injection of 20 mg monthly for 6 months. Moreover, a 2014 meta-analysis appears to confirm the value of octreotide and its analogs as medical therapy in small bowel angioectasias.[108]

Thalidomide

Thalidomide is an antiangiogenic agent, thought to be due to its inhibition of vascular endothelial growth factor.[116] It is also an antitumor necrosis factor agent and an immune modulator.

In a randomized, controlled open label trial, including patients with at least six or more bleeding episodes (measured by positive immunoassay fecal occult blood test), subjects received thalidomide 25 mg (four times/day) or 100 mg of daily oral iron.[117] Over a 12-month follow-up period, 20/28 (71%) of patients on thalidomide versus only 1/27 (4%) of patients receiving oral iron had a reduction in bleeding episodes by 50% or more (p < 0.001). Adverse events including fatigue, constipation, and somnolence were reported by 73% of the thalidomide group and 34% of the iron cohort. Levels of vascular endothelial growth factor were consistently and significantly lower in the thalidomide treated group. The benefit of thalidomide for patients with small bowel angioectasia failing endoscopic therapy was demonstrated in 9/12 (75%) patients in a study published in 2012 where patients received 200 mg of thalidomide per day for 4 months.[118] Routine use of thalidomide in cases of resistant small bowel bleeding requires further investigation and its use is mostly restricted because of its known teratogenicity.

Surgical Treatment

Surgical treatment of small intestinal bleeding should be guided by careful IOE whenever possible or by a combination of VCE, deep enteroscopy, and/or angiographic techniques. A combined radiological and surgical option has been reported involving angiographic localization of small bowel vascular lesions.[119] The angiographic catheter is left in place and the patient is transferred to the operating room. At laparotomy, methylene blue is injected via the angiographic catheter. The dye highlights the vasculature and mesentery related to the intestinal lesion allowing for identification and resection of the involved small bowel. Surgery demonstrates excellent results with discrete small bowel lesions, such as tumors or localized arteriovascular malformations. More diffuse lesions, such as multiple angioectasias, are usually treated endoscopically.

KEY REFERENCES

1. Pennazio M, Spada C, Eliakim R, et al: Small bowel capsule endoscopy and device-assisted enteroscopy for diagnosis and treatment of small bowel disorders: European Society of Gastrointestinal Endoscopy Clinical Guideline, *Endoscopy* 47:352–376, 2015.
2. Gerson LB, Fidler JL, Cave DR, Leighton JA: ACG clinical guideline: diagnosis and management of small bowel bleeding, *Am J Gastroenterol* 110:1265–1287, 2015.
3. Fry LC, Bellutti M, Neumann H, et al: Incidence of bleeding lesions within reach of conventional upper and lower endoscopes in patients undergoing double-balloon enteroscopy for obscure gastrointestinal bleeding, *Aliment Pharmacol Ther* 29:342–349, 2009.
10. Teshima CW, Kuipers EJ, van Zanten SV, et al: Double balloon enteroscopy and capsule endoscopy for obscure gastrointestinal bleeding: an updated meta-analysis, *J Gastroenterol Hepatol* 26:796–801, 2011.
11. Liao Z, Gao R, Xu C, et al: Indications and detection, completion, and retention rates of small-bowel capsule endoscopy: a systematic review, *Gastrointest Endosc* 71:280–286, 2010.
12. Triester SL, Leighton JA, Leontiadis GI, et al: A meta-analysis of the yield of capsule endoscopy compared to other diagnostic modalities in patients with obscure gastrointestinal bleeding, *Am J Gastroenterol* 100:2407–2418, 2005.
15. Koh SJ, Im JP, Kim JW, et al: Long-term outcome in patients with obscure gastrointestinal bleeding after negative capsule endoscopy, *World J Gastroenterol* 19:1632–1638, 2013.
20. Pennazio M, Santucci R, Rondonotti E, et al: Outcome of patients with obscure gastrointestinal bleeding after capsule endoscopy: report of 100 consecutive cases, *Gastroenterology* 126:643–653, 2004.

36. Liao Z, Gao R, Xu C, et al: Indications and detection, completion, and retention rates of small-bowel capsule endoscopy: a systematic review, *Gastrointest Endosc* 71:280–286, 2010.

39. Zhang W, Han ZL, Cheng Y, et al: Value of the patency capsule in pre-evaluation for capsule endoscopy in cases of intestinal obstruction, *J Dig Dis* 15:345–351, 2014.

44. Yamamoto H, Sekine Y, Sato Y, et al: Total enteroscopy with a nonsurgical steerable double-balloon method, *Gastrointest Endosc* 53:216–220, 2001.

50. May A, Nachbar L, Schneider M, et al: Push-and-pull enteroscopy using the double-balloon technique: method of assessing depth of insertion and training of the enteroscopy technique using the Erlangen Endo-Trainer, *Endoscopy* 37:66–70, 2005.

51. Moschler O, May A, Muller MK, et al: Complications in and performance of double-balloon enteroscopy (DBE): results from a large prospective DBE database in Germany, *Endoscopy* 43:484–489, 2011.

52. Messer I, May A, Manner H, et al: Prospective, randomized, single-center trial comparing double-balloon enteroscopy and spiral enteroscopy in patients with suspected small-bowel disorders, *Gastrointest Endosc* 77:241–249, 2013.

61. May A, Farber M, Aschmoneit I, et al: Prospective multi-center trial comparing push-and-pull enteroscopy with the single- and double balloon techniques in patients with small-bowel disorders, *Am J Gastroenterol* 105:575–581, 2010.

64. Akerman PA, Agrawal D, Cantero D, et al: Spiral enteroscopy with the new DSB overtube: a novel technique for deep per-oral small-bowel intubation, *Endoscopy* 40:974–978, 2008.

69. Akerman PA, Cantero D: Severe complications of spiral enteroscopy in the first 1750 patients, *Gastrointest Endosc* 69:5, 2009.

72. May A, Farber M, Aschmoneit I, et al: Prospective multi-center trial comparing push-and-pull enteroscopy with the single- and double-balloon techniques in patients with small-bowel disorders, *Am J Gastroenterol* 105:575–581, 2010.

81. Zaman A, Sheppard B, Katon RM: Total per-oral intraoperative enteroscopy for obscure GI bleeding using a dedicated push enteroscope: diagnostic yield and patient outcome, *Gastrointest Endosc* 50:506–510, 1999.

84. Wang Z, Chen JQ, Liu JL, et al: CT enterography in obscure gastrointestinal bleeding: a systematic review and meta-analysis, *J Med Imaging Radiat Oncol* 57:263–273, 2013.

85. Leighton JA, Triester SL, Sharma VK: Capsule endoscopy: a meta-analysis for use with obscure gastrointestinal bleeding and Crohn's disease, *Gastrointest Endosc Clin N Am* 16:229–250, 2006.

106. Laine L, Sahota A, Shah A: Does capsule endoscopy improve outcomes in obscure gastrointestinal bleeding? Randomized trial versus dedicated small bowel radiography, *Gastroenterology* 138:1673–1680, 2010.

107. Junquera F, Feu F, Papo M, et al: A multicenter, randomized, clinical trial of hormonal therapy in the prevention of rebleeding from gastrointestinal angiodysplasia, *Gastroenterology* 121:1073–1079, 2001.

108. Jackson CS, Gerson LB: Management of gastrointestinal angiodysplastic lesions (GIADs): a systematic review and meta-analysis, *Am J Gastroenterol* 109:474–483, 2014.

112. Goddard AF, James MW, McIntyre AS, et al: Guidelines for the management of iron deficiency anaemia, *Gut* 60:1309–1316, 2011.

A complete reference list can be found online at ExpertConsult .com

18

Occult and Unexplained Chronic Gastrointestinal Bleeding

Maite Betés Ibáñez and Miguel Muñoz-Navas

CHAPTER OUTLINE

INTRODUCTION

Chronic gastrointestinal (GI) hemorrhage may be overt or occult. Overt bleeding is defined as chronic if it is persistent but not severe enough to cause circulatory compromise. It may be seen in the form of melena or red rectal bleeding. If bleeding is occult, patients may present with symptomatic anemia and evidence of occult bleeding with stool testing. In some patients, chronic hemorrhage may be clinically interspersed with acute episodes.[1] Acute GI bleeding is discussed in detail in Chapters 14–17.

Chronic GI bleeding includes common clinical scenarios, yet the meaning and diagnostic criteria for the different terms are not well delineated.[2] Chronic bleeding from the gut is always significant; in particular, malignant tumors of the gut that are curable may be present. There is no universal agreement regarding the nomenclature of GI lesions that can cause chronic bleeding. Development of new technology, mainly wireless video capsule endoscopy (CE) and balloon-assisted enteroscopy, has provided an opportunity to revisit the traditional classifications of the source of GI bleeding into upper or lower GI bleeding based on the location of the bleeding, either proximal or distal to the ligament of Treitz.[3]

Some authors propose reclassifying GI bleeding into three categories: upper GI, mid-GI, and lower GI bleeding. Bleeding above the ampulla of Vater, within the reach of esophagogastroduodenoscopy (EGD), is defined as upper GI bleeding; small intestinal bleeding from the ampulla of Vater to the terminal ileum, best investigated by CE and balloon-assisted enteroscopy, is defined as mid-GI bleeding; and colonic bleeding, which can be evaluated by colonoscopy, is defined as lower GI bleeding. A simple classification is presented in Table 18.1. This chapter discusses the evaluation and some of the most frequent causes of occult or unexplained chronic GI bleeding.

Vascular lesions are a common cause of chronic GI bleeding. Arteriovenous malformations (AVMs) of the small bowel account for 30% to 40% of unexplained chronic GI bleeding and are the most common source in older patients. The categorization of vascular abnormalities in the GI tract has been inconsistent and a source of confusion.[4,5] It can be based on histologic characteristics, gross appearance, or association with systemic diseases. These considerations permit categorization into three broad groups, as follows:

1. *Vascular tumors,* which can be benign (e.g., hemangiomas) or malignant (e.g., Kaposi's sarcoma or angiosarcoma).
2. *Vascular anomalies associated with congenital or systemic diseases,* such as blue rubber bleb nevus syndrome, Klippel-Trénaunay-Weber syndrome, Ehlers-Danlos syndrome, pseudoxanthoma elasticum, the CREST (calcinosis, *R*aynaud's phenomenon, *e*sophageal dysmotility, *s*cleroderma, and *t*elangioectasias) variant of scleroderma, and hereditary hemorrhagic telangiectasia.
3. *Acquired or sporadic lesions,* such as angiodysplasias, gastric antral vascular ectasia, portal hypertensive enteropathy, radiation-induced vascular ectasias, and Dieulafoy's lesions. Younger individuals (< 40 years of age) most commonly have chronic unexplained bleeding due to Crohn's disease or Meckel's

TABLE 18.1 Causes of Chronic Gastrointestinal Bleeding

Gastrointestinal Lesions

Within Reach of Upper Endoscope	May Be Beyond Reach of Upper Endoscope
Esophagitis	Celiac sprue
Cameron lesions	Crohn's disease
Peptic ulcer disease	Intestinal lymphoma
Gastritis and erosions	Small bowel angiodysplasia
Duodenitis and erosions	Small bowel tumors
Angiodysplasia	Small bowel ulcers and erosions, including NSAID- and other drug-induced lesions
Portal hypertensive gastropathy	Small bowel diverticulosis
Gastroesophageal cancer	Small bowel varices
Gastric or duodenal polyps	Lymphangioma
Gastroduodenal lymphoma	Radiation enteritis
Partial gastrectomy	Blue rubber bleb nevus syndrome
GAVE	Osler-Weber-Rendu syndrome
Dieulafoy's lesion	Small bowel polyposis syndromes Gardner's syndrome Amyloidosis Meckel's diverticulum Hemosuccus pancreaticus, hemobilia Klippel-Trénaunay-Weber syndrome

Colonic Lesions

Colon polyps
Colon cancer
Angiodysplasia
Colonic ulcers
Colitis and IBD
Parasitic infestation
Hemorrhoids
Diverticular bleeding

GAVE, Gastric antral vascular ectasia; *IBD,* inflammatory bowel disease; *NSAID,* nonsteroidal antiinflammatory drug.

diverticulum–associated ulceration(s). Small bowel neoplasms (e.g., GI stromal tumor, lymphoma, carcinoid, adenocarcinoma, or other polypoid lesions) and Dieulafoy's lesions can occur in both younger and older patients. Nonsteroidal antiinflammatory drug (NSAID) enteropathy has been associated with mucosal erosions, ulcers, and strictures of the small bowel. Less common causes of unexplained GI bleeding include hemosuccus pancreaticus, *Strongyloides stercoralis* infection, radiation-induced enteritis, and pseudoxanthoma elasticum.

INVESTIGATING CHRONIC UNEXPLAINED GASTROINTESTINAL BLEEDING

Patient age, symptoms, medical/surgical history, physical examination findings, and laboratory data may all provide clues and help guide diagnostic investigations. Recurrent hematemesis indicates bleeding proximal to the ligament of Treitz, whereas recurrent passage of hematochezia without hemodynamic instability usually suggests a colonic source. Melena can originate from a bleeding site located anywhere from the upper GI tract to the right colon.

Thus, a history of melena provides only limited value in terms of localization of obscure GI bleeding. A thorough review of medications may reveal inadvertent use of NSAIDs. A family history of cancer occurring at an early age, particularly colorectal or endometrial, may suggest the presence of hereditary nonpolyposis colorectal cancer. Skin, nail, and oral mucosal changes may suggest the presence of several disorders associated with obscure GI bleeding or iron deficiency anemia, including telangiectasias, which may reflect hereditary hemorrhagic telangiectasia (Osler-Weber-Rendu syndrome); other conditions with cutaneous and GI manifestations include Kaposi's sarcoma, Peutz-Jeghers syndrome, tylosis, pseudoxanthoma elasticum, Ehlers-Danlos syndrome, blue rubber bleb nevus syndrome, Henoch-Schönlein purpura, neurofibromatosis, malignant atrophic papulosis, and Klippel-Trénaunay-Weber syndrome.[6]

Endoscopic Investigations
Repeat EGD and Colonoscopy
Second-look upper endoscopy may be helpful in identifying bleeding lesions potentially overlooked or unrecognized at the time of the initial endoscopic evaluation.[7,8] Data suggest that 2% to 25% of lesions causing obscure gastrointestinal bleeding may be overlooked and are within reach of a standard upper endoscope. More recent studies using double-balloon enteroscopy (DBE) and CE have also confirmed these findings.[9–11] Commonly overlooked lesions in the upper GI tract include Cameron's erosions or ulcerations in large hiatal hernias, isolated gastric fundal varices, peptic ulcers, AVMs including gastric antral vascular ectasia (watermelon stomach), and Dieulafoy's lesion. An aorto-enteric fistula should always be considered in patients with prior abdominal aortic aneurysm repair. If second-look upper endoscopy is selected, push enteroscopy may be the chosen method to more thoroughly examine the distal duodenum and proximal jejunum in addition to the more proximal upper GI tract.

Although the reported yield of repeat colonoscopy is low (6%–23%), it may be helpful in selected patients when the original colonoscopy examination was documented to have had a mediocre or poor preparation, the extent of the examination was not to the cecum, the patient is older and risk of a previously missed neoplastic lesion is considered, or the terminal ileum was not previously evaluated. Lesions missed or unrecognized during colonoscopy may include AVMs, polyps, solitary rectal ulcers, rectal varices, and neoplasms.[12]

ANGIODYSPLASIA OF THE GASTROINTESTINAL TRACT

Vascular ectasia of the GI tract, also referred to as angiodysplasia (AD) or less accurately as AVM, is a distinct clinical and pathologic entity.[13–15] It is the most common vascular abnormality of the GI tract and probably the most frequent cause of lower intestinal bleeding in patients older than 60 years. Although the terms *angiodysplasia* and *arteriovenous malformation* have been used synonymously, the term *angiodysplasia* (Greek *angeion,* "vessel"; *dys,* "bad" or "difficult"; *plasis,* "a molding") means a poorly formed vessel but with a lesser connotation of congenital origin than with the word *malformation.* AD are usually distinguished from telangiectasias, which, although anatomically similar, are usually referred to in the context of systemic or hereditary diseases. Because most vascular abnormalities are detected during endoscopy, a classification based on endoscopic appearance has been proposed.[16] The classification system recognizes the location, size, and number of AD.

Pathogenesis

AD are composed of ectatic, dilated, thin-walled vessels that are lined by endothelium alone or by only small amounts of smooth muscle. Arteriovenous communications are present because of incompetence of the precapillary sphincter. Enlarged arteries are also present in bigger AD and may be associated with arteriovenous fistulas, which explains why bleeding can be a risk in some patients. Histologic examination shows dilated vessels in the mucosa and submucosa, sometimes covered by a single layer of surface epithelium. The pathogenesis of AD is not well understood. Several theories have been proposed, as follows:

1. AD may develop in response to chronic partial, intermittent, low-grade obstruction of the submucosal veins at the point where they penetrate the muscle layers of the colon.[17] Following this logic, the prevalence of vascular ectasias in the right colon can be attributed to a greater tension in the cecal wall compared with other parts of the colon, according to LaPlace's principle. Over many years, repeated contraction and distention of the cecum results in dilation and tortuosity of the submucosal vein and, later, the venules and capillaries draining into it. Finally, the capillary rings dilate, the precapillary sphincters become incompetent, and a tiny arteriovenous fistula develops.
2. AD may be a complication of chronic mucosal ischemia, which can occur during episodes of bowel obstruction or straining stools.[18]
3. AD may be a complication of local ischemia associated with cardiac, vascular, or pulmonary disease.[19,20]
4. AD may be congenital, which is probably more likely in young patients or patients who have angiodysplasias associated with congenital diseases.
5. Increased expression of angiogenic factors, namely vascular endothelial growth factor (VEGF) and basic fibroblast growth factor, has been demonstrated in human colonic AD and is therefore likely to play a very important role in the development of these lesions as well as in modifying the risk of bleeding.

Epidemiology and Natural History

The prevalence of GI angiodysplasias in the overall population is not well known, but angioectasiases have been seen in 0.2% to 2.9% of "nonbleeding persons"[21,22] and in 2.6% to 6.2% of patients evaluated specifically for occult blood in the stool, anemia, or hemorrhage.[21-23] AD occur most often in the colon, where they are an important cause of lower GI bleeding, particularly in patients older than 60 years of age,[24-26] although presentation in patients in their 30s has been described.[27] There is no gender predilection.

Clinical Manifestations

AD can remain clinically silent or cause bleeding. The estimated incidence of active GI bleeding in patients with AD is less than 10%. These lesions may be located throughout the GI tract with a variable rate of bleeding associated with them and presentation ranging from hematemesis or hematochezia to occult anemia.[3,28,29] Bleeding is usually chronic or recurrent and, in most cases, low grade and painless.

AD of the stomach have been found to be the cause of blood loss in 4% to 7% of patients with GI bleeding.[24,30] AD in the stomach or duodenum are found incidentally in approximately 50% of cases.[31] The risk that an incidentally found gastric or duodenal AD will subsequently bleed is uncertain. Patients who have bled from gastric or duodenal AD do rebleed. This rebleeding was illustrated in a series of 30 patients with gastric or duodenal AD; 77% had experienced at least one episode of overt bleeding before diagnosis.[24] Approximately 5% of patients presenting with GI hemorrhage have no source found by upper endoscopy and colonoscopy. In approximately 75% of these patients, responsible lesions can be detected in the small bowel. In patients presenting with obscure overt bleeding (defined as the presence of recurrent melena or hematochezia with normal evaluation by upper endoscopy and colonoscopy), small bowel angioectasias are detected in 30% to 60% of examinations.[3,20,32]

The colon is the most common site of AD in the GI tract; colonic lesions are most often found in the cecum and ascending colon. In some reported experiences, AD of the colon account for approximately 20% to 30% of cases of acute lower GI bleeding, approaching the frequency of acute colonic diverticular bleeding.[33] Foutch et al (1995)[34] noted the prevalence of AD to be 0.83% from three prospective studies in which screening colonoscopies were performed in 964 asymptomatic individuals (mean age 61 years) and none of them developed bleeding over a mean follow-up of 3 years.

Conditions With Increased Prevalence
End-Stage Renal Disease

AD is the second most common cause of GI bleeding in patients with end-stage renal disease.[35] These lesions account for approximately 20% of upper GI bleeds and 30% of lower GI bleeds,[35] and approximately 50% of recurrent upper GI bleeds.[36] In a prospective study of upper GI hemorrhage over a 50-month period, vascular ectasia was the etiology of upper GI hemorrhage in 13% of patients with renal insufficiency and was the etiology of bleeding more often in patients with renal insufficiency than in patients with normal renal function.[37] The prevalence of vascular ectasia as a cause of upper GI bleeding was related to the duration of renal failure and the requirement of hemodialysis. Although the reason for the increased prevalence among patients with end-stage renal disease is unknown, a possible explanation is that there is an increased risk of bleeding associated with uremia-induced platelet dysfunction (aggregation and adhesion).

von Willebrand's Disease

von Willebrand's disease is a bleeding disorder that results from a qualitative or quantitative defect in von Willebrand factor (vWF). vWF is a complex multimeric glycoprotein present in platelets, plasma, and subendothelium, and is essential to platelet adhesion and aggregation at the site of vascular injury. In a study of patients with both bleeding and nonbleeding angioectasias of the GI tract and control patients with colonic diverticular hemorrhage, Veyradier et al (2001)[38] showed that most patients with bleeding angioectasias of the GI tract lack the largest multimers of vWF induced by a latent acquired form of von Willebrand's disease. Because these specific multimers are the most effective in inducing platelet aggregation in high shear stress that is commonly present in the microcirculation of angioectasias, it was concluded their deficiency contributes to active bleeding.

Aortic Stenosis

Approximately 50% of patients with bleeding vascular ectasias have evidence of cardiac disease, and 25% have been reported

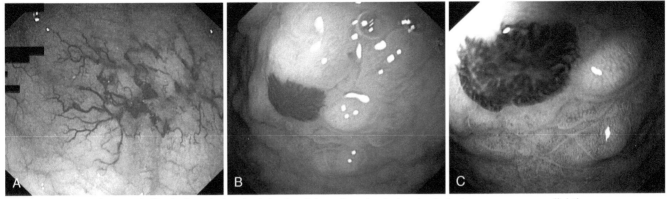

FIG 18.1 A, Typical angiodysplasia in the right colon. Angiodysplastic lesions are seen as slightly dilated tortuous vessels. **B,** Angiodysplasia in the stomach. **C,** Narrow-band imaging of the same lesion.

to have aortic stenosis (AS). Bleeding from angiodysplasias in patients with AS (Heyde's syndrome) has been repeatedly reported but is highly controversial.[39] Support for this hypothesis comes from evidence of improvement or cessation of chronic GI bleeding in the vast majority of patients with AS after aortic valve replacement. This effect was sustained for up to 12 years after surgery in the largest case series of 91 patients.[20]

Two possible explanations have been proposed to explain this observation. Patients with AS may develop an acquired form of von Willebrand's disease, which can be reversed after aortic valve replacement.[38,40,41] Patients with AS may be more likely to bleed from existing AD. Another explanation is that existing AD may bleed as a result of ischemic necrosis in patients who have a low cardiac output.[18,42,43] However, this explanation is inconsistent with the observations that bleeding AD have not been observed with other forms of heart disease associated with a low cardiac output and that a low cardiac output is a late complication of AS.

Several retrospective, uncontrolled studies[44,45] and a prospective, controlled investigation[46] do not substantiate a causative role or association of aortic valve diseases with colonic angioectasias. Replacement of the aortic valve for control of bleeding secondary to these vascular lesions is not universally accepted.[29] A logical approach to patients with both lesions is to treat the colonic lesion first endoscopically, regardless of whether the patient's cardiac status warrants surgery. If valve replacement is necessary and endoscopic therapy is unsuccessful, further endoscopic or surgical treatment of the colonic AD should be delayed until after cardiac surgery. Further attempts at endoscopic treatment or surgical resection are indicated if bleeding recurs.[47]

Progressive Systemic Sclerosis

Vascular lesions are a prominent feature of progressive systemic sclerosis, especially in the CREST variant.[48] In patients with progressive systemic sclerosis, sites most frequently affected by telangioectasias are the hands, lips, tongue, and face, but gastric, intestinal, and colorectal lesions have been reported. These lesions may be the source of occult or clinically significant bleeding and are best treated by endoscopic coagulation.[49]

Left Ventricular Assist Devices

Patients with left ventricular assist devices have higher rates of GI bleeding, most commonly from angioectasias in the upper digestive tract and small bowel.[50]

TABLE 18.2 Lesions Confused With Angioectasias on Endoscopy

Vascular	Nonvascular	Colitis
Arteriovenous malformations	Trauma	Ischemic
Angiomas	Polyps	Infectious
Phlebectasia	Adenomatous	Radiation (acute)
Varices	Hyperplastic	Inflammatory bowel disease
Venous stars	Lymphoid	

Diagnosis
Endoscopic Imaging: Standard Upper Endoscopy and Colonoscopy

Angioectasias have a characteristic appearance of a cherry-red, fern-like pattern of arborizing, ectatic blood vessels radiating from a central vessel (Fig. 18.1). This pattern should be specifically looked for because angioectasias may be confused with other erythematous mucosal lesions or with normal vessels (Table 18.2).[29,51] Because traumatic and endoscopic suction artifacts may resemble vascular lesions, all lesions must be evaluated immediately on insertion, rather than during withdrawal. "Anemic halos" are often seen surrounding angioectasias of the bowel. Although these halos do not differentiate the various types of vascular lesions, they distinguish true vascular lesions from artifacts.[47] Newer alternative imaging options, such as narrow-band imaging, allow precise discrimination of vascular structures from artifactual mucosal hemorrhage. Punch biopsy samples of vascular lesions obtained during endoscopy are usually nonspecific; the bleeding induced by performing biopsies of these abnormalities is not justified.

Angioectasias may be difficult to visualize during colonoscopy in patients who do not have an optimal bowel cleaning. Because the appearance of angioectasias is influenced by blood pressure, blood volume, and state of hydration, these lesions may not be evident in patients with severely reduced blood volumes or who are in shock until red blood cell and volume deficits are corrected. Cold water lavage of the colon, as is sometimes done to clean the luminal surface from debris during colonoscopy, reportedly may mask these lesions.[52] Meperidine also has been implicated in masking lesions because of a transient decrease in mucosal blood flow. Minimizing use of meperidine and reversal with naloxone to increase the yield of detection has been advocated by some clinicians. Naloxone has been reported to enhance the appearance of normal vasculature in approximately 10% of patients and to cause angioectasias to appear (2.7%) or increase in size (5.4%).[53] Reversal of narcotic analgesia may affect the comfort of an examination, particularly if therapeutics are performed.

Assessment of the Small Bowel

Some patients presenting with GI bleeding have no source found by upper endoscopy and colonoscopy, even after second-look endoscopy.[3] In these cases of unexplained chronic GI bleeding, endoscopic examination of the small bowel has been limited by several factors. The length of the small intestine, in addition to its free intraperitoneal location, vigorous contractility, and overlying loops, confounds the usual diagnostic techniques, including barium studies, endoscopic intubation, and identification of specific sites by special imaging techniques of nuclear medicine scans and angiography. The bleeding rate may be slow or intermittent, not allowing identification by either angiography or radionuclide bleeding scan. Because of the inability to localize a bleeding site in the small bowel, patients with obscure GI bleeding from a small bowel source typically presented with prolonged occult blood loss or recurrent episodes of melena or maroon stool without a specific diagnosis. In this group of patients, previous noninvasive tests, such as small bowel follow-through, radioisotope-labeled red blood cell scan, and push enteroscopy, have had suboptimal diagnostic yields of 20% to 40%. Invasive methods, such as laparotomy or intraoperative enteroscopy, may improve the yield up to 70%.[54]

An early diagnosis of the bleeding site has become possible recently with the development of several endoscopic modalities for assessment of the small bowel that include wireless CE and deep small bowel enteroscopy (DBE, single-balloon enteroscopy, and spiral enteroscopy [SE]).

When performing a second-look endoscopy, useful adjunctive diagnostic maneuvers include use of a cap-fitted endoscope to examine blind areas, such as the high lesser curve, under the incisura angularis, and the posterior wall of the duodenal bulb; use of a side-viewing endoscope to examine the ampulla in patients with suspected pancreaticobiliary pathology; and use of a push enteroscope to examine the C-loop of duodenum carefully after injection of glucagon. Although the yield is low (6%), repeat colonoscopy may be useful in the setting of prior poor bowel preparation. Use of naloxone may improve the detection of colonic angioectasias that were not obvious at the index examination.[3] When all the findings on standard examinations (upper endoscopy and colonoscopy) are negative, the small bowel may be presumed to be the source of blood loss. CE should be the third test in the evaluation of patients with GI bleeding (Fig. 18.2). CE, balloon, and spiral enteroscopy, as well as other diagnostic modalities for suspected small bowel bleeding, are discussed in detail in Chapter 17: Middle Gastrointestinal Bleeding.

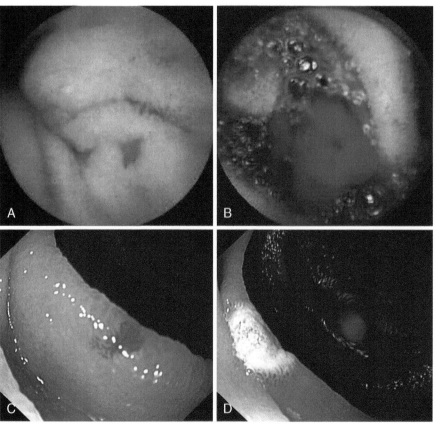

FIG 18.2 Small bowel angiodysplasias in patients with obscure gastrointestinal bleeding. **A,** Nonbleeding angiodysplasia diagnosed by wireless capsule endoscopy. **B,** Active bleeding angiodysplasia visualized by capsule endoscopy. **C,** Small bowel angiodysplasia seen with balloon enteroscopy. **D,** Same lesion treated with argon plasma coagulation.

Diagnostic Algorithm for Endoscopy in Suspected Middle Gastrointestinal Bleeding

Similar to other authors, we recommend[55–57] CE as a first-line investigation over balloon-assisted enteroscopy in view of its convenience, higher chance to visualize the entire small intestine, and similar diagnostic yield. A recent updated and revised meta-analysis of 10 studies involving 642 patients demonstrated that the pooled overall diagnostic yield for video CE (VCE) and DBE was 62% and 56%, respectively.[58] The diagnostic yield of DBE was significantly higher when performed after a positive VCE compared with negative VCE (75% vs. 27.5%). No test substitutes for good clinical judgment, however, and all small bowel diagnostic studies must be considered in difficult cases of obscure GI bleeding, particularly in a young patient.[59]

In the setting of unexplained overt GI bleeding, CE should be performed close to the bleeding episode. In case of negative CE, we recommend that a second endoscopist reread the CE study. We also recommend a second-look EGD with special attention to areas less optimally examined by CE, especially the duodenum, before concluding with a final diagnosis of obscure GI bleeding. Second-look CE has also been suggested for patients with a prior nondiagnostic CE. Bar-Meir et al (2004)[60] reported that 7 out of 20 patients (35%) who underwent second-look CE had positive or suspicious findings. Another study showed that patients with a nondiagnostic CE test would benefit from a second-look CE if the bleeding presentation changed from occult to overt, or if the hemoglobin value decreased 4 g/dL or more.[61]

Management

The natural history of colonic angioectasias is benign in healthy, asymptomatic individuals, and the risk of bleeding is small.[34] It is estimated that only approximately 50% of colonic lesions ever bleed. There is a risk of bleeding and perforation following attempts at endoscopic obliteration. For all these reasons, in incidentally found angioectasias at all levels of the gut, endoscopic therapy is not warranted.[62]

Pharmacologic Treatment

Pharmacotherapy should be considered whenever endoscopic therapy, surgical intervention, or angiographic therapy is impractical or ineffective, such as in patients in whom the source and the etiology of bleeding are unknown or the pathology is too diffuse to be amenable to ablative therapies.

Nonbleeding AD detected during evaluation of occult bleeding or iron deficiency anemia should be considered to be causative, if no other cause is found. In patients with occult bleeding, bleeding from AD may be more likely in patients who have multiple lesions and a bleeding diathesis (e.g., anticoagulation). As a result, a graduated approach with primary or adjunctive iron-replacement therapy may be initiated, with pursuit of more aggressive therapeutic options guided by the clinical circumstances.[62–64] The aims of iron-replacement therapy should be to restore hemoglobin levels and mean corpuscular volume to normal, and to replenish body stores.

Numerous oral iron preparations are available, although ferrous sulfate and ferrous gluconate are the preferred forms because of low cost and high bioavailability. A liquid preparation is often tolerated better. Ascorbic acid enhances iron absorption. Parenteral iron should be used when there is intolerance to at least two oral iron preparations or noncompliance, when there is a suboptimal clinical response secondary to suspected iron malabsorption, and when blood transfusion becomes difficult to achieve because of excessive antibodies that challenge crossmatching.

Estrogen-progesterone combination hormonal therapy has been used to treat patients with angioectasias of the GI tract.[65,66] The effect, which is not immediate, seems to be estrogen dose–dependent. Hormonal therapy acts by enhancing microvascular circulation, coagulation, and vascular endothelial integrity. The most common combination schedule has been ethinyl estradiol 0.01 to 0.05 mg and norethisterone 1 to 3 mg. This therapy should be used in 6-month courses with pauses to reduce the incidence of adverse effects, mostly secondary to the estrogen component. The results of several prospective, controlled trials examining hormonal therapy have been divergent.[67–70] In a long-term observational study, combination hormonal therapy was shown to stop bleeding in patients with occult GI bleeding of obscure origin, likely to have resulted from small bowel AD.[69] Although uncontrolled studies suggest that combination estrogen-progesterone therapy prevents bleeding episodes secondary to AD, the evidence from the largest placebo-controlled trial to date suggests that this therapy is ineffective.[71] These authors considered that efficacy of hormonal therapy in these patients remains to be proven by a large, randomized, placebo-controlled trial with long-term follow-up.

Reports of efficacy of octreotide in the treatment of AD have been limited to case reports and small series in which a response has been reported in some patients.[66,72–74] Octreotide produces vasoconstriction secondary to inhibitory effects on growth hormone and multiple GI vasodilator hormones, and markedly reduces splanchnic blood flow. Its antiangiogenic properties have been shown in different tissues (eye, placenta, liver, and GI neuroendocrine tumors); however, applicability and utility in obscure GI bleeding remain unknown.

The dosage of octreotide can be tapered to the lowest quantity that prevents rebleeding. Response is immediate, and the drug can be administered intravenously (50 µg/hr) or subcutaneously (50–100 µg two or three times a day).[66] Its subcutaneous administration and its longer half-life (90–100 minutes) make octreotide superior to somatostatin and allow use in the outpatient setting. A 6-month course of therapy has been used to treat most patients. A meta-analysis reported by Jackson and Gerson in 2014 including four studies with a total sample size of 77 patients concluded that there is a significant effect on bleeding cessation rates for the somatostatin analogs with a pooled odds ratio of 14.52 (95% confidence interval [CI]: 5.9–36).[75] The standard mean reduction in number of transfusions after 1 year of therapy was 0.55 (95% CI: 0.29–0.82). However, it is difficult to ascertain whether this represents the true effect of octreotide, as this meta-analysis had some inherent weaknesses.[20]

Sandostatin LAR Depot (Novartis Pharmaceuticals Corporation, East Hanover, NJ) is a depot formulation of octreotide for long-term maintenance therapy currently approved for acromegaly and GI and pancreatic neuroendocrine tumors. Compared with conventional octreotide, Sandostatin LAR Depot is administered at a dose of 20 mg intramuscularly once a month with a similar efficacy and safety profile.[66,73,76–78] Sandostatin LAR Depot does not require hospital admission, which makes it an attractive outpatient option for long-term therapy in patients with chronic GI bleeding, but is more expensive than conventional octreotide.

Thalidomide is a drug with powerful immunomodulatory, antiinflammatory, and antiangiogenic effects that was withdrawn from the market in the 1960s because of its teratogenicity. It has been reintroduced more recently and has been demonstrated to inhibit VEGF-dependent angiogenesis. Thalidomide administered orally at a variable dose of 100 to 300 mg/day is an innovative and promising therapeutic option for GI bleeding associated with AD and can be used in refractory cases or when other drugs or therapies are contraindicated.[66] Thalidomide is contraindicated in patients with peripheral neuropathy and pregnant women and women with childbearing potential because of its teratogenic effects, and it should be used cautiously in patients with cardiovascular or neurologic disorders and hepatic or renal impairment. Owing to its immunosuppressant activity by blocking tumor necrosis factor, use of thalidomide may also be discouraged in patients at risk for infection or chronic infectious disease, especially patients with HIV infection. In all these clinical settings, Sandostatin LAR Depot may be safer than thalidomide.

Two recent studies explore the use of thalidomide for gastrointestinal angiodysplastic lesions (GIADs) in a series of patients. The first study from China in 2011 randomized patients to 100 mg of thalidomide versus iron therapy for 4 months and demonstrated efficacy when rebleeding rates and transfusional requirements were analyzed.[79] The second study from Spain treated 12 refractory patients and demonstrated an increase in hemoglobin values after 4 months.[80]

Other agents that have been used for management of angioectasias with limited available data include tranexamic acid, danazol, desmopressin, and recombinant activated factor VII.

Endoscopic Treatment

The goal of endoscopic therapy is thrombosis of the bleeding vessel. Studies directly comparing the effectiveness of the different approaches have not been performed. The approach depends on the location of the lesion, the experience of the endoscopist, and the availability of equipment.

Bipolar or heater probe coagulation. Bipolar devices deliver heat via a current that flows between the two electrodes at the tip of the probe. This limits the maximum temperature generated, as well as the depth and surface area of tissue injury. Bipolar or heater probe coagulation is said to be effective for treatment of AD,[81,82] and these modalities have replaced monopolar coagulation.[19] The choice between argon plasma coagulation (APC) and bipolar coagulation depends on availability and local expertise.[20] Both techniques should be used with caution in the duodenum and ascending colon.

Sclerotherapy. Injection of a sclerosant, such as ethanolamine, has been used to obliterate lesions.[83] Epinephrine injection works by volume tamponade of the bleeding vessel and transient vasoconstriction, but should probably be avoided, however, because of the risk of bleeding, ulceration and perforation.[47,84]

Band ligation. Band ligation has been used to treat angioectasias of the stomach.[85,86] The walls of the small and large intestine above the rectum (especially the right colon) are thinner than the stomach. For this reason, band ligation therapy cannot be advocated owing to the recognized risk for perforation.[87,88]

Endoscopic resection. There are some cases reported of polypoid colonic AD treated by polypectomy using a polyloop ligation device in one case with no complications.[20]

Lasers. Argon and neodymium:yttrium-aluminum-garnet (Nd:YAG) lasers have been used in the past.[89–91] These techniques require expensive equipment and specific training. More convenient and safer coagulation options have replaced laser therapy.

Endoscopic clips. This approach has shown safety and efficacy in few case reports using endoscopic clipping for bleeding colonic AD[20] either as a monotherapy or in combination with thermal ablation using APC and contact probes. Clipping may be particularly useful in cases of isolated and relatively large lesions to obliterate the feeding vessel and reduce the risk of precipitating bleeding from subsequent electrocoagulation. It can also be useful in patients with high risk of bleeding due to drugs or coagulation defects.

Argon plasma coagulation. APC is a monopolar electrosurgical procedure in which electrical energy is transferred to the target tissue using ionized and conductive argon gas (argon plasma).[92] APC seems to be most effective in the treatment of vascular lesions.[93,94] Its great advantage is the limited depth of tissue injury and low cost. Shallow tissue injury is due to the fact that the argon stream always seeks electrically conductive areas of tissue, avoiding the coagulated zones, which have lost their electrical conductivity as a result of desiccation. Before APC, it is recommended to collapse the lumen partially while maintaining the treatment site in view. It is important to avoid thinning of the colonic wall with excessive air insufflation because this increases the risk for perforation during therapy, especially in the cecum.[84]

Cryotherapy. Endoscopic cryotherapy allows circumscribed tissue destruction by freezing. Three- to four-second impacts create a 2- to 10-mm large ice layer around the probe tip on the surface of the mucosa. Safety and efficacy of cryotherapy have been reported for treatment of diffuse mucosal lesions of the GI tract.[95]

Tips to get the best results with endoscopic treatment of GIAD. The effectiveness of endoscopic treatment of angioectasias is difficult to assess owing to the absence of prospective controlled trials. Endoscopic treatment of vascular lesions in patients known to have coagulation disorders carries an increased risk of procedure-induced hemorrhage.

When treating large lesions, some experienced endoscopists recommend[47] to first ablate the periphery of the lesion to create a collar of edema that theoretically reduces the vascular supply to the lesion and diminishes the potential for immediate or delayed hemorrhage. Some clinicians have placed mechanical clips around the margins of large lesions also to reduce the blood supply and facilitate effective coagulation. Others typically target the central portion of the AD because ensuing coagulation and edema obstruct the peripheral branches and limit the extent of coagulation needed. In addition, for a very large AD, epinephrine injection may contract the lesion and reduce the amount and area of coagulation needed for eradication.[84] In our experience, prior submucosal injection of normal saline can prevent unexpected deep thermal injury from coagulation therapy, especially in areas with a thin wall. Recurrent bleeding can be expected in approximately 20% of patients with colonic angioectasias and in a greater percentage of patients with associated coagulopathies, renal failure, portal hypertension, or additional upper GI vascular lesions.[47] It is reasonable to attempt endoscopic therapy in patients with accessible lesions despite various coexisting morbidities that may allow only short-term success. Patients with multiple lesions or an underlying bleeding diathesis are less likely to benefit long term from endoscopic therapy and are at increased risk of complications, especially delayed bleeding from treatment site thermally induced ulceration. Such patients benefit from any attempts to improve their underlying bleeding tendency.

In preparation for endoscopic ablation of vascular lesions, aspirin, NSAIDs, anticoagulants, and antiplatelet agents should be withdrawn at least 1 week to 10 days before the procedure, when feasible. After therapy, patients must be cautioned not to resume full doses of anticoagulants or antiplatelet agents for at least 1 week if clinically possible. Coagulated tissues are at their

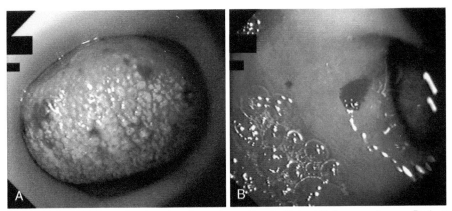

FIG 18.3 Hereditary hemorrhagic telangiectasia or Rendu-Osler-Weber syndrome. Patient with multiple telangioectasias involving **A,** the tongue and **B,** the stomach.

maximum of thermal injury by 5 to 10 days, and the onset of hemorrhage may be delayed.

HEREDITARY HEMORRHAGIC TELANGIECTASIA

Hereditary hemorrhagic telangiectasia, or Rendu-Osler-Weber disease, is an uncommon, autosomal dominant disorder characterized by telangioectasias and AVMs that affect many organs, including the skin, periungual areas, lips, oral and nasopharyngeal membranes, tongue (Fig. 18.3A), lungs, GI tract (see Fig. 18.3B), liver, and brain,[96,97] and can result in bleeding. In these vessels, no elastic lamina or muscular tissue is present, so they cannot contract; this property may explain why these lesions tend to bleed.[29]

Mucocutaneous and GI telangioectasias develop progressively with age.[98] Severe GI bleeding is unusual before the 5th or 6th decade[99]; occurs in 25% to 33% of patients with hereditary hemorrhagic telangiectasia; is challenging to treat; and can cause significant morbidity, resulting in severe anemia and high blood transfusion requirements.[100,101]

Endoscopy may reveal telangioectasias in the stomach (see Fig. 18.1B), duodenum, small bowel, or colon that are punctiform, discrete, red spots or with a classic fern-like border similar to all other angioectasias. Lesions are usually flat, although they may be slightly raised 1 to 3 mm, similar in size and appearance to angioectasias of the nasal and oral mucosa.[99] Telangioectasias are more common in the stomach, duodenum, or jejunum than in the colon.[98] They may also have a characteristic pale mucosal halo. CE contributes significantly to defining the extent of small intestinal telangioectasias and can be used to stage the disease to decide on the extent and form of endoscopic therapy.[97] Endoscopic therapy is the most effective form of treatment in stopping hemorrhage from actively bleeding lesions and has reduced the need for emergency bowel resection. Because of the multiplicity of lesions and the redevelopment of lesions, sometimes within weeks, bleeding recurs at varying intervals after therapy, depending on the extent and thoroughness of ablative therapies.[102] Selective mesenteric arteriography may localize the precise bleeding site, but in most cases this is unnecessary.[103]

GASTRIC VASCULAR LESIONS IN PATIENTS WITH CIRRHOSIS

After variceal bleeding, hemorrhagic gastritis is the most frequent cause of upper GI bleeding in cirrhotic patients with portal hypertension.[104] The term *hemorrhagic gastritis* has included bleeding from various nonvariceal mucosal lesions, such as multiple ulcerations, portal hypertensive gastropathy (PHG), and gastric antral vascular ectasia (GAVE).[104–106] PHG and GAVE can cause acute and chronic upper GI blood loss.[107] These conditions frequently, but not invariably, are diagnosed by upper endoscopy. Although they are fairly prevalent, only 15% to 20% of affected individuals experience symptomatic GI blood loss.

Portal Hypertensive Gastropathy

PHG describes the endoscopic appearance of gastric mucosa, with a characteristic mosaic-like pattern with or without red spots, seen in patients with cirrhotic or noncirrhotic portal hypertension. The mosaic-like pattern appears as a white reticular network separating areas of raised red or pink mucosa, resembling the skin of a snake (*snakeskin appearance*). PHG is seen mainly in the body and the fundus of the stomach, but is also seen rarely in the gastric antrum (Fig. 18.4). When PHG is severe, it can include discrete cherry-red spots, fine pink speckling, or scarlatina-type rash, collectively called *red marks*.[108] The characteristic histologic finding of PHG is dilated capillaries and venules in the mucosa and submucosa without erosion, inflammation, or fibrinous thrombi.[109]

Classification

There is no general consensus on the endoscopic classification of PHG. The most widely used classification is the one recommended by McCormack et al (1985),[109] who classified PHG into mild and severe (Table 18.3). Mild PHG is defined by the presence of only a mosaic-like pattern, whereas severe PHG is diagnosed when red point lesions, cherry-red spots, or black-brown spots are present. The popularity of this classification relates in part to its simplicity and its ability to predict the risk of bleeding, with an increased risk of gastric hemorrhage in severe cases (38%–62%) compared with mild cases (3.5%–31%).[105,106] Observed endoscopic findings are often of an intermediate severity, however, and are not well represented as being either mild or severe. Tanoue et al (1992)[110] and the New Italian Endoscopy Club[111] have described a more detailed scoring system. Tanoue et al (1992)[110] classified PHG into four grades (grade 0 = none, grade 1 = mild, grade 2 = moderate, grade 3 = severe). This grading permits more informative description of the observed endoscopic findings. A simpler classification system such as recommended by McCormack et al (1985)[109] has a better intraobserver and interobserver agreement and reproducibility.[112]

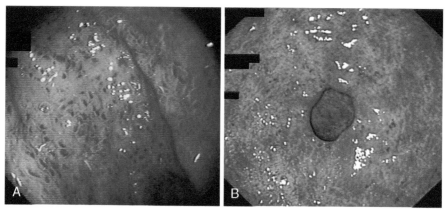

FIG 18.4 Portal hypertensive gastropathy with mosaic pattern and cherry-red spots in **A,** the body of the stomach and **B,** localized in the antrum of a cirrhotic patient.

McCormack et al[161]	Tanoue et al[162]	Primignani et al (NIEC)[163]
Mild	**Grade I**	**Mosaic Pattern**
Fine pink speckling (scarlatina-type rash)	Mild reddening	Mild—diffuse pink areola
Superficial reddening	Congestive mucosa	Moderate—flat red spot
Mosaic pattern		Severe—diffuse red areola
Severe	**Grade II**	**Red Mark Lesion**
Discrete red spots	Severe redness and fine reticular pattern separating areas of raised edematous mucosa	Discrete
Diffuse hemorrhagic lesion		Confluent (diffuse)
	Grade III Point bleeding + grade II	**Black-Brown Spot**

NIEC, New Italian Endoscopic Club.

Further work needs to be done to improve the currently available grading system.

Prevalence and Risk Factors

The reported prevalence varies widely in patients with portal hypertension (20%–75%) and also in patients with cirrhosis (35%–80%) because of patient selection, absence of uniform criteria and classification, and, more importantly, the differences in interobserver and intraobserver variation.[113,114] Although different studies have yielded mixed results, sometimes contradictory, the preponderance of data[113] suggest that (1) the severity of portal hypertension is associated with the severity or frequency of PHG; (2) the frequency of PHG is higher in portal hypertension with cirrhosis than in portal hypertension without cirrhosis; (3) the underlying etiology of cirrhosis does not affect PHG frequency

or severity; (4) duration of liver disease positively correlates with development of PHG; (5) severity of cirrhosis, as measured by Child-Pugh score, is correlated with frequency of PHG. There is general agreement that the prevalence of PHG increases with variceal obliteration.[115] However, some investigators believe that the higher rate of PHG in patients undergoing endoscopic variceal sclerotherapy merely reflects a longer duration of portal hypertension, more advanced liver disease, or more severe portal hypertension in patients selected to undergo variceal sclerotherapy compared with controls rather than the performance of sclerotherapy per se.[116,117]

Natural History and Complications

The overall incidence of acute bleeding from PHG is low, and acute bleeding is seen mostly in patients with more severe PHG. Bleeding is often mild, and transfusion requirement is usually limited to 1 to 2 units of blood. The prevalence of chronic bleeding cannot be reliably estimated because of the uncertainty of making a firm diagnosis. Major determinants of bleeding from PHG are length of time the patient had PHG and the extent and severity of lesions. The mortality associated with bleeding from PHG is very low because most bleeds are minor compared with variceal bleeding. Screening for PHG is currently not recommended in patients with liver disease.[113]

Management

Management of PHG is centered on reduction in portal pressure, largely through the use of medical rather than endoscopic means.

Pharmacologic treatment. The aim of pharmacologic treatment is (1) to control hemorrhage in patients with actively bleeding PHG and (2) to prevent rebleeding in patients with known PHG. Primary prophylaxis of bleeding from PHG is not recommended.[113]

Nonselective β-blockers. Nonselective β-blockers, such as propranolol and nadolol, have been shown to reduce portal pressure and gastric mucosal blood flow. In small studies, propranolol has been shown to reduce bleeding related to PHG.[118,119] The use of propranolol in PHG leads to endoscopic improvement, a cessation of bleeding in acutely hemorrhaging patients, and a decreased incidence of rebleeding from severe PHG. Therefore, nonselective β-blockers are a first-line therapy for secondary prophylaxis of PHG bleeding.[120,121] At the current time, there are not enough data to recommend β-blockers for

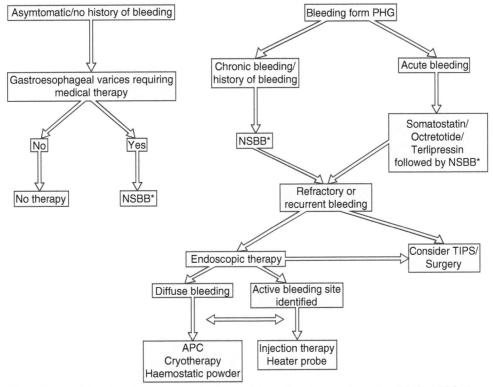

FIG 18.5 Algorithm for the treatment of portal hypertensive gastropathy (PHG). *APC,* Argon plasma coagulation; *NSBB,* nonselective β-blocker; *TIPS,* transjugular intrahepatic portosystemic shunt.

primary prophylaxis of bleeding from PHG in patients with cirrhosis who do not require β-blockers for other reasons. Nonresponse to β-blockers, defined as continued bleeding despite this therapy and transfusion dependency despite iron-replacement therapy, should prompt consideration of interventional therapies.[113] Other medications, such as prednisone, estrogen, and progesterone, are ineffective for bleeding-related PHG.

Vasoactive agents. Given the proven beneficial effects of vasoactive agents such as somatostatin, octreotide, and terlipressin in variceal bleeding, their role in the management of PHG has also been evaluated. In patients with acute bleeding, an uncontrolled study showed efficacy with somatostatin and octreotide.[122] A more recent study (2001) showed that the decrease in portal pressure is only transient, however, and use of somatostatin or octreotide is unlikely to benefit patients with chronic PHG bleeding.[123] Use of these agents should be limited to patients with acute bleeding. There are no clinical trials directly comparing the efficacy of propranolol versus octreotide for active hemorrhage related to PHG. We recommend the use of octreotide first in patients with acute bleeding because it is better tolerated than propranolol in this setting.[124] The results with vasopressin and terlipressin may be inferior to that achieved with octreotide, possibly because vasopressin does not inhibit release of peptides, including glucagon and vasoactive intestinal polypeptide, and does not inhibit gastric acid secretion.[113] Proton pump inhibitors may indirectly stop bleeding from the stomach by raising intraluminal gastric pH and thereby stabilizing blood clots.

Endoscopic treatment. Endoscopic treatment does not have a significant role in the management of PHG bleeding because the bleeding is often mild and diffuse. If an active bleeding site is identified, it could be managed by injection of sclerosant or cauterization using the heater or bipolar probe. APC or hemospray, a rapid hemostatic agent, are experimental endoscopic therapies for PHG. These therapies can treat a larger bleeding surface area than cauterization or sclerotherapy. Hemospray has recently shown promise in halting active PHG bleeding while long-term therapy is being initiated.[125,126] Endoscopic cryotherapy has been used for PHG bleeding after all other modalities failed.[127] Transjugular intrahepatic portosystemic shunt (TIPS) and shunt surgery have also been shown to be effective for PHG bleeding. A treatment algorithm for patients with PHG is described in Fig. 18.5.

Gastric Antral Vascular Ectasia

GAVE was first described in 1984 by Jabbari and colleagues.[128] These authors coined *watermelon stomach* to describe GAVE because of its resemblance to the skin of a watermelon. GAVE describes vascular lesions of the antrum organized in a linear array on top of raised convoluted folds radiating outward from the pylorus, similar to spokes from a wheel, and resembling the dark stripes on the surface of a watermelon (Fig. 18.6A). The typical histologic appearance of GAVE includes marked dilation of capillaries and collecting venules in the gastric mucosa and submucosa with areas of intimal thickening characterized by fibromuscular hyperplasia, fibrohyalinosis, and thrombi.[105,106,128] Diffuse antral vascular ectasia or *honeycomb stomach* is recognized as the same entity as watermelon stomach, and both are regarded as GAVE (see Fig. 18.6B).[31]

The diffuse form is the predominant pattern in patients with cirrhosis. Noncirrhotic patients with GAVE are typically middle-aged or older women; in these patients, GAVE is associated with achlorhydria, atrophic gastritis, CREST syndrome, autoimmune

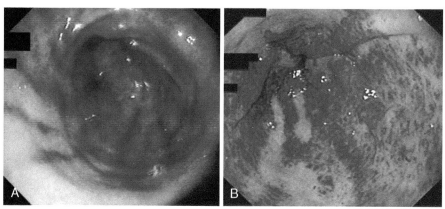

FIG 18.6 Two different forms of gastric vascular antral ectasia: **A,** "watermelon stomach" and **B,** diffuse vascular antral ectasia.

diseases, chronic renal failure, cardiac diseases, and post–bone marrow transplantation.[31,48,120,129]

Management

Bleeding from gastric mucosal lesions in patients with portal hypertension is a serious complication, although bleeding is usually slow and insidious, and rarely massive and life threatening. However, multiple transfusions may be required during follow-up. In patients with GAVE, the reduction of portal pressure by using drugs (β-blockers, somatostatin, octreotide), TIPS, or surgery (portocaval shunts) are not effective. Endoscopic therapy is generally preferred because of its efficacy, but pharmacologic treatment may be used as adjunct therapy or in patients with persistent bleeding from mucosal areas not amenable to endoscopic therapy. The aim of endoscopic therapy is to eliminate completely or significantly reduce the blood transfusion requirements of a patient with bleeding.

Many studies have demonstrated the efficacy of APC; however, most have been single-center trials with a low number of subjects.[130,131] The tangential approach to the vascular lesions, especially along the posterior wall of the antrum, makes APC an attractive tool. Among noncontact thermal endoscopic treatments for GAVE, APC has gained popularity in recent years and is now widely available in endoscopy units. The results from several small series and case reports so far have been similar to the results achieved with the Nd:YAG laser but with a superior safety profile.[132] Long-term efficacy remains suboptimal, however, with a 22% incidence of recurrent bleeding and with up to 31% of patients requiring ongoing transfusions.[106,133,134] Long-term sequelae of ablation include antral scarring and hyperplastic polyps.[135] Most rebleeding episodes respond to repeated treatment, but these patients may require multiple sessions and commitment to ongoing endoscopic treatments.[132]

Higher power settings should be used for patients with GAVE to provide ablation of the mucosal and submucosal vascular abnormalities. Generally, a mean of 2.5 sessions are needed to achieve complete eradication, with repeated sessions every 2 to 6 weeks.[136] Generally, Nd:YAG laser and APC are preferred over heater probe for the treatment of GAVE because of their ability to cover a greater surface area. The endoscopic therapeutic modality chosen also depends on the individual experience of the endoscopist and local availability.[124] The underlying pathophysiology is unclear, and endoscopic ablative methods do not affect the origins of the problem, so there is a long-term potential for recurrent vascular lesions and bleeding.

The rationale for recurrent bleeding following thermal treatment for GAVE is that GAVE commonly involves deeper structures than the superficial epithelium, including the submucosa, which may not be treated adequately with coagulation. It has been postulated that endoscopic band ligation (EBL) may more reliably obliterate vascular structures in the deep mucosa and submucosa, thus reducing the need for further treatments.[120] A retrospective study of thermal therapy (APC or multipolar electrocoagulation probe) compared with band ligation found that band ligation may offer a more definitive option.[137] Endoscopists banded vascular ectasias in the most distal antrum closest to the pylorus and then moved proximally until the entire affected areas were treated (up to 12 bands placed in a single session). Patients required between 2 and 4 sessions of EBL for resolution of GAVE. Other studies have also reported similar results.[120,138,139] At the present time, this form of therapy cannot be advocated as superior to existing therapies, but is an attractive option for health facilities with limited financial resources.

Cryotherapy is based on the rapid decrease of temperature due to the rapid expansion of carbon dioxide (CO_2) released by the spray catheter; such sudden decrease of temperature causes superficial necrosis of the mucosa and of the superficial submucosal, with eradication of antral telangiectasias, and subsequent re-epithelialization. In 2003 Kantsevoy et al reported a study of 26 patients with various bleeding lesions including GAVE that were treated with cryotherapy with a mean of 3.6 sessions.[95] These patients had previously undergone treatment with multipolar electrocoagulation and heater probe, but continued to have bleeding. Cryotherapy was efficacious in causing hemostasis in 77% overall, with follow-up of 6 months. Preliminary data suggest that cryotherapy may be a reasonable option for diffuse GAVE lesions. Cryotherapy seems to work in GAVE by causing a deeper injury compared with APC with necrosis of mucosa and superficial submucosa, followed by re-epithelialization. A major advantage of cryotherapy over APC is its ability to treat large areas of mucosa relatively quickly because ice formation occurs after 2 to 3 seconds of spraying the mucosa and is quickly followed by thawing.[95]

Additional modalities that have been investigated for GAVE include radiofrequency ablation (RFA) and endoscopic mucosal resection, but are considered more investigational and cannot

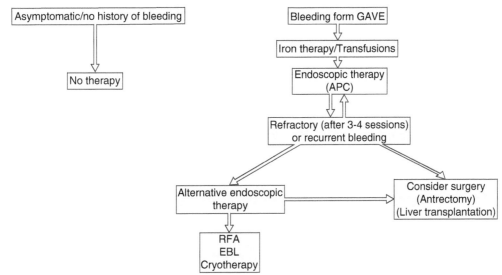

FIG 18.7 Algorithm for the treatment of gastric antral vascular ectasia (GAVE). *APC*, Argon plasma coagulation; *EBL*, endoscopic band ligation; *RFA*, radiofrequency ablation.

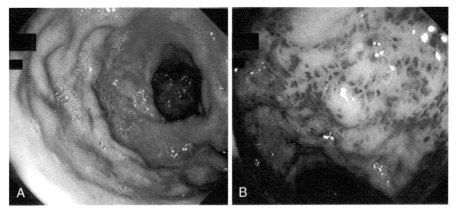

FIG 18.8 Portal colopathy. **A,** Portal hypertension causing collateral circulation in the rectum. **B,** Colitis with granularity, erythema, friability, and cherry-red spots.

be considered as part of a more routine treatment modality.[131,140,141,142] A treatment algorithm for patients with GAVE is described in Fig. 18.7.

Lesions Resembling PHG in Other Gastrointestinal Regions

Portal hypertensive gastropathy-like lesions can occur in other parts of the GI tract and are named according to the involved segment[113] as portal hypertensive duodenopathy, portal hypertensive biliopathy, small intestinal vasculopathy, and portal hypertensive colopathy[143] (Fig. 18.8). Standardized management of these lesions does not exist due to limited available data. Broadly speaking, management options are similar to those of PHG.

HEMANGIOMAS

Clinical Manifestations

Hemangiomas are the second most common vascular lesion of the colon. They are generally thought to be hamartomas because most are present at birth. They may be solitary or multiple lesions limited to one segment of the GI tract, or they may be part of diffuse GI or multisystem angiomatosis. Most are small (Fig. 18.9), ranging from a few millimeters to 2 cm, but larger lesions do occur, especially in the rectum (see later section on Cavernous Hemangioma of the Rectum). In the presence of GI bleeding, hemangiomas of the skin should suggest the possibility of associated bowel lesions.[47] Hemangiomas causing upper GI hemorrhage are most commonly identified in the proximal small bowel. These benign vascular tumors, almost all of which are cavernous hemangiomas, appear as single or multiple red, purple, or blue nodular lesions.

Bleeding from colonic hemangiomas is usually low in volume, producing occult blood loss with anemia or melena. Hematochezia is less common except in large, cavernous hemangiomas of the rectum, which may cause massive hemorrhage. Diagnosis is best established by endoscopy, including enteroscopy, because radiologic studies, including angiography, are frequently normal.

Management

Hemangiomas that are small, solitary, or few in number can be treated by endoscopic coagulation using laser or other thermal

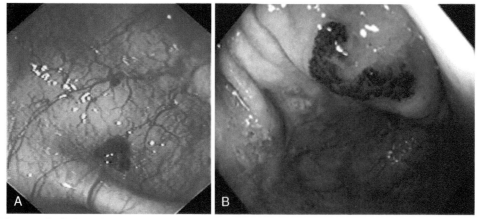

FIG 18.9 **A,** Solitary hemangioma of the colon. **B,** Narrow-band imaging of hemangioma of the colon.

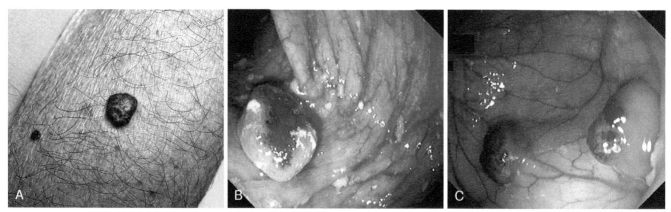

FIG 18.10 Multiple hemangiomas of blue rubber bleb nevus syndrome. **A,** Typical dark blue nodular lesions of the skin and **B** and **C,** involving the colon.

mode. Colonoscopic excision of small lesions has been described,[144] including removal of small lesions for the purpose of diagnosis in patients with multiple hemangiomas.[145,146] Although complications of colonoscopic excision of hemangiomas seem to be rare, the number of reports is small, and it is difficult to determine the safety of colonoscopic treatment. Angiographic therapy or surgical resection may be required for large or refractory bleeding lesions.

Cavernous Hemangioma of the Rectum

A distinct form of colonic hemangioma is cavernous hemangioma of the rectum.[47] These lesions are usually not associated with other GI hemangiomas and are extensive, involving the entire rectum or portions of the rectosigmoid colon. The massive bleeding resulting from these rectal hemangiomas often necessitates excision of the rectum by either abdominal-perineal or low-anterior resection; ligation and embolization of major feeding vessels have been employed successfully. Attempts at local control have been valuable in some instances, but mostly these have been only temporarily effective.

BLUE RUBBER BLEB NEVUS SYNDROME

Blue rubber bleb nevus syndrome, also known as Bean's syndrome, is a rare entity, characterized by cutaneous hemangiomas and

vascular tumors of the GI tract, that can also involve other organs such as the brain, kidneys, lungs, eyes, oronasopharynx, parotids, liver, spleen, heart, pleura, peritoneum, pericardium, skeletal muscles, bladder, penis, and vulva.[147–149] Although a familial history is infrequent, a few cases of autosomal dominant transmission have been reported,[29] and one analysis identified a responsible locus on chromosome 9. The lesions were thought to be hemangiomas, but they are now considered to be venous malformations,[29,150] which usually appear in early childhood and tend to increase in size and number with age. They are usually blue and raised, vary from 0.1 to 5 cm in diameter, have a wrinkled surface, and are easily compressible with light palpation. The contained blood can be emptied by direct pressure, leaving a wrinkled blue sac that slowly refills over several seconds or minutes.[29] Skin lesions may be present throughout the body, particularly predominating on the upper limbs (Fig. 18.10A), trunk,[151] and face.

GI lesions are usually multiple and may involve any portion of the GI tract, but are most common in the small bowel and in the distal part of the colon.[29] The characteristic GI lesion is a discrete mucosal nodule with an overlying central bluish-red cap resembling a nipple, but a lesion may be a flat, macular, dark bluish-red spot or a frankly polypoid nodule with a central venous colored portion (see Fig. 18.10B and C).[148,152] Most patients are asymptomatic. The onset of GI bleeding may be at any time from early childhood to middle age.[103] The lesions can also cause intestinal intussusception[153] and are associated with a variety of extraintestinal problems. Most patients respond to supportive therapy, such as iron supplementation and blood transfusion when required.[152] For recurrent bleeding, medical, endoscopic, and surgical therapies have been used. Medical therapy includes the use of corticosteroids,[154,155] γ-globulin,[154] interferon,[150,155] octeotride,[156] and sirolimus.[157,158]

Endoscopic management seems to be safe and useful, although the lesions can be transmural, which implies a theoretical increase in risk for bowel perforation as a complication. There are several reports of endoscopic therapy, including sclerotherapy with absolute alcohol,[159] sodium morrhuate,[160] epinephrine and polidocanol,[161] band ligation,[161–163] polypectomy,[151,162,164] bipolar coagulation,[165] and laser therapy.[165,166] Angiographic embolization and surgical excision have also been used.[150,163,167,168]

KLIPPEL-TRÉNAUNAY-WEBER SYNDROME

Klippel-Trénaunay-Weber syndrome, also known as nevus vasculosus hypertrophicus, is a rare congenital vascular malformation, secondary to a generalized mesodermal development abnormality.[169] Originally described by Klippel and Trénaunay in 1900, it is characterized by bony or soft tissue hypertrophy, usually affecting one extremity (Fig. 18.11A); hemangiomas or lymphangiomas or both; and varicosities or venous malformations, appearing at birth or in childhood. Visceral hemangiomas have been described involving organs such as the GI tract (see Fig. 18.11B and C), liver, spleen, bladder, kidney, lung, and heart.[170,171] Involvement of the GI tract may be more common than previously believed, occurring in 20% of patients.[171] GI bleeding usually begins in the first decade of life and may be recurrent and mild or severe.[170] The severity may be enhanced by a consumption coagulopathy owing to intravascular clotting within the venous sinusoids of the hemangiomas.[47] The most common reported cause of GI bleeding is attributed to diffuse cavernous hemangiomas of the distal colon and rectum,[172] found in 1% to 12.5% of cases.[170,173] Less frequent causes of GI bleeding are rectal or rectovaginal varices caused by obstruction of the internal iliac system, esophageal varices secondary to prehepatic portal hypertension owing to cavernous transformation or hypoplasia of the portal vein,[174] and jejunal hemangiomas.[175] Colonic obstruction and ascites secondary to

massive hemangiomatous-lymphangiomatous retroperitoneal masses may occur.[176]

At colonoscopy, the rectum and the lower part of the colon may show visible mucosal vessels or compressible nodules and extensive bluish angiomatous submucosal lesions. Biopsy of the lesions should be avoided because it may precipitate severe hemorrhage.[170] Lesions in deeper layers of the wall can be assessed by endoscopic ultrasound.[177] Doppler transrectal ultrasonography could be very important for sphincter-saving surgery in patients with rectal hemangioma.[178] Endoscopic therapy has a limited role because of the commonly diffuse nature of the intestinal hemangiomas[179] and is reserved for management of localized lesions or ablation of postoperative residual disease. The use of argon[180] and Nd:YAG laser,[179] sclerosis with formaldehyde and absolute alcohol,[181] and placement of hemostatic clips in the rectum combined with arterial embolization[182] have been reported with success.

RADIATION INJURY OF THE GASTROINTESTINAL TRACT

Radiation Proctopathy

Clinical Manifestations

Radiotherapy is a common treatment modality used for several pelvic malignancies. Despite progress in radiation techniques, adjacent organs are still exposed to chronic radiation injury, which occurs in 2% to 25% of patients.[183]

The rectum, a fixed organ in the pelvis, has a glandular-type epithelium in which the cells undergo a rapid turnover. This organ is particularly vulnerable to ionizing radiation and to radiation-induced complications. The incidence of such complications is proportional to the dose and its degree of spreading, and to the volume and method of irradiation (external or by brachytherapy).[183] Intracavitary radiation delivery has been shown to increase the risk of developing chronic radiation proctopathy (CRP).[184] Risk factors for radiation-induced damage include history of abdominal surgery, arteriosclerosis, obesity, diabetes, and concomitant chemotherapy.[183,185,186]

Radiation injury to the intestine has acute and chronic phases. Acute radiation injury occurs during or immediately after treatment and results from direct cellular damage. This injury inhibits

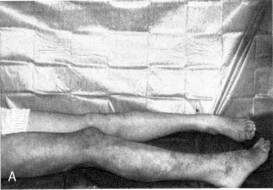
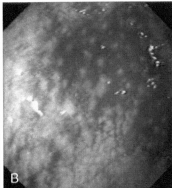
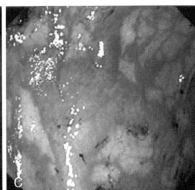

FIG 18.11 Klippel-Trénaunay-Weber syndrome involving gastrointestinal tract. **A,** Hypertrophic leg caused by venous hypertension and stasis. **B,** Rectal hemangioma in the same patient. **C,** Rectal hemangiomas and venous varicosities in another patient with Klippel-Trénaunay-Weber syndrome.

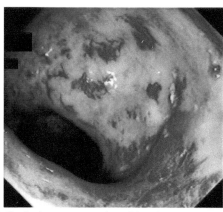

FIG 18.12 Radiation proctopathy with pale mucosa, edema, and angioectasias.

division of the intestinal crypt stem cells, and the lamina propria becomes infiltrated with inflammatory cells resulting in loss of cellular function and mucosal inflammation. Clinical symptoms of acute radiation proctitis, diarrhea and tenesmus, are usually self-resolving, requiring only symptomatic treatment and are not typically therapeutic challenges.[187] CRP is histologically characterized by submucosal collagen proliferation, endarteritis of arterioles, and thrombi in vessel lumens, leading to submucosal fibrosis, chronic mucosal ischemia, and progressive epithelial atrophy.[188] Clinical symptoms of chronic radiation usually begin months to years after the initial radiation exposure, with a median of 8 to –16 months[188,189] but with latencies as long as 30 years.[190] Symptoms include rectal bleeding, diarrhea, rectal pain, fecal urgency, tenesmus, obstructed defecation (in patients who have developed stenosis), and less commonly fecal incontinence and fistulas.[187] Bleeding may be severe enough to require frequent hospitalizations and blood transfusions; 55% of patients may require support with blood transfusions before undergoing definitive therapy.[191] Flexible sigmoidoscopy and colonoscopy aid in diagnosis and determine the extent and severity of radiation injury. The findings include distinctive angioectasias accumulated in the distal rectum, extending to and often including the dentate line, along with friability and spontaneous bleeding (Fig. 18.12). Less frequently, there may be ulceration, stenosis, and fistulas. There is often a distinct margin between normal and abnormal tissue that relates to the edge of the radiation field.[191] In some patients, especially women who have undergone radiation therapy after surgery for a gynecologic malignancy, there may be an associated segment of sigmoid colon with identical findings.

Treatment

Medical therapies. The traditional approach to treatment of CRP has been directed toward decreasing any inflammation with the use of antiinflammatory agents such as aminosalicylic acid derivatives and corticosteroids.[187] The response to such agents is disappointing. Other approaches, such as promoting healing in damaged tissue with short-chain fatty acid enemas,[192] oral and rectal sucralfate,[189,193] antioxidants and vitamins,[187] or hormonal therapy with an estrogen-progesterone combination,[194] have been tried. At the moment, just a few treatments have shown, in randomized controlled trials, to be effective for the treatment of radiation-induced rectal bleeding[195]: metronidazole and sucralfate enemas. Small, randomized trials have shown a beneficial effect of topical rectal treatment with butyrate and

short-chain fatty acids (which exert a trophic effect on the rectal and colonic mucosa and stimulate mucosal blood flow) only for acute-onset radiation-induced bleeding but not for chronic, late-onset symptoms. The use of hyperbaric oxygen has been shown to be helpful in patients who are not controlled with endoscopic techniques. The response rate was 68%.[196] The response rate for bleeding was 70% to 76%; 48% showed complete resolution of bleeding, and 28% reported significantly fewer bleeding episodes.[197] Although this therapy is expensive and inconvenient, requiring 20 to 40 treatment sessions,[198,199] it could be offered to patients who fail conventional treatments.[200]

Endoscopic therapies

Topical formalin. Topical formalin application for radiation injury was first reported in radiation-induced cystitis.[201] Its mechanism of action is likely to be due to a local chemical cauterization of the inflamed or fragile telangiectatic rectal mucosa.[191] The treatment is inexpensive and easy to perform. The technique involves the direct application of 4% formalin to the affected area in the rectum, either with formalin-soaked gauze[202] or by direct instillation and timed retention (typically approximately 10 minutes).[203] The application continues until mucosal blanching occurs, usually within 2 to 3 minutes.[204] The perianal area should be protected with careful draping and the application of petroleum jelly around the anus and perianal skin to avoid formalin injury.[205] The rectum is irrigated liberally after topical application to remove residual formalin. Formalin is contraindicated in the presence of fissures or ulceration. The short-term success of the technique with complete cessation of bleeding ranges from 59% to 100%.[191,206] Recurrent symptomatic relapses have been treated successfully with repeated applications.

In patients with severe CRP, the administration of topical formalin may be more effective than APC.[207] Complications have been described in 27% to 57% of patients.[206,208] According to an email survey with members of the American Society of Colon Rectal Surgeons, formalin is the most popular method to treat radiation proctitis.[209] However, some authors think that this technique should be reserved for severe hemorrhagic proctitis refractory to medical or endoscopic treatment, and that it should be thoroughly discussed in cases of anorectal radiation-induced stricture, prior anal incontinence, or treated anal cancer.[206] Formalin offers an excellent option for patients who are on anticoagulation and have increased risk for bleeding from thermally induced ulceration after conventional coagulation therapies.

Laser. Argon,[210] Nd:YAG,[211] and potassium titanyl phosphate (KTP) laser[212] have been reported to be effective, with a marked decrease in bleeding in 87% of treated patients.[191] Repeated treatments were needed in the long-term because symptoms tended to recur.[210] Laser therapy has the advantage of being a precise technique that does not involve tissue contact, is well tolerated, and improves activities of daily life. Disadvantages include its high cost, the need for protective precautions, and the risk of rectal ulcer,[212] bowel perforation, and rectovaginal fistulas.[191]

Argon plasma coagulation. APC is the best studied technique in the management of this disease and it is considered to be first-line therapy for CRP.[213,214] Nevertheless, APC settings, including gas flow rate and power, have not been standardized across publications. When the lesions are circumferential and numerous, a staged treatment may be useful, allowing a sufficient period for healing of the previously treated area. APC session intervals range from every 4 to every 8 weeks. A mean of 1.7 to 3.7 treatment sessions is necessary for control of bleeding.[191]

APC improves rectal bleeding in 80% to 90% of cases, as well as symptoms of tenesmus, diarrhea, and urgency in 60% to 75% of cases.[214] In the presence of significant oozing, adrenaline solution (1:10,000) should be sprayed over the mucosal surface,[214] as APC is relatively ineffective in patients with excessive bleeding owing to the absorption of current by blood on the surface. It is important to minimize contact-induced bleeding during endoscopy to maximize access to the vascular lesions. Complete anterograde bowel preparation is recommended for all treatment sessions, as good bowel preparation is crucial for endoscopic therapy.

Care must be taken not to overdistend the bowel with argon gas insufflation.[191] In the case of low rectal lesions, the use of a transparent cap at the tip of the colonoscope allows direct viewing of these lesions and of the upper part of the anal canal without requiring retroflexion of the endoscope. Because of its limited depth of penetration, morbidity is usually minor and consists of gas bloating, tenesmus, transient abdominal or anal pain, and diarrhea in approximately 20% of cases. Major complications are exceptional but include rectovaginal fistula,[215] chronic rectal ulceration, anal or rectal stricture,[183] and perforation.[216] Deliberate care should be taken to use the lowest power setting that provides a coagulum and to avoid overtreating, especially with persistent oozing after initial coagulation.

Only four studies have compared APC with other therapy for CRP.[214] Two compared APC with formalin, one with hyperbaric oxygen, and another study assessed APC versus bipolar circumactive probe (BiCAP). The results of these preliminary studies show that APC is at least as effective and safer than other treatments. However, more comparative studies with larger series, especially between APC and the newest techniques (radiofrequency ablation [RFA] and cryotherapy), are needed for definite conclusions.

Endoscopic cryotherapy. Few studies have evaluated endoscopic cryoablation as a treatment for CRP.[95,214] The initial case reports support the use of cryotherapy. Cryotherapy was applied every 2 to 3 days until all lesions were ablated. The average number of therapeutic sessions needed to stop the bleeding was 3.6. Cryotherapy resulted in superficial tissue necrosis that was usually completely healed within 3 months after the final treatment sessions. Cryotherapy was remarkably safe with only benign self-limited adverse events. However, there has been no prospective study comparing cryotherapy with other methods such as APC, regarding the durability of results, safety, and efficacy.

Radiofrequency ablation. Recently, a number of studies have evaluated the safety and efficacy of RFA for CRP treatment, the largest one including 39 consecutive cases.[217] RFA is generally performed on outpatients using a single-use HALO90 electrode catheter (BARRx/Covidien, Sunnyvale, CA) that is passed through a standard gastroscope. A gastroscope is used instead of a colonoscope because HALO devices are designed for a gastroscope, and because retroflexion is easier using a gastroscope, especially with the RFA catheter attached. During the ablation procedure, the HALO90 catheter is mounted in the 6 o'clock position (as opposed to the 12 o'clock location usually used for the ablation of Barrett's esophagus). To promote hemostasis, the coagulum in treated areas is not scraped off. The endoscope and device are removed for cleaning every eight applications to preserve electrode surface effectiveness for subsequent areas treatment. Ablations are performed approximately 1 mm proximal to the dentate line (to prevent sensory injury to the anal mucosa) and restricted to a short length (less than 6 cm to the dentate line).

The procedure is repeated as needed until complete rectal mucosa ablation is achieved. Based on prior studies, an energy density of 12 to 15 J/cm² at a power density of 40 W/cm² can be selected, which has shown no transmural damage at these settings.

RFA units deliver a consistent energy to the surface by using a well-defined and reproducible ramp-up of energy, thereby diminishing the likelihood of overtreatment and operator dependence that may lead to ulcerations or perforations. However,[214] the published studies are retrospective and conclusions are limited by the lack of a control group. They are also nonpowered, and even considering all published works, only a few dozen patients with CRP have been treated with RFA. Another important limitation is that no sigmoid or proximal rectal lesions were ablated, thus safety in those areas (with a thinner wall) remains uncertain. Therefore, additional controlled studies are required to compare RFA to other therapeutic modalities for CRP.

Radiation Gastropathy

Gastric complications secondary to radiotherapy are uncommon, but injury can occur when the stomach lies within the radiation field of an adjacent extragastric tumor.[218] A high total dose, usually greater than 5000 rad, and a high daily fraction seem to be the main risk factors.[219] There have been reports of chronic gastroduodenal ulcerations, gastritis, and duodenitis being diagnosed days to months after selective internal radiation therapy with resin-based microspheres loaded with yttrium-90. It is possible to find small spheres located inside the vessels in the biopsy specimens.[220-222] Acute vasculopathy may progress to a prolonged and progressive endarteritis obliterans, vasculitis, and endothelial proliferation, leading to mucosal ischemia, ulceration, mucosal angioectasias, and fibrosis.[223]

In contrast to radiation proctopathy, GI bleeding from chronic radiation gastropathy is rare, with very few cases reported.[223-225] When present, there are multiple friable angioectasias. These lead to melena and significant blood loss requiring multiple blood transfusions, prolonged hospitalizations, and repeated endoscopies. Endoscopically, the mucosa of the affected stomach (usually antrum) is friable and with multiple angioectasias (Fig. 18.13). Other possible severe complications are perforation and gastric outlet obstruction.[188]

Treatment

There is very little information in the literature on the management of radiation-induced complications in the stomach.[188]

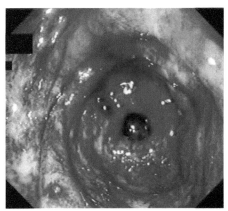

FIG 18.13 Radiation-induced gastritis with erythema, friability, and ulcerated mucosa.

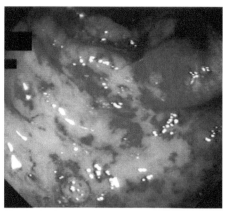

FIG 18.14 Radiation-induced duodenopathy with edema, friability, and diffuse angioectasias.

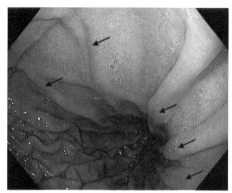

FIG 18.15 Cameron lesions with long linear erosions *(black arrows)* on the crests of gastric folds in a patient with a large hiatal hernia.

Prolonged blood loss needs to be treated with iron and folic acid supplements and with transfusions. Aminocaproic acid,[223] hyperbaric oxygen,[224] growth hormone,[226] and oral prednisolone[227] have been reported to be effective in control of bleeding in a few patients or case reports. Bleeding can be controlled by any endoscopic coagulation technique, with APC preferred[225,228,229] and cryotherapy.[95] Surgery may be necessary if other treatment fails,[219,230] but is associated with high morbidity.[223]

Radiation Injury of the Small Bowel

The small intestine is particularly susceptible to radiation injury (Fig. 18.14).[218] Radiation injury to the small intestine most often occurs in the clinical setting of radiotherapy for rectal, urologic, gynecologic, or retroperitoneal malignancies. The degree of injury seems to be proportional to radiation dosage delivered to the segment of small bowel that lies within the radiation field. The relative fixed position of the duodenum and distal ileum within the abdominal cavity make these portions particularly vulnerable to radiation-induced injury. Predisposing factors in the progression of radiation injury include excessive radiation, previous abdominal surgery that fixes loops of bowel in place, underlying cardiovascular disease, and a slender build.[231] The mechanism of injury is vascular damage with progressive localized ischemia. The ischemia leads to angioectasias and ulceration of the mucosa, fibrosis with stricturing, and, less frequently, fistula formation or perforation.

The clinical manifestations of chronic radiation typically occur 1 to 2 years after exposure and can include malabsorption, hemorrhage, bowel obstruction, fistulas, and abscess formation secondary to perforation.[232] Bleeding can be managed with the same endoscopic techniques that are used in radiation proctitis. Balloon enteroscopy may be needed to access distal small bowel involvement and perform dilation of the diaphragm-like strictures, which resemble strictures seen with long-standing use of NSAIDs. The treatment is difficult, and often surgery is necessary.[231] Resection of the involved small bowel segment is preferable to bypass.[233]

CAMERON ULCERS AND EROSIONS

Patients with large hernias may develop Cameron ulcers or erosions. These mucosal lesions are usually located on the crest of the mucosal folds that make up the distal hiatal hernia rosette, on the lesser curve of the stomach, or at the level of the diaphragmatic hiatus (Fig. 18.15).[234] Cameron lesions can be found in 5% of all patients with hiatal hernias.[235] The cause of Cameron lesions is still unclear, but it is thought that mechanical trauma secondary to diaphragmatic contraction from respiratory excursions and, perhaps, ischemia and acid mucosal injury, play a primary role in their pathogenesis.[236] Cameron lesions manifest clinically with chronic occult GI bleeding and associated iron deficiency anemia. These lesions can also manifest as acute upper GI bleeding in one-third of cases.[235] Treatment includes antisecretory therapy and supplemental iron. In approximately one-third of patients, Cameron lesions may persist or recur despite antisecretory medication, in which case surgical repair of the hiatal hernia is required.[235]

KEY REFERENCES

3. Raju GS, Gerson L, Das A, et al: American Gastroenterological Association: American Gastroenterological Association (AGA) Institute technical review on obscure gastrointestinal bleeding, *Gastroenterology* 133:1697–1717, 2007.

16. Schmit A, Van Gossum A: Proposal for an endoscopic classification of digestive angiodysplasias for therapeutic trials. The European Club of Enteroscopy, *Gastrointest Endosc* 48:659, 1998.

20. Sami S, Al-Araji S, Ragunath K: Review article: gastrointestinal angiodysplasia–pathogenesis, diagnosis and management, *Aliment Pharmacol Ther* 39:15–34, 2014.

29. Brandt LJ, Aroniadis OC: Vascular lesions of the gastrointestinal tract. In Feldman M, Friedman LS, Brandt LJ, editors: *Sleisenger and fordtran's gastrointestinal and liver disease: pathophysiology, diagnosis, management*, ed 10, Philadelphia, 2016, Elsevier, pp 617–635.

47. Brandt LJ, Boley SJ: Vascular disorders of the colon. In Sivak MVJ, editor: *Gastroenterologic endoscopy*, ed 2, Philadelphia, 2000, Saunders, pp 1324–1350.

55. ASGE Standards of Practice Committee, Khashab MA, Pasha SF, et al: The role of deep enteroscopy in the management of small-bowel disorders, *Gastrointest Endosc* 82:600–607, 2015.

66. Molina Infante J, Perez Gallardo B, Fernández Bermejo M: Update on medical therapy for obscure gastrointestinal hemorrhage, *Rev Esp Enferm Dig* 99:457–462, 2007.

75. Jackson CS, Gerson LB: Management of gastrointestinal angiodysplastic lesions (GIADs): a systematic review and meta-analysis, *Am J Gastroenterol* 109:474–483, 2014.

98. Begbie ME, Wallace GM, Shovlin CL: Hereditary haemorrhagic telangiectasia (Osler-Weber-Rendu syndrome): a view from the 21st century, *Postgrad Med J* 79:18–24, 2003.

103. Spencer J, Camillieri M: Chronic gastrointestinal haemorrhage. In Bouchier IAD, Allan RN, Hodgson HJF, Keighley MRB, editors:

Gastroenterology: Clinical Science and Practice, London, 1993, Saunders, pp 988–1003.

113. Gjeorgjievski M, Cappell MS: Portal hypertensive gastropathy: a systematic review of the pathophysiology, clinical presentation, natural history and therapy, *World J Hepatol* 8:231–262, 2016.

116. Shah VH, Kamath PS: Portal hypertension and variceal bleeding. In Feldman M, Friedman LS, Brandt LJ, editors: *Sleisenger and fordtran's gastrointestinal and liver disease: pathophysiology, diagnosis, management*, ed 10, Philadelphia, 2016, Elsevier, pp 1549–1552.

117. Kamath PS, Shah VH: Portal hypertension and bleeding esophageal varices. In Boyer TD, Manns MP, Sanyal AJ, editors: *Zakim and boyer's hepatology: a textbook of liver disease*, ed 6, Philadelphia, 2012, Elsevier, pp 296–326.

120. Patwardhan V, Cardenas A: Review article: the management of portal hypertensive gastropathy and gastric antral vascular ectasia in cirrhosis, *Aliment Pharmacol Ther* 40:354–362, 2014.

131. Naidu H, Huang Q, Mashimo H: Gastric antral vascular ectasia: the evolution of therapeutic modalities, *Endosc Int Open* 2:e67–e73, 2014.

136. Fuccio L, Mussetto A, Laterza L, et al: Diagnosis and management of gastric antral vascular ectasia, *World J Gastrointest Endosc* 5:6–13, 2013.

143. Urrunaga NH, Rockey DC: Portal hypertensive gastropathy and colopathy, *Clin Liver Dis* 18:389–406, 2014.

171. Cha SH, Romeo MA, Neutze JA: Visceral manifestations of Klippel-Trénaunay syndrome, *Radiographics* 25:1694–1697, 2005.

186. Cho LC, Antoine JE: Radiation injury to the gastrointestinal tract. In Feldman M, Friedman LS, Brandt LJ, editors: *Sleisenger and fordtran's gastrointestinal and liver disease: pathophysiology, diagnosis, management*, ed 8, Philadelphia, 2006, Saunders, pp 813–826.

214. Lenz L, Rohr R, Nakao F, et al: Chronic radiation proctopathy: a practical review of endoscopic treatment, *World J Gastrointest Surg* 8:151–160, 2016.

A complete reference list can be found online at ExpertConsult .com

19

Esophageal Motility Disorders

John O. Clarke and George Triadafilopoulos

CHAPTER OUTLINE

INTRODUCTION

Esophageal motility disorders are ubiquitous in gastroenterology practice today, and developments in technology have led to a revolution in both their diagnosis and treatment. This chapter focuses on clinically significant esophageal motility disorders relevant to gastrointestinal endoscopy practice, primarily achalasia, but also on other potentially related disorders, including esophagogastric junction (EGJ) outflow obstruction, distal esophageal spasm, hypercontractile esophagus, and ineffective esophageal motility (IEM). For each disorder, we will review what is known regarding etiology and pathophysiology, followed by an exploration of diagnostic options available (both endoscopic and non-endoscopic) and review therapy. We will examine other potential areas in which endoscopic techniques could be employed in the management of esophageal dysmotility, including deep tissue acquisition and potentially endoscopic implantation applications. Finally, we will speculate as to what the near future may hold in the endoscopic management of these challenging conditions.

ACHALASIA

Achalasia is characterized by loss of inhibitory neurons in the esophagus, leading to tonic contraction of the lower esophageal sphincter (LES) and altered or absent peristalsis. The term *achalasia* itself is derived from the Greek words *a* and *Khalasis*, meaning "not loosening or relaxing." The first clinical case was described by Sir Thomas Willis in 1674, where he described successfully treating a patient with associated dysphagia with a sponge-tipped whalebone, which was applied as needed after meals for approximately 15 years. The first pneumatic dilatation was performed in 1898, and the first surgical myotomy was described in 1913 by Ernst Heller. Therapies for achalasia were relatively quiescent thereafter for much of the 20th century; however, the past 25 years have seen significant diagnostic and therapeutic advancements.

Etiology and Pathophysiology

Achalasia is a rare disorder with a traditionally reported incidence of approximately 1:100,000.[1,2] However, two reports from early 2017 suggest a two- to fourfold increase in incidence.[3,4] In the vast majority of cases, no underlying etiology is found to explain disease onset, and it is labeled as idiopathic. Achalasia can also be labeled as secondary (pseudoachalasia) if there is a defined underlying etiology leading to degeneration of the myenteric plexus due to local invasion by neoplasia or other causes, such as amyloidosis or sarcoidosis. This is relatively rare, however, and believed to account for only 2% to 4% of patients with suspected achalasia.[5] Chagas disease, or infection with *Trypanosoma cruzi*, is endemic in parts of South America and can also present with an indistinguishable clinical picture (at least from the esophageal standpoint). Other cases of pseudoachalasia may occur, resulting from circulating antibodies in the setting of non-local malignancy (usually small-cell lung cancer). Achalasia can also be seen rarely in certain systemic syndromes, such as Allgrove syndrome (familial adrenal insufficiency with alacrima and achalasia), Down's syndrome, and familial visceral neuropathy.[1,2] We will focus our discussion primarily on idiopathic achalasia, as this is by far the most commonly encountered in clinical practice.

The pathogenesis of achalasia is still unclear, but it affects the myenteric neurons that mediate and coordinate esophageal peristalsis and relaxation. The pathologic hallmark of achalasia is a functional loss of these neurons resulting in tonic contraction of the LES and discoordinated or absent peristalsis.[2] The trigger for this neuronal degeneration is not entirely clear, but there are data to suggest a potential autoimmune process triggered by infection in the context of genetic susceptibility.

Prior to the 1990s, the leading hypothesis with regard to pathogenesis was the degeneration of the myenteric plexus.[6] In the early 1990s, pathology from patients with early achalasia showed inflammatory infiltration, with subsequent studies showing T-cell predominance (in particular CD8[+]).[7–9] The question remained, however, as to what prompted this inflammation. An autoimmune hypothesis was suggested, based on evidence of circulating antibodies to myenteric neurons in patients with achalasia,[10] links to specific HLA subtypes in affected patients,[11,12] and the observation that patients with achalasia were also more likely to have other perceived autoimmune disorders.[13] However, data have not been universally supportive of this theory, as myenteric antibodies have been found to be present equally in patients with achalasia and reflux (arguing that these antibodies are not causative, but simply a marker of esophageal injury).[14] Arguments have also been made in favor of a potential infection. This was supported by early case reports linking achalasia to varicella, measles and polio[15–18]; however, subsequent detailed analyses of esophageal tissue for potential viral infection/inclusions have been negative in most affected patients, while HSV-1 has also been found in analysis of control subjects.[19,20] Interestingly, parrots (and over 50 other tropical birds) suffer from proventricular dilatation disease, which is histopathologically indistinguishable from achalasia, but in contrast to human disease, it occurs in outbreaks. Recently, avian bornavirus was identified as the cause,[21] but it does not have any human equivalent. At present, most authorities subscribe to a combination of the aforementioned theories, that prior viral infection triggers immune-mediated ganglionitis, resulting in loss of myenteric neurons in a genetically-susceptible host.

Clinical Manifestations

The most common symptoms of achalasia are dysphagia and regurgitation. Dysphagia occurs with both solids and liquids, and is seen in over 90% of patients. Of note, a proportion of patients will not have dysphagia in both consistencies, and a distinct minority (< 5%) will not report dysphagia at all. Regurgitation of undigested foods is reported in 59% to 91% of patients and may be the dominant symptom at presentation. Chest pain occurs to a variable degree (17%–64%) and is more pronounced in spastic variants and perhaps in younger patients. Patients may also report heartburn (18%–75%), which, although counterintuitive, is likely related to stasis of ingested contents or intraesophageal reflux. Weight loss and aspiration are more worrisome but fortunately are seen less frequently (10%–30%).[1,2]

Symptoms associated with achalasia can be non-specific and the diagnosis is often not straightforward. Dysphagia is reported in approximately 4% of American adults on a weekly basis[22] and achalasia has an incidence of approximately 1:100,000,[1,2] so, not surprisingly, the vast majority of patients who present with dysphagia will not have achalasia, nor is it at the top of the differential diagnosis given its relatively rarity. Dysphagia is not seen in all patients with achalasia, and the presence of heartburn and chest pain can often sway presumptive management toward more common entities, such as gastroesophageal acid reflux. Despite the colloquial association of achalasia with weight loss, it is not unusual to see obese patients with achalasia. At tertiary

facilities, a small percentage (< 3%) of patients referred for evaluation of refractory reflux will eventually be diagnosed with achalasia. Because of these factors, many series report a relatively long delay (up to 5 years) between symptom onset and establishment of a final diagnosis.[23,24] With regard to other key demographics, men and women are affected evenly, and there is no reported gender discrepancy. Achalasia has increasing incidence with age, with an estimated incidence of greater than 10:100,000 above 80 years of age and less than 1:100,000 below 16 years of age; however, it can be reported at any age, and in our practice we have seen patients diagnosed at both younger than 1 year of age and older than 90 years.

Diagnosis

Accurate diagnosis of achalasia depends on recognition of associated symptoms and careful employment of diagnostic modalities to identify the underlying etiology and exclude mimicking conditions. For those patients who present with dysphagia, the key first step is to exclude a mechanical or infiltrative process using endoscopy or barium esophagraphy. Due to improvement in endoscopic technology and the clinical emergence of eosinophilic esophagitis, endoscopy is often the first-line study employed for evaluation of dysphagia in community and academic practices; however, there are no guidelines that specifically recommend endoscopy over a barium esophagraphy in the initial evaluation of dysphagia, and either approach would be reasonable, based on local practice patterns and expertise.

Endoscopy

Patients presenting with dysphagia and suspicion for achalasia should undergo endoscopy for evaluation and exclusion of potential neoplasms masquerading as pseudoachalasia. Esophageal biopsies to exclude eosinophilic esophagitis or other infiltrative disorders should be performed. In many patients with achalasia, especially early cases without significant esophageal dilatation, the endoscopy is unremarkable. Subtle endoscopic findings include frothy secretions in the esophagus and subjective feeling of tightness to the passage of the endoscope at the EGJ. In more advanced cases, esophageal distention, tortuosity, retention of pooled liquid or food, or frank food impaction can be seen; however, these are usually later findings denoting advanced disease. Due to stasis, it is also not unusual to see associated Candidiasis and, in the absence of immunosuppression, this finding on endoscopy should raise warning with regards to potentially significant dysmotility (Fig. 19.1). Endoscopy cannot definitively establish the diagnosis of achalasia and additional evaluation is required.

Radiology

A barium esophagram allows objective assessment of esophageal emptying, diameter, and contour, and can provide information relative to structural abnormalities, including epiphrenic diverticula, that may not be appreciated on endoscopy. In early cases or cases not associated with esophageal dilatation, it is important to recognize that the barium study may be interpreted as normal, and in fact some series report that almost half of early achalasia cases may be missed if relying on barium study alone.[25,26] However, although not sensitive, esophageal fluoroscopy can be quite specific in advanced cases. Characteristic findings include a dilated esophagus with retained food or an air-fluid level, and narrowing at the EGJ, often referred to as a *bird-beak*. Other findings seen in advanced cases include a large intragastric air bubble and

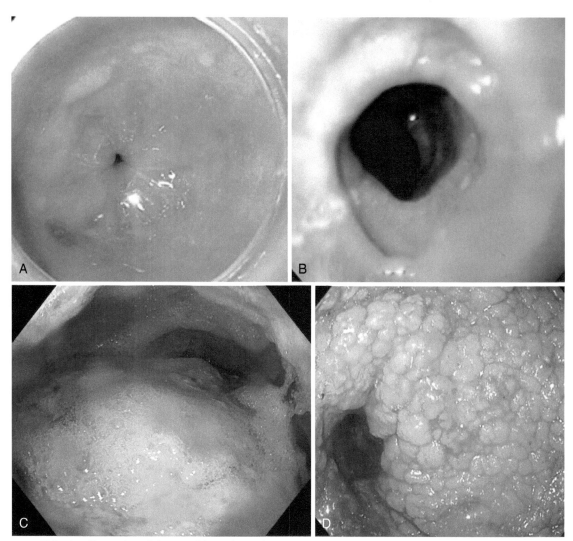

FIG 19.1 Examples of the possible endoscopic appearance of a spectrum of patients with achalasia. **A,** A subjectively tight esophagogastric junction is visualized, which, albeit subtle, may be an early marker of diagnosis. **B,** A spastic esophagus is visualized, typical of what is occasionally seen with type III (spastic) achalasia. **C,** A dilated atonic esophagus is seen with stasis and retained food, which is a more specific finding and generally associated with more chronic disease. **D,** An end-stage esophagus is seen with massive dilatation and characteristic mucosal change.

severe esophageal dilatation with a sigmoid-like appearance (Fig. 19.2). A timed barium esophagram can also be employed, where the patient ingests a fixed amount of barium and then retention is measured at 5 minutes while the patient is upright. This allows objective assessment of functional esophageal emptying and can be followed longitudinally after therapy.

Esophageal fluoroscopy remains an invaluable part of the diagnostic evaluation due to its unique ability to visualize anatomy and diameter. It is our practice to always obtain a barium esophagram before proceeding with more invasive treatment options in a patient with suspected achalasia.

In select cases, one could also consider other imaging modalities, including computed tomography (CT). CT scans in achalasia had characteristic findings highlighted by esophageal dilatation with normal wall thickness; however, patients with suspected achalasia who were found to have secondary achalasia had atypical radiographic manifestations.[27] CT is useful in separating primary and secondary achalasia, with nodular/lobulated or asymmetric distal wall thickening, mediastinal lymphadenopathy, or a soft-tissue mass being supportive of a secondary process.[28] We do not routinely obtain cross-sectional imaging on all patients with achalasia; however, for complicated cases or patients with atypical features there may be a role.

Manometry

Esophageal manometry is considered the gold standard for the diagnosis of achalasia and has the highest sensitivity for detection of early disease. The past decade has seen the emergence of high-resolution esophageal manometry (HRM) with esophageal pressure topography, which is now the standard of care in most institutions. The concept of HRM stems from Clouse (1998)[28a] at Washington University, who speculated that, by increasing the number of monitoring channels and decreasing the distance between those channels, diagnostic yield would be

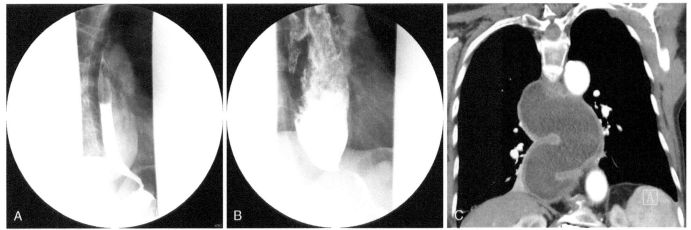

FIG 19.2 Examples of the possible radiographic appearance of a spectrum of patients with achalasia. **A,** The esophageal diameter appears relatively normal and an air-fluid level or significant esophagogastric junction (EGJ) narrowing is not appreciated. As sensitivity of fluoroscopy for detection of achalasia is significantly lower than manometry in early disease, this is not an unusual finding in patients with early disease. **B,** A dilated esophagus is seen with an air-fluid level and narrowing at the EGJ consistent with a classic "bird-beak" appearance. **C,** A mega-esophagus with sigmoidization is shown on chest computed tomography. Unfortunately, in the context of an end-stage esophagus, therapies directed at amelioration of lower esophageal sphincter pressure alone may not be effective and esophagectomy is often required.

TABLE 19.1 The Chicago Classification for Esophageal Motility Disorders

Diagnosis	HRM Chicago Classification (v.3) Criteria
Disorders of Outflow Obstruction	
Achalasia	
Type I	Elevated median IRP with 100% failed peristalsis
Type II	Elevated median IRP with 100% failed peristalsis and intermittent pan-esophageal pressurization (≥ 20% swallows)
Type III	Elevated median IRP, premature (spastic) contractions (≥ 20% swallows), no normal peristalsis
EGJ outflow obstruction	Elevated median IRP with preserved peristalsis (not meeting criteria for achalasia)
Major motility disorders	Never encountered in healthy subjects
Absent contractility	Normal median IRP with 100% failed peristalsis
Distal esophageal spasm	Normal median IRP; premature (spastic) contractions (≥ 20% swallows)
Hypercontractile esophagus (jackhammer esophagus)	Hypercontractile esophagus with DCI > 8000 mm Hg/s per cm (≥ 20% swallows)
Minor motility disorders	Seen in some healthy asymptomatic controls and of uncertain clinical significance
Ineffective esophageal motility	Intermittent weak or failed contractions (≥ 50% swallows) with periodic normal peristalsis (DCI: > 450 mm Hg/s per cm)
Fragmented peristalsis	≥ 50% fragmented contractions with normal DCI (> 450 mm Hg/s per cm)
Normal	Not meeting any of the previous criteria

DCI, Distal contractile integral; *EGJ,* esophagogastric junction; *HRM,* high-resolution esophageal manometry; *IRP,* integrative relaxation pressure.
Adapted from Kahrilas PJ, Bredenoord AJ, Fox M, et al: The Chicago Classification of esophageal motility disorders, v3.0. *Neurogastroenterol Motil* 27(2):160–174, 2015.

enhanced. Pinnacle work in HRM was performed by investigators in Europe and at Northwestern University in the early 2000s, and their combined work eventually led to the Chicago Classification for Esophageal Motility Disorders, widely considered the core reference for esophageal manometry interpretation today and currently on its third rendition (Table 19.1).[29–31]

When interpreting HRM using the Chicago Classification, the diagnosis of achalasia relies on the identification of impaired LES relaxation (as defined by an elevated integrative relaxation pressure [IRP]) in tandem with identification of absent or aberrant peristalsis. One of the key advantages to HRM has been the ability to recognize clinically meaningful achalasia subtypes that

predict clinical course and response to therapy. In 2008, Pandolfino and colleagues at Northwestern University described three distinct manometric achalasia subtypes (types I, II, and III) (Fig. 19.3). In all three, there was abnormal relaxation of the LES/EGJ, defined by an elevated IRP. In type I achalasia, the esophageal body displayed absent peristalsis. In type II, the esophageal body displayed simultaneous, pan-esophageal pressurization with wet swallows. In type III, the esophageal body displayed (for at least some swallows) disorganized contractility akin to spasm. These investigators showed that outcomes to therapeutic intervention varied depending on manometric subtype and, specifically, that patients with a type II pattern (characterized by pan-esophageal

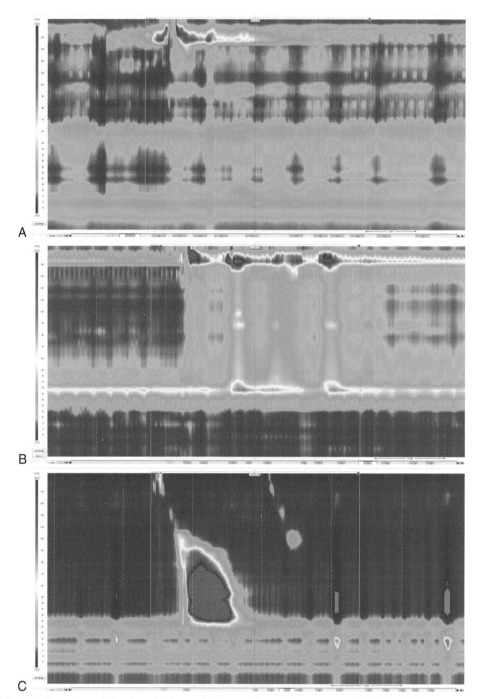

FIG 19.3 Examples of the three high-resolution esophageal manometry (HRM) achalasia subtypes. **A,** Type I (or classic) achalasia is characterized by impaired esophagogastric junction (EGJ) relaxation with absent contractility in the esophageal body. **B,** Type II achalasia is characterized by impaired EGJ relaxation in tandem with pan-esophageal pressurization in the esophageal body. This is the phenotype with the best prognostic implications. **C,** Type III (or spastic) achalasia is characterized by impaired EGJ relaxation with evidence of rapid distal latency/spasm in at least 20% of wet swallows.

pressurization) had excellent outcomes to therapy, whereas patients with a type I pattern required more definitive sphincter disruption and patients with a type III pattern did not respond as well to intervention aimed solely at the LES.[32] This work has now been replicated by others, confirming robust therapeutic response for those with type II achalasia.

The sensitivity of manometry is, however, imperfect, and there are cases that fall outside conventional diagnostic paradigms.[33] The Chicago Classification relies on the IRP as a marker of deglutitive EGJ relaxation; however, there are some patients with achalasia who may have true sphincteric dysfunction with a technically normal IRP. In cases where the manometry is not classic but clinical suspicion for achalasia is high, other complementary tests (such as barium or the Functional Lumen Imaging Probe [FLIP; Crospon, Galway, Ireland]) will need to be employed. Likewise, there are patients who have manometric impairment of deglutitive relaxation but preservation of peristalsis. These patients are currently defined by the Chicago Classification as having EGJ outflow obstruction, a diagnosis of uncertain clinical significance, that in fact could be an achalasia variant or achalasia in transition.[34] Although HRM is considered the most sensitive test for recognition of early achalasia, it is not perfect and there will be some patients (albeit rarely) who clinically have achalasia but may not meet current manometric definitions.

Impedance

Impedance refers to opposition to current within a closed circuit and, when applied to esophageal physiology, it can measure movement of bolus (air, liquid, or food) throughout the esophageal body. Achalasia is characterized by aberrant bolus transit, which can be measured directly via impedance. This was first demonstrated elegantly by Castell and colleagues from Medical University of South Carolina in 2004.[35] However, impedance measurements alone do not distinguish achalasia from other conditions, such as scleroderma, which also result in impaired bolus transit. Likewise, some patients with type III achalasia on HRM may have relative preservation of bolus transit despite a clear manometric diagnosis. For these reasons, impedance serves only a complementary role at present in the diagnosis of achalasia.

There have been two developments with regard to impedance, however, which are worth mention. To begin with, investigators from Northwestern (2014) have evaluated bolus clearance via impedance in comparison to the traditional timed barium swallow.[36] The hypothesis is that monitoring bolus clearance via impedance in conjunction with manometry would be technically simple and may provide similar information regarding functional emptying of the esophagus to that of the timed barium swallow, but would obviate the requirement for radiation and perhaps be more acceptable as a long-term option. Initial data appear promising; however, it should be noted that timed impedance monitoring will only assess functional emptying of the esophagus and will not provide the same information regarding esophageal diameter and anatomy that is provided via fluoroscopy. Whether that gain is worth periodic radiation exposure, however, remains uncertain. The second key development with impedance relates to the use of mucosal impedance as a diagnostic marker for esophageal mucosal integrity. This has been found to be abnormal in esophageal disease states, including achalasia; however, it is not specific enough to reliably separate achalasia from other entities that may impact mucosal integrity and at present remains only a complementary test.[37]

Functional Lumen Imaging Probe

Clinical characterization of esophageal motility disorders has become increasingly multimodal and existing technologies rely primarily on assessment of pressure patterns or bolus flow; however, biomechanical properties of the esophageal wall are likely also an important component in many patients. FLIP has proved to be a novel key addition. The concept of FLIP is based on the use of impedance measurements within a fluid-filled, high-compliance balloon. By knowing the volume of fluid instilled in the balloon and the conductance of that fluid, it is possible to determine the diameter of the balloon between each set of impedance rings; when combined with a pressure sensor, the distensibility of the lumen can be calculated. Development of the device was based on the work of Gregersen in the early 1990s, leading to its commercialization and eventual approval in the United States and Europe.[38,39]

FLIP offers a unique vantage point for the evaluation of patients with potential achalasia, in that it allows direct measurement of EGJ distensibility and diameter. Not surprisingly, research has suggested that distensibility at the EGJ is decreased in the setting of achalasia and reliably improves after mechanical therapy. This was initially demonstrated elegantly in a study of 30 patients with achalasia and 15 healthy controls, showing a marked difference in distensibility between patients with untreated achalasia (distensibility index [DI]: 0.7 ± 0.9 mm^2/mm Hg) and healthy controls (DI: 6.3 ± 0.7 mm^2/mm Hg); moreover, changes in distensibility after therapy predicted clinical response, with patients with good clinical outcome showing increased distensibility (DI: 4.4 ± 0.5 mm^2/mm Hg) compared with those who had unsuccessful treatment (DI: 1.6 ± 0.3 mm^2/mm Hg). Of interest, over half the patients with persistent symptoms after achalasia therapy were noted to have an adequate posttherapy manometry, suggesting that the FLIP measurements provided additive benefit over traditional means of assessment.[40] In a subsequent analysis of 54 achalasia patients and 20 healthy controls, investigators from Northwestern University reported very similar findings, noting a gradient of distensibility between untreated achalasia (0.7–1.1 mm^2/mm Hg), treated achalasia with poor response (1.1–1.5 mm^2/mm Hg), treated achalasia with good response (1.8–3.5 mm^2/mm Hg), and healthy controls (4.2–8.2 mm^2/mm Hg).[41] A 2017 study from investigators in Amsterdam (The Netherlands) has raised the question of whether FLIP may in fact be a more sensitive test for the detection of achalasia than manometry.[42] In our practice, FLIP is an important complementary test to evaluate those patients with symptoms suggestive of achalasia, but conflicting data from other diagnostic modalities or, more frequently, as a means to assess sphincter dynamics in the context of ongoing symptoms after treatment. A clinical example highlighting the use of FLIP in the evaluation of a patient with achalasia is shown in Fig. 19.4.

A key recent development with regard to FLIP has been the formulation of FLIP topography and incorporation of this modality in the evaluation of dysphagia. This has been championed by the Northwestern Group, who have compared FLIP topography to HRM. In their patients with dysphagia (approximately half of whom had achalasia by manometry), FLIP topography showed aberrant contractility patterns in 95% of patients with a major motility disorder characterized by HRM, but also provided additional information in 50% of patients with significant clinical symptoms and an unremarkable HRM.[43,44] At present, data regarding FLIP topography remain limited to a few academic centers; however, with commercialization, this modality is expected to be much more widely available in the near future.

The final role of FLIP in the evaluation of patients with suspected achalasia, patients with established achalasia and symptoms despite therapy, and in the intra-procedural tailoring of achalasia therapy remains to be determined; however, the published data look promising, and the ability to measure EGJ distensibility and diameter directly are compelling arguments for future use and development. Moreover, this test has the capability of being performed during endoscopy, which is invariably already being performed for these patients, rather than as a separate standalone procedure, such as manometry. Where

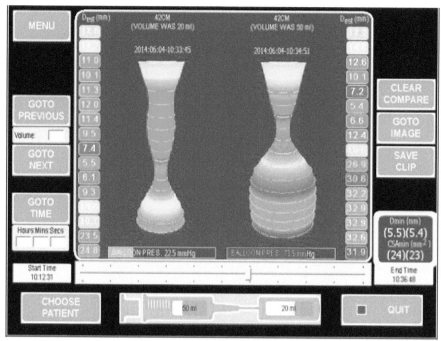

FIG 19.4 A Functional Lumen Imaging Probe (FLIP) study performed on a patient referred for evaluation of persistent dysphagia. Achalasia was clinically suspected, but prior endoscopy, barium esophagram, and several manometry studies had not confirmed the diagnosis. The FLIP procedure was performed and the figure shown is with the balloon placed across the esophagogastric junction. The image on the left represents the balloon with 20 cc of fluid instilled, whereas the image on the right represents the balloon with 30 cc of fluid instilled. With increased fluid, there was minimal change in diameter and cross-sectional area, but pressure markedly increased. The distensibility index for this patient was 0.3. This study confirmed a diagnosis of achalasia and the patient was treated with peroral endoscopic myotomy (POEM) with excellent clinical results.

FLIP ultimately is placed in the diagnostic algorithm for achalasia remains to be determined; however, it clearly will have a role.

Therapy

The physiologic hallmarks of achalasia are impaired LES relaxation and absent or aberrant esophageal peristalsis. As achalasia is a chronic degenerative condition, there is no cure per se; however, most patients will respond effectively to therapy aimed at disruption of the LES and effective removal of the esophageal outlet barrier. Current treatment options include observation, medical therapy, botulinum toxin injection, pneumatic dilatation, Heller myotomy with or without partial fundoplication, peroral endoscopic myotomy (POEM), stent placement, and esophagectomy. Observation is generally viewed as a poor option because untreated achalasia can lead to progressive esophageal dilatation with aspiration, less robust response to the aforementioned therapies, and potentially the need for esophagectomy. For this reason, early treatment is recommended once the diagnosis is established, both to improve symptoms and to prevent progression to an end-stage mega-esophagus.

Medical Therapy

Medical therapy for achalasia is of limited utility. Three classes of agents have been studied: calcium channel blockers,[45–48] nitrates,[45,48,49] and phosphodiesterase inhibitors.[50] The hypothesis is that smooth muscle relaxation will reduce LES pressure, reduce esophageal contractility if spastic achalasia is present, and assist in esophageal emptying. Nifedipine, given in sublingual doses of 10–20 mg prior to meals, is the most widely used medical agent and can decrease LES pressure by 30% to 60% with modest improvement in dysphagia; however, side effects associated with hypotension (headache, dizziness) are significant. Furthermore, there are no data to suggest that medical therapy in any way changes the natural history of achalasia. Moreover, the temporal effects of this therapy on LES dynamics are relatively brief. Tachyphylaxis is noted, and even the marginal initial benefit observed often reaches a plateau after which drug efficacy wanes. In addition, absorption of these medications can be difficult to predict in the context of significant achalasia and delayed esophageal emptying, further compounding the issue. Phosphodiesterase inhibitors may offer similar benefits without as much hypotension as nitrates and calcium channel blockers; however, data are limited. All published series represent short-term use, and there are no long-term trials available to support efficacy of this approach. In our practice, medical therapy for achalasia is employed solely as a bridge to more definitive therapy directed at sphincter disruption.

Botulinum Toxin

The use of botulinum toxin injection of the EGJ for treatment of achalasia was first proposed by Pasricha et al at Johns Hopkins in 1994. Botulinum toxin A is a neurotoxin that blocks the release of acetylcholine from excitatory nerve terminals, leading to decreased muscle contraction and effective reduction in LES pressure. After promising animal experiments, a pilot study was conducted in patients with achalasia and revealed short-term success.[51] This led to a double-blind, placebo-controlled trial wherein 90% of patients with achalasia treated with botulinum toxin reported improvement at 1 week, with approximately two-thirds still reporting improvement at 6 months.[52] However, the effect is temporary and eventually reversed with axonal regeneration. Duration of benefit is typically approximately 9 months, although individual patients may report shorter or longer duration of benefit. Published data suggest decreased efficacy with repeated injection, and fibrosis can be seen with repeated injections, potentially worsening future surgical outcomes.[53]

The initial publications by Pasricha and colleagues employed a dose of 80 units, divided in a circular fashion and injected under endoscopic visualization into the presumed LES. As botulinum toxin is dispensed typically in 100-unit vials, most subsequent publications have utilized this dose. The conventional approach is to mix the botulinum toxin in 4 cc of saline and then inject 1 cc in four quadrants approximately 1 cm proximally to the z-line under endoscopic visualization. Higher doses of botulinum toxin have not been shown to be more effective for treatment of achalasia.[54] Some centers have proposed use of endoscopic ultrasound to aid in placement of the neurotoxin in the LES directly, rather than blind endoscopic injection[55]; however, there are no randomized trials to show that this results in superior outcomes, and in our practice endoscopic ultrasound is not employed for this procedure.

Because of the short duration of benefit, the question of injection-related fibrosis potentially complicating future therapies, and decreased efficacy with time, botulinum toxin is not generally viewed as an ideal first-line therapy for most patients with newly diagnosed achalasia. However, it can be an excellent option for some patients. In our practice, we often employ botulinum toxin in four distinct patient subgroups: (a) those who are either elderly or generally too frail to undergo more definitive therapy (pneumatic dilatation, surgical myotomy, or POEM). Botulinum toxin has a generally good safety profile and in the short-term is a safer option than the other more invasive definitive therapies; (b) those in whom the diagnosis remains in question despite appropriate testing. Between endoscopy, fluoroscopy, manometry, impedance, and FLIP there are multiple means by which esophageal motility can be interrogated and it is not rare that the results of the diagnostic evaluation are incongruent, with some studies suggestive of achalasia and others arguing against. In this situation, we often employ botulinum toxin as a diagnostic test, with the hypothesis that the safety profile is good and if they have significant clinical improvement, they would be amenable to more invasive definitive therapies; (c) those with recurrent symptoms after achalasia therapy, where the pertinent question is whether their symptoms stem from continued sphincteric impairment versus a combination of hyperawareness, hypersensitivity, and aperistalsis. We find this particularly useful for patients who have had a prior Heller myotomy or POEM but may have a short residual remnant sphincter; (d) those patients with predominant chest pain and evidence of spasm. Given that chest pain may not respond as well to mechanical disruption of the LES, we may try botulinum toxin in that subgroup specifically. For most patients with achalasia, however, we do not recommend botulinum toxin as the first-line therapy for the reasons detailed previously.

Pneumatic Dilatation

The concept behind pneumatic balloon dilation is to partially tear the LES by forceful balloon expansion, usually, although not always, utilizing air. Early literature with pneumatic dilatation quoted high perforation rates (> 5%); however, with adoption of the newer Rigiflex balloons (Boston Scientific, Marlborough, MA), those rates are decidedly lower. In a systematic review of 24 studies encompassing 1144 patients with an average follow-up of approximately 3 years, the overall clinical response to pneumatic dilatation was 78%; however, there was a graded response rate based on the balloon size employed. Dilatation using a 3.0-cm balloon alone resulted in a clinical improvement rate of 74%, versus 86% with a 3.5-cm balloon and 90% with a 4.0-cm balloon. Approximately one-third of patients were noted to have recurrence of symptoms requiring additional intervention, usually a repeat pneumatic dilatation. The perforation rate was 1.9%.[56,57] Predictors of decreased response include age over 40 years, male gender, dilated esophagus, small-size balloon, a single dilatation procedure, LES pressure greater than 10 to 15 mm Hg within a year of the procedure, poor esophageal emptying via barium swallow following treatment, and a type III HRM pattern.[1]

Since this series, two large, multicenter trials have provided additional information. The European Achalasia Trial compared pneumatic dilatation versus laparoscopic Heller myotomy for idiopathic achalasia in 201 patients. In the initial protocol, a 35-mm balloon was employed for the first dilatation; however, perforation occurred in 4 of the first 13 patients, and the protocol was subsequently changed so that all patients started with a 30-mm balloon. All patients included in the trial analysis underwent dilatation using a 30-mm balloon followed by dilatation using a 35-mm balloon 1 to 3 weeks later. If they were still symptomatic thereafter (defined by an Eckardt score > 3), then they underwent a subsequent third pneumatic dilatation using a 40-mm balloon. Using this protocol, the investigators achieved a 90% 1-year success rate, 86% 2-year success rate, and 82% 5-year success rate, all of which were statistically similar to those achieved via laparoscopic Heller myotomy.[58,59] However, the rate of perforation for pneumatic dilatation was higher than typically reported in the achalasia series (4.1%), even after discounting the initial four perforations utilizing a 35-mm balloon alone. Recently, a large multicenter study evaluating POEM versus pneumatic dilatation for treatment of therapy-naïve achalasia was presented. In this protocol, all patients randomized to pneumatic dilatation underwent initial dilatation utilizing a 30-mm balloon and then subsequently underwent dilatation utilizing a 35-mm balloon if they remained symptomatic (defined by an Eckardt score > 3) or had evidence of stasis on barium esophagram. Utilizing this less aggressive protocol, 1-year success was reported in 78.8% of patients, with a perforation rate of 1.5%.[60] Putting this information together with prior reports, one can surmise a response rate with pneumatic dilatation of approximately 70% to 80% with an estimated rate of perforation of less than 2% if a conservative approach is employed, starting with a 30-mm balloon and then increasing to a 35-mm balloon if the patient remains symptomatic or has objective evidence of continued impairment in emptying. If one is willing to employ a more aggressive approach (as was done in the European Achalasia Trial), then success rates will be higher (approaching 90% at 1 year), but with the trade-off of an increased perforation risk. Regardless of the approach taken, it is important to recognize that success will wane with time and patients may require additional intervention, usually with a repeat dilatation.

Pneumatic dilatation is typically performed in the endoscopy suite utilizing fluoroscopic guidance. If the risk of aspiration is significant (e.g., if the patient has food or liquid retention on prior endoscopy or imaging), then a liquid diet may be employed for a few days and a longer preprocedure fasting period may be utilized. Efforts should be made to perform these procedures in the morning, as patients may require extended postprocedure monitoring. Either conscious sedation in the left lateral position or anesthesia with airway protection can be employed, based on aspiration risk and local practice patterns. During endoscopy, a Savary guidewire is placed in the stomach under endoscopic guidance, and the endoscope is subsequently removed. A Rigiflex balloon (Boston Scientific) is then passed over the guidewire and fluoroscopically positioned across the narrowed EGJ region. The balloon is then inflated until the radiographic waist from the LES (located ideally in the middle of the balloon) is flattened. If utilizing air, the pressure needed is typically 7 to 15 psi. The balloon can be held in place for 60 seconds if desired, although there is no convincing evidence that keeping the balloon inflated longer than what is required to achieve initial waist flattening improves outcomes. The balloon is then deflated and removed. In some centers, radiographic contrast may be used instead of air to enhance radiographic visualization. The patient is then typically monitored for 2 to 6 hours postprocedure. A gastrografin esophagram can be employed to evaluate for perforation if there is significant pain. Some centers obtain this routinely after pneumatic dilatation to exclude perforation, but this is controversial, and in our practice formal radiographic studies are only obtained postprocedure if there are symptoms that suggest a possible complication. Clinical response should be seen within 1 week following the procedure, although there is some patient heterogeneity. Some centers have published on pneumatic dilatation without fluoroscopy; however, we believe fluoroscopy aids in optimal balloon placement, and we always utilize it. Of note, a 30-mm dilator has been recently released using the FLIP system. Data regarding this dilator are limited, but utilization of this balloon may potentially obviate the need for fluoroscopy.

Heller Myotomy

The idea behind surgical myotomy is to identify the impaired muscle region and to cut the LES and adjacent regions, affecting both the longitudinal and circular fibers, such that the mechanical obstruction is eliminated. The first minimally invasive approach to achalasia was reported by Pellegrini in 1992 using thorascopy; however, a laparoscopic approach has since become the standard of care. A systematic review of data from over 3000 laparoscopic Heller myotomies reported an overall clinical success rate of approximately 90%.[61] More recently, Boeckxstaens et al (2014) reviewed all laparoscopic myotomy series with a sample size of more than 100 patients. In their review of 2264 patients with a mean follow-up of 42 months, clinical efficacy was reported to be 84%.[1] This is in line with the recent 5-year data from the European Achalasia Trial, which also reported a 5-year clinical success rate of 84% in their series of 105 patients who underwent laparoscopic Heller myotomy.[59] Laparoscopic Heller myotomy is clearly superior to pneumatic dilatation if a single balloon dilatation session is employed, but the European Achalasia Trial suggests that the two approaches are equivalent if an aggressive graded balloon dilatation approach is pursued.[58,59]

Although debated in the literature, the addition of a partial fundoplication to the myotomy results in similar efficacy but reduced rates of reflux, with rates of 31.5% after a myotomy alone versus 8.8% when combined with a partial fundoplication.[61] This was echoed in a small, prospective randomized trial showing reflux rates after a Heller myotomy of 47.6% versus rates after

a Heller combined with (anterior) Dor fundoplication of 9.1%, with similar clinical efficacy for the two procedures.[62] However, a complete fundoplication (Nissen) combined with myotomy is not recommended, as rates of dysphagia were significantly higher postoperatively in a prospective trial evaluating this approach.[63]

Peroral Endoscopic Myotomy

POEM is the newest treatment option available for achalasia and was first conceived by Pasricha in 2007[64] and first performed by Inoue[65] in a human subject shortly thereafter. The concept is to create a submucosal tunnel that allows direct visualization of the circular muscle layer in the esophagus, to advance the submucosal tunnel to below the gastroesophageal junction, and then to perform a selective myotomy beginning approximately 3 cm distal to the EGJ (to include the gastric sling and clasp fibers), extending proximally as needed. The endoscope is then removed from the submucosal tunnel and the mucosal defect is closed using endoscopic clips (Videos 19.1–19.4).[66] POEM has the theoretical advantage of allowing direct access to the circular muscle layer of the esophagus without the need to enter the abdominal or thoracic cavities, resulting in no skin incisions and faster recovery. POEM also has the benefit of not being limited to either above or below the diaphragm, as is the problem if either a laparoscopic or thorascopic surgical approach is chosen. However, the two disadvantages of POEM are (a) lack of true long-term data, as this is a relatively novel procedure, and (b) higher reported rates of reflux, as the endoscopic procedure cannot currently be combined with an anti-reflux procedure. Although well over 5000 procedures have been performed worldwide, most of these have been performed in Asia. POEM is currently limited to specialty centers and is not as widely available as the other therapies mentioned earlier.

The published efficacy and safety of POEM have been evaluated in several recent systematic reviews, many including outcomes from over 1000 cases.[67–70] Efficacy is difficult to quantify because of study heterogeneity, but one systematic review evaluating 16 studies with a total of 551 patients reported technical and clinical success rates of 97% and 93%, respectively.[69] However, most of the included patients were published in retrospective analyses and no randomized controlled trials were included. Published short-term results have invariably been very good, with most centers reporting a greater than 90% clinical success rate.[71] Long-term data are more limited. Inoue (2015) published long-term outcome data for his first 500 POEM cases, with an overall success rate of 88.5% at a minimum interval follow-up of 3 years.[72] A 24-month outcomes study of 205 patients with achalasia who underwent POEM at 10 tertiary care centers across the world reported clinical success (defined by an Eckardt score < 3) in 98% at 6 months, 98% at 12 months, and 91% at 24 months or more.[73] Less optimistically, a 2-year follow-up study of 85 patients treated with POEM at three academic centers reported an initial clinical response in 96.3%, but recurrence in a 2-year period in an additional 18% of patients (resulting in a total success rate of 79% at 2 years).[74] A multicenter randomized, prospective study (2017) comparing POEM with pneumatic dilatation in 133 patients with treatment-naïve achalasia reported POEM success rates of 98.4% at 12-week follow-up and 92.2% at 1 year.[60] To our knowledge, this is the first prospective randomized controlled trial evaluating POEM versus another treatment modality for achalasia.

Safety of POEM appears to be excellent. In a recent evaluation of 1826 patients who underwent POEM at 12 tertiary care centers between 2009 and 2015, adverse events were noted in 137 patients (7.5%); however, the bulk of these were judged to be mild, and severe adverse events were only seen in 9 patients (0.5%). The most commonly reported adverse events were inadvertent mucosotomy and adverse events related to insufflation. Only four patients (0.2%) required surgery for bleeding during tunneling, mucosotomy, esophageal leak, or empyema, and no fatalities were reported.[75]

Perhaps the most significant concern regarding POEM is the potential for abnormal gastroesophageal reflux following the procedure, given that it certainly seems effective at LES disruption without being combined with an anti-reflux procedure. A study of 100 treated patients after POEM reported a short-term clinical success of 94%, but 24-hour pH monitoring demonstrated pathologic esophageal acid exposure in 53.4% of patients, a minority of them with heartburn (24.3%) or esophagitis (27.4%).[76,77] Of note, all the symptomatic patients were well controlled with medical therapy. In two systematic reviews, the post-POEM reflux rates were estimated to range from 10% to 19%[67,68,71]; however, relatively few of these studies performed pH monitoring, and these numbers were largely based on symptoms and endoscopic appearance for those few patients who underwent postprocedure endoscopy. In the 2017 multicenter randomized prospective study comparing POEM to pneumatic dilatation, all subjects underwent pH monitoring and endoscopy at 1-year post-POEM. In this series, abnormal esophageal acid exposure was noted in 49.1% of POEM patients versus 38.6% of pneumatic dilatation patients. However, significantly more patients with severe reflux esophagitis (Los Angeles C or D) were seen in the post-POEM group.[60] Whether this higher acid exposure has clinical relevance is unknown, but is worth following as more data become available in the future.

Whereas POEM can be considered as a treatment option for all patients with achalasia, it may have a special niche for treatment of those patients with type III, or spastic, achalasia. As POEM is not limited by the diaphragm, one has the option of creating a long myotomy in conjunction with a standard sphincter-disruption procedure. In a retrospective analysis of 49 patients with type III achalasia who underwent POEM at eight academic centers versus 26 patients who underwent laparoscopic Heller myotomy at a single center, POEM resulted in clinical success in 98% of patients versus 80% with surgical myotomy. The average POEM myotomy length was 16 cm, versus an average Heller myotomy length of 8 cm.[78]

The data regarding POEM for treatment of achalasia is rapidly emerging, and its role is evolving. At present, POEM is a reasonable option for any patient with achalasia if local expertise exists. For those with type III achalasia, POEM may be preferable to other modalities because a long myotomy is appealing and makes physiologic sense. For those patients with type II achalasia, POEM remains a very reasonable option, but there are no data at present to suggest that POEM is superior to surgery in terms of efficacy. For this reason, the decision as to which modality to employ for those patients with type I or type II achalasia depends on many factors, including local expertise, patient preference, and likelihood of postprocedure reflux.

Stent Placement

Placement of an esophageal self-expanding metal stent is not typically considered in the treatment algorithm; however, based on data from China, it is a potential option that can be considered in extenuating circumstances.[79–82] In 2009, Zhao and colleagues reported a series of 75 patients with achalasia who were treated with a 30-mm esophageal stent. Stents were placed under fluoroscopic guidance and removed approximately 5 days later. Clinical response was reported to be 100% at 1 month and 83% at 10 years.[79] No perforations were reported. Investigators from Italy utilized temporary placement of a 30-mm stent in 7 patients with achalasia, and reported complete symptom resolution in 5 and marked symptom improvement in 2, without complications.[83] Most recently, investigators from Shanghai (2016) evaluated stent placement versus balloon dilatation in 77 patients with achalasia, and reported increased short-term efficacy and decreased recurrence in patients treated with stent placement in comparison to balloon dilatation.[84] More data are needed to support this thought-provoking and apparently efficacious approach.

Esophagectomy

Approximately 5% of achalasia patients will eventually require esophagectomy either because of pronounced esophageal dilatation, severe dysphagia despite appropriate therapy directed at the LES, a peptic stricture that is not amenable to dilatation, or complications related to esophageal dilatation/aspiration or surgical intervention, or esophageal cancer. Several options are available for patients who reach this point, including a distal segmental esophagectomy, vertical esophagectomy and myotomy, vagal-sparing esophagectomy, and subtotal esophagectomy. Each of these procedures has pros and cons, with subtotal esophagectomy being the most commonly performed today for end-stage achalasia.[85] Although certainly a reasonable option in the appropriate patient, esophagectomy has greater morbidity and mortality than other therapies and is generally viewed as a last resort. In a 2014 analysis of 963 patients with achalasia who underwent esophagectomy, the median length of hospital stay was 13 days, with a cost of $115k and a mortality rate of 2.7%.[86]

OTHER MOTILITY DISORDERS

There are many patients who have significant symptoms suggestive of dysmotility with abnormal objective testing, but who do not meet the current Chicago criteria for achalasia. These patients are typically classified by their manometry pattern into the following categories: EGJ outflow obstruction, distal esophageal spasm, and hypercontractile esophagus. Each of these is seen frequently in practice, but treatment options are less well defined than for achalasia. Although not considered a major motility disorder, we will also touch on IEM, which is frequently seen in evaluation and is of uncertain clinical significance (Fig. 19.5).

EGJ Outflow Obstruction

EGJ outflow obstruction is defined by the Chicago Classification as impaired relaxation of the LES (defined by an elevated IRP > 15 mm Hg) with preserved peristalsis.[31] This pattern has uncertain clinical significance and appears to be a clinically heterogeneous rather than a uniform process. The first significant description of EGJ outflow obstruction came from Scherer et al at Northwestern University in 2009, who identified 16 patients from 1000 consecutive manometries. They noted that these patients had dysphagia and/or chest pain and responded to sphincteric disruption therapy, specifically Heller myotomy. They concluded that in some cases, functional EGJ outlet obstruction may represent a variant of achalasia with incomplete manometric manifestations.[87] In a series of 34 patients, Van Hoeij et al (2015) from Amsterdam (The Netherlands) reported that 82% required

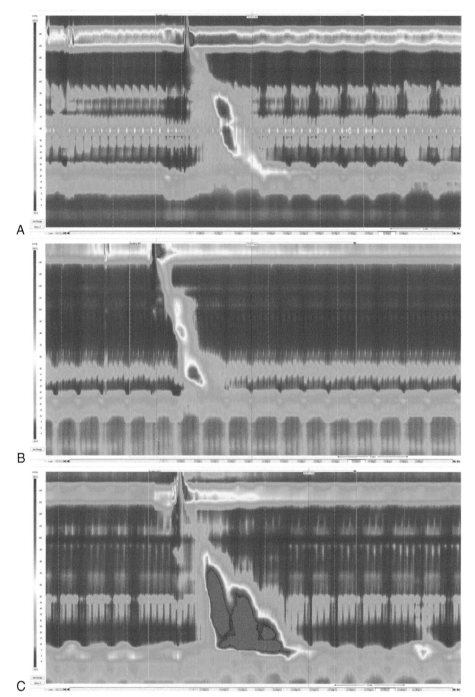

FIG 19.5 High-resolution manometry examples of major motility disorders. **A,** Typical image of esophagogastric junction (EGJ) outflow obstruction (with impaired EGJ relaxation but preserved peristalsis). **B,** Typical image of distal esophageal spasm (with a short distal latency and rapid contraction). Of note, this can be relatively subtle and may be missed if not looking at the distal latency specifically. In this swallow, the distal latency was 3.9 seconds (normal < 4.5 seconds). **C,** Typical image of a hypercontractile esophagus, with classic jackhammer appearance.

no treatment and over half of the patients had symptoms judged unrelated to the manometric obstruction. Three patients progressed to achalasia on subsequent evaluation. They concluded that the clinical significance of EGJ outflow obstruction was unclear, that a substantial subset has unrelated symptoms, and that spontaneous improvement is not uncommon.[88] In another

series of 44 patients, over 30% had spontaneous resolution of symptoms without treatment directed at the EGJ and cautioning that invasive treatments may not be needed.[89] In 2016, investigators from South Florida evaluated 49 patients with EGJ outflow obstruction, noting that 27 patients had functional issues, whereas 22 patients had an anatomic abnormality (most commonly strictures and hiatal hernias). Manometry and barium esophagram studies did not distinguish the two groups, but they behaved distinctly due to their different underlying etiologies.[90] In the largest series yet, patients who met criteria for EGJ outflow obstruction were a hodgepodge of different clinical subgroups, including patients with unrelated symptoms (identified incidentally, for instance, on a manometry performed to evaluate for reflux), anatomic abnormalities (particularly hiatal hernias), and patients with potential variant achalasia.[34] Interestingly, EGJ outflow obstruction was more frequently seen in patients who had used opiates within the past 24 hours (27%) compared with controls (7%).[91]

When all these series are taken in context, one is left with the question of how to approach a symptomatic patient with EGJ outflow obstruction identified by manometry. In our practice, we generally take the following steps. First, given the known association with opiate use and EGJ outflow obstruction, we ensure that patients are not taking opiates and there are no potential medicinal causes for the manometric finding. Second, due to recognition that EGJ outflow obstruction is a mixture of patients with anatomic abnormalities and functional issues, we perform complementary testing (endoscopy with biopsies, barium esophagography, FLIP) to evaluate for hiatal hernias, subtle strictures, and infiltrative processes, particularly eosinophilic esophagitis. Third, due to reports linking EGJ outflow obstruction to neoplasm in rare cases, we ensure that there has been appropriate imaging (either via CT/magnetic resonance imaging or endoscopic ultrasound) if no alternative etiology is found to explain the findings and it is clinically appropriate. If, after the aforementioned, no underlying etiology is found to explain the manometric findings, abnormality is corroborated on complementary testing, and the patient has symptoms significant enough to warrant intervention, then we consider therapy aimed at reduction in LES pressure (smooth muscle relaxants, botulinum toxin injection, pneumatic dilatation, myotomy). As symptoms and findings may abate spontaneously, we start with less invasive options upfront (medical therapy or botulinum toxin injection), with other interventions reserved for those with persistent findings and significant symptoms. We have referred select patients with EGJ outflow obstruction for definitive intervention (pneumatic dilatation, POEM, and Heller myotomy) with excellent outcomes, but only after careful deliberation and extensive evaluation.

Distal Esophageal Spasm

Esophageal spasm is commonly considered as a diagnosis for patients with dysphagia and chest pain but rarely proven on manometry. Esophageal spasm was first described clinically in 1889 and first documented by manometry in 1958.[92,93] Utilizing conventional manometry, spasm was defined by the presence of rapid conduction velocity, simultaneous contractions, or multi-peaked contractions.[94] However, with the advent of HRM, these findings have been found to be non-specific. In 2011, Pandolfino and colleagues proposed that spasm be diagnosed based solely on distal latency (essentially the time between upper esophageal sphincter relaxation and when the deglutitive contraction reaches the distal esophagus) after showing that this was a more specific finding than the contractile front velocity. A cutoff of 4.5 seconds for 20% or more of wet swallows was proposed.[95] This quantification of spasm was subsequently adopted in the Chicago Classification and is the basis of the manometric diagnosis of distal esophageal spasm today.[31]

Medical options for treatment of esophageal spasm are relatively limited. To compound the issue, most published studies rely on conventional manometric criteria for esophageal spasm, which in the days prior to HRM, likely represented a heterogeneous collection of different manometric phenotypes (as classification could be based on velocity, simultaneous contractions, and multiphasic contractions). The mainstay of medical therapy for distal esophageal spasm has been smooth muscle relaxants, specifically calcium channel blockers,[96] nitrates,[97,98] and phosphodiesterase inhibitors.[99] However, data are limited to small case series and there are no randomized controlled trials that show efficacy at the present time. Anecdotally, pharmacologic therapy for spasm has been disappointing; however, it is still a reasonable first-line treatment for symptomatic patients with documented or suspected esophageal spasm. In our practice, we often start with low-dose calcium channel blockers taken 15 minutes before meals or sublingual nitroglycerin taken as needed during episodes.

If symptoms persist despite medical therapy, then botulinum toxin injection is a reasonable next step, with the hypothesis that blockage of acetylcholine release from excitatory neurons will weaken esophageal contractions and improve symptoms. This was evaluated in a randomized controlled trial of 22 patients with either distal esophageal spasm or a hypercontractile esophagus. Patients underwent injection in two regions, immediately proximal to the EGJ and in the esophageal body. Fifty percent of patients responded to botulinum toxin, as opposed to only 10% of controls at 1 month, and in the subgroup analysis the distal esophageal spasm patients were noted to have significant improvement in dysphagia and symptoms scores.[100] However, it should be noted that there are no long-term studies evaluating the efficacy of repeated botulinum toxin injection for spasm, and botulinum toxin, although considered relatively safe, is not risk free. In a 2017 analysis of 386 patients undergoing 661 botulinum toxin injections for treatment of esophageal motility disorders (51% achalasia, 30% spasm), 7.9% developed mild complications (chest pain, heartburn, or epigastric pain in the majority of cases), and 1 patient developed a fatal acute mediastinitis.[101]

Finally, POEM has been evaluated as a potential option. This has been proposed for patients with significant symptoms in the context of well-documented spasm refractory to medical intervention. POEM offers the theoretical ability to cut esophageal musculature and prevent contractions in a more durable fashion than achieved with botulinum toxin injection. A 2017 systematic review and meta-analysis evaluated 8 observational studies including 179 patients with spastic esophageal disorders. Of that group, 18 were identified to have distal esophageal spasm. The weighted pool rate for clinical success of POEM in these patients was 88%, and the weighted pool rate for adverse events was 14%.[102] Long surgical myotomy has also been reported for treatment of esophageal spasm,[103,104] but data are limited and this appears to have fallen out of favor with the advent of POEM. More data are needed to better stratify which patients require and benefit from more invasive intervention.

Hypercontractile Esophagus

Hypertensive peristaltic contractions are commonly encountered at manometry. These were initially labeled as *nutcracker esophagus* based on seminal work from Castell et al (1987, 2006), and were hypothesized to cause chest pain and dysphagia.[105,106] However, data regarding symptom causality were contradictory, and these values were also found in patients with reflux and healthy asymptomatic controls. With the advent of HRM, terminology changed to provide greater specificity. Initially the terms *hypertensive peristalsis* and *spastic nutcracker* were used to signify patients who may have been previously labeled as nutcracker esophagus.[29] However, investigators from Northwestern University subsequently coined the label *jackhammer esophagus* to signify a degree of hypercontractility never seen in healthy controls. In their seminal publication, they evaluated 72 healthy asymptomatic controls in comparison to 2000 patients. Using the distal contractile integral (DCI) as a marker of esophageal contractile vigor, they found that a cutoff of more than 8000 mm Hg/s per cm for a single swallow exceeded the peak DCI of any healthy control and seemed pathologic. As most of these hypertensive aberrant contractions were multi-peaked, they coined the term *jackhammer esophagus* as a visual description of the contraction. To qualify for this diagnosis, patients had to have a single swallow with a DCI greater than 8000 mm Hg/s per cm in the context of normal LES relaxation and normal distal latency (excluding achalasia or spasm).[107] The term *nutcracker esophagus* was used in the second version of the Chicago Classification to refer to hypertensive peristaltic contractions not fulfilling criteria for jackhammer esophagus, but then was subsequently removed.[30,31] In the most recent third version of the Chicago Classification, the criteria for a hypercontractile esophagus were tightened to include a DCI greater than 8000 mm Hg/s per cm for at least 20% of wet swallows to increase specificity.

Treatment options for a hypercontractile esophagus are the same as those for esophageal spasm. Most publications evaluating treatment for esophageal hypercontractility were published before the term *jackhammer esophagus* was coined and likely included numerous manometric subgroups. Specifically, the multi-peaked contractions seen frequently in jackhammer esophagus previously would have satisfied criteria for distal esophageal spasm using conventional manometric criteria.[94] As such, nitrates, calcium channel blockers, and sildenafil can all be considered, but there are no randomized controlled trials evaluating any medical options for the treatment of jackhammer esophagus. Botulinum toxin injection has also been employed with some success, similar to that reported for spasm. Marjoux et al (2015) reported clinical success in 5 out of 7 patients with jackhammer esophagus at greater than 6 months.[108] In the randomized trial detailed earlier showing efficacy of botulinum toxin in spastic disorders, Vanuytsel et al (2013) included 7 patients with a hypercontractile esophagus; however, subgroup analysis of these 7 patients was not reported.[100,109] POEM has also been employed with some success. In a 2017 systematic review evaluating POEM in the context of spastic esophageal disorders, 8 observational studies with 179 patients were identified. In the 37 patients with jackhammer esophagus who underwent POEM, the weighted pooled rate for clinical success was 72%, and the weighted pooled rate for postprocedure adverse events was 16%.[102] Akin to distal esophageal spasm, more data are needed to make concrete recommendations as to the best management for these patients.

Ineffective Esophageal Motility

IEM was defined by the third Chicago Classification as low-amplitude contractions (DCI < 450 mm Hg/s per cm) in 50% or more of wet swallows, and is synonymous with weak peristalsis.[31] Although the manometric criteria for this diagnosis are clearly defined, etiology, pathophysiology, and clinical significance remain uncertain. As opposed to the major motility disorders detailed earlier, IEM is labeled as a minor motility disorder,

meaning that, whereas it may be associated with symptoms in some patients, the pattern also can be found in healthy asymptomatic controls. Recently, Castell et al (2017) reviewed their experience with 231 IEM patients, relating an association with abnormal esophageal acid exposure and suggesting different clinical subgroups within the broader IEM umbrella.[110] Although a significant impairment of bolus clearance is seen in symptomatic patients with gastroesophageal reflux disease and IEM, such patients are otherwise indistinguishable from those with acid reflux symptoms and normal motility.[111]

Patients with IEM can pose a significant clinical challenge, and data on specific treatments is limited. Given the uncertain clinical significance of this manometric finding, lifestyle modifications are a reasonable first step. Proposed modifications include ensuring an upright position during mealtime, sufficient chewing, intake of carbonated beverages, effortful swallowing, and decreased bolus consistency. If reflux-related symptoms are dominant, then lifestyle, medical, and interventional therapy directed at reflux are recommended. The role of anti-reflux mechanical interventions in the context of IEM is controversial and outside the scope of this chapter. There are no medical options that have been clinically studied specifically for IEM; however, several medications have been shown to enhance esophageal contractility, including bethanechol, pyridostigmine, metoclopramide, domperidone, prucalopride, and buspirone.[112] At present, however, usage of all these medications for IEM would be off label and there are no published studies showing long-term efficacy for symptoms related to IEM with any specific medical therapy at present. There are no data to suggest benefit with either endoscopic or surgical approaches.

NOVEL ENDOSCOPIC APPLICATIONS

Improvements in endoscopic technology have opened frontiers previously unknown. POEM has evolved from conceptualization to full implementation around the globe in under a decade. In addition, submucosal tunneling has become more widely available, making the submucosal space more readily accessible for interventions beyond a simple myotomy. Biopsies are now feasible during POEM, allowing direct access to the muscularis propria. In addition, novel diagnostic tools that may be less invasive, such as endocytoscopy, are also potential additions to the diagnostic armamentarium.[113] Given how much is still unknown regarding the etiology and pathophysiology of achalasia and other motility disorders, the ability to get directed samples from the affected tissues via submucosal tunneling offers great potential to hopefully increase our understanding of these disorders, and potentially suggest future therapies that will be disease modifying rather than palliative.

In addition to directed deep-biopsy acquisition and in vivo evaluation, the other key potential offered by esophageal submucosal tunneling is the ability to directly implant devices and drugs in the deep layers of the esophagus. Investigators from Johns Hopkins evaluated the blind insertion of a microstimulator in the distal esophagus of a canine model approximately a decade ago.[114] However, with the advent of submucosal tunneling, targeted delivery of these devices will become feasible and may potentially be less invasive and safer than surgically implanted devices that run the risk of lead migration. Likewise, targeted drug delivery (presently speculative) may allow local action of select medications, leading to potentially greater efficacy and less systemic side effects.

FUTURE DIRECTIONS

The past decade has seen rapid development in the use of diagnostic technologies including HRM, impedance, and FLIP, as well as rapid expansion in endoscopic therapies, and, in particular, POEM. However, there are still many basic questions regarding esophageal motility disorders that have not yet been answered. FLIP topography seems poised to change the diagnostic landscape of esophageal motility disorders within the next few years, and may lead to greater understanding of physiology and symptom pathogenesis. Long-term data regarding POEM are emerging, and we expect a greater understanding regarding the relative pros and cons (particularly with regard to acid reflux) of this approach compared with other modalities. Randomized controlled trials comparing POEM with laparoscopic Heller myotomy are currently underway. Ultimately, however, many big questions remain regarding disease pathogenesis and etiology, and with increased technology and the accessibility of the submucosal space we are hopeful that some of those questions can be answered.

CONCLUSION

Esophageal motility disorders are frequently encountered in gastroenterology practices today, with achalasia being the most prominent. Utilizing endoscopy, fluoroscopy, and manometry, most patients can be successfully diagnosed and receive prognostic information regarding optimal treatment. For a handful of patients with conflicting information, FLIP and, potentially, impedance may offer additive information. For most patients, treatment of achalasia should be with definitive therapy, specifically pneumatic dilatation, Heller myotomy, or POEM, all of which have their selling points and are reasonable options based on patient specifics and local expertise. Other major motility disorders of the esophagus, including EGJ outflow obstruction, distal esophageal spasm, and the hypercontractile esophagus, have less defined treatment algorithms and should be evaluated on a case-by-case basis.

KEY REFERENCES

1. Boeckxstaens GE, Zaninotto G, Richter JE: Achalasia, *Lancet* 383:83–93, 2014.
2. Pandolfino JE, Gawron AJ: Achalasia: a systematic review, *JAMA* 313:1841–1852, 2015.
29. Pandolfino JE, Fox MR, Bredenoord AJ, et al: High-resolution manometry in clinical practice: utilizing pressure topography to classify oesophageal motility abnormalities, *Neurogastroenterol Motil* 21: 796–806, 2009.
30. Bredenoord AJ, Fox M, Kahrilas PJ, et al: Chicago classification criteria of esophageal motility disorders defined in high resolution esophageal pressure topography, *Neurogastroenterol Motil* 24(Suppl 1):57–65, 2012.
31. Kahrilas PJ, Bredenoord AJ, Fox M, et al: The Chicago Classification of esophageal motility disorders, v3.0, *Neurogastroenterol Motil* 27: 160–174, 2015.
32. Pandolfino JE, Kwiatek MA, Nealis T, et al: Achalasia: a new clinically relevant classification by high-resolution manometry, *Gastroenterology* 135:1526–1533, 2008.
34. Okeke FC, Raja S, Lynch KL, et al: What is the clinical significance of esophagogastric junction outflow obstruction? evaluation of 60 patients at a tertiary referral center, *Neurogastroenterol Motil* 29(6): 2017.
38. Gregersen H, Djurhuus JC: Impedance planimetry: a new approach to biomechanical intestinal wall properties, *Dig Dis* 9:332–340, 1991.
40. Rohof WO, Hirsch DP, Kessing BF, et al: Efficacy of treatment for patients with achalasia depends on the distensibility of the esophagogastric junction, *Gastroenterology* 143:328–335, 2012.
41. Pandolfino JE, de Ruigh A, Nicodeme F, et al: Distensibility of the esophagogastric junction assessed with the functional lumen imaging probe (FLIP) in achalasia patients, *Neurogastroenterol Motil* 25:496–501, 2013.
43. Carlson DA, Lin Z, Rogers MC, et al: Utilizing functional lumen imaging probe topography to evaluate esophageal contractility during volumetric distention: a pilot study, *Neurogastroenterol Motil* 27: 981–989, 2015.
44. Carlson DA, Kahrilas PJ, Lin Z, et al: Evaluation of esophageal motility utilizing the functional lumen imaging probe, *Am J Gastroenterol* 111: 1726–1735, 2016.
51. Pasricha PJ, Ravich WJ, Hendrix TR, et al: Treatment of achalasia with intrasphincteric injection of botulinum toxin. A pilot trial, *Ann Intern Med* 121:590–591, 1994.
52. Pasricha PJ, Ravich WJ, Hendrix TR, et al: Intrasphincteric botulinum toxin for the treatment of achalasia, *N Engl J Med* 332:774–778, 1995.
56. Richter JE: Update on the management of achalasia: balloons, surgery and drugs, *Expert Rev Gastroenterol Hepatol* 2:435–445, 2008.
58. Boeckxstaens GE, Annese V, des Varannes SB, et al: Pneumatic dilation versus laparoscopic Heller's myotomy for idiopathic achalasia, *N Engl J Med* 364:1807–1816, 2011.
59. Moonen A, Annese V, Belmans A, et al: Long-term results of the European achalasia trial: a multicentre randomised controlled trial comparing pneumatic dilation versus laparoscopic Heller myotomy, *Gut* 65:732–739, 2016.
60. Ponds FA, Fockens P, Neuhaus H, et al: Peroral endoscopic myotomy versus pneumatic dilatation in therapy-naive patients with achalasia: results of a randomized controlled trial, *Gastroenterology* 152:S139, 2017.
64. Pasricha PJ, Hawari R, Ahmed I, et al: Submucosal endoscopic esophageal myotomy: a novel experimental approach for the treatment of achalasia, *Endoscopy* 39:761–764, 2007.
65. Inoue H, Minami H, Kobayashi Y, et al: Peroral endoscopic myotomy (POEM) for esophageal achalasia, *Endoscopy* 42:265–271, 2010.
72. Inoue H, Sato H, Ikeda H, et al: Per-oral endoscopic myotomy: a series of 500 patients, *J Am Coll Surg* 221:256–264, 2015.
74. Werner YB, Costamagna G, Swanstrom LL, et al: Clinical response to peroral endoscopic myotomy in patients with idiopathic achalasia at a minimum follow-up of 2 years, *Gut* 65:899–906, 2016.
87. Scherer JR, Kwiatek MA, Soper NJ, et al: Functional esophagogastric junction obstruction with intact peristalsis: a heterogeneous syndrome sometimes akin to achalasia, *J Gastrointest Surg* 13:2219–2225, 2009.
95. Pandolfino JE, Roman S, Carlson D, et al: Distal esophageal spasm in high-resolution esophageal pressure topography: defining clinical phenotypes, *Gastroenterology* 141:469–475, 2011.
107. Roman S, Pandolfino JE, Chen J, et al: Phenotypes and clinical context of hypercontractility in high-resolution esophageal pressure topography (EPT), *Am J Gastroenterol* 107:37–45, 2012.

A complete reference list can be found online at ExpertConsult .com

20

Endoscopic Diagnosis and Management of Zenker's Diverticula

Ryan Law and Todd H. Baron

INTRODUCTION

Zenker's diverticulum (ZD) is a posterior pharyngoesophageal mucosal outpouching that forms through Killian's triangle. Poor upper esophageal sphincter (UES) compliance is the acknowledged pathophysiologic mechanism of action, leading to creation of a high-pressure zone, ultimately resulting in diverticulum formation. This entity most commonly presents in the elderly, and can be associated with a plethora of potential symptoms, most commonly dysphagia. Cricopharyngeal myotomy is usually performed alone or in combination with diverticulectomy (when open surgery is performed) to improve symptoms and prevent recurrence.

CLINICAL PRESENTATION AND DIAGNOSIS

ZD most frequently occurs between the seventh and eighth decades of life, predominantly in men.[1-4] ZD is rarely identified before the age of 40 years. The overall prevalence in the general population is between 0.01% and 0.11%, and varies markedly throughout the world. However, these data reflect symptomatic patients, and the number of asymptomatic patients with ZD remains unknown. Anatomical differences or life expectancy may account for the varying prevalence between geographic areas.[5] In the United Kingdom, the incidence of ZD is approximately 2 per 100,000 people per year.[6] It has been described more commonly in the United States, Canada, and Australia than in Japan and Indonesia.[7] Symptoms may be present for weeks to years before diagnosis.[8] Cervical borborygmus, in the presence of a palpable lump in the neck, is nearly pathognomonic for ZD. Although a multitude of symptoms have been attributed to ZD, 80–90% of patients suffer from dysphagia. Dysphagia occurs secondary to incomplete opening of the UES and extrinsic compression of the cervical esophagus by the diverticulum itself. As the pouch enlarges and dysphagia increases, symptoms often worsen, leading to resultant weight loss and malnutrition. A sudden increase in symptom severity and/or the development of alarming symptoms such as local pain, hemoptysis, or hematemesis may signal the presence of ulceration[9] or squamous cell carcinoma within the diverticulum. Squamous cell carcinoma arising in a ZD is said to have an incidence of 0.4–1.5%,[10] though these older data might reflect more long-standing, untreated disease. Presumably, therapy decreases stasis and risk of cancer. Additional symptoms such as hoarseness/dysphonia, regurgitation, halitosis, cough, and aspiration pneumonia have been described in 30–40% of patients.[11] It is unclear if pneumonia occurs due to direct aspiration of diverticular contents or aspiration of contents pooled within the pharynx.[12] Medications (i.e., capsules, tablets) can become entrapped in the diverticulum, leading to decreased efficacy and, potentially, ulceration with bleeding.[13] Entrapment of a video capsule within a ZD has also been reported.[4,14] Gastrointestinal bleeding within the diverticulum can occur, and is amenable to endoscopic management.[15,16]

A variety of other conditions have been associated with ZD. These include laryngocele, leiomyoma, polymyositis, cervical esophageal web, carotid body tumor, postanterior cervical discectomy and fusion, upper esophageal stenosis, hiatal hernia, and gastroesophageal reflux disease.[17]

PATHOPHYSIOLOGY

The UES is composed of the posterior surface of the thyroid and cricoid cartilage, as well as three muscles: the inferior pharyngeal constrictor, cricopharyngeus (CP), and cervical esophagus.[5] Of these three muscles, the CP provides for the dominant portion of UES function. It forms a muscular sling around the upper esophagus between the two sides of the cricoid cartilage and extends posteriorly to mesh with the inferior pharyngeal constrictor. Two sets of CP muscle fibers have been identified: the horizontally oriented fibers that occlude the esophageal introitus, and an oblique band of fibers that are responsible for propulsion of the bolus.

The inciting pathophysiologic mechanism of ZD is inadequate UES sphincter compliance with failure to open completely.[18] This failure to achieve adequate diameter for effective bolus clearance leads to increased intraluminal pressure with outpouching in an area of relative wall weakness in the hypopharynx

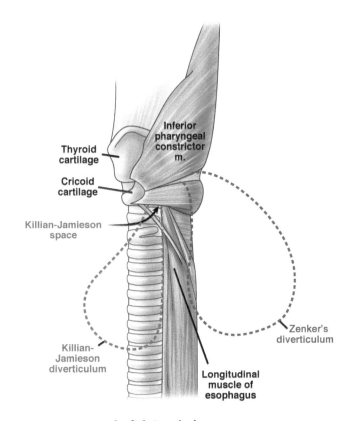

Left lateral view

FIG 20.1 Illustration of Zenker's diverticulum as a herniation through Killian's triangle. *m,* muscle. (From Law R, Katzka DA, Baron TH: Zenker's diverticulum. *Clin Gastroenterol Hepatol* 12[11]:1773–1782, 2014.)

BOX 20.1   Bromberg Classification of Zenker's Diverticulum

Stage I: Thorn-like with longitudinal axis of 2–3 mm visible during the contraction phase of the upper esophageal sphincter after deglutition but not during deglutition

Stage II: Club-shaped with longitudinal axis of 7–8 mm visible during the contraction phase of the upper esophageal sphincter

Stage III: Bag-shaped with a caudally-oriented axis of more than 1 cm but without compression of the esophagus

Stage IV: Large with compression of the esophagus

---

between the CP and inferior pharyngeal constrictor. This area, known as Killian's Triangle, is adjacent to the retropharyngeal space and thus leads to pouch formation posteriorly (Fig. 20.1). The diverticulum may be posterior, posterolateral, or lateral (pharyngocele), but the most common subtype is the posterior pulsion diverticulum.[19] ZD most commonly forms posteriorly on the left side. This is important for determination of the neck incision site during an open surgical approach and when performing endoluminal therapy, as division of the common wall between the diverticulum and the esophageal lumen is necessary for complete symptom relief. It should be noted that this posterior pouch includes only mucosa and submucosa; therefore a ZD should be considered a "pseudo-diverticulum." Several other factors may contribute to pharyngoesophageal pouch formation. For example, increased intrabolus pressures have been well documented, and likely occur due to stiffness of the CP and hypopharynx. Increased intrabolus pressure is also increased in older patients who perform multiple swallows to achieve bolus clearance. Moreover, as the diverticulum enlarges, it may compress the pharyngoesophageal segment and lead to increased intrabolus pressure secondary to extrinsic compression. Finally, incoordination of pharyngeal contraction and UES opening has also been variably demonstrated by some investigators.[1,8] Video fluoroscopy is a valuable tool, particularly for diagnosis, but precise determination of abnormal function is limited by variation in interpretation and quality. Furthermore, useful manometric data are exceedingly difficult to obtain in this area, due to asymmetry in sphincter pressures and wide variations in sphincter motility during swallowing.

DIAGNOSTIC EVALUATION

A diagnosis of ZD is most commonly obtained via radiography in conjunction with videofluoroscopy (Fig. 20.2). The defect is best seen during the act of swallowing in the lateral view. Evidence of aspiration may be seen as contrast is cleared from the diverticulum. Static images are often inadequate in patients with a small diverticulum. The size of the diverticulum may vary considerably. Early stage diverticula may be 1 cm or less and difficult to appreciate; however, ZDs as large as 6 cm have been reported.[20]

The Brombart classification scheme (Box 20.1) defines four types of ZD based on findings from barium esophagography. The original concept of this little-known staging system was that patients progressed from one stage to another.[21] Although this hypothesis has not been validated, the scheme has been used to assess response to therapy, with postprocedural residual diverticulum and contrast retention strongly associated with prolonged dysphagia in the early postoperative period.

ZD may also be diagnosed by transcutaneous ultrasonography. This technique may be useful in elderly patients who cannot tolerate barium esophagography, and in patients with a palpable neck mass on physical examination. During ultrasound, ZD appears as a pouch-shaped structure posteriorly at the level of the pharyngoesophageal junction.[22] Similar to videofluoroscopy, contrast can be given to the patient, but is not mandatory. Retention of contrast for longer than 3 minutes during ultrasound is consistent with a ZD. Other ultrasonographic findings include an increase in the lesion's size with water ingestion and focal heterogeneous echogenicity secondary to retained contents (i.e., fluid, retained food, etc.) within the diverticular sac. In the future, neck ultrasonography may play a more prominent role during assessment of the UES. In a 2013 study, transcutaneous ultrasound was able to identify the normal diameter of the closed UES, mean duration of opening and mean duration of displacement in the anterior and lateral directions.[23]

Differentiation from the Killian-Jamieson diverticulum is important. Killian-Jamieson diverticula are smaller and less common, and arise from the proximal anterolateral cervical esophagus, lying inferior to the CP. Endoscopic treatment of Killian-Jamieson diverticula has been reported.[24] It remains unclear if the efficacy and safety profile of endoscopic therapy parallel those seen with ZD. It should be noted that the recurrent laryngeal nerve often runs in close proximity to the base of a Killian-Jamieson diverticulum.

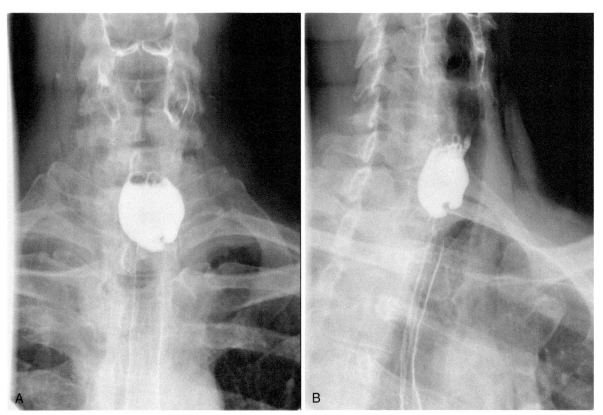

FIG 20.2 Radiographic images of Zenker's diverticulum. **A,** Frontal view; **B,** Lateral view.

THERAPEUTIC OPTIONS

For decades, the treatment of ZD entailed an open surgical approach through a neck incision with subsequent myotomy of the UES and removal or suspension of the diverticulum.[25] Over the past four decades, alternative incisionless transoral approaches have been developed that utilize both rigid and flexible endoscopy. Most commonly performed by otorhinolaryngologists, rigid endoscopic therapy became popularized after a landmark study published by Dohlman and Mattson in 1960.[26] More recently, an increasing body of literature has demonstrated similar efficacy and safety using a flexible endoscopic approach, performed predominately by surgical endoscopists and gastroenterologists.[27]

Open Surgical Approach

Open surgery resolves symptoms in 90–95% of patients.[25] For the open surgical approach, an external neck incision is made along the anterior border of the sternocleidomastoid muscle, typically on the left side, given the propensity of the pouch to emerge in this location. Frequently, this incision readily exposes the diverticulum. Dissection is performed to achieve adequate visualization of the neck of the diverticulum just below the inferior pharyngeal constrictor and the CP muscle. A myotomy is performed to access the proximal esophagus, thereby allowing treatment using one of three methods: inversion, resection or diverticulopexy. Larger diverticula (> 5 cm) typically require excision with closure of the defect using a linear stapling device. Moderate-sized diverticula can be treated with combined diverticulopexy and CP myotomy, whereas smaller diverticula are more frequently treated with CP myotomy alone. Potential adverse events of open surgery occur in 11% of patients, and include fistula formation, abscess,

hematoma, recurrent laryngeal nerve paralysis, difficulties in phonation, and Horner's syndrome.[25]

Transoral Endoscopic Approaches

There are two types of endoscopic therapies for ZD: rigid and flexible. The common goal of both approaches is to sever the CP muscle (Fig. 20.3). The transoral endoscopic treatment for ZD was developed to mitigate the relatively high frequency (> 10%) of adverse events and mortality associated with the open approach. Although some adverse events are secondary to the frailty of elderly patients who frequently develop a pharyngeal diverticulum, many adverse events (i.e., leaks, fistulae, abscesses, etc.) are surgically related due to dehiscence/disruption of the suture/staple line with an inadvertent breach of the mucosa. Recent data from a meta-analysis and systematic review found that the endoscopic approach resulted in shorter procedure times, earlier diet introduction and lower rates of adverse events when compared to the open surgical approach.[28] However, higher rates of symptom recurrence were noted in patients undergoing endoscopic therapy.

Rigid Endoscopic Approach

The rigid endoscopic approach is performed by passing a rigid (i.e., Weerda) diverticuloscope (Fig. 20.4), followed by dividing the common wall. Methods used to divide the common wall have evolved from electrocautery (known as Dohlman's technique) to CO_2 laser therapy to the now more commonly performed stapling, which cuts the septum and seals without causing tissue damage. Reports have also emerged on the use of ultrasonic scalpels to perform diverticulotomy.[25] These devices use ultrasonic energy to coagulate the septal tissue prior to division. Outcomes

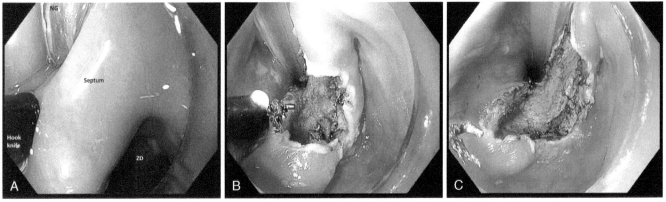

FIG 20.3 Flexible endoscopic cricopharyngeal myotomy for Zenker's diverticulum therapy. **A,** Endoscopic view with short, clear cap attached to endoscope tip. Nasogastric tube is in place and hook knife sheath is seen. **B,** Midpoint of the cricopharyngeal myotomy procedure. **C,** Completion myotomy. (From Law R, Katzka DA, Baron TH: Zenker's diverticulum. *Clin Gastroenterol Hepatol* 12[11]:1773–1782, 2014.)

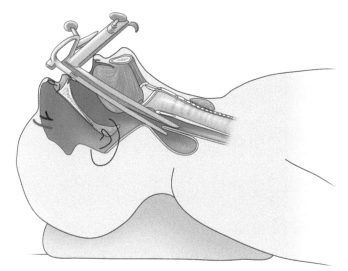

FIG 20.4 Illustration of rigid endoscopic approach for Zenker's therapy. The patient's neck is hyperextended. A rigid diverticuloscope is inserted into the esophagus and Zenker's pouch to expose the septum. (From Law R, Katzka DA, Baron TH: Zenker's diverticulum. *Clin Gastroenterol Hepatol* 12[11]:1773–1782, 2014.)

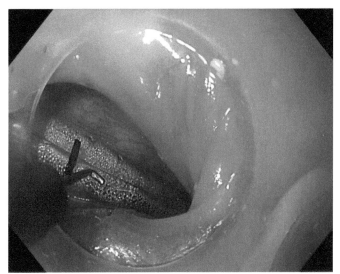

FIG 20.5 Flexible endoscopic Zenker's diverticulotomy using a hook knife (Olympus America, Center Valley, PA).

of rigid endoscopic therapy, regardless of the incising device, demonstrate greater than 90% overall symptom improvement and a decreased rate of adverse events (< 10%) when compared to the open surgical approach. Adverse events specific to the rigid endoscopic approach include sore throat and gingival/mucosal laceration.

Transoral rigid endoscopic therapy cannot be performed in all patients due to inadequate exposure of the diverticulum. Historic data suggests that an open surgical approach is required in 15%–68% of cases when upper teeth protrusion, inadequate jaw opening, or insufficient neck mobility preclude rigid endoscopic therapy.[29,30]

Flexible Endoscopic Approach

Due to the inherent limitations of the open surgical approach and the rigid endoscopic approach, a variety of techniques and methods have been developed to perform flexible endoscopic transoral cricopharyngeal myotomy (Video 20.1). Similar to other presented treatment options, the endoscopic technique aims to reduce cricopharyngeal sphincter pressure by dividing the CP muscle to the level of the diverticular apex.[31] Various dissection methods have been presented, including the use of endoscopic submucosal dissection (ESD) techniques and the creation of a diamond-shaped incision.[32,33] The septum (CP muscle) is commonly divided using needle-knives designed for pancreaticobiliary use and other electrocautery devices designed for ESD, such as a hook knife (Fig. 20.5).[34] Other methods used to divide the septum include monopolar and bipolar forceps, argon plasma coagulation, endoscopic scissor forceps (stag beetle knife, clutch cutter), harmonic scalpels, and stapling devices, the latter two of which are passed alongside a slim, flexible endoscope and not through the standard-diameter flexible endoscope working channel.[35–39] The optimal cutting device remains unclear, as comparative trials in this arena are lacking. The key advantages

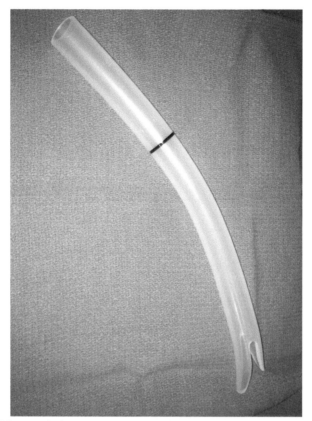

FIG 20.6 Soft diverticuloscope (ZD overtube, ZDO-22-30, Cook Endoscopy, Winston-Salem, NC).

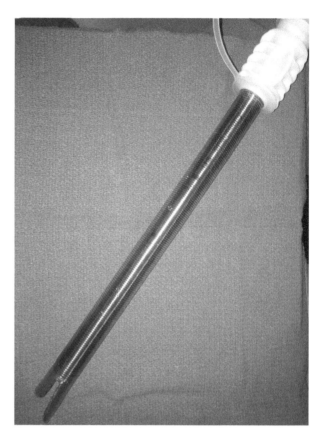

FIG 20.7 Modified esophageal overtube for Zenker's diverticulotomy (Guardus, US Endoscopy, Mentor, OH).

of the flexible endoscopic approach lie in the flexibility and smaller diameter of the gastroscope as compared to the large, rigid scopes, features that are vitally important for treating patients with limited neck extension and/or jaw retraction. Flexible endoscopic intervention may be most suitable for elderly patients with comorbid medical conditions limiting surgical intervention. In rare instances, patient comorbidities limit even flexible endoscopic diverticulotomy. Finally, flexible endoscopic therapy can be performed without the use of general anesthesia. However, the use of anesthesia support is recommended, due to the potential need for acute airway protection. Some authors have noted that an average of 60 minutes is required to perform flexible cricopharyngeal myotomy.[27]

Although not Food and Drug Administration–approved in the United States, a soft diverticuloscope (Cook Medical, Cork, Ireland) can be used to stabilize the septum, improve visualization, and further guide the instrument of incision (Fig. 20.6). This overtube-like device is designed to mimic the rigid diverticuloscope and has duckbill flanges at the distal aspect: one short flange that is seated within the diverticulum, and one longer flange that is placed within the true esophageal lumen. The cricopharyngeal septum is then exposed and stabilized between the flanges. Positioning of a diverticuloscope may be challenging or impossible in patients with small diverticula. Other alternative accessories used to enhance visualization include transparent hoods or caps attached to the tip of the endoscope, which are readily available and used for other endoscopic interventions such as mucosal resection. Various attempts to modify an esophageal overtube or the clear distal attachment cap for the

purpose of Zenker's diverticulotomy have been previously described (Fig. 20.7).[40,41]

When the soft diverticuloscope is not used, we recommend the preprocedural placement of a nasogastric (NG) tube. The NG tube serves two purposes. Firstly, it serves as a guide to continually orient the endoscopist to the true esophageal lumen during the procedure. Secondly, the NG tube provides a method to deliver enteral nutrition in the event of an adverse procedural event such as perforation. Blind passage of an NG tube is not recommended. Our protocol is to pass a small-caliber endoscope transnasally to facilitate guidewire placement into the stomach. The endoscope is then removed, leaving the guidewire in place. A small hole is made in the distal tip of the NG tube using an 18G needle to allow guidewire passage, and the NG tube is passed into the stomach. This technique avoids the need for oral-to-nasal transfer of the guidewire.

Treatment of ZD using a transoral flexible endoscopic approach was first described more than 20 years ago.[42,43] Many case series of flexible endoscopic therapy have since been published, comprising more than 650 patients.[44] Available studies have demonstrated safety and efficacy using various techniques and devices, comparable to the observed outcomes using a rigid transoral approach.[45] A high rate of durable symptom relief (> 90%) with a low rate of endoscopically-evident diverticular recurrence/persistence can be achieved after one to two treatment sessions. The recurrence or persistence of clinical symptoms appears to be less than 20%, though no consensus definition of postprocedural clinical success exists. Logically, clinical success should be based solely on symptom improvement, and not on radiographic or endoscopic findings, as evidence of a refractory septum and/or residual diverticulum does not correlate with symptom persistence or recurrence after intervention.

Based on the available literature, the median adverse event rate following flexible endoscopic therapy is approximately 5% (range 0%–38%). Postprocedural throat pain is nearly uniform and may require narcotic analgesics, usually for up to 72 hours. Bleeding is the most common intraprocedural event. This is generally self-limited, but if persistent can be controlled endoscopically using standard therapies (i.e., electrocautery devices, endoclip placement, epinephrine injection). Uncomplicated subcutaneous emphysema may represent a microperforation; however, this can also be seen due to air tracking within the submucosal plane in the absence of a perforation.[46] We recommend the use of CO_2 for insufflation in all patients undergoing therapy for ZD. Overall, patients should be followed closely, though subcutaneous emphysema in an asymptomatic patient does not mandate surgical intervention. The most dreaded adverse event is perforation, a relatively uncommon adverse event that can occur during flexible endoscopic therapy even when performed by skilled endoscopists. Data compilations have demonstrated a median rate of perforation and/or leak of 4%, regardless of whether or not endoclips are placed at the diverticular apex following myotomy.[47,48] Concern for frank perforation should prompt an oral contrast study using water-soluble contrast to document the presence or absence of extravasation. Alternatively, a computed tomography scan of the neck with oral contrast can be performed.

TRAINING IN FLEXIBLE ENDOSCOPIC CRICOPHARYNGEAL MYOTOMY

Incorporation of the flexible endoscopic approach into clinical practice should only be undertaken by expert therapeutic endoscopists with training in advanced endoscopy and experience in advanced endoscopic techniques, and only after careful consideration of the risks and benefits of the procedure on a patient-to-patient basis. This is especially true because the relative rarity of patients does not allow inexperienced endoscopists to pass the learning curve. Specifically, expertise in the use of various electrocautery devices is necessary when performing Zenker's diverticulotomy. Many of the techniques and devices used during flexible endoscopic cricopharyngeal myotomy overlap with ESD and peroral endoscopic myotomy.[27] Therapeutic endoscopists with advanced training in these procedures may be best equipped to perform transoral flexible endoscopic therapy for ZD.

Preclinical training using an animal model is recommended to gain familiarity with the procedural nuances, such as the unique endoscopic view, gastroscope positioning and stability, and the correct identification of esophageal wall layers during dissection. An animal model using domestic pigs has been previously described in the literature.[49] Pigs are an ideal model for flexible endoscopic cricopharyngeal myotomy using the devices listed previously, due to their normal anatomic pharyngeal pouch that closely resembles a ZD.

CONCLUSIONS

The principles in diagnosis and treatment of a ZD have remained largely unchanged for decades. Rigid transoral endoscopic therapy remains the most often used treatment modality, likely due to historical treatment and referral patterns; however, the continued development of flexible endoscopic treatment allows select therapeutic endoscopists the opportunity to participate in the care of patients with symptomatic ZD. An abundance of available data on the flexible endoscopic approach has demonstrated equivalent efficacy when compared to the traditional open and rigid endoscopic approaches, with an acceptable adverse event profile. Nevertheless, the flexible endoscopic procedure demands considerable endoscopic skill and mastery of neck anatomy, as well as a thorough knowledge of the indications and contraindications of this approach.

KEY REFERENCES

1. Ferreira LE, Simmons DT, Baron TH: Zenker's diverticula: pathophysiology, clinical presentation, and flexible endoscopic management, *Dis Esophagus* 21:1–8, 2008.
2. Baron TH: Role of endoscopy in the management of esophageal diseases, *Minerva Gastroenterol Dietol* 54:415–427, 2008.
4. Watemberg S, Landau O, Avrahami R: Zenker's diverticulum: reappraisal, *Am J Gastroenterol* 91:1494–1498, 1996.
7. van Overbeek JJ: Meditation on the pathogenesis of hypopharyngeal (Zenker's) diverticulum and a report of endoscopic treatment in 545 patients, *Ann Otol Rhinol Laryngol* 103:178–185, 1994.
8. van Overbeek JJ: Pathogenesis and methods of treatment of Zenker's diverticulum, *Ann Otol Rhinol Laryngol* 112:583–593, 2003.
18. Cook IJ, Gabb M, Panagopoulos V, et al: Pharyngeal (Zenker's) diverticulum is a disorder of upper esophageal sphincter opening, *Gastroenterology* 103:1229–1235, 1992.
21. Mantsopoulos K, Psychogios G, Karatzanis A, et al: Clinical relevance and prognostic value of radiographic findings in Zenker's diverticulum, *Eur Arch Otorhinolaryngol* 271:583–588, 2014.
22. Lixin J, Bing H, Zhigang W, et al: Sonographic diagnosis features of Zenker diverticulum, *Eur J Radiol* 80:e13–e19, 2011.
25. Yuan Y, Zhao YF, Hu Y, et al: Surgical treatment of Zenker's diverticulum, *Dig Surg* 30:207–218, 2013.
26. Dohlman G, Mattsson O: The endoscopic operation for hypopharyngeal diverticula: a roentgencinematographic study, *AMA Arch Otolaryngol* 71:744–752, 1960.
27. Katzka DA, Baron TH: Transoral flexible endoscopic therapy of Zenker's diverticulum: is it time for gastroenterologists to stick their necks out?, *Gastrointest Endosc* 77:708–710, 2013.
28. Albers DV, Kondo A, Bernardo WM, et al: Endoscopic versus surgical approach in the treatment of Zenker's diverticulum: systematic review and meta-analysis, *Endosc Int Open* 4:E678–E686, 2016.
32. Kedia P, Fukami N, Kumta NA, et al: A novel method to perform endoscopic myotomy for Zenker's diverticulum using submucosal dissection techniques, *Endoscopy* 46:1119–1121, 2014.
33. Lara LF, Erim T, Pimentel R: Diamond-shaped flexible endoscopic cricopharyngeal myotomy for treatment of Zenker's diverticulum, *Gastrointest Endosc* 82:403, 2015.
34. Halland M, Grooteman KV, Baron TH: Flexible endosopic management of Zenker's diverticulum: characteristics and outcomes of 52 cases at a tertiary referral center, *Dis Esophagus* 29:273–277, 2016.
35. Rieder E, Martinec DV, Dunst CM, et al: Flexible endoscopic Zenkers diverticulotomy with a novel bipolar forceps: a pilot study and comparison with needleknife dissection, *Surg Endosc* 25:3273–3278, 2011.
40. Seaman DL, de la Mora Levy J, Gostout CJ, et al: A new device to simplify flexible endoscopic treatment of Zenker's diverticulum, *Gastrointest Endosc* 67:112–115, 2008.
41. Tang SJ: Flexible endoscopic Zenker's diverticulotomy: approach that involves thinking outside the box (with videos), *Surg Endosc* 28:1355–1359, 2014.
42. Ishioka S, Sakai P, Maluf Filho F, et al: Endoscopic incision of Zenker's diverticula, *Endoscopy* 27:433–437, 1995.
43. Mulder CJ, den Hartog G, Robijn RJ, et al: Flexible endoscopic treatment of Zenker's diverticulum: a new approach, *Endoscopy* 27:438–442, 1995.

44. Law R, Katzka DA, Baron TH: Zenker's diverticulum, *Clin Gastroenterol Hepatol* 12:1773–1782, quiz e111–e112, 2014.

45. Repici A, Pagano N, Fumagalli U, et al: Transoral treatment of Zenker diverticulum: flexible endoscopy versus endoscopic stapling. A retrospective comparison of outcomes, *Dis Esophagus* 24:235–239, 2011.

46. Baron TH, Wong Kee Song LM, Zielinski MD, et al: A comprehensive approach to the management of acute endoscopic perforations (with videos), *Gastrointest Endosc* 76:838–859, 2012.

48. Sakai P: Endoscopic myotomy of Zenker's diverticulum: lessons from 3 decades of experience, *Gastrointest Endosc* 83:774–775, 2016.

49. Seaman DL, de la Mora Levy J, Gostout CJ, et al: An animal training model for endoscopic treatment of Zenker's diverticulum, *Gastrointest Endosc* 65:1050–1053, 2007.

A complete reference list can be found online at ExpertConsult.com

21

Benign Esophageal Strictures

Michael W. Rajala and Michael L. Kochman

INTRODUCTION

In this chapter, we describe the evaluation, treatment, and subsequent long-term management for patients with benign esophageal strictures.

Patients with clinically significant esophageal strictures present with symptoms of dysphagia, typically first to solid foods. Symptoms may then progress in frequency and severity and some patients may develop dysphagia to liquids. Patients often modify their diets to avoid foods that lead to symptoms, and a thorough history is required to parse out the true severity of their symptoms. In the past, the most common etiology for esophageal strictures were peptic causes: however, the widespread use of proton pump inhibitor (PPI) therapy has markedly reduced the incidence of this etiology. Anastomotic and radiation-induced strictures are now the most common encountered overall, but the incidence of eosinophilic esophagitis associated strictures is increasing and being recognized more frequently in all age groups.

INITIAL EVALUATION

The diagnosis of an esophageal stricture, both benign and malignant, commences with a clinical suspicion based on symptoms of esophageal dysphagia and is supported by elucidating a history of a known risk factor (Box 21.1). The maximal inner diameter of an esophageal stricture that will typically result in symptoms of dysphagia is 13 mm. Use of a validated dysphagia score allows for an objective measurement of symptoms and may be used to gauge response to treatment and inform research studies (Table 21.1).

When an esophageal stricture is suspected as the etiology of the dysphagia, the initial evaluation may begin with either a contrast esophagram or an upper endoscopy. In cases of mild, intermittent symptoms of dysphagia to certain foods (dysphagia score of 1 or less), most gastroenterologists will proceed to endoscopy, as this pathway allows for both diagnosis and treatment with one procedure. In the presence of more significant dysphagia to most solid food (dysphagia score of 2 or above) or indeterminate symptoms, a barium swallow with optional 12.7 mm barium tablet should be considered, as it may provide additional information regarding the location, likely severity, and characteristics of the stricture. Knowledge of stricture characteristics is helpful when planning for the therapeutic endoscopic procedure, including appropriate endoscope selection (standard versus pediatric endoscope or bronchoscope) and assessing the potential need for fluoroscopy and adjunctive endoscopic accessories. For example, if the luminal diameter is less than 10 mm, but greater than 6 mm, a pediatric endoscope (5.9 mm) may be more likely to traverse the stricture endoscopically and would be advantageous to have on hand at the start of the procedure. Likewise, for narrower or more complex (long, angulated, or irregular) strictures, fluoroscopy may be required and preprocedure arrangements completed beforehand. An esophagram may also provide information on gross esophageal dysmotility, findings suggestive of achalasia, or the presence of proximal lesions such as esophageal bars or diverticuli that may be difficult to definitively visualize during endoscopy.

Strictures are typically classified as simple or complex. Simple strictures are focal (< 2 cm), straight, and easily traversed by an endoscope. These strictures are typically easily treated with standard dilation techniques.[1] Examples include Schatzki rings (Fig. 21.1), esophageal webs (Fig. 21.2), and some reflux-induced strictures (Fig. 21.3). Complex strictures are defined as angulated, multiple, or longer (> 2 cm), and typically cannot be traversed with a standard endoscope. Examples of typical complex strictures include those that may be the result of surgical anastomosis (Fig. 21.4), radiation therapy (Fig. 21.5), caustic ingestion (Fig. 21.6), ablative therapy, or neoplasm.

TABLE 21.1   Dysphagia Score

Score	Symptom Severity
0	Able to consume normal diet
1	Dysphagia with certain solid foods
2	Able to swallow semi-solid soft foods
3	Able to swallow liquids only
4	Unable to swallow saliva

Adapted from Sharma P, Kozarek R, Practice Parameters Committee of the American College of Gastroenterology: role of esophageal stents in benign and malignant diseases. *Am J Gastroenterol* 105(2):258–273, 2010.

Treatment of esophageal inflammation with a PPI is recommended as inflammation may contribute to symptoms of dysphagia just as much as luminal strictures.[2] The main etiologies of inflammation in the esophagus are reflux, ischemia from prior surgery, caustic ingestion, and radiation-induced injury. If the stricture is due to inflammation from reflux, acid suppression is essential to promote a durable response to dilation and to prevent stricture recurrence. If a patient has persistent dysphagia despite normal upper endoscopy and a trial of PPIs, a dedicated esophagram with a barium tablet should be obtained to rule out a subtle luminal narrowing that may have been missed on endoscopy, and/or esophageal manometry to assess for motility disorders including achalasia. Moreover, extrinsic compression of the esophagus by mediastinal tumors, lymph nodes, or vascular structures may lead to dysphagia and may be more easily diagnosed by contrast esophagram than by upper endoscopy. Symptoms due to extrinsic compression are not typically amenable to long-term remediation by endoscopic dilation and may require endoprosthetic placement.

In some cases, history alone can be strongly suggestive of both the presence and etiology of an esophageal stricture, such as those patients with a prior history of caustic injury, radiation therapy, esophagectomy, or onset of symptoms following endoscopic therapy for Barrett's esophagus or squamous dysplasia. If symptoms arise within the early postoperative period following esophagectomy, anastomotic narrowing may be related to inflammation that will resolve with time or, alternatively, may be due

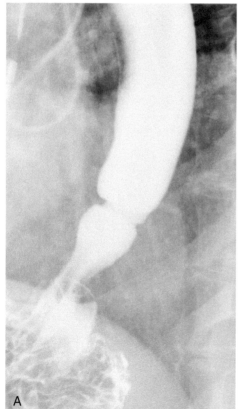

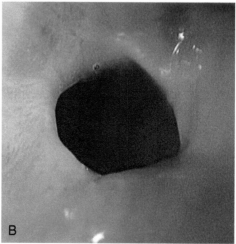

FIG 21.1 **A,** Schatzki ring above hiatal hernia on prone single contrast esophagram. Note short vertical height of ring (seen as smooth, relatively symmetric area of ring-like narrowing) versus greater length of peptic strictures. **B,** Endoscopic appearance of typical Schatzki ring. (**A,** Courtesy of Marc S. Levine, MD.)

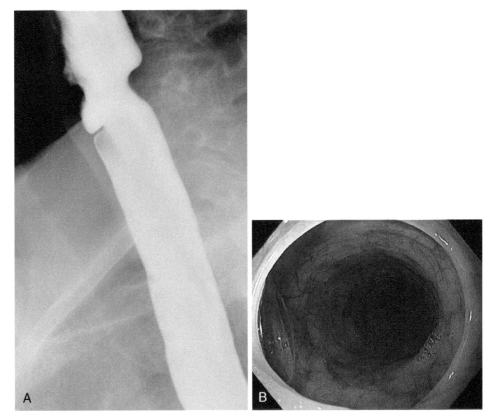

FIG 21.2 **A,** Anterior cervical web on steep oblique (near lateral) view of pharyngoesophageal region and upper esophagus. Note thin, weblike indentation on anterior wall of upper cervical esophagus (cervical webs are typically seen as incomplete anterior structures and are less frequently circumferential). This patient also has a smooth, broad-based indentation on the posterior wall (the side the spine is on) secondary to mild cricopharyngeal dysfunction with incomplete opening of cricopharyngeus. **B,** Endoscopic appearance of esophageal web. Note the thin, smooth contour of the ring. (**A,** Courtesy of Marc S. Levine, MD.)

to early ischemia that would carry significant risk for wound dehiscence if aggressively dilated.

PREPROCEDURE PLANNING

Preparation prior to upper endoscopy with the potential for dilation includes anticoagulation management, obtaining informed consent, sedation planning, selection of the equipment anticipated to be utilized, and determination of the appropriate venue for the procedure.

The American Society for Gastrointestinal Endoscopy (ASGE) recommendations on the management of antithrombotic agents for patients undergoing gastrointestinal (GI) endoscopic procedures rate the risk of bleeding related to dilation of benign esophageal strictures as low.[3] Despite the overall low risk of bleeding, the safety of dilation on anticoagulants remains unknown. Given the potential for bleeding at sites that are relatively difficult to access postdilation, dilation is categorized as a higher risk procedure as far as the use of antithrombotic agents. It is recommended that, when possible, anticoagulants and antiplatelet agents be held for sufficient time to allow for their effects to dissipate prior to dilation.[3]

The 2015 ASGE Standards of Practice committee guideline on the use of prophylactic antibiotics for GI endoscopy does not recommend use of antibiotics prior to esophageal dilation.[4] Patients with vascular anomalies such as a prosthetic heart valve, history of endocarditis, or congenital defect repairs in the absence of prior vascular infection, do not require antibiotics. Despite esophageal dilation having a high rate of transient bacteremia (12% to 22%) in several prospective trials, the degree and duration of the transient bacteremia associated does not differ significantly from that resulting from routine activities such as brushing one's teeth.[4]

For most simple strictures, a standard upper endoscope without fluoroscopy is sufficient for a safe and successful dilation. For those patients with suspected complex esophageal strictures or high dysphagia scores (dysphagia score of 2 or above), having additional equipment available prior to the start of the procedure is recommended. Useful adjunctive equipment includes pediatric endoscope, bronchoscope, fluoroscopy, endoscopic retrograde cholangiopancreatography (ERCP) guidewires, and ERCP catheters for contrast injection. Whereas through-the-scope dilation balloons will not fit through the accessory channel of pediatric endoscopes, standard stainless-steel guidewires with flexible tips used for Savary wire-guided bougie dilation will pass.

In general, endotracheal intubation is not necessary prior to esophageal dilation. However, in the case of complete obstruction with a history raising the possibility of retained food or fluid in

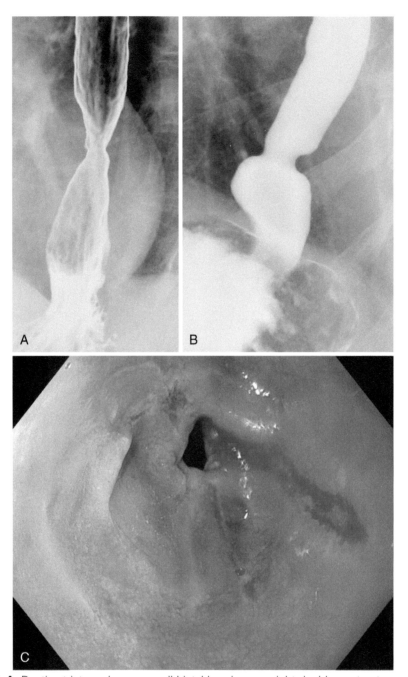

FIG 21.3 **A,** Peptic stricture above a small hiatal hernia on upright double contrast esophagram. Note relatively long segment of narrowing that has smooth, tapered proximal and distal margins, the classic radiographic findings of a peptic stricture. **B,** Short peptic stricture in distal esophagus above hiatal hernia on prone single contrast esophagram. Note short segment of smooth, asymmetric narrowing with tapered margins in distal esophagus. **C,** Endoscopic appearance of classic short peptic stricture. Note the presence of active esophagitis. (**A** and **B,** Courtesy of Marc S. Levine, MD.)

the esophagus, endotracheal intubation may be prudent. Most patients with simple strictures can be safely dilated in the ambulatory setting.

RISKS/ADVERSE EVENTS

The overall rate of adverse events of esophageal dilation is estimated to be between 0.1% and 0.4%.[1,5,6] Perforation and bleeding are the most common adverse events with lower incidences for pain, aspiration, and infection.

Risk factors for adverse events related to dilation include the presence of a complex stricture, prior radiation therapy, caustic ingestion, esophageal pseudodiverticulum, and possibly chronic steroid use and surgically altered anatomy.[7] Although there was initially concern for an increased risk for perforation in patients with eosinophilic esophagitis (EoE), more recent data (2010)

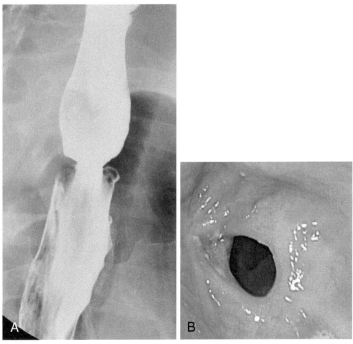

FIG 21.4 A, This patient has had an esophagogastrectomy and gastric pull-through with an end-to-end esophagogastric anastomosis in the upper thorax below the thoracic inlet on upright esophagram. There is a benign anastomotic stricture seen as a short segment of smooth, symmetric narrowing without significant obstruction to flow of barium (though this patient had solid food dysphagia). **B,** Endoscopic appearance of esophagogastric anastomotic stricture. Note the presence of the surgical staple at the anastomosis. (**A,** Courtesy of Marc S. Levine, MD.)

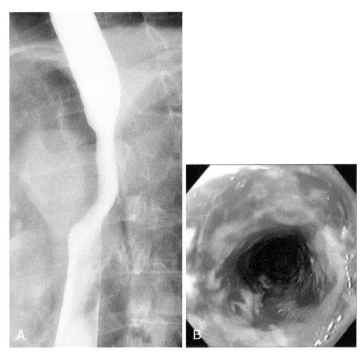

FIG 21.5 A, Radiation stricture in upper thoracic esophagus at level of aortic arch on prone single contrast esophagram. Note smooth contour and tapered margins of stricture, findings characteristic of scarring from radiation. **B,** Endoscopic appearance of radiation stricture with active inflammation. Note the long segment of stenosis that correlates with radiation therapy. (**A,** Courtesy of Marc S. Levine, MD.)

does not appear to support this.[8] Despite the absence of an increased risk of perforation in patients with EoE, the risk of postdilation pain is greater in these patients and the patient and physician should be aware of this.

Likely risk factors for clinically significant bleeding following dilation are radiation induced strictures and complex strictures.

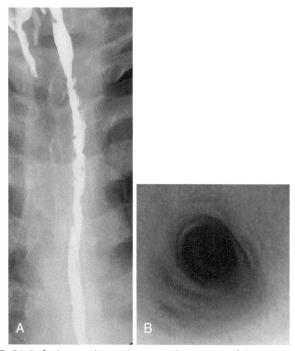

FIG 21.6 A, Lye stricture seen as long area of irregular and marked narrowing in thoracic esophagus on upright single contrast esophagram. Note irregularity of contour, most likely secondary to multiple intramural dissections. **B,** Endoscopic appearance of chronic stricture due to prior lye ingestion. Note the long, significantly narrowed lumen. (**A,** Courtesy of Marc S. Levine, MD.)

Most mucosal tears will stop bleeding spontaneously; however, if significant bleeding requiring transfusion is observed or suspected after the procedure, a repeat endoscopy to evaluate for utility of endoscopic therapy should be considered. Bleeding following dilation of complex strictures that cannot be traversed with an adult endoscope may be more challenging, or even impossible to treat endoscopically due to lack of access to the bleeding site. Pediatric endoscopes may be useful in this setting to assess and treat. Some patients may have a gastrostomy that would make retrograde endoscopy another potential approach for hemostasis.

Although a full discussion of the management of dilation-related esophageal perforation is beyond the scope of this chapter, it is critical to be aware of the signs of, and initial evaluation of, a suspected perforation. Early recognition and steps to avoid gross mediastinal contamination are of paramount importance and vital to reducing the risk of death. In 390 patients with acute esophageal perforation, when comparing the mortality rate of those who received care either within 24 hours or those treated after 24 hours, it was demonstrated that the mortality rate was twice as high (27% vs. 14%) in those treated after 24 hours.[9] Perforations may occur in the cervical, intrathoracic, or subdiaphragmatic regions following dilation. Clinical manifestations of perforation include pain in the neck, ear, chest, or abdomen, odynophagia, dysphagia, fever, tachycardia, and the finding of subcutaneous emphysema. Lack of any of these signs and symptoms does not definitely exclude perforation; clinical suspicion plays an important role to lead to further investigation and early diagnosis (Fig. 21.7).

If there is any question of perforation, the patient should be kept NPO until either the pain subsides or studies are done to exclude perforation and the concern for perforation is resolved. Broad-spectrum antibiotics should be instituted and a nasogastric (NG) tube placed for decompression of the stomach to minimize reflux of contents into any potential esophageal defect. The NG tube may require additional modalities (e.g., fluoroscopy) to ensure that it is intragastric and not exiting through a potential site of perforation. Although a chest x-ray is frequently the initial

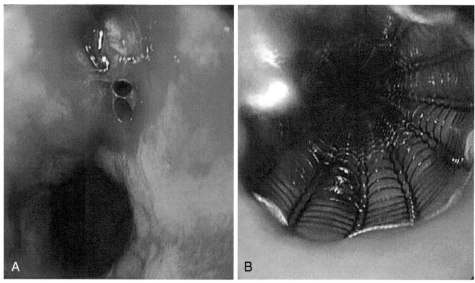

FIG 21.7 A and **B,** Suspected esophageal perforation of a radiation stricture following Savary dilation. Note the air bubbles and appearance of muscle tissue at site of the rent. Due to concern for a leak, a fully covered esophageal stent was deployed during the procedure.

test ordered when there is concern for perforation, extraluminal air alone is not associated with significant morbidity, except in cases of significant pneumothorax. The major concern is leakage of fluid and particulate matter into the mediastinum. Assuming the perforation was not directly visualized during the endoscopy, the initial study should be a water-soluble esophagram to evaluate for extravasation of contrast into the mediastinum. If demonstrating a leak, a computed tomography scan should be considered to evaluate for fluid collections that may require separate drainage; a surgical consultation should be obtained.

Often mature anastomotic strictures or those resulting from radiation are fibrotic, and tissue planes are obliterated such that free uncontained perforations are less common even in the setting of a significant esophageal wall defect. Contained perforations (Fig. 21.8) can often be managed conservatively; surgical teams should be consulted to assist as patients with esophageal perforation may become septic and unstable early in the course.

Attempts at closure of the esophageal defect with hemoclips or an over-the-scope (OTS) clip can be considered and is more likely to be successful when the perforation is within the chest and not at or extending across the gastroesophageal (GE) junction. If the stricture is relatively fibrotic, closure with clips can be challenging due to a lack of flexibility of the esophageal wall. If an OTS clip is used, one should use caution not to compromise the lumen of the esophagus, which would effectively make matters significantly worse. Endoscopic treatment options also include bridging the defect with a fully covered, self-expanding stent. Esophageal stents have been shown to be relatively effective in managing esophageal perforations in several case series and prospective studies[10–12]; however, the Practice Parameters Committee of the American College of Gastroenterology felt the quality of evidence to be low and strength of recommendation for their use weak.[13] If endoscopic closure is attempted, efforts

to close the leak to limit mediastinal contamination should be performed expeditiously. An esophagram to ensure effective diversion around the defect following stent placement should be obtained. Fully covered stents have a relatively high rate of migration and a chest x-ray may be obtained to ensure lack of migration for the first few days or if concern for displacement occurs. Repeat endoscopy to remove the covered stent in 4 to 6 weeks should again be typically followed by an esophagram to ensure remediation of the defect.

INITIAL INSPECTION

Relative contraindications to dilation include recent esophageal perforation and malignant appearing strictures. If, upon initial inspection of an esophageal stricture, an underlying malignancy or infectious etiology is suspected, the lesion should be biopsied prior to aggressive therapeutic intervention. Tissue sampling should also be considered if there are findings consistent with eosinophilic esophagitis, concurrent inflammation, or ischemia. As biopsies are almost always mucosal with very rare exception, biopsy prior to dilation is considered safe.

TYPES OF DILATORS

There are three primary types of dilators used for esophageal dilation: (1) metal filled rubber bougies with either a blunt (Hurst) or tapered tip (Maloney) used without a guidewire, (2) polyvinyl wire-guided bougies, and (3) through-the-scope (TTS) balloon dilators. With the exception of the indication of patient self-dilation, liquid metal filled bougies have been largely supplanted by wire-guided and balloon dilators. Wire-guided bougies range in size from 5 mm to 20 mm (15 Fr to 60 Fr) and dilation balloons are available in a comparable range of sizes (Table 21.2).

Selection of Dilating Devices: Balloons Versus Bougies

Stricture dilation can be achieved with either a rigid, wire-guided bougie or a balloon dilator, either wire-guided or without a wire. These dilation methods differ in their manner of delivery of dilating force to the stricture. Wire-guided bougies are mechanical dilators that exert both longitudinal and radial shear forces. Theoretically the radial dilating force increases within the stricture as the tapered dilator is advanced. Balloon dilators deliver nearly pure radial shear force over the length of the stricture with significantly less longitudinally shear stress.[14,15] Despite mechanistic differences between the two, there has been no data to suggest superiority of either type of dilator in regard to complication rates or significant superiority for symptomatic relief of dysphagia.[1,16–19] In a study comparing the perforation rates

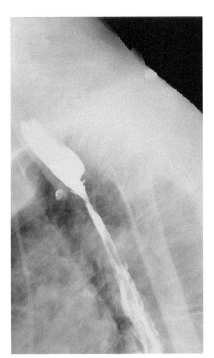

FIG 21.8 Esophagram of a contained esophageal perforation following dilation of a radiation induced stricture. Note the limited extravasation of contrast due to extensive fibrosis.

TABLE 21.2 Esophageal Dilators	
Mercury- or tungsten filled bougies	Maloney (tapered tip) Hurst (blunt tip)
Wire-guided polyvinyl bougies	Savary-Gilliard American Endoscopy Celestin (stepwise diameter increase)
Balloon dilators	Through-the-scope (TTS) Controlled radial expansion (CRE) through-the-scope Over-a-wire fluoroscopic control

between Maloney, balloon and wire-guided bougie dilation of complex esophageal strictures, blind (non–wire-guided) passage of a Maloney dilator was associated with increased risk of perforation when compared to the other dilator types, despite endoscopic evaluation immediately before Maloney dilation in three of the four perforations reported.[6] We therefore advocate the use of wire-guided or balloon dilators for all esophageal strictures, with the notable exception of self-dilation for recurrent esophageal strictures in carefully selected patients.

Selection of a type of dilator should then be based on the comfort level and experience of the operator, although there are clinical scenarios where we advocate preferential use of one type of dilator over the other. The ability to have direct visualization endoscopically and fluoroscopically combined with lack of longitudinal shear stress make balloons preferable for dilation of anastomotic strictures in the immediate postoperative period, as well as for selected caustic and radiation strictures, due to the potential risk for proximal perforation (above the stricture) with the longitudinal force that bougie dilators exert in difficult to dilate strictures. In cases in which the standard endoscope, or pediatric endoscope, cannot pass beyond the stricture, or if visualization beyond the stricture is not clear, we advocate for the use of fluoroscopy with passage of a guidewire into the gastric lumen. Bougies are preferred in some cases as they are more likely to effect dilation to the stated diameter of the dilator in scirrhous strictures. This is demonstrated in cases where increasing balloon diameter may not correlate with the maximal diameter obtained within the stricture despite appropriate pressure registered on the inflation device, which is observed as a "waist" on the balloon when under fluoroscopy with contrast (Fig. 21.9). In addition, balloon dilators may not dilate fully in a 360-degree circumferential manner. Wire-guided dilators may also be easier to use for proximal strictures, cricopharyngeal bars, and webs, as endoscope position above the upper esophageal sphincter during dilation may not be well tolerated. Finally, bougie dilators are reusable and therefore may be more cost-effective in the long run, though local costs for reprocessing are variable.

Fluoroscopy is not needed to safely perform most esophageal dilations as most are simple strictures and may be traversed. In a study of over 300 patients having wire-guided bougienage, fluoroscopy was only required in 8% of cases.[20]

DILATION

One of the major tenets for a safe and successful dilation is both proximal and distal localization and control of the stricture (i.e., the endoscopist should have knowledge of the proximal and distal extents, as well as assurance that the dilator will effectively be able to engage the full length of the stricture). For bougie dilation, a guidewire is first passed through the residual lumen of the stricture distally via the accessory channel of the endoscope under direct endoscopic and/or fluoroscopic visualization. The endoscope is then withdrawn over the guidewire, which is maintained stable in a constant wire position. Standard guidewires have distance markers marking 20 cm increments; the inserted length of guidewire should be confirmed after withdrawal of the endoscope to confirm that the wire was maintained through the stricture in a stable position.

A general guide for safely dilating esophageal strictures with a rigid bougie dilator, known as the rule of threes, dictates that once moderate resistance is felt with passage of the dilator across the stricture, the diameter of the dilator is then increased by no more than two dilators of 1 mm ($\cong$ 3-Fr) increments. Although a common practice, there have not been prospective studies validating that the rule of three reduces the risk of perforation. In fact, a 2017 study retrospectively examined adverse events when they were nonadherent to the rule of three and found no increased risk of perforation or other adverse events.[21] In a study of over 400 patients with single session dilation in which either multiple bougie dilators or a single >45-Fr dilator was used, there was only one perforation.[20] If larger diameters are desired, sequential repeat dilation at intervals ranging from 24 hours to 4 weeks may be efficacious and safe to achieve adequate dilation. It is generally safe to dilate a Schatzki ring directly to 18 mm with a single rigid dilator.

As resistance will not be transmitted to the operator, the rule of three does not apply with balloon dilation. The maximal expansion planned for a session should be reasonable for the suspected etiology and starting size of the stricture. In patients who are undergoing repeat dilations, it is reasonable to dilate to the maximal diameter plus one millimeter from the prior session if safely done in the previous few weeks, even if the diameter has decreased significantly. Once a size is selected, the balloon is typically inflated and held in place for 30 to 60 seconds, although the exact duration and number of dilations has not been validated. Water or contrast, and not air, should be used for inflation, as liquids are less compressible than air.

It is important to assess the response to dilation intraprocedurally. Without evidence of trauma, meaningful durable dilation is unlikely. A mucosal rent is a sign of satisfactory dilation and remediation of a mucosal-based stricture (Fig. 21.10). Visual inspection may also raise awareness of a perforation prompting further evaluation.

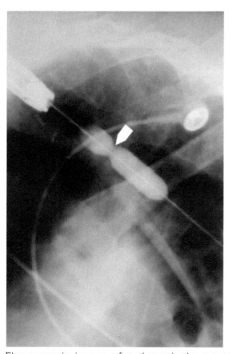

FIG 21.9 Fluoroscopic image of a through the scope balloon dilation of an esophageal stricture with persistent waist *(arrow)*. Note that without fluoroscopy, the postdilation diameter of the stricture may be less than anticipated based on diameter of the controlled radial expansion (CRE) balloon.

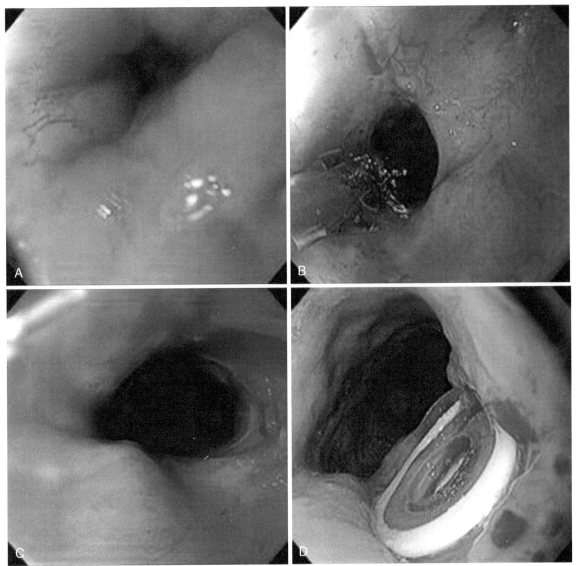

FIG 21.10 Combined radiation and anastomotic stricture in a patient after radiation and laryngectomy with tracheoesophageal voice prosthesis. Note the stricture **A,** before, **B,** during, and **C,** immediately after dilation. Note the presence of a mucosal rent after dilation suggestive of a satisfactory dilation. **D,** Care must be taken to avoid displacement of the prosthesis during endoscopic therapy.

Foreign Body Removal

Protruding surgical staples or visible suture at anastomotic strictures can often be visualized prior to or after successful dilation. It has been suggested that the presence of either may impair stricture remediation by contributing to inflammation and scarring and removal with forceps or endoscopic scissors is speculated to decrease stricture recurrence.[1] In a study by Mendelson et al (2015), removal of staples or sutures at surgical anastomotic strictures trended, but did not reach statistical significance, toward decreasing time to initial patency. There was additionally no effect on the total number of dilations required to achieve clinical response.[22] Despite this common albeit low-risk practice, no studies have conclusively shown removal of surgical staples or sutures to alter the clinical course, and the decision to do so is at the discretion of the endoscopist.

POSTDILATION FOLLOW-UP

The goal of treatment is to reduce or eliminate symptoms of dysphagia to allow sufficient and gratifying oral nutrition. Depending on the etiology, length, and complexity of a stricture, completely ameliorating symptoms is not always possible. However, if a systematic approach is followed, the likelihood of success is increased. The patient should be aware that symptomatic relief is often possible but will require active involvement on their part. This involves following dietary and medication recommendations, understanding the potential for frequent dilations every 1 to 2 weeks initially, with decreasing intervals pending response, and acceptance of an increasing level of risk for complications if standard therapies are ineffective and alternative techniques are employed. The risks of therapeutic interventions should be considered prior to every intervention and weighed against the response already achieved by the patient and the overall goals of therapy.

Whereas some characteristics, including complexity of stricture and etiology, may portend a lower response rate to mechanical dilation, ultimately there is no validated method to accurately a priori predict response to dilation. As such, a trial of mechanical dilation remains the mainstay of initial therapy for the management of benign esophageal strictures. The need for repeat dilation will depend partly on symptomatic response to therapy, as well as anticipated need to return based on suspected etiology of the stricture, diameter of prior dilation, presence of active inflammation, and postdilation appearance. Symptomatic relief is generally not achieved until stricture remediation to at least a diameter of 13 mm. This may not always be the case and routinely pursuing a dilation target size in the face of symptomatic relief reported by the patient is not advised. Conversely, if a patient continues to have significant dysphagia despite successful stricture remediation to a diameter greater than 15 mm, other confounding etiologies, such as dysmotility related to neuromuscular damage from radiation, surgical intervention, prior cerebrovascular accident, or connective tissue disorders, should be considered. A barium esophagram may be informative in theses instances, often in conjunction with a speech pathology evaluation.

Presence of inflammation will hinder, if not prevent, successful remediation of an esophageal stricture. Adequate acid suppression is therefore critical in successful remediation of a stricture. In a study by Patterson et al (1983) prior to the widespread use of PPI therapy, 43% of patients with benign strictures responded to only one session of dilation.[23] Now with effective acid suppression, only 30% of patients with peptic strictures will require repeat dilations in 1 year, most commonly in patients with hiatal hernias or persistent symptomatic heartburn following dilation.[24] In a study of 140 patients (57% postsurgical, 26% peptic, 9% caustic, 8% other), adequate response to mechanical dilation to a diameter of 14 mm was achieved in 94% of patients. The authors found that peptic strictures needed one to three dilation sessions, whereas patients with postsurgical or caustic strictures required more dilations, with a maximum of five sessions in 95% of patients.[25] In this study, only 25% to 30% of patients with simple strictures required any repeat dilation.

If a simple stricture, such as a Schatzki ring, web, or peptic stricture, is dilated to a diameter expected to relieve symptoms of dysphagia, it is then reasonable to have the patient return if, or when, symptoms of dysphagia recur. If they have recurrent symptoms within a short period of time (< 6 months), compliance with a PPI should be discussed prior to repeat endoscopy.

If the underlying mechanism of injury resulted from deep ulceration or chronic inflammation, such as caustic or radiation injury, it should be anticipated that it will require multiple dilation sessions and possibly adjunctive therapy in order to achieve adequate clinical response.[13,22] Rana et al (2015) evaluated the relationship between wall thickness, depth of involvement, and the need for multiple dilations using endoscopic ultrasound.[26] They demonstrated that the depth of involvement, specifically deeper lesions involving the muscularis propria, and not the thickness of the esophageal wall, predicted a need for more dilation sessions.[26] This is congruent with data that caustic and radiation-induced strictures, which may involve the submucosa or in some instances be transmural, require more sessions. Although of interest, the use of endoscopic ultrasound for evaluation of benign esophageal strictures is not currently recommended as it does not change standard management, specifically,

a trial of serial mechanical dilation. However, knowing the likely inciting injury may have caused deeper injury (i.e., caustic, radiation therapy) can be useful for early patient discussions regarding the likely need for repeated dilation and for tempering expectations as to the degree at which resolution of symptoms will occur. Anastomotic strictures following surgery for esophageal or head and neck cancer are also typically more difficult to remediate and will often require multiple dilations for sustained clinical response.[25,27–29] Strictures related to cap-assisted endoscopic mucosal resection are more likely to form with an increasing percentage of circumferential treatment area. Fortunately, these strictures often respond to one treatment with a dilator.[30]

REFRACTORY OR RECURRENT STRICTURES

It can often take several sessions of dilation before a satisfactory long-term response is seen. Definitions for both refractory and recurrent strictures have been developed: a refractory esophageal stricture is defined as a stricture that could not be successfully remediated to a diameter of 14 mm over five sessions at 2-week intervals. A recurrent stricture is a stricture that does not maintain a satisfactory luminal diameter for 4 weeks once the target diameter of 14 mm has been achieved.[31] Exceptions to either of these definitions are patients with inflammatory strictures or underlying neuromuscular dysfunction as a result of surgery or radiation. Inflammatory strictures are not expected to respond significantly to dilation until the underlying inflammation has been treated. Furthermore, patients with underlying neuromuscular dysfunction can have continued dysphagia despite achieving a luminal diameter of greater than 14 mm. In these patients, it is reasonable to remediate the stricture to 14 mm and evaluate for clinical response. If symptoms of dysphagia persist, motility studies could be considered; however, further dilation to greater luminal diameters would likely have minimal clinical response coupled with an increased risk of complication. Other considerations for continued dysphagia include poor mastication of food due to neuromuscular dysfunction or ill-fitting dentures related to accompanying weight loss.

When complete resolution of dysphagia is not possible through stricture remediation, a consultation with a speech pathologist coupled with a combination of a modified diet and deliberate chewing will often allow the patient to maintain normal daily and social function without succumbing to complications of additional dilation, endoprosthetic, or surgical intervention. There should be frequent communication with the patient regarding symptomatic improvement and the goals of therapy, especially in the setting of multiple comorbidities.

ADJUNCTIVE THERAPIES

Once a stricture has been deemed to be either refractory or recurrent, successful remediation, if obtainable, will typically require adjunctive techniques. This section includes intralesional steroid injection, incisional therapy, and transient placement of an endoprosthetic.

Intralesional Steroid Injection

Intralesional steroid injection is thought to reduce remodeling and fibrosis following mechanical dilation to prevent or reduce stricture recurrence. Literature supporting the efficacy of steroid injection with concurrent dilation for refractory or recurrent strictures is not definitive with variable results reported. A prospective, randomized, double-blind, placebo-controlled trial evaluated the effect of intralesional steroid injection followed by balloon dilation of peptic strictures and showed that 2 out of 15 patients treated with steroids compared with 9 out of 15 patients with sham therapy required repeat dilation in one year.[32] The efficacy of intralesional steroid injection has been more variable for other types of benign esophageal strictures. For example, delayed radiation-induced strictures are less likely to respond to steroid injection because these strictures are due to extensive fibrosis.[33]

A multicenter, double-blind trial tested whether untreated cervical anastomotic strictures following esophagectomy were more effectively treated with intralesional steroid injection combined with bougie dilation to 16 mm than placebo with dilation. In this study, there was no statistical difference in the dysphagia-free interval up to 6 months, complications or quality of life. Although this study saw no reduction in repeat dilations or prolongation of dysphagia-free intervals, it should be noted that these were treatment naïve patients and not in patients with refractory strictures for which adjunctive steroid injection is normally considered.[34] Conversely, benefits were seen in a nonrandomized study of 19 patients with refractory anastomotic strictures following esophagectomy with a significant decrease in the periodic dilation index following steroid injection.[35] A positive benefit was also seen in a retrospective study of 30 patients with subtotal esophagectomy complicated by an anastomotic stricture who were either treated with intralesional steroid injection and endoscopic balloon dilation (10 patients) or balloon dilation alone (20 patients). The patients in the steroid group required less repeat endoscopies with balloon dilation (2.5 [1-6] vs. 4.5 [1-20]) and had a significantly shorter interval between first treatment and resolution of stenosis (58.5 days [0–142 days] vs. 94.5 days [0–518 days]).[36]

In a study of 14 patients with caustic strictures, intralesional steroid injection combined with dilation significantly decreased the interval between dilations as compared with prior dilation regimen alone.[37] In one randomized study of only 14 patients comparing steroid versus saline injection,[38] there was improvement in maximal diameter reached, but not in dysphagia score or frequency of dilation. In another study of 29 patients with caustic strictures, there was again a decrease in the periodic dilation index and associated significant improvement in the dysphagia score.[35]   ·

The dose and steroid used for treatment is also variable in practice. Triamcinolone (Kenalog, Bristol-Myers Squibb Company, Princeton, NJ) is the most commonly used, with four to eight circumferential injections of 0.5 to 1.0 mL/injection for a total dose of 40 to 80 mg. There is also variable practice regarding injection before or after dilation. Injection before dilation allows adequate submucosal delivery with potential for both loss due to compression and for deeper and more extensive tissue dispersion during dilation. Injection after dilation can make injection difficult, with steroid leakage at mucosal tears and reduced visibility due to active oozing, although it does allow for injection within longer complex strictures that are not accessible prior to dilation. It is our preference to inject 4×10 mg from the proximal aspect into the stricture prior to dilation for focal strictures and following dilation for longer strictures.

In summary, the likelihood of response varies depending on the etiology of the stricture. Given the low risk of steroid injection and the increased risks of alternative approaches following failed mechanical dilation, we recommend a trial of intralesional steroid injection combined with dilation for strictures that fail to respond to dilation or those that rapidly return to near predilation diameter. The practice is considered safe and low risk with few reports of adverse events, such as increased Candida esophagitis.[34] Inflammation at the stricture should be managed and reduced prior to considering adjunctive steroid therapy. If after three sessions, there is no significant improvement in the either the response of dilation or frequency of dilations required, it is unlikely to provide any additional benefit and other adjunctive methods should be employed.

Endoscopic Incisional Therapy

Endoscopic incisional therapy is a technique of making 8 to 12 radial incisions of the intraluminal stricture longitudinally oriented to the esophageal lumen. The incised stricture is then either dilated with a bougie or balloon dilator or, in some instances, the tissue between cuts excised off circumferentially with a needle knife. No studies have shown superiority of one approach over the other. The method of incision has been described using a number of tools including endoscopic scissors[39] (Fig. 21.11) and needle knives[40] either with or without an insulated tip.

Evidence best supports incisional therapy in patients with short segment (< 1 cm) strictures due to either refractory Schatzki rings or anastomotic strictures.[41] A study comparing incisional therapy to mechanical dilation as primary therapy for anastomotic strictures in treatment naïve patients was shown to have a similar safety and response to mechanical dilation, although not a superior response rate at 6 months when compared to dilation alone.[42] In another prospective study, 24 patients underwent incisional therapy as primary treatment; at 24 months follow-up, 21 out of 24 patients had no symptoms of dysphagia after having received only one treatment session. Of those that responded, 21 of 22 patients had a stricture less than 1 cm, whereas only one out of three patients with strictures greater than 1 cm responded. No significant bleeding or perforations were reported.[43] In a study of 20 patients with anastomotic strictures who failed repeated bougie dilation, incisional therapy with electrocautery was performed. All the patients with strictures of less than 1 cm were dysphagia free at 1 year (12/20). Most of the remaining patients with longer strictures (1.5 to 5 cm) responded to therapy but required a mean of three additional treatment sessions. There were no immediate or delayed complications.[44] A retrospective study by Muto et al (2012)[45] described the clinical response of the "radial incision and cutting (RIC)" method of incisional therapy for 54 patients with refractory anastomotic esophageal strictures compared with continued management with repeat balloon dilation. Approximately 63% of patients were able to eat solids after 12 months compared with only 20% of patients treated with balloon dilation alone. In another study of nine patients with anastomotic strictures that did not respond to mechanical dilation, needle-knife incision reduced dysphagia symptoms in eight out of nine, with a reduced need for endoscopic dilation during follow-up 90 to 420 days compared with a mean of 13 days prior. No complications occurred.[46]

Although studies have not shown significantly higher complication rates of incisional therapy in expert hands, we recommend that endoscopic incisional therapy be reserved for management of refractory or recurrent strictures that have already failed dilation with adjunct intralesional steroid injection and that it be performed by experienced endoscopists. Strictures less than 1 cm in diameter are most likely to have a positive response to incisional therapy.

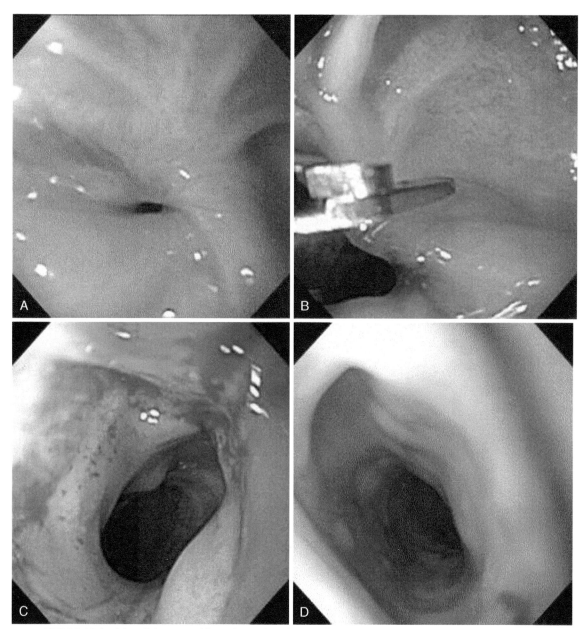

FIG 21.11 Incisional therapy with endoscopic scissors. **A,** A severe esophageal stricture refractory to bougie dilation. The stricture is treated by **B,** cutting the fibrotic stricture with endoscopic scissors, followed by **C,** bougie dilation. **D,** At 4-week follow-up, the appearance was satisfactory with good clinical response. (From Beilstein MC, Kochman ML: Endoscopic incision of a refractory esophageal stricture: novel management with an endoscopic scissors. *Gastrointest Endosc* 61[4]:623–625, 2005.)

Endoprosthetics

Once a benign refractory esophageal stricture fails to respond to dilation with adjunctive steroid injection and/or incisional therapy, endoprosthetic placement should be considered prior to referral to surgery or declaring a failure of remediation. Available stents used for treatment of benign esophageal strictures include self-expanding fully covered metal stents (SEMS), plastic stents (SEPS), and biodegradable stents (BDS). Uncovered metal stents should never be used for benign strictures and, despite reports of partially covered stents being used to prevent migration, we do not recommend their use due to concern that the uncovered portions of the stents will embed in the esophageal wall.

Common adverse events related to stent placement include migration, mediastinal pain, nausea, and vomiting. Nausea may be severe, and patients should be warned prior to placement, with a plan for antiemetics and pain control as needed following placement, though this is less frequent than for patients with malignant esophageal obstruction. Location of the stricture is also important as patients with very proximal strictures can often feel a foreign body sensation in addition to pain following placement. Esophageal stents also increase the risk for aspiration, especially if they cross the GE junction. Long-term complications include potential fistula formation and tissue overgrowth at the ends of the stent, creating partial obstruction and making removal challenging. Finally, symptoms of dysphagia can recur following stent removal, as stent placement often does not treat the underlying etiology of the stricture.

A retrospective study by Repici et al (2016)[47] studied 70 consecutive patients at two tertiary institutions over a 15-year span to evaluate the outcomes of patients with benign esophageal strictures refractory to dilation treated with esophageal endoprosthetics. Patients were treated either with serial dilations or with dilations and esophageal stent placement (SEMS, SEPS, or BDS). Clinical success was defined as no need for additional endoscopic procedures for 6 months after endoprosthetic removal or from the time of the last dilation. In this study, only one out of three patients (approximately 31%) with refractory benign esophageal strictures (RBES) achieved clinical success. It was concluded that endoprosthetics failed to improve clinical response rates and were of limited value.

A European multicenter randomized study of 66 patients with RBES compared biodegradable endoprosthetics with ongoing dilation. There was a longer time to recurrent dysphagia (95 days vs. 30 days), as well as improved quality of life, with placement of an endoprosthetic. Complications of stent placement included two perforations and two fistulas. Hirdes et al (2012) used sequential biodegradable stents in patients with refractory strictures and demonstrated a similar clinical response rate with 25% dysphagia free at 6 months and with major complications occurring in 29%.[48]

Finally, a recent systematic review and meta-analysis by Fuccio et al (2016)[49] combined 18 studies (444 patients) and found a slightly higher rate of response, with stent placement effective in approximately 40% of patients with RBES. There were no differences in response rate, migration rate (28.6%), or adverse events (20.6%) when comparing SEMS, SEPS, and BDS.

Mortality rates associated with treating RBES ranged from 1.7% to 2.8% in studies with 168 and 70 patients, respectively.[50,47] Although relatively high, it was noted by Siersema (2016) that these rates were similar to that of esophagectomy. Additional studies are required to determine which stricture characteristics are most likely to durably respond to dilation therapy. Furthermore, it is anticipated that improvements in endoprosthetics to achieve a balance between sufficient radial force to prevent migration and characteristics to decrease perforation or fistula formation will improve the overall response to therapy.

In summary, treatment of benign esophageal strictures is effective in the majority of patients, but not without risk that increases with adjunctive therapies for those patients with recurrent strictures or those refractory to dilation. Although placement of endoprostheses for benign esophageal strictures can be an effective adjunctive therapy, it is not without significant associated adverse events, and long-term clinical response is questionable. Based on current data, placement of an endoprosthetic should be considered as a last resort for patients with benign refractory strictures who have failed all other therapeutic options. Finally, for those who have strictures that transiently respond to therapy, daily self-dilation may be considered. For all the remaining, surgical referral can be considered.

Self-Dilation

In a select group of patients with stenosis with transient response to dilation requiring frequent dilations to maintain luminal patency, daily esophageal self-dilation with a bougie dilator can be learned. Although this technique requires active patient participation, it can increase a patient's quality of life by decreasing dependence on frequent procedures. We reserve this technique for patients who require frequent dilation to maintain patency over a prolonged period. We typically ensure that the patient is dilated to 15 mm and teach self-bougienage with a 13-mm dilator. This technique is effectively demonstrated on an ASGE video entitled *Esophageal self-dilation: a teaching guide for physicians (DV049).*

Esophageal Luminal Reconstitution

Surgical procedures and radiation to the esophagus may result in complete loss of the esophageal lumen, making standard dilation techniques ineffective due to the inability to pass even guidewires. Techniques for luminal reconstitution of completely obstructing complex radiation induced esophageal strictures have been described by a number of groups.[51-54] We confirm that there is total stenosis as tight complex strictures can usually be endoscopically remediated via a gastrostomy if wire passage via the oropharynx is unsuccessful. We use a combined retrograde endoscopic and anterograde laryngoscopic approach. The combined technique involves the passage of an endoscope through a gastrostomy tube site retrograde up the esophagus to the level of the obstruction. Using wires, catheters, scissors, and endoscopic dissectors, a track is made in the cephalad direction to the oropharynx. Visible transillumination, and at times fluoroscopy, are used to guide passage of a guidewire. Once the guidewire is passed proximally through the stricture, it is then used for anterograde passage of wire guided bougie and balloon dilators (Fig. 21.12). The esophagus is typically dilated to 15 mm and an NG tube bridled in place to maintain patency. Repeated dilation is then performed over the ensuing days and weeks to maintain the newly established tract and to allow it to epithelialize.[52]

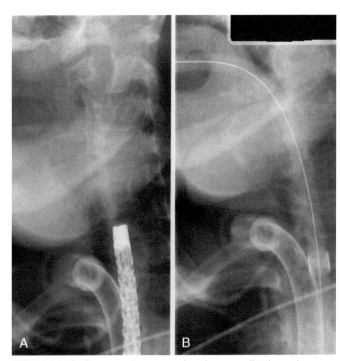

FIG 21.12 A, Retrograde approach using a pediatric endoscope introduced through a dilated PEG tube site and up the esophagus to the stricture. **B,** A wire was advanced through the stricture and out the mouth, followed by the retrograde passage of a wire guided bougie dilator.

SUMMARY

Most esophageal strictures can be effectively and safely managed with esophageal dilation techniques. For strictures that recur at short intervals, repeat dilation with adjunctive therapies such as intralesional steroid injection and incisional therapy can be effective. If these techniques fail to maintain patency, then endoprosthetic placement may be considered, but a refractory stricture is not likely to respond well to intermittent placement and may require nearly continuous indwelling endoprosthetic treatment. It is important to remember the goal of therapy is to improve the patient's quality of life. As patients' risk tolerances differ, the escalation and order of therapy should be individualized.

KEY REFERENCES

1. Lew RJ, Kochman ML: A review of endoscopic methods of esophageal dilation, *J Clin Gastroenterol* 35(2):117–126, 2002.

3. ASGE Standards of Practice Committee, Acosta RD, Abraham NS, et al: The management of antithrombotic agents for patients undergoing GI endoscopy, *Gastrointest Endosc* 83(1):3–16, 2016.

4. ASGE Standards of Practice Committee, Khashab MA, Chithadi KV, et al: Antibiotic prophylaxis for GI endoscopy, *Gastrointest Endosc* 81(1):81–89, 2015.

5. ASGE Standards of Practice Committee, Ben-Menachem T, Decker GA, et al: Adverse events of upper GI endoscopy, *Gastrointest Endosc* 76(4):707–718, 2012.

7. Kochman ML: Minimization of risks of esophageal dilation, *Gastrointest Endosc Clin N Am* 17(1):47–58, vi, 2007.

8. Jacobs JW, Jr, Spechler SJ: A systematic review of the risk of perforation during esophageal dilation for patients with eosinophilic esophagitis, *Dig Dis Sci* 55(6):1512–1515, 2010.

13. Sharma P, Kozarek R, Practice Parameters Committee of American College of Gastroenterology: Role of esophageal stents in benign and malignant diseases, *Am J Gastroenterol* 105(2):258–273, quiz 274, 2010.

17. Shemesh E, Czerniak A: Comparison between Savary-Gilliard and balloon dilatation of benign esophageal strictures, *World J Surg* 14(4):518–521, discussion 521–522, 1990.

18. Saeed ZA, Winchester CB, Ferro PS, et al: Prospective randomized comparison of polyvinyl bougies and through-the-scope balloons for dilation of peptic strictures of the esophagus, *Gastrointest Endosc* 41(3):189–195, 1995.

21. Grooteman KV, Wong Kee Song LM, Vleggaar FP, et al: Non-adherence to the rule of 3 does not increase the risk of adverse events in esophageal dilation, *Gastrointest Endosc* 85(2):332–337.e1, 2017.

22. Mendelson AH, Small AJ, Agarwalla A, et al: Esophageal anastomotic strictures: outcomes of endoscopic dilation, risk of recurrence and refractory stenosis, and effect of foreign body removal, *Clin Gastroenterol* 13(2):263–271.e1, 2015.

30. Lewis JJ, Rubenstein JH, Singal AG, et al: Factors associated with esophageal stricture formation after endoscopic mucosal resection for neoplastic Barrett's esophagus, *Gastrointest Endosc* 74(4):753–760, 2011.

31. Kochman ML, McClave SA, Boyce HW: The refractory and the recurrent esophageal stricture: a definition, *Gastrointest Endosc* 62(3):474–475, 2005.

32. Ramage JI, Jr, Rumalla A, Baron TH, et al: A prospective, randomized, double-blind, placebo-controlled trial of endoscopic steroid injection therapy for recalcitrant esophageal peptic strictures, *Am J Gastroenterol* 100(11):2419–2425, 2005.

34. Hirdes MM, van Hooft JE, Koornstra JJ, et al: Endoscopic corticosteroid injections do not reduce dysphagia after endoscopic dilation therapy in patients with benign esophagogastric anastomotic strictures, *Clin Gastroenterol Hepatol* 11(7):795–801.e1, 2013.

35. Kochhar R, Makharia GK: Usefulness of intralesional triamcinolone in treatment of benign esophageal strictures, *Gastrointest Endosc* 56(6):829–834, 2002.

39. Beilstein MC, Kochman ML: Endoscopic incision of a refractory esophageal stricture: novel management with an endoscopic scissors, *Gastrointest Endosc* 61(4):623–625, 2005.

40. Hagiwara A, Togawa T, Yamasaki J, et al: Endoscopic incision and balloon dilatation for cicatricial anastomotic strictures, *Hepatogastroenterology* 46(26):997–999, 1999.

44. Hordijk ML, Siersema PD, Tilanus HW, Kuipers EJ: Electrocautery therapy for refractory anastomotic strictures of the esophagus, *Gastrointest Endosc* 63(1):157–163, 2006.

46. Simmons DT, Baron TH: Electroincision of refractory esophagogastric anastomotic strictures, *Dis Esophagus* 19(5):410–414, 2006.

47. Repici A, Small AJ, Mendelson A, et al: Natural history and management of refractory benign esophageal strictures, *Gastrointest Endosc* 84(2):222–228, 2016.

49. Fuccio L, Hassan C, Frazzoni L, et al: Clinical outcomes following stent placement in refractory benign esophageal stricture: a systematic review and meta-analysis, *Endoscopy* 48(2):141–148, 2016.

50. Siersema PD: Treatment of refractory benign esophageal strictures: it is all about being "patient", *Gastrointest Endosc* 84(2):229–231, 2016.

52. Lew RJ, Shah JN, Chalian A, et al: Technique of endoscopic retrograde puncture and dilatation of total esophageal stenosis in patients with radiation-induced strictures, *Head Neck* 26(2):179–183, 2004.

53. van Twisk JJ, Brummer RJ, Manni JJ: Retrograde approach to pharyngo-esophageal obstruction, *Gastrointest Endosc* 48(3):296–299, 1998.

A complete reference list can be found online at ExpertConsult.com

22

Ingested Foreign Objects and Food Bolus Impactions

Mark Benson and Patrick R. Pfau

CHAPTER OUTLINE

INTRODUCTION

Gastrointestinal foreign bodies (GIFBs) and food impactions are a common problem encountered by endoscopists, and, next to gastrointestinal bleeding, are the second most common endoscopic emergency encountered. Previous studies have suggested that between 1500 and 2750 deaths occurred in the United States secondary to GIFBs.[1–3] More recently, mortality from GIFBs has been shown to be significantly lower, with no GIFB reported deaths reported in over 850 adults and only one death in approximately 2200 children.[4–10] However, regardless of imprecise morbidity and mortality rates, serious complications and deaths occur as a consequence of foreign body ingestions.[11–13] Thus, because of their frequent occurrence and potential for negative consequences, it is important to understand which patients are in need of treatment, which techniques best treat GIFBs, and how to manage related complications.

Flexible endoscopy has become the treatment of choice for GIFBs and food impactions because it is safe and highly efficacious. Knowledge of the indications for endoscopic treatment, patient preparation, and accessory selection to achieve treatment success is crucial in the management of GIFBs. In addition, the specific techniques to safely and successfully treat food impactions, true ingested foreign bodies, and colorectal foreign bodies will be covered in detail in this review.

NONENDOSCOPIC THERAPIES

A number of medical therapies have been considered as treatment of esophageal foreign bodies and food impactions. The smooth muscle relaxant glucagon is the most widely used and studied drug for the treatment of esophageal foreign bodies. Glucagon, given in doses of 0.5 to 2.0 mg, can produce relaxation of esophageal smooth muscle and lower esophageal sphincter by as much as 60%, with the potential to permit passage of the impacted food or foreign body.[14,15] Success with primary glucagon therapy ranges from 12% to 58% in treating food impactions.[16–18]

However, a small randomized study showed no benefit with the administration of glucagon over placebo.[19] Glucagon used in conjunction with endoscopy has shown that glucagon given at the time of endoscopy promotes clearance of the food bolus.[20] Glucagon may cause nausea, vomiting, and abdominal distention. Glucagon has little effect when a fixed obstruction is present, preventing passage of the foreign body. In a retrospective study, glucagon was ineffective in treating food impactions in patients with eosinophillic esophagitis.[21] Nifedipine and nitroglycerin are not recommended because of side effects and lack of efficacy.

The use of effervescent agents such as carbonated beverages have been described for treating esophageal impactions. These agents are purported to release carbon dioxide gas to distend the lumen and act as a piston to push the object from the esophagus into the stomach.[22] However, the effectiveness of this method is doubtful with perforations and aspirations having been reported associated with the use of gas-forming objects.[23] Similarly, the meat tenderizer papain is not recommended for the treatment of esophageal meat impactions because of risk of complications, including perforation and mediastinitis.[24,25]

Radiologic methods have been described for the treatment of esophageal foreign bodies. Under fluoroscopic guidance, Foley catheters, suction catheters, wire baskets, and magnets have been used to retract objects.[26] The most commonly described device is the Foley catheter; the balloon tip of the catheter is passed distal to the object, inflated, and then the object is withdrawn into the oropharynx. Success of Foley catheter extraction of esophageal foreign bodies under fluoroscopy has been described as more than 90%. However, all radiographic methods suffer from lack of control of the object, particularly at the level of the upper esophageal sphincter and hypopharynx. Complications may include nosebleeds, laryngospasm, aspiration, perforation, and even death.[27] Data on radiologic methods for foreign body removal is primarily limited to the esophagus. Radiographic methods are generally recommended only if flexible endoscopy is not available.

ENDOSCOPIC METHODS

Multiple large series have reported the success rate for endoscopic treatment of GIFBs to be more than 95%, with complication rates of less than 5%.[4,28–33] Timing and indication for the treatment of GIFBs should always be planned with the knowledge that 80% to 90% will spontaneously pass through the GI tract without complication.[4,7] Although conservative management may be effective in many cases of GIFB, it is most appropriate to perform selective endoscopy for treatment based on the location, size, and type of foreign body ingested.[28,34]

Generally, all foreign bodies, including food impactions lodged in the esophagus, require urgent intervention. The risk for an adverse outcome from an esophageal foreign body or food impaction is directly related to how long the object or food dwells in the esophagus.[35] Ideally, no object should be left in the esophagus longer than 24 hours, and preferably the endoscopy should be performed within 12 hours of presentation. In particular, if the patient is in severe distress and unable to handle secretions, the risk for aspiration increases, and endoscopy should be done in the first 6 to 12 hours within presentation. It is not unusual, especially in children and in impaired adults, that there is a significant delay from ingestion to presentation.

Once in the stomach, most ingested objects will pass spontaneously and the risk of complications is much lower, thus making observation acceptable and endoscopic intervention may not be necessary. There are notable exceptions that will almost always require endoscopic intervention due to their increased likelihood of causing a complication or, with some objects, the likelihood that they will not pass from the stomach. Sharp and pointed objects are associated with perforation rates as high as 15% to 35%.[35] Sharp objects should be removed in an urgent fashion due to the risk of complication; removal may not be possible once the object is past the ligament of Treitz. Objects longer than 5 cm and round objects wider than 2 cm may not pass spontaneously and should be removed from the stomach with an endoscope at presentation or if they have not progressed in three to five days.

With the increasing use of device-assisted enteroscopy, case reports have detailed the use of these scopes to retrieve foreign bodies from the small bowel safely and effectively.[36,37] Balloon enteroscopy has been frequently used for removal of entrapped video endoscopy capsules, as well as migrated esophageal and enteric metal stents.[38,39] Furthermore, balloon enteroscopy has been shown to be safe and effective in objects that have been present in the small bowel a number of weeks after the objects were observed and given an opportunity to pass spontaneously.[40] Accessories including baskets, hoods, and forceps have been designed for the balloon enteroscopes to enable foreign body retrieval.

The type of sedation selected to facilitate endoscopy for the management of food impactions and ingested foreign objects should be individualized. Moderate sedation is adequate for the treatment of the majority of food impactions and simple foreign bodies in the adult population. Monitored anesthesia care or general anesthesia assistance may be required for uncooperative patients or patients who have swallowed multiple complex objects. This is due to the prolonged time associated with some cases, the necessity to protect the airway, and the need for repetitive esophageal intubation. The possibility of anesthesia assistance should be available even for cases that are initiated with moderate sedation due to potential failure to not complete the case or

respiratory complications in these cases. Endoscopy for treatment of foreign bodies in the pediatric population is usually performed with the aid of anesthesia and endotracheal intubation.[41]

For management of impactions and ingestions below the level of the laryngopharynx (esophagus, stomach, small intestine), flexible endoscopy is almost always preferred.[42] Rigid esophagoscopy and flexible nasoendoscopes can be used for esophageal foreign bodies, but provide no additional benefit and are often available to only a few endoscopists.[6,43] A comparison of rigid versus flexible endoscopes in the treatment of esophageal foreign bodies found significantly less perforations with flexible endoscopes.[42] Use of rigid endoscopes and laryngoscopes is usually performed by otolaryngologists. Rigid esophagoscopy will almost always require general anesthesia with endotracheal intubation. Laryngoscopes with the aid of a Kelly or McGill forceps can be useful for proximal foreign bodies and small sharp objects in the hypopharynx. An anesthesia video laryngoscope can be used for objects at the hypopharynx and upper esophageal sphincter when gastroenterology and otolaryngology flexible scopes have failed to identify and remove the object.[44]

Availability of and familiarity with multiple endoscopic retrieval devices for the removal of foreign bodies and food impactions is critical (Table 22.1). An endoscopy suite and/or travel cart should be equipped with at least the following to allow successful treatment of a variety of GIFBs: a rat tooth or alligator grasping forceps, polypectomy snare, Dormia basket, and retrieval net[45] (Fig. 22.1). Use of a double channel therapeutic endoscope can allow passage of two retrieval devices simultaneously if needed. Removal of foreign bodies with standard forceps is rarely successful and not recommended. A transparent vacuum cap similar to that used for esophageal banding or endoscopic mucosal resection may be used in challenging food impactions. Overtubes of 45 and 60 cm in length should be available to the endoscopist (Fig. 22.2). An overtube allows protection of the airway, multiple exchanges of the endoscope, and mucosal protection from sharp objects.[46] The longer 60-cm overtube is designed to be advanced into the stomach, thereby enabling the retrieval of sharp and complex objects from the stomach without injuring the lower esophageal sphincter. Due to the size of overtubes and potential trauma upon insertion, their use is limited in the pediatric population and patients with suspected eosinophillic esophagitis. An alternative adjunct for extraction of sharp objects is a latex protection hood, which fits onto the tip of the endoscope[47,48] (Fig. 22.3).

When planning for extraction of complex objects, it may be valuable to go through an ex vivo dry run on a similar object

TABLE 22.1   Equipment for Treatment and Removal of Gastrointestinal Foreign Bodies and Food Impactions

Endoscopes	Overtubes	Accessory Equipment
Flexible endoscope	Standard esophageal overtube	Retrieval net
Rigid endoscope		Grasping forceps
Laryngoscope	45- to 60-cm foreign body overtube	Dormia basket
		Polypectomy snare
		Transparent vacuum cap
		Inflatable balloons
		Latex protector hood
		Kelly or McGill forceps

when considering retrieval devices and extraction technique.[4] Success and speed of retrieval of the foreign body have been shown to be directly related to endoscopist experience.[49] When personnel or facilities are not available to accomplish success endoscopically, consideration should be given to transferring the patient to another more experienced center.

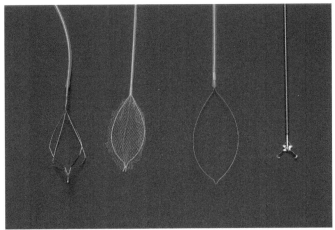

FIG 22.1 Endoscopic accessory and retrieval devices necessary for treatment of food impactions and foreign bodies. (*Left to right:* Basket, retrieval net, snare, rat-tooth forceps).

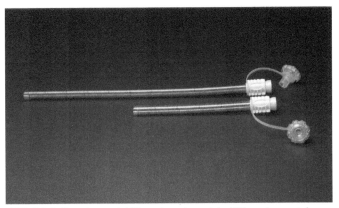

FIG 22.2 Esophageal (45 cm) and gastric (60 cm) overtubes.

Prior to endoscopic therapy, assessment of the patient's airway, ventilatory status, and risk for aspiration are crucial. A neck and chest examination looking for crepitus, erythema, and swelling can suggest a proximal perforation. Lung examination should be performed to detect the presence of aspiration or wheezing. An abdominal examination should be performed to evaluate for signs of perforation or obstruction. If physical exam evidence of aspiration or perforation is present, chest and/or abdominal radiographs should be performed.

SPECIFIC FOREIGN BODIES

Food Impaction

Given that food boluses may pass spontaneously, the need for endoscopic intervention is often based on the persistence of symptoms. Patients with clinical signs of complete or near-complete esophageal obstruction who are unable to swallow their own oropharyngeal secretions should undergo urgent upper endoscopy. The endoscopic intervention should be completed at least within 24 hours of symptom onset and ideally within the first 6 to 12 hours. Performing an endoscopy in the first 6 to 12 hours after symptom onset may allow for endoscopic removal of the food bolus in one piece before it has a chance to soften and break down, making extraction more challenging and time consuming.[50] An increased risk for complications is proportional to the duration of esophageal food impaction.[51–53] Patients who have procedures completed after 24 hours of symptoms onset are more likely to develop esophageal ulcerations and prolonged odynophagia.[54] Furthermore, patients with esophageal impactions for more than 24 hours have more than a 14-fold risk of developing a major complication, such as perforation.[55]

The primary method to endoscopically treat food impaction is the push method, with success rates well over 90% and minimal complication rates.[56] Before the food impaction is pushed into the stomach, an attempt to maneuver the endoscope around the food into the stomach should be made. Generally, if the endoscope can be advanced around the food impaction into the stomach, the food impaction can be then safely pushed with gentle pressure using the tip of the endoscope into the stomach without difficulty. This technique allows assessment of any obstructive esophageal pathology distal to the impacted food. If the endoscope cannot maneuver around the food impaction, gentle pushing pressure can be safely attempted. However, if significant resistance is

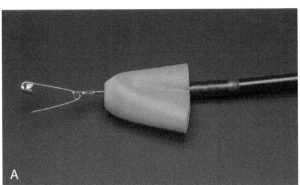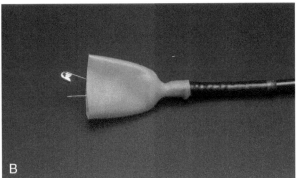

FIG 22.3 **A,** Use of a protector hood wherein the hood is flipped back allowing visualization and grasping of a sharp object. **B,** When the protector hood is pulled through the lower esophageal sphincter, it flips forward covering the sharp object and protecting the mucosa.

encountered, the pushing should not continue as this can lead to a tear and perforation. Particularly in patients with a hiatal hernia, the gastroesophageal junction may have a left turn, thus pushing the food bolus from the right side may allow easier and safer passage of the obstructing bolus into the stomach. Larger boluses of impacted meat can be broken apart with the endoscope or an accessory prior to pushing the smaller pieces into the stomach safely. When the endoscope cannot first pass the food bolus, a method has been described wherein a Savary wire is passed into the stomach and the food is subsequently pushed into the stomach through the use of Savary-Gillard dilators (Cook Medical, Bloomington, IN).[57] This method has been shown to be successful but should be used with caution because of the lack of visualization.

Eosinophilic esophagitis has increasingly been associated with esophageal food impactions and is thought to be the leading cause for patients presenting to emergency departments with impacted food boluses.[58,59] Reports indicate that food impaction in patients with eosinophilic esophagitis can be treated effectively and safely with the push method.[60] However, care should be taken to minimize inducing mucosal tears.[61] Particular care should be taken when using rigid endoscopes if eosinophilic esophagitis is suspected as perforation rates with rigid scopes in this patient population has been reported as high as 20%.[62] If eosinophillic esophagitis is suspected, mucosal biopsies can be obtained after removal of the food bolus (Fig. 22.4). Many patients with eosinophilic esophagitis do not have esophageal biopsies obtained after food bolus removal leading to a delay in treatment and possible underestimation of disease prevalence.[63]

Food impactions that cannot be pushed into the stomach must be dislodged and removed proximally. Proximal removal can be achieved with various endoscopic retrieval devices, including snares, baskets, nets, and alligator, shark, rat-tooth or tripod forceps. When grasping the food bolus with a snare, basket, or forceps, the food should be pulled tight against the endoscope and then the device, scope, and food impaction should be withdrawn simultaneously to limit the risk of releasing the food at the proximal esophageal sphincter or posterior oropharynx.

Use of a net may reduced the risk of a food bolus dislodging in the hypopharynx. In addition, using a retrieval net has been shown to result in fewer passes and shorten overall procedure duration.[64] A dedicated food bolus retrieval net can be useful for removing large pieces of food without the use of an overtube because the food can be satisfactorily secured within the net, thus reducing the risk of aspiration of the ingestate.[65] For food impactions that are difficult to dislodge, a novel technique using a through-the-scope balloon passed distal to the impacted food then inflated and withdrawn proximally has been reported.[65] For lengthy or complex esophageal food impactions, an esophageal overtube should be used as it protects the airway and allows multiple exchanges of the endoscope during retrieval.

Transparent plastic hoods or caps, such as those used to perform variceal band ligation and endoscopic mucosal resection, have been used successfully for the removal of large, tightly impacted meat boluses. With the cap secured to the tip of the endoscope, the device can be used to suction the food into the cap and to withdraw the bolus retrograde with constant suction applied.[66,67] Use of a Dormia basket within a transparent cap has also been used in the extraction of food impactions.[68] Two large Asian studies demonstrated that sharp food impactions, usually fish or chicken bones, are best retrieved with a rat-tooth forceps.[69,70] Ideally, the sharp food should be grasped at one end with the most sharp end trailing as the item is removed to limit the risk of tear or perforation.

More than 75% of patients with food impactions have associated esophageal pathology with strictures being the most common finding.[4,71,72] In addition, approximately half of patients with food bolus impactions have abnormal 24-hour pH studies and/or esophageal manometry. If an esophageal stricture or Schatzki's ring is present after the food bolus is cleared, it can be safely and effectively dilated after the food impaction is removed if circumstances allow. More often, mucosal abrasions, erosions, or erythema exist due to the impacted food for an extended period and the dilation is delayed for 2 to 4 weeks, during which patients should be prescribed proton pump inhibitor therapy. When endoscopic findings such as longitudinal furrows, multiple

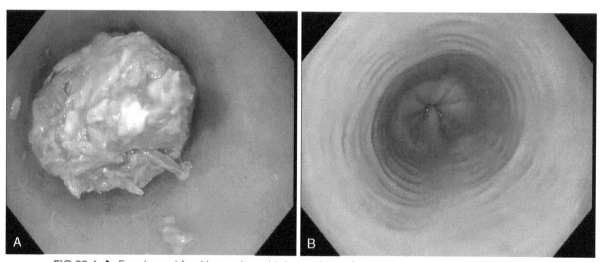

FIG 22.4 A, Esophageal food impaction with large piece of meat that was treated with the push method. **B,** More proximal esophagus in the same patient demonstrating rings. Esophageal mucosa biopsied at same time of treatment of food impaction with biopsies consistent with eosinophillic esophagitis.

rings, and white exudates are present, biopsies should be obtained from throughout the esophagus to evaluate for eosinophilic esophagitis.[73] Lack of appropriate follow-up for patients, particularly those with strictures or rings, has been shown to be a predictor for recurrent food impactions.[74]

True Foreign Bodies

True foreign bodies (nonfood ingestions) can occur from either intentional or unintentional ingestion. Children between the ages of 6 months and 6 years are the most common cohort to intentionally ingest true foreign bodies.[4,75] In adults, true foreign body ingestion is more common in patients who are acutely intoxicated with alcohol, have a psychiatric disorder, developmental delay, seek secondary gain, or are edentulous.[4,76,72] Once ingested, a higher rate of recurrent ingestion is found in males, prisoners, and patients with a psychiatric disorder.[77]

Sharp and Pointed Objects

The ingestion of sharp and pointed objects carries a significant risk of complications, including perforation. Perforation can occur in up to 15% to 35% of patients and accounts for one-third of all perforations from GIFBs.[78]

Sharp and pointed objects retained in the esophagus are thus considered a medical emergency and should be removed within 6 to 12 hours.[79] Objects at the cricoopharyngeus may be best visualized and removed with a laryngoscope. Due to risk of complications, any sharp and pointed object within reach of the endoscope should be removed urgently if this can be done safely. Prior to the removal of sharp objects, Chevalier Jackson's axiom should be remembered; "advancing points puncture, trailing points do not."[80] To accomplish this, the foreign body should be grasped and oriented so that the sharp end trails on withdrawal to reduce the risk of perforation and mucosal laceration upon removal.[80] This sometimes entails pushing the object into the stomach with the endoscope and then orientating the sharp edge to be the trailing point upon withdrawal. For sharp and pointed objects, retrieval is best achieved with grasping forceps such as rat tooth, shark tooth, or alligator forceps, tripod forceps, a polypectomy snare, or biliary stone retrieval basket.[49] Retrieval nets tend to shear in the removal of sharp objects and may compromise visualization.

In some circumstances, use of an overtube should be considered to protect the esophagus and oropharynx from the sharp object. Long, pointed objects in the esophagus and stomach can be grasped and withdrawn into the overtube; the entire assembly, including the sharp object, the endoscope, and the overtube can then be removed in unison. An alternative device to an overtube, for the extraction of sharp objects, is a retractable latex hood attached to the tip of the endoscope. The flexible latex trails the endoscope tip. Thus, as the endoscope is being advanced the hood is pointed proximally. When the endoscope is pulled back through the lower esophageal sphincter, the hood flips over the grasped object and protects the mucosa during withdrawal[47,81] (see Fig. 22.3).

Although associated with an increased risk of perforation, most sharp or pointed objects beyond reach of the endoscope will pass unimpeded and be eliminated through the GI tract without complication. Because of the increased risk of perforation, sharp and pointed objects should be followed by serial daily radiographs to ensure progression (Fig. 22.5). If a sharp or pointed object fails to progress over three days, or if there is evidence of a complication such as abdominal pain, fever, nausea, bleeding,

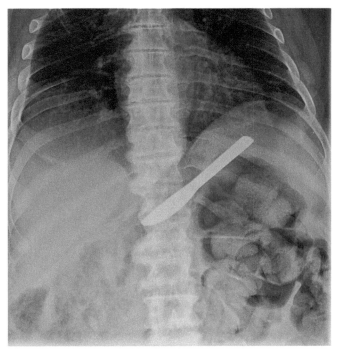

FIG 22.5 Radiograph of large, ingested knife located within the stomach.

or overt signs of perforation, surgical intervention should be considered. Balloon assisted enteroscopy is a viable option when a sharp object has passed the duodenum.[40,82]

Long Objects

Ingested objects longer than 5 cm (2 inches), and especially those longer than 10 cm (4 inches), such as toothbrushes, forks, and spoons, have difficulty passing through the pylorus and duodenal sweep. This can lead to an obstruction or perforation at these locations. Removal is best attempted while the object remains in the stomach, as duodenal removal is more difficult given the smaller diameter and tortuous lumen. The most commonly ingested long objects are pens, pencils, toothbrushes, and eating utensils. Removal of these objects is sometimes challenging and caution to avoid mucosal injury or perforation should be taken. Grasping forceps and polypectomy snares are commonly used to secure and remove long objects. Long objects should be grasped at one end and oriented longitudinally to permit removal (Fig. 22.6). Grasping a long object near the middle will not allow it to be withdrawn safely through the upper gastrointestinal tract sphincters. For extraction of long sharp objects, a 60 cm overtube can be used, which will cross the lower esophageal sphincter when introduced. The object can be grasped with the endoscope and a retrieval device and then brought into the overtube to make it align in a vertical position without causing mucosal injury.

Blunt Objects: Coins, Batteries, and Magnets

Small blunt objects, such as pieces of toys, disc or button batteries, and coins, are the most commonly ingested objects by children younger than 4 years old.[83] Blunt objects in the esophagus should be removed promptly with the use of grasping forceps, snare, retrieval basket, or net. Coins impacted in the esophagus can result in pressure necrosis of the esophageal wall and lead to perforation or fistulization. A coin of any size can become lodged

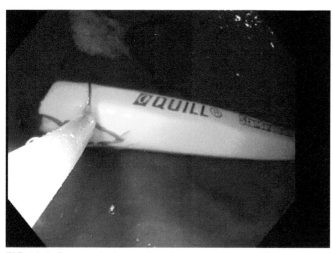

FIG 22.6 Removal of pencil with snare. The pencil is grasped on the very end with the sharp point trailing.

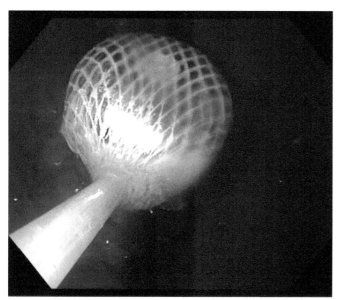

FIG 22.7 Retrieval net used in the removal of a blunt object (lip gloss) that was pushed from the esophagus into the stomach and then removed without difficulty.

in the esophagus of children, but ingested coins, in particular dimes and pennies measuring 17 and 18 mm, will usually pass through the adult esophagus. Coins located in the distal esophagus on imaging are twice as likely to pass spontaneously then coins in the proximal esophagus.[84]

Retrieval nets are the preferred retrieval device as they allow capture and secure removal of coins and most small blunt objects (Fig. 22.7).[49] This allows for additional airway protection as the object is pulled past the oropharynx. Grasping forceps and biliary stone retrieval baskets are also effective but the objects are often slightly less secure. Standard biopsy forceps and snares are not recommended because they fail to secure coins reliably during extraction and can lead to airway compromise. If it is difficult to capture a blunt object in the esophagus, it is generally safe to gently push the object into the stomach, where there is more room to negotiate. If there is concern of airway compromise, particularly for removal of coins in the esophagus, endotracheal

intubation should be considered. An overtube can also be used for airway protection.

Once a small blunt object enters the stomach, conservative outpatient management is appropriate for many patients.[85] Exceptions to this include patients with surgically altered digestive tract anatomy, those with symptoms, and those who have ingested large blunt objects. In adults, the pylorus will allow passage of most blunt objects up to 25 mm in diameter, which includes all coins except half-dollars (30 mm) and silver dollars (38 mm). Otherwise, once in the stomach, a regular diet is appropriate, with radiographic monitoring every 1 to 2 weeks to confirm progression or elimination. If after 3 to 4 weeks a blunt object has not passed, endoscopic removal should be performed.[86]

The incidence of small disc battery ingestion is increasing due to the increased use of lithium button batteries in electronics.[87] Disc batteries are of special concern because they may contain an alkaline solution that can rapidly cause a liquefaction necrosis of esophageal tissue resulting in perforation or fistula formation. The disc batteries can also lead to additional mucosal damage due to the local electrical current. Disc batteries are present in many small toys, watches, calculators, and other electronic devices that are accessible to young children. Disc battery ingestion occurs most commonly in younger children, with approximately 10% becoming symptomatic.[88] Therefore any clinical suspicion of a disc battery in the esophagus should prompt emergent endoscopy. Grasping forceps and snares are generally ineffective for disc battery removal, but use of a retrieval net permits successful removal in almost 100% of cases.[89] Protection of the airway with an overtube or, in pediatric patients, endotracheal intubation, is crucial in retrieval of disc batteries. Once in the stomach or small intestine, disc batteries rarely cause clinical problems and can be observed radiographically. Once in the duodenum, 85% will pass through the GI tract within 72 hours.[90] Batteries located beyond the esophagus require endoscopy if the patient develops symptoms or the battery remains in the stomach for 48 hours on repeat radiograph.[90]

Cylindrical batteries appear to cause symptoms less frequently with no reports of major life-threatening injuries and only approximately 20% having some minor symptoms after ingestion.[90] Due to their size, cylindrical batteries do not have the same risks of electrical discharge compared to disc batteries. Cylindrical batteries should be removed from the esophagus within 24 hours if possible. If in the stomach, batteries larger than 20 mm or those that have not progressed in 48 hours should be removed endoscopically (Fig. 22.8).

Small coupling magnets have become popular as children's toys. Ingested magnets within the reach of the endoscope should also be removed on an urgent basis. Although a single magnet will rarely be a cause of symptoms, concern exists if multiple magnets are ingested or if magnets were ingested with other metal objects. This can result in magnetic attraction between the objects and coupling between interposed loops of bowel with subsequent pressure necrosis, fistula formation, and bowel perforation.[91,92] Removal should be performed urgently when the magnets are more likely to be within reach of a standard endoscope; this can be achieved with grasping forceps, retrieval net, or basket. Magnetic attraction to metallic retrieval devices may ease the task of removal.[93,94] If multiple magnets have been ingested, a postprocedure x-ray can be performed to ensure that all have been retrieved. If more than one magnet is not within endoscopic reach, surgical removal versus enteroscopy should be performed.

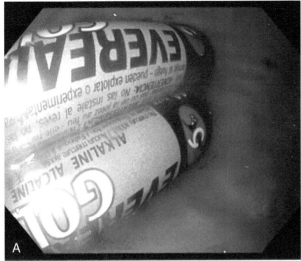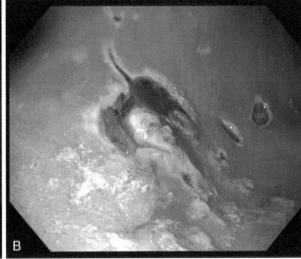

FIG 22.8 A, Cylindrical batteries in stomach that did not pass after 48 hours of observation. Removed with snare with endotracheal intubation. **B,** Stomach ulceration caused by cylindrical batteries.

Narcotic Packets

Narcotic packets are often filled with cocaine, amphetamines, or heroin and endoscopic removal is contraindicated because of the high risk of package perforation with resultant drug overdose, which can be fatal.[51] Observation on a clear liquid diet is recommended with serial radiographs. Operative intervention is indicated when bowel obstruction, failure to progress, or drug leakage/toxicity is suspected. A large study indicated that up to 45% may require surgery with gastrostomy, enterotomy, or colotomy performed based on the location of the packages.[95]

Colorectal Foreign Bodies

Ingested objects uncommonly become lodged in the colorectum. More commonly, colorectal foreign bodies are inserted into the rectum intentionally or unintentionally. Males are much more likely than females to present with a rectal foreign body, with a ratio of 37:1.[96] The initial assessment should include an evaluation for signs of peritonitis and need for a laparotomy. Radiographs should be obtained prior to attempting removal of colorectal foreign bodies for better visualization of the location, orientation, and configuration of the object. To avoid health care provider injury, attempts at manual removal or digital rectal examination should be deferred until the presence of a sharp or pointed object has been excluded.

Most objects (76%) can be removed nonsurgically.[96] Manual digital extraction may be successful for the removal of small, blunt objects in the distal rectum that are palpable on rectal examination.

Nonpalpable and sharp or pointed objects should be removed under direct visualization with the use of a rigid proctoscope or flexible sigmoidoscope.[97] Standard retrieval devices can be used as described earlier for the upper digestive tract. The use of obstetric tools has also been reported.[98] A latex hood or overtube can be particularly useful in removing long, sharp, pointed objects to protect the rectal mucosa from laceration and to overcome the tendency of the anal sphincter to contract on attempted removal of objects. Although conscious sedation will often facilitate removal, general anesthesia can allow maximum dilation of the anal sphincter to help remove larger and more complex objects.[99]

Operative intervention is indicated for any suspected complications secondary to a rectal or colon foreign body, including perforation, abscess, and obstruction, and for failure of endoscopic removal. Patients with objects retained within the sigmoid colon are more than twofold more likely to require an operative intervention compared to those with objects within the rectum.[100] Furthermore, complications are more common when the object is proximal to the rectum.[100]

PROCEDURE-RELATED COMPLICATIONS

Although the reported complication rate associated with endoscopic removal of gastrointestinal foreign bodies and food impactions is low (0% to 1.8%), it is thought to be much higher in practice (more than 5%).[4,8,30,31,56,101] Perforation is the most feared complication, although aspiration and sedation-related cardiopulmonary complications may also occur. Factors that increase the risk for complications include removal of sharp and pointed objects, an uncooperative patient, multiple and/or deliberate ingestions, and extended duration of time from food impaction or foreign body ingestion to endoscopy.[11]

KEY REFERENCES

4. Webb WA: Management of foreign bodies of the upper gastrointestinal tract: update, *Gastrointest Endosc* 41:39–51, 1995.

11. Tokar B, Cevik AA, Ilhan H: Ingested gastrointestinal foreign bodies: Predisposing factors for complications in children having surgical or endoscopic removal, *Pediatr Surg Int* 23:135–139, 2007.

21. Thimmapuram J, Oosterveen S, Grim R: Use of glucagon in relieving food bolus impaction in the era of eosinophillic esophageal infiltration, *Dysphagia* 28:212–216, 2013.

29. Mosca S: Management and endoscopic techniques in cases of ingestion of foreign bodies, *Endoscopy* 32:232–233, 2000.

30. Wong KKY, Fang CX, Tam PHK: Selective upper endoscopy for foreign body ingestion in children: an evaluation of management protocol after 282 cases, *J Pediatr Surg* 41:2016–2018, 2006.

31. Katsinelos P, Kountouras J, Paroutoglou G, et al: Endoscopic techniques and management of foreign body ingestion and food bolus impaction in the upper gastrointestinal tract: a retrospective analysis of 139 cases, *J Clin Gastroenterol* 40:784–789, 2006.

32. Conway WC, Sugawa C, Ono H, et al: Upper GI foreign body: an adult urban emergency hospital experience, *Surg Endosc* 21:455–460, 2007.

34. O'Sullivan ST, McGreal GT, Reardon CM, et al: Selective endoscopy in management of ingested foreign bodies of the upper gastrointestinal tract: is it safe?, *Int J Clin Pract* 51:289–292, 1997.

40. Chen WC, Bartel M, Kroner T, et al: Double ballon enteroscopy is a safe and effective procedure in removing entrapped foreign objects in the small bowel for up to 3 months, *J Laparoendosc Adv Surg Tech A* 25: 392–395, 2015.

43. Weissberg D, Refaely Y: Foreign bodies in the esophagus, *Ann Thorac Surg* 84:1854–1857, 2007.

49. Faigel DO, Stotland BR, Kochman ML, et al: Device choice and experience level in endoscopic foreign object retrieval: an in vivo study, *Gastrointest Endosc* 45:490–492, 1997.

50. Smith MT, Wong RK: Esophageal foreign bodies: types and techniques for removal, *Curr Treat Options Gastroenterol* 9:75–84, 2006.

51. ASGE Standards of Practice Committee, Ikenberry SO, Jue TL, et al: Management of ingested foreign bodies and food impactions, *Gastrointest Endosc* 73:1085–1091, 2011.

52. Smith MT, Wong RKH: Foreign bodies, *Gastrointest Endosc Clin N Am* 17:361–382, 2007.

54. Wu WT, Chiu CT, Kuo CJ, et al: Endoscopic management of suspected esophageal foreign body in adults, *Dis Esophagus* 24(3):131–137, 2011.

56. Vicari JJ, Johanson JF, Frakes JT: Outcomes of acute esophageal food impaction: success of the push technique, *Gastrointest Endosc* 53: 178–181, 2001.

58. Kerlin P, Jones D, Remedios M, et al: Prevalence of eosinophilic esophagitis in adults with food bolus obstruction of the esophagus, *J Clin Gastroenterol* 41:356–361, 2007.

63. Sperry SL, Crockett SD, Miller CB, et al: Esophageal foreign-body impactions: epidemiology, time trends, and the impact of the increasing prevalence of eosinophilic esophagitis, *Gastrointest Endosc* 74(5): 985–991, 2011.

72. Sugawa C, Ono J, Taleb M, Lucas CE: Endoscopic management of foreign bodies in the upper gastrointestinal tract: a review, *World J Gastrointest Endosc* 6:475–481, 2014.

74. Prasad GA, Reddy JG, Boyd-Enders FT, et al: Predictors of recurrent esophageal food impaction: a case control study, *J Clin Gastroenterol* 42:771–775, 2008.

77. Grimes IC, Spier BJ, Swize LR, et al: Predictors of recurrent ingestion of gastrointestinal foreign bodies, *Can J Gastroenterol* 27:e1–e4, 2013.

78. Chen T, Wu HF, Shi Q, et al: Endoscopic management of impacted esophageal foreign bodies, *Dis Esophagus* 26:799–806, 2013.

84. Waltzman ML, Baskin M, Wypij D, et al: A randomized clinical trial of the management of esophageal coins in children, *Pediatrics* 116: 614–619, 2005.

91. Alzakem AM, Soundappan SSV, Jefferies H, et al: Ingested magnets and gastrointestinal complications, *J Pediatr Child Health* 40:497–498, 2007.

96. Kurer MA, Davey C, Khan S, Chintapatla S: Colorectal foreign bodies: a systematic review, *Colorectal Dis* 12(9):851–861, 2010.

100. Lake JP, Essani R, Petrone P, et al: Management of retained colorectal foreign bodies: predictors of operative intervention, *Dis Colon Rectum* 47(10):1694–1698, 2004.

A complete reference list can be found online at ExpertConsult .com

23

Eosinophilic Esophagitis

Leila Kia and Ikuo Hirano

INTRODUCTION

Eosinophilic esophagitis (EoE) is a chronic, immune-mediated clinicopathological disease characterized by esophageal symptoms, eosinophilic inflammation localized to the esophagus, and the absence of other causes of eosinophilia.[1,2] This evolving definition, devised after multiple iterations by a consensus panel, excludes endoscopic findings as part of the diagnostic criteria. Nonetheless, such findings are often the first clue to the gastroenterologist that a patient may have EoE. Moreover, endoscopic features provide important clinical information regarding the underlying phenotype of the disease, which can have both prognostic and therapeutic implications. A comprehensive assessment of endoscopic features, alongside clinical and histopathological data, can therefore provide a more comprehensive assessment of the patient's overall disease activity and severity, thereby informing management decisions.

LIMITATIONS TO ENDOSCOPIC ASSESSMENT OF EOE

The relevance of endoscopic features in EoE has historically been challenged by concerns of inadequacies, including reports of limited sensitivity and interobserver agreement. Moreover, early retrospective studies reported a normal endoscopic appearance in approximately one-third of children with EoE.[2] Studies evaluating interobserver agreement among gastroenterologists who were shown still images demonstrated poor to fair agreement, which was independent of practice setting, patient volume, or use of narrow-band imaging, suggesting that perhaps we are not all "seeing the same things."[3,4] A meta-analysis reviewing 80 original articles and 20 abstracts found a pooled prevalence of 44% for rings, 21% for strictures, 9% for narrow-caliber esophagus, 48% for linear furrows, 27% for white plaques, and 41% for edema.[5] The diagnostic sensitivity for these features ranged from 15% to 48%. Interestingly, when only prospective studies were included, one or more endoscopic abnormalities were found

in 93% of patients. These findings highlight important inadequacies in reporting endoscopic features.

IMPORTANCE OF STANDARDIZED NOMENCLATURE AND DEFINITIONS

The primary endoscopic features reported in EoE include longitudinal furrows (vertical lines), white exudates (plaques), rings (trachealization), strictures, edema (mucosal pallor or decreased vascularity), narrow-caliber esophagus, and "crêpe-paper" mucosa[2,5–7] (Table 23.1). Variable terminology has been used to describe these findings and this has led to inconsistency in reporting features attributable to EoE. Rings have been referred to as *trachealization*, *corrugation*, and *felinization*. Although some use these terms interchangeably, there are differences among these descriptors. Felinization traditionally refers to transient plications in the esophageal mucosa that occur during short-duration, axial shortening events such as retching, belching, or swallows. The "ripples" are often visualized by radiologists during barium swallows and completely efface spontaneously within seconds or with luminal distension with air. Such transient plications should not be confused with the fixed rings seen in EoE, which do not efface and are accentuated with air insufflation (Videos 23.1 and 23.2).[4] Appreciating this distinction between transient and fixed rings is important in establishing consistency among endoscopists. Multiple fixed rings of the esophagus have been confused with congenital esophageal stenosis. However, most cases of congenital esophageal stenosis do not produce a trachealization pattern, but instead a single fixed stenosis of the esophageal body.

Endoscopically characterized inflammatory features of EoE include edema, furrows, and exudates (Video 23.3). Edema is another term that has shown variability in reporting across endoscopists, in part because visualization of loss of vascular findings is highly dependent upon the contractile state of the esophagus and degree of luminal distension. Moreover, it may be neglected during routine reporting of esophagogastroduodenoscopy (EGD)

TABLE 23.1   Primary Endoscopic Features Reported in Eosinophilic Esophagitis

Endoscopic Feature	Comment
Edema	Mucosal pallor or decreased vascularity. Best assessed either in real-time or with video assessment as vascular markings are diminished during esophageal contractions.
Rings	Often confused with feline esophagus (transient plications). Best appreciated when esophagus is fully insufflated.
Exudates	Often confused with *Candida* esophagitis infection. Often track along furrows.
Furrows	Longitudinal "track marks" or lines along the esophagus. Blood from biopsies can fill the indentations and aid in detection.
Strictures	Can be focal or diffuse. Distal strictures best appreciated on retroflexion. Precise determination of diameter is difficult.
Crêpe-paper esophagus	Fragile mucosa with disruption or sloughing from passage of an endoscope.
Narrow-caliber esophagus	Difficult to appreciate with endoscopy. Better defined by barium esophagram or functional luminal imaging probe.
"Tug" sign	Subjective resistance or "stiffness" appreciated when taking biopsies (suggests underlying fibrosis).

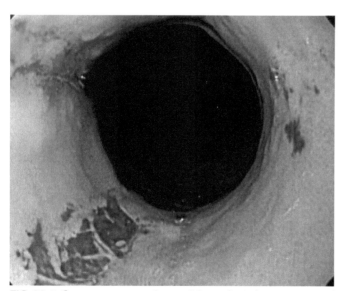

FIG 23.1 Crepe paper esophagus (also referred to as mucosal fragility or laceration upon passage of an endoscope).

examinations. Lower resolution imaging on older generation endoscopes or transnasal endoscopes may impair detection of vascular markings. Exudates, which often track along longitudinal furrows, may be confused with white plaques from *Candida* esophagitis, and thus may be misdiagnosed. Crepe paper esophagus has been described as sloughing of esophageal mucosa during passage of an endoscope, perhaps secondary to subepithelial fibrosis or mucosal fragility[7] (Fig. 23.1). A "tug" sign, described

as stiffness or resistance when taking esophageal biopsies, is inherently difficult to standardize due to its subjective nature.[8]

Endoscopic assessment of strictures of the esophagus in EoE is often challenging. *Narrow-caliber* esophagus is often difficult to consistently report on endoscopy given the absence of a standardized definition. The degree of radial narrowing and axial involvement that characterizes an esophageal stricture as narrow-caliber esophagus has not been specified. Recently, a luminal diameter of less than 17 to 20 mm involving more than 50% of the length of the esophagus has been proposed as diagnostic criteria.[9] Accurate assessment of luminal diameter is, however, imprecise, particularly in patients with proximal or diffuse involvement. A 2014 study evaluating the sensitivity and specificity of identifying narrow-caliber esophagus (in this case defined as < 21 mm in diameter) on EGD compared with barium esophagram revealed poor sensitivity (14.7%) and modest specificity (79.2%) of endoscopy.[10] The same limitation applies for measurement of discrete strictures, wherein stenoses between 12 and 20 mm may be overlooked due to lack of focality or superimposed constriction by the lower esophageal sphincter and crural diaphragm.

EOE ENDOSCOPIC REFERENCE SCORE (EREFS)

Due to the variability and heterogeneity of endoscopic findings, a standardized classification and grading system was developed and subsequently validated to describe the endoscopic findings of EoE.[6] This system, referred to as the EoE Endoscopic Reference Scoring system, or EREFS, provides standardized nomenclature for five major features of EoE (edema, rings, exudates, furrows, and strictures) and includes a grading system to define severity of these individual findings (Fig. 23.2). In the original validation study, this grading system demonstrated good agreement for edema, rings, exudates, and furrows ($\kappa = 0.40$–0.54, 71%–81% pairwise agreements) and for strictures and crêpe-paper esophagus ($\kappa = 0.52$ and 0.58, 79% and 92% agreement). Despite good agreement, crêpe-paper esophagus was excluded from the final scoring system due to its low prevalence. Narrow-caliber esophagus was excluded due to lack of an operational definition.

Since its introduction, the EREFS grading system has been independently validated in a European study. Inter- and intra-observer agreement between four expert and four trainee endoscopists using an atlas of still images from 30 patients was assessed.[11] The authors found good interobserver agreement for rings ($\kappa = 0.70$), exudates ($\kappa = 0.63$), and crêpe-paper esophagus ($\kappa = 0.62$), moderate for furrows ($\kappa = 0.49$) and strictures ($\kappa = 0.54$), and poor for edema ($\kappa = 0.12$). Intraobserver agreement was substantial for rings, furrows, and crêpe-paper esophagus, moderate for exudates and strictures, and less than chance for edema. The low agreement for edema was likely affected by the use of still rather than video images. No difference was noted between expert and trainee endoscopists.

Compared to prior studies, where endoscopic identification of esophageal abnormalities was 83% to 93% as reported in a meta-analysis, prospective utilization of the EREFS system has identified abnormalities in over 95% of patients with EoE.[5,12,13] This suggests that this system may also have utility as a diagnostic tool given its high sensitivity. Moreover, the clinical relevance of endoscopic severity assessment has also recently been ascertained. The severity of EREFS subscores has been associated with patient-reported global symptom activity, and food impaction risk has been linked to ring severity.[14,15] A 2015

EoE **E**ndoscopic **ReFe**rence **S**core (EREFS)

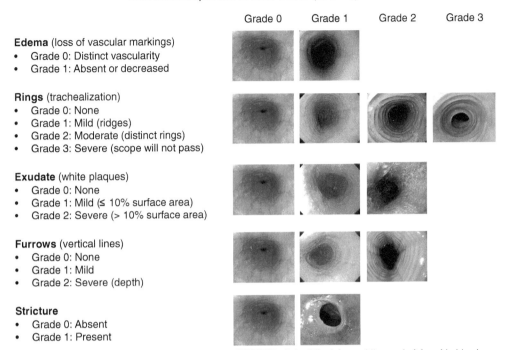

Edema (loss of vascular markings)
- Grade 0: Distinct vascularity
- Grade 1: Absent or decreased

Rings (trachealization)
- Grade 0: None
- Grade 1: Mild (ridges)
- Grade 2: Moderate (distinct rings)
- Grade 3: Severe (scope will not pass)

Exudate (white plaques)
- Grade 0: None
- Grade 1: Mild (≤ 10% surface area)
- Grade 2: Severe (> 10% surface area)

Furrows (vertical lines)
- Grade 0: None
- Grade 1: Mild
- Grade 2: Severe (depth)

Stricture
- Grade 0: Absent
- Grade 1: Present

FIG 23.2 EoE endoscopic reference score (EREFS). (Modified from Hirano I, Moy N, Heckman MG, et al: Endoscopic assessment of the oesophageal features of eosinophilic oesophagitis: validation of a novel classification and grading system. *Gut* 62[4]:489–495, 2013.)

study evaluating physicians' judgment of overall disease activity found that EoE activity assessment by gastroenterologists is largely based on endoscopic findings and symptoms, rather than histopathology.[16]

ENDOSCOPIC FINDINGS AS THERAPEUTIC ENDPOINTS

Therapeutic trials in EoE currently utilize symptomatic and histopathological endpoints as the primary determinants of successful therapy.[17] Symptoms of dysphagia, however, may improve as a result of behavioral changes, such as avoidance of hard texture foods, excessive mastication, and prolonged meal times, and thus may not accurately reflect disease activity. This type of adaptive behavior may explain the placebo response in terms of dysphagia. Using a validated patient-reported outcome instrument (eosinophilic esophagitis symptom activity index, or EESAI), symptoms were shown to have modest accuracy as an indicator of disease activity as determined by endoscopy and histology.[18] Further evidencing this symptom-histology dissociation is the observation that dysphagia responds dramatically to esophageal dilation, without affecting disease histology.[19] For these reasons, symptomatic improvement, although certainly an important goal of treatment, is not a reliable marker of disease activity as a therapeutic endpoint. Histologic improvement is also limited as a therapeutic marker, as correlation with patient-reported symptoms and physician-reported disease activity has been shown to be poor.[12,18]

The utility of grading endoscopic findings to predict response to treatment may have value, particularly in identifying various phenotypes of disease. Patients who have a predominantly "fibro-stenotic" pattern of injury with high-grade stenoses benefit from esophageal dilations, irrespective of disease activity as measured by eosinophilic inflammation.[19] These patients demonstrate the consequence of remodeling changes in EoE, wherein lamina propria fibrosis is believed to be a primary determinant. Those with an "inflammatory" phenotype, characterized by presence of exudates and furrows with predominant eosinophilic inflammation, typically respond well to topical corticosteroid therapy and may not require esophageal dilations.[20,21] Topical therapy, however, does not appear to affect underlying fibrostenotic disease activity. A 2016 retrospective study found that the presence of severe esophageal strictures was a negative predictor of histologic response to topical steroids.[22] However, topical therapy is likely playing some role in modulating remodeling changes, as demonstrated by a study wherein the thickness of the esophageal wall in patients undergoing treatment with nebulized budesonide was measured via endoscopic ultrasonography. In this randomized, controlled trial, the authors found that when compared to controls, EoE patients demonstrated significant thickening of the esophageal submucosa and muscularis propria, which improved, but did not normalize after treatment.[23]

The use of EREFS as a grading tool also has important clinical implications in determining responsiveness to treatment. A 2016 study demonstrated that EREFS had a high degree of accuracy not only for diagnosis of EoE, but also for responsiveness to treatment.[13] This prospective study evaluated 67 patients with EoE who were treated with either topical steroids or dietary elimination, and compared their endoscopic findings to 144 controls. Not surprisingly, EREFS scores (0–9) were greater in EoE patients versus controls (3.88 vs. 0.42, $p > 0.001$), and the authors were able to define a threshold score of two or greater to identify EoE patients with 88% sensitivity and 92% specificity. After treatment, the scores decreased significantly in EoE patients. Another recent study (2017) presented the first randomized, placebo-controlled trial of topical steroids that included endoscopic outcomes as defined by EREFS. In this study, oral budesonide suspension resulted in significant reduction in EREFS scores compared with placebo (where scores were unchanged), and improvement in all subscores with the exception of strictures.[12]

In discussing the advantages of using endoscopic features, one also has to consider their limitations. First, not all patients have every endoscopic feature, so using endoscopic grading systems to measure improvement is limited in patients that do not display all features. Secondly, the role of endoscopic features in predicting histologic remission may be limited. A 2016 study evaluated the predictive values of endoscopic features in assessing disease activity (peak eosinophil count) in a review of endoscopic still images and histopathology by a blinded endoscopist and pathologist.[24] The authors found that individual endoscopic findings did not correlate with peak eosinophil count, though a composite score of fibrotic signs, inflammatory signs, and total EREFS correlated weakly to moderately, without high positive or negative predictive values. Though technically a negative study, one can glean that a global clinical and endoscopic assessment, as determined by the composite scores, is likely more clinically relevant than the correlation of one endoscopic feature with peak eosinophil count. Furthermore, the use of still images may have been a limitation, and future studies using video images are needed to control for this limitation.

ALTERNATIVES AND ADJUNCTS TO ENDOSCOPIC ASSESSMENT

Identifying adequate targets for treatment has become an important goal in therapeutic trials and clinical practice. The ability of medical and dietary therapies to improve endoscopically visible inflammatory and structural alterations correlates with improvements in patient-reported outcomes and histologic assessments. As in inflammatory bowel disease, endoscopic mucosal healing, along with histologic and clinical improvement, will likely become the new therapeutic target for trials and clinical practice. Incorporating a validated grading system for endoscopic features will be paramount in standardizing therapeutic trials going forward. The role of other tools to assess remodeling changes is also yet to be determined. Although initially promising, endoscopic ultrasonography has been abandoned as a tool to assess remodeling, but measurements of mural compliance via the functional luminal imaging probe (FLIP) has yielded promising results. By using a multichannel electrical impedance catheter and manometric sensor surrounded by an infinitely compliant bag, the mechanical properties of the esophagus can be measured. Initial studies showed a significant reduction in esophageal distensibility in EoE patients when compared with controls.[25] A subsequent study found that patients with a history of food impactions exhibited lower esophageal distensibility when compared to those with dysphagia alone, and that the need for follow-up dilation also correlated with lower distensibility.[26] Finally, studies have also shown that higher grades of ring severity, as graded using EREFS, correlated stepwise with reduced distensibility metrics.[15,27] The same study, however, found that severity of exudates, furrows, and degree of eosinophilia was not associated with distensibility parameters, which may be a reflection of the inflammatory phenotype. Though not yet widely available, FLIP technology may play an important role in identifying adequate therapeutic goals, particularly in those patients with fibrostenotic phenotypes.

Other less invasive techniques have also been the focus of ongoing research, in attempts to identify tools for assessment of disease severity that do not require sedation and/or endoscopy. One such technology is the Cytosponge, an ingestible gelatin capsule comprising of compressed mesh attached to a string, which, in a small study of 20 patients, identified 11 of 13 patients with active EoE (defined at greater than 15 eosinophils/high power field) when compared to standard endoscopy.[28] Similarly, a swallowed esophageal string test has identified eosinophil-derived protein biomarkers in children with EoE.[29] Use of unsedated transnasal endoscopy has also been evaluated in both adult and pediatric populations, and has been found to be effective, lower-cost, and well tolerated by patients.[30,31] Finally, the use of esophageal brushings has been studied as a cheaper and more convenient alternative to esophageal biopsies, but has shown limited sensitivity and specificity for the detection of esophageal eosinophilia in a prospective study.[32]

CONCLUSION

There have been significant advances in our understanding of the mechanisms that drive the inflammatory and remodeling consequences of EoE. We have learned that standardizing definitions has helped clinicians and researchers define adequate therapeutic goals, allowing for a common language to be spoken among physicians. Although not a part of the diagnostic criteria, endoscopic findings play a critical role in the global assessment of disease severity, and are often the first hint to a physician that a patient has EoE. Moreover, initial severity of endoscopic findings has important clinical implications with regard to treatment options, including the need for dilations and predicting the effectiveness of medical therapies. Finally, given the discord between patient-reported symptoms and histologic outcomes, endoscopic features may serve as a more reliable therapeutic marker. Therefore a comprehensive assessment of a patient's symptoms, histology, and endoscopic findings is critical in ascertaining a global assessment of a patient's disease phenotype to determine an adequate treatment plan.

KEY REFERENCES

2. Dellon ES, Gonsalves N, Hirano I, et al: ACG clinical guideline: evidenced based approach to the diagnosis and management of esophageal eosinophilia and eosinophilic esophagitis (EoE), *Am J Gastroenterol* 108(5):679–692, quiz 693, 2013.

6. Hirano I, Moy N, Heckman MG, et al: Endoscopic assessment of the oesophageal features of eosinophilic oesophagitis: validation of a novel classification and grading system, *Gut* 62(4):489–495, 2013.

10. Gentile N, Katzka D, Ravi K, et al: Oesophageal narrowing is common and frequently under-appreciated at endoscopy in patients with oesophageal eosinophilia, *Aliment Pharmacol Ther* 40(11-12):1333–1340, 2014.

11. van Rhijn BD, Warners MJ, Curvers WL, et al: Evaluating the endoscopic reference score for eosinophilic esophagitis: moderate to substantial intra- and interobserver reliability, *Endoscopy* 46(12):1049–1055, 2014.

12. Dellon ES, Katzka DA, Collins MH, et al: Budesonide oral suspension improves symptomatic, endoscopic, and histologic parameters compared with placebo in patients with eosinophilic esophagitis, *Gastroenterology* 152(4):776–786, 2017.

13. Dellon ES, Cotton CC, Gebhart JH, et al: Accuracy of the eosinophilic esophagitis endoscopic reference score in diagnosis and determining response to treatment, *Clin Gastroenterol Hepatol* 14(1):31–39, 2016.

16. Schoepfer AM, Panczak R, Zwahlen M, et al: How do gastroenterologists assess overall activity of eosinophilic esophagitis in adult patients?, *Am J Gastroenterol* 110(3):402–414, 2015.

18. Safroneeva E, Straumann A, Coslovsky M, et al: Symptoms have modest accuracy in detecting endoscopic and histologic remission in adults with eosinophilic esophagitis, *Gastroenterology* 150(3):581–590 e4, 2016.

19. Schoepfer AM, Gonsalves N, Bussmann C, et al: Esophageal dilation in eosinophilic esophagitis: effectiveness, safety, and impact on the underlying inflammation, *Am J Gastroenterol* 105(5):1062–1070, 2010.

20. Dohil R, Newbury R, Fox L, et al: Oral viscous budesonide is effective in children with eosinophilic esophagitis in a randomized, placebo-controlled trial, *Gastroenterology* 139(2):418–429, 2010.

21. Straumann A, Conus S, Degen L, et al: Budesonide is effective in adolescent and adult patients with active eosinophilic esophagitis, *Gastroenterology* 139(5):1526–1537, 37 e1, 2010.

22. Eluri S, Runge TM, Cotton CC, et al: The extremely narrow-caliber esophagus is a treatment-resistant subphenotype of eosinophilic esophagitis, *Gastrointest Endosc* 83(6):1142–1148, 2016.

23. Straumann A, Conus S, Degen L, et al: Long-term budesonide maintenance treatment is partially effective for patients with eosinophilic esophagitis, *Clin Gastroenterol Hepatol* 9(5):400–409 e1, 2011.

24. van Rhijn BD, Verheij J, Smout AJ, et al: The Endoscopic Reference Score shows modest accuracy to predict histologic remission in adult patients with eosinophilic esophagitis, *Neurogastroenterol Motil* 28(11):1714–1722, 2016.

25. Kwiatek MA, Hirano I, Kahrilas PJ, et al: Mechanical properties of the esophagus in eosinophilic esophagitis, *Gastroenterology* 140(1):82–90, 2011.

26. Nicodeme F, Hirano I, Chen J, et al: Esophageal distensibility as a measure of disease severity in patients with eosinophilic esophagitis, *Clin Gastroenterol Hepatol* 11(9):1101–1107 e1, 2013.

27. Chen JW, Pandolfino JE, Lin Z, et al: Severity of endoscopically identified esophageal rings correlates with reduced esophageal distensibility in eosinophilic esophagitis, *Endoscopy* 48(9):794–801, 2016.

A complete reference list can be found online at ExpertConsult.com

24

Gastroesophageal Reflux Disease

David A. Leiman and David C. Metz

CHAPTER OUTLINE

INTRODUCTION

Gastroesophageal reflux (GER) occurs when there is retrograde movement of gastric contents into the esophagus. It occurs primarily after meals, and is part of a normal venting process to prevent excessive gastric distension and dyspepsia (the so-called "burp or belch" reflex). In contrast, gastroesophageal reflux disease (GERD) is defined as an abnormally elevated frequency of reflux and/or volume of refluxate, and typically presents as troublesome symptoms including heartburn and regurgitation.[1] Other atypical and extra-esophageal symptoms like chest pain, cough, and hoarseness can also occur.[2] Although chronic, GERD is generally not progressive. The majority of patients with GERD will not manifest endoscopically identifiable mucosal damage; others may present with esophagitis, esophageal stricture, or Barrett's esophagus (BE).[3]

GERD is one of the most common diseases worldwide and, whereas its incidence has increased over time, its prevalence is unequally distributed across the world. There is a substantially higher burden of GERD in the United States and Europe than in Asia. Recent data (2014) demonstrate that typical GERD symptoms occurring at least once weekly can be found in up to 27.8% of individuals in Western populations, but only 7.8% of individuals in East Asian populations.[4] There are some data linking GERD to genetic factors, particularly within families, but there are no known genetic risk factors.[5] Rather, this discrepancy across populations is likely due to both environmental factors like *Helicobacter pylori* infection, as well as lifestyle and dietary discrepancies.[6] Nonetheless, GERD is a frequent cause for referral to the gastroenterologist, and accounts for billions of dollars of health care costs annually.[7]

ETIOLOGY

The search for a single etiologic factor for the development of GERD has been met with frustration. Instead, GERD can be considered a multifactorial disease, and our understanding of its pathogenesis has evolved, and continues to evolve, over time.

Although it is clearly associated with exposure to gastric acid and pepsin, and occasionally worsened in the setting of esophageal dysmotility, the underlying mechanism of GERD relates to a disorder at the level of the gastroesophageal junction (GEJ).

The GEJ is comprised of several components, including the extrinsic skeletal muscle of the diaphragm, the intrinsic smooth muscle of the distal esophagus, and the angle of His created by the specialized gastric sling fibers and connective tissue that includes the phrenoesophageal ligament.[8] As early as 1956, Code et al described a high pressure zone between the esophagus and the stomach.[9] It became clear over time that this zone was actually the combination of two integral parts, which includes a 4 cm-long lower esophageal sphincter (LES) and a 2 cm-long portion of the crural diaphragm. The GEJ is the barrier to reflux, and the intraluminal pressure at this level is a measure of the antireflux barrier.[10]

Although a low GEJ pressure and/or a dissociated GEJ region (such as occurs in patients with a hiatal hernia) permits GER if the gastric pressure rises higher than the GEJ resistance, a more important and far more common cause of GERD is transient relaxation across this barrier. In 1964, McNally et al described how belching is facilitated by LES relaxation, and in 1980, Dent et al reported on LES relaxation in reflux disease.[11,12] Transient lower esophageal sphincter relaxations (TLESRs) are a vagally mediated normal physiologic mechanism that facilitates the retrograde flow of gastric contents, including eructation and vomit, in the presence of gastric distension. However, in patients with GERD, TLESRs are the single most important mechanism underlying reflux, and they can be influenced by several factors.[13] During a TLESR, there is equalization of pressure between the stomach and esophagus, along with contraction of longitudinal esophageal muscle in a reverse peristaltic fashion (Fig. 24.1). TLESRs are increased during pharyngeal stimulation and with increasing gastric distension, both of which occur during the prandial and postprandial states, when most reflux events occur.[14,15] Patients with disordered sleep are at higher risk of GERD and, simultaneously, GERD increases the risk of disordered sleep in a positive feedback loop.[16,17] In contrast, the supine

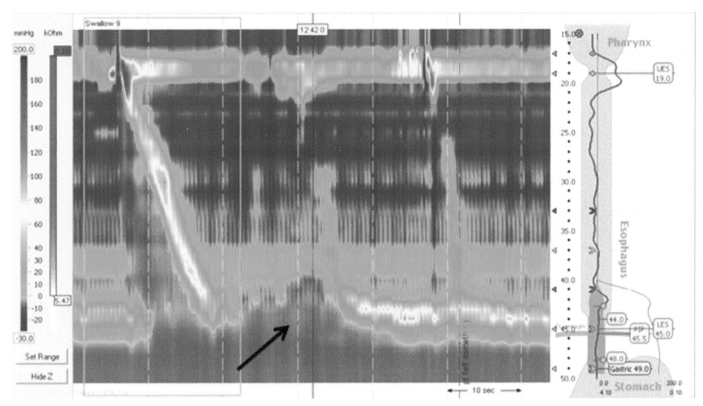

FIG 24.1 High-resolution manometry with impedance demonstrating a transient lower esophageal sphincter relaxation (TLESR, identified by the *black arrow*) following a normal swallow. *LES*, lower esophageal sphincter; *PIP*, pressure inversion point; *UES*, upper esophageal sphincter.

position generally, and stable sleep specifically, can reduce the number of TLESRs.

The presence of a hiatal hernia also increases the frequency of TLSESRs, though this phenomenon alone does not explain the higher number of total reflux episodes in patients with GERD.[18] It is clear that a weakening of the GEJ is mechanistically related to pathologic reflux in other ways as well. Having several constituent parts, in the normal state the GEJ can respond rapidly and dynamically to changes in both intraabdominal and intrathoracic pressures. In patients with a hiatal hernia, there is a relative or fixed dissociation between the LES and the crural diaphragm, limiting the capacity for preventing reflux. With an incompetent diaphragmatic component, gastric contents may flow more easily into the hernia sac and ultimately reflux into the esophagus across a weakened LES, especially during a TLESR.[19] As the hernia sac size increases, there is additional dilation of the esophageal hiatus, leading to further incompetence.[20] As expected, the severity of erosive esophagitis is predicted by hernia size and LES pressure.[21]

External factors that lead to hiatal hernia may therefore influence the presence of GERD. Instigating events causing an increase in intraabdominal pressure, like pregnancy, obesity, and trauma, are associated with the development of a hiatal hernia. Age, too, plays a role, as increased "wear and tear" results in loosening of the phrenoesophageal ligament.[22] Finally, there is evidence that the layer of highly acidic gastric juice in the postprandial proximal stomach (the so-called "acid pocket") also contributes to GERD.[23] The pH of this area is lower relative to the remainder of the gastric juices, which are buffered by the ingested food. Its clinical relevance was noted when GERD patients were shown to have longer acid pockets compared to healthy

patients due to the presence of hiatal hernia. When the acid pocket is located above the level of the diaphragm, as much as 85% of TLESRs are associated with reflux.[24]

Eventually, refluxed gastric contents are buffered, and must ultimately be cleared from the esophagus.[25] In patients with weak esophageal peristaltic strength (as determined by ineffective esophageal motility on high resolution manometry) there is reduced esophageal clearance capacity.[26] It is also possible that frequent reflux and pathologic acid exposure can in themselves lead to ineffective esophageal motility, thus creating another positive feedback loop contributing to GERD.[27]

A current conceptual model (Fig. 24.2) accounts for all these components that influence the development of GERD symptoms, as well as the mucosal changes or complications that are frequently associated with these factors. There are likely intrinsic and extrinsic factors that lead to a mechanically impaired GEJ and the development of a hiatal hernia, that both allow and cause increased frequency of reflux events and increased volume of refluxate. This cycle may cause ineffective esophageal clearance and lead to prolonged acid exposure, symptoms, and mucosal disease.

Injury to the esophageal mucosa is likely a multistep process. Experimental data demonstrate that repeated exposure to acid and pepsin in combination can lead to reduced distal esophageal motor contractions, reduced GEJ competence, and reduced compliance.[28] Although exposure to very high doses of acid alone may cause esophagitis, the addition of the proteolytic enzyme pepsin leads to an increasing degree of mucosal injury and permeability.[29] Although elevated acid exposure is correlated with the development of esophagitis, it is not a good predictor of the severity of the esophagitis or mucosal complications like BE.[30] Therefore other factors aside from acid and pepsin

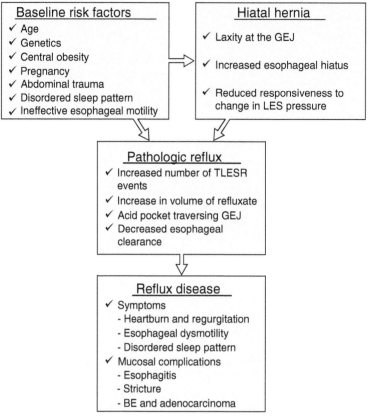

FIG 24.2 A conceptual model of gastroesophageal reflux disease. *BE,* Barrett's esophagus; *GEJ,* gastroesophageal junction; *LES,* lower esophageal sphincter; *TLESR,* transient lower esophageal sphincter relaxation. (Adapted from Boeckxstaens G, El-Serag HB, Smout AJ, et al: Symptomatic reflux disease: the present, the past and the future. *Gut* 63[7]:1185–1193, 2014.)

alone are thought to be related to the development of GERD. Duodenogastroesophageal reflux (DGER) of bile acids and pancreatic enzymes are both implicated in the development of GERD symptoms. The precise role of these components depends on whether the bile acids are conjugated or unconjugated; both of these processes occur in different pH environments.[31] DGER and bile acids have a putative role in the development of BE and esophageal adenocarcinoma and may be associated with the development of symptoms in patients with nonerosive reflux disease (NERD).[32] Esophageal mucosa exposed to bile acids in acidic conditions develop dilated intercellular spaces (DISs), a marker of mucosal permeability that can be seen in patients with NERD.[33] Even in neutral pH environments, the pancreatic enzyme trypsin can damage the esophageal mucosa.[34]

Intriguing new evidence is further modifying our understanding of the pathogenesis of mucosal injury in GERD. In addition to acid and pancreaticobiliary reflux, a cytokine-mediated inflammatory cascade may prime the mucosa for injury from acid. As first reported in animal studies, acid exposure may trigger cytokine production, leading to lymphocytic infiltration that starts in the submucosa and progresses toward the epithelial surface. The corresponding inflammatory reaction may make later acid-mediated injury possible.[35] These findings have been reproduced in a small human tissue study.[36] Although preliminary, these data suggest that our understanding of the pathogenesis of GERD continues to grow, and further reveal the complex nature of this common disease.

DIAGNOSIS

The diagnosis of GERD can be made clinically based on typical symptoms responding to treatment with acid suppression. Indeed, current guidelines recommend an empiric 4–8 week trial with acid-suppressive proton pump inhibitors (PPIs) for patients with typical symptoms, as well as for other common GERD presentations like dyspepsia or epigastric pain.[37] However, this approach is limited, as PPI trials show only 78% sensitivity and 54% specificity for accurately diagnosing GERD.[38] Therefore even in patients with typical symptoms, and especially in patients with atypical symptoms like cough, specific physiologic testing may be required to establish or confirm a diagnosis. Mucosal changes like erosive esophagitis (EE) or BE are the *sine qua non* of GERD, and no additional confirmatory testing is needed, but these findings are rather infrequent, and endoscopy is not considered necessary for the diagnosis of GERD in patients with typical symptoms.[37] In fact, esophagogastroduodenoscopy (EGD) would miss the presence of GERD in many patients, as the esophagus may appear completely normal despite the presence of symptomatic GERD.[3] Endoscopic findings can be characterized as signs of severe disease and are actually complications of GERD (the endoscopic evaluation of GERD is described further later). Although historically included as part of the diagnostic testing algorithm for GERD, barium esophagography findings do not correlate with the incidence or extent of reflux seen on physiologic testing.[39] Although

TABLE 24.1   Symptoms and Complications of Gastroesophageal Reflux Disease

Esophageal Symptoms	Extra-Esophageal Symptoms	Complications
Heartburn	Pulmonary reflux	Reflux esophagitis
Regurgitation	Asthma	Stricture
Chest pain	Cough	Barrett's esophagus
Dysphagia	Laryngeal reflux	Adenocarcinoma
	Globus	
	Throat clearing	
	Hoarseness	

potentially helpful in evaluating or excluding other causes of esophageal symptoms, barium esophagography has no role in diagnosing GERD.

Symptoms

The symptoms of GERD should be classified as either typical or atypical, which correlate roughly with esophageal and extraesophageal symptoms, respectively (Table 24.1). Heartburn is a burning sensation in the retrosternal area, and regurgitation is the perception of flow of refluxed gastric contents into the mouth or hypopharynx.[1] In the United States, heartburn is more common than regurgitation (13.2%–25.2% vs. 6.3%–14.9%), and this same relationship also holds in Western Europe.[4] These typical symptoms respond better to acid-suppressive therapy than atypical symptoms, but even when they are the only symptoms present, they are not sensitive for the diagnosis of GERD.[40] Clinical evaluation alone is not good at predicting erosive esophagitis, with only 30%–76% sensitivity and 62%–96% specificity in the presence of typical symptoms.[41] However, in patients with typical symptoms who do respond to PPI therapy, no additional testing is needed.[42]

GERD can also manifest as chest pain, and it is thought to be a major cause of noncardiac chest pain syndrome.[43] Pulmonary symptoms like nonallergic asthma may also be attributed to GERD.[44] Complaints of chest pain, cough, or dyspnea in the absence of typical GERD symptoms warrant further diagnostic investigation (at least physiologic testing) after exclusion of primary cardiopulmonary disease. Dysphagia is also a possible presentation of GERD, especially if esophagitis is present, and is a red flag symptom that deserves initial endoscopic evaluation (discussed in further detail later).

The correlation between acid reflux and atypical, or extraesophageal, symptoms is less clear. Patients with atypical symptoms frequently present to otorhinolaryngologists.[45] However, only 54% of patients diagnosed with laryngoesophageal reflux disease (LERD) have abnormal acid exposure (confirming a diagnosis of GERD), despite up to 93% of patients with posterior laryngeal inflammation having symptoms.[46] As such, these complaints are less responsive to acid suppression or antireflux surgery.[47] Prolonged trials of even high (off-label) doses of acid suppressors have not shown a benefit for empiric therapy in this population.[48] Recent data (2016) demonstrate no ability to distinguish between healthy subjects and those with laryngoesophageal symptoms using salivary pepsin and oropharyngeal reflux testing.[49]

Endoscopy

EGD diagnostic testing is not recommended initially for GERD symptoms unless red flag signs are present.[37] In fact, EE will only be present in approximately one-third of patients with reflux

symptoms, and only 20%–60% of patients with abnormal reflux testing, which therefore limits its utility.[3] Instead, EGD should be used to avoid misdiagnosing patients who have failed initial therapy or to identify and/or treat patients with complications of GERD. The role of endoscopy in patients with GERD, therefore, is limited to the evaluation of those patients with persistent symptoms despite adequate PPI therapy, those who have multiple risk factors for BE because of its premalignant nature, those who require pre- or postoperative evaluation for antireflux procedures, or those with symptoms (especially dysphagia) suggestive of complicated disease (Fig. 24.3).[50] Patients who fail to respond adequately to empiric PPI therapy should be counseled regarding how best to take their PPI therapy to optimize the trial before EGD is considered, and in those who respond to PPIs, the lowest effective PPI dose should be sought for chronic administration to limit the potential for long-term side effects of therapy.[37] In addition, consideration should be given to pulmonary or otorhinolaryngology (ENT) evaluation in patients with atypical symptoms prior to resorting to EGD because atypical manifestations of GERD are often confounded with other more common non-gastrointestinal conditions, such as asthma, postnasal drip, or allergies.[37] If ENT and/or pulmonary evaluation fails to identify an alternative cause for the symptoms, EGD often fails to identify any abnormalities, so many authorities will often forego EGD altogether and proceed directly to pH testing instead.[37] However, EGD should always be considered, especially in young males with dysphagia, in order to distinguish GERD from eosinophilic esophagitis (EoE) or PPI-responsive eosinophilia; this should generally be done in the presence of PPI therapy to permit exclusion of the latter condition.[51]

There are multiple endoscopic findings that can occur in GERD. Early changes include edema and friability.[52] These are nonspecific findings, but in the presence of persistent acid exposure, erosions can develop that are characterized by shallow mucosal breaks. These usually occur at the squamocolumnar junction (SCJ) and extend proximally. Identified as linear streaks extending from and/or present between the folds, these erosions are often bordered by white exudate and erythema. In severe cases, there may be ulceration, but this finding is not pathognomonic for GERD, and may also be seen in infectious, pill-induced, or stasis esophagitis.[53] In addition to revealing normal mucosa or EE, the endoscopic appearance of the esophagus may mimic other disorders. Most importantly, there can be substantial overlap between the appearance of GERD and EoE, including with the presence of so-called ringed or feline esophagus.[54] Late findings of chronic reflux include peptic strictures, BE, and esophageal adenocarcinoma.[55] Schatzki, or type B, rings are always associated with a hiatal hernia and mark the inferior margin of the esophagus; they can also be seen in conjunction with GERD, although a direct correlation is controversial.[56] The endoscopic findings and management of these topics are discussed in detail in Chapters 21, 25, and 27.

Several endoscopic grading systems have been developed to standardize reporting and interpretation of endoscopic findings of GERD (Table 24.2). In Europe, the Savary-Miller schema has been favored, whereas the most commonly used method in the United States is the Los Angeles (LA) Classification (Fig. 24.4).[57,58] In Japan, a modified version of the LA grading scale is sometimes used that includes normal mucosa as well as minimal changes, although there is poor inter-rater reliability with milder findings of esophagitis.[59]

In typical EE, endoscopic tissue sampling is generally not indicated. Routine biopsies of normal tissue may reveal basal

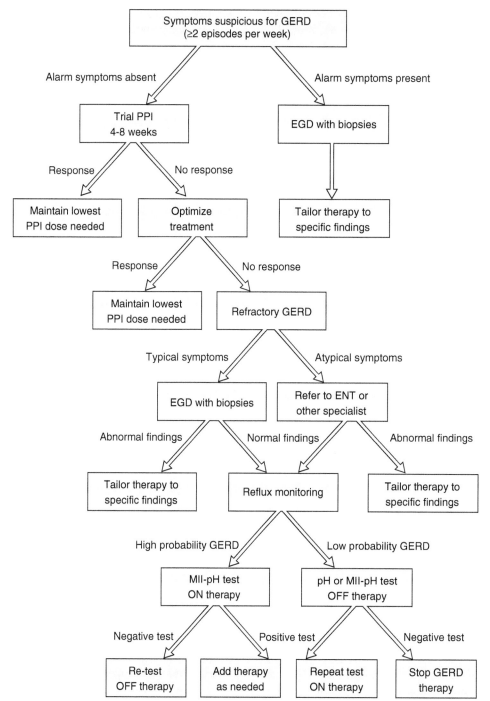

FIG 24.3 A proposed diagnostic approach for the management of symptoms of gastroesophageal reflux disease (GERD). In this schema, the use of multichannel intraluminal impedance-pH (MII-pH) probes on or off proton pump inhibitor (PPI) therapy in patients who remain undiagnosed despite a trial of empiric PPI therapy and esophagogastroduodenoscopy (EGD) or targeted specialist referral is determined by the type of presenting symptom complex. *ENT,* otolaryngology. (Modified from Katz PO, Gerson LB, Vela MF: Guidelines for the diagnosis and management of gastroesophageal reflux disease. *Am J Gastroenterol* 108[3]:308–328, 2013.)

cell hyperplasia, papillary elongation, and DIS.[60] In the setting of inflammation, a neutrophilic and/or eosinophilic infiltrate may be present. None of these histologic findings are sensitive or specific for GERD.[61] Therefore the main indications for tissue sampling are to exclude EoE in patients with reflux despite therapy, confirm the presence of BE, or exclude infectious etiologies. All

these topics, including specific sampling techniques, are discussed in further detail in Chapters 23 and 25.

Although an esophageal capsule endoscopy device has been developed, its performance compared to standard endoscopy for diagnosing esophagitis, hiatal hernia, and BE is poor, and therefore it has not gained widespread clinical use.[62,63]

TABLE 24.2   Endoscopic Grading Schemes for Esophagitis

Modified Los Angeles Classification

Grade N	Normal mucosa
Grade M	Minimal changes to the mucosa (such as erythema)
Grade A	One or more mucosal breaks < 5 mm in length, confined to folds
Grade B	One or more mucosal breaks > 5 mm in length, confined to folds and not continuous between folds
Grade C	Mucosal breaks between folds, but affecting < 75% of luminal circumference
Grade D	Mucosal breaks between folds, but affecting > 75% of luminal circumference

Savary-Miller Classification

Grade 0	No esophagitis
Grade I	Single erosion on one longitudinal fold
Grade II	Multiple erosions on multiple folds
Grade III	Circumferential erosions
Grade IV	Ulcer, stricture, or short esophagus with or without Grades I-III
Grade V	Barrett's esophagus with or without Grades I-III

Data from Lundell LR, Dent J, Bennett JR, et al: Endoscopic assessment of oesophagitis: clinical and functional correlates and further validation of the Los Angeles classification. *Gut* 45(2):172–180, 1999; Ollyo J, Lang F, Fontolliet C, et al: Savary-Miller's new endoscopic grading of reflux-oesophagitis: a simple, reproducible, logical, complete and useful classification. *Gastroenterology* 1990;98:A100.

Esophageal pH Testing

There are several physiologic tests currently available to aid in the diagnosis of GERD. Because up to 40% of patients with GERD symptoms have no endoscopic evidence of reflux, these tests can be helpful to "rule in" patients with NERD, as well as to exclude those patients with esophageal hypersensitivity or functional heartburn if medical therapy and EGD have both been nondiagnostic.[3,64]

Catheter-based testing includes both pH-only probes and multichannel intraluminal impedance-pH testing (MII-pH). Reflux testing has evolved since 1960, when Tuttle et al developed a glass tube probe to identify a pH gradient between the esophagus and the stomach.[65] Initial catheters were cumbersome, until DeMeester et al (1974) created a device with an external electrode, though even this test still required hospitalization.[66] More practical means of outpatient ambulatory testing became available in the 1980s.

Current reflux testing takes advantage of the same principles. In pH-only probes, a catheter with one to three electrodes along the catheter length is passed transnasally through the esophagus into the stomach. The reference electrode is located 5 cm proximal to the LES, which is typically identified first by manometry and, if present, additional probes can be placed higher in the esophagus (usually 10–15 cm proximally) to evaluate for proximal reflux, or lower into the stomach (usually 15 cm below the reference electrode) to evaluate therapeutic efficacy. Patients usually keep this probe in place for 24 hours and are instructed to carry out their normal activities without restrictions other than bathing (which can damage the probe), exercising vigorously (which can dislodge the probe), and ingestion of acidic substances such as wine (which can lead to false positive results). Patients are also asked to maintain a log or diary of their position (upright or supine), eating, medication administration, and symptoms during monitoring, the latter to provide a measure of the correlation of reflux events with symptoms.[67]

Although useful, catheter-based pH testing has a disadvantage in that it may discourage patients from performing their usual activities during the study period because of discomfort and or aesthetic concerns.[68] A significant development occurred with the introduction of the Bravo wireless pH monitoring system (Medtronic, North Haven, CT). Compared to patients undergoing catheter-based testing, patients using the Bravo system have fewer nasopharyngeal side effects and are more likely to perform usual daily activities like going to work, sleeping, and eating, thereby more closely matching their general activities during reflux events.[69] Although not required, this system is often deployed in conjunction with endoscopy to help identify the SCJ so that accurate manometric identification of the proximal border of the LES is not required (Fig. 24.5). When the capsule is placed endoscopically, it is attached to the esophageal mucosa 6 cm above the SCJ (which correlates closely with the proximal border of the LES) and deployed using a specialized delivery system that includes a vacuum pump and firing pin. Less discomfort and fewer migrations occur with this device compared with catheter-based systems. Additionally, Bravo monitoring allows for prolonged monitoring for 48–96 hours, and even permits "on" and "off" therapy periods of monitoring to potentially improve the sensitivity and specificity of testing.[70,71]

Nonetheless, both catheter and wireless pH tests only provide information on esophageal acid exposure. In contrast, MII-pH probes allow for the detection of acid as well as intraluminal bolus presence. This technique was first described by Silny in 1991, and is based on the principle of measuring the difference in the electrical conductivity of air and liquid.[72] With the addition of multiple impedance sensors spaced several centimeters apart along the length of the catheter, it is possible to determine the presence of liquid versus air and its direction of flow.[73] As a result, one can determine if acid or nonacid refluxate is present. As with the pH-only probe, though, this test is limited by duration, the presence of an indwelling catheter, and accurate patient-reported symptoms. Nonetheless, this technique correlates well with barium studies and manometry to confirm bolus movement, and is considered the most sensitive tool for detecting GERD independent of refluxate acidity.[72,74] In addition, MII-pH testing can arguably also be performed in patients on antisecretory therapy to distinguish incompletely treated GERD from GERD-like symptoms arising from another cause (see Fig. 24.3).

Normative data exist for pH and reflux testing to aid in the diagnosis of GERD. The exact cutoff values may vary depending on the center, but the most relevant parameter is esophageal acid exposure, i.e., the time for which the pH is less than 4.0 at a reference point located 5 cm above the LES.[75,76] This value reliably correlates with the presence of heartburn in patients with GERD, and it is also an excellent way to differentiate between patients with EE or BE and those with NERD.[77] Several other variables can be identified with combined impedance/pH testing, including the total number of reflux episodes, esophageal acid clearance times, and composite indices like the DeMeester score. Additional symptom association analyses have been devised to predict the likelihood that reported symptoms are related to GERD. The most straightforward to calculate is the symptom index (SI). This is determined by dividing the number of reflux-related symptoms by the total number of symptoms reported and multiplying by

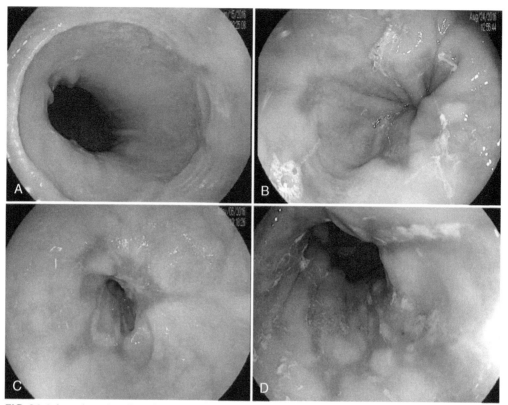

FIG 24.4 Los Angeles (LA) Classification. Clockwise from the top left: **A,** LA A (one or more mucosal breaks < 5 mm in length, confined to folds). **B,** LA B (one or more mucosal breaks > 5 mm in length, confined to folds and not continuous between folds). **C,** LA C (mucosal breaks between folds, but affecting < 75% of luminal circumference). **D,** LA D (mucosal breaks between folds, but affecting > 75% of luminal circumference). (From Lundell LR, Dent J, Bennett JR, et al: Endoscopic assessment of oesophagitis: clinical and functional correlates and further validation of the Los Angeles classification. *Gut* 45[2]:172–180, 1999.)

100. If the SI value is greater than or equal to 50%, it is considered positive, with greater than 90% sensitivity and over 70% specificity.[78] Fig. 24.6 demonstrates a symptom-associated acidic reflux event identified by MII-pH testing. Unfortunately, there are scant data correlating the SI, or other symptom association scales, with outcomes in patients who have failed a PPI trial.[79]

Substantial debate also exists over whether testing should optimally be done on or off PPI therapy. Although many factors may influence baseline normal levels, there are standard ranges for abnormal acid exposure on and off acid suppression.[80,81] The esophageal acid exposure is lower with a wireless pH probe, and may justify a modified threshold, but there is very good concordance between this and catheter-based pH testing.[82] Current guidelines recommend that the decision to test on versus off therapy should be based on the pretest probability of GERD. Specifically, patients with a low likelihood of GERD should be evaluated off therapy, whereas a test should be done on PPI if there is a high likelihood of GERD.[37]

Although all forms of current reflux monitoring are reliable in patients with erosive esophagitis, in patients with nonerosive disease, or who are at least endoscopy negative, both sensitivity and specificity are decreased.[83] This creates a clinical conundrum because patients with EE are most likely to have typical symptoms and least likely to need confirmatory testing. As a result, direct mucosal impedance measurement has gained increasing attention, particularly for patients with NERD. Traditional reflux testing

provides data over only a short study period, and due to the brief study duration, there is the possibility of missed events or false negative results. Directly measuring mucosal impedance attempts to evaluate chronic mucosal changes, and is theoretically more sensitive. The basis for this approach is the DISs that are known to be present within the esophageal mucosa. This finding occurs even in the absence of esophagitis, and it may be a marker for chronic GERD.[84] The presence of DISs leads to increased permeability in animal models, and may be measured using a through-the-scope catheter to evaluate impedance between two points along the esophageal mucosa.[85] Compared to wireless pH monitoring, direct mucosal impedance had superior positive predictive value (96% vs. 40%) for identifying GERD patients[86] in the limited number of studies that have been performed to date. This represents an exciting development in GERD testing and warrants further study.

TREATMENT

Medical acid suppression remains the cornerstone of GERD treatment. As discussed previously, patients with typical symptoms or EE on endoscopy demonstrate the best response to acid inhibition. In those patients with atypical symptoms or those who fail to respond to initial therapy, adjunctive therapies like lifestyle modification, including weight loss and smoking cessation, are recommended.[37] Elevating the head of the bed and avoiding late night eating is effective in patients with nocturnal GERD.[87]

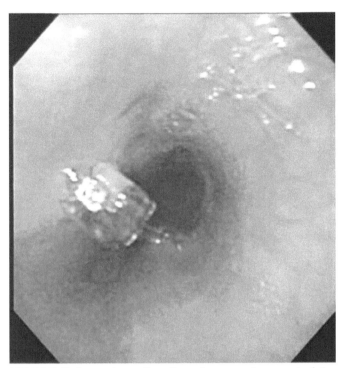

FIG 24.5 Endoscopic confirmation of proper placement of the Bravo (Medtronic, North Haven, CT) pH monitoring system approximately 6 cm proximal to the squamocolumnar junction, which correlates closely with the proximal border of the lower esophageal sphincter (LES).

Atypical symptoms often prove more difficult to resolve, and can require combination therapy with other agents. In patients requiring long-term medical therapy for complete symptom control, particularly those with typical symptoms responsive to PPIs but unwilling to take them long term, traditional antireflux surgery remains an option. The laparoscopically placed LINX device (Torax Medical, Shoreview, MN) is another Food and Drug Administration (FDA)-approved option for patients who continue to experience GERD symptoms despite maximum medical therapy.[88] Emerging endoscopic technologies such as the transoral incisionless fundoplication (TIF) have received substantial interest as possible nonoperative procedural interventions for GERD.

Medical Management

Prior to the approval of PPIs, histamine-2 receptor antagonists (H2RAs) were the most potent therapies available for GERD management.[89] Traditional antacids like calcium carbonate do not provide any long-term benefit for patients with GERD. In contrast, H2RAs are superior to placebo and are effective in the management of mild, intermittent GERD (with symptoms occurring 1 day or less per week). Unfortunately, tachyphylaxis can occur with this class of medications, and therefore they have relatively limited utility in patients with chronic moderate to-severe GERD (with symptoms occurring 2 or more days per week).[90]

However, in the modern era, the mainstay of medical therapy for GERD is PPI therapy. These drugs were initially developed in the 1980s, and omeprazole, first approved by the FDA for the treatment of Zollinger-Ellison Syndrome, was initially marketed in the United States in 1989.[91] Since that time, three additional

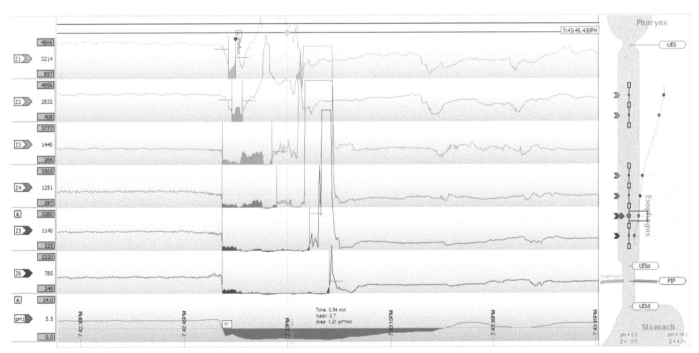

FIG 24.6 Tracing of a multichannel intraluminal impedance with pH testing. In this example, there is excellent symptom correlation with chest pain recorded by the patient during the acid reflux event. *LES,* lower esophageal sphincter; *PIP,* pressure inversion point; *UES,* upper esophageal sphincter.

compounds and two enantiomers have become available that are currently indicated for healing and maintenance of EE, as well as treatment of GERD symptoms.[92]

Antisecretory therapy with PPIs targets the final common pathway for acid secretion into the gastric lumen. PPIs effectively and consistently raise intragastric pH and decrease gastric acid secretion.[93] In these ways, PPIs reduce both the acid content and volume of gastric refluxate. All PPIs are superior to H2RAs for healing of EE, as well as for treatment of nonerosive disease.[94,95] For maximum efficacy, it is recommended that all delayed-release PPIs should be taken 30–60 minutes prior to meals[21] (with the exception of dexlansoprazole and omeprazole–sodium bicarbonate combination therapy). Although a common cause of failing to respond to PPI therapy is incorrect dosing administration,[96] GERD is chronic, and symptoms are likely to recur after discontinuing medical therapy, even when PPIs have been used correctly.[57] There are no significant differences between PPIs that warrant switching medications in patients with inadequate response to one PPI.[97]

Although these drugs have been available and used safely for several decades, there are now numerous reports of potential side effects. In addition to pathologic bone fractures, idiosyncratic electrolyte disturbances, and renal injury, more recent data (2016) have shown long-term PPI treatment to be potentially associated with micronutrient deficiencies, infections, cardiovascular disease, and dementia.[98] The studies that generated these alarms are retrospective and correlational in nature, but have generated substantial concern among patients. As a result, in addition to using the lowest effective doses of PPIs for adequate GERD symptom management, alternative therapies can be considered alone or in combination with traditional PPI treatment.[42] Among these alternatives are alginate-based medications, which are often combined with typical antacids. These medications treat GERD via a unique mechanism by creating a mechanical barrier that displaces the postprandial acid pocket.[99] They are superior to both placebo and antacids in treating symptomatic GERD.[100] Although further studies are needed, this represents a potentially attractive option as an adjunctive therapy in patients who respond incompletely to PPI therapy, particularly as it relates to the acid pocket.[101]

Another medical alternative to PPIs is a novel class of medications called potassium competitive acid blockers (PCABs). These drugs are neither acid-activated nor affected by genetic variants, which are both drawbacks of PPIs; they also have very rapid onset and offset, which may allow for as-needed (i.e., PRN) usage even for more severe forms of GERD.[102] Their use in GERD may be an area of future investigation, although initial trials did not reveal improved symptomatic management of NERD or healing of EE compared to traditional PPIs.[103,104] Moreover, PCABs are extremely potent inhibitors of acid production, leading to higher gastrin levels than occur with PPIs, and there may be some safety concerns regarding this effect if therapy use is prolonged. Therapies that target other pathways involved in the development of GERD are also available. Baclofen, which effectively decreases TLESR frequency and increases LES pressure, has shown some clinic benefit, but is not FDA-approved for treatment of GERD.[105] Prokinetics like metoclopramide have a limited role and only in patients with evidence of delayed gastric emptying.[37] There are multiple other compounds under investigation that aim to modulate pain perception or provide mucosal protection.[106]

Surgical Treatment

Historically, the primary alternative to treatment with acid suppression has been surgical treatment by gastric fundoplication.

Reproducing a functioning antireflux barrier by wrapping the LES with the proximal stomach was first described by Nissen in the 1950s.[107] His approach has undergone several iterations since that time, including modifications to the degree of wrap (e.g., 270-degree posterior, or Toupet, fundoplication). Enthusiasm for performing antireflux surgery, on the other hand, has waxed and waned. The number of antireflux surgical procedures performed in the United States has varied dramatically over the last several decades, often in response to the availability of new medications and concerns over cancer risks associated with GERD, as well as side effects from antireflux surgery.[108]

The Nissen fundoplication, as originally described, required an open incision and substantially longer hospitalization time than its modern iteration. The laparoscopic Nissen approach gained popularity in the early 1990s, but it was around this time that a randomized control trial demonstrated superior efficacy of open Nissen in controlling GERD than H2RA medical therapy.[109] Importantly, this study compared an open surgical procedure to treatment with H2RAs at a time when the laparoscopic approach had already been reported and PPIs were already available. Long-term follow-up data from this same cohort demonstrated no significant differences between the groups with respect to esophagitis, need for subsequent antireflux surgery, or satisfaction with their antireflux therapy.[110] The accompanying video (Video 24.1) discusses the endoscopic appearance of a surgical Nissen fundoplication.

It has become clear that carefully selected patients (those with typical symptoms who have responded to PPIs) are most likely to benefit from antireflux surgery.[111] Indeed, the laparoscopic approach has also been demonstrated to be superior to open surgery, with similar treatment outcomes and fewer complications.[112] This approach results in more durable long-term healing of esophagitis compared to PPIs, and fewer patients need PPIs after surgery, though remission rates are high in both groups.[110,113,114] Nonetheless, patients undergoing antireflux surgery risk perioperative complications that include death, and face other side effects like dysphagia, gas-bloat syndrome, disruption of the fundoplication, as well as unmet expectations.[115] On balance, there is general equivalence between these approaches for patients with typical symptoms, with surgery being favored for patients with volume regurgitation and intolerance of PPIs. In patients with GERD as a complication of morbid obesity, however, Roux-en-Y gastric bypass provides symptomatic improvement and is the preferred operative approach.[116]

The most recent surgical advance is magnetic LES sphincter augmentation using the LINX (Torax Medical) device. Composed of a circle of magnetic iron beads enclosed in a titanium case and connected by titanium arms, this is a laparoscopically-placed antireflux device (Fig. 24.7). It fits around the outside of the esophagus and, through magnetic forces, provides baseline LES sphincter augmentation that also accommodates the passage of food aborally and retrograde belching or vomiting. Developed by Ganz and colleagues, this device aims to provide a physical antireflux barrier without the troublesome side effects of migration or new onset bowel symptoms.[117] First described in 2008, this device now has longer-term safety and efficacy. Use of the device appears to result in significant and durable improvement in symptomatic response and a decreased need for medical acid suppression, and there have been no device migrations, erosions, or malfunctions reported in the device trials; however, postmarketing and surveillance data do demonstrate that these adverse events have occurred.[118] Symptoms that have often discouraged referral

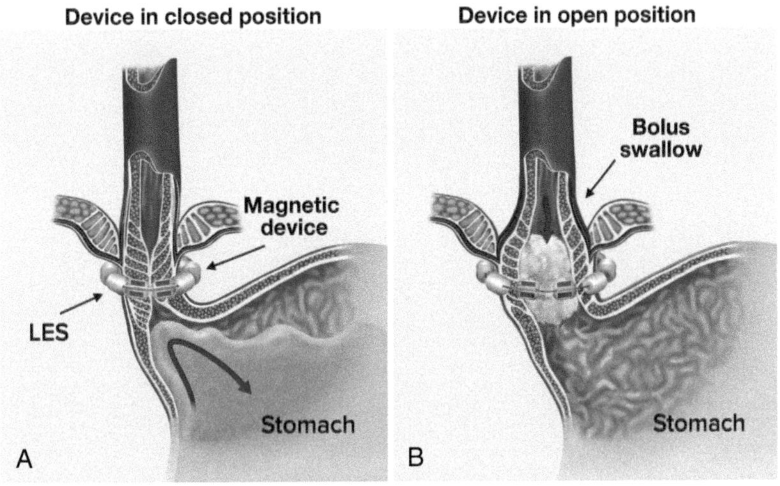

FIG 24.7 Diagrammatic representation of the LINX device (Torax Medical, Shoreview, MN) **A,** in the closed position (providing baseline resistance to reflux of gastric contents) and **B,** in the open position (accommodating for the passage of ingested material into the stomach). *LES,* lower esophageal sphincter. (From Ganz RA, Edmundowicz SA, Taiganides PA, et al: Long-term outcomes of patients receiving a magnetic sphincter augmentation device for gastroesophageal reflux. *Clin Gastroenterol Hepatol* 14[5]:671–677, 2016.)

to surgery, including gas-bloat and dysphagia, occurred in 8.3% and 6% of patients, respectively, at five years.[119] These data are intriguing, but to date, no randomized controlled trials have been conducted comparing the device to traditional surgery or medical acid suppression. Current procedures have been conducted only in patients with small hiatal hernias (< 3 cm) and without esophageal dysmotility; therefore the data may not be generalizable, and it remains to be seen whether there is a specific patient for which this operation is ideal.

Emerging Treatments

As neither surgery nor PPIs satisfactorily treat all GERD patients, there remains a strong incentive to develop alternative therapies. Endoscopic therapy is highly effective for many complications of GERD, and remains appealing as a potential therapeutic avenue for treating GERD itself. Such therapy should be safe, effective, and easy to apply. Multiple endoscopically placed devices and sphincter augmentation injectates have been developed over the last several decades. However, these have been troubled by serious adverse events, and currently there are no such devices available for use.[120] The Stretta technique, which involves the delivery of radiofrequency energy across the LES via a balloon-based array, has been advocated by surgical societies.[121] However, the data supporting such an approach are mixed. The exact mechanism by which this treats GERD patients is unclear, but is thought to be through a combination of provoking a local fibrotic process and disrupting the neural feedback pathway to blunt the noxious sensory response. Unfortunately, a systematic review and meta-analysis demonstrated no significant change in LES pressure, need for PPI use, or occurrence of GERD symptoms overall.[122]

An alternative approach has been to endoscopically recreate an antireflux barrier. Two endoscopic fundoplication devices are undergoing development and study. The concept of endoscopic suturing dates to the 1980s, but has improved over time. TIF has yielded equivocal results. This technique uses a device that is advanced over an endoscope into the stomach. It is composed of several components that bring gastric tissue into abutment with the esophageal lumen, after which H-shaped fasteners are deployed to create a valve-shaped antireflux barrier (Fig. 24.8).[123] Use of this device is associated with temporary improvements in pH scores, but its durability is less clear.[124] Importantly, a randomized controlled trial comparing TIF to PPIs did show improvement in regurgitation symptoms.[125] The patients selected were highly restricted, and could not have a hiatal hernia larger than 2 cm. Nonetheless, regurgitation is the main symptom that would otherwise prompt surgical fundoplication and, although these data need to be replicated, TIF might be a potential future substitute for laparoscopic fundoplication in some patients. Fewer data are available for another endoscopic fundoplication system that uses ultrasound guidance for the deployment of an endostapler. A relatively small study did demonstrate improvement in symptom scores and the need for PPIs, but these data only reflected a short follow-up interval.[126] Endoscopic fundoplication is an exciting prospect, but currently only preliminary data exist, and these need to be recreated and demonstrated over a longer timeframe prior to more widespread use of either of these techniques.

In the future, additional therapeutic options may include surgically implanted electronic LES pacing with the EndoStim system (EndoStim, The Hague, Netherlands). Although no randomized control trial data are available yet, there are uncontrolled data to support improvement in symptoms and a decreased need for medical therapy.[127] This approach has the possible advantages of having a minimal impact on the underlying anatomy and potentially being reversible.

Treatment Summary

The primary and initial long-term treatment modality for patients with GERD is acid suppression with a PPI at the lowest effective dose. However, some of these patients will be inadequately controlled, and alternative therapies can be considered. Antireflux surgery with laparoscopic fundoplication is a good alternative to medical therapy for those with volume regurgitation or intolerance to medications, but is otherwise not superior and comes with attendant complications, and should thus be reserved for patients who respond to PPIs. On the basis of current data,

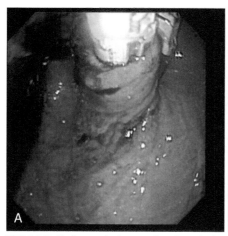
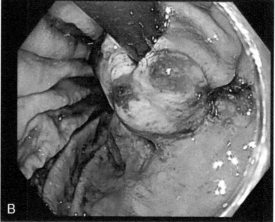

FIG 24.8 Endoscopic image **A,** taken during the creation of a transoral incisionless fundoplication. An over-the-endoscope device is attached and advanced into the stomach. Several components bring gastric tissue into abutment with the esophageal lumen, and a series of H-shaped fasteners are deployed to **B,** create a valve-shaped antireflux barrier. (Photos courtesy Kenneth J. Chang, MD.)

the use of the magnetic sphincter augmentation device appears to be an acceptable alternative to fundoplication in a highly-restricted cohort of patients with nonerosive disease and minimal hiatal herniation, though side effects may become a concern in the future. Future options for the treatment of GERD might include novel medical therapies and incorporate new technology to allow for the endoscopic creation or augmentation of antireflux barriers.

KEY REFERENCES

1. Vakil N, van Zanten SV, Kahrilas P, et al: The Montreal definition and classification of gastroesophageal reflux disease: a global evidence-based consensus, *Am J Gastroenterol* 101(8):1900–1920, 2006.
4. El-Serag HB, Sweet S, Winchester CC, Dent J: Update on the epidemiology of gastro-oesophageal reflux disease: a systematic review, *Gut* 63(6):871–880, 2014.
13. Mittal RK, Holloway RH, Penagini R, et al: Transient lower esophageal sphincter relaxation, *Gastroenterology* 109(2):601–610, 1995.
17. Schey R, Dickman R, Parthasarathy S, et al: Sleep deprivation is hyperalgesic in patients with gastroesophageal reflux disease, *Gastroenterology* 133(6):1787–1795, 2007.
19. Bredenoord AJ, Weusten BL, Timmer R, Smout AJ: Intermittent spatial separation of diaphragm and lower esophageal sphincter favors acidic and weakly acidic reflux, *Gastroenterology* 130(2):334–340, 2006.
22. Boeckxstaens G, El-Serag HB, Smout AJ, Kahrilas PJ: Symptomatic reflux disease: the present, the past and the future, *Gut* 63(7):1185–1193, 2014.
28. Zhang X, Geboes K, Depoortere I, et al: Effect of repeated cycles of acute esophagitis and healing on esophageal peristalsis, tone, and length, *Am J Physiol Gastrointest Liver Physiol* 288(6):G1339–G1346, 2005.
30. Avidan B, Sonnenberg A, Schnell TG, Sontag SJ: Acid reflux is a poor predictor for severity of erosive reflux esophagitis, *Dig Dis Sci* 47(11):2565–2573, 2002.
37. Katz PO, Gerson LB, Vela MF: Guidelines for the diagnosis and management of gastroesophageal reflux disease, *Am J Gastroenterol* 108(3):308–328, quiz 329, 2013.
38. Numans ME, Lau J, de Wit NJ, Bonis PA: Short-term treatment with proton-pump inhibitors as a test for gastroesophageal reflux disease, *Ann Intern Med* 140(7):518–527, 2004.
39. Saleh CM, Smout AJ, Bredenoord AJ: The diagnosis of gastro-esophageal reflux disease cannot be made with barium esophagograms, *Neurogastroenterol Motil* 27(2):195–200, 2015.

41. Moayyedi P, Talley NJ, Fennerty MB, Vakil N: Can the clinical history distinguish between organic and functional dyspepsia? *JAMA* 295(13):1566–1576, 2006.
48. Vaezi MF, Richter JE, Stasney CR, et al: Treatment of chronic posterior laryngitis with esomeprazole, *Laryngoscope* 116(2):254–260, 2006.
50. Muthusamy VR, Lightdale JR, Acosta RD, et al: The role of endoscopy in the management of GERD, *Gastrointest Endosc* 81(6):1305–1310, 2015.
57. Lundell LR, Dent J, Bennett JR, et al: Endoscopic assessment of oesophagitis: clinical and functional correlates and further validation of the Los Angeles classification, *Gut* 45(2):172–180, 1999.
69. Wong WM, Bautista J, Dekel R, et al: Feasibility and tolerability of transnasal/per-oral placement of the wireless pH capsule vs. traditional 24-h oesophageal pH monitoring–a randomized trial, *Aliment Pharmacol Ther* 21(2):155–163, 2005.
74. Sifrim D, Castell D, Dent J, Kahrilas PJ: Gastro-oesophageal reflux monitoring: review and consensus report on detection and definitions of acid, non-acid, and gas reflux, *Gut* 53(7):1024–1031, 2004.
86. Ates F, Yuksel ES, Higginbotham T, et al: Mucosal impedance discriminates GERD from non-GERD conditions, *Gastroenterology* 148(2):334–343, 2015.
87. Ness-Jensen E, Hveem K, El-Serag H, Lagergren J: Lifestyle intervention in gastroesophageal reflux disease, *Clin Gastroenterol Hepatol* 14(2):175–182.e3, 2016.
96. Dickman R, Boaz M, Aizic S, et al: Comparison of clinical characteristics of patients with gastroesophageal reflux disease who failed proton pump inhibitor therapy versus those who fully responded, *J Neurogastroenterol Motil* 17(4):387–394, 2011.
98. Laine L, Nagar A: Long-term PPI use: balancing potential harms and documented benefits, *Am J Gastroenterol* 111(7):913–915, 2016.
101. Kahrilas PJ, McColl K, Fox M, et al: The acid pocket: a target for treatment in reflux disease? *Am J Gastroenterol* 108(7):1058–1064, 2013.
110. Spechler SJ, Lee E, Ahnen D, et al: Long-term outcome of medical and surgical therapies for gastroesophageal reflux disease, *JAMA* 285(18):2331–2338, 2001.
115. Wileman SM, McCann S, Grant AM, et al: Medical versus surgical management for gastro-oesophageal reflux disease (GORD) in adults, *Cochrane Database Syst Rev* (3):CD003243, 2010.
117. Ganz RA, Peters JH, Horgan S, et al: Esophageal sphincter device for gastroesophageal reflux disease, *N Engl J Med* 368(8):719–727, 2013.

A complete reference list can be found online at ExpertConsult .com

25

Barrett's Esophagus: Diagnosis, Surveillance, and Medical Management

Gary W. Falk and Sachin Wani

INTRODUCTION

Barrett's esophagus (BE) is an acquired condition resulting from severe esophageal mucosal injury. It is unclear why some patients with gastroesophageal reflux disease (GERD) develop BE whereas others do not. The diagnosis of BE is established if the squamocolumnar junction is displaced more than 1 cm proximal to the esophagogastric junction, and intestinal metaplasia is detected by biopsy.[1] BE would be of little importance if not for its well-recognized association with esophageal adenocarcinoma (EAC). The incidence of EAC continues to increase, and the 5-year survival rate for this cancer remains very poor.[2] However, the overall disease burden of esophageal cancer and cancer risk for an individual patient with BE remains low.

Current strategies for improved survival in patients with EAC focus on cancer detection at an early and potentially curable stage. Early detection can be accomplished either by screening more patients for BE, or with endoscopic surveillance of patients with known BE. However, current screening and surveillance strategies are inherently expensive, inefficient, and of unproven benefit. New techniques to improve the efficiency of cancer surveillance continue to evolve and hold promise to change clinical practice in the future. Treatment options include aggressive acid suppression, antireflux surgery, and chemoprevention with endoscopic eradication therapy reserved for patients with dysplasia or early EAC.

EPIDEMIOLOGY

The incidence of BE has increased markedly since the 1970s. This increase was previously thought to be due to the increased use of diagnostic upper endoscopy combined with the change in the definition of BE to include shorter segments of columnar-lined epithelium. However, more recent data from a Northern Ireland population based study found that the incidence of BE has increased from 23.9/100,000 between 1993 and 1997 to 62.0/100,000 between 2002 and 2005.[3] These findings have also been encountered in the Netherlands and Australia.[4,5]

It is estimated that BE is found in approximately 5% to 15% of patients undergoing endoscopy for symptoms of GERD. Population-based studies suggest that the prevalence of BE is approximately 1.3% to 1.6%.[6] Interestingly, most of these patients in the general population have short segments of BE, and approximately 45% have no reflux symptoms. The prevalence of BE in white men increases with age until a plateau is reached at approximately age 50.[7]

Various risk factors have been identified for the presence of BE, including frequent and long-standing reflux episodes, erosive esophagitis, smoking, male gender, white race, older age, central obesity, absence of *H. pylori* infection and absence of statin use.[8–13] Familial aggregation of BE is seen in less than 10% of patients with BE and is felt to be caused by an incompletely penetrant autosomal dominant genetic variant.[14] Genome wide association studies have also identified several candidate susceptibility loci for BE.[15]

DIAGNOSIS

BE is currently best defined as a metaplastic change in the lining of the tubular esophagus extending more than 1 cm above the gastroesophageal junction with biopsy confirmation of intestinal metaplasia.[1] Endoscopically, this metaplastic change is characterized by displacement of the squamocolumnar junction proximal to the esophagogastric junction defined by the proximal margin of gastric folds (Fig. 25.1). At the time of endoscopy, landmarks should be carefully identified, including the diaphragmatic pinch, the esophagogastric junction as best defined by the proximal margin of the gastric folds seen on partial insufflation of the

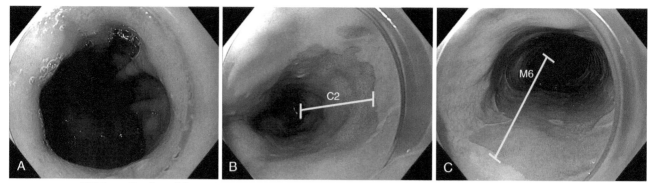

FIG 25.1 Grading of Barrett's esophagus using Prague criteria. **A,** Identification of gastroesophageal junction (top of the gastric folds); **B,** defining the circumferential extent; and **C,** maximal extent of the columnar lined esophagus.

esophagus, and level of the squamocolumnar junction. It is commonly accepted that the proximal margin of the gastric folds is the most useful landmark for the junction of the stomach and the esophagus.[16] However, the precise junction of the esophagus and the stomach may be difficult to determine endoscopically because of the presence of a hiatal hernia, the presence of inflammation, and the dynamic nature of the esophagogastric junction, all of which may make targeting of biopsy specimens problematic.

Endoscopists identify landmarks necessary for the diagnosis of the columnar-lined esophagus inconsistently (see Fig. 25.1)[17]; this leads to inconsistencies in the diagnosis of BE. The Prague classification was developed to standardize the description of BE. This classification scheme describes the circumferential extent (C value) and maximum extent (M value) of columnar mucosa above the proximal margin of the gastric folds (see Fig. 25.1).[18] The Prague classification does not include columnar islands; however, reliability coefficients for both criteria for segments greater than 1 cm in length, as well as for other endoscopic landmarks, including the diaphragmatic hiatus and proximal margin of the gastric folds, are excellent. Recognition of less than 1 cm of columnar metaplasia even with this scoring system is still problematic, pointing out the difficulties in measuring such short segments. The Prague classification has been validated in clinical settings in North America, Europe, and Asia.[19–21]

If the squamocolumnar junction is 1 cm or more above the level of the esophagogastric junction, as defined by the proximal margin of the gastric folds using partial insufflation, biopsy specimens should be obtained for confirmation of intestinal metaplasia. There is ongoing debate regarding the need for intestinal metaplasia for the diagnosis of BE. The professional societies of North America all require intestinal metaplasia for the diagnosis of BE, whereas the British Society of Gastroenterology does not require the presence of intestinal metaplasia for the diagnosis.[22] Although one study suggested that nongoblet cell columnar metaplasia shows DNA content abnormalities indicative of neoplastic risk similar to neoplasia encountered in intestinal metaplasia, a large population based study from Northern Ireland found that the risk of EAC was higher in patients with intestinal metaplasia than in those without.[23,24]

How many biopsy specimens are needed to detect intestinal metaplasia? Detection of intestinal metaplasia is related to several factors, including location of biopsies, length of columnar-lined segment, number of biopsy specimens obtained, male gender, and increasing age.[25,26] Intestinal metaplasia is more commonly found in biopsy specimens obtained in the proximal portion of the columnar-lined esophagus where goblet cell density is also greater.[27] Data suggests that the detection of intestinal metaplasia increases with increasing number of biopsy specimens per endoscopy; four biopsy specimens have a yield of 34.7%, whereas eight biopsy specimens have a yield of 94% for intestinal metaplasia.[28] Taking more than eight biopsy specimens does not seem to enhance the yield of intestinal metaplasia. This has led the current iteration of the American College of Gastroenterology Barrett's Esophagus (ACG BE) guidelines to suggest obtaining a minimum of eight biopsies to maximize the yield of intestinal metaplasia.[1]

It may be difficult to determine endoscopically where the esophagus ends and the stomach begins for the reasons outlined earlier. It is impossible to reliably distinguish columnar metaplasia of the distal esophagus from columnar metaplasia of the stomach. All current practice guidelines and quality metrics recommend that biopsy specimen of the normal squamocolumnar junction should not be routinely obtained in clinical practice if it is at the level of the esophagogastric junction.[29] Several studies indicate that cancer risk of intestinal metaplasia of the normal gastroesophageal junction is substantially lower compared to those with BE and thus that routine biopsies should not be obtained.[30,31]

SCREENING

Only 5% to 7% of patients newly diagnosed with EAC have undergone endoscopy and received a prior diagnosis of BE.[32,33] As such, surveillance of patients with BE would be expected to have limited impact on the 95% of EAC patients who are not known to have BE. One potential strategy to decrease the mortality rate of EAC is to identify more patients at risk, namely those with BE. Population-based studies suggest that in patients with newly diagnosed EAC, a prior endoscopy and diagnosis of BE are associated with both early stage cancer and improved survival.[34] Current professional society practice guidelines now all recommend considering screening for BE in selected patients at high risk for BE. The target population includes patients with chronic GERD symptoms and one or more risk factors including male gender, age over 50 years, Caucasian ethnicity, central obesity, and a positive family history of BE or EAC.[1,22,35,36]

High-definition white light endoscopy (HD-WLE) with biopsy is still the only validated technique to diagnose BE. However, it has clear limitations as a screening tool, including cost, risk, complexity, and diagnostic inconsistencies. For example, a 2014 study found that only 68% of patients diagnosed with BE in the community had confirmed BE, whereas the remainder had the diagnosis of BE reversed due to the absence of a columnar lined esophagus, intestinal metaplasia, or both.[37] If screening with endoscopy and biopsy were applied to the estimated 20% of the population with regular GERD symptoms, the cost implications would be staggering. Unsedated upper endoscopy using small-caliber instruments still has the potential to change the economics of endoscopic screening because this technique may decrease sedation-related complications and costs. Unsedated small-caliber endoscopy detects BE and dysplasia with sensitivity comparable to conventional endoscopy.[38] Although both procedures are well tolerated by patients, a major hurdle for unsedated endoscopy is continued patient resistance to undergoing a test without sedation. Otherwise, there are still no validated alternative techniques to screen for BE that overcome the cost and risks associated with conventional upper endoscopy.

There is clearly a need to develop either a better profile of patients at high risk for BE or a far less expensive tool to provide mass population screening. A variety of risk prediction models have been studied to accomplish this by examining risk factors such as frequency and duration of GERD symptoms, age, smoking, waist to hip ratio, *H. pylori* status, and inflammatory cytokines.[39,40] Models that include variables in addition to GERD frequency show encouraging performance characteristics but need further validation prior to application into clinical practice.

A variety of alternatives to both sedated and unsedated endoscopy are also now under investigation around the world. Much interest is directed at a nonendoscopic Cytosponge currently undergoing clinical trials. This Cytosponge capsule, administered by a nonphysician in an outpatient setting, had a sensitivity of 80% for BE and a specificity of 92% in a United Kingdom trial.[41] Another nonendoscopic device under study is tethered endomicroscopy, but data to date are limited.[42] Exciting new screening strategies based on the microbiome and exhaled volatile organic compounds are also under study.[43,44]

After a normal initial upper endoscopy, some clinicians wonder if a repeat screening upper endoscopy should be undertaken in symptomatic GERD patients at a later date. Several studies have addressed this point with consistent results. In patients with nonerosive reflux disease at the index endoscopy, BE is rarely found if the repeat endoscopy is performed within 5 years.[45,46] BE may be present in 9% to 12% of patients with erosive esophagitis at the time of index endoscopy, and higher grades of esophagitis are associated with a higher case finding rate of BE on repeat endoscopy.[47,48] Screening for BE in GERD patients should take place only after initial therapy with a proton pump inhibitor (PPI). A negative endoscopy at baseline makes it highly unlikely to find BE if endoscopy is repeated.

There are still no data from randomized controlled trials or observational studies to evaluate the strategy of screening. A decision analysis model by Inadomi et al (2009) examined screening of 50-year-old white men with chronic GERD symptoms for BE and found that one-time screening is probably cost-effective if subsequent surveillance is limited to patients with dysplasia on initial examination.[49] This strategy would result in a cost of $10,440 per quality-adjusted life year saved compared with a strategy of no screening or surveillance. Other modeling studies support screening in patients with chronic GERD symptoms as well, but only if the following conditions are met: patients at high risk for BE, high-grade dysplasia (HGD), or EAC; high sensitivity and specificity of endoscopy with biopsy; and little sensitivity and specificity of endoscopy with biopsy; and little

or no reduction in quality of life with esophagectomy.[50,51] Any variation of these ideal conditions quickly made this strategy cost-ineffective. Problems inherent in showing the utility of a screening program, such as healthy volunteer bias, lead time bias, and length time bias, all need to be addressed.

SURVEILLANCE

Rationale for Surveillance

Current practice guidelines recommend endoscopic surveillance of patients with BE in an attempt to detect cancer at an early and potentially curable stage.[1,22,52] Numerous observational studies suggest that patients with BE in whom EAC was detected in a surveillance program have their cancers detected at an earlier stage with markedly improved 5-year survival compared with similar patients not undergoing routine surveillance.[53-57] Because survival in EAC is stage-dependent, these studies suggest that survival may be enhanced by endoscopic surveillance. Several decision-analysis models support the concept of endoscopic surveillance.[49,58] Four recent population-based studies (2013–16) evaluated the impact of surveillance in patients with BE. A large Northern Ireland population-based study showed that in patients with EAC and a prior diagnosis of BE, survival was improved and tumor stage and grade was lower compared with patients without a prior diagnosis of BE.[33] Similarly, a large Dutch population-based study confirmed survival advantage for EAC in patients who were in surveillance programs compared with patients who were not a part of surveillance programs.[59] A cohort study of patients with BE diagnosed in the National Veterans Affairs hospitals showed that surveillance endoscopy was associated with an early stage diagnosis of EAC, longer survival, and decreased overall and cancer-related mortality.[60] On the other hand, a case-control study from the Northern California Kaiser Permanente population found no evidence that endoscopic surveillance improved survival from EAC.[61] Despite the variable results and lack of data from randomized controlled trials comparing surveillance versus no surveillance (not likely to be performed in the future), surveillance of BE patients is recommended.

Candidates for Endoscopic Surveillance

Patients with documented BE are candidates for surveillance. Before entering a surveillance program, patients should be advised about risks and benefits, including the limitations of surveillance endoscopy and the importance of adhering to appropriate surveillance intervals.[1] Other considerations include age, likelihood of survival over the next 5 years, and ability to tolerate either endoscopic/surgical interventions or medical/radiation oncologic treatments for EAC.

Surveillance Technique

The aim of surveillance is to detect dysplasia. The revised Vienna classification for gastrointestinal (GI) mucosal neoplasia and the World Health Organization (WHO) classification of GI tumors are the most commonly utilized grading systems to categorize patients with and without dysplasia in BE.[62,63] Dysplasia is described as negative for dysplasia, indefinite for dysplasia, low-grade dysplasia (LGD), HGD, and carcinoma. Active inflammation makes it more difficult to distinguish dysplasia from reparative changes. It is essential that surveillance endoscopy is performed only after any active inflammation related to GERD is controlled with antisecretory therapy. The presence of ongoing erosive esophagitis is a contraindication to performing surveillance biopsies. Current guidelines suggest obtaining systematic four-quadrant biopsies at 2-cm intervals along the entire length of the Barrett's segment after inflammation related to GERD is controlled.[1] A systematic biopsy protocol clearly detects more dysplasia and early EAC compared with ad hoc random biopsies.[64] The "turn and suction" technique allows acquisition of biopsy specimens that are significantly larger than the specimens obtained by the traditional techniques of advancing an open biopsy forceps into the lumen and then closing it to obtain the biopsy sample.[65] The safety of systematic endoscopic biopsy protocols has been demonstrated.[66] Separate biopsies of subtle mucosal abnormalities, no matter how trivial, such as ulceration, erosion, plaque, nodule, stricture, or other luminal irregularity in the BE segment should be performed, given the association of such lesions with underlying cancer.[67] Patients with mucosal abnormalities should undergo endoscopic mucosal resection (EMR). EMR will change the diagnosis in approximately 50% of patients when compared with endoscopic biopsies, given the larger tissue sample available for review, and will result in an improvement in interobserver agreement among pathologists.[68,69] The role of wide-area transepithelial sampling using a minimally invasive brush biopsy technique for acquiring wide-area sampling of BE followed by computer-assisted analysis needs to be further elucidated in future trials.[70]

Surveillance Intervals

Surveillance intervals are determined by the presence and grade of dysplasia and based on expert opinion given the limited understanding of the biology of EAC. Current guidelines recommend surveillance endoscopy at 3 to 5 year intervals in patients with BE without dysplasia given the low risk of progression of BE to EAC.[1,22,24,52,71,72] In BE patients diagnosed with LGD, the diagnosis of LGD should be confirmed by an expert GI pathologist given the significant interobserver variability among pathologists.[73] Patients in whom the diagnosis of LGD is downgraded to nondysplastic BE should be managed as nondysplastic BE. In patients with confirmed LGD, repeat upper endoscopy using HD-WLE should be performed under maximal acid suppression in 8 to 12 weeks. Surveillance biopsies should be performed in a 4-quadrant fashion every 1 to 2 cm with targeted biopsies from visible lesions. Ideally, EMR should be performed in patients with endoscopically visible lesions (no matter how subtle). In patients with confirmed BE with LGD that persists on a second endoscopy, risks and benefits of management options of endoscopic eradication therapy and ongoing surveillance should be discussed and documented. Patients with LGD undergoing surveillance rather than endoscopic eradication therapy should undergo surveillance every 6 months (×2), then annually unless there is reversion to BE without dysplasia.[73] If HGD is found, the diagnosis should first be confirmed by an expert GI pathologist. EMR should be performed if a visible lesion is identified. If HGD is confirmed, endoscopic eradication therapy is recommended.

Limitations of Surveillance

As currently practiced, endoscopic surveillance of BE has numerous shortcomings. Dysplasia and early EAC may be endoscopically indistinguishable from BE without dysplasia. The distribution of dysplasia and early EAC is highly focal and variable, and even the most thorough biopsy surveillance program has the potential for sampling errors. Current surveillance programs are expensive

and time-consuming. Although survey data indicate that surveillance is widely practiced, there is considerable variability in the technique and interval of surveillance and practice guidelines are not widely followed in the community.[74–77] In addition, there is significant interobserver and intraobserver variability among community and expert pathologists in the interpretation of dysplasia.[68,78–80]

Potential Strategies to Enhance Surveillance
Uniform Grading Systems

For patients with BE, standardized reporting and grading systems such as the Prague C&M criteria based on the circumferential (C) and (M) extent of the columnar-lined esophagus should be utilized. This system has been extensively validated among experts, nonexperts and trainees.[18,20] All visible lesions identified within the Barrett's segment should be recorded using the Paris classification; protruded lesions are recorded as: 0-Ip (pedunculated) or 0-Is (sessile) and flat lesions are recorded as: 0-IIa (superficially elevated), 0-IIb (flat), 0-IIc (superficially depressed), and 0-III (excavated). Lesions classified as 0-Is, 0-IIc, and 0-III are most likely to harbor invasive cancer, whereas 0-IIa and 0-IIb are unlikely to contain invasive cancer (Fig. 25.2).[81] However, the use of the Paris classification as a prognostic tool has not been extensively evaluated in Barrett's related neoplasia. The use of uniform grading systems such as the Prague and Paris criteria help improve communication between endoscopists during endoscopic follow-up and potentially in predicting the presence of invasive cancer and considering endoscopic therapies in appropriate candidates.

Cognitive Knowledge, Learning Curves, and Training

The cognitive knowledge regarding endoscopic appearance of subtle lesions during surveillance endoscopy is critical. These are lesions that harbor esophageal neoplasia at an early stage and are amenable to early, minimally invasive therapies. The appearance of subtle lesions varies widely and can include slight polypoid protrusion or nodularity, ulceration, areas of depression, superficial plaques, or mucosal discoloration. It is important to spend adequate time during upper endoscopy to detect subtle lesions. It has been suggested that inspecting the Barrett's segment for more than one minute per centimeter length of BE is associated with detection of more patients with suspicious lesions, with a trend toward a higher detection rate of HGD or EAC.[82] These findings need to be validated in future studies, especially in low-risk populations undergoing surveillance endoscopy. There are limited data on the learning curves and impact of training in the detection of early neoplasia (with or without advanced imaging techniques). A 2015 study showed that endoscopists trained in BE surveillance (training in Prague classification, Seattle protocol biopsy technique, and lesion detection) with dedicated time slots or lists had higher dysplasia detection rates than a nontrained/specialist cohort.[83] Recent studies have also demonstrated that endoscopists at community hospitals detect neoplastic lesions at a significantly lower rate compared to endoscopists at expert centers.[84,85] These data suggest that surveillance should be performed by trained endoscopists in dedicated endoscopy blocks.

Imaging Modalities to Enhance Surveillance

Several imaging modalities have been investigated to improve detection and identification of patients with early neoplastic lesions during routine screening and surveillance endoscopy

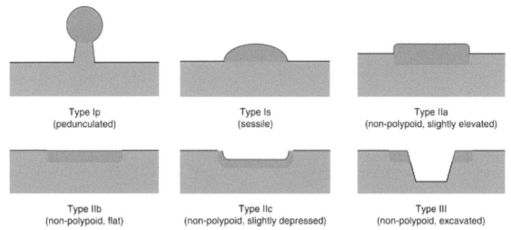

FIG 25.2 Paris Classification for Gastrointestinal Neoplasia. (Modified from Endoscopic Classification Review Group: the Paris endoscopic classification of superficial neoplastic lesions: esophagus, stomach, and colon: November 30 to December 1, 2002. *Gastrointest Endosc* 58[6]: S3–S43, 2003.)

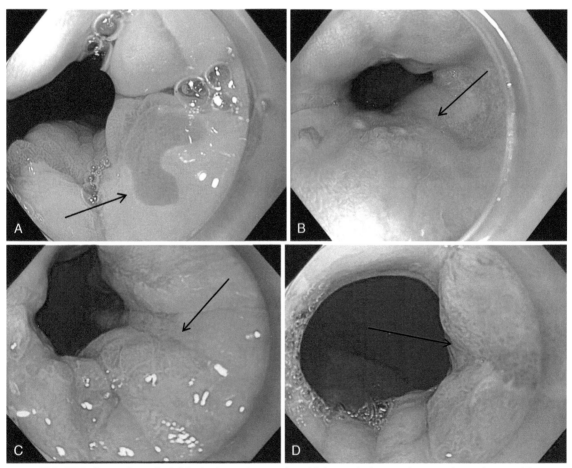

FIG 25.3 Examples of visible lesions detected at high resolution endoscopy in patients with Barrett's esophagus (*arrows* pointing to the visible lesions within the Barrett's segment).

and prediction of histology and real-time diagnosis during endoscopy.

High-definition white light endoscopy. Technologic advancements have allowed the creation of smaller charge-coupled device chips that are capable of producing images with high resolution (over 850,000 to 2.1 million pixels) displayed on monitors with a 16:9 aspect ratio and resulting in superior imaging quality compared to standard definition (SD) WLE. High definition magnification endoscopes can optically magnify images up to 150 times (not available in the United States).[86] The use of HD-WLE should be considered the standard of care and the first critical step in the evaluation of BE patients undergoing surveillance or being considered for endoscopic eradication therapies (Fig. 25.3).[87] Although there is no level 1 evidence in the form of a randomized controlled trial comparing HD-WLE to SD-WLE, this recommendation has been endorsed by guidelines and consensus documents.[22,52,88] Indirect evidence from three prospective trials and a single retrospective study suggests that HD-WLE is more sensitive compared to SD-WLE in the detection of Barrett's related neoplasia.[89–92]

Optical electronic chromoendoscopy. This diagnostic modality provides enhanced visualization of the mucosa using light filters and computer processing technology without the need to spray dye. There are three available platforms for optical chromoendoscopy: narrow band imaging (NBI; Olympus, Center Valley, PA), Fujinon intelligent color enhancement (FICE; Fujinon, Wayne, NJ), and i-Scan (Pentax Medical, Montvale, NJ). NBI is an imaging technique that is based on the optical phenomenon that the depth of light penetration into tissue depends on the wavelength; the shorter the wavelength, the more superficial the penetration. Use of blue light with narrow band filters enables detailed imaging of the mucosal and vascular surface patterns with a high level of resolution and contrast without the need for chromoendoscopy.[93] FICE and i-Scan use proprietary post-image acquisition processing technology to modify the white light image, enhancing the superficial mucosal and vascular pattern. Optical chromoendoscopy is easy to use, utilizes "push button" technology, and frequently used as an adjunctive tool to HD-WLE (although the additional benefit in some situations has been debated).

NBI is the most widely studied electronic chromoendoscopy technique and has been evaluated as a tool to predict histology during surveillance, improve detection of dysplasia, and guide endoscopic eradication therapies. Characteristic patterns associated with nondysplastic BE (regular mucosal and vascular pattern) and BE with early neoplasia (irregular mucosal and vascular pattern) have been described using NBI (Figs. 25.4 and 25.5).[94,95] However, no standardized classification system for BE exists. In a 2016 study, an international working group of experts established a classification system (regular vs. irregular mucosal and vascular pattern based on NBI features; Table 25.1) that had an overall accuracy rate of 85.4% (95% confidence interval [CI] 82.6%–87.9%) with higher accuracy rates in images where the endoscopist had a high confidence diagnosis (92.2% [95% CI 89.3%–94.5%]). The overall strength of interobserver agreement was substantial ($\kappa = 0.68$).[96] A prospective tandem study that compared HD-NBI targeted biopsy with SD-WLE targeted with random biopsy showed that NBI increased the per-patient yield of dysplasia, identified higher grades of dysplasia, and required fewer biopsies.[89] This classification system requires external validation among nonexperts and trainees during real-time endoscopy or using video-based assessment. A recent, randomized, multicenter study comparing NBI to HD-WLE demonstrated a comparable detection rate of intestinal metaplasia and early neoplasia with fewer biopsies required in the NBI arm.[96a] In contrast, a 2013 systematic review and meta-analysis showed that advanced imaging techniques

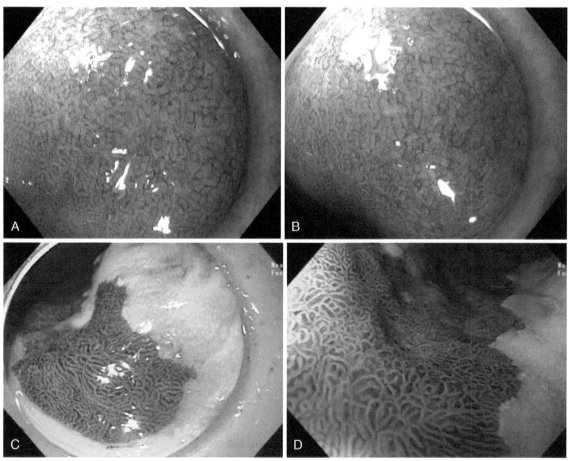

FIG 25.4 Detailed close (**A** and **B**) and overview imaging (**C** and **D**) using NBI demonstrating regular mucosal and vascular patterns in patients with nondysplastic Barrett's esophagus.

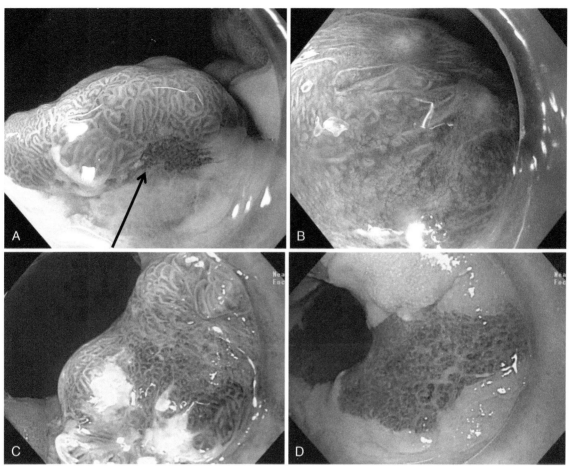

FIG 25.5 Examples of early neoplastic lesions demonstrating irregular mucosal and vascular patterns using NBI.

TABLE 25.1 Consensus-Driven NBI Classification for Identification of High-Grade Dysplasia and Esophageal Adenocarcinoma in Barrett's Esophagus

Morphologic Characteristics	Classification
Mucosal Pattern	
Circular, ridged/villous, or tubular patterns	Regular
Absent or irregular patterns	Irregular
Vascular Pattern	
Blood vessels situated regularly along or between mucosal ridges and/or those showing normal, long, branching patterns	Regular
Focally or diffusely distributed vessels not following normal architecture of the mucosa	Irregular

From Sharma P, Bergman JJ, Goda K, et al: Development and validation of a classification system to identify high-grade dysplasia and esophageal adenocarcinoma in Barrett's esophagus using narrow-band imaging. *Gastroenterology* 150(3):591–598, 2016.

(optical chromoendoscopy and chromoendoscopy) increased dysplasia or cancer detection by 34% (95% CI 20%–56%, $p < 0.0001$).[97]

Chromoendoscopy. Chromoendoscopy is a technique that involves the spraying of dyes to improve characterization of the mucosa resulting in selective uptake (vital staining: methylene blue, Lugol's solution) or enhancement of mucosal surface pattern (contrast staining: indigo carmine, acetic acid). It is frequently used in combination with high-resolution and high-magnification endoscopes.[93] A number of initial studies suggested that chromoendoscopy with magnification endoscopy reveals mucosal patterns that correlate with intestinal metaplasia and early neoplasia and may improve detection of the latter. However, a meta-analysis of nine studies concluded that chromoendoscopy with methylene blue did not increase the yield of detecting intestinal metaplasia and dysplasia compared to standard four-quadrant biopsies.[98] Problems associated with the use of chromoendoscopy in clinical practice include the need for dye spraying equipment, difficulty in achieving complete and uniform coating of the mucosal surface with the dye, inability to detect superficial vascular patterns, the time consuming nature of the procedure, conflicting published data, the need for magnification endoscopy, and lack of a standardized classification system. These issues have led to this technique being largely supplanted by optical chromoendoscopy.

Confocal laser endomicroscopy. Confocal laser endomicroscopy (CLE) is a technology that has the potential to provide real time histologic visualization of the GI tract. The probe-based system (pCLE) is available commercially with the most extensive published literature. This technology requires the injection of intravenous fluorescein and provides a 240 μm field of view with a range of depth of 55 to 65 μm. Studies have demonstrated

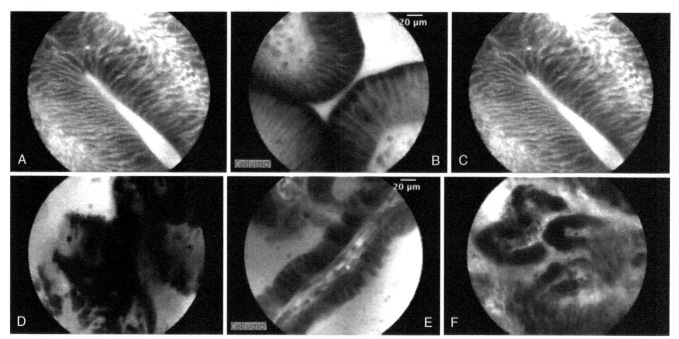

FIG 25.6 Representative images of confocal laser endomicroscopy in nondysplastic Barrett's esophagus (**A** to **C**) and Barrett's with high grade dysplasia (**D** to **F**).

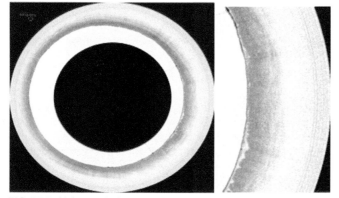

FIG 25.7 Volumetric laser endomicroscopy: second generation optical frequency domain imaging that provides high speed and high-resolution images of the entire Barrett's segment, 6 cm at a time, using a balloon imaging catheter.

an improved diagnostic yield for dysplasia in BE patients compared to standard four-quadrant biopsies (Fig. 25.6).[99,100] However, there are several issues with this technology that have limited its widespread adoption in routine clinical practice, such as sampling error associated with the small visual field, increased procedure time and possible decreased efficiency, associated equipment costs, as well as the inconclusive impact of pCLE findings on guiding endoscopic management.

Future emerging technologies. Volumetric laser endomicroscopy (VLE, optical frequency domain imaging) is an emerging broad-field imaging technology that provides high-speed real time high resolution images of the entire Barrett's segment (Fig. 25.7). It scans 6 cm of the esophagus over 90 seconds and provides a resolution of 10 μm and an imaging depth of 3 mm.[86,101] The safety and feasibility of this technology was demonstrated in a multicenter trial.[102] A revised scoring system for detection of

dysplasia in BE improved the overall diagnostic characteristics (sensitivity 86%, specificity 88%, and accuracy 87%) using EMR specimens.[103] In a 2017 study that utilized high-quality, ex vivo VLE-histology correlation, the VLE features independently and significantly associated with BE-related neoplasia included layering, surface signal, and irregular glands/ducts. A VLE prediction score for BE neoplasia was developed and validated, with receiver operating curve showing an area under curve of 0.81 (95% CI 0.71–0.90).[104] Future iterations of this device will incorporate laser marking to accurately sample abnormalities seen on imaging. In addition, objective measures such as computer-aided detection are currently being investigated to assist in HD-WLE and VLE and interpretation.[104,105]

High-resolution microendoscopy is a novel imaging modality that allows real-time epithelial imaging at subcellular resolution, and its use has been suggested in conjunction with red flag technologies.[106] Finally, the role of advanced imaging platforms that risk stratify BE patients using fluorescently labeled peptides or lectins needs to be evaluated in future studies.[107,108]

Current Status of Real-Time Imaging-Assisted Endoscopic Targeted Biopsy During Surveillance

The American Society for Gastrointestinal Endoscopy (ASGE) Preservation and Incorporation of Valuable Endoscopic Innovations (PIVI) document outlined performance thresholds for an imaging technology with targeted biopsies to eliminate the need for random biopsies during endoscopic surveillance of BE.[109] The established thresholds were as follows: (1) imaging technology with targeted biopsies should have a per-patient sensitivity of 90% or higher and a negative predictive value (NPV) of 98% or greater for detecting HGD or early EAC, compared with the current standard protocol; and (2) the imaging technology should have a specificity that is sufficiently high (80%) to allow a reduction in the number of biopsies (compared with random biopsies). A 2016 meta-analysis assessed the diagnostic characteristics of

BOX 25.1 Basic Principles and Practical Tips to Improve Detection of Subtle Lesions During Upper Endoscopy

Technical

1. Ensure that the procedure is performed under adequate sedation
2. Use of high-definition endoscopes is the minimum standard for adequate inspection
3. Clean the mucosa using water and/or mucolytic agent (e.g., N-acetylcysteine)
4. Spend adequate time for inspection during endoscopy and obtain multiple endoscopy images
5. Follow a systematic and meticulous approach during inspection
6. Carefully scrutinize the right side of the esophagus (12 to 6 o'clock position) during inspection of the Barrett's segment
7. Inspect gastric mucosa after adequate air insufflation in en-face and retroflexed views
8. Consider the use of a distal attachment cap
9. Clearly document landmarks, location of lesions and use standardized grading systems such as the Prague C&M criteria and Paris classification
10. Biopsies should be based on published guidelines (e.g. Seattle protocol for surveillance of Barrett's esophagus)

Cognitive

1. Knowledge of standardized grading systems
2. Training and familiarity of key signs for detecting early neoplasia
3. Training in the use of high-definition white light endoscopy and optical chromoendoscopy

TABLE 25.2 Current Status of Biomarkers for Diagnosis, Risk Stratification, and Prediction of Response to Therapy

Biomarker	Current Status
Trefoil factor 3 (TFF3)	• Phase 4 study showed significant promise for diagnosis
FISH	• Phase 3 and 4 studies showed promise for risk stratification, potential candidates studied alone or in combination [8q24 (C-MYC), 9p21 (p16), 17q12 (HER2), 17p13.1 (p53), 20q13, and ZNF217] • Phase 3 and 4 studies showed p16 loss and multiple gains to hold promise for prediction of response to therapy
DNA content abnormalities/ aneuploidy	• Useful for risk stratification, possibly a late biomarker • Somatic gene diversity can be quantified
Methylation	• Phase 2 studies show promise for diagnosis given the different methylation signatures between squamous and BE tissues (potential candidates – p16, RUNX3, MGMT, SFRP1, TIMP3, and CDH13 among others) • No dominant marker for risk stratification based on phase 3 and 4 studies
MicroRNA	• Phase 2 studies show promise for diagnosis (miRNAs – 192, -215, -194, -205, and -203 different between squamous and BE tissue) • No dominant miRNA for risk stratification
P53	• Only biomarker recommended to clarify histologic diagnosis of dysplasia • P53 mutational analysis feasible on cytologic specimens • Phase 4 data support use of p53 analysis for risk stratification • Not a predictor for response to therapy in a phase study
Clonal diversity	• Phase 2 studies suggest predictive ability
Proliferation markers	• Limited utility for risk stratification

BE, Barrett's esophagus; *FISH,* fluorescent in-situ hybridization.
From Bansal A, Fitzgerald RC: Biomarkers in Barrett's esophagus: role in diagnosis, risk stratification, and prediction of response to therapy. *Gastroenterol Clin North Am* 44(2):373–390, 2015.

chromoendoscopy using acetic acid and methylene blue, and electronic chromoendoscopy by using NBI and CLE for the detection of dysplasia.[110] This meta-analysis showed that targeted biopsies obtained by expert endoscopists using acetic acid chromoendoscopy (sensitivity 96.6%, NPV 98.3%, specificity 84.6%), NBI (sensitivity 94.2%, NPV 97.5%, specificity 94.4%) and CLE (sensitivity 90.4%, NPV 98.3%, specificity 92.7%) meet the thresholds set by the ASGE PIVI document. That being said, several challenges need to be addressed before these technologies can become part of routine clinical practice and include (1) establishing training programs for detection of early neoplasia that are acceptable and applicable to the broader gastroenterology community; (2) demonstrating that these results can also be obtained by nonexperts; (3) standardization of classification systems for advanced imaging techniques; and finally (4) to set quality indicators for image-guided target biopsies. Until these endpoints are achieved, endoscopists should follow the basic principles outlined in Box 25.1 for improving detection of early neoplasia in BE (see also Video 25.1).

Biomarkers of Increased Risk of Progression

Biomarkers have the potential to predict the risk of progression to cancer in patients with BE. The Early Detection Research Network, established by the National Cancer Institute, has defined five phases of biomarker development and validation analogous to phases of drug development.[111] To become a useful screening/risk-stratification tool, biomarkers must pass through each phase of research, starting at identification and culminating in an understanding of the impact of screening/surveillance on reducing the burden of disease in the population. Phase 1 involves identification of a biomarker (exploratory phase) followed by development of a clinical assay (phase 2). Phases 3 and 4 entail validation in retrospective and prospective studies, respectively.

This is followed by phase 5 studies that evaluate the impact of a biomarker on the population disease burden and primary outcomes, such as costs and mortality rates.[112] Although many biomarkers have been identified and evaluated in phase 3 and a few in phase 4 studies, none have progressed through and been validated in a phase 5 trial. Several biomarkers have been studied to improve the current risk stratification approach and identification of patients at the highest risk for progression. These include detection of DNA content abnormalities (aneuploidy or increased 4N fraction), mutation or loss of heterozygosity of the p53 and p16 genes, chromosomal abnormalities, and methylation-based biomarkers among others (Table 25.2).[112a–118] The use of biomarkers in clinical practice has been limited by a lack of prospective data, differences in reproducibility of results, cost, and complexity of testing: current US guidelines recommend against the use of individual or a panel of biomarkers.[35] An ideal biomarker or panel of biomarkers needs to be validated in prospective trials, be inexpensive, easily administered and accessible, and highly accurate in risk stratification (superior to the current gold standard of dysplasia grade on histology). The goal of identifying such a biomarker or panel of biomarkers ready for clinical application remains elusive.

Risk Stratification and Prediction Tools

Clinical and endoscopic predictors of progression. Advanced age and increasing length of the BE segment are known predictors for the presence and progression of BE to HGD/EAC.[71,119–122] A multicenter study that included 1175 patients with nondysplastic BE showed that the risk of progression to HGD/EAC increased with an increase in BE segment length (28% increase in risk for every 1-cm increase in BE length, $p = 0.01$). After adjusting for confounding variables, BE length was a significant predictor of progression with an odds ratio (OR) of 1.2 (95% CI 1.1–1.3).[122] Similarly, another prospective study of 713 patients with BE showed that for every 1 cm increase in BE length segment, the relative risk of progression to HGD/EAC was 1.11 (95% CI 1.01–1.2).[123] Presence of visible endoscopic lesions is a predictor for prevalent HGD/EAC and a risk factor for progression to EAC.[123–126]

Dysplasia and risk of progression. Currently, despite all the advances in the field of molecular markers to predict progression to EAC in patients with BE, dysplasia is used as the standard marker of progression risk. The progression of BE to EAC is believed to occur in a probabilistic manner through recognizable histologic steps of intestinal metaplasia, LGD, (HGD, intramucosal cancer, and finally, invasive EAC. Several contemporary studies have demonstrated a low rate of progression to EAC in patients with nondysplastic BE, and this estimate ranges from 0.1% to 0.3% per year.[71,72,127] Results from a multicenter study demonstrated that persistence of nondysplastic BE identifies patients who are at low risk for development of EAC.[128] These findings need to be reproduced in other larger cohorts before lengthening or discontinuation of surveillance can be recommended in patients with persistent nondysplastic BE. Variable rates of progression of LGD to endpoints of HGD/EAC and EAC alone have been reported with progression rates ranging from 0.4% to 13.4% per year.[73,126,129–141] These variable rates stem from inclusion of a relatively small number of patients with LGD in the vast majority of the studies, lack of expert or central pathology panel review which limited reliability of LGD diagnosis, variability in pathologic diagnosis of LGD, analyses not distinguishing prevalent from incident dysplasia, referral and selection bias, and limited endoscopic follow-up data, especially for survival analyses.[142,143] A systematic review and meta-analysis that included 24 studies with 2694 LGD patients reported a pooled annual incidence rate of 1.73% (95% CI 0.99%–2.47%) for the endpoint of HGD/EAC and 0.54% (95% CI 0.32%–0.76%) for EAC.[144] However, substantial heterogeneity in the results was a major limitation of this study. A noteworthy feature, as demonstrated in several studies, in the natural history data of LGD patients, is the phenomenon of regression where follow-up endoscopic biopsies after an initial diagnosis of LGD do not demonstrate LGD and the diagnosis is downgraded to nondysplastic BE.[126,140,141,145,146] The potential reasons for this phenomenon include interobserver variability among pathologists, sampling errors, misdiagnosis, removal of the dysplastic focus by biopsies, and perhaps even true regression of the dysplastic area. The diagnosis of HGD is associated with a high yearly rate of progression to EAC (approximately 7% based on a meta-analysis) making this an actionable diagnosis.[147] Two randomized controlled trials have reported even higher rates of progression to EAC in BE patients with HGD.[148,149]

Predictors of progression in patients with low-grade dysplasia. Review of pathology slides by an expert GI pathologist has been shown to "purify" the group of LGD patients by downgrading the vast majority of cases to nondysplastic BE. Studies have demonstrated that individuals with confirmed LGD (defined by confirmation of diagnosis by an expert GI pathologist or panel) are at a higher risk of progression to EAC and HGD/EAC.[130,134,150] In addition, patients with LGD confirmed by multiple pathologists instead of a single pathologist diagnosis may be associated with a higher risk of progression to HGD/EAC.[151,152] Persistent LGD (defined by the presence of LGD on two consecutive endoscopies) has also been identified as a risk factor for progression, or as a risk factor for failure to regress subsequently. A 2017 study showed that the number of pathologists confirming the diagnosis of LGD (OR 47.14, 95% CI 13.1–169.7 when all three pathologists agreed) and persistent LGD (OR 9.28, CI 4.39–19.64 for individual pathologists) were predictors associated with progression of LGD.[153] Similarly, another Dutch study showed a statistically significant difference in the rates of progression to HGD/EAC between cases with and without confirmed LGD (confirmed incidence rate: 5.18 [95% CI 3.63–7.19]/100 person-years vs. 1.85 [95% CI 1.52–2.22]/100 person-years, $p < 0.001$). Persistent LGD was the only independent risk factor for the development of HGD/EAC (hazard ratio [HR] 3.5, 95% CI 1.48–8.28).[154] Aside from pathologist confirmation of LGD and persistent LGD, no other factor appears to be reproducibly associated with progression.

Prediction models. There is growing interest in the development of risk-prediction models to identify patients with BE at risk for the development of HGD/EAC. Models described have incorporated demographic and clinical factors such as age, sex, smoking status, body mass index, waist:hip ratio, frequency of GERD, frequency of use of acid suppressive medications, and nonsteroidal antiinflammatory drugs (NSAIDs), along with endoscopic findings such as BE length, presence of nodularity in combination with histology, and relevant biomarkers.[116,155,156] Currently available models need to be validated prior to clinical application. Until clinically applicable biomarkers are available, there is significant interest in validating models that incorporate clinical, endoscopic, and histologic factors in risk stratification.

MANAGEMENT

Medical Therapy

Because BE has the most severe pathophysiologic abnormalities of GERD, PPIs are the cornerstone of medical therapy for BE. Studies show that PPIs consistently result in symptom relief and heal esophagitis in patients with BE.[157–159] However, even at high doses, PPIs result in either no regression of the Barrett's segment or modest regression that is of uncertain clinical importance.[160–162] PPIs typically increase squamous islands in the Barrett's segment, but biopsy specimens taken from such islands often show underlying intestinal metaplasia.[163]

Alleviation of reflux symptoms in BE is not equivalent to normalization of esophageal acid exposure, despite the use of high-dose PPI therapy. Persistent abnormal acid exposure is encountered in approximately 25% of patients with BE despite use of twice-daily PPIs.[164,165] The importance of complete control of esophageal acid exposure in patients with BE is unknown. A 2014 meta-analysis found that PPI use was associated with a reduction in the risk of EAC and/or HGD (OR 0.29; 95% CI

0.12–0.79).[166] Furthermore, longer duration of PPI use (> 2–3 years) was associated with a greater protective effect.

Antireflux Surgery

Antireflux surgery effectively alleviates GERD symptoms in patients with BE. The LOTUS randomized controlled trial that compared laparoscopic antireflux surgery to esomeprazole found that the outcome of laparoscopic antireflux surgery was similar in GERD patients with and without BE and comparable to use of esomeprazole for symptom control and quality of life measures, although antireflux surgery afforded better intraesophageal acid control.[167] The indications for surgery in patients with BE are the same as the indications for GERD patients without BE.

It has long been hypothesized that antireflux surgery provides protection from progression of BE to EAC. However, two randomized clinical trials found no attenuation of the risk for developing EAC in BE patients treated surgically compared with patients treated medically.[168,169] However a 2016 meta-analysis of surgical versus medical therapy of BE found that in a subgroup of four studies published after 2000, antireflux surgery was associated with a decreased risk of developing EAC when compared to medical therapy.[170] The best available evidence suggests that antireflux surgery has outcomes equivalent to medical therapy for symptom control in BE and surgery should not be chosen solely as an intervention to decrease cancer risk in BE patients.

Chemoprevention

Chemoprevention is a pharmacologic intervention for either the prevention of cancer or the treatment of identifiable precancerous lesions. Various chemoprevention agents have been proposed for patients with BE, including PPIs, NSAIDs, aspirin, lyophilized black raspberries, antioxidants, green tea, retinoids, ursodeoxycholic acid, statins, and curcumin.

Multiple observational studies suggest that NSAIDs, including aspirin, may play a protective role against BE by inhibiting the cyclooxygenase 1 and 2 enzymes, which regulate PGE_2 production. A 2012 pooled analysis of six population-based studies in the Barrett's and Esophageal Adenocarcinoma Consortium (BEACON) group examined the association between NSAID use and risk of EAC and found that when compared to nonusers, NSAID users had a reduced risk of EAC, and almost identical effects were seen for both aspirin and nonaspirin NSAIDs.[171] Furthermore, higher frequency and longer duration use were associated with a decreased risk of cancer in this study. A 2014 meta-analysis of nine observational studies likewise found that both aspirin and NSAIDs were associated with a decreased risk of HGD/EAC in BE patients.[172] Despite the consistent evidence from observational studies, limited clinical trial data are available to address this issue. A single clinical trial has examined the effect of celecoxib at a dose of 200 mg twice daily given for 48 weeks in patients with LGD/HGD on change in proportion of biopsy samples with dysplasia between patients treated with celecoxib compared to those treated with a placebo.[173] No differences were found between the two groups. A clinical trial of esomeprazole in conjunction with low and high dose aspirin found that only high dose aspirin (325 mg daily) was able to decrease mucosal PGE_2 content in mucosal biopsies from BE patients.[174] The results of a large randomized clinical trial in the United Kingdom (ASPECT) are awaited to see if chemoprevention with aspirin in conjunction with a PPI is a useful clinical strategy in BE patients. Currently, it is premature to use aspirin or NSAIDS for chemoprevention in BE patients.

> ## BOX 25.2 Relevant Quality Indicators Pertinent to the Diagnosis, Surveillance and Medical Management of Barrett's Esophagus
>
> 1. For patients in whom Barrett's esophagus (BE) is being considered, the squamocolumnar junction, the gastroesophageal junction, and the location of the diaphragmatic hiatus (if there is a hiatal hernia present) should be recorded on each endoscopy
> 2. If BE is suspected on an endoscopy, the endoscopist should document the extent of suspected BE using a standardized grading system (Prague criteria)
> 3. Inspection of the BE segment should be performed using high-definition white light endoscopy
> 4. Biopsies should be obtained in patients with suspected BE
> 5. The normal-appearing and normally located squamocolumnar junction should not be biopsied
> 6. In a patient with BE undergoing surveillance endoscopy, systematic biopsies should be obtained from every 1 to 2 cm in a four-quadrant fashion throughout the extent of the Barrett's segment
> 7. In a patient with BE undergoing surveillance endoscopy, biopsies from any visible lesion should be obtained and processed separately from the systematic biopsies
> 8. The diagnosis of dysplasia should be confirmed by an expert GI pathologist
> 9. If surveillance biopsies in a patient with BE show no evidence of dysplasia, surveillance endoscopy should be recommended in no sooner than 3 to 5 years

Statins, a class of drugs well known for cholesterol lowering effects, also have antiproliferative, proapoptotic, antiangiogenesis, and immunomodulatory effects which could provide chemoprevention potential in BE.[175] A systematic review and meta-analysis of five studies of Barrett's patients demonstrated a 43% reduction in the risk of progressing to the combined endpoints of HGD/adenocarcinoma after adjustment for potential confounders.[175] Taken together, these data suggest the potential for statins in chemoprevention of BE, but this has not yet been addressed in clinical trials.

QUALITY INDICATORS IN DIAGNOSIS AND MANAGEMENT

The recent shift from volume-based to value-based practice in the United States and variability in quality of care have provided the impetus for defining quality indicators in the diagnosis and management of patients with BE. The quality of health care delivered can be measured by comparing the performance of an individual or a group of individuals with an ideal or benchmark, and nonadherence to a quality indicator reflects suboptimal care. Three recent documents have addressed this important issue.[29,176,177] Relevant quality indicators pertinent to this chapter are highlighted in Box 25.2. Adherence to these quality indicators has the potential to improve quality of care, reduce variability in health care, and ultimately improve patient outcomes.

KEY REFERENCES

1. Shaheen NJ, Falk GW, Iyer PG, et al: ACG clinical guideline: diagnosis and management of barrett's esophagus, *Am J Gastroenterol* 111:30–50, 2016; quiz 51.
9. Cook MB, Shaheen NJ, Anderson LA, et al: Cigarette smoking increases risk of Barrett's esophagus: an analysis of the Barrett's and Esophageal Adenocarcinoma Consortium, *Gastroenterology* 142:744–753, 2012.

18. Sharma P, Dent J, Armstrong D, et al: The development and validation of an endoscopic grading system for Barrett's esophagus: the Prague C & M criteria, *Gastroenterology* 131:1392–1399, 2006.

22. Fitzgerald RC, di Pietro M, Ragunath K, et al: British Society of Gastroenterology guidelines on the diagnosis and management of Barrett's oesophagus, *Gut* 63:7–42, 2014.

35. American Gastroenterological Association, Spechler SJ, Sharma P, et al: American Gastroenterological Association medical position statement on the management of Barrett's esophagus, *Gastroenterology* 140:1084–1091, 2011.

39. Rubenstein JH, Morgenstern H, Appelman H, et al: Prediction of Barrett's esophagus among men, *Am J Gastroenterol* 108:353–362, 2013.

49. Inadomi JM, Sampliner R, Lagergren J, et al: Screening and surveillance for Barrett esophagus in high-risk groups: a cost-utility analysis, *Ann Intern Med* 138:176–186, 2003.

53. Corley DA, Levin TR, Habel LA, et al: Surveillance and survival in Barrett's adenocarcinomas: a population-based study, *Gastroenterology* 122:633–640, 2002.

59. Verbeek RE, Leenders M, Ten Kate FJ, et al: Surveillance of Barrett's esophagus and mortality from esophageal adenocarcinoma: a population-based cohort study, *Am J Gastroenterol* 109:1215–1222, 2014.

68. Wani S, Mathur SC, Curvers WL, et al: Greater interobserver agreement by endoscopic mucosal resection than biopsy samples in Barrett's dysplasia, *Clin Gastroenterol Hepatol* 8:783–788, 2010.

71. Wani S, Falk G, Hall M, et al: Patients with nondysplastic Barrett's esophagus have low risks for developing dysplasia or esophageal adenocarcinoma, *Clin Gastroenterol Hepatol* 9:220–227, 2011; quiz e26.

72. Hvid-Jensen F, Pedersen L, Drewes AM, et al: Incidence of adenocarcinoma among patients with Barrett's esophagus, *N Engl J Med* 365:1375–1383, 2011.

73. Wani S, Rubenstein JH, Vieth M, et al: Diagnosis and management of low-grade dysplasia in Barrett's esophagus: expert review from the Clinical Practice Updates Committee of the American Gastroenterological Association, *Gastroenterology* 151:822–835, 2016.

76. Abrams JA, Kapel RC, Lindberg GM, et al: Adherence to biopsy guidelines for Barrett's esophagus surveillance in the community setting in the United States, *Clin Gastroenterol Hepatol* 7:736–742, 2009; quiz 710.

78. Wani S, Falk GW, Post J, et al: Risk factors for progression of low-grade dysplasia in patients with Barrett's esophagus, *Gastroenterology* 141:1179–1186, 1186 e1, 2011.

96. Sharma P, Bergman JJ, Goda K, et al: Development and validation of a classification system to identify high-grade dysplasia and esophageal adenocarcinoma in Barrett's esophagus using narrow-band imaging, *Gastroenterology* 150:591–598, 2016.

97. Qumseya BJ, Wang H, Badie N, et al: Advanced imaging technologies increase detection of dysplasia and neoplasia in patients with Barrett's esophagus: a meta-analysis and systematic review, *Clin Gastroenterol Hepatol* 11:1562–1570 e1-2, 2013.

110. ASGE Technology Committee, Thosani N, Abu Dayyeh BK, et al: ASGE Technology Committee systematic review and meta-analysis assessing the ASGE Preservation and Incorporation of Valuable Endoscopic Innovations thresholds for adopting real-time imaging-assisted endoscopic targeted biopsy during endoscopic surveillance of Barrett's esophagus, *Gastrointest Endosc* 83:684–98 e7, 2016.

112a. Bansal A, Fitzgerald RC: Biomarkers in Barrett's esophagus: role in diagnosis, risk stratification, and prediction of response to therapy, *Gastroenterol Clin North Am* 44:373–390, 2015.

149. Shaheen NJ, Sharma P, Overholt BF, et al: Radiofrequency ablation in Barrett's esophagus with dysplasia, *N Engl J Med* 360:2277–2288, 2009.

150. Duits LC, Phoa KN, Curvers WL, et al: Barrett's oesophagus patients with low-grade dysplasia can be accurately risk-stratified after histological review by an expert pathology panel, *Gut* 64:700–706, 2015.

153. Duits LC, van der Wel MJ, Cotton CC, et al: Patients with Barrett's esophagus and confirmed persistent low-grade dysplasia at increased risk for progression to neoplasia, *Gastroenterology* 152:993–1001, e1, 2017.

171. Liao LM, Vaughan TL, Corley DA, et al: Nonsteroidal anti-inflammatory drug use reduces risk of adenocarcinomas of the esophagus and esophagogastric junction in a pooled analysis, *Gastroenterology* 142:442–452 e5, 2012; quiz e22-e23.

176. Park WG, Shaheen NJ, Cohen J, et al: Quality indicators for EGD, *Am J Gastroenterol* 110:60–71, 2015.

177. Wani S, Muthusamy VR, Shaheen N, et al: Development of quality indicators for endoscopic eradication therapies in Barrett's esophagus: the TREAT-BE (Treatment with Resection and Endoscopic Ablation Techniques for Barrett's Esophagus) Study, *Gastointest Endosc* 2016; [in press].

A complete reference list can be found online at ExpertConsult .com

26

Screening for Esophageal Squamous Cell Carcinoma

Chin Hur and Patrick S. Yachimski

CHAPTER OUTLINE

INTRODUCTION AND EPIDEMIOLOGY

Esophageal cancer is the eighth most common cancer and the sixth leading cause of cancer death in the world. There are two major histologic subtypes of esophageal cancer: adenocarcinoma and squamous cell cancer. Globally, more than 400,000 deaths were estimated attributable to esophageal cancer in 2012.[1] There is considerable geographic variability in the incidence of esophageal cancer, with the majority of cases (80%) occurring in less-developed parts of the world.[1] Based on recent incidence data, nearly 17,000 new cases of esophageal cancer will be diagnosed in the United States in 2016 (13,460 cases in men and 3,450 cases in women), and there will be 15,690 esophageal cancer-related deaths.[2] On the other hand, more than 290,000 new esophageal cancer diagnoses and more than 218,000 esophageal cancer deaths were estimated in China in 2011.[3]

Overall survival rates for esophageal cancer are poor, with highest mortality rates observed in regions with highest disease incidence, including Eastern Asia, Southern Africa, and Eastern Africa[1] (Fig. 26.1). Even within regions there is substantial geographic heterogeneity in the incidence of disease. Data published nearly four decades ago from the Caspian Cancer Registry, originating from the Caspian Littoral region on the rim of the Caspian Sea, reported annual age-adjusted incidence rates ranging from a low of 20.1 cases per 100,000 population in subregions of lowest incidence to a high of 165.5 cases per 100,000 population in subregions of highest incidence.[4]

Of the two major histologic subtypes of esophageal cancer, the majority of diagnosed cases worldwide are classified as esophageal squamous cell carcinoma (ESCC). A unique trend in Western countries, including the United States, has been a dramatic increase in the incidence of esophageal adenocarcinoma over the past several decades, to the extent that proportionally the majority of esophageal cancers diagnosed currently in the United States are adenocarcinoma rather than ESCC.[5]

Nonetheless, due to the significant morbidity of ESCC, the potential for prevention through early detection and treatment of ESCC and precursor lesions, and the nuances of endoscopic diagnosis of ESCC (with particular attention to the role of chromoendoscopy), understanding and implementing an evidence-based approach to screening for ESCC is essential for health care providers, and particularly the practicing gastrointestinal endoscopist.

Risk Factors for ESCC and Unique Populations at Risk

Common to the pathogenesis of many types of neoplasia, development of ESCC is often a consequence of the interplay between nonmodifiable (genetic) and modifiable (environmental) risk factors for disease.

Worldwide, ESCC incidence rates are more than twofold higher for men than for women.[1] In many countries, including relatively lower-incidence countries in the developed world, alcohol and tobacco use are major risk factors for ESCC. For instance, in a case control study of African-American men in an urban location, the relative risk of esophageal cancer associated with alcohol consumption was 6.4 (95% confidence interval [CI] 2.5–16.4) and the relative risk associated with tobacco use (not controlling for alcohol consumption) was 1.9 (95% CI 1.0–3.0).[6] In this study, consumption of hard liquor was associated with a higher risk of esophageal cancer than beer or wine consumption.[6] In addition, the race-specific incidence of ESCC among US men with exposure to alcohol and tobacco is highest among African-American men compared to other racial and ethnic groups.[7]

The combined effects of alcohol and tobacco are synergistic. In a case control study from Italy, with individuals who were nonsmokers and with moderate weekly alcohol consumption as the reference standard, odds ratios for development of esophageal cancer were 2.6 (95% CI 4–29) for nonsmokers with very heavy alcohol consumption, 8.4 (95% CI 16–41) for heavy smokers with moderate alcohol consumption, and 21.8 (95% CI 6–15)

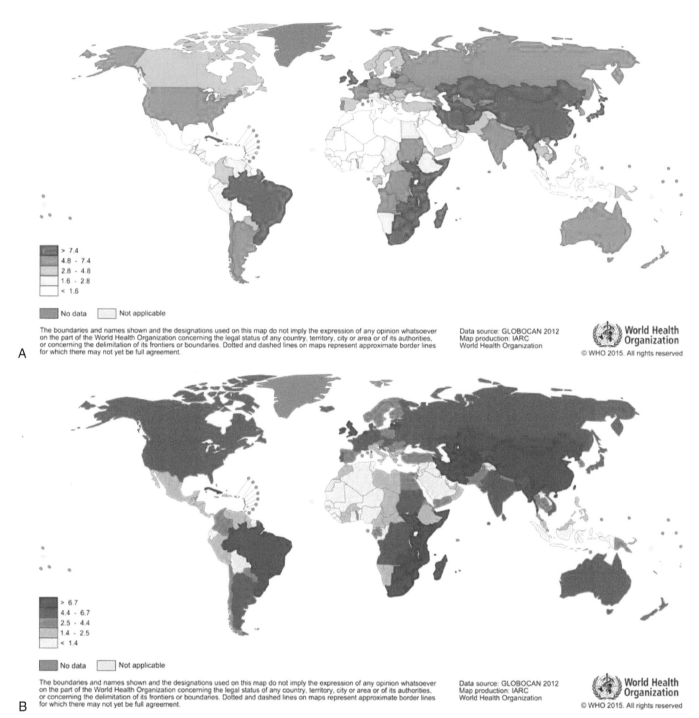

> 7.4
4.8 - 7.4
2.8 - 4.8
1.6 - 2.8
< 1.6

☐ No data ☐ Not applicable

The boundaries and names shown and the designations used on this map do not imply the expression of any opinion whatsoever on the part of the World Health Organization concerning the legal status of any country, territory, city or area or of its authorities, or concerning the delimitation of its frontiers or boundaries. Dotted and dashed lines on maps represent approximate border lines for which there may not yet be full agreement.

Data source: GLOBOCAN 2012
Map production: IARC
World Health Organization

World Health Organization
© WHO 2015. All rights reserved

A

> 6.7
4.4 - 6.7
2.5 - 4.4
1.4 - 2.5
< 1.4

☐ No data ☐ Not applicable

The boundaries and names shown and the designations used on this map do not imply the expression of any opinion whatsoever on the part of the World Health Organization concerning the legal status of any country, territory, city or area or of its authorities, or concerning the delimitation of its frontiers or boundaries. Dotted and dashed lines on maps represent approximate border lines for which there may not yet be full agreement.

Data source: GLOBOCAN 2012
Map production: IARC
World Health Organization

World Health Organization
© WHO 2015. All rights reserved

B

FIG 26.1 A, Esophageal cancer incidence in men (2012 data). **B,** Esophageal cancer mortality in men (2012 data). (From International Agency for Health Research on Cancer; World Health Organization: GLOBOCAN 2012: estimated cancer incidence, mortality and prevalence worldwide in 2012. 2015. Available at globocan.iarc.fr. Accessed February 1, 2017.)

for heavy smokers with very heavy alcohol consumption.[8] Even in higher-incidence regions for ESCC, such as China, smoking has been implicated as a significant risk factor for esophageal cancer as tobacco consumption has increased across the population.[9] And in a case control study from Uganda, the age- and gender-adjusted percentage of cases of ESCC attributable to alcohol and smoking was 13%.[10] Smokeless tobacco use has also been implicated as a risk factor for ESCC. In a study on the global burden of disease, smokeless tobacco use was implicated as the cause of more than 24,000 deaths worldwide due to ESCC, with the majority of these deaths (> 20,000) occurring in Southeast Asia.[11]

Consumption of alcohol and/or tobacco can significantly influence host factors contributing to baseline ESCC risk. For instance, an increased risk of ESCC has been reported in individuals with a family history of esophageal cancer, yet this risk increases substantially for individuals with a family history of esophageal cancer and who are also current smokers and heavy drinkers.[12] In addition, whereas the incidence of ESCC is higher in men than in women, an increasing prevalence of female smokers in the United States can result in comparable incidence between women and men smokers in smoking-related cancers, including ESCC.[13]

Throughout the world, dietary and nutritional factors have been implicated in the pathogenesis of ESCC. Multiple studies have suggested that populations with low dietary intake of fruits and vegetables are at increased risk for ESCC.[14,15] Micronutrient deficiencies including zinc[16] and selenium[17] may also be associated with increased risk for ESCC. Dietary folate consumption was reported to be inversely associated with risk for ESCC in a European population with high alcohol consumption.[18] On a population health scale, alterations in nutritional habits represent an opportunity to modify ESCC risk. Long-term decline in ESCC mortality in China has been attributed to changes in diet.[19]

Other specific environmental exposures reported to be associated with ESCC risk include exposure to polycyclic aromatic hydrocarbons from not only tobacco smoke but sources including indoor coal stoves[20] and the Brazilian beverage maté;[21] hot tea consumption (in a northern Iranian region);[22] poor oral hygiene;[23,24] and infection with certain serotypes of human papillomavirus infection.[25,26]

Unique populations of patients with comorbid illness are at increased risk for ESCC and may be candidates for targeted screening programs. The rare genetic condition tylosis, characterized by cutaneous hyperkeratosis associated with a chromosome 17 abnormality, is associated with a high cumulative lifetime risk of ESCC.[27] Current American Society for Gastrointestinal Endoscopy (ASGE) guidelines recommend screening for ESCC among patients with tylosis beginning at age 30 and repeated at 1 to 3 year intervals thereafter.[28] Targeted screening for ESCC is also recommended in patients who have sustained caustic esophageal injury, typically following lye ingestion, beginning 10 to 20 years after exposure and repeated at 2 to 3 year intervals.[28]

Other populations at increased risk for ESCC include patients with upper aerodigestive (head and neck) squamous cell cancers, among whom high rates of synchronous and metachronous ESCC have been reported,[29,30] as well as patients with achalasia.[31,32] However, current ASGE guidelines recommend against screening in patients with upper aerodigestive cancers or achalasia due to a lack of sufficient evidence to suggest that screening confers a benefit with respect to early cancer detection or survival.[28]

RATIONALE FOR POPULATION SCREENING FOR ESCC

The high mortality rates observed for ESCC[1] reflect the fact that most patients diagnosed with ESCC have advanced disease at the time of diagnosis. The development of luminal obstruction sufficient to cause the cardinal symptom of dysphagia is typically indicative of the presence of invasive carcinoma. A rationale for implementation of a screening program aimed at early cancer detection and, ultimately, improved cancer-specific prognosis and survival must be interpreted in this context. In general, several criteria must be fulfilled for a screening test to be recommended for routine clinical practice:

1. Screening should enable early detection of an unrecognized (asymptomatic) disease or precursor lesion which, if left undetected and untreated, has the potential to progress and result in significant morbidity and/or burden of suffering.
2. The test utilized for screening should be accurate, cost-effective, safe, and acceptable to both clinicians and patients undergoing screening.
3. Effective and acceptable treatment options should be available for patients found to have disease as a result of the screening examination.

Each of these criteria can be examined with respect to ESCC.

Precursors of ESCC

Squamous dysplasia has been recognized as a precursor lesion to ESCC (Fig. 26.2). Squamous dysplasia can be detected in a substantial proportion of patients in regions with high prevalence of ESCC. A study in Linzhou, China, subjecting more than 700 adult volunteers to screening upper endoscopy, detected a 32% prevalence of squamous dysplasia.[33] Risk factors for squamous dysplasia in this study mirrored risk factors for ESCC.[33] A 2016 prospective study in a high-risk region of Kenya detected a 14% prevalence of squamous dysplasia; the prevalence was greater than 20% in men older than age 50 and women older than age 60.[34]

Risk of progression from dysplasia to ESCC can be stratified according to grades of dysplasia. In a cohort of Chinese individuals diagnosed with squamous dysplasia and followed for 13.5 years, ESCC developed in 17%.[35] Relative risk (RR) of progression was lowest for patients with dysplasia classified as mild at baseline study entry (RR 2.9, 95 % CI 1.6–5.20), intermediate for patients with moderate dysplasia (RR 9.8, 95% CI 5.3–18.3), and highest for patients with severe dysplasia (RR 28.3, 95% CI 15.3–52.3) or carcinoma in situ (RR 34.4, 95% CI 16.6–71.4).[35]

Histopathologic grading of dysplasia associated with esophageal intestinal metaplasia (Barrett's esophagus), the major precursor lesion for esophageal adenocarcinoma, is subjective and notoriously fraught with high rates of interobserver variability.[36] There are no data available to estimate either the interobserver or intraobserver variability in grading of esophageal squamous dysplasia. In the esophageal adenocarcinoma context, when histopathologic assessment of Barrett's esophagus suggests the presence of dysplasia, the standard practice recommendation is to obtain additional review from a second expert pathologist for confirmation of the diagnosis of dysplasia. No equivalent recommendation exists with respect to the diagnosis of squamous dysplasia, nor would such a practice be feasible in a resource-limited setting. A potential further confounder in the assessment and grading of dysplasia is inconsistency in descriptive terminology, with World Health Organization guidelines, for instance, preferring the term *intraepithelial neoplasia* (classified as either low grade or high grade) over dysplasia.[37]

Novel tissue biomarkers may, in the future, facilitate detection, diagnosis, and risk stratification for ESCC and precursor lesions. For instance, a recent screen of candidate genes found overexpression of two genes (TNFAIP3 and CHN1) with differential overexpression in squamous dysplasia and ESCC compared to normal esophagus.[38] On the other hand, cytologic assessment of DNA ploidy and p53 loss of heterozygosity appears to offer no additional benefit to endoscopically obtained biopsies in detection of ESCC.[39] Absent further validation and rigorous assessment of the performance characteristics of novel tissue biomarkers, at this time the presence of squamous dysplasia remains the only clinically relevant and accepted precursor lesion for ESCC capable of predicting future cancer risk and a target

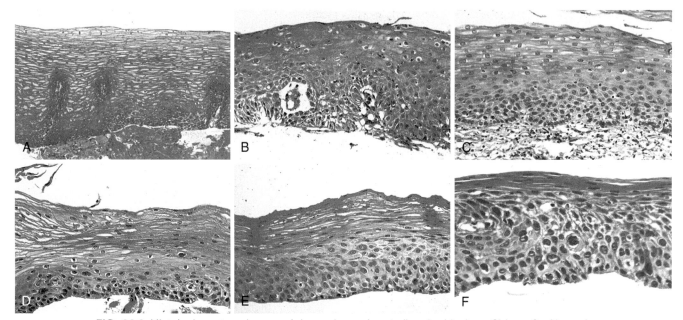

FIG 26.2 Histologic categories used in endoscopic studies in Linxian, China. **A,** Normal. **B,** Esophagitis. The epithelium is infiltrated by polymorphonuclear leukocytes. **C,** Basal cell hyperplasia. The basal zone is greater than 15% of the epithelial thickness, without cellular atypia. **D,** Mild squamous dysplasia. There is cellular atypia, confined to the lower third of the epithelium. **E,** Moderate squamous dysplasia. There is cellular atypia involving the lower two-thirds of the epithelium. **F,** Severe squamous dysplasia. The cellular atypia involves all thirds of the epithelium, without invasion of the lamina propria.

for potential intervention during screening and surveillance examinations.

Endoscopic Screening

Upper gastrointestinal endoscopy has emerged in the United States and much of the developed world as the primary test for screening for foregut malignancy. The capabilities of endoscopy for this purpose have been progressively influenced by generational technological advantages, as flexible endoscopes have evolved from fiber optics, to high definition white light imaging, to platforms capable of offering real-time image modification and enhancement.

ESCC has a predilection for the upper and mid esophagus, which should be inspected carefully during both endoscopic intubation and withdrawal from the esophagus. Early-stage ESCC may be detectable on careful white light inspection as a focal endoscopic abnormality such as a nodule or superficial ulceration (Figs. 26.3 and 26.4A). Variants of ESCC such as verrucous carcinoma may have a uniquely identifiable morphology (Video 26.1).

In many instances, however, detection of early ESCC and precursors lesions may prove elusive. Chromoendoscopy has therefore played a fundamental role in endoscopic screening for ESCC. The principle of chromoendoscopy consists of topical application of a liquid substance, typically a vital dye, to elicit subtle mucosal morphology and abnormalities. In ESCC screening, the agent of choice for endoscopic screening has been Lugol's iodine solution. Iodine binds to glycogen, a substance that is present in squamous epithelial cells throughout the body. Normal squamous epithelial cells will have a characteristic brown ("stained") appearance following topical application of Lugol's iodine. In contrast, atypical squamous cells, including areas

containing dysplasia or cancer, contain less glycogen, have less cellular uptake of iodine, and therefore exhibit a characteristic "unstained" appearance on inspection following application of Lugol's iodine (see Figs. 26.3 and 26.4C; Video 26.2).

The practice of chromoendoscopy for detection of neoplasia using Lugol's iodine is not unique to the esophagus, and was initially described for evaluation of the cervix.[40] Reports describing use of Lugol's iodine for esophageal examination emerged in the late 1960s and early 1970s.[41–43] Since that time, an extensive and robust experience with use of Lugol's iodine for diagnosis of ESCC has been reported. Misumi and colleagues reported the use of this technique in 1990 for detection of 17 lesions in a Japanese cohort with ESCC. Endoscopic inspection was initially performed using conventional (white light) endoscopy. After administration of mucolytics, 20 mL of 1.5% Lugol solution was applied under direct visualization. The iodine solution was aspirated through the scope 30 to 60 seconds later, followed by irrigation with 40 to 60 mL of water prior to endoscopic inspection. Whereas only 14 of 17 lesions were detected using white light endoscopy, all 17 lesions were detected following application of Lugol's iodine. Moreover, the size and margin of the lesions as estimated by Lugol's chromoendoscopy correlated reliably with the histopathologic assessment of the size of the lesion, an important consideration if an endoscopic resection is to be entertained with the goal of achieving an R0 resection[44] (see Chapter 27).

Also in 1990, Shiozaki and colleagues reported the results of endoscopic examination of the esophagus, first with conventional endoscopy, and then with chromoendoscopy following application of Lugol's iodine, in 178 patients with known head and neck cancer but no esophageal symptoms. Unstained lesions were identified in 69 patients. Biopsy of unstained lesions detected

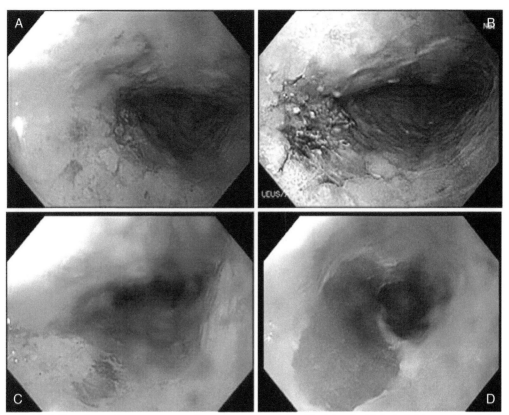

FIG 26.3 Esophageal squamous cell carcinoma as identified by **A,** high-definition white light, **B,** narrow band imaging, **C,** chromoendoscopy with Lugol's iodine, and **D,** following mucosal resection.

13 cancerous lesions in 9 patients (5% of the cohort) and squamous dysplasia in 22 patients (12% of the cohort); the remainder of the unstained lesions demonstrated pathology consistent with either inflammation or what was described as parakeratosis. The majority of ESCC lesions detected by chromoendoscopy were undetectable by conventional endoscopy or esophagram.[45]

In a 1998 study reported by Dawsey and colleagues, 225 patients with known esophageal dysplasia or cancer detected initially by nonendoscopic cytologic evaluation underwent endoscopy, including chromoendoscopy following application of a 1.2% Lugol's solution. The sensitivity of endoscopy for detection of high-grade dysplasia or cancer without Lugol's chromoendoscopy was 62%; the sensitivity for detection of high-grade dysplasia or cancer by identification of unstained lesions on Lugol's chromoendoscopy was 96%. All cases of invasive cancer were detected by conventional endoscopy; however, 55% of cases of moderate dysplasia and 23% of cases of severe dysplasia would have been missed without chromoendoscopy.[46]

Practical aspects of Lugol's use include appropriate dilution to the desired concentration, followed by application under direct visualization using a spray catheter or cannula. Potential adverse events include postprocedure chest discomfort,[47] allergic reaction,[48] and esophagitis.[49]

Additional agents that have been utilized for chromoendoscopic detection of ESCC include toluidine blue. In series of 18 patients with head and neck cancer reported by Hix et al (1987), esophagoscopy following toluidine blue staining detected esophageal cancer in 17% of subjects.[50] In a larger series of 103 patients

with head and neck cancer, vital staining with 1% toluidine blue resulted in detection of two neoplastic lesions not detected by standard endoscopy.[51]

Advances in endoscopic technology have provided the opportunity for increasingly accurate endoscopic detection and diagnosis of mucosal pathology, potentially including ESCC. Many modern endoscope processors are equipped with proprietary technologies capable of image modification/enhancement to assist in endoscopic detection of mucosal pathology. One such technology is narrow band imaging (NBI) (Olympus, Tokyo, Japan), which filters white light to two wavelengths (450 nm and 514 nm) specific for hemoglobin absorption. The rationale behind this image enhancement is that accentuation of the mucosal vasculature will allow detection of unique vascular morphology present in neoplastic lesions (see Figs. 26.3, 26.4B, 26.5).

Multiple early studies designed to assess the ability of NBI to detect ESCC used the combination of NBI with magnification endoscopy capabilities. White light endoscopy and NBI were compared head to head in a multicenter randomized controlled trial. Three hundred and twenty patients with histologically confirmed ESCC were randomized to undergo either white light endoscopy followed by NBI or NBI followed by white light endoscopy. In addition, the imaging platform utilized for the study enabled 80× optical magnification. Fifty-five percent of ESCC were detected by primary white light endoscopy, whereas 97% of lesions were detected by primary NBI. Forty-eight lesions were detected by NBI only (and not white light); one lesion was detected by white light only (and not NBI). Overall procedure

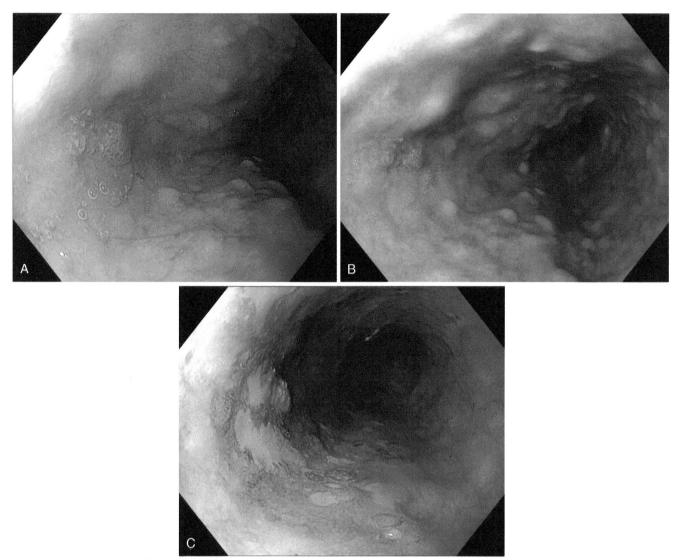

FIG 26.4 Esophageal squamous cell carcinoma visualized with **A,** high definition white light imaging, **B,** narrow band imaging, and **C,** Lugol's chromoendoscopy.

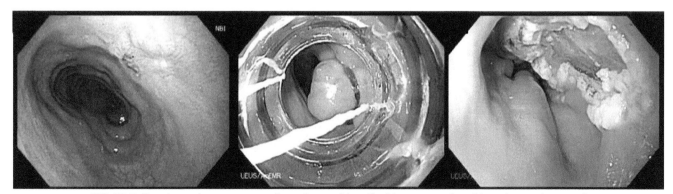

FIG 26.5 Esophageal squamous cell carcinoma identified by narrow band imaging and treated with mucosal resection using a band ligator device.

time was longer for primary NBI versus primary white light examinations (135 seconds vs. 95 seconds, $p < 0.001$).[52]

In a study by Takenaka et al (2009) comparing NBI with chromoendoscopy, 142 patients with head and neck cancer underwent NBI endoscopy (with magnification) followed by Lugol chromoendoscopy. Twenty-one lesions were detected in 16 patients with NBI. All lesions were subsequently evaluated by Lugol chromoendoscopy; 20 of 21 lesions measured greater than 5 mm in diameter and were biopsied. Histopathology confirmed ESCC in 4 lesions, high-grade intraepithelial neoplasia in 11 lesions, and low-grade intraepithelial neoplasia in 4 lesions. Lugol chromoendoscopy detected four additional lesions in patients with NBI findings, two of which proved to be low-grade intraepithelial neoplasia. With histopathology as the gold standard, the sensitivity of endoscopy for detection of ESCC was 91% using NBI versus 100% using Lugol chromoendoscopy. Performance characteristics of NBI were superior to Lugol's chromoendoscopy with respect to specificity (95% vs. 85%, $p < 0.001$) and overall accuracy (95% vs. 86%, $p < 0.01$).[53]

In a prospective study of NBI without magnification endoscopy, 202 patients deemed at high risk for ESCC underwent endoscopy with white light, followed by NBI inspection, then followed by chromoendoscopy. Biopsies were obtained following complete endoscopic inspection. In analysis using propensity score matching, the accuracy and specificity of NBI were superior to chromoendoscopy, whereas the sensitivity of NBI and chromoendoscopy were comparable.[54]

Additional enhanced endoscopy techniques that have been investigated for the detection of ESCC include autofluoroescence imaging (AFI).[55,56] Whereas at least one study reported acceptable test performance characteristics (sensitivity 97% and specificity 95%),[55] large-scale validation of AFI for ESCC screening has not been performed, and this technology is not in routine clinical use at this time.

Disruptive and Nonendoscopic Screening Techniques

Potential disadvantages of endoscopic screening as currently practiced include: 1) the invasive nature of endoscopic examination and need for administration of procedural sedation; 2) potential for adverse events as a consequence of endoscopic examination and/or procedural sedation; 3) direct costs to the health care system, chiefly in the form of physician and facility reimbursement; and 4) indirect costs incurred via missed work time (by patient and driver/chaperone) on the date of endoscopic examination. Additionally, whereas endoscopy may be viewed by health care providers as a minimally invasive, low-risk procedure, patient willingness to undergo endoscopy as an "acceptable" screening test may be limited. In a high-risk region for ESCC in Iran, only 18% of adult individuals contacted by phone for a screening program agreed to a clinic visit and only 16% underwent endoscopy.[57]

An option for addressing some of these disadvantages would include unsedated endoscopy, which would conceivably allow the patient to return to work following an office-based examination and eliminate the need for a chaperone. In a study of patients undergoing inspection for upper aerodigestive cancers, including the esophagus, using a standard endoscope under topical pharyngeal anesthesia and given the choice of either propofol sedation or no sedation, 123 patients opted for no sedation. The examination was reported as acceptable by 68% (84/123) of unsedated patients; however a complete (pharyngeal) examination was achieved in only 60% (74/123). ESCC was detected in 21% (26/123) of the no sedation group compared to 19% (25/132) of the propofol group.[58]

An alternative to standard peroral esophagoscopy is performance of unsedated transnasal endoscopy using a narrow-caliber endoscope. In a study of 248 patients with established head and neck cancer, unsedated transnasal endoscopy was performed to evaluate for synchronous esophageal neoplasia. Topical nasal decongestive and oropharyngeal anesthesia was administered. Complete esophageal examination was achieved in 244 out of 248 subjects, and esophageal lesions were detected in 46%

(111/244), including 36 patients with ESCC and 23 patients with squamous dysplasia.[59]

Wireless capsule endoscopy for ESCC screening has been described in at least one study, in which esophageal examination with a swallowed pill camera was followed by upper gastrointestinal endoscopy including Lugol chromoendoscopy. Compared to lesions detected by Lugol chromoendoscopy as the gold standard, the sensitivity of capsule endoscopy for the detection of dysplasia or cancer was less than 50%.[60]

Yet, whereas endoscopy may be considered as the standard and reflexive screening test in the developed world, there are well-established means for ESCC screening with nonendoscopic, peroral cytologic sampling. The general principle of this technique involves asking the patient to swallow a tethered cellular acquisition device, which can then be withdrawn from the stomach and through the esophagus, with the goal of cytologic sampling of the esophageal mucosa.

Several iterations of balloon-based cytologic sampling devices have been developed and used for ESCC screening (Figs. 26.6 and 26.7). A tethered, uninflated balloon is swallowed and then inflated with a small volume (20–30 mL) of air before being withdrawn from the stomach. The balloon is covered with a cotton mesh, and some versions also allow for aspiration of samples through the lumen of the catheter. In a study of more than 12,000 subjects in Linxian, China, balloon-based cytologic screening detected cancer in 2% and dysplasia in more than a quarter of subjects.[61] Among more than 10,000 subjects without cancer at initial screening, 747 incident cancers and 322 cancer-related deaths were identified during 7.5 years of subsequent follow-up. Relative risk of cancer correlated with grade/severity of cytologic dysplasia at baseline.[62]

The other principal category of devices utilized for nonendoscopic cytologic screening for ESCC consists of sponge-based brush biopsy devices (see Fig. 26.6). These devices are enclosed in a gelatin capsule which dissolves in the stomach within a few minutes following ingestion, thereby permitting expansion of the sponge. In a study using an esophageal brush biopsy capsule for screening of subjects in southern Africa, satisfactory specimens were obtained from 96% of subjects screened. Subjects were allocated to subgroups deemed as low-risk, intermediate-risk,

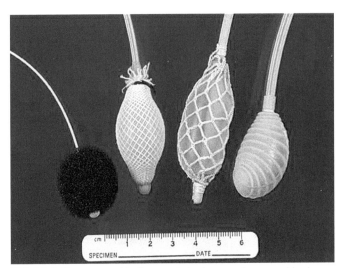

FIG 26.6 Sponge and balloon cytologic samplers used in Japan and China.

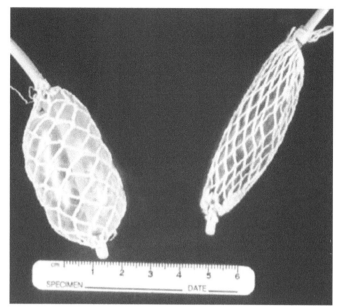

FIG 26.7 Balloon cytologic samplers. (From Roth MJ, Liu SF, Dawsey SM, et al: Cytologic detection of esophageal squamous cell carcinoma and precursor lesions using balloon and sponge samplers in asymptomatic adults in Linxian, China. *Cancer* 80[11]:2047–2059, 1997.)

TABLE 26.1	Detection of Esophageal Squamous Neoplasia by Cytologic and Endoscopic Sampling	
	Balloon Cytology (%) N = 434	Sponge Cytology (%) N = 378
LGSIL	42 (10)	23 (6)
HGSIL	5 (1)	0
Suspicious for carcinoma	4 (1)	3 (1)
Carcinoma	7 (2)	0

LGSIL, low grade squamous intraepithelial lesion; *HGSIL,* high grade squamous intraepithelial lesion.
Data from Roth MJ, Liu SF, Dawsey SM, et al: Cytologic detection of esophageal squamous cell carcinoma and precursor lesions using balloon and sponge samplers in asymptomatic adults in Linxian, China. *Cancer* 80(11):2047–2059, 1997.

or high-risk, respectively, for esophageal cancer based on geographic location. Among subjects in the high-risk location, this screening technique detected cancer in 2% of subjects; dysplasia was detected in 9% of subjects older than age 35.[63] In a study of 334 subjects with previously treated upper aerodigestive tract malignancy, brush biopsy capsule screening had a sensitivity of 89% and specificity of 91% for detection of recurrent malignancy during a 3-year follow-up period; approximately one-third of malignancies were esophageal, while the remainder were oropharyngeal.[64] In a 2014 study, more than 300 subjects in Iran underwent screening with a new iteration of a sponge-based device. The sensitivity for detection of high-grade squamous dysplasia was 100% and the specificity was 100%. Addition of p53 immunohistochemistry to cytology resulted in a diagnostic accuracy of 100% for detection of high-grade dysplasia. Ninety-three percent of subjects reported the sponge examination as "acceptable" on a 6-point visual analog scale.[65]

Balloon-based and sponge-based cytologic sampling devices were compared head-to-head, followed by standard endoscopy with Lugol chromoendoscopy, in a study of asymptomatic, previously unscreened individuals in Linxian, China. The order of nonendoscopic cytologic sampling (balloon vs. sponge) was randomized. A complete examination was achieved in 99% of 625 subjects using the balloon and in 86% of 538 subjects using the sponge. Thirty-one percent of subjects reported preference for the balloon technique, 43% reported preference for the sponge, and 26% reported no preference. Adequate squamous cells for analysis were obtained in 99% of 434 cases using the balloon and 86% of 378 cases using the sponge.[66] The comparative yield for detection of squamous dysplasia/ESCC by these two techniques is depicted in Table 26.1.

Four hundred and fifty-nine subjects then underwent standard endoscopy with Lugol chromoendoscopy and biopsy, following administration of topical oropharyngeal anesthesia but no other

sedation. Endoscopy with biopsy detected pathology in nearly a third of subjects: mild squamous dysplasia in 12% (52/459), moderate dysplasia in 10% (45/459), severe dysplasia in 6% (26/459), and ESCC in 4% (16/459).[66] With endoscopic diagnosis as the comparative standard, the sensitivity of nonendoscopic cytologic sampling for detection of ESCC was 44% using the balloon and 18% using the sponge, and the sensitivity for detection of the combined diagnoses of dysplasia and/or ESCC was 47% using the balloon and 24% using the sponge. Specificity for detection of cancer was 99% using the balloon and 100% using the sponge; specificity for detection of dysplasia or cancer was 81% using the balloon and 92% using the sponge.[66]

Endoscopic Treatment of Superficial ESCC

The final criteria for implementation of a screening program is the requirement that effective and acceptable treatment options should be available for patients found to have disease as a consequence of screening examination. Esophageal malignancy, when detected at an asymptomatic or otherwise advanced stage, is associated with a poor prognosis. Treatment regimens may be multimodal and entail systemic chemotherapy, radiation therapy, and/or surgical esophagectomy (if therapeutic intent is curative rather than palliative).

The endoscopic techniques of endoscopic mucosal resection (EMR) (see Fig. 26.5) and endoscopic submucosal dissection (ESD) have revolutionized treatment for superficial gastrointestinal tract neoplasia, including esophageal neoplasia. The ability to offer EMR/ESD techniques provides a strong rationale for early detection of ESCC with the goal of endoscopic therapy for durable disease remission/cure. These techniques are described in detail elsewhere in this textbook (see Chapter 27).

SUMMARY OF CURRENT RATIONALE FOR SCREENING: EFFECTIVENESS AND COST-EFFECTIVENESS

Individuals at high risk for ESCC can be identified based on factors including residence in a high-risk geographic location and health-associated factors including alcohol and tobacco use. Squamous dysplasia is a precursor lesion to ESCC, and both squamous dysplasia and ESCC can be detected at an asymptomatic stage by nonendoscopic cytologic or endoscopic screening. Endoscopic biopsy, particularly following Lugol chromoendoscopy, is highly accurate for detection of dysplasia/ESCC. Individuals detected with esophageal neoplasia as a consequence of screening at an early, asymptomatic stage may be candidates for endoscopic, esophagus-preserving therapy with minimal associated morbidity.

It must be recognized that the detection of dysplasia and even ESCC is, to some degree, a surrogate endpoint. Each of the criteria requisite for the justification of an ESCC screening program can be supported by data. Ultimately, however, the metric by which an ESCC screening program should be judged is the extent to which a program aimed at early detection and prevention reduces ESCC-associated mortality. For instance, relatively recent data reported 10-year follow-up data of 3,319 patients from fourteen villages in a high-risk area of China who underwent one time screening endoscopy. Patients found to have lesions amenable to endoscopic intervention were treated with endoscopic resection and/or fulguration; treatment for invasive/advanced disease included surgery and systemic therapy when appropriate. Comparison was made to a control group of 23,733 subjects who did not undergo endoscopic screening. Cumulative incidence of ESCC was 4.17% in the screening group compared to 5.92% in the control group. Mortality due to ESCC was 3.35% in the screening group compared to 5.05% in the control group. The adjusted hazard ration for ESCC mortality was 0.51 in the screening group.[67]

Whereas the effectiveness of a program is one measure, cost may be an equally important measure within the constraints of any given health system, particularly in a region or setting that may be resource-limited. Formal cost-utility analysis (often referred to as cost-effectiveness analysis) is a technique in which a mathematical model is created to allow a simulated patient to transition between varying health and disease states. A "utility" score can be used to assign a relative value for any given health or disease state, with reference values ranging from 1 for perfect health and 0 for death. Actual or estimated costs can be assigned to interventions (such as screening tests or treatments) that affect the likelihood of transitioning between health and disease states or for the costs associated with treatment of various health states. For instance, costs for management of esophageal cancer are generally high and are dominated by costs of surgery and chemotherapy.[68] At final analysis, for any given intervention an incremental cost effectiveness ratio (ICER) can be calculated; for instance, in a typical cost-effectiveness analysis the ICER is reported as dollars spent for quality adjusted life year saved ($/QALY). Based on this calculation, a screening test might be deemed acceptable from a societal standpoint if the ICER is below an accepted willingness to pay threshold (WTP), usually $50,000–$100,000/QALY in the United States. Other commonly performed health interventions (mammogram for breast cancer screening, colonoscopy for colorectal cancer screening, etc.) fulfill this criterion as their ICER is below the accepted WTP.

Numerous cost-effectiveness analyses have been published to examine the rationale for endoscopic prevention of esophageal adenocarcinoma in the United States and Western populations via screening endoscopy among patients with gastroesophageal reflux disease and surveillance endoscopy among patients with established Barrett's esophagus. Similar analysis of ESCC screening is limited.

General population screening for ESCC via endoscopy cannot be justified in a region of low prevalence. One study estimated that the prevalence rate of ESCC in the United States would have to increase 1948% from current levels to justify endoscopic screening at a WTP of less than $50,000/QALY.[69] On the other hand, the cost utility calculation for ESCC screening in a highly endemic area may be much more favorable. It has been suggested that 100 adults in a high-risk region of China could undergo endoscopic screening with Lugol chromoendoscopy and biopsy at a cost equivalent to the cost of treating one patient with advanced stage cancer.[70]

Disruptive technologies that offer new mechanisms for screening can be assessed by cost-utility analysis. As an example, emerging endoscopic technologies with "optical biopsy" capabilities offer the promise of real-time histopathologic assessment, and potential cost savings by reducing the number of unnecessary biopsies, or conceivably even by allowing the endoscopist to proceed immediately from diagnostic assessment to therapeutic intervention in a single endoscopy session. High-resolution microendoscopy (HRME) technology used as an adjunct to Lugol's chromoendoscopy may improve the diagnostic accuracy for detection of squamous neoplasia[71] (Fig. 26.8), and cost-effectiveness analysis has demonstrated that incorporation of HRME into an endoscopic screening program for a high-risk population could be cost-effective at an ICER of $8173/QALY.[72]

Additional technologies that offer the promise of optical biopsy include confocal laser endomicroscopy (Fig. 26.9). In this technique, fluorescein is administered intravenously. Following cellular uptake of fluorescein, the esophageal mucosa is examined with a specially equipped endoscope or accessory probe, permitting evaluation of cellular and capillary architecture as histopathologic correlates. Whereas the ability of this technique to discriminate between normal mucosa and early ESCC has been reported,[73,74] and the learning curve and interobserver variability appear reasonable,[75] formal cost-utility analysis has not been reported.

FUTURE DIRECTIONS FOR NONINVASIVE SCREENING: SEROLOGIC AND STOOL TESTING; MICROBIOTA

Future advances in early detection and diagnosis of ESCC may be facilitated by emerging insights into risk factors and disease pathogenesis, allowing for risk stratification and identification of individuals and groups at risk for ESCC. An active area of current investigation is the role of the microbiome in health and disease through the gastrointestinal tract. The most well-known example is that of *Helicobacter pylori*, which is strongly associated with gastric cancer and inversely associated with esophageal adenocarcinoma, but not associated with ESCC.[76] Data suggest that salivary microbiota may be altered in patients with ESCC[77] and squamous dysplasia[78] compared to nonaffected controls.

Noninvasive stool sample assays have been a staple of colorectal cancer screening, and newer generation tests include options for fecal DNA testing. Whether fecal DNA testing (or other assays) could be an option for ESCC screening will require investigation, which to date has not been reported. Elevated fecal calprotectin levels have been described in patients with esophageal and gastric cancer,[79] although the specificity of this marker, which can be elevated in benign conditions including inflammatory bowel disease, is uncertain. Elevated serum microRNA levels can be detected in patients with ESCC,[80,81] raising the prospect that novel biomarkers may offer a future opportunity for serologic screening.

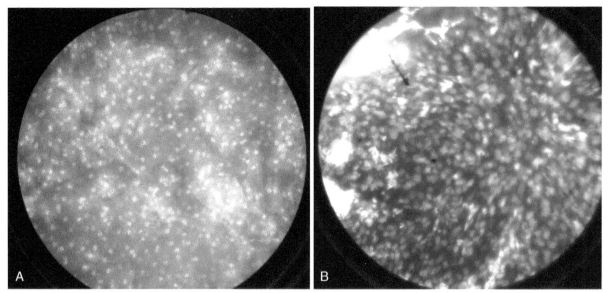

FIG 26.8 High-resolution microendoscopy (HRME) demonstrating **A,** benign esophageal squamous epithelium, and **B,** neoplastic esophageal squamous epithelium.

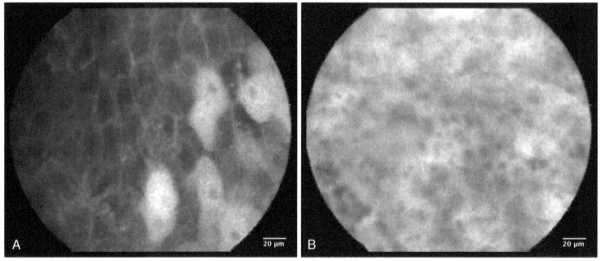

FIG 26.9 Confocal laser microscopy. **A,** Confocal image of normal squamous epithelium shows normal cellular structure. **B,** Image of esophageal cancer shows disorganized cells with enlarged and hyperchromatic nuclei. (Photographs courtesy Dr Cuong Nguyen and Dr. Ananya Das.)

Targeted mucosal assessment with molecular probes may allow optimized endoscopic detection and localization of ESCC. Use of fluorescent-labeled, topically administered probes may assist in this fashion. Probes whose ligand is an aminopeptidase expressed and activated in ESCC have been described in ex vivo use.[82]

CONCLUSIONS

ESCC is a leading cause of cancer death worldwide. When diagnosed at a symptomatic phase, ESCC is often already at an advanced stage with attendant poor prognosis. Detection of esophageal squamous dysplasia or early stage ESCC when in a latent, asymptomatic phase can offer opportunities for curative, endoscopic, esophagus-preserving treatment. For each of these reasons, screening for ESCC is an intuitively attractive option. Endoscopic examination, particularly with Lugol's chromoendoscopy, has high performance characteristics as a screening test for squamous dysplasia/ESCC. This is, however, a costly, resource-intensive examination, which is on one hand not cost-effective in relatively affluent Western countries with low ESCC prevalence, and on the other hand not cost feasible in many resource-limited areas of the world with high ESCC prevalence. Nonendoscopic cytologic screening has proven efficacy in regions of high prevalence. Future disruptive screening technologies may expand opportunities for reduction in mortality from the global ESCC epidemic.

KEY REFERENCES

1. International Agency for Health Research on Cancer; World Health Organization: GLOBOCAN 2012: Estimated cancer incidence, mortality and prevalence worldwide in 2012. Available at globocan.iarc.fr. Accessed 1 February 2017.

4. Mahboubi E, Kmet J, Cook PJ, et al: Oesophageal cancer studies in the Caspian Littorial of Iran: the Caspian cancer registry, *Br J Cancer* 28: 197–214, 1973.

7. Prabhu A, Obi K, Lieberman D, Rubenstein JH: The race-specific incidence of esophageal squamous cell carcinoma in individuals with exposure to tobacco and alcohol, *Am J Gastroenterol* 111(12):1718–1725, 2016.

8. Baron AE, Francheschi S, Barra S, et al: A comparison of the joint effects of alcohol and smoking on the risk of cancer across sites in the upper aerodigestive tract, *Cancer Epidemiol Biomarkers Prev* 2:519–523, 1993.

11. Siddiqi K, Shah S, Abbas SM, et al: Global burden of disease due to smokeless tobacco consumption in adults: analysis of data from 113 countries, *BMC Med* 13:194, 2015.

14. Tran GD, Sun XD, Abnet CC, et al: Prospective study of risk factors for esophageal cancer and gastric cancers in the Linxian general population trial cohort in China, *Int J Cancer* 113:456–463, 2005.

15. Cook-Mozaffari PJ, Azordegan F, Day NE, et al: Oesophageal cancer studies in the Caspian Littoral of Iran: results of a case-control study, *Br J Cancer* 39:293–309, 1979.

19. Guo P, Huang ZL, Yu P, Li K: Trends in cancer mortality in China: an update, *Ann Oncol* 23:2755–2762, 2012.

20. Roth MJ, Strickland KL, Wang GQ, et al: High levels of carcinogenic polycyclic aromatic hydrocarbons present within food from Linxian, China may contribute to that region's high incidence of oesophageal cancer, *Eur J Cancer* 34:757–758, 1998.

21. Fagundes RB, Abnet CC, Strickland PT, et al: Higher urine 1-hydroxy pyrene glucuronide (1-OHPG) is associated with tobacco smoke exposure and drinking maté in healthy subjects from Tio Grande do Sul, Brazil, *BMC Cancer* 6:139, 2006.

28. ASGE Standards of Practice Committee, Evans JA, Early DS, et al: The role of endoscopy in Barrett's esophagus and other premalignant conditions of the esophagus, *Gastrointest Endosc* 76:1087–1094, 2012.

29. Muto M, Hironaka S, Nakane M, et al: Association of multiple Lugol-voiding lesions with synchronous and metachronous esophageal squamous cell carcinoma in patients with head and neck cancer, *Gastrointest Endosc* 56:517–521, 2002.

30. Petit T, Georges C, Jung GM, et al: Systematic esophageal endoscopy screening in patients previously treated for head and neck squamous-cell carcinoma, *Ann Oncol* 12:643–646, 2001.

33. Wei WQ, Abnet CC, Lu N, et al: Risk factors for oesophageal squamous dysplasia in adult inhabitants of a high risk region of China, *Gut* 54: 759–763, 2005.

35. Wang GQ, Abnet CC, Shen Q, et al: Histological precursors of oesophageal squamous cell carcinoma: results from a 13 year prospective follow up study in a high risk population, *Gut* 54:187–192, 2005.

37. Gabbert HE, Shimoda T, Hainaut P, et al: Squamous cell carcinoma of the esophagus. In Hamilton SR, Alltonen LE, editors: *World Health Organization classification of tumours. Pathology and genetics. Tumours of the digestive system*, Lyon, 2000, IARC Press, pp 8–19.

44. Misumi A, Harada K, Murakami A, et al: Role of Lugol dye endoscopy in the diagnosis of early esophageal cancer, *Endoscopy* 22:12–16, 1990.

45. Shiozaki H, Tahara H, Kobayashi K, et al: Endoscopic screening of early esophageal cancer with the Lugol dye method in patients with head and neck cancers, *Cancer* 66:2068–2071, 1990.

46. Dawsey SM, Fleischer DE, Wang GQ, et al: Mucosal iodine staining improves endoscopic visualization of squamous dysplasia and squamous cell carcinoma of the esophagus in Linxian, China, *Cancer* 83:220–231, 1998.

52. Muto M, Minashi K, Yano T, et al: Early detection of superficial squamous cell carcinoma in the head and neck region and esophagus by narrow band imaging: a multicenter randomized controlled trial, *J Clin Oncol* 28:1566–1572, 2010.

53. Takenaka R, Kawahara Y, Okada H, et al: Narrow-band imaging provides reliable screening for esophageal malignancy in patients with head and neck cancers, *Am J Gastroenterol* 104:2942–2948, 2009.

61. Shen O, Liu SF, Dawsey SM, et al: Cytologic screening for esophageal cancer: results from 12,877 subjects from a high-risk population in China, *Int J Cancer* 54:185–188, 1993.

A complete reference list can be found online at ExpertConsult .com

27

Endoscopic Treatment of Early Esophageal Neoplasia

Kavel Visrodia, Kenneth K. Wang, and Prasad G. Iyer

CHAPTER OUTLINE

INTRODUCTION

Esophageal cancer remains the eighth most common cancer and the sixth leading cause of cancer-related mortality worldwide.[1] Two main subtypes exist: esophageal adenocarcinoma (EAC) and esophageal squamous cell carcinoma (ESCC). EAC predominates in North America and Europe, and there has been a steep rise in its incidence over the last several decades.[2] ESCC is most prevalent in Asia and Africa, and accounts for over 90% of esophageal cancers worldwide.[3] The prognosis for esophageal cancer is poor, with an overall 5-year survival of less than 20%.[4] This stems in large part from challenges related to early detection, as the majority of cancers present at advanced stages (T3 and T4) for which effective treatments do not yet exist. However, when esophageal cancer is encountered early (i.e., stage Tis or T1a), survival can be dramatically improved with therapy. Until recently, the only curative treatment option was esophagectomy, which carries substantial risk and may not be advised in patients with significant comorbidities.[5] Improvements in endoscopic resection techniques, namely endoscopic mucosal resection (EMR) and endoscopic submucosal dissection (ESD), devised to procure larger amounts of tissue for accurate staging, have also enabled endoscopists to curatively treat early esophageal cancers.[3] Moreover, residual mucosa that could become neoplastic is treated with ablative therapies that can be applied with less morbidity than previously.[6] Endoscopic methods to treat cancer have become an important tool for the gastroenterologist, and their mechanisms, techniques, and evidence are reviewed in this chapter. Screening and surveillance for Barrett's esophagus is covered in Chapter 25.

ESCC is believed to follow a stepwise process of neoplastic progression. Established risk factors include alcohol, tobacco, exposure to environmental toxins such as polycyclic aromatic hydrocarbons, and potentially nutritional deficiencies.[7] Recent studies (2015) suggest a cost benefit for screening endoscopy or balloon brush cytology in areas of high incidence such as northern and rural areas of China.[8] At this time, however, there are no widely accepted guidelines for ESCC screening.

ENDOSCOPIC DETECTION AND DIAGNOSIS

At an early stage, esophageal cancer is usually asymptomatic (without dysphagia, weight loss, or anemia, which tend to reflect advanced disease), and is typically detected during screening or surveillance endoscopy or during the endoscopic evaluation of unrelated abdominal symptoms. Moreover, both histologic subtypes may appear subtle and be easily missed during endoscopy, underscoring the importance of a careful, systematic endoscopic evaluation. EAC is predominantly detected in the distal third of the esophagus, arising from a background of Barrett's epithelium, possibly in the form of an ulceration, an altered mucosal pattern, or a nodularity (Fig. 27.1). EAC may also be detected during random biopsies in the absence of any apparent endoscopic abnormality. Enhanced techniques can be used to complement white light endoscopy (WLE) for a more detailed inspection of Barrett's mucosa and abnormalities. Dye-based chromoendoscopy involves the topical application of methylene blue or acetic acid using a catheter spray.[9,10] These techniques are detailed in Chapter 25.

ESCC is more commonly found in the middle and proximal third of the esophagus. Early signs of ESCC may be as subtle as a mucosal irregularity, sometimes with a thin white coating or a reddish hue. Dye chromoendoscopy, specifically using Lugol solution, can aid in the detection of early ESCC. Lugol solution is sprayed over the esophageal mucosa during endoscopy, and within minutes preferentially stains normal squamous epithelium brown/black. Demarcated, unstained tissue may represent dysplasia, carcinoma, or inflammation (Fig. 27.2). In a study investigating the detection of high-grade dysplasia (HGD) or cancer in a high-risk population from China, the application of Lugol solution improved the sensitivity of WLE from 62% to 96%, while retaining a specificity of 63% (79% prior to staining).[11]

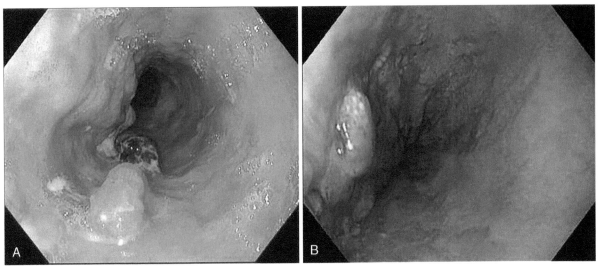

FIG 27.1 **A,** Early esophageal adenocarcinoma. **B,** Squamous cell carcinoma.

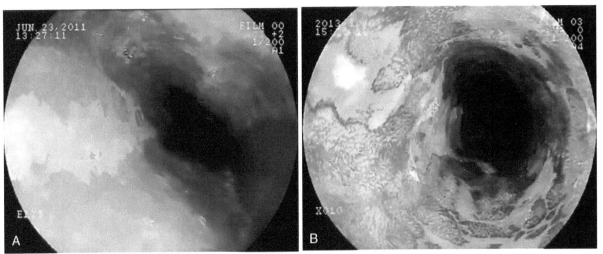

FIG 27.2 **A,** Before and **B,** after application of iodine-containing Lugol solution.

In another study, the additional finding of reddish or rose-pink appearance (so-called pink sign) was helpful in differentiating ESCC and HGD from low-grade dysplasia (LGD) or inflammation, with a sensitivity and specificity of 92% and 94%, respectively.[12] Thus, Lugol chromoendoscopy is generally recommended during screening for ESCC. The utility of virtual chromoendoscopy in improving ESCC detection has also been investigated. Using narrow band imaging (NBI), ESCC or dysplasia may appear as a well-demarcated brownish area with distorted patterns of intrapapillary capillary loops (Fig. 27.3). In a prospective, randomized controlled study, virtual chromoendoscopy significantly improved the detection of head, neck, and esophageal squamous cell cancer compared to WLE alone (97% vs. 55%).[13] A 2015 randomized noninferiority trial comparing Lugol and virtual chromoendoscopy concluded there was no significant difference in diagnostic yield.[14]

STAGING OF EARLY ESOPHAGEAL CANCER

The depth of esophageal cancer invasion (i.e., T staging) is critical in determining the risk of lymph node involvement and whether

a patient is a candidate for curative endoscopic treatment or will need esophagectomy and/or (neo)adjuvant chemoradiotherapy. To understand why, it is helpful to remember that the esophageal mucosal layer is comprised of epithelium, lamina propria, and muscularis mucosa layers. The mucosa is separated from the underlying submucosa by the basement membrane. The esophageal cancer staging system most commonly used is outlined by the American Joint Committee on Cancer.[15] The staging system was updated in 2010, at which time separate staging systems were developed for EAC and ESCC. However, they remain identical with respect to staging of early esophageal cancers. Early esophageal cancers (i.e., stage Tis and T1a) are characterized by confinement to the esophageal mucosal layer. Specifically, stage Tis is characterized by HGD limited to the epithelium (formerly known as carcinoma in situ), and stage T1a by lamina propria or muscularis mucosa involvement (intramucosal cancers). Later-stage tumors, beginning with T1b, invade the submucosa (Fig. 27.4).

Submucosal tumor involvement marks an important distinction because it confers a higher risk of lymph node metastasis and usually precludes endoscopic treatment with curative intent.

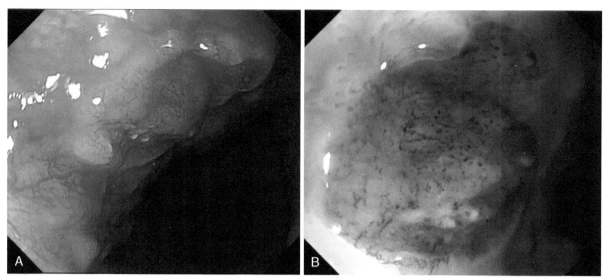

FIG 27.3 The added utility of virtual chromoendoscopy (**B**) to white-light endoscopy (**A**) in evaluating for dysplasia or squamous cell cancer. Using virtual chromoendoscopy (**B**), neoplasia may appear as a well-demarcated, brownish area with distorted patterns of intrapapillary capillary loops.

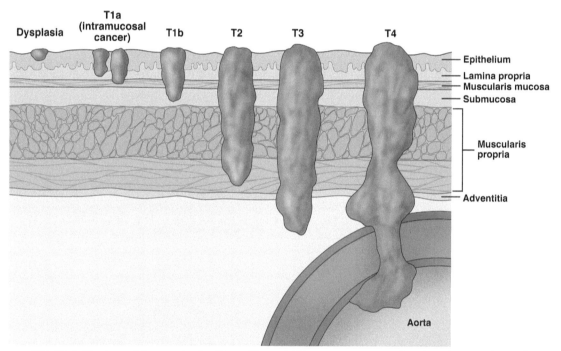

FIG 27.4 Staging of tumor depth. Stage Tis and T1a tumors are confined to the esophageal mucosa, whereas stage T1b and more advanced tumors invade the esophageal submucosa. (From Rubenstein JH and Shaheen NJ: Epidemiology, diagnosis, and management of esophageal adenocarcinoma. *Gastroenterology* 149[2]:302–317.e1, 2015.)

In a large systematic review of 70 studies including 1874 patients undergoing esophagectomy with lymph node dissection for HGD or intramucosal adenocarcinoma, lymph node metastasis was found in 0% of 524 patients with HGD and 1.9% of patients with intramucosal cancer.[16] In another study reviewing the outcomes of the National Cancer Database, the risk of nodal metastasis for T1a disease in patients undergoing esophagectomy for EAC and ESCC was 6.4% and 6.9%, whereas for T1b disease it was 19.6 and 20%, respectively.[17] Hence, the risk of nodal metastasis is much greater for submucosally invasive tumors,

and patients with T1b disease should be referred for consideration of esophagectomy. A subset of patients with T1b disease limited to the superficial third of submucosa (i.e., T1b sm1) and well-differentiated histology without lymphovascular invasion who are not good candidates for surgery may still be treated endoscopically with encouraging outcomes,[18] but this decision should involve a multidisciplinary surgical and oncology discussion.

Staging of potential early esophageal cancers is best achieved by endoscopic methods of tissue acquisition (discussed later). If confinement to mucosa is confirmed, imaging modalities such as endoscopic ultrasound (EUS) and computed tomography (CT) with or without positron-emission tomography (PET) do not appear to impact the management of early esophageal cancer.[19]

Endoscopic Inspection

Although tissue acquisition is the gold standard for early esophageal cancer staging, inspection for macroscopic clues may be helpful in predicting tumor depth, particularly for superficial ESCC. Various classification schemes have been described. The Paris classification categorizes superficial-appearing esophageal carcinoma accordingly: type 0-I (protruding), 0-II (without definite protrusion or depression), and 0-III (excavated).[20] Type 0-I and 0-III lesions carry a high likelihood of submucosal invasion (94.7% and 100%, respectively) consistent with stage T1b disease. Type 0-IIa (slightly elevated) and 0-IIb (completely flat) tumors suggest stage Tis or T1a disease. Type 0-IIc (slightly depressed) may be either stage Tis, T1a, or T1b (Fig. 27.5).[7] The utility of NBI magnification in detecting microvascular irregularities such as intrapapillary capillary loops (to differentiate T1a from T1b tumors) has also been reported to have high sensitivity (78%) and specificity (95%).[21] It is worth remembering that documentation of the shape, size, and location (with respect to the gastroesophageal junction) of all potential tumors can aid in planning, if surgery is recommended.

Endoscopic Resection

The presence of an esophageal nodule or mucosal irregularity in patients with risk factors, especially Barrett's esophagus (BE), should immediately raise concern, due to the high probability of harboring cancer.[22] Biopsies alone have been found to underestimate the degree of dysplasia because of difficulty in judging the extent of invasion, and therefore have been largely supplanted by EMR and ESD, which enable acquisition of larger amounts of tissue for histology. Studies have demonstrated that EMR alters the final histological stage in 30% to 50% of cases when compared to biopsies alone.[23,24] Given the low rate of lymph node metastasis in early esophageal cancer, endoscopic resection has the potential to be simultaneously curative in patients. Resection also has the potential to spare the cost, patient anxiety, and delays in care stemming from other staging modalities in this low-yield setting. Histology from EMR or ESD also provides information on prognostic factors for the survival of patients with early stage esophageal cancer, such as lymphovascular invasion and deep margin involvement (Fig. 27.6).[25] For these reasons, endoscopic resection should be the initial step in the evaluation of visible esophageal nodules or lesions suspicious for early esophageal cancer.

Endoscopic Ultrasound and PET/CT

EUS can be performed with either dedicated echoendoscopes or high-frequency ultrasound probes to assess the esophageal wall layers and assess tumor depth of invasion, as well as regional lymph node involvement. However, EUS may not be very accurate in staging early esophageal cancers, and may overstage cancers as T1b (due to tumor-associated inflammation), resulting in the exclusion of lesions amenable to endoscopic therapy.[26,27] In a meta-analysis of 12 studies including 292 patients with HGD or early esophageal cancer, EUS had a T-stage concordance of 67% when compared to surgical or EMR pathology.[27] PET/CT has not been demonstrated to be of benefit in patients with established intramucosal cancer. EUS and PET/CT may best be reserved for lymph node evaluation in patients with at least T1b

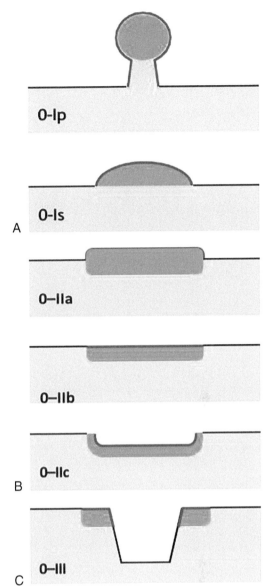

FIG 27.5 The Paris classification categorizes superficial-appearing esophageal carcinoma as **A,** type 0-I (protruding), **B,** type 0-II (without definite protrusion or depression), or **C,** type 0-III (excavated). Type 0-I and 0-III lesions carry a high likelihood of submucosal invasion, suggesting stage T1b disease, whereas type 0-IIa (slightly elevated) and 0-IIb (completely flat) tumors suggest stage Tis or T1a disease. Type 0-IIc (slightly depressed) lesions may be stage Tis, T1a, or T1b. (Adapted from Endoscopic Classification Review Group: Update on the Paris classification of superficial neoplastic lesions in the digestive tract. *Endoscopy* 37[6]:570–578, 2005.)

disease, particularly if being considered for endoscopic resection, which, in the presence of lymph node metastasis, would necessitate esophagectomy and chemoradiation for the chance of a cure.

METHODS OF ENDOSCOPIC TREATMENT OF ESOPHAGEAL CANCER

Endoscopic treatment can be broadly divided into tissue-acquiring and tissue ablative therapies. Tissue-acquiring strategies, namely

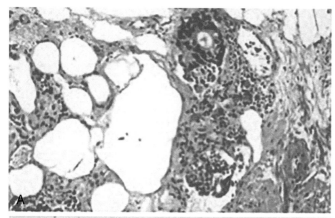

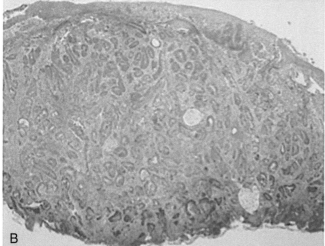

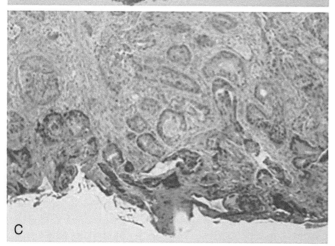

FIG 27.6 **A,** Lymphovascular invasion. **B,** Deep margin involvement with **C,** magnification.

EMR and ESD, as mentioned previously, are not only diagnostic but also potentially therapeutic. Ablative therapies induce tissue injury via heat (radiofrequency ablation or argon plasma coagulation [APC]), cold (cryotherapy), or photochemical energy (photodynamic therapy [PDT]), and do not yield tissue for histology. The principle of ablation is based on the concept of inducing squamous re-epithelialization with acid reflux control following ablation of the metaplastic mucosa.

In patients with BE and intramucosal adenocarcinoma treated with endoscopic resection, the risk of metachronous or recurrent cancer remains substantial (approximately 30%).[28] Thus, ablative therapies are recommended in an effort to eradicate the background of premalignant BE and promote neosquamous re-epithelialization. Additionally, the presence of residual BE mucosa has been shown to be predictive of recurrent cancers.[28,29] If HGD or intramucosal cancer is detected on random biopsies in the absence of visible abnormalities, despite careful examination, ablative therapies should be directly pursued following careful evaluation for any visible abnormalities, which should be endoscopically resected. An algorithmic approach to patients with BE found to have focal lesions, HGD, or cancer is shown in Fig. 27.7.

Endoscopic Resection
Endoscopic Mucosal Resection
EMR was pioneered in Japan for the management of gastric cancer, and has since been successfully applied to the treatment of various other lesions in the gastrointestinal tract. The main indications for performing esophageal EMR are the evaluation and staging of potentially malignant nodular lesions and treatment of established early esophageal cancer.

The two main methods of performing EMR are the cap and snare technique (Cap EMR) following saline injection, and band ligation (Band EMR) with snare resection. Both techniques are considered equally effective, and are demonstrated in Videos 27.1 and 27.2.[30] The cap is available in two styles; one is completely level or straight, whereas the other is oblique. The cap also varies in terms of the consistency of the material from which it is made. Generally, hard plastic caps are favored when there is a need to try to suction more scarred tissue, whereas soft caps are more useful when passing the caps through the upper pharynx, particularly in the presence of stenosis. The oblique cap is favored in resection of larger pieces of tissue, whereas the straight cap may be more favored when precision is required in the amount of tissue targeted for resection. Submucosal injection of a saline-epinephrine solution to lift the lesion may assist with resection and avoid deeper tissue layers. Depending on the visibility of the lesion, the borders may need to be marked using a cautery device (such as a multipolar coagulator) before injection, to ensure that the area to be removed can be visualized after injection. The area of carcinoma may have previously been established by biopsy, and the area is lifted by positioning an injection needle proximal to the lesion. The sequence of an injection with adequate lifting of the target lesion is shown in Fig. 27.8C.

Once the target lesion is lifted by the injection, it can be removed with resection. If removal is not accomplished immediately, inflammation induced by the injection may cause the cancer to become adherent to the submucosa or muscularis propria, which would make resection challenging. The mucosal resection component of this technique is similar to a standard polypectomy, except that suction is needed to create a pseudopolyp for mucosal removal. The endoscope with the resection cap attached is advanced into the stomach. It is generally recommended that the snare be positioned in the antrum of the stomach because the mucosa there is smoother and allows easier deflection of the snare around the diameter of the cap. Individuals experienced in this technique can position the snare using mucosa from the esophagus or proximal stomach, although this can be challenging.

The sequence of positioning a snare around the lip of a mucosal resection cap is shown in Fig. 27.8D. This is often the most difficult portion of the mucosal resection because, if the snare

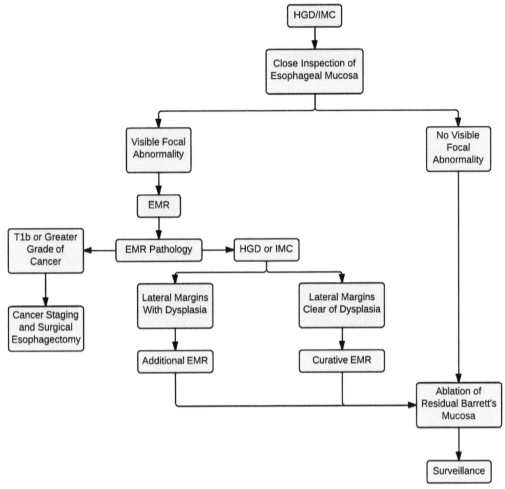

FIG 27.7 An algorithmic approach to patients with Barrett's esophagus found to have lesions, HGD, or cancer. *EMR,* endoscopic mucosal resection; *HGD,* high-grade dysplasia; *IMC,* intramucosal cancer. (From Blevins CH, Iyer PG: Endoscopic therapy for Barrett's oesophagus. *Best Pract Res Clin Gastroenterol* 29[1]:167–177, 2015.)[63]

is not properly formed, suctioning the tissue into the cap can result in dislodgment of the snare. In addition, the snare is easily deformed, and can be twisted during the process of forming the loop around the lip of the resection cap, resulting in the need for a new snare.

The tissue resection is completed by suctioning the tissue into the cap, as shown in Fig. 27.8E. When sufficient tissue is suctioned into the cap, the snare is closed, and cautery is applied until the tissue is transected. The average diameter of the resected specimen is approximately 1 cm. The resection and the residual ulcer are shown in Fig. 27.8F. Because lesions may be larger than the size of a single EMR, a second resection can be performed directly adjacent to the first resection; care must be taken not to suction the tissue exposed at the site of the first resection into the cap. Multiple resections in the same area should be attempted only by endoscopists familiar with the mucosal resection technique.

Band EMR is similar, but with some key differences. This technique uses a banding device, much like that used in esophageal variceal band ligation, which contains six bands and allows up to six resections to be performed without removal of the endoscope (Fig. 27.9). Saline injection is often not necessary if the

lesion can be adequately suctioned into the banding cap. A band is then released around the tissue, effectively creating a pseudo-polyp. A hexagonal electrocautery snare inserted through the working channel is used to resect the lesion. EMR fragments are then retrieved using a net-like device. In some centers, the specimens are pinned onto cork boards to orient the pathologists and aid in margin identification. Inking of margins may also be helpful in this regard.

The efficacy of EMR is well established, particularly when the tumor is of a moderate or well-differentiated grade, free of lymphovascular invasion, and confined to the mucosa.[31] In a study of 100 patients with early adenocarcinoma and no high-risk features undergoing EMR, the 5-year survival rate was 98%.[32] In the absence of BE ablative therapy, metachronous cancers were detected in 11% of patients during a mean 37-month follow-up period, but were treated successfully with additional endoscopic therapy. Although no randomized controlled trials comparing EMR with esophagectomy exist, observational studies suggest equivalent rates of cure and survival between the two.[28,29] These data have resulted in the recommendation that endoscopic resection supplant esophagectomy as first-line therapy for mucosal esophageal cancer.[33] Nonetheless, each patient should

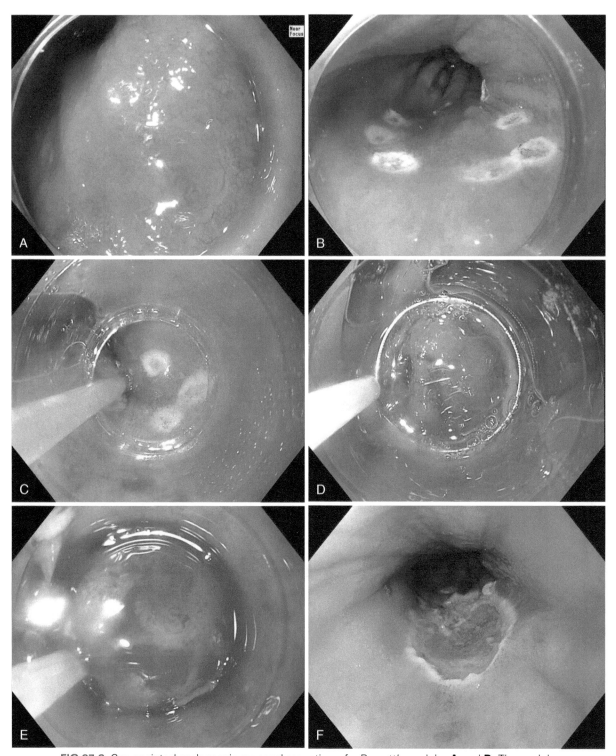

FIG 27.8 Cap-assisted endoscopic mucosal resection of a Barrett's nodule. **A** and **B,** The nodule is identified. It may be helpful to outline the nodule using cautery. **C,** The area is lifted via submucosal saline injection. **D,** A snare is carefully deployed and seated in the inner lip of the cap. **E,** Continuous suction is applied to gather adequate tissue within the cap. **F,** The snare is closed to excise the tissue, leaving behind a typical endoscopic mucosal resection defect.

be approached in a multidisciplinary manner in an effort to provide a full understanding of surgical and oncological treatment options before proceeding with any one therapy.

EMR is very safe. Early complications of EMR include major bleeding (1%–2%) and, rarely, perforation,[34,35] whereas the main late complication is delayed stricture (approximately 1%), which can typically be managed by dilation. EMR may be used to eradicate residual BE via piecemeal circumferential resection, although the risk of stricture formation is much higher compared to radiofrequency ablation (RFA) (discussed later).

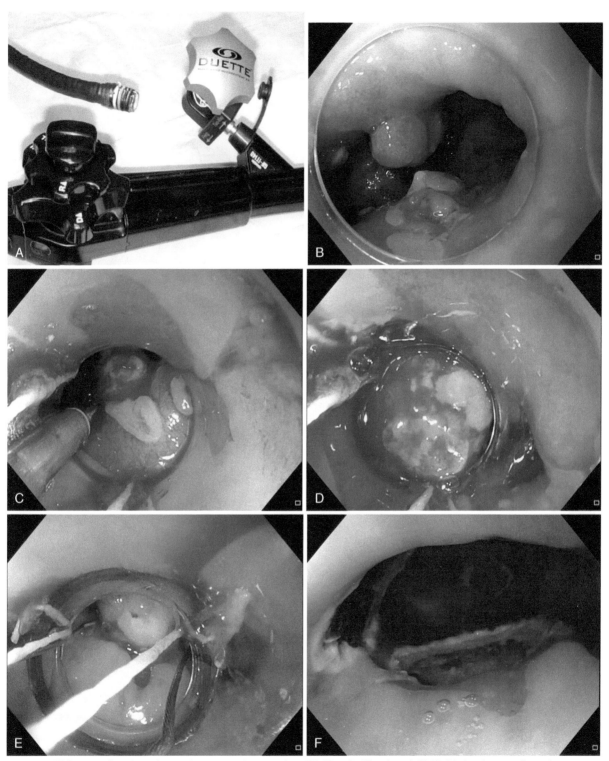

FIG 27.9 Band endoscopic mucosal resection (EMR). **A,** The band EMR kit is shown. **B** and **C,** As with cap-assisted EMR, the lesion is identified and lifted with submucosal injection of saline. **D,** The lesion is suctioned to allow deployment of a band around its base. **E,** An electrocautery snare is used to excise the "pseudopolyp" above or below the band. **F,** The EMR defect is seen (along with others) following multiband mucosectomy.

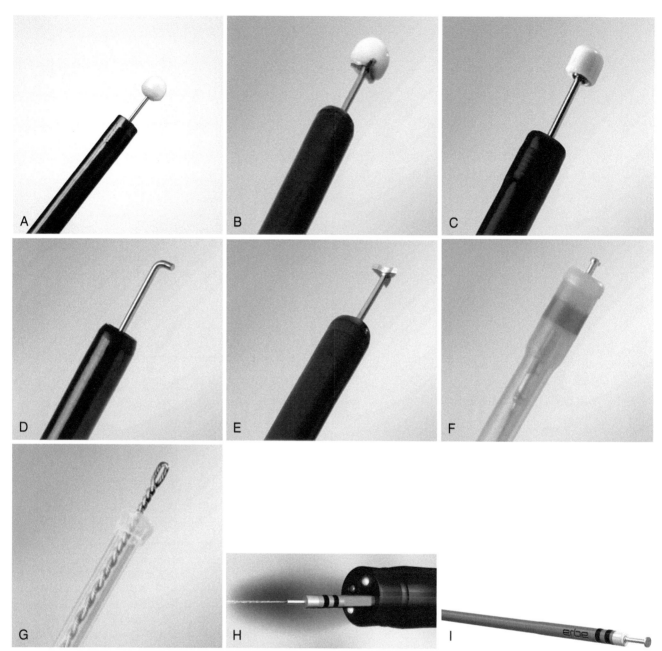

FIG 27.10 Various endoscopic "knives" are available for performing endoscopic submucosal dissection. **A,** ITKnife; **B,** ITKnife2; **C,** ITKnife nano; **D,** HookKnife; **E,** TTKnife; **F,** DualKnife; **G,** FlexKnife; **H,** HybridKnife I type; **I,** HybridKnife T type. (**A** to **G,** Courtesy of Olympus Corporation of the Americas, Center Valley, PA; **H** and **I** courtesy of Erbe USA, Inc., Marietta, GA.)[64]

If circumferential or widefield EMR of the residual BE segment is pursued, a stepwise approach is generally recommended over multiple endoscopic treatment sessions, to reduce the risk of stricturing.

Endoscopic Submucosal Dissection

A disadvantage of EMR has been the inability to obtain en bloc resection in larger lesions, rendering lateral margins uninterpretable in piecemeal EMR and raising the possibility of residual disease, which may increase the risk of recurrence.[36] ESD has been popularized in Asia as a method to mitigate this risk by allowing en bloc resections, and may be preferred over EMR in lesions larger than 2 cm.

The target lesion is first identified and marked 3 to 5 mm beyond its perimeter using cautery or APC. A submucosal bleb is formed as in EMR by injecting saline, 0.5% hyaluronate, or epinephrine diluted in glycerin. The goal is to allow en bloc dissection in the submucosal plane utilizing "knives." Several such knives with varying morphologies are now available for ESD (Fig. 27.10).

Initially, a circular incision is made around the lesion with a knife to free the lesion completely from the rest of the normal mucosa. Sharp-edged knives, such as the Hook knife or Triangle tip knife (Olympus Corporation of the Americas, Center Valley, PA), have an advantage in that they allow easier application through the tissue. The cut is made carefully to avoid penetrating

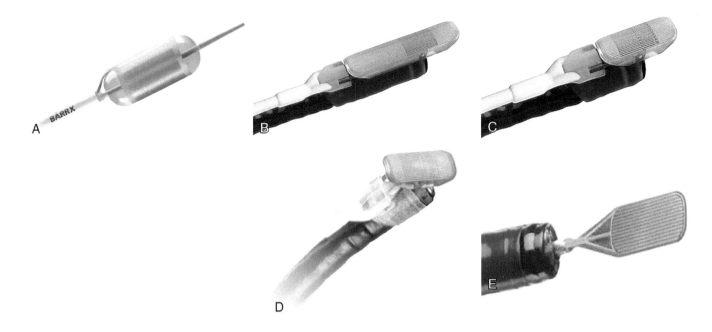

FIG 27.11 Radiofrequency ablation can be delivered circumferentially (**A**) or focally using various kits (**B** through **E**). (From Blevins CH, Iyer PG: Endoscopic therapy for Barrett's oesophagus. *Best Pract Res Clin Gastroenterol* 29[1]:167–177, 2015.)[63]

the entire wall, and once the defect is made, a knife similar to the IT knife (Olympus) is used, as the tip is not sharp enough to penetrate through the muscularis propria. The submucosal dissection is performed using a small dissection cap to lift the mucosa and cut the fibrous tissue that is underneath. This is the most challenging part of the dissection, and requires careful control. The hook knife has an advantage because the knife can "hook" the fibrous tissue from underneath the mucosa, and the cutting can be done more in the endoscopic field of vision. The dissection is a substantial undertaking, although a typical lesion can be removed in 1 to 2 hours by an experienced endoscopist.

Much of the data regarding ESD for esophageal cancer originates from Japan and involves the treatment of ESCC. In a meta-analysis of eight studies comparing ESD with EMR for the treatment of intramucosal cancers, the rates of en bloc resection (97.1% vs. 49.3%) and curative resection (92.3% vs. 52.7%) were superior for ESD.[37] A recent randomized controlled trial compared EMR and ESD for resection of Barrett's-related lesions smaller than 3 cm in 40 patients.[37a] Among those specimens revealing HGD and EAC, the rate of R0 resection (tumor-free resection margins) was higher in the ESD group (10/17) compared to the EMR group (2/17), but there was no significant difference in the rates of complete remission from neoplasia at 3 months. Moreover, ESD was noted to be technically more difficult, and was more time-consuming than EMR (mean procedure duration: 55 vs. 22 minutes). ESD was also associated with two perforations.

Ablative Therapies
Radiofrequency Ablation

RFA employs a bipolar electrode array located on circumferential (balloon) or focal devices that deliver precise amounts of thermal energy in a controllable fashion to the superficial 0.5 to 1.0 mm of mucosa. Necrosis ensues, and allows re-epithelialization with normal squamous mucosa. RFA is indicated in patients following endoscopic resection of intramucosal adenocarcinoma or HGD in the setting of BE due to the high risk of recurrent and/or metachronous lesions. RFA should also be considered to treat flat dysplasia (HGD and LGD) detected in the absence of a visible lesion.

RFA can be delivered in two ways: circumferentially or focally (Fig. 27.11). Typically, the initial treatment involves circumferential delivery, while follow-up sessions involve focal treatment for residual BE. Preparation for RFA involves cleansing the esophageal wall of mucus using either 1% acetylcysteine or the water jet channel. Next, endoscopic landmarks are identified, specifically noting the distances to the proximal extent of contiguous and circumferential BE and the top of the gastric folds. Time should be taken to exclude the presence of any structures that may compromise balloon expansion, such as strictures or nodularity.

A guidewire is then passed through the working channel into the gastric antrum. Using the original technique, the endoscope is then removed over the guidewire and exchanged for a sizing balloon catheter. The balloon is positioned in the esophagus approximately 3 cm proximal to the top of contiguous BE. Serial balloon diameter measurements are then taken, advancing the balloon distally to the top of the gastric folds in 1 cm intervals. The balloon with the smallest suggested diameter is selected for ablation. The sizing balloon catheter is then exchanged for the appropriately sized balloon catheter and positioned 1 cm proximal to the top of the proximal extent BE, which should be confirmed by parallel endoscopic intubation. The balloon is inflated, and ablation is initiated by pressing the foot pedal for approximately 1 second. The treated area (3 cm in length) is then examined by deflating the balloon, followed by balloon advancement with minimal overlap of the treated area (less than 1 cm). This sequence is repeated until the entire region of BE is treated (Fig. 27.12).

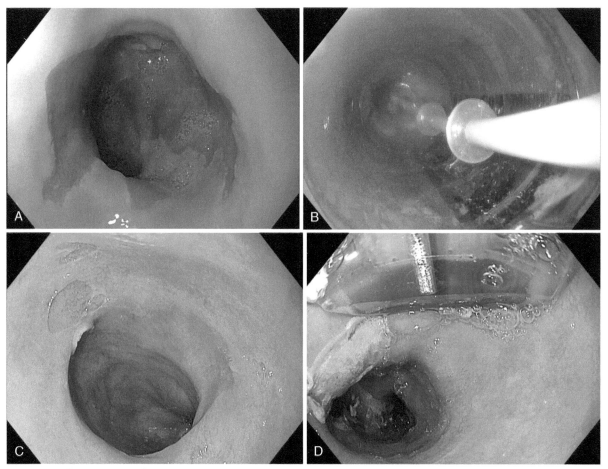

FIG 27.12 Radiofrequency ablation delivered **A** and **B,** circumferentially using a balloon system and **C** and **D,** focally during follow-up in the same patient for residual Barrett's epithelium.

The balloon is decompressed, removed, and reinflated to allow cleaning of any adherent coagulum. Coagulum should also be gently sloughed from the ablated BE area using the provided soft cap fixed to the end of the endoscope. Ablation of the BE area is then repeated once more in a similar fashion. A balloon ablation device that unfurls to conform to the shape and diameter of the esophagus, eliminating the need for sizing the esophagus before ablation, has recently become available. This device also allows ablation of 4 cm segments in one application instead of the previous 3 cm.

Patients should return in 8 to 12 weeks for follow-up endoscopy, at which time any residual BE can be treated using focal ablation. This technique delivers an electric current through an electrode array stationed on an over-the-scope distal attachment. After a careful endoscopic inspection has been performed and landmark measurements have been obtained, as described previously, the endoscope is removed, and the electrode array is positioned at 12 o'clock in the endoscopic image, followed by careful reintubation. Any residual BE should be held in the 12 o'clock position corresponding to the electrode array, followed by upward tip deflection, causing contact with the mucosa. The energy is activated using the foot pedal at 12 to 15 J/cm^2 (typically 12 J/cm^2), followed by a second pulse. This technique is then repeated for all areas of residual BE. Coagulum adherent to treated BE mucosa should then be sloughed using the provided cap, and the electrode cleaned externally using wet gauze. The

procedure is completed by performing another round of treatment in a similar fashion.

The efficacy of RFA was established in the Ablation of Intestinal Metaplasia with Dysplasia trial.[38] This was a multicenter, sham-controlled randomized trial in which 127 patients with dysplastic BE (LGD and HGD) were randomized to RFA or sham procedure every 2 months. At 12 months of follow-up, 81.0% of patients with HGD in the ablation group experienced complete eradication of dysplasia and metaplasia (with squamous re-epithelialization), compared with 19.0% in the sham group. Moreover, the rate of progression from HGD to cancer was significantly lower in the group treated with RFA compared to sham (2% vs. 19%, respectively). At 3 years of follow-up, 98% of all patients treated with RFA remained free of dysplasia, and 91% were free of recurrent intestinal metaplasia (accounting for repeat treatments).[39] Several studies have since reported similar findings.[40] RFA can also be effective in treating flat HGD and intramucosal cancer. In a retrospective study assessing the efficacy of RFA in 104 patients with BE who were determined to have HGD or intramucosal cancer in the absence of a visible lesion, the rates for eradication of dysplasia and intestinal metaplasia were 82.7% and 77.6%, respectively.[41]

RFA is a safe procedure with relatively few complications when administered alone, likely secondary to its minimal depth of mucosal penetration and injury. Bleeding, perforation, and death are all rare occurrences. Postprocedurally, chest pain and dysphagia are common, but typically resolve spontaneously within a few days. Stricture formation is uncommon (at a rate of 5%), and is usually managed with endoscopic dilatation.[6] Its favorable side effect profile, combined with its excellent efficacy and ease of delivery, has resulted in its endorsement as first-line ablative therapy.

Cryoablation

Cryoablation is an alternative technique for the ablation of BE. Cryoablation is characterized by cycles of rapid cooling (via liquid nitrogen or carbon dioxide) and thawing, resulting in tissue injury needed to promote healing by the squamous epithelium in a background of acid reflux control. The optimal dosimetry is still under investigation, but increased treatment durations are associated with a greater depth of tissue injury. Its advantage over RFA lies in its noncontact application, which facilitates its use in areas of mucosal irregularity. Moreover, cryoablation may cause less distortion of underlying tissue architecture, resulting in less fibrosis and a lower risk of stricture formation.

In preparation for cryoablation with liquid nitrogen, a decompressive gastric tube is inserted into the distal esophagus and antrum to prevention perforation secondary to overinsufflation from evaporated liquid cryogen. A cryotherapy spray catheter is then passed through the working channel of the endoscope and used to spray the liquid cryogen on the affected area (Fig. 27.13). This is delivered by an external console that stores the liquid nitrogen and controls application. The cryogen portion of the cycle lasts 20 seconds (range: 10–30), and is followed by a thawing period of 60 seconds. Typically, 3 to 4 endoscopic sessions are needed to treat long segment BE, and the procedure can be repeated every 6 to 8 weeks until eradication is achieved. A more recent approach involves a conforming balloon that is inflated and internally cooled by a small handheld unit, while a catheter is used for the treatment of focal lesions.

In an initial pilot study involving the monthly application of cryoablation until BE was eliminated, Johnston et al (2005) reported the complete healing of BE in 9 of 11 patients by 6 months of follow-up.[42] In a 2010 multicenter cohort study involving 98 patients with HGD, complete eradication of HGD (with persistent LGD) and complete eradication of all dysplasia in patients with HGD was reported in 97% and 87% of patients,

respectively.[43] Recent studies suggest good durability of eradication at 2 years post-treatment.[44] However, there is concern that recurrent dysplasia may be localized to the area just distal to the neosquamocolumnar junction, and therefore surveillance biopsies of this region may be advised.[45] The utility of cryoablation in treating intramucosal tumors is less well-known, but in a small series of 24 patients, 18 (75%) achieved complete eradication.[46] Cryoablation appears to be comparably effective to RFA in eradicating dysplasia, with lower rates of eradication of all intestinal metaplasia, although no direct comparison trials exist. Major complications from cryoablation are rare, although postprocedural chest pain and dysphagia are common.[47] Currently, cryotherapy is being offered to patients who have failed RFA (salvage therapy), are poor candidates for surgery, or are seeking palliative management.[48]

Photodynamic Therapy

PDT has been investigated as a treatment for cancer since its origins in 1961.[49] The therapy has traditionally involved the use of a combination of a photosensitizer drug and light of a specific wavelength that is required to activate the drug. The typical practice is to administer the drug days or hours before light delivery to allow the photosensitizer to concentrate into the neoplastic tissue. Light from a laser is applied to the mucosa, which causes general tissue destruction and cell death.

Photoradiation is usually performed by placing an optical fiber through the biopsy channel of the endoscope. The tip of this optical fiber has a cylindrical diffusing fiber that can be placed in the lumen of the esophagus. Generally, in the case of an early tumor, the fiber is placed next to or pressed against the tumor (Fig. 27.14). Treatment parameters for PDT for BE–associated neoplasia using porfimer sodium involve a drug dosage of 2 mg/kg body weight. The drug is given 48 hours before PDT. Red light is delivered through a diffusing fiber at a power output of 400 mW/cm fiber, for a total energy of approximately 300 J/cm fiber. If there is no endoscopically apparent disease, and mucosal resection has completely removed the lesion, a smaller dose of light, such as 200 J/cm fiber, can be used to treat the remaining Barrett's mucosa.

The overall results for PDT show good efficacy for early cancers. In a multicenter study comparing PDT to omeprazole, PDT improved the rates of complete eradication of HGD (77%

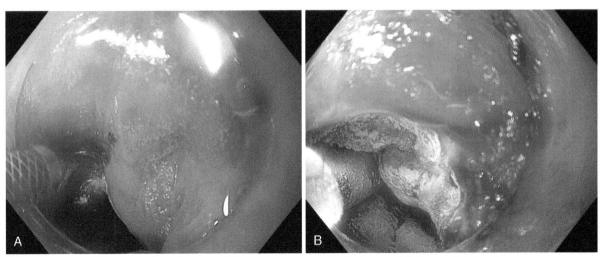

FIG 27.13 Cryoablation of Barrett's mucosa. **A,** Before and **B,** immediately after.

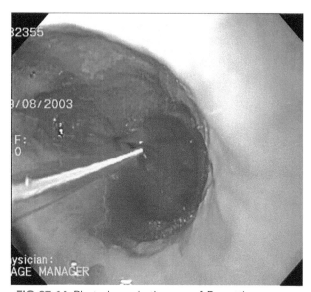

FIG 27.14 Photodynamic therapy of Barrett's mucosa.

vs. 39%) and intestinal metaplasia (52% vs. 7%), as well as progression to cancer (13% vs. 28%).[50] During 5 years of follow-up, 15% of the PDT group progressed to cancer, versus 29% in the omeprazole group. In another long-term study of 66 patients with HGD and early adenocarcinoma undergoing PDT, the 5-year survival rate was 97% for patients with HGD and 80% for patients with early adenocarcinoma.[51]

Complications include a cutaneous photosensitivity reaction, chest pain, dehydration due to the inability to obtain adequate fluid intake, and nausea. Rare side effects include injury of organs that are located near the esophagus, resulting in atrial fibrillation or pleural effusions.[52,53] Esophageal strictures are a major problem, as they occur in approximately one-third of patients treated.[54] These strictures are often quite fibrotic, and require multiple dilations to large diameters to resolve the constriction. PDT is currently listed as an option for ablative therapy by all three major US gastrointestinal societies, but should involve careful patient selection.

Argon Plasma Coagulation

APC involves the use of a hemostatic device in a noncontact fashion to cauterize bleeding lesions that are awkward to reach with traditional probes. APC has the ability to treat superficially, and has been thought to present a decreased risk of perforation. Mucosal ablative therapy for BE has been investigated, with good to excellent results.[55,56]

The primary goal of APC is to apply a current to the target lesion without producing a perforation. The argon gas is released under pressure. The endoscopist must be vigilant against allowing the tip of the probe to become embedded in the mucosa during treatment; this could result in the introduction of air into the submucosa or, worse, a perforation. For this reason, coagulation performed with the argon plasma coagulator should be done only while the probe is being withdrawn toward the endoscope; this should ensure that the tip of the probe is not embedded in the mucosa. Settings for treating adenocarcinoma should be in the higher power ranges; a range of 80 to 90 W has been cited in the literature. Higher output powers seem to be associated with improved outcomes in BE with HGD, although complications such as perforation and strictures are also seen at these dosages.

Treatment of intraepithelial carcinoma in BE has been reported in a limited series of patients. In one series of only three intraepithelial cancers, treatment with APC was ineffective and resulted in invasive disease.[57] These cancers also failed treatment with subsequent PDT. Similar results were observed in another small series of three patients with early esophageal cancers who were treated with APC; one recurrence was noted, and was subsequently treated with PDT.[58] Early ESCC and HGD have been treated with APC in Asian populations with good results.[59,60] In one series, 29 patients with ESCC and 42 patients with HGD were first treated with EMR, with any residual disease treated with APC.[60] The early results seem promising, as only three of the cancers (10%) recurred after 4 months. Esophageal strictures were found in four of the cases after EMR of most of the diameter of the esophagus. Overall, it seems that, although APC is well-tolerated with few described complications, its efficacy in the elimination of early esophageal cancer is limited, with significant (33%) failure rates in small numbers of BE–related cancers and lower failure rates (10%) in superficial squamous cell carcinomas. This finding is not surprising, given the decreased depth of injury associated with this treatment.

Combined EMR and Ablation

Treatment of early EAC in patients with BE frequently involves EMR for the removal of nodular lesions, followed by RFA for the eradication of underlying intestinal metaplasia, given the high risk of metachronous lesions. In a study including mostly patients with HGD and intramucosal cancer, EMR followed by RFA until complete ablation of BE was achieved resulted in complete eradication of dysplasia in 81% of patients, and clearance of HGD in 86% of patients.[61] This is now the preferred regimen for treating nodular BE, and is endorsed by major gastroenterological societies.

FOLLOW-UP

Patients undergoing endoscopic resection with or without ablative therapy for intramucosal EAC require close follow-up for surveillance of metachronous or recurrent lesions.[62] Evidence-based guidelines are lacking, but expert recommendations are to perform surveillance every 3 months for the first year, every 6 months during the second year, and annually the following years.[3]

Similarly, patients whose ESCC has been treated endoscopically require continued endoscopic surveillance, given the risk of head and neck squamous cell carcinoma. Moreover, additional resection and/or ablation may be necessary for recurrent or metachronous ESCC. Surveillance can be performed every 3 months for the first year after treatment, and every 3 to 6 months the following year.[7]

KEY REFERENCES

1. Arnold M, Soerjomataram I, Ferlay J, et al: Global incidence of oesophageal cancer by histological subtype in 2012, *Gut* 64:381–387, 2015.

3. Rubenstein JH, Shaheen NJ: Epidemiology, diagnosis, and management of esophageal adenocarcinoma, *Gastroenterology* 149:302–317 e1, 2015.

4. Hur C, Miller M, Kong CY, et al: Trends in esophageal adenocarcinoma incidence and mortality, *Cancer* 119:1149–1158, 2013.

6. Qumseya BJ, Wani S, Desai M, et al: Adverse events after radiofrequency ablation in patients with Barrett's esophagus: a systematic review and meta-analysis, *Clin Gastroenterol Hepatol* 14:1086–1095 e6, 2016.

7. Ohashi S, Miyamoto S, Kikuchi O, et al: Recent advances from basic and clinical studies of esophageal squamous cell carcinoma, *Gastroenterology* 149:1700–1715, 2015.

11. Dawsey SM, Fleischer DE, Wang GQ, et al: Mucosal iodine staining improves endoscopic visualization of squamous dysplasia and squamous cell carcinoma of the esophagus in Linxian, China, *Cancer* 83:220–231, 1998.

15. Edge SB, American Joint Committee on Cancer: *AJCC cancer staging manual*, New York, 2010, Springer.

16. Dunbar KB, Spechler SJ: The risk of lymph-node metastases in patients with high-grade dysplasia or intramucosal carcinoma in Barrett's esophagus: a systematic review, *Am J Gastroenterol* 107:850–862, quiz 863, 2012.

17. Dubecz A, Kern M, Solymosi N, et al: Predictors of lymph node metastasis in surgically resected T1 esophageal cancer, *Ann Thorac Surg* 99:1879–1885, discussion 1886, 2015.

18. Manner H, Pech O, Heldmann Y, et al: Efficacy, safety, and long-term results of endoscopic treatment for early stage adenocarcinoma of the esophagus with low-risk sm1 invasion, *Clin Gastroenterol Hepatol* 11:630–635, quiz e45, 2013.

19. Shaheen NJ, Falk GW, Iyer PG, et al: ACG clinical guideline: diagnosis and management of Barrett's esophagus, *Am J Gastroenterol* 111:30–50, quiz 51, 2016.

23. Moss A, Bourke MJ, Hourigan LF, et al: Endoscopic resection for Barrett's high-grade dysplasia and early esophageal adenocarcinoma: an essential staging procedure with long-term therapeutic benefit, *Am J Gastroenterol* 105:1276–1283, 2010.

25. Leggett CL, Lewis JT, Wu TT, et al: Clinical and histologic determinants of mortality for patients with Barrett's esophagus-related T1 esophageal adenocarcinoma, *Clin Gastroenterol Hepatol* 13:658–664 e1–3, 2015.

27. Young PE, Gentry AB, Acosta RD, et al: Endoscopic ultrasound does not accurately stage early adenocarcinoma or high-grade dysplasia of the esophagus, *Clin Gastroenterol Hepatol* 8:1037–1041, 2010.

28. Pech O, Behrens A, May A, et al: Long-term results and risk factor analysis for recurrence after curative endoscopic therapy in 349 patients with high-grade intraepithelial neoplasia and mucosal adenocarcinoma in Barrett's oesophagus, *Gut* 57:1200–1206, 2008.

29. Prasad GA, Wu TT, Wigle DA, et al: Endoscopic and surgical treatment of mucosal (T1a) esophageal adenocarcinoma in Barrett's esophagus, *Gastroenterology* 137:815–823, 2009.

33. Bennett C, Vakil N, Bergman J, et al: Consensus statements for management of Barrett's dysplasia and early-stage esophageal adenocarcinoma, based on a Delphi process, *Gastroenterology* 143:336–346, 2012.

34. Tomizawa Y, Iyer PG, Wong Kee Song LM, et al: Safety of endoscopic mucosal resection for Barrett's esophagus, *Am J Gastroenterol* 108:1440–1447, quiz 1448, 2013.

35. Pech O, May A, Manner H, et al: Long-term efficacy and safety of endoscopic resection for patients with mucosal adenocarcinoma of the esophagus, *Gastroenterology* 146:652–660 e1, 2014.

36. Prasad GA, Buttar NS, Wongkeesong LM, et al: Significance of neoplastic involvement of margins obtained by endoscopic mucosal resection in Barrett's esophagus, *Am J Gastroenterol* 102:2380–2386, 2007.

38. Shaheen NJ, Sharma P, Overholt BF, et al: Radiofrequency ablation in Barrett's esophagus with dysplasia, *N Engl J Med* 360:2277–2288, 2009.

39. Shaheen NJ, Overholt BF, Sampliner RE, et al: Durability of radiofrequency ablation in Barrett's esophagus with dysplasia, *Gastroenterology* 141:460–468, 2011.

40. Orman ES, Li N, Shaheen NJ: Efficacy and durability of radiofrequency ablation for Barrett's Esophagus: systematic review and meta-analysis, *Clin Gastroenterol Hepatol* 11:1245–1255, 2013.

43. Shaheen NJ, Greenwald BD, Peery AF, et al: Safety and efficacy of endoscopic spray cryotherapy for Barrett's esophagus with high-grade dysplasia, *Gastrointest Endosc* 71:680–685, 2010.

61. Haidry RJ, Dunn JM, Butt MA, et al: Radiofrequency ablation and endoscopic mucosal resection for dysplastic barrett's esophagus and early esophageal adenocarcinoma: outcomes of the UK National Halo RFA Registry, *Gastroenterology* 145:87–95, 2013.

A complete reference list can be found online at ExpertConsult .com

28

Palliation of Malignant Dysphagia and Esophageal Fistulas

Andrea Anderloni, Gianluca Lollo, and Alessandro Repici

INTRODUCTION

The incidence of new cases of esophageal and gastroesophageal junction (GEJ) cancer is estimated to be 450,000 per year worldwide. Esophageal cancer is the eighth most frequent malignancy and has the sixth-highest cancer-specific mortality. The estimated 5-year survival rate in Western countries is less than 20% after the diagnosis.[1] In the past, squamous cell carcinoma (SCC) was responsible for more than 90% of cases of esophageal carcinoma, but currently, adenocarcinoma is by far the leading esophageal malignancy, representing more than 60% of overall esophageal cases.[2] This change in the histologic trend probably comes from the modification of risk factors for esophageal cancer, with several risk factors for adenocarcinoma (such as gastroesophageal reflux disease [GERD], Barrett's esophagus, cigarette smoking, obesity, hiatal hernia, and age > 50 years) being very globally distributed.[3] Esophageal SCC is more frequently associated with smoking and alcohol intake. In patients with head and neck cancer, the risk of developing esophageal cancer is increased 3 to 10 times, with incidence ranging from 1% to 8%.[4] SCC is located predominantly in the upper and middle parts of the esophagus.[5] However, there are other nonesophageal cancers that can cause dysphagia, including primary lung cancer, proximal gastric cancer, and mediastinal lymphadenopathy.[6] Adenocarcinoma of the esophagus, on the other hand, is located primarily in the distal esophagus. The poor prognosis of esophageal cancer is mainly due to the late diagnosis of advanced neoplasia, which allows only palliative treatments. The most common clinical symptom at presentation is dysphagia; other symptoms include drooling, thoracic pain, anemia, nausea, and weight loss usually associated with severe malnutrition. Moreover, advanced esophageal neoplasia may be associated in a limited number of cases with the presence of tracheal or bronchoesophageal fistula. Thus, the main goal of the palliative measures is the treatment of dysphagia and eventually the treatment of esophagorespiratory fistulas.[7,8] Significant weight loss and malnutrition as a consequence of malignant dysphagia, as well as cachexia, are predominant symptoms in esophageal neoplastic strictures. To diagnose nutritional imbalances at an early stage, the European Society for Clinical Nutrition and Metabolism (ESPEN) recommends regular evaluation of nutritional intake, weight change, and body mass index (BMI) at the time of cancer diagnosis and repeated according to the stability of the clinical situation.[9] Esophageal stenting is currently the most effective method for this aim and is used in approximately 50% of patients with inoperable esophageal carcinoma. Tracheoesophageal or bronchoesophageal fistulas usually develop quite late in the context of advanced cancer of the esophagus, lung, or mediastinum, either as a consequence of progressive tumoral invasion or as an adverse event of cancer therapies, in particular chemoradiotherapy. Unfortunately, the clinical condition of such patients has often already significantly worsened at the time they develop a fistula, and the remaining life expectancy is quite short (within weeks to months). Rapid relief of life-threatening symptoms related to the fistula, preferably by minimally invasive treatment such as esophageal stenting, is thus of pivotal importance to improve quality of life. In this chapter, we will address the endoscopic management of malignant dysphagia due to advanced cancer that is not suitable for surgery.

ESOPHAGEAL STENTS

Thanks to the technologic improvements of the last 20 years, different types of stents have been introduced to the market. Multiple types of self-expandable stents are available. They differ in terms of design, luminal diameter, radial force, flexibility, and degree of shortening after deployment. Available stents can be divided in two main categories: self-expandable metal stents (SEMSs) and self-expandable plastic stent (SEPSs). SEMSs are further subdivided into fully covered (FCSEMS), partially covered (PCSEMS), or uncovered SEMS.[10] SEMS are mainly made of nitinol, a nickel and titanium alloy. In clinical practice, covered stents (partially or full covered) are usually preferred to the uncovered ones. It has been demonstrated that covered stents may delay tumor ingrowth without increasing the risk of

TABLE 28.1 Characteristics of Currently Available Types of Metal Stents

Stent Type	Covering	Length (cm)	Diameter (mm)	Release System	Degree of Shortening	Flexibility	Stent Material	Manufacturer
Alimaxx-ES	Full	7, 10, 12	12, 14, 16, 18, 22	Distal	0%	Moderate to high	Nitinol/polyurethane	Merit, South Jordan, UT
SX-Ella	Full	8.5, 11, 13.5, 15	20, 25	Distal	10%–20%	Low	Nitinol/polyethylene	Ella, Hradec Kralove, Czech Republic
Evolution	Partial/full	8, 10, 12, 12.5,15	23, 25	Distal	10%–20%	Moderate	Nitinol/Silicone	Cook Medical, Limerick, Ireland
Niti-S	Full/partial	6, 8, 10, 12, 14, 15	16, 18, 20, 22, 24, 28	Proximal/ distal	10%	High	Nitinol/polyurethane	Taewoong, Pusan, South Korea
Wallflex	Full/partial	10, 12, 15	18, 23	Distal	30%–40%	Moderate	Nitinol/silicone	Boston Scientific, Marlborough, MA
Ultraflex	Partial/ uncovered	10, 12, 15	18, 23	Proximal/ distal	30%–40%	High	Nitinol/polyurethane	Boston Scientific, Marlborough, MA
Polyflex	Full (plastic stent)	9, 12, 15	16, 18, 21	Distal	0%	Low	Polyester/silicone	Boston Scientific, Marlborough, MA

migration.[11] The most common metal stents currently available are listed in Table 28.1.

Of course, an ideal stent that can perfectly fit all clinical situations does not exist. However, all available covered metal stents meet some of the criteria required to palliate malignant dysphagia and to provide temporary relief from refractory esophageal strictures. Some FCSEMS and plastic stents are also approved for temporary stenting in patients with benign recurrent or refractory esophageal strictures.[11]

MANAGEMENT OF NONOPERABLE ESOPHAGEAL MALIGNANCY

The European Society of Gastrointestinal Endoscopy (ESGE) guidelines suggest:

- Placement of PCSEMSs or FCSEMSs for palliative treatment of malignant dysphagia over laser therapy, photodynamic therapy, and esophageal bypass.
- For patients with longer life expectancy, brachytherapy can be considered a valid alternative, or used in addition, to stenting in esophageal cancer patients with malignant dysphagia. Brachytherapy may provide a survival advantage and possibly a better quality of life compared to SEMS placement alone.
- Esophageal SEMS placement is the preferred treatment for sealing tracheoesophageal or bronchoesophageal fistulas.
- The use of concurrent external radiotherapy and esophageal stent treatment is not recommended.
- SEMS placement is also not recommended as a bridge to surgery or prior to preoperative chemoradiotherapy because it is associated with a high incidence of adverse events, and alternative satisfactory options, such as placement of a feeding tube, are available.[10]

TECHNIQUES OF STENT PLACEMENT

Stent placement should be performed in the endoscopic room by an experienced endoscopist, preferably under deep sedation and fluoroscopy control, and with the support of personnel who are familiar with stent placement and related devices, such as guidewires and catheters. The length and diameter of the stent should be adequately chosen before stent placement according to stricture size and length: stent length should be 2 cm longer than the distal and proximal border of the neoplasia. Marking of proximal tumor borders is of paramount importance to properly deploy the stent under fluoroscopic control. Some experts prefer to use internal markers as clips or submucosal injection of Lipiodol (Guerbet, Villepinte, France) to achieve a better radiological identification of tumor localization. After proper definition of stricture characteristics (length, size, borders), a super-stiff steel guidewire, such as the Savary guidewire (Cook Medical, Bloomington, IN), is introduced through the stricture under fluoroscopic guidance, with the distal tip placed deeply into the stomach. Occasionally, in cases of very tight strictures, an endoscopic retrograde cholangiopancreatography (ERCP)-like technique with catheters and hydrophilic guidewires may be required to safely cannulate the stricture and advance the guidewire down into the stomach. In such a case the hydrophilic guidewire is then replaced with a stiffer one (i.e., Amplatz, Boston Scientific, Marlborough, MA), which is better able to support the proper advancement of the stent catheter through the stricture. Once the stent is advanced through the esophagus over the guidewire, it should be released slowly and carefully under fluoroscopic and/or endoscopic visualization. Stent deployment can also be performed under pure endoscopic control with results that are comparable in terms of efficacy and safety to stents released under fluoroscopic control. In such a case, a small-caliber scope is usually advanced alongside the stent catheter and used to monitor stent deployment, keeping it a few centimeters proximal to the stricture.[12,13] At the end of the procedure, contrast medium may be injected through the working channel of the scope to confirm the correct positioning of the stent and to exclude complications, such as perforation. After the procedure, the patient should be closely observed in the recovery room to quickly diagnose early procedural-related complications such as hemorrhage, aspiration, perforation, and respiratory failure.

Once immediate complications are excluded, it is possible to restart feeding with fluids and then progressively with semisolids. A special mention should be made on the positioning of the stent in esophageal cancers located close to the upper esophageal sphincter (UES) (Fig. 28.1). These tumors represent only 7% to 10% of all esophageal carcinomas. However, they are considered the most difficult to treat because of possible complications such

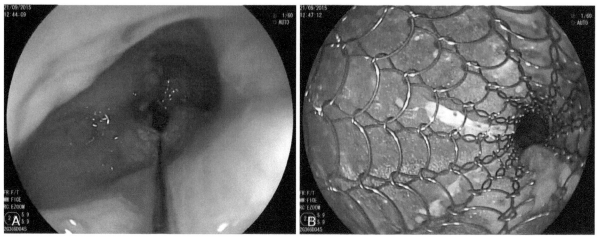

FIG 28.1 **A,** Proximal esophageal cancer immediately distal to the upper esophageal sphincter (UES). **B,** Post successful self-expandable metal stent (SEMS) placement distal to the UES.

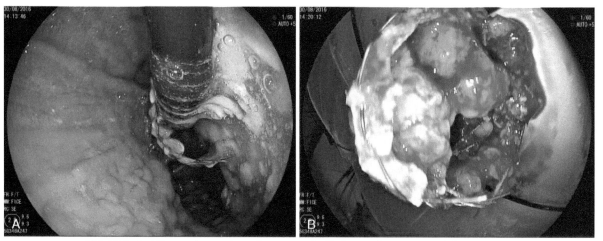

FIG 28.2 **A,** Migrated stent into the stomach. **B,** Stent after successful extraction.

as aspiration pneumonia and proximal migration, as well as the complaint of foreign body sensation and quite relevant local pain in some cases.[14] Several studies have shown that treatment with stents is possible without major complications compared with middle/distal esophageal tumors.[14] In these cases, it is better to perform the procedure under endoscopic and fluoroscopic control using a stent with proximal deployment to allow a more precise release and placement.

STENT COMPLICATIONS

The placement of esophageal stents as a palliative treatment can cause complications, such as pain, bleeding, migration of the stents, perforations, or the onset of esophageal fistula,[2,3,15,16] with an overall mortality rate of 2.2%.[17] These complications are usually divided according to their appearance, either early (within one week) or late (after 1 week). The most frequently reported complications are stent migration, stent obstruction, and esophageal perforation.[12]

Stent Migration

Stent migration occurs in approximately 20% of patients and is often reported in noncircumferential esophageal tumors, or with use of a stent which has too small a caliber (Fig. 28.2).

The removal of a migrated stent can be performed endoscopically with foreign body forceps, but it may be challenging due to a number of anatomical and stent-related factors.

Indication for removal must be carefully considered in each patient because most patients do not develop symptoms directly related to a stent residing in the stomach, but have symptoms due to recurrent dysphagia.

Endoscopic removal will depend on the type of stent and the site of migration. When the stent is migrated distally but still in the esophagus, removal is indicated. Those with a proximal lasso can be easily pulled back by grasping the lasso with forceps, which allows constriction of the upper flange, permitting repositioning or removal. Endoscopic traction of plastic or metallic stents that do not have a proximal lasso might be more difficult (Fig. 28.3). Failure in esophageal stent removal rarely causes other complications, such as satiety.

Perforation

Perforation may occur in 2% to 8% of cases.[12,13] Early diagnosis of esophageal perforation is essential to avoid a disastrous outcome. Patients who experience pain or crepitus in the neck and chest should be evaluated immediately by chest radiography followed by computed tomography. Confined perforation may be managed conservatively with nothing by mouth, aspiration

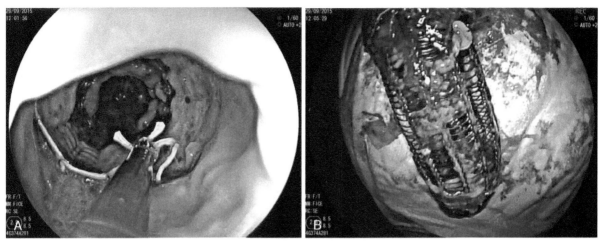

FIG 28.3 A, Esophageal stent removal using forceps to grab a proximal lasso. **B,** Stent after being removed from the individual using traction technique.

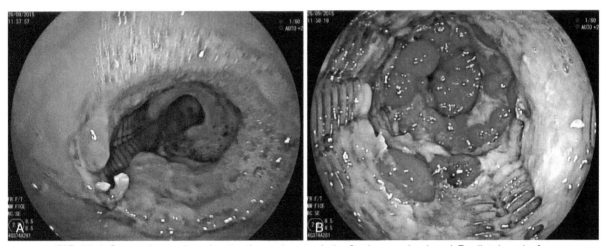

FIG 28.4 Stent obstruction due to tissue ingrowth in **A,** the proximal and **B,** distal end of a self-expandable metal stent (SEMS).

of the upper esophagus, antibiotics, and parenteral nutrition. If perforation is noted to occur during the procedure, it is reasonable to attempt to complete stent placement because this may seal the perforation. Aggressive covered stent preinsertion esophageal dilatation, prior esophageal surgery, and necrotic, angulated tumor characteristics may increase the risk of perforation. Perforation during deployment can be caused by the guidewire itself, application of excessive force to the endoscope during attempts to pass the stricture, or excessive dilation of the stricture. If a small perforation is recognized, it will usually seal if a covered stent is placed in the proper position, assuming the stricture can be traversed. Delayed perforation is less common and may be associated to concomitant radiation or chemotherapy. Moreover, pressure necrosis caused by the proximal or distal edge of the stent on the healthy esophageal mucosa may result in the development of a fistula. Delayed perforation and fistula formation are life-threatening complications, with a mortality rate of up to 50%.[13]

Bleeding

Bleeding may be caused by stent placement but, in most cases, does not require any further intervention. In patients with aortic involvement (i.e., stents are placed either before or after radiation

therapy), fatal bleedings are frequent.[18,19] Other possible causes of bleeding are mechanical ulcers due to the positioning of the esophageal stent with the distal end at the level of the gastric greater curvature. Therefore it is recommended to choose a stent with a suitable length, short enough to avoid ulceration but long enough to fully traverse the tumor. Finally, a stent located in proximity to the GEJ can cause reflux esophagitis with bleeding; in these cases, treatment with gastroprotective agents is sufficient.

Stent Obstruction

Another possible complication is stent obstruction, including tumor ingrowth/overgrowth, nonneoplastic tissue hyperplasia, and food impaction (Fig. 28.4). This complication has been reported in 30% to 40% of cases.[12] Tumor ingrowth is usually treated with the "stent-in-stent technique," or the positioning of an additional stent inside the previously placed stent. Multiple sessions of endoscopic treatments with argon plasma coagulation (APC) for tissue ablation and debulking have also been used. It is important with this condition to recommend diet adjustments and the selection of liquid foods to facilitate food transit until stent obstruction has been resolved; in addition, the consumption of drugs in liquid form reduces the risk of stent obstruction.[20]

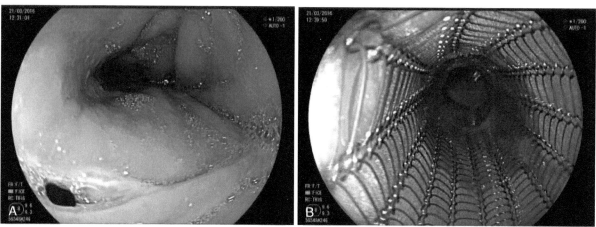

FIG 28.5 **A,** Esophagorespiratory fistula **B,** successfully treated with covered self-expandable metal stent (SEMS) placement.

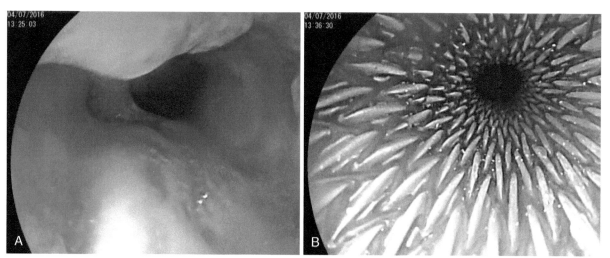

FIG 28.6 **A,** Partial esophageal stenosis due to persistent bulky tumor after radiation therapy. **B,** After self-expandable metal stent (SEMS) placement.

ESOPHAGORESPIRATORY FISTULA

Progressive infiltration of the primary esophageal tumor or late effects of previous radiation therapy can be the main causes of an esophagorespiratory fistula or, more rarely, of a fistula between the esophagus and the aorta, the mediastinum, or the pleura. Esophagorespiratory fistulae have been reported in 5% of patients with malignant esophageal strictures treated with stent placement.[21] Fistula formation can result in serious pulmonary infections from aspiration pneumonia. In these cases, it is important to assess the exact location of the fistula by using multiple imaging modalities. In most cases, the best therapeutic option for these types of fistulas is the use of a covered stent (Fig. 28.5).

However, a bronchoscopy is recommended prior to the second stent placement; sometimes it is necessary to place a tracheal stent before the esophageal stent to balance the compression caused by the esophageal stents and consequently avoid acute respiratory failure. Several retrospective and prospective series on endoscopic placement of a covered stent reported a complete sealing of the fistula in more than 90% of patients.[22,23] Aortic

erosion after stent placement is a life-threatening complication that comes with massive bleeding and rapid deterioration of the patient's condition due to shock and anemia. Most of the reported cases have led to patient death before any possible attempt at treatment.

STENT PLACEMENT AFTER RADIOTHERAPY AND/OR CHEMOTHERAPY

Physicians have historically avoided placing stents in patients with esophageal cancer before chemotherapy and radiotherapy to avoid the risk of complications such as esophageal fistulas.[24] Recent data are quite contradictory with regard to the risk of serious adverse events in patients receiving a stent after radiotherapy alone or in combination with chemotherapy (RTCT). Some studies show an increased risk, whereas other studies, including a meta-analysis, do not report any relationship between SEMS placement after RTCT and the incidence of life-threatening adverse events or survival[25] (Fig. 28.6). It has been reported that the potential increased risk, if any, of developing major complications in patients with prior radiation or chemotherapy may be mainly related to the radiation-induced damage on the esophageal wall, potentiated by chemotherapy. However, it is difficult to discern whether such stent-related adverse events are due to stents and radiation effects, the advanced nature of the disease process, or both. In general, the decision to place a stent in such situations must be carefully balanced in a multidisciplinary context, with due consideration given to other palliative modalities, and after having specifically informed the patient about the potential risk of life-threatening adverse events. Tailored therapy is the mainstay in challenging patients with recurrent dysphagia and disease progression despite previous attempts with radiation and chemotherapy. However, the ESGE guidelines suggest that the placement of an esophageal stent during concurrent external radiotherapy is not recommended.

CLINICAL OUTCOMES

Palliative stenting for malignant dysphagia is associated with a technical success of approximately 95%, a very low risk of early major complications (< 5%), and early clinical success of 80%. The median and mean survival after stent placement range from 78 to 83 days and 120 to 126 days, respectively. Survival has not been associated with the type of stent used.[26,27] Reintervention rate is approximately 25% to 35% and is mostly related to tumor ingrowth/overgrowth and stent migration/dislocation. Late complications after placement of esophageal stents may occur in 53% to 65% of patients, with almost half of these patients requiring some form of additional reintervention.[28,29] Procedure-related causes of death are seen in 0.5%–2% of patients, with an increased risk of mortality in those patients who have been previously treated with radiation or chemotherapy.[30,31]

CONCLUSION

Esophageal stenting is the most frequently used method of treating dysphagia caused by esophageal cancer. Physicians have several choices regarding esophageal stents and should choose the right stent based on the indication and the precise dimension and anatomic characteristics of the stricture, as well as the physician's personal experience. Even though stents are effective in improving dysphagia, the complication rate and the number of reinterventions for recurrent dysphagia are still rather high. Fortunately, many of these complications are within the endoscopist's control and can be successfully managed.

KEY REFERENCES

1. Ferlay J, Steliarova-Foucher E, Lortet-Tieulent J, et al: Cancer incidence and mortality patterns in Europe: estimates for 40 countries in 2012, *Eur J Cancer* 49:1374–1403, 2013.
5. Miller C: Carcinoma of the thoracic esophagus and cardia: a review of 405 cases, *Br J Surg* 49:507–522, 1962.
7. Van Heel NC, Haringsma J, Spaander MC, et al: Esophageal stents for the palliation of malignant dysphagia and fistula recurrence after esophagectomy, *Gastrointest Endosc* 72:249–254, 2010.
8. Van Heel NC, Haringsma J, Spaander MC, et al: Esophageal stents for the relief of malignant dysphagia due to extrinsic compression, *Endoscopy* 42:536–540, 2010.
9. Arends J, Bachmann P, Baracos V, et al: ESPEN guidelines on nutrition in cancer patients, *Clin Nutr* 36(1):11–48, 2017.
10. Spaander MC, Baron TH, Siersema PD, et al: Esophageal stenting for benign and malignant disease: European Society of Gastrointestinal Endoscopy (ESGE) Clinical Guideline, *Endoscopy* 48:939–948, 2016.
11. Schembre DB: Recent advances in the use of stents for esophageal disease, *Gastrointest Endosc Clin N Am* 20:103–121, 2010.
12. Baron TH: Minimizing endoscopic complications: endoluminal stents, *Gastrointest Endosc Clin N Am* 17:83–104, 2007.
13. Siersema P: Treatment options for esophageal strictures, *Nat Clin Pract Gastroenterol Hepatol* 5:142–152, 2008.
14. Verschuur EM, Kuipers EJ, Siersema PD: Esophageal stents for malignant strictures close to the upper esophageal sphincter, *Gastrointest Endosc* 66:1082–1090, 2007.
15. Homs MY, Steyerberg EW, Eijkenboom WM, et al: Single-dose brachytherapy versus metal stent placement for the palliation of dysphagia from oesophageal cancer: multicenter randomised trial, *Lancet* 364:1497–1504, 2004.
17. Simmons DT, Baron TH: Endoluminal palliation, *Gastrointest Endosc Clin N Am* 15:467–484, 2005.
18. Sumiyoshi T, Gotoda T, Muro K, et al: Morbidity and mortality after self-expandable metallic stent placement in patients with progressive or recurrent esophageal cancer after chemoradiotherapy, *Gastrointest Endosc* 57:882–885, 2003.
19. Yakami M, Mitsumori M, Sai H, et al: Development of severe complications caused by stent placement followed by definitive radiation therapy for T4 esophageal cancer, *Int J Clin Oncol* 8:395–398, 2003.
20. Repici A, Rando G: Expandable stents for malignant dysphagia, *Tech Gastrointest Endosc* 10:175–183, 2008.
22. Bethge N, Sommer A, Vakil N: Treatment of esophageal fistulas with a new polyurethane-covered, self-expanding mesh stent: a prospective study, *Am J Gastroenterol* 90:2143–2146, 1995.
23. May A, Ell C: Palliative treatment of malignant esophagorespiratory fistulas with Gianturco-Z stents. A prospective clinical trial and review of the literature on covered metal stents, *Am J Gastroenterol* 93:532–535, 1998.
24. Nishimura Y, Nagata K, Katano S, et al: Severe complications in advanced esophageal cancer treated with radiotherapy after intubation of esophageal stents: a questionnaire survey of the Japanese Society for Esophageal Diseases, *Int J Radiat Oncol Biol Phys* 56(5):1327–1332, 2003.
25. Sgourakis G, Gockel I, Radtke A, et al: The use of self-expanding stents in esophageal and gastroesophageal junction cancer palliation: a meta-analysis and meta-regression analysis of outcomes, *Dig Dis Sci* 55:3018–3030, 2010.
26. Christie NA, Buenaventura PO, Fernando HC, et al: Result of expandable metal stents for malignant esophageal obstruction in 100 patients: short-term and long-term follow-up, *Ann Thorac Surg* 71(6):1797–1802, 2001.
27. Yakoub D, Fahmy R, Athanasious T, et al: Evidence-based choice of esophageal stent for the palliative management of malignant dysphagia, *World J Surg* 32(9):1996–2009, 2008.
28. Johnson E, Enden T, Noreng HJ, et al: Survival and complications after insertion of self-expandable metal stents for malignant oesophageal stenosis, *Scand J Gastroenterol* 41(3):252–256, 2006.
29. Lowe AS, Sheridan MB: Esophageal stenting, *Semin Intervent Radiol* 21(3):157–166, 2004.
30. Wang MQ, Sze DY, Wang ZP, et al: Delayed complications after esophageal stent placement for treatment of malignant esophageal obstructions and esophagorespiratory fisulas, *J Vasc Interv Radiol* 12(4):465–474, 2001.
31. Baron TH: Expandable metal stents for the treatment of cancerous obstruction of the gastrointestinal tract, *N Engl J Med* 334(22):1681–1687, 2001.

A complete reference list can be found online at ExpertConsult .com

29

Endoscopic Approaches for Gastroparesis

John O. Clarke and Richard W. McCallum

CHAPTER OUTLINE

INTRODUCTION

The word *gastroparesis* is derived from the Greek words *gastro* and *pa'resis,* and translates to partial paralysis of the stomach. The diagnosis of gastroparesis is defined as delayed gastric emptying in the absence of mechanical obstruction, associated with one or more of the following symptoms: postprandial fullness, early satiety, nausea, vomiting, and bloating.[1] Whereas gastroparesis can be associated with diabetes mellitus, neuromuscular and connective tissue diseases, vagal injury, or some medications, in the majority of patients, no underlying etiology is identified, and they are presumed to be idiopathic. For reasons that are not entirely clear, there is a marked gender discrepancy in all subgroups, with women being affected far more often than men. True prevalence data are unclear, with estimates of up to 3%. One large study performed at the Mayo Clinic estimated a community prevalence of 1.8%.[2] However, this may be a significant underestimate of true prevalence, as approximately 40% of patients with functional dyspepsia have delayed gastric emptying on evaluation, and the prevalence of functional dyspepsia has been suggested to be approximately 10% to 15% worldwide.[3] In addition, the societal impact of gastroparesis is significant. Worsening symptoms are accompanied by poor food intake, weight loss, malnutrition, impaired function, and more emergency room visits. Data suggest that hospital admissions for gastroparesis in the United States now exceed those for gastroesophageal reflux, peptic ulcer disease, gastritis, and nausea.[4]

One of the most frustrating aspects of gastroparesis is the paucity of treatment options that are currently available. The only medication that is approved by the Food and Drug Administration (FDA) at present is metoclopramide, which also has an associated black box warning related to tardive dyskinesia. Other drugs that have shown efficacy in controlled trials are either not available in the United States (domperidone) or have been pulled from the market due to safety concerns (cisapride). Gastric electrical stimulation (GES) was given a Humanitarian Device Exemption by the FDA in 2000 based on the results of a double-blind controlled trial.[5] The lack of established treatment options, in tandem with the significant symptom burden associated with gastroparesis, has led to intense interest in alternative diagnostic and treatment paradigms. In particular, endoscopic options for both diagnosis and therapy have risen to the forefront in recent years, driven by a number of factors: (1) the paucity of accepted medical treatment options, (2) increased understanding regarding the pathophysiology of gastroparesis, and (3) technical advances in endoscopy that have expanded the feasibility of interventional endoscopic options. In this chapter, we will present our understanding of the current role of endoscopy in the diagnosis and treatment of gastroparesis, and will speculate on what the near future holds.

PHYSIOLOGY OF GASTROPARESIS

Although delayed gastric emptying is the *sine qua non* of gastroparesis, it is well-recognized that multiple mechanisms are at play in addition to gastric emptying with regards to symptom pathogenesis. The National Institutes of Health (NIH) Gastroparesis Clinical Research Consortium, consisting of six Academic Motility Centers, has played an integral role in advancing our understanding of pathogenesis, but much remains to be learned.

In addition to objective impairment of gastric emptying, subsets of affected patients have also been shown to have impaired fundic accommodation, gastric dysrhythmias, impaired gastroduodenal coordination, abnormal duodenal signaling, autonomic dysfunction, visceral hypersensitivity, and abnormal central processing of peripheral stimulation.[6] Each of these mechanisms may play a role in the clinical presentation of subsets of affected patients, and it is unlikely that symptoms can be attributed to a uniform origin.

This recognition of gastroparesis as a heterogeneous process is perhaps best exemplified through the lens of histopathology. Recent studies undertaken through the NIH gastroparesis consortium have utilized full-thickness gastric biopsies to evaluate for histopathologic changes that may provide evidence as to underlying mechanisms. These investigations have led to intriguing observations, including loss of interstitial cells of Cajal (ICCs), abnormal macrophage-related immune infiltrates, and decreased nerve fibers.[7-10] One common theme that has emerged is that the histopathologic pattern observed in these patients can be variable. For example, a depletion of ICC numbers in the smooth muscle of the antrum or gastric body has been recognized in up to 40% of severe gastroparetics not responding to medical therapies and requiring surgery to place a gastric electrical stimulator device (Enterra, Medtronic, Minneapolis, MN). However, approximately 50% of such severely symptomatic patients had a normal number of ICCs.[11]

Recent research (2016) has also expanded our understanding of the role of pylorus in gastroparesis through looking at the histopathology of this region in patients with severe disease who underwent surgery to insert a gastric electric stimulator and/or perform a pyloroplasty. In one series, approximately 70% of gastroparetic patients had pyloric ICC loss. Moreover, collagen fibrosis was observed in the pylorus of more than 80% of these patients. These findings may help explain pyloric dysfunction in gastroparesis, making interventions in the pyloric region a reasonable therapeutic approach in these patients. This study also identified eosinophilic inclusion bodies in the antrum and/or the pylorus, which were limited to diabetic gastroparetic patients. The clinical role of these inclusion bodies remains unclear, and further investigation is needed.[12]

Studies of the histopathology of the stomach in gastroparesis have relied on patients with severe cases who underwent surgery, which allowed full-thickness biopsies of the gastric wall to be taken. Therefore, a knowledge gap still remains in regard to patients with mild or moderate symptoms who are treated medically. Minimally invasive techniques such as percutaneous endoscopically assisted transenteric full-thickness gastric biopsy[13] or biopsies utilizing endoscopic ultrasound guidance[14] may allow us to study the gastric tissue in patients with less severe gastroparesis and provide further insight into the potential mechanisms of disease pathogenesis and progression.

Overall, there does not appear to be any single gold standard histopathologic marker for gastroparesis as the disorder is currently defined. It is likely that our current definition of gastroparesis, which relies on symptoms in tandem with gastric emptying, lumps many related subgroups under the same umbrella. As data emerge, there will be refinement of the underlying mechanisms of symptom pathogenesis and the relative importance of each mechanism in the development of individual symptoms, and there will also likely be a change in disease nomenclature based on recognition of clinically meaningful subgroups.

THE ROLE OF ENDOSCOPY

The role of endoscopy in the diagnosis and management of gastroparesis has evolved in the past decade. Endoscopy has always been required to exclude gastric outlet obstruction, peptic ulcer disease, malignancy, or significant inflammation prior to establishment of the diagnosis of gastroparesis, a functional disorder of gastric emptying. However, the role of endoscopy has recently expanded to include more in-depth diagnostic investigations, as well as novel treatment options. In this chapter, we will focus on the numerous primary roles endoscopy plays in the diagnosis and management of gastroparesis. Specifically, we will review the data regarding endoscopic therapeutic advances in subsets of patients who may have primary pyloric dysfunction (either in isolation or in tandem with other defects); examine the role of endoscopy in the acquisition of full-thickness biopsies; evaluate the role of endoscopic temporary GES; and review the data regarding endoscopic venting/feeding options for patients with refractory symptoms. This is by no means an exhaustive account of all the ways in which endoscopy can be of benefit in gastroparesis; however, we have tried to highlight recent advances and the state of the art as we see it today.

PYLORIC DYSFUNCTION

Whereas multiple mechanisms may be responsible for symptom pathogenesis in affected patients, pyloric dysfunction has received significant attention. Pyloric involvement in symptom pathogenesis has been speculated for some time, with the first report of successful intrapyloric botulinum toxin injection for gastroparesis appearing as an abstract at the annual meeting of the American College of Gastroenterology almost 20 years ago.[15] However, recent developments in diagnostic technology and endoscopic therapeutic options have brought this issue to the forefront.[16]

Endoscopic Diagnostic Options for Pyloric Dysfunction

There are multiple means by which pyloric function can be assessed endoscopically, but no true gold standard, as each available modality assesses a different aspect of pyloric function. Traditional investigation relied on fluoroscopy and routine endoscopy to assess for pyloric outlet obstruction. Although both these investigations are adequate for detection of obstruction, neither assesses muscular function reliably enough to guide definitive treatment, and they certainly cannot quantify pyloric dysfunction. Scintigraphy is considered a gold standard for assessment of motility, but it does not evaluate pyloric function as an isolated component of the emptying process. When further diagnostic information is needed with regards to pyloric function, there are four additional modalities available for investigation, some of which are accessible via endoscopy, and some of which require more specialized motility equipment. At present, all are complementary, and there is not a true gold standard amongst the group; however, that may change in upcoming years as additional data emerge.

Antroduodenal or pyloric manometry (ADM) involves the placement, either via endoscopy or fluoroscopy, of a manometry catheter with multiple pressure sensors across the pylorus such that sensors are present in both the gastric antrum, the duodenum, and the small bowel. The initial papers evaluating the role of ADM in the assessment of pyloric pressure in health and disease stemmed from investigators at the University of

Southern California and the Mayo Clinic in the mid-1980s.[17,18] Investigators at the Mayo Clinic showed that some patients with gastroparesis had prolonged pyloric pressurization and more intense contraction, which they labeled "pylorospasm." ADM may identify a subset of patients who are more likely to have pyloric dysfunction; however, this technology has not been widely adopted, as the pylorus is relatively short, migration of the catheter is common, the technique is cumbersome and resource-intensive, and few companies produce the necessary equipment. At present, ADM is largely limited to only a few tertiary referral centers. One potential change in recent years has been the development of high-resolution manometry catheters with shorter interval spacing of pressure sensors, which could lead to less risk of migration over the course of the study. Researchers from Temple University investigated the role of a high-resolution ADM catheter in 10 patients, but data using this technology in clinical care are extremely limited at present, and it is unclear how much of an inroad high-resolution ADM will be able to make, given the high cost of the equipment and the significant risk for sensor injury in the course of endoscopic placement. Whereas ADM is the traditional means for assessment of pyloric function, it has not achieved a strong clinical foothold in its three decades of availability (largely for the reasons mentioned previously), and likely will not in the future, unless a low-cost high-resolution dedicated ADM catheter is developed for routine clinical use.

The wireless motility capsule is a wireless, ingestible medical device that measures pH, pressure, and temperature throughout the gastrointestinal tract. This was approved by the FDA in 2006 for the evaluation of gastric emptying in patients with suspected gastroparesis. Given the relative ease of this technology as compared to ADM, there has been speculation that perhaps similar information could be derived with regards to pyloric pressurization without the hassle of performing ADM. However, there are also reasons why this may not be feasible, as (a) the wireless motility capsule is not fixed in space, but rather allowed to move with contractions (perhaps making it less reliable for detection of contractile amplitude and frequency at a single or specific site) and (b) passage of the capsule through the pylorus itself would be relatively brief, perhaps giving only limited information with regards to pyloric function. Data with regards to antroduodenal pressure patterns in patients with gastroparesis are very limited. There has only been one direct comparison between ADM and the wireless motility capsule,[19] and only one key paper investigating gastric motility recordings in patients with gastroparesis versus healthy controls.[20] However, neither of these papers evaluated pyloric function specifically. Investigators from Johns Hopkins evaluated the role of the wireless motility capsule in the assessment of intrapyloric pressure and suggested a correlation between this measurement and gastric emptying as detected by scintigraphy.[21] However, the utilization of the wireless motility capsule to evaluate pyloric function is still in the research phase, and progress seems unlikely. This could change with further models or improvements on the wireless motility capsule principles, and as additional data emerge.

Impedance planimetry, otherwise known as the functional lumen imaging probe (FLIP), has recently emerged as a legitimate means by which to measure pyloric diameter and distensibility. This device was approved by the FDA in 2010, but has only recently entered routine clinical practice. Most studies to date have utilized FLIP in the assessment of esophageal disorders; however, there is a growing body of literature reporting on the use of FLIP in the assessment of pyloric distensibility. Gourcerol et al (2015) recently evaluated pyloric compliance in healthy controls and patients with gastroparesis and reported that patients with gastroparesis had lower pyloric compliance versus healthy controls. They also noted that pyloric compliance correlated with symptom severity, quality of life, and gastric emptying, and potentially predicted clinical response to pyloric dilatation.[22] Investigators from Temple University evaluated FLIP in 54 patients with gastroparesis, and reported a wide range of values in symptomatic patients. They noted correlation between pyloric diameter and symptoms of early satiety and postprandial fullness. Most interestingly, however, their data suggested that FLIP could be used to identify a distinct subset of patients with decreased pyloric distensibility. Finally, Snape et al (2016) at the California Pacific Medical Center utilized FLIP, sleeve manometry, and gastric emptying studies in 114 patients with symptoms suggestive of gastroparesis. Similar to the findings from the Temple University group, they reported a correlation between symptoms and pyloric distensibility, as well as the ability of FLIP to potentially identify a clinically meaningful subset with possible pyloric dysfunction.[23] Whereas data are still emerging with regards to FLIP and gastroparesis, what has been published to date is encouraging, and suggests that FLIP can be utilized to identify a subgroup of patients with decreased pyloric distensibility. Whether this information will lead to more tailored therapy and the identification of a clinical subset that may more readily benefit from pyloric-directed therapy remains to be seen, and further investigation is ongoing.

With regards to logistics, FLIP is commonly, though not always, performed in conjunction with endoscopy. The catheter has a 3-mm outer diameter. While different balloon lengths are available, a length of 8 cm seems to be most often employed for evaluation of the pylorus. Different investigators have utilized various means of placement. Gourcerol and colleagues placed the catheters transnasally and positioned the device across the pylorus using videofluoroscopy; however, both studies from the United States utilized endoscopic placement. The device is too wide to fit in the working channel of a standard diagnostic endoscope; however, it can fit in the working channel of a large-channel therapeutic endoscope, and this is likely the easiest means to secure appropriate placement. Other options include tying a suture to the end of the device and pulling it across the pylorus with biopsy forceps, or trying to direct passage of the catheter past the pylorus with the endoscope; however, both these approaches add time and complexity to the procedure. Moreover, it is theoretically possible that using a biopsy forceps to drag the catheter across the pylorus before measurement may impact the recorded parameters (as opposed to passing the catheter directly across the pylorus from a therapeutic endoscope). In our experience, utilizing the working channel of a large-channel therapeutic endoscope appears to be the easiest means of quickly and reliably measuring pyloric distensibility.

Finally, any discussion of pyloric functional assessment would not be complete without a brief mention of EGG. EGG involves the placement of cutaneous leads to record gastric rhythm, and is performed at certain tertiary referral centers. It is not an endoscopic technique, nor does it evaluate pyloric function per se. However, there was a recent report by Wellington et al (2017) at Wake Forest evaluating EGG as a means to predict response to pyloric intervention. The normal gastric electrical rhythm (or slow wave frequency) is three cycles per minute, and the investigators noted that patients with documented gastric emptying delay and symptoms consistent with gastroparesis would invariably have a disorganized, dysrhythmic pattern. However, if pyloric dysfunction (as opposed to another etiology for symptom pathogenesis) is a major component of the gastroparesis, then the gastric rhythm as measured by EGG would be regular, and the amplitude of the three-cycles-per-minute rhythm could be more pronounced. They reported that, in patients with a normal EGG and suspected pyloric dysfunction, the clinical response rate to pyloric intervention (botulinum toxin or balloon dilatation) was 78%.[24] Although these data are from only one center, they do raise the question of whether EGG, which is not interventional, easy to perform, and low-risk, could help stratify patients for targeted therapy aimed at pyloric intervention.

Endoscopic Therapeutic Options for Pyloric Dysfunction

Given the paucity of treatment options available for gastroparesis, there has been significant interest in therapy aimed at pyloric disruption. This generally has fallen into five distinct subgroups: balloon dilatation, botulinum toxin injection, transpyloric stent placement, surgical pyloroplasty, and endoscopic pyloromyotomy. The data with regards to balloon dilatation are quite limited, and even the appropriate balloon size is not agreed upon. Most data suggest an 18- to 20-mm size with a 1 minute duration of distention. There are no reports of long-lasting benefit with this intervention, although several small studies do report transient symptom improvement.[22,24]

Botulinum toxin is a potent neurotoxin that inhibits acetylcholine release from presynaptic cholinergic receptors, and has been utilized in the treatment of multiple gastrointestinal motility disorders, most prominently achalasia. The first case report of prepyloric botulinum toxin use for gastroparesis was in 1988 by Sharma and colleagues.[15] This was followed by a number of small case series showing significant improvement in select patients.[25-30] Given the increasing use of botulinum toxin injection for the clinical treatment of gastroparesis, two randomized, double-blind, placebo-controlled trials were conducted. The first was by investigators at Leuven University in Belgium. They evaluated 23 patients with gastroparesis using a crossover protocol. Patients received 100 units of botulinum toxin or saline every 4 weeks, with symptom scores and gastric emptying assessed at baseline and after each intervention. Gastric emptying and symptom improvement were recorded after both interventions (botulinum toxin injection and saline injection) and were noted to be improved; however, there was no statistically significant difference between the two treatments.[31] The second randomized trial was performed by investigators at Temple University. Thirty-two patients were randomized to receive either botulinum toxin (200 units) or placebo (saline injection). Similar to the Belgium trial, both groups were noted to have improvement in symptoms and gastric emptying after 1 month; however, there was no significant difference between the two groups.[32]

The negative findings from these two randomized placebo-controlled trials tempered the excitement about prior case reports. A systematic review published in 2010 incorporating the data to date concluded that "there is no evidence to recommend botulinum toxin injection for the treatment of gastroparesis,"[33] and the American College of Gastroenterology Clinical Guideline on the Management of Gastroparesis stated with a high level of evidence that botulinum toxin was not recommended for patients with gastroparesis.[34] However, there are some important caveats that need to be mentioned to round out the botulinum toxin story. To begin with, both randomized controlled trials were

small, and perhaps not adequately powered to detect a significant difference in a small subgroup of patients with pyloric dysfunction. Secondly, larger case reports have since emerged that suggest that, in a carefully selected group of patients, the benefit may be more significant. The largest series to date is from investigators at the University of Michigan. They evaluated 179 patients receiving botulinum toxin injections between 2001 and 2007. Overall, there was improvement in 51.4% of patients; however, when a higher dose of botulinum toxin was used (200 units), the percentage that derived improvement increased to 76.7%. Other factors that predicted response in that series included female gender, age less than 50, and a nondiabetic, nonsurgical etiology.[35] Finally, it is important to note that neither of the randomized trials evaluating botulinum toxin specifically stratified patients based on suspicion for pyloric dysfunction. Given that pyloric dysfunction affects a subset of patients with gastroparesis, the jury is still out regarding the efficacy of botulinum toxin administration to patients with high suspicion for pyloric dysfunction. This point is evidenced by the good responses to pyloric botulinum toxin injection reported in the subset of patients with gastroparesis secondary to accidental vagotomy (usually accompanying a surgical fundoplication). It is known that a vagotomy inhibits pyloric relaxation and coordination with antral motility.

Given the suspicion that pyloric dysfunction may play a role in some patients with gastroparesis, and the development of temporary through-the-scope stents, investigators at Johns Hopkins evaluated the use of temporary transpyloric stent placement as salvage therapy in patients with refractory gastroparesis. In the initial report of three patients, placement of a double-layered, fully covered Niti-S self-expandable metal stent (Taewoong Medical, Gyeonggi-do, South Korea) across the pylorus resulted in both clinical and scintigraphic improvement.[36] This was followed by a retrospective evaluation of 30 patients treated with stent placement as salvage therapy. Over half of the patients were treated in the midst of hospitalization, and all had failed conventional therapy to date. Clinical response was reported in 75% of patients, although the duration of follow-up was relatively short. Stent migration was a persistent problem, and occurred in 48% of patients despite the use of endoscopic suturing techniques during stent placement. The authors proposed that stent placement could be used as a potential salvage therapy and also, potentially, as a means to select which patients may benefit from more definitive pyloric intervention.[37] However, it should be noted that, although these results seem encouraging, all the data to date with regards to transpyloric stent placement have been from one center, and at present, there are no prospective trials available to evaluate this modality. With that caveat, transpyloric stent placement is a tool in the armamentarium of the therapeutic endoscopist, and further study is needed to determine the prospective efficacy, duration of benefit, predictors of response, and whether clinical response to stent placement predicts response to pyloroplasty/myotomy.

Surgical pyloroplasty has been used as a drainage procedure after elective vagotomy and for the treatment of mechanical obstruction for over 40 years, but has recently returned to the forefront for treatment of patients with gastroparesis. Investigators from Oregon reviewed their experience with 28 patients and reported improvement in symptoms, gastric emptying via scintigraphy, and prokinetic use, with 83% of patients overall reporting improvement at 1 month follow-up.[38] This was followed by a second report evaluating 175 patients who underwent

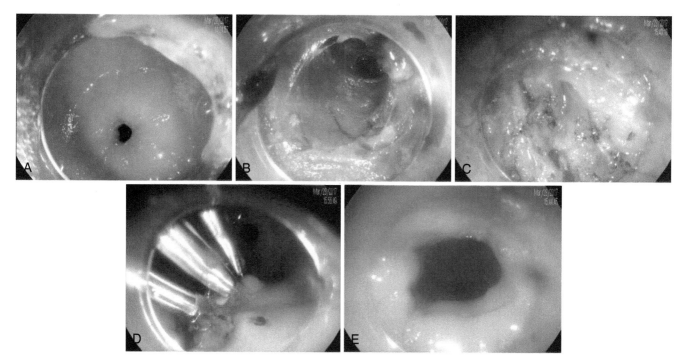

FIG 29.1 These images depict several key stages of a gastric peroral endoscopic myotomy procedure in a patient with refractory gastroparesis. **A,** Pylorus before intervention. **B,** Tunnel created by submucosal dissection. **C,** Myotomy. **D,** Clips used to close the mucosal entry site. **E,** Postprocedure pylorus, with clear widening as compared to the initial image. (See also Video 29.1.) (Images courtesy of Dr. Mohamed O. Othman, Assistant Professor of Medicine in the Division of Gastroenterology and Hepatology, and Director of Advanced Endoscopy, Baylor College of Medicine, Houston, TX.)

laparoscopic pyloroplasty. Gastric emptying time significantly improved in 86% of patients and normalized in 77%, with corresponding symptom improvement. Of note, however, 105 of the patients had a concurrent fundoplication for reflux, and a number of patients went on to require additional surgical intervention.[39] Investigators from Texas Tech University have evaluated the clinical efficacy of pyloroplasty combined with GES, and found that patients who received both interventions had significantly accelerated gastric emptying, as well as symptom improvement, compared to patients receiving GES alone.[40] Investigators at Emory University reported on pyloroplasty in 50 patients from 2006 through 2013. Symptom improvement was reported in 82%, although it should be noted that the majority of the patients in this series had prior foregut surgical intervention. There are no reported prospective randomized trials comparing surgical pyloroplasty with other interventions for gastroparesis, although currently there is a randomized blinded trial at Texas Tech University, El Paso, comparing surgical pyloroplasty to the combination of GES and surgical pyloroplasty.

The success of surgical pyloroplasty combined with the clear efficacy of peroral endoscopic myotomy for the treatment of achalasia has fueled interest in endoscopic pyloromyotomy for treatment of refractory gastroparesis. The first feasibility studies were performed in a porcine model in 2012 by Kawai and colleagues.[41] The first human report emerged from Johns Hopkins University in late 2013.[42] This has been followed by a wave of reports from multiple groups showing efficacy in small numbers of patients.[43–47] Gonzalez et al (2017) from Aix-Marseille University, France investigated the role of endoscopic pyloromyotomy in 12 children with refractory gastroparesis and reported a technical success rate of 100% with no adverse events, significant symptom improvement in 85%, and normalization of gastric emptying in 75% of cases.[48] Dacha et al (2017) from Emory University School of Medicine, Atlanta recently reported their experience with endoscopic pyloromyotomy in 16 patients with refractory gastroparesis. They reported clinical improvement of symptoms in 81%, significant improvement in gastric emptying, and no adverse events.[49] Finally, Khashab et al (2017) recently reported on the results of a multicenter international study involving 30 patients with refractory gastroparesis. They reported a clinical response in 86% of patients during a median follow-up of 5.5 months, with lack of response seen in only four of 30 patients. Normalization of gastric emptying was seen in 47%, and an additional 35% were noted to have objective improvement. Two adverse events were noted (capnoperitoneum and a prepyloric ulcer)[50] (Fig. 29.1 and Video 29.1).

Summing this data in aggregate, the published responses to pyloric intervention in open-label and retrospective reports are impressive. However, these results should be interpreted cautiously, given the negative results from the only two randomized controlled trials (both utilizing botulinum toxin). Whereas the favorable reports of pyloric stent placement, surgical pyloroplasty, and endoscopic pyloromyotomy raise optimism regarding the future of pyloric treatments for gastroparesis, there is an urgent need for prospective randomized studies to evaluate these techniques. Given the heterogeneous nature of gastroparesis, we also strongly advocate for use of pyloric diagnostic techniques (in particular impedance planimetry) to select patients who may benefit from more invasive pyloric intervention. Not all patients with gastroparesis will be expected to have pyloric dysfunction, and the exact size of this subset is unclear. Tailoring appropriate therapy to the appropriate patient is going to be a key part of adequately evaluating these techniques. This is a rapidly changing field, and one that is likely to see evolving expansion in the upcoming years as techniques become more streamlined and more technologic advances are made.

FULL-THICKNESS GASTRIC BIOPSY

One of the major advances produced by the NIH gastroparesis consortium has been the identification of clear histopathologic changes in select patients with gastroparesis and the recognition that these changes are not uniform, but rather heterogeneous, with identification of clear histopathologic subsets. To date, there are no convincing data that identification of histopathologic subsets leads to improvement in clinical care; however, these data are relatively new, and the expectation of the authors is that future research will attempt to tailor specific mechanism-based therapies to specific histopathologic subsets. As such, there will likely be an increasing need for biopsy acquisition deeper than the mucosal and submucosal layers. This has colloquially been referred to as full-thickness gastric biopsy.

Initial reports of full-thickness gastric biopsy relied solely on surgical acquisition of tissue, either during a dedicated surgical procedure for tissue acquisition, or concurrently with another indicated procedure such as GES.[51–53] In 2008, the Mayo Clinic reported on endoscopic deep tissue acquisition in a porcine model using a double endoscopic mucosal resection technique. Whereas adequate tissue was obtained for staining of myenteric ganglia, delayed perforation was reported, limiting enthusiasm for this technique.[54] In 2010, investigators from the University of Calgary evaluated the role of a percutaneous, endoscopically assisted transenteric approach in a canine model, using a spring-loaded 14-gauge biopsy needle inserted through a 3-mm abdominal wall incision into the antrum under endoscopic guidance.[55] This was followed by a pilot study in 10 patients in 2011 that reported technical success, although smaller tissue samples were obtained than via surgery.[13]

In part due to the rapid expansion of the use of peroral endoscopic myotomy, the development of submucosal endoscopic access techniques has fueled development of this technique. Investigators from the Mayo Clinic reported on their experience of using submucosal endoscopy to obtain full-thickness gastric biopsies in a porcine model in 2012.[56] These investigators subsequently reported on a novel technique for gastric endoscopic muscle biopsy using a double resection clip-assist technique, in which endoscopic mucosal resection was performed to unroof and expose the muscularis propria, after which the muscalaris propria was retracted into the cap of an over-the-scope clip. The clip was then deployed, creating a pseudopolyp of muscularis mucosa, which was then resected. Although the report describes the technique as "easy to perform," it should be noted that the paper included only three patients.[57]

Othman et al (2016) from Texas Tech University also reported on tissue acquisition from the muscularis propria of the gastric wall in patients with gastroparesis using endoscopic ultrasound (EUS)-guided fine-needle acquisition (FNA) biopsies (using a 19-gauge needle). They evaluated 11 patients from whom samples were taken via this approach in comparison to surgical biopsy acquisition during gastric electrical stimulator placement within

24 hours. They noted adequate histologic assessment of ICCs in 81% of patients and adequate assessment of the myenteric plexus in 54% of patients. There were no adverse effects noted during the study.[14]

At present, the ideal way to obtain full-thickness gastric biopsies is not clear. EUS-guided FNA certainly may be the easiest approach, and, as detailed previously, may provide adequate information in a majority of patients. Although submucosal dissection and the double resection clip-assist technique will likely provide more substantial tissue samples, these procedures are also more time-consuming, and require significantly more technical expertise. Surgical tissue acquisition remains the gold standard, although it is our hope that, as endoscopic techniques become more refined, surgical tissue acquisition will only be required in cases where a concurrent surgery is being performed for other clinical indications. In addition, it should be noted that all of these publications have reported on a relatively small number of patients. With that caveat, however, we envision nonsurgical methods for deep tissue acquisition as a key component of endoscopic care for gastroparesis going forward. If these techniques can provide information on the spectrum of ICC-opathy and other tissue abnormalities in mild, moderate, and severe patient settings, they will hopefully lead to guided treatment algorithms and better outcomes.

TEMPORARY GASTRIC ELECTRICAL STIMULATION

GES was approved by the FDA under a Humanitarian Device Exemption for treatment of patients with chronic, intractable nausea and vomiting secondary to gastroparesis in 2000. Although there are significant data suggesting clinical improvement in patients after GES,[58] the role of and place for GES in gastroparesis has not been established. Two randomized controlled trials evaluating the efficacy of GES for gastroparesis did not meet their primary endpoints; however, both studies had methodologic issues that may explain these results. In the initial double-blind trial conducted in 2000, the period of activation/inactivation was only 1 month, but the study showed significant improvement at 12 months of follow-up. In the second randomized trial, all patients were activated for 6 weeks following surgery before randomization to "off" or "on" treatment periods. However, in both studies (one of which involved diabetic gastroparesis patients and the other of which involved patients with idiopathic gastroparesis), patients who continued to have GES activation were significantly improved at the end of the study (12 months after implantation) as compared to baseline.[5,58]

GES traditionally requires surgical implantation of the device. As clinical response is not universal, there has been interest in potential diagnostic studies that may predict which patients will respond to surgical implantation. With that background, temporary endoscopic GES has garnered favor as a potential predictor of surgical response. Initial reports of temporary placement involved the use of a concurrent gastrostomy tube; however, in 2005, Abell and colleagues first reported on endoscopic implantation without the need for a concurrent gastrostomy. They used a temporary cardiac pacing lead that was passed through the working channel of an endoscope, screwed into place in the gastric mucosa, and then secured with placement of three to five clips. The lead was passed through the mouth or nose and attached to an external GES device, and the patient received temporary pacing via this arrangement. An initial report indicated a rapid improvement in vomiting frequency scores.[59]

Since this initial report, Abell and colleagues pursued a randomized, placebo-controlled crossover trial of temporary electrical stimulation for 72 hours, involving 58 patients. Vomiting decreased in both groups after the index endoscopy, with greater response seen in the group receiving active stimulation. Although the overall treatment effects in the study did not meet statistical significance, differences in favor of stimulation were suggested.[60] A further report evaluated temporary stimulation in 379 patients with gastroparesis-like syndrome. During this study, there was significant improvement in gastric emptying, for patients with both delayed and rapid gastric emptying, and significant improvement in symptoms (nausea, vomiting, and total symptom scores).[61]

Although using temporary gastric stimulation as a tool for predicting the success of a surgically implanted permanent device is a very appealing concept, there are many concerns: (1) the ability to reverse vomiting that has been present for months and years in 3 days does not seem likely, and is not borne out by using the same GES parameters in a permanently implanted device; (2) normalized gastric emptying in both slow and rapid settings has not been found in other reports; (3) the parameters used have been shown not to affect the electrical dysrhythmias present in gastroparesis patients; and (4) adoption of this technique has been limited by the unpredictable duration of electrode attachments to gastric mucosa, as well as the new understanding that the pylorus must also be addressed to improve gastroparesis. Both from a gastric emptying endpoint and a symptom resolution standpoint, better predictive testing will be needed. However, the pioneering work of Dr. Abell in this field may lead to better electrode recording methods in patients, helping study pathophysiology and response to treatment.

ENTERAL TUBES

For patients with severe disease, enteral tubes can be considered as a therapeutic option for either gastric venting (with the hypothesis that gastric distention is contributing to symptoms) or postpyloric feeding. With regards to venting procedures, there are several options, including a nasogastric tube, gastrostomy, and gastrojejunostomy. Placement of a nasogastric tube is often preferred in the acute setting, as it is less invasive; however, this can be associated with patient discomfort, and cannot be tolerated for long-term use. Placement of a gastrostomy tube is one way to address gastric decompression, and can be used intermittently for venting of secretions to decrease vomiting and fullness when patients are symptomatic. However, placement of a gastric tube may complicate future interventions (including gastric electrical stimulator placement), and can lead to cosmetic issues, leakage, infection, and other complications, while also setting a very negative precedent that decompression of gastric contents is condoned with any threshold of discomfort. This actually limits the normal fundic/proximal stomach relationship, and can also lead to serious potassium deficiency. A gastrojejunostomy tube has the potential to combine venting and postpyloric feeds in one device; however, migration from the proximal jejunum with coughing and/or retching is a frequent complication.[34,62]

Postpyloric feeding has a clear role in patients with severe symptoms who are unable to support their nutritional needs. In patients with isolated gastroparesis, placement of a feeding jejunostomy tube has been shown to reduce hospitalization, maintain nutrition, and improve symptoms.[1,63] Several options exist for postpyloric feeding. Placement of a nasoduodenal or nasojejunal tube is often the first avenue explored to ensure that postpyloric feeding is tolerated, as gastroparesis is often linked with extensive gastrointestinal dysmotility. However, nasoduodenal or nasojejunal tubes are not a long-term option. Direct endoscopic placement of a jejunostomy tube or a gastrojejunostomy tube is usually the more definitive long-term option, but the former can be associated with leakage, cosmetic issues, and infection, whereas the latter frequently migrates.[34] The gastrojejunostomy tube also partially blocks the pyloric opening, and hence may theoretically compromise resumption of oral intake. We believe a surgically placed jejunostomy tube (J tube) is the best option when long-term (3 months or more) use is being contemplated. The usual size is a 14- to 16-Fr diameter, which can also permit medications to be administered through the tube once they are dissolved. Infections are not generally an issue, and the tube is typically well-tolerated by the patient. Nocturnal J-tube feeding is recommended, with patients trying to eat during the day with no concurrent J-tube feedings. The laparoscopically placed surgical J tube also allows the surgeon to obtain a biopsy of gastric antral smooth muscle and thus histologically examine the ICCs, neurons, and smooth muscle for diagnostic and/or prognostic applications.

FUTURE DIRECTIONS

The role of endoscopy in the management of gastroparesis has changed, and is due to shift further in upcoming years. There is increasing recognition that gastroparesis, as defined today, is a heterogeneous disorder, and that neither the presence of specific symptoms nor the time course of gastric emptying is a true gold standard for diagnosis. Histopathology may be the missing link that allows more finite classification of these patients and better identification of underlying mechanisms, with the end result of tailored patient-specific care. We envision an increasing role for endoscopy in the acquisition of deep tissue in a minimally invasive fashion, and see this resulting in a paradigm shift for this disorder, consistent with the well-accepted statement that "tissue is the issue." With easier tissue acquisition and an increased ability to visualize the myenteric plexus and ICCs, we hope to see the identification of clinically meaningful subsets. For those patients with pyloric dysfunction, endoscopic techniques will continue to expand, aimed both at the identification of pyloric dysfunction, as well as further refinement of pyloric disruption techniques.

Gastroparesis can now be viewed in a similar light to achalasia, where loss of esophageal motility in the body of the esophagus is accompanied by impaired relaxation of the lower esophageal sphincter. In gastroparesis, there is impaired electrical and motor function in the antrum, accompanied by pyloric sphincter dysfunction and poor opening/compliance of the pylorus. In any given gastroparesis patient, both aspects need to be recognized and therapeutically addressed, although in some patients one aspect may be more dominant.

High-resolution EGG has identified multiple variants of gastric dysrhythmia, and there is no reason to think that treatment of these entities via endoscopic approaches may not be feasible in the future. In addition, as GES devices become more compact and submucosal dissection techniques become more refined, we predict that GES devices could be inserted through endoscopes. Targeted endoscopic drug or stem cell delivery (specifically ICC stem cells) may also be an option in the future, specifically with endoscopic delivery into the antral smooth muscle.

CONCLUSIONS

Endoscopy plays a key role in the diagnosis and management of gastroparesis. In a conventional sense, endoscopy is required to both establish and confirm the diagnosis of gastroparesis. Postpyloric feeding may be required to stabilize patients nutritionally while diagnostic studies and therapy proceed. Recent reports have highlighted the identification of a subset of patients with prominent pyloric dysfunction, and endoscopy plays a role in both the identification of this subset and the treatment of these patients. Impedance planimetry has emerged as a novel tool for assessing pyloric distensibility and compliance, and could potentially be used to identify a subgroup of patients in whom endoscopic techniques for pyloric disruption can be utilized. Advances in endoscopic techniques have led to the development of numerous methods by which full-thickness gastric biopsy can be obtained and clear histopathologic subsets can be identified, with the hope of identifying subgroups for which treatment decisions can be based on these histologic features. Finally, endoscopy may play a role in placing both temporary and permanent electrical stimulation devices, and certainly in facilitating electrical recording of gastric smooth muscle. We predict that the role for endoscopy should only continue to expand in the future, and that a revolution in this area is clearly underway.

KEY REFERENCES

1. Parkman HP, Hasler WL, Fisher RS, et al: American Gastroenterological Association technical review on the diagnosis and treatment of gastroparesis, *Gastroenterology* 127:1592–1622, 2004.
3. Tack J, Talley NJ: Functional dyspepsia—symptoms, definitions and validity of the Rome III criteria, *Nat Rev Gastroenterol Hepatol* 10:134–141, 2013.
5. Abell T, McCallum R, Hocking M, et al: Gastric electrical stimulation for medically refractory gastroparesis, *Gastroenterology* 125:421–428, 2003.
8. Farrugia G: Histologic changes in diabetic gastroparesis, *Gastroenterol Clin North Am* 44:31–38, 2015.
10. Grover M, Farrugia G, Lurken MS, et al: Cellular changes in diabetic and idiopathic gastroparesis, *Gastroenterology* 140:1575–1585.e8, 2011.
12. Moraveji S, Bashashati M, Elhanafi S, et al: Depleted interstitial cells of Cajal and fibrosis in the pylorus: novel features of gastroparesis, *Neurogastroenterol Motil* 28:1048–1054, 2016.
16. Clarke JO, Snape WJ, Jr: Pyloric sphincter therapy: botulinum toxin, stents, and pyloromyotomy, *Gastroenterol Clin North Am* 44:127–136, 2015.
19. Cassilly D, Kantor S, Knight LC, et al: Gastric emptying of a non-digestible solid: assessment with simultaneous SmartPill pH and pressure capsule, antroduodenal manometry, gastric emptying scintigraphy, *Neurogastroenterol Motil* 20:311–319, 2008.
22. Gourcerol G, Tissier F, Melchior C, et al: Impaired fasting pyloric compliance in gastroparesis and the therapeutic response to pyloric dilatation, *Aliment Pharmacol Ther* 41:360–367, 2015.
23. Snape WJ, Lin MS, Agarwal N, et al: Evaluation of the pylorus with concurrent intraluminal pressure and EndoFLIP in patients with nausea and vomiting, *Neurogastroenterol Motil* 28:758–764, 2016.
24. Wellington J, Scott B, Kundu S, et al: Effect of endoscopic pyloric therapies for patients with nausea and vomiting and functional obstructive gastroparesis, *Auton Neurosci* 202:56–61, 2017.
31. Arts J, Holvoet L, Caenepeel P, et al: Clinical trial: a randomized-controlled crossover study of intrapyloric injection of botulinum toxin in gastroparesis, *Aliment Pharmacol Ther* 26:1251–1258, 2007.
32. Friedenberg FK, Palit A, Parkman HP, et al: Botulinum toxin A for the treatment of delayed gastric emptying, *Am J Gastroenterol* 103:416–423, 2008.
34. Camilleri M, Parkman HP, Shafi MA, et al: Clinical guideline: management of gastroparesis, *Am J Gastroenterol* 108:18–37, quiz 38, 2013.
35. Coleski R, Anderson MA, Hasler WL: Factors associated with symptom response to pyloric injection of botulinum toxin in a large series of gastroparesis patients, *Dig Dis Sci* 54:2634–2642, 2009.
36. Clarke JO, Sharaiha RZ, Kord Valeshabad A, et al: Through-the-scope transpyloric stent placement improves symptoms and gastric emptying in patients with gastroparesis, *Endoscopy* 45(Suppl 2):UCTN:E189–E190, 2013.
37. Khashab MA, Besharati S, Ngamruengphong S, et al: Refractory gastroparesis can be successfully managed with endoscopic transpyloric stent placement and fixation (with video), *Gastrointest Endosc* 82:1106–1109, 2015.
38. Hibbard ML, Dunst CM, Swanstrom LL: Laparoscopic and endoscopic pyloroplasty for gastroparesis results in sustained symptom improvement, *J Gastrointest Surg* 15:1513–1519, 2011.
40. Sarosiek I, Forster J, Lin Z, et al: The addition of pyloroplasty as a new surgical approach to enhance effectiveness of gastric electrical stimulation therapy in patients with gastroparesis, *Neurogastroenterol Motil* 25:134–e80, 2013.
42. Khashab MA, Stein E, Clarke JO, et al: Gastric peroral endoscopic myotomy for refractory gastroparesis: first human endoscopic pyloromyotomy (with video), *Gastrointest Endosc* 78:764–768, 2013.
50. Khashab MA, Ngamruengphong S, Carr-Locke D, et al: Gastric per-oral endoscopic myotomy for refractory gastroparesis: results from the first multicenter study on endoscopic pyloromyotomy (with video), *Gastrointest Endosc* 85:123–128, 2017.
57. Rajan E, Gostout CJ, Wong Kee Song LM, et al: Innovative gastric endoscopic muscle biopsy to identify all cell types, including myenteric neurons and interstitial cells of Cajal in patients with idiopathic gastroparesis: a feasibility study (with video), *Gastrointest Endosc* 84:512–517, 2016.
58. McCallum RW, Lin Z, Forster J, et al: Gastric electrical stimulation improves outcomes of patients with gastroparesis for up to 10 years, *Clin Gastroenterol Hepatol* 9:314–319.e1, 2011.
60. Abell TL, Johnson WD, Kedar A, et al: A double-masked, randomized, placebo-controlled trial of temporary endoscopic mucosal gastric electrical stimulation for gastroparesis, *Gastrointest Endosc* 74:496–503.e3, 2011.
61. Singh S, McCrary J, Kedar A, et al: Temporary endoscopic stimulation in gastroparesis-like syndrome, *J Neurogastroenterol Motil* 21:520–527, 2015.

A complete reference list can be found online at ExpertConsult.com

30

Gastric Polyps and Thickened Gastric Folds

Pari M. Shah and Hans Gerdes

CHAPTER OUTLINE

INTRODUCTION

Examination of the stomach by upper endoscopy often results in the incidental finding of gastric polyps or thickened gastric folds. Gastric polyps are estimated to be identified in 6% to 8% of all upper endoscopy exams.[1] Most series report that the most common type of polyp encountered is the fundic gland polyp (FGP) (77% to 80%), followed by the hyperplastic polyp (17% to 19%),[1,2] though series differ through time and based on the series of patients being evaluated. Generally, patients with gastric polyps are asymptomatic but polyps may cause clinical manifestations, including gastrointestinal (GI) bleeding, iron deficiency anemia, and gastric outlet obstruction. Many of these lesions are benign, whereas others have malignant potential; understanding and recognizing the various diagnoses and malignant risk may impact endoscopic treatment, future management, and surveillance recommendations.

Gastric polyps are generally defined as lesions in the lumen of the stomach with protrusion above the mucosal plane.[3] These lesions may be epithelial or subepithelial at their presentation. This chapter reviews the most common etiologies of epithelial gastric polyps and discusses the endoscopic approach to management of these lesions. Subepithelial lesions are discussed in Chapter 31 of this text. At the conclusion of this chapter, we discuss the evaluation of thickened gastric folds and outline the endoscopic approach to these entities.

GASTRIC POLYPS

There are several types of epithelial gastric polyps encountered, including those that are generally benign (FGPs, hyperplastic polyps, hamartomatous polyps/juvenile polyposis), those that have malignant potential (gastric adenomas, gastric carcinoids types 1, 2, 3), and those that are malignant (gastric cancer). Endoscopic features may suggest the diagnosis, but histology is generally necessary to confirm the type of polyp encountered. Recommendations for further management may be based on the size, symptoms, and type of polyp identified.

Fundic Gland Polyps

The most common gastric polyp encountered during upper endoscopy is the FGP (Fig. 30.1), which account for greater than 70% of all polyps identified during upper endoscopy and have a prevalence of 3% in the general population. FGPs are generally incidentally identified and are most often asymptomatic in patients. FGPs may occur as single or multiple epithelial lesions often clustered with a grape-like appearance. They are predominantly located in the gastric fundus or proximal body of the stomach, and are generally small, varying from 1 mm to occasionally up to 2 cm.

Endoscopic appearance is generally suggestive of these lesions with bland overlying glistening mucosa of pale color; however, diagnosis of these lesions is confirmed by histology after biopsy or removal of representative lesions. Histology reveals the classic appearance of dilated oxyntic glands with flattened parietal cells forming a microcystic appearance.[4]

The pathogenesis of FGPs is unknown. Sporadic FGPs are more commonly seen in women than in men.[5] They may be frequently seen in conjunction with *Helicobacter pylori* (*H. pylori*) infection.[5] FGPs have been thought to occur more frequently in patients taking proton pump inhibitors (PPIs), though a causal relationship has not been demonstrated. A 2016 meta-analysis of 12 papers found an increased odds ratio of PPI use with the development of FGPs.[4] Overall, sporadic FGPs are benign entities with no clinical consequence.[5]

Multiple FGPs are seen in association with familial adenomatous polyposis (FAP) syndrome (Fig. 30.2). Patients with FAP will have hundreds to thousands of FGPs in the gastric fundus and body, and may have no such polyps in the antrum. In patients with FAP, FGPs have a similar benign natural history, but there are reports of conversion of benign FGPs to dysplastic lesions in as many as up to 40% of cases.[6]

For patients without FAP, FGPs usually require no intervention. Biopsies on initial endoscopy to confirm the diagnoses are standard. Once diagnosed as FGPs, no surveillance is recommended; however, because of the risk of neoplastic transformation,

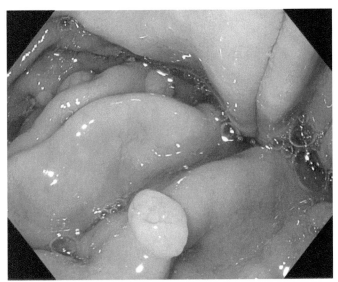

FIG 30.1 Fundic gland polyp.

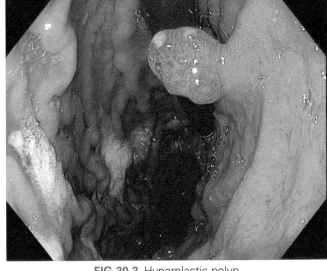

FIG 30.3 Hyperplastic polyp.

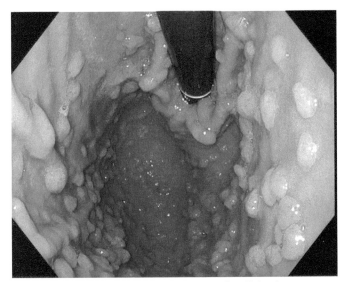

FIG 30.2 Fundic gland polyps seen in familial adenomatous polyposis (FAP).

surveillance with biopsies of these lesions in FAP patients is recommended.

Hyperplastic Polyps

Hyperplastic polyps are the second most common type of polyps encountered in routine upper endoscopy (Fig. 30.3). These polyps are generally felt to be benign; however, several series have identified the presence of dysplasia (0.2% to 10%) or adenocarcinoma (0.6% to 3%) within these lesions.[7–12] Endoscopically, hyperplastic polyps have a wide range of appearances. There may be one or multiple. They can arise in any part of the stomach. They may be small, starting at a few millimeters in size, to large, mimicking the appearance of carcinoma. They may be sessile or pedunculated. The overlying mucosa may appear normal or may appear erythematous and with patches of exudate as the size increases.

Hyperplastic polyps have been associated with *H. pylori* gastritis and chronic gastritis, noted in association with autoimmune or atrophic gastritis with pernicious anemia.[7,11,13] Histology reveals submucosal edema, prominent foveolar hyperplasia, and inflammation of the lamina propria.

The approach to endoscopic management of hyperplastic polyps is debated. Biopsy of representative lesions to establish the diagnosis is recommended. Removal of polyps is generally individualized based on the size, appearance, histology, and clinical presentation. Some authors advocate for removal of all hyperplastic polyps above 5 mm because of the potential for development of dysplasia.[14] Generally, though, authors believe the risk of malignant transformation is low. Thus, large polyps should be sampled or removed depending on safety and feasibility of doing so. Bleeding polyps or those thought to be contributing to symptomatic anemia should be considered for polypectomy. Whether surveillance endoscopy should be performed after biopsy of hyperplastic polyps is also unclear. In our practice, hyperplastic polyps are not generally surveyed unless dysplasia has been established on first endoscopy. The presence of *H. pylori* should also be assessed and treated as this has been associated with reduced polyp recurrence and reduced progression to cancer.[14]

Gastric Adenoma

Adenomatous polyps of the stomach are less common and constitute approximately 10% of polyps identified (Fig. 30.4).[2,3] Gastric adenomas are premalignant, with an increasing risk of developing into adenocarcinoma based on the size and degree of dysplasia of the lesion. Sporadic gastric adenomas may be found arising from normal or atrophic mucosa. Patients with genetic predisposition to gastric cancer, including FAP or hereditary nonpolyposis colon cancer syndrome (HNPCC), have an increased risk of developing gastric adenomas that are likely to progress to cancer. These lesions may be found anywhere in the stomach but have a predisposition to the antrum.

Endoscopically, these lesions can range in size from a few millimeters to centimeters. They may be single or multiple. The mucosal surface generally contains a cerebriform mucosal pattern. These lesions may be polypoid or sessile, raised, or flat.

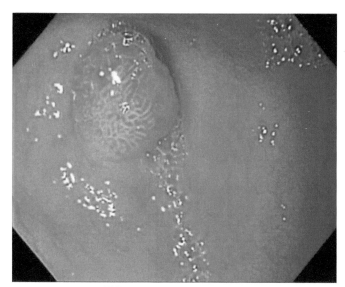

FIG 30.4 Gastric adenoma.

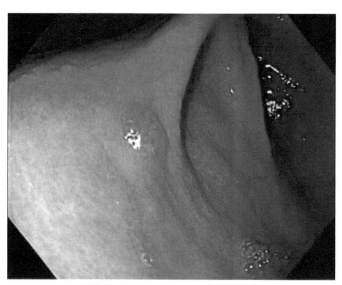

FIG 30.5 Gastric carcinoid Type 1.

Histologically, gastric adenomas exhibit columnar epithelium with elongated atypical nuclei and increased mitotic activity. Adenomas may have varying degrees of tubular, villous, or tubulovillous architecture. Dysplasia and carcinoma are more frequently noted in villous or tubulovillous adenoma histologies. Similarly, the presence of increasing degrees of villous features correlate with increased risk of progressing to cancer. Adenomas may be associated with more advanced lesions in other areas of the stomach and necessitates a thorough exam of the entire gastric mucosa. One 2009 study noted 7% of adenomas had high grade dysplasia, and 3.7% of patients with adenomas had synchronous lesions with adenocarcinoma.[2]

Because of the malignant potential of these lesions, all gastric adenomas should be completely removed endoscopically if feasible, and surgically if needed. After resection, surveillance endoscopy is warranted to evaluate for residual or metachronous lesions.

Gastric Carcinoma

Gastric carcinoma can be identified as a gastric polyp or a gastric mass. Differentiation between gastric adenoma and gastric carcinoma can be difficult endoscopically and often requires histology for determination. The epidemiology, endoscopic appearance, and management of early or polypoid gastric carcinomas is discussed in detail in Chapter 32.

Gastric Carcinoid

Gastric carcinoid can be incidentally identified in the stomach on routine endoscopy or may be identified after presentation with symptoms. Gastric carcinoids represent 2% of all gastric polyps identified on endoscopy.[15] They may appear as an epithelial or subepithelial lesion. Gastric carcinoids are subdivided into three different types.

Type 1 lesions are the most common and represent 70% of gastric carcinoids (Fig. 30.5). They are usually asymptomatic and are identified in patients with prolonged hypergastrinemia, usually associated with autoimmune chronic atrophic gastritis. Type 1 gastric carcinoid lesions are generally small, multiple, and benign with a low risk of progression to malignancy. They

are often clustered in the gastric body or fundus, with a smooth erythematous surface. Histology reveals sheets of neuroendocrine enterochromaffin-like cells (ECLs). Diagnostic confirmation of Type 1 gastric carcinoids usually requires identification of serum hypergastrinemia, the presence of serum parietal cell and intrinsic factor antibodies, and the histologic presence of diffuse atrophic gastritis in the flat mucosa of the fundus, body, and antrum. Type 1 gastric carcinoids have a low risk of growth or progression and can generally be monitored with annual surveillance endoscopy with endoscopic or surgical intervention reserved for large or progressive lesions.

Type 2 gastric carcinoids are similar to the type 1 lesions histologically, and are also caused by the unabetting stimulation by gastrin hormone in patients with Zollinger-Ellison Syndrome (ZES), or functional gastrinoma. Such patients may also have multiple carcinoids in the fundus and body, in association with hypertrophied gastric epithelium. There is usually no evidence of parietal cell and intrinsic factor antibodies, nor atrophy of the gastric epithelium in such patients. Similar to type 1 lesions, the risk of metastatic spread of these carcinoids is low and patients can generally be monitored with annual surveillance endoscopy.

Type 3 gastric carcinoids usually present as isolated lesions that are similar in histology to type 1 and 2 lesions, but develop autonomously, without underlying hypergastrinemia (Fig. 30.6). These lesions often appear to be larger at presentation, have deeper penetration into the stomach wall, and are more likely to be associated with metastases to lymph nodes or distant organs at the time of diagnosis.

The management of patients with gastric carcinoids is usually tailored to the type and underlying stimulus. In the case of type 1 and 2 carcinoids, the ongoing stimulation of gastric epithelium by gastrin hormone will result in recurrent formation of these lesions. Because of the low risk of metastases with these lesions, the management usually consists of endoscopic resection for lesions larger than 1 cm and annual surveillance. An alternative strategy is to perform a surgical intervention to reduce the gastrin level. In type 1 carcinoid, the most effective surgical strategy is antrectomy as it removes the source of high gastrin secretion from the antral G cells, which are overactive as a result of the

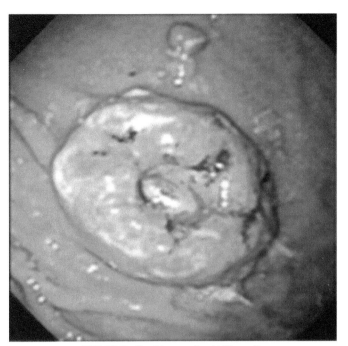

FIG 30.6 Gastric carcinoid Type 3.

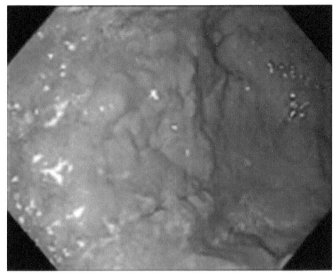

FIG 30.7 Thickened gastric folds due to gastric adenocarcinoma.

achlorhydria caused by parietal cell destruction. In Type 2 carcinoid, surgical removal of the gastrinoma, if feasible, will likewise remove the source of gastrin hormone and result in the complete cessation of gastric carcinoid growth.

For type 3 carcinoid, which is completely autonomous of gastrin stimulation, complete excision of the primary lesion prior to development of metastases via endoscopic or surgical resection is warranted and should result in long-term cure.

ENDOSCOPIC RESECTION

Endoscopic resection of gastric polyps is generally performed via similar techniques despite the etiology or histology of the gastric polyp. The general approach to endoscopic technique begins with a complete assessment of the type of polyp to be removed and the malignant potential of the polyp. For polyps less than 1 cm in size, snare polypectomy with or without cautery techniques are often effective at complete removal of benign gastric polyps. For polyps that are greater than 1 cm in size and with histology suggestive of a premalignant or malignant condition, endoscopic ultrasound (EUS) can be a supplemental tool to aid in the determination of whether endoscopic resection is feasible for curative intent. EUS evaluation can confirm that the abnormality visualized endoscopically is limited to the superficial or deep mucosal layers without demonstration of submucosal invasion. For polyps limited to the mucosal layers, saline injection lift technique with subsequent endoscopic mucosal resection (EMR) can generally be employed for complete removal of gastric polyps. Depending on the size and location of the lesion, EMR may be performed with the aid of a band ligator device. EMR is ideally performed en bloc with one piece but can be removed in a piecemeal fashion if necessary, with the goal being to eliminate all abnormal tissue. Additional endoscopic techniques have been developed to target lesions, including endoscopic submucosal dissection for lesions involving the submucosa or lesions suspected

to harbor malignancy. Chapter 32 in this text provides a greater discussion of these techniques.

THICKENED GASTRIC FOLDS

Thickened gastric folds are often identified on endoscopy, barium upper GI series, and computed tomography (CT) scanning of the abdomen as part of a work-up for symptoms, or may be identified incidentally during routine examinations (Fig. 30.7). The differential diagnosis is broad, including malignancies such as adenocarcinoma and lymphoma, or benign conditions such as hypertrophic gastritis or chronic *H. pylori* associated gastritis.[16] Less common causes include Menetrier's disease, infiltrative diseases such as amyloidosis and anisakiasis, lymphoid hyperplasia, and ZES. Rarely, metastatic cancer from a distant primary site (breast cancer, lung cancer, and melanoma) may present as large gastric folds.[17]

Work-up of thickened gastric folds generally starts with mucosal biopsy, but mucosal biopsies are often unable to provide a diagnosis and biopsy of deeper layers through several different methods must be considered. Standard endoscopic biopsy specimens usually contain superficial mucosa ranging in size from 2 to 4 mm. Large fragment biopsies have been proposed using snare electrocautery. This technique provides the ability to obtain full thickness or deeper specimens in an effort to increase the diagnostic yield, but has not been widely accepted because of the perceived risk of major complications, most notably hemorrhage or perforation.[18–20] When repeated attempts at endoscopic biopsy are inconclusive and the index of suspicion for malignancy is high, EUS-guided fine-needle aspiration (FNA) may be attempted for diagnosis. Laparotomy or laparoscopy may be indicated to obtain a full-thickness biopsy of the stomach wall when repeated endoscopic biopsies have been inconclusive.

The differential diagnosis of thickened gastric folds varies widely from entirely benign etiologies to diffuse malignant processes, and a prompt diagnosis is important for the appropriate triage of the patients. In the work-up of this finding, EUS evaluation is often warranted and can be particularly useful in providing diagnostic information that would help determine the best

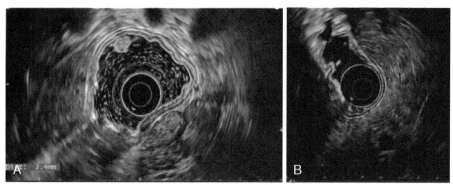

FIG 30.8 **A** and **B,** Endoscopic ultrasound (EUS) demonstrating a normal gastric wall layer pattern.

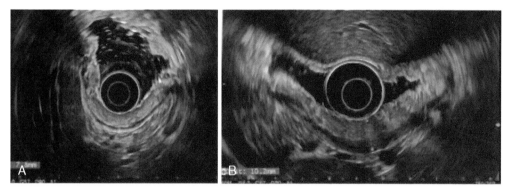

FIG 30.9 **A** and **B,** Endoscopic ultrasound (EUS) demonstrating a thickened gastric wall due to linitis plastica gastric adenocarcinoma.

approach to achieve an accurate diagnosis. EUS has been shown to primarily aid in identifying which layer of the gastric wall is thickened for targeted approaches at that layer. The normal gastric wall has a thickness of 3 to 5 mm. Most of the gastric wall layers are distinctly visualized on EUS examination (Fig. 30.8): layer 1, superficial mucosa; layer 2, deep mucosa and muscularis mucosa; layer 3, submucosa; layer 4, muscularis propria; and layer 5, subserosa and serosa. The thickness of each particular layer tends to be similar in the normal state, so an increase in size of any individual or multiple layers is easily recognized during EUS examination and can help formulate a differential diagnosis and guide further diagnostic work-up targeting the thickened layers. Specifically, loss of wall layer pattern or thickening in the muscularis propria (layer 4) has been shown to be most concerning for malignant involvement (Fig. 30.9).[21,22] Additionally, thickening in the mucosal layer or the muscularis mucosa can generally be diagnosed by forceps biopsies, "well biopsies" (where the forceps are placed repeatedly at the same site to obtain deeper sampling), or large particle biopsies using snare cautery. Thickening of deeper layers of the stomach wall, namely the submucosa and/or muscularis propria, has been a challenge for standard endoscopic techniques and may need to be approached by the large particle snare cautery biopsy technique, or with EUS-guided FNA of the specific thickened layer. If these approaches fail to determine the cause of thickening, then a surgical full thickness biopsy may be required.

Malignancy

The differential diagnosis for thickened gastric folds often includes malignancy. The most common type of malignancy that presents

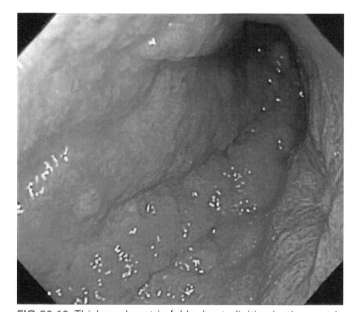

FIG 30.10 Thickened gastric folds due to linitis plastica gastric adenocarcinoma.

in this fashion is gastric adenocarcinoma, which can present in some patients as linitis plastica (Fig. 30.10). Linitis plastica represents a diffuse process within the gastric body of enlarged, often edematous and erythematous, folds with poor distensibility of the gastric wall with insufflation. A high index of suspicion must be present when this appearance is identified, as mucosal

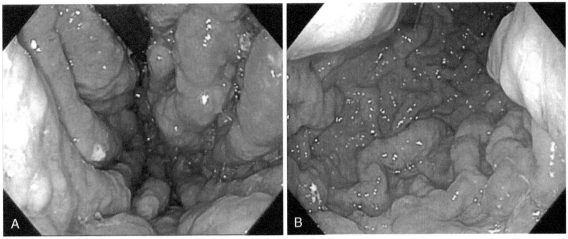

FIG 30.11 **A** and **B,** Thickened gastric folds due to mantle cell lymphoma.

biopsies are often negative and deeper biopsies are required to make the diagnosis, as described earlier.

Lymphoma is another malignancy that can present as diffuse thickening of gastric folds (Fig. 30.11). There are various subtypes of non-Hodgkin's lymphoma that may infiltrate into the gastric wall and result in diffusely thickened folds. The mucosa is similarly often edematous and erythematous, but generally distensibility of the stomach may be maintained.

Finally, other malignancies on rare occasions may spread to the stomach and cause thickened gastric folds. Lobular breast cancer, lung cancer, and melanoma have been described in cases to involve the stomach. Similar to gastric adenocarcinoma, this may present as a linitis plastica appearance, or may be diffuse in the stomach. Metastatic malignancy may be difficult to diagnose on mucosal biopsies alone and may require deeper tissue sampling.

When malignancy is causing the presentation of thickened gastric folds, symptoms such as early satiety, weight loss, or anemia are often present. Additionally, in patients with malignancy, other corroborating examinations, including CT scans, may suggest the finding of thickened gastric folds prior to the patient's presentation for endoscopy. Patients with symptoms secondary to thickened gastric folds require management targeted at their underlying malignancy and often are unable to maintain nutrition because of the diffuse nature of malignancy involving the stomach. As such, these patients are sometimes sent to gastroenterologists for supplemental treatment, such as placement of percutaneous endoscopic jejunostomy tubes.

Menetrier's Disease

Menetrier's disease is a rare disease that can result in diffusely thickened or giant gastric folds. Menetrier's disease generally presents with a clinical syndrome of weight loss, edema, and diarrhea secondary to protein losing enteropathy.[23,24] The diagnosis is made by endoscopy, which reveals the appearance of thickened or giant gastric folds diffusely and most pronounced in the fundus and the body. There are often mucosal changes, including erosions or ulcerations. EUS examination of these folds generally reveals thickening in layers 2 and 3 of the gastric wall and mucosal biopsies are often insufficient to make the diagnosis. Histology of these areas reveal pronounced foveolar hyperplasia, cystic dilation, and glandular atrophy. The cystic glands may also extend into the superficial submucosa, causing gastritis cystica profunda.

The clinical pattern of symptoms in conjunction with the histology is used to make the diagnosis of Menetrier's disease. Treatment of this entity is often challenging and various medical therapies have been tried, including treatment of any coexisting infection such as *H. pylori*. In patients refractory to medical management or with severe symptoms, gastrectomy is often indicated and can be curative. Publications have shown effective treatment with monoclonal antibodies to the epidermal growth factor receptor.[25]

CONCLUSION

Gastric polyps and thickened gastric folds are commonly encountered during routine endoscopy or as part of work-up of symptoms including nausea, early satiety, vomiting, weight loss, or anemia. Diagnosis often requires histology in the form of biopsies and occasionally requires EUS for further evaluation. Once histology is established, endoscopic treatment with polypectomy or EMR is often warranted for certain premalignant or early malignant lesions.

KEY REFERENCES

1. Nelson M, Ganger D, Keswani R, et al: Endoscopic resection is effective for the treatment of bleeding gastric hyperplastic polyps in patients with and without cirrhosis, *Endosc Int Open* 4:E874–E877, 2016.
2. Carmack SW, Genta RM, Schuler CM, Saboorian MH: The current spectrum of gastric polyps: a 1-year national study of over 120,000 patients, *Am J Gastroenterol* 104:1524–1532, 2009.
3. Vatansever S, Akpinar Z, Alper E, et al: Gastric polyps and polypoid lesions: retrospective analysis of 36650 endoscopic procedures in 29940 patients, *Turk J Gastroenterol* 26:117–122, 2015.
4. Tran-Duy A, Spaetgens B, Hoes AW, et al: Use of proton pump inhibitors and risks of fundic gland polyps and gastric cancer: systematic review and meta-analysis, *Clin Gastroenterol Hepatol* 14:1706–1719, 2016.
5. Genta RM, Schuler CM, Robiou CI, Lash RH: No association between gastric fundic gland polyps and gastrointestinal neoplasia in a study of over 100,000 patients, *Clin Gastroenterol Hepatol* 7:849–854, 2009.
6. Bianchi LK, Burke CA, Bennett AE, et al: Fundic gland polyp dysplasia is common in familial adenomatous polyposis, *Clin Gastroenterol Hepatol* 6:180–185, 2008.
7. Salomao M, Luna AM, Sepulveda JL, Sepulveda AR: Mutational analysis by next generation sequencing of gastric type dysplasia occurring in

hyperplastic polyps of the stomach: mutations in gastric hyperplastic polyps, *Exp Mol Pathol* 99:468–473, 2015.

8. Diabo M, Itabashi M, Hirota T: Malignant transformation of gastric hyperplastic polyps, *Am J Gastroenterol* 82:1016–1025, 1987.

9. Orlowska J, Jarosz D, Pachlewski J, Butruk E: Malignant transformation of benign epithelial gastric polyps, *Am J Gastroenterol* 90:2152–2159, 1995.

10. Zea-Iriarte WL, Sekine I, Itsuno M, et al: Carcinoma in gastric hyperplastic polyps. A phenotypic study, *Dig Dis Sci* 41:377–386, 1996.

11. Abraham SC, Singh VK, Yardley JH, Wu TT: Hyperplastic polyps of the stomach: associations with histologic patterns of gastritis and gastric atrophy, *Am J Surg Pathol* 25:500–507, 2001.

12. Terada T: Malignant transformation of foveolar hyperplastic polyp of the stomach: a histopathological study, *Med Oncol* 28:941–944, 2011.

13. Torbenson M, Abraham SC, Boitnott J, et al: Autoimmune gastritis: distinct histological and immunohistochemical findings before complete loss of oxyntic glands, *Mod Pathol* 15:102–109, 2002.

14. Markowski AR, Markowska A, Guzinska-Ustymowicz K: Pathophysiological and clinical aspects of gastric hyperplastic polyps, *World J Gastroenterol* 22:8883–8891, 2016.

15. Gencosmanoglu R, Sen-Oran E, Kurtkaya-Yapicier O, et al: Gastric polypoid lesions: analysis of 150 endoscopic polypectomy specimens from 91 patients, *World J Gastroenterol* 9:2236–2239, 2003.

16. Reeder MM, Olmsted WW, Cooper PH: Large gastric folds, local or widespread, *JAMA* 230:273–274, 1974.

17. Okanobu H, Hata J, Haruma K, et al: Giant gastric folds: differential diagnosis at US, *Radiology* 226:686–690, 2003.

18. Bjork JT, Geenen JE, Soergel KH, et al: Endoscopic evaluation of large gastric folds: a comparison of biopsy techniques, *Gastrointest Endosc* 24:22–23, 1977.

19. Komorowski RA, Caya JG, Geenen JE: The morphologic spectrum of large gastric folds: utility of the snare biopsy, *Gastrointest Endosc* 32:190–192, 1986.

20. Martin TR, Onstad GR, Silvis SE, Vennes JA: Lift and cut biopsy technique for submucosal sampling, *Gastrointest Endosc* 23:29–30, 1976.

21. Mendis RE, Gerdes H, Lightdale CJ, Botet JF: Large gastric folds: a diagnostic approach using endoscopic ultrasonography, *Gastrointest Endosc* 40:437–441, 1994.

22. Ginès A, Pellise M, Fernández-Esparrach G, et al: Endoscopic ultrasonography in patients with large gastric folds at endoscopy and biopsies negative for malignancy: predictors of malignant disease and clinical impact, *Am J Gastroenterol* 101:64–69, 2006.

23. Sundt TM, 3rd, Compton CC, Malt RA: Ménétrier's disease. A trivalent gastropathy, *Ann Surg* 208:694–701, 1988.

24. Lim JK, Jang YJ, Jung MK, et al: Ménétrier disease manifested by polyposis in the gastric antrum and coexisting with gastritis cystica profunda, *Gastrointest Endosc* 72:1098–1100, 2010.

25. Coffey RJ, Washington MK, Corless CL, Heinrich MC: Ménétrier disease and gastrointestinal stromal tumors: hyperproliferative disorders of the stomach, *J Clin Invest* 117:70–80, 2007.

A complete reference list can be found online at ExpertConsult .com

31

Subepithelial Tumors of the Esophagus and Stomach

Kristian Wall and Nicholas Nickl

CHAPTER OUTLINE

INTRODUCTION

Neoplasms of nonepithelial origin, although uncommon, are lesions that a gastrointestinal (GI) endoscopist can expect to encounter with some regularity. Although the number of such pathologic entities is manageably small, the spectrum of clinical behavior manifested by these lesions spans from trivial to life-threatening. The difficulty in managing patients with such lesions is that the tumor originates from within the GI tract wall and often appears as a mass beneath otherwise normal mucosa. Encountering such a seemingly innocent façade behind which lurks a range of ominous possibilities, the GI endoscopist is challenged to use additional diagnostic tools appropriately to direct the patient's care.

EPIDEMIOLOGY

The clinical starting point for patients with lesions of nonepithelial origin is the discovery of a mass impinging on the GI tract mucosa from beneath, the so-called submucosal tumor (Fig. 31.1). In its classic form, a discrete tumorous appearance is present with overlying mucosa that, although most commonly bland, may be erythematous, pale, dimpled, or ulcerated. Lesions are often initially identified at esophagogastroduodenoscopy (EGD), but the patient may also be referred to an endoscopist for evaluation of an abnormal radiograph (e.g., barium contrast examination).

Applied literally, the term *submucosal* would imply the presence of an intramural mass originating in the submucosal layer of the GI wall. Therefore, the term *subepithelial* tumor or lesion is the preferred nomenclature for describing a range of lesions that create a similar appearance, including intramural and extramural structures. Such subepithelial tumors (SETs) may include both neoplastic and non-neoplastic masses, and even mucosal neoplasms have been reported to exhibit a submucosal appearance.[1] Examples of nonepithelial lesions in all four categories are listed in Table 31.1. This discussion centers on neoplasms that primarily originate from nonepithelial GI tract cell lines, but all types of pathology must be considered when developing a management plan.

Depending on the clinical circumstances and type of tumor, the lesion may cause symptoms such as bleeding, obstruction, or pain. However, such lesions are commonly serendipitously found during evaluation for a different, unrelated problem. Because most such lesions are asymptomatic, epidemiologic data are skewed by the nature of their discovery incidental to a different, usually unrelated condition. In one study of 15,104 EGD reports, SETs were identified in 0.36%.[2] As most in this series were life-threatening tumors, the study database likely underreported less serious lesions. Many such lesions turn out to be normal extramural organs. Allgayer (1995)[3] found that among 30 patients referred for subepithelial lesions (SELs), normal extramural structures were present in 14 (47%). Motoo et al (1994)[4] also reported normal organs in 16 of 19 SELs, as did Caletti et al (1989)[5] in 10 of 25 tumors; organs identified include the spleen, liver, splenic vessels, and pancreas.

Because SETs are often left in situ, the pathologic distribution among tumors is unknown. It is reported that 1% to 3% of resected gastric tumors are stromal cell tumors[6]; it can be inferred that the actual incidence, when including tumors that were not resected, is considerably higher. In a small prospective study[7]

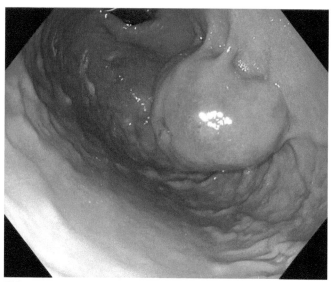

FIG 31.1 Endoscopic view of a proximal gastric subepithelial tumor in the retroflexed view.

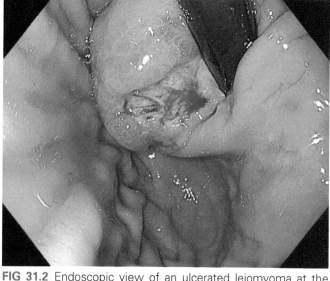

FIG 31.2 Endoscopic view of an ulcerated leiomyoma at the gastroesophageal junction.

TABLE 31.1   Types of Masses Causing Esophageal and Gastric Subepithelial Tumors

	Neoplastic Masses	Non-Neoplastic Masses
Intramural masses	Stromal cell tumor	Varices
	Lipoma	Duplication cyst
	Granular cell tumor	Inflammatory granuloma
	Lymphoma	Foreign body (e.g., surgical suture or clip)
	Fibrovascular polyp	Pancreatic rest
	Hemangioma/ hemangiosarcoma	
	Lymphangioma/ lymphangiosarcoma	
	Metastatic neoplasm	
Extramural masses	Primary neoplasm of adjacent organs (benign and malignant)	Benign lymph node
	Metastatic lymph node	Inflammatory mass of adjacent organs (e.g., pancreas, spleen)
		Organomegaly (e.g., spleen, liver)

among 45 SETs, most were found to have a benign appearance that required no follow-up. From these available data, it may be cautiously concluded that SETs are found in less than 1% of routine upper endoscopy examinations, half of such lesions are found to be normal extramural structures, most remaining lesions are benign, and stromal cell tumors constitute most such neoplasms.

CLINICAL FEATURES

Lumps and bumps of all sorts are regularly encountered in endoscopic examinations; the decision regarding which to evaluate further depends on the endoscopic appearance, the clinical circumstances, and the inclination of the endoscopist. A 2015

American Society for Gastrointestinal Endoscopy (ASGE) guideline[8] on the role of endoscopy in the management of premalignant conditions of the stomach focuses primarily on mucosal lesions, but does include that endoscopic ultrasound (EUS) with or without fine-needle aspiration (FNA) is the preferred technique to characterize subepithelial gastric lesions. Symptoms attributed to the mass nearly always drive further investigation, but our own EUS study of a subset of such lesions found that nearly 90% were asymptomatic.[9] GI bleeding may be seen in many SELs, most commonly in the form of slow blood loss causing iron-deficiency anemia. The surface of the tumor may be ulcerated in such cases (Fig. 31.2). Malignant tumors may be more prone to ulceration and bleeding[10]; this might be taken as a sign of a potentially malignant form that compels definitive treatment. However, benign lesions may also cause severe bleeding,[11] and occasionally rapid hemorrhage may occur.[12] Less often, GI tract obstruction may be caused by such masses,[13] especially if the lesion is located in a narrow area such as the esophagogastric junction or pylorus; intussusception caused by such masses has been reported.[14] Pain may be a presenting complaint, especially if the SET is neoplastic or malignant.[15]

Because most lesions are incidentally found during endoscopic examination for another problem, the clinical features of subepithelial masses are primarily those that, in the endoscopist's opinion, compel further evaluation. Size greater than 2 cm has been proposed as an ominous finding,[16] and lesions with an ulcerated or irregular (lumpy) surface often undergo additional testing or treatment. Patients with SETs who have a prior history of malignancy should receive further evaluation to exclude metastatic disease. Finally, patients with SETs that change appearance on serial examination are usually directed by an alert clinician to further testing.

PATHOLOGY

Extramural masses compose half of suspected SELs and include normal organs, non-neoplastic masses, and extramural neoplasms. Normal liver, spleen, pancreas, gallbladder, colon, and kidney all have been reported to appear as suspected SELs.[4–6] Vascular

TABLE 31.2 Classification of Gastrointestinal Mesenchymal Tumors

Tumor Type	Examples
Stromal tumors	GIST, smooth muscle tumors (leiomyoma, leiomyosarcoma), glomus tumors, leiomyomatosis, pleomorphic sarcoma
Neural tumors	Neuroma/neurofibroma, paraganglioma, ganglioneuromatosis
Endothelial and vascular tumors	Hemangioma, hemangiosarcoma, Kaposi's sarcoma, lymphangioma
Lipocytic tumors	Lipoma, liposarcoma, lipohyperplasia (ileocecal valve), lipomatosis (colon)
Granular cell tumor	Granular cell tumor
Inflammatory fibroid polyp	Inflammatory fibroid polyp
Fibrohistiocytic tumors	Fibrovascular polyp, fibrous histiocytoma, desmoid tumors (mesentery), fibroepithelial polyp
Striated muscle tumors	Rhabdomyosarcoma

GIST, gastrointestinal stromal tumor.
Data from Lewin K, Riddel RH, Weinstein WM: Mesenchymal tumors. In *Gastrointestinal Pathology and Its Clinical Implications,* New York, 1992, Igaku-Shoin, pp 284–341.

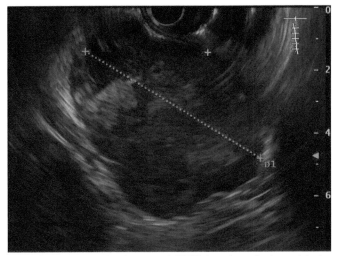

FIG 31.3 Endoscopic ultrasound (EUS) imaging of a large lobular gastric gastrointestinal stromal tumor (GIST) arising from the fourth wall layer (demarcated with a +).

structures often produce the appearance of a discrete tumor, including normal vessels of the spleen[17] and abnormal vessels such as varices and aneurysms.[18] Neoplasms and non-neoplastic masses involving these same organs can also produce this appearance, as can such masses involving the peritoneum, mediastinum, and the lymph nodes adjacent to the upper GI tract. The various malignancies, cysts, and inflammatory masses of these structures need no further elaboration here because a large variety of such findings have been noted in the case report literature.

Masses that arise within the wall of the esophagus and stomach require further discussion, particularly because many are peculiar to the GI tract. Most neoplasms in this category are mesenchymal tumors, meaning that they arise from cells of mesodermal origin. Most such neoplasms are clinically benign, although, as discussed subsequently, tumor histology may not provide reliable clues to malignant behavior. A large variety of such neoplasms have been described (Table 31.2), but most are exceedingly rare. The SETs most likely to be encountered in the esophagus and stomach in a routine clinical setting are discussed here.

Gastrointestinal Stromal Tumor

Most mesenchymal GI tumors are pale, firm, spherical, or ovoid structures embedded in the wall of the affected organ. The microscopic appearance of muscle-like eosinophilic, spindle-shaped cells in uniform sheets and the proximity of the tumors to the muscular wall layers led early observers to believe that these tumors were of myogenic origin,[19] hence the name "leiomyoma" and its variations (e.g., leiomyosarcoma, leiomyoblastoma). However, it later became clear that these neoplasms not only are not of obvious myogenic origin but also often lack any specific markers of differentiation whatsoever.[20] Immunohistochemical analyses showed variable expression of smooth muscle features such as desmin and actin, and neural proteins such as S-100.[21] For the sake of clarity, these lesions came to be referred to as gastrointestinal stromal tumors (GISTs), an acknowledgment

that they originate in mesenchymal stroma. Endoscopically, GISTs appear as a dome-shaped, firm subepithelial mass. Central umbilication or frank ulceration is common, and there may be a lobulated or irregular appearance (see Fig. 31.1; Video 31.1). GISTs are noted to arise from the fourth wall layer with EUS imaging (Fig. 31.3).

A significant breakthrough occurred with the discovery that most GI stromal tumors stain positive for a specific membrane protein, designated CD117.[22] The protein was subsequently identified as one of a class of stem cell factor (SCF) receptors. SCF receptors can exist as either soluble or transmembrane receptors; CD117 was subsequently identified as KIT, a transmembrane tyrosine kinase receptor[23] first found in a feline sarcoma (hence "kit" for kitten).[24]

Abnormal cell growth is a fundamental element of cancer physiology, and hyperfunction of the KIT receptor can lead to neoplasia. This concept is supported by the observation that nearly all GISTs express KIT. It has further been observed that the interstitial cells of Cajal (ICC) share some phenotypic and ultrastructural similarities with GIST and normally express the KIT receptor; this observation has led to the current hypothesis that GISTs arise from ICC[29] or from ICC precursor cells. This hypothesis is bolstered by the observation that ICC cells are seen outside the GI tract, and likewise extra-intestinal GIST have been described[30,31] Finally, it has been noted that this gain-of-function mutation is not found in true leiomyomas.[32] Some pathologists have suggested that CD117 positivity is required to confirm a diagnosis of GIST.[33] It is now known, however, that a few otherwise obvious GISTs do not express KIT. Many of these tumors have been identified as expressing platelet-derived growth factor receptor α (PDGFRα), another distinct tyrosine kinase receptor that also mediates many of the same growth and antiapoptotic proliferation pathways.[34] Several gain-of-function mutations have been reported in the PDGFRα gene, and the resulting tumors are otherwise indistinguishable from GISTs that are KIT-positive. There also remains a small subset of GISTs that express neither KIT nor PDGFRα; presumably other pathophysiologic pathways exist to account for these, including other tyrosine kinase gain-of-function mutations.

Nearly all upper GI tumors of this type occur in the stomach, but duodenal lesions have been described.[35] Most esophageal stromal tumors lack the CD117 protein and may be true leiomyomas.[33] The tumors are most often solitary except in the case of specific disease entities such as Carney's triad (GIST, pulmonary chondroma, and extra-adrenal paraganglioma). Germline KIT mutation kindreds have been described,[36] however, in which case multiple GISTs are seen. Giant sizes of greater than 10 cm have been noted, but most tumors are less than 3 cm.

Pathologically, the tumor usually consists of uniform pale tissue, although hemorrhagic and necrotic areas may be seen. Microscopically, the cells are spindle shaped with uniform nuclei and general cytologic uniformity. Some cell groups may show epithelioid configurations (closely packed polygonal cells), and there may be nuclear pleomorphism. It has been observed more recently that the histologic pattern is sometimes related to the nature of the underlying genetic abnormality; KIT mutations at exon 13 or 17 more often show spindle cell morphology,[37] whereas PDGFRα GISTs often exhibit epithelioid histology.[38] Ultrastructural cellular abnormalities have also been linked to specific gene mutations.[39] Recent research (2015) has linked some specific mutations with clinical features and outcomes; for instance, KIT exon 9 mutations show higher risk of progression and lower 5-year relapse-free survival than those with exon 11 mutations.[40] It has long been known that malignant behavior in GISTs is difficult to predict given the relatively bland cytology and slow growth of these neoplasms. It has been reported that even small, benign-appearing stromal tumors have been known to metastasize.[41] This discovery led to considerable confusion about the appropriate criteria to categorize these tumors as benign or malignant. Older pathologic scoring systems relied on numerous histologic features[20] and were plagued with problems. More recent attention has focused on the size of the tumor and the number of mitoses observed (mitotic index), at least in part because these are easily quantifiable findings. In one study of 100 cases, tumors with more than 5 mitoses per 10 high-power fields (HPFs) were significantly more likely to metastasize, although 40% of malignant lesions in that study had fewer mitoses.[42] In another study, multivariate analysis of various clinical and pathologic features in 122 specimens showed that more than 10 mitoses/50 HPFs correlated with poor outcome, whereas site, epithelioid histology, and tumor size were not independently predictive.[43]

Attempts to correlate tumor marker status such as CD117 positivity with malignant behavior have produced generally confusing or negative results,[44] as have studies of specific KIT mutations[32,45] and other tumor markers.[46,47] Older GIST scoring systems have been abandoned following a National Institutes of Health (NIH) consensus conference, which defined malignancy risk based on size and mitotic index alone.[48,49] The NIH criteria divide tumors into four categories of malignant risk (Table 31.3), an acknowledgment that even the most innocent lesion poses a slight but definite risk of malignant behavior.

If all such neoplasms entail malignant risk, prudence might dictate that they should always be resected. However, more recent data suggest that GISTs are more common than previously thought. Up to 10% of resection and autopsy specimens contain such tumors,[50] and microscopic GISTs (also called seedling GISTs, minimal GISTs, or GIST tumorlets) can be seen in 35% of some patient groups.[51,52] These incidental and microscopic GISTs display the same KIT and PDGFRα mutations as their larger counterparts. The finding that synchronous GISTs from the same patient

TABLE 31.3 National Institutes of Health Criteria for Malignant Risk in Gastrointestinal Stromal Tumors

Risk Level	Size (cm)	Mitoses/50 HPF
Very low risk	< 2	< 5
Low risk	2–5	< 5
Intermediate risk	< 5	6–10
	5–10	< 5
High risk	> 5	> 5
	> 10	Any
	Any	> 10

HPF, high-power field.
Data from Berman JJ, O'Leary TH: Gastrointestinal stromal tumor workshop. *Hum Pathol* 32:578–582, 2001; Toquet C, Le Neel JC, Guillou L, et al: Elevated (> or = 10%) MIB-1 proliferative index correlates with poor outcome in gastric stromal tumor patients: A study of 35 cases. *Dig Dis Sci* 47:2247–2253, 2002; Hedenbro JL, Ekelund M, Wetterberg P: Endoscopic diagnosis of submucosal gastric lesions: the results after routine endoscopy. *Surg Endosc* 5:20–30, 1991.

regularly show different gene mutations (and are independent sporadic GISTs) confuses the picture further.[53] GISTs that were earlier classified as metastatic or recurrent may have been distinct neoplastic events. If it turns out that most small and asymptomatic GISTs stay that way, a conservative approach may be the most prudent.

A second breakthrough in GISTs has been the development of tyrosine kinase inhibitors such as imatinib mesylate, which are effective in reducing KIT enzyme activity and are useful for tumor treatment. Imatinib targets the specific abnormal enzyme activity in the neoplasm and does not rely on generalized cytotoxicity for its effect. In an open-label study of 147 patients with unresectable malignant GISTs, an overall response rate of 38% was seen.[54] Among responders, results are often dramatic. A number of newer compounds with similar tyrosine kinase inhibitory function have been examined in GISTs and have been found to be effective. Sunitinib and regorafenib have shown effectiveness, particularly in imatinib-resistant tumors, as have a variety of agents that target downstream oncogenetic proteins.[55] The recognition of the malignant potential of GIST, combined with the availability of effective treatment even for unresectable disease, has compelled new thinking in the accurate diagnosis of this neoplasm.

Glomus Tumors

Glomus tumors are mesenchymal tumors that generally occur in the skin; a morphologically similar lesion has long been known in the stomach.[56] They arise from modified cells of the glomus body that regulate arteriolar blood flow. They are typically located in the antrum and are generally small, although they can range up to 5 cm.[57] These usually appear as circumscribed hypoechoic masses in the third or fourth layer and can have a characteristic peripheral halo around them. There may have arterial enhancement on computed tomography (CT) scanning similar to hemangiomas. An immunohistochemical study of 32 cases showed that all examined glomus tumors were negative for desmin, S-100, CD34, and KIT,[58] suggesting a different histogenesis from leiomyomas, neuromas, and GISTs. They will typically stain positive for actin. A larger retrospective study of 1894 resected gastric mesenchymal tumors revealed 11 gastric glomus tumors.[59]

This same study showed that all glomus tumors examined stained positive for α-smooth muscle actin, laminin, collagen type IV, and vimentin. No C-kit mutations were present. Previous studies have suggested a malignancy risk that is low but not zero. Another study[60] suggested that metastases were found in 38% of glomus tumors (52 cases) and that the possible risk factors for malignancy included deep location, size greater than 2 cm, atypical mitotic figures, moderate-to-high nuclear grade, and greater than 5 mitotic figures per 50 HPFs. Typically, the main goals in diagnosing glomus tumors of the stomach have been to differentiate them from other tumors such as GISTs.

Neural Tumors

Technically, most tumors that appear to be of neural origin continue to be classified as stromal tumors, although the more recent revolution in GIST understanding brought about by the discovery of CD117 mutations has led to confusing terminology in some cases, including neural tumors. Many experts consider stromal tumors that are positive for S-100 and negative for CD117 to be of neural origin.

Neural tumors may represent glial cell proliferation, sometimes in combination with other neural elements. *Neuroma, neurofibroma*, and *schwannoma* are largely interchangeable terms, although some pathologists observe differences among these lesions. When ganglion cells are present, the term *ganglioneuroma* is often applied. They seem to arise from ganglion cells in either the myenteric plexus or submucosal plexus. Schwannomas are slow-growing tumors derived from Schwann cells, which are typically found in the subcutaneous tissue of the distal extremities or head/neck. They are extremely rare in the GI tract, but the stomach is the most common site. Typical histology reveals atypical spindle cells in a microtrabecular pattern, S-100 positivity, negative glial fibrillary acidic protein, and negative c-KIT,[61] as well as negative staining for CD34, desmin, and smooth muscle actin. Previous studies have found no malignant variants.[62] Incidence of Schwannomas is predominantly based on case reports, but has been estimated to be 0.2% of all gastric tumors.

Neuroma and Neurofibroma

Neuroma and neurofibroma are well-circumscribed, nonencapsulated tumors arising from either the submucosa or the muscularis propria layer. Except in the case of von Recklinghausen's neurofibromatosis, they are usually solitary nodules. They consist of bland spindle-shaped cells and are often classified as neuromas (as opposed to GISTs) if neural markers are identified on immunohistochemical stain.

Gangliocytic Paraganglioma

Gangliocytic paragangliomas are rare tumors that range from 0.5 to 4 cm in size and are found in the periampullary duodenum. They may be present in either the submucosa or the muscularis propria layers and consist of a combination of ganglion cells, columnar or polymorphic epithelioid cells, and spindle cells (staining positive for S-100) with a cord-like arrangement that may be of neural derivation[63]; they usually also contain a component resembling carcinoid tumor or neuroendocrine cells. Immunocytochemically, somatostatin is usually present, and other neuropeptides may also be seen, including chromogranin A. They are always benign but may be locally infiltrative and can present as bleeding from surface ulceration/erosion. Diagnosis is typically focused on differentiating this from neuroendocrine tumors that could have some malignant potential.

Endothelial and Vascular Tumors

Cavernous hemangiomas are vascular neoplasms that rarely occur in the GI tract and even more rarely in the upper tract. They appear as sessile red or blue nodules and can be difficult to distinguish from vascular ectasias (which are not neoplastic). A malignant counterpart, hemangiosarcoma, is exceedingly rare but has been described in nearly all parts of the GI tract.[64] Lymphatic tumors are also exceedingly rare in the GI tract, primarily being reported in the duodenum. They are described as having a smooth, sessile, or polypoid translucent appearance endoscopically.[65] Histologically, they are mucosal or submucosal and contain hamartomatous rather than true neoplastic elements[64]; they are always benign.

Lipocytic Tumors: Lipoma and Liposarcoma

Lipomas are usually harmless neoplasms arising from submucosal adipocytes. They are most common in the colon but may appear in any part of the GI tract, particularly the gastric antrum.[66] The typical endoscopic appearance is a pale yellowish, soft submucosal tumor; usually a solitary lesion is seen. The overlying mucosa can sometimes be tented up with a biopsy forceps, and the lesion deforms easily when pushed with the forceps (pillow sign). Histologically, such tumors are encapsulated and consist of typical benign mature lipocytes. When they contain a large number of blood vessels, they are sometimes called angiolipomas. It is rarely necessary to evaluate them further or remove them unless they cause bleeding or obstruction. They are normally small, but giant lipomas have been described[67] that can cause obstruction or intussusception.[68] The clinically aggressive malignant form, liposarcoma, is exceedingly rare.[69]

Granular Cell Tumor

The esophagus is the most common site of granular cell tumors (approximately 75% of granular cell tumors were esophageal in one study), but they may be found throughout the GI tract. They are most often located in the submucosa and often have a polypoid shape. Multiple tumors are common. They are of Schwann cell origin and consist of masses of histiocytes-like cells containing periodic acid–Schiff-positive cytoplasmic granules. A literature review of 117 cases found dysphagia to be the most common symptom in roughly half of patients; three-fourths were smaller than 2 cm.[70] Malignancy appears rare and in the same review four cases were locally invasive, but distant metastases were not noted. In another study,[71] 1% to 2% of cases were reported as malignant. They generally appear as yellowish, plaque-like, round or oval lesions less than 2 cm across.[72] The overlying squamous epithelium of the esophagus may show pseudoepitheliomatous hyperplasia.[73] If this is misinterpreted as metaplastic mucosal transformation, confusion may lead to additional investigations in search of an epithelial neoplasm. Another recent study published in 2015 reviewed 98 granular cell tumors from 95 patients.[74] They found a 2.2:1 male predominance and also noted that gastric and colonic granular cell tumors were larger and their growth pattern was more infiltrative. One colonic tumor in this study had infiltration to pericolonic soft tissue and lymph node metastasis. High expression of S-100 protein, CD56, CD68, and SOX-10 was also seen.

Inflammatory Fibroid Polyp

Inflammatory fibroid polyps are uncommon tumors that can occur anywhere in the GI tract; the stomach is the most common site,[20] but they have been described elsewhere.[75] Pathologically, they consist of nonencapsulated myxoid stroma that includes blood vessels, inflammatory cells, and invariably eosinophils. The eosinophilic infiltrate had previously led to the (now discarded) designation of this tumor as localized eosinophilic gastroenteritis. They are often small, but giant tumors have been described that can cause (as usual) bleeding, obstruction, or intussusception.[76] Current theories of their pathogenesis focus on myofibroblasts or fibroblasts,[77] but the cell of origin is unknown. They tend to originate in the muscle layers of the GI tract wall, beginning as an intramural bulge but later assuming a polypoid shape; there may often be a significant extramural (subserosal) extension. There seems to be no malignant potential.

Fibrous (Fibrovascular) Polyp

Fibrous polyps are esophageal tumors that can grow to an enormous size. They occur predominantly in male patients, usually originate in the upper esophagus, and often assume a polypoid shape.[78] Tumors up to 20 cm have been described[79] and can cause dysphagia, globus, bleeding, and asphyxiation from laryngeal impaction.

Although these tumors may have ulcerated overlying mucosa, the sheer size of the lesion may make it difficult to identify endoscopically.[80] Histologically, a large variety of cytologic elements are seen, including spindle cells, lipocytes, mononuclear inflammatory cells, and vascular connective tissue. However, because some typical characteristics of inflammatory fibroid polyps are lacking and because of differing epidemiology and location, these lesions are classified separately from inflammatory fibroid polyps and should not be confused with them, despite the similar names. They are of uncertain histogenesis but do not seem to possess malignant potential. Nevertheless, because fatal outcomes have been described arising from the mechanical size of these tumors, removal is considered prudent, which can either be via endoscopic or surgical techniques.

Metastatic Tumors

Intramural metastases to the GI tract are less common than compression or invasion from extramural cancer. In a study of gastric mural metastases, the most common primary sites were lung, breast, and esophagus, but malignant melanoma was the most frequent tumor to metastasize to the stomach. Half appeared endoscopically as SETs, and the rest were ulcerated or fungating; one-third showed multiple lesions.[81]

Cystic Tumors

Various cystic intramural lesions may manifest as SELs. In an individual patient, it may be unclear until EUS is performed that these tumors are cystic. However, it is worth collectively listing lesions (some of which have already been discussed) that can assume such an appearance. Small lymphatic ectasias are a common endoscopic finding,[64] particularly in the duodenum, and represent cystic structures less than 5 mm in size; they are not neoplasms. Duplication cysts are another non-neoplastic intramural cyst that may be seen as SELs. These are very rarely encountered lesions in the upper GI tract[82,83] and are caused by embryonic epithelial nodules that fail to regress. Brunner's gland hamartomas and heterotopic pancreas have also been described as having a cystic appearance.[84] Among neoplastic cysts, lymphangiomas[85] and hemangiomas[86] (and hemangiosarcomas) assume a cystic appearance. In addition, any malignant neoplasm with central necrosis may appear as a cystic intramural lesion.

DIFFERENTIAL DIAGNOSIS

As has been shown, SELs may represent the full spectrum of symptoms and pathology from innocent to critical. Various diagnostic tools are available to sort out the possibilities.

Conventional Endoscopy, Computed Tomography, and Transabdominal Ultrasound

Confronted with a SEL, the alert endoscopist should not permit the presence of mucosa between the endoscopic camera and the mass to preclude preliminary conclusions about the nature of the unseen tumor. Despite the multitude of possibilities already discussed, a short list of half a dozen lesions covers nearly everything likely to be found in all but the largest referral centers. Each has distinctive clinical and endoscopic features (Table 31.4) to provide an adequate preliminary assessment, which can be used to direct further management.

Routine endoscopic pinch biopsies are often performed but rarely yield diagnostic material, even when large size (jumbo) pinch forceps are used.[87] Other efforts to obtain tissue during routine endoscopy have been described, including standard FNA needles,[88] a special guillotine aspiration biopsy needle,[89] and mucosal stripping followed by forceps biopsy[90]; these show variable success but have not yet gained widespread acceptance.

Conventional CT has traditionally been unhelpful in evaluating intramural tumors because of their small size, but new CT methods show promise. Multidetector high-resolution CT scanners can identify most tumors larger than 1 cm, although further characterization may be difficult.[91] Three-dimensional computerized reconstruction techniques are also able to detect intramural tumors reliably and may provide useful images.[92] Ongoing improvements in CT resolution may yet result in clinically important images and allow diagnosis radiologically. CT scanning can reveal large lesions, and National Comprehensive Cancer Network (NCCN) guidelines have recommended using CT for monitoring for recurrent or metastatic disease, as well as to gauge the response to therapy.[93] FDG (fluorodeoxyglucose)-positron emission tomography/CT can also be useful in staging of GISTs and can help diagnose, stage, and monitor.

Conventional transabdominal ultrasound has likewise been unhelpful in this setting, but similar to CT, useful progress is being reported. High-resolution transabdominal ultrasound, using transducer frequencies of 5 MHz or 7.5 MHz, and a

TABLE 31.4 Endoscopic Appearance of Typical Upper Gastrointestinal Subepithelial Lesions

Clinical Characteristics	Most Likely Tumor
Lower esophagus: < 2 cm, plaque-like, firm, yellowish, sometimes multiple	Granular cell tumor
Upper esophagus: firm, large, polypoid	Fibrous (fibrovascular) polyp
Stomach: ovoid, firm, any size, single lesion	GIST
Stomach: < 1 cm, firm, dimpled	Heterotopic pancreas
Any organ: translucent, soft	Lymphangioma
Any organ: soft, yellowish, soft, compressible, any size, single lesion	Lipoma

GIST, gastrointestinal stromal tumor.

water-filled stomach, provides remarkable imaging of tumors 10 mm in size and their relationship to the five-layer GI tract wall.[94] Although unsuitable for obese patients or many anatomic tumor locations, this technique could potentially supplement many EUS examinations of such tumors at centers where such equipment is available.

Endoscopic Ultrasound

High-resolution scanning from an intraluminal position makes EUS ideally suited for evaluation of SELs and for complete characterization of intramural masses that are identified. Extramural impression from normal and abnormal structures can be reliably shown, and intramural masses can be readily characterized. The ability to relate intramural tumors to the five-layer wall structure of the GI tract permits conclusions about the origin of the lesion (and its probable histology) and, where appropriate, the degree of local invasion (T stage). Table 31.5 lists some important features that can be derived from EUS and which are usually helpful in diagnosing the lesion and directing further management.

Several studies have documented the ability of EUS to characterize such lesions accurately. Yasuda et al (1990)[95] reported their experience with 308 patients, including 210 SELs. Characteristic echo features of benign and malignant stromal tumors, varices, cysts, lipomas, lymphoma, and aberrant pancreas were described. Rösch et al (2002)[96] described the appearance of 102 SELs collected in a multicenter German study group. Characterizing the accuracy of EUS for this purpose is difficult and depends on the question being asked. The ability of EUS to measure tumor size accurately has been documented[97] as has reliability in identifying extramural structures. However, distinguishing among different classes of lesions (e.g., cystic, fatty, stromal) or pathologic entities (e.g., stromal tumor, carcinoid) is hampered by the fact that pathologic confirmation is not uniformly available in these research subject groups. Rösch and coworkers[96] reported sensitivity and specificity figures of 64% to 92% and 80% to 100%, for various types of pathologic distinctions being examined.

These and other authors have characterized the typical appearance of several intramural lesions. Lipomas (Fig. 31.4) are brightly echogenic structures with uniform echotexture and

well-demarcated margins (Video 31.2), and they are generally associated with the submucosal layer (layer 3). They are easily deformed by compression from the transducer tip. Because they are virtually always benign, identifying continuity of the muscularis propria layer behind the tumor is helpful in confirming the diagnosis. Varices (Fig. 31.5) are also easy to recognize as anechoic vermiform structures. They are nearly always in groups,

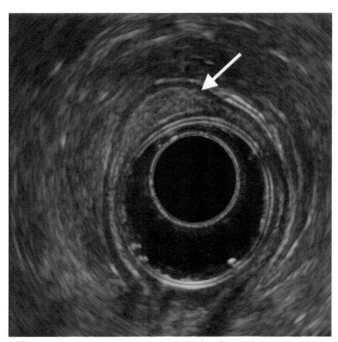

FIG 31.4 Endoscopic ultrasound (EUS) of gastric lipoma. Note uniform hyperechoic echogenicity and submucosal position with intact muscularis propria layer *(arrow).*

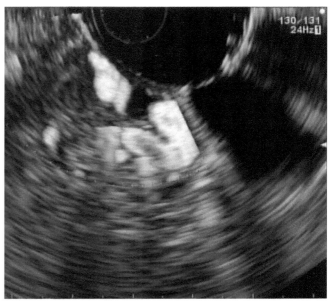

FIG 31.5 Endoscopic ultrasound (EUS) of gastric varices. Note anechoic serpiginous structures; that demonstrate blood flow with on real-time Doppler imaging.

TABLE 31.5	**Important Endoscopic Ultrasound Features in Intramural Masses**
Attribute	**Attribute Values**
Location	Organ (e.g., stomach) and position (e.g., greater curve)
Size	Measured (in three dimensions if possible)
Background echogenicity	Hypoechoic, hyperechoic, or anechoic
Focal echogenicity	Hypoechoic foci, hyperechoic foci, both, or neither
Shape/margin shape	Round, oval; smooth margins, irregular margins
Margin definition	Well-defined margins, poorly defined margins
Position/origin relative to wall layers	Involves mucosa, submucosa, muscularis propria
Tumor extension or invasion	T stage relative to site organ

and extramural varices can usually be seen. When a variceal structure is seen in isolation, a hemangioma or lymphangioma should be considered because these may have a similar appearance (Video 31.3). Cysts such as duplication cysts also have an anechoic internal structure (Fig. 31.6), although debris may be seen as hyperechoic foci within the cyst structure. Aberrant pancreas (Fig. 31.7) is usually suspected by the endoscopic appearance, and the EUS structure of a hypoechoic lesion associated with the submucosal layer is confirmatory. Internal echogenic spots are often observed with this lesion.

The most frequent finding is of a hypoechoic intramural structure (Figs. 31.8 and 31.9). Various tumors, mostly neoplasms, can have this appearance, including GISTs, carcinoids, granular cell tumors, lymphomas, and metastatic tumors. These lesions all show generally hypoechoic (ground-glass) background echotexture, often containing hyperechoic foci or hypoechoic and anechoic foci (or both hyperechoic and hypoechoic foci).

The tumor margins are typically well defined and smooth, and the overall shape is round or oval. Despite the similarities, some EUS clues may help distinguish among these lesions. Granular cell tumors, usually located in the esophagus, are typically seen within the third (submucosal) echo layer and are generally smaller than 2 cm (see Fig. 31.8A). Carcinoid tumors are most common in the mucosal and submucosal layers (see Fig. 31.8B), as are lymphomas (see Fig. 31.8C), whereas metastatic tumors (see Fig. 31.8D) may occupy any layer in any organ.

Stromal tumors (see Fig. 31.9) are typically located in the muscularis propria layer and indistinguishably blend into it. Their most innocent appearance is of rounded, well-circumscribed, smooth tumors of 1 to 2 cm with uniform echogenicity (see Fig. 31.9A). Other EUS features may be seen, however, and significant effort has been expended to determine whether those features can distinguish benign from malignant behavior. Giant size (see Fig. 31.9B) and irregular or knobby margins (see Fig. 31.9C) have been imputed to predict malignancy, as have internal foci that are hyperechoic or hypoechoic (see Fig. 31.9D).

Early proposals that all these features were ominous[98] have been investigated further with mixed results. Tsai et al (2001)[99] showed a correlation of each of these features with malignant histology, but no single factor or combination of factors yielded satisfactory diagnostic accuracy. Chak et al (1997)[100] showed sensitivity figures of 80% to 100% for malignancy in a retrospective videotape study using these factors, but there was only fair-to-moderate intraobserver agreement for the factors themselves, especially for hyperechoic and hypoechoic foci; specificity was 80%. A multicenter prospective study of 198 tumors attempted to validate these criteria further and found that tumor size, surface ulceration, non-oval shape, and irregular or indistinct margins were associated with malignancy, whereas hyperechoic and hypoechoic internal foci were not correlated.[9] The authors also reported that serial surveillance of initially innocent lesions by repeat EUS provided a very low yield of additional malignant neoplasms. Reviewing the literature on the subject collectively, most experts agree that size greater than 3 cm and irregular or indistinct margins are worrisome features.

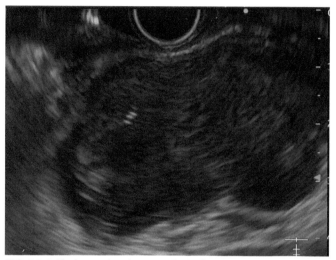

FIG 31.6 Endoscopic ultrasound (EUS) of a large esophageal duplication cyst.

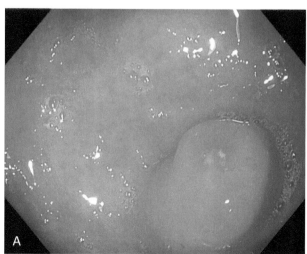 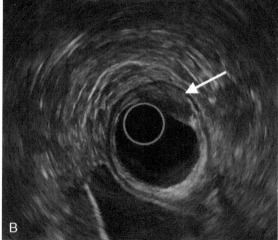

FIG 31.7 **A,** Endoscopic and **B,** endoscopic ultrasound (EUS) imaging of an ectopic pancreas (i.e., pancreatic rest) in the gastric antrum. Note the central umbilication with imaging and on EUS; this appears as a heterogeneous structure located in the mucosal layer and submucosal layer (arrow).

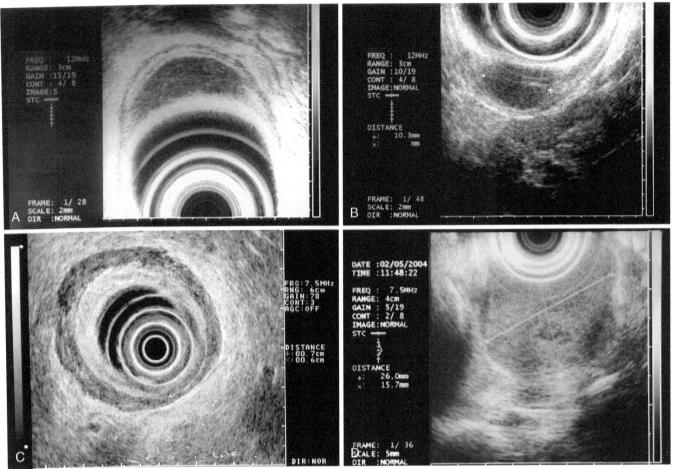

FIG 31.8 Endoscopic ultrasound (EUS) appearance of intraepithelial neoplasms. **A,** Granular cell tumor of the esophagus, seen as a hypoechoic structure located within the submucosal layer (note intact muscularis propria layer). **B,** Carcinoid tumor of the duodenum, a hypoechoic tumor in the submucosa. **C,** Infiltrating lymphoma causing thickening of both the third and the fourth echo layers. **D,** Large metastatic tumor that mostly replaces the entire wall locally.

Fine-Needle Aspiration

Given the ambiguous predictive value of EUS morphology in identifying tissue histology or predicting malignant behavior when considering hypoechoic intramural tumors, efforts to obtain diagnostic tissue assume greater importance. Transcutaneous sampling under CT or ultrasound guidance is possible for some lesions and can yield diagnostic material in up to three-fourths of lesions.[101] Likewise, endoscopic FNA by direct puncture or under EUS guidance has been reported to yield adequate diagnostic material in up to 90%[88] and, when combined with immuno-histochemical stains, can distinguish GIST from leiomyoma.[102] However, anecdotal reports suggest that a large number of FNA passes may be needed to secure adequate diagnostic tissue. Such specimens may be adequate to distinguish other neoplasms from GISTs, but they are unable to reliably distinguish benign from malignant GISTs. The fact that the cellularity is insufficient to obtain a mitotic index is a major obstacle, but the addition of immunohistochemical stains in biopsy specimens, including c-KIT and Ki-67, improves the diagnostic accuracy of stromal tumors[103] and can suggest malignant risk. Case series of an "unroofing" technique for tissue acquisition from lesions of the muscularis propria has been described.[104] A 2000 modeling study suggested that biopsy can improve clinical management of hypoechoic tumors,[105] lending support to the routine performance of needle biopsy of hypoechoic tumors, with immunostaining when appropriate. Recently there have been advances in needle design, with fine-needle biopsy (FNB) needles becoming more commonly used to hopefully improve tissue acquisition and thus improve definitive diagnosis with fewer passes. Previous studies using Trucut biopsy showed improved diagnostic yield (77.8% vs. 38.7%, $p < 0.001$) compared with standard FNA with fewer non-diagnostic specimens.[106] A 2017 article showed improved adequacy of tissue acquisition determined by immunohistochemi-cal staining (64.8% of FNA group and 100% in FNB group, $p = 0.006$) with no significant change in safety, although the sample size for the FNB group was small (15 patients).[107]

TREATMENT

The initial management of intramural tumors typically involves a decision as to whether the lesion will be resected and how that will be accomplished. New diagnostic and therapeutic options make the decision easier. The use of EUS appearance combined with FNA or FNB specimens and immunostaining provides important information to direct the choice. Similarly, new options for removing the tumors have emerged to supplant or replace the traditional choice of open laparotomy or thoracotomy.

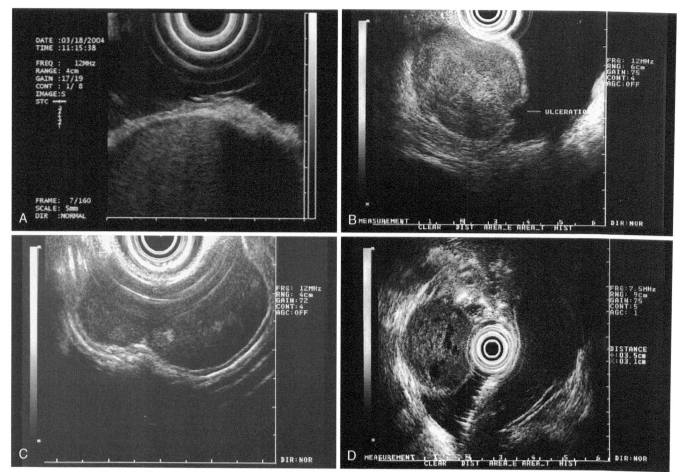

FIG 31.9 Endoscopic ultrasound (EUS) appearance of gastrointestinal stromal tumors (GISTs). **A,** Benign-appearing GIST. Note small size, layer four (muscularis propria) location, and smooth and well-defined margins. **B,** Large gastric GIST greater than 3 cm with surface ulceration and hyperechoic internal foci. **C,** GIST with multilobed irregular margins and hyperechoic foci. **D,** Hypoechoic (anechoic) foci within large GIST.

Indications and Contraindications

Several clear-cut indications have emerged to direct resection of intramural tumors. Most obvious is the presence of symptoms that are caused by the lesion, such as bleeding, obstruction, or intussusception. Beyond this, lesions that are malignant or pose a significant risk of becoming malignant require resection, whereas clearly benign tumors, such as granular cell tumors and lipomas, pose no meaningful malignant risk and may be safely left in situ. Because GISTs comprise most intramural tumors, it remains to identify which hypoechoic lesions are GISTs and how high the malignant risk is for a given GIST. For this reason, EUS combined with FNA or FNB and immunostaining is emerging as the diagnostic procedure of choice. In a 2002 study, 71% of resected hypoechoic tumors were GISTs; 12% of these were malignant GISTs, and another 41% were GISTs of indeterminate malignant potential.[9] Given what seems to be a significant malignant risk among such tumors, criteria to direct resection should have high sensitivity, even at the expense of low specificity. It seems reasonable to perform resection of hypoechoic tumors with size greater than 3 cm, irregular or indistinct margins, ulceration, or non-oval shape. Rapid growth on serial examination, although not a validated criterion, is nevertheless a sufficiently alarming finding also to direct removal of the tumor.

Preoperative History and Considerations

In selecting patients with GISTs who should be directed to surgical resection, it is important to maintain perspective on the actual level of malignant risk compared with the surgical risk. Despite the suggestion that the proportion of GISTs containing a meaningful malignant risk may approach 50%, it remains widely accepted that most GISTs, if left alone, remain benign and asymptomatic. Among patients with an average surgical risk, it is reasonable to maintain a low threshold for resection of tumors with alarming EUS or histologic features. EUS features that have previously been described as being predictive of malignant risk include irregular extraluminal margin, cystic spaces, and lymph nodes with a malignant pattern.[108] A review of 14 patients found that EUS features including tumor size, irregular extraluminal border, local invasion, and heterogenicity correlated with intermediate- or high-risk malignant potential.[109] However, for patients with advanced age or significant comorbidities that render surgical resection risky, a higher threshold is warranted. In such patients, a more diligent search for immunohistochemical markers of malignancy, such as MIB-1 or Ki-67, would be prudent in directing surgery, as the presence of staining for Ki-67 in particular may point to a more aggressive lesion. Studies have suggested that GISTs larger than 2 cm or with EUS features associated with malignant potential such as greater size, lobulated forms, irregular borders, and echogenic foci should be considered for resection. A retrospective review of 75 patients with surgically resected 2- to 5-cm GISTs found that tumor size and EUS features (heterogeneity, hyperechoic foci, calcification, cystic change, hypoechoic foci, lobulation, and ulceration) could not be used to preoperatively predict the risk of malignancy.[108] Previous NCCN guidelines from 2007 recommended resection for all GISTs larger than 2 cm.[93] Recent ASGE guidelines recommended annual EUS surveillance of GISTs smaller than 2 cm if surgical resection is not performed.[8]

Description of Techniques

Some SETs are appropriate for endoscopic removal. Numerous reports document success in removal of tumors of the mucosa or submucosa, including lipomas, inflammatory fibroid polyps, carcinoids,[110] and granular cell tumors.[111] Stromal cell tumors that do not involve the muscularis propria can also be successfully removed endoscopically.[112] Generally, a snare or injection-assisted snare technique is described, although newer techniques of endoscopic submucosal dissection (ESD) may be required for larger lesions. Bleeding is the most common complication and may require transfusion, endoscopic therapy,[110] or surgery.[113] Despite the reported success of this technique, the number of tumors appropriate for endoscopic removal is limited. The most problematic intramural tumors are tumors that show EUS features of GIST (see Video 31.1); because most of these involve the muscularis propria, they were previously thought to be unsuitable for endoscopic treatment. Recent advances in ESD techniques

have shown that small SELs arising from the muscularis propria can be removed, but techniques that include closure of the muscularis propria (and possibly the serosa) will be required for endoscopic removal of tumors involving that layer.[114,115] There have also been advancements in developing endoscopic full-thickness resection (EFTR) with the aid of over-the-scope clips, and a recent study (article in press) of nine patients undergoing EFTR for subepithelial and epithelial lesions (five lesions in the stomach or duodenum) demonstrated an effective procedure (R0 resection confirmed in all cases) with no reported adverse events.[116]

Advances in minimally invasive surgery have made laparoscopic removal possible for many such tumors. Several small case series describe successful laparoscopic removal of GISTs in various gastric sites,[117,118] including the posterior wall of the stomach.[119] Tumors up to 7 cm in size can be removed.[120] Surgical techniques described include tumor enucleation, wedge resection, and partial gastrectomy. A combined endoscopic and laparoscopic approach may be required when the tumor cannot be readily identified from the serosal surface.[121] In these small series, few complications are reported,[117] but conversion to open resection may be required.[119] A more recent (2002) retrospective study comparing open and laparoscopic resection of GISTs found a shorter mean hospital stay for the latter (3.8 days vs. 6.2 days) but otherwise comparable technical and safety outcomes,[122] and a smaller prospective study found a similar decrease in hospital stay but also noted hospital costs to be 31% less in the laparoscopy group.[123] It has been emphasized that such resections require a high degree of technical skill in laparoscopic surgery.[122] As experience widens,

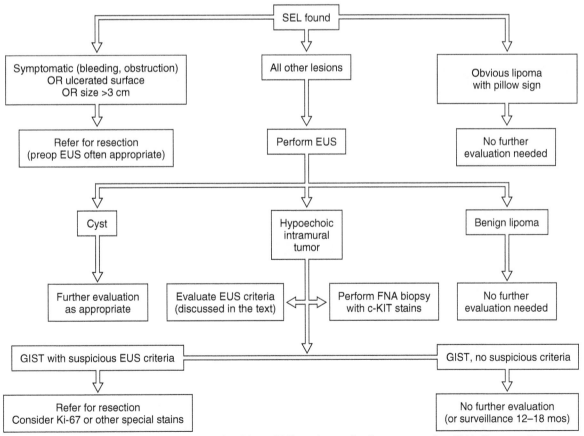

FIG 31.10 Provisional treatment algorithm. *EUS,* endoscopic ultrasonography; *FNA,* fine-needle aspiration; *GIST,* gastrointestinal stromal tumor; *SEL,* subepithelial lesion.

it is likely that laparoscopic resection will become the procedure of choice in the near future for GISTs requiring removal; the convenience and patient acceptance of this method may lead to decreased resistance to resection of GISTs of equivocal malignant potential.

FUTURE TRENDS

An alert reader perusing the literature on the subject must be struck by the extremely variable quality of the data available. It cannot be otherwise: all the lesions discussed here range from "uncommon" to "never in my lifetime," and even the largest of case series rarely contains more than a few dozen individuals. Developing a management algorithm, or even a reasonable plan for a single patient, based on such scant data is a hazardous undertaking.

Despite the dearth of clinical material, great strides have been made. The advance in the understanding of stromal tumors by the discovery of KIT and its dovetailing with other known oncogenic markers has provided great insight into the histogenesis and growth mechanism of these neoplasms and has pioneered treatment agents, such as imatinib, of novel therapeutic action. Extending this work will provide exciting new insights and therapies, and the "Grail" of GISTs, a reliable test of benign versus malignant behavior, may be right around the corner. Another revolution has been in the development of advanced endoscopic and laparoscopic surgical approaches to these tumors. The ability to remove intramural masses safely and reliably in what may soon become an outpatient procedure enormously increases the management options. However, the pressure on GI endoscopists to establish efficacy and cost efficiency in endoscopic management is also substantially increased. Multiple endoscopic evaluations and serial surveillance of SELs, by either EGD or EUS, makes little sense when the tumor can be easily and conveniently dispensed with altogether.

More recent modeling suggests that the GI endoscopist who cannot establish definitive patient management in an average of 1.7 EUS examinations may not be cost effective.[8] This suggestion leads to what is, from the GI endoscopist's perspective, a critical need. Clinical studies that reliably define SETs that require further investigation and that establish the performance characteristics of EUS and other diagnostic modalities would permit the endoscopist to direct further management of SETs safely and reliably. A provisional treatment algorithm is proposed here (Fig. 31.10), but substantial work remains to be done to validate the steps that would translate this provisional algorithm into a reliable management tool.

KEY REFERENCES

2. Hedenbro JL, Ekelund M, Wetterberg P: Endoscopic diagnosis of submucosal gastric lesions: the results after routine endoscopy, *Surg Endosc* 5:20–30, 1991.

3. Allgayer H: Cost-effectiveness of endoscopic ultrasonography in submucosal tumors, *Gastrointest Endosc Clin N Am* 5:625–629, 1995.

8. Evans J, Chandrasekhara V, Chathadi K, et al: The role of endoscopy in the management of premalignant and malignant conditions of the stomach, *Gastrointest Endosc* 82(1):1–8, 2015.

15. Sanders L, Silberman M, Rossi R, et al: Gastric smooth muscle tumors: diagnostic dilemmas and factors affecting outcome, *World J Surg* 20:992–995, 1996.

33. Miettinem M, Sobin LH, Sarlomo-Rikala M: Immunohistochemical spectrum of GISTs at different sites and their differential diagnosis with reference to CD117 (KIT), *Mod Pathol* 13:1134–1142, 2000.

34. Heinrich MC, Corless CL, Duensing A, et al: PDGFRA activating mutations in gastrointestinal stromal tumors, *Science* 299:708–710, 2003.

35. Miettinen M, Kopczynski J, Makhlouf HR, et al: Gastrointestinal stromal tumors, intramural leiomyomas, and leiomyosarcomas in the duodenum: a clinicopathologic, immunohistochemical, and molecular genetic study of 167 cases, *Am J Surg Pathol* 27:625–641, 2003.

36. Graham J, Debiec-Rychter M, Corless CL, et al: Imatinib in the management of multiple gastrointestinal stromal tumors associated with a germline KIT K642E mutation, *Arch Pathol Lab Med* 131: 1393–1396, 2007.

41. Evans HL: Smooth muscle tumors of the gastrointestinal tract: a study of 56 cases followed for a minimum of 10 years, *Cancer* 56:2242–2250, 1985.

47. Toquet C, Le Neel JC, Guillou L, et al: Elevated (> or = 10%) MIB-1 proliferative index correlates with poor outcome in gastric stromal tumor patients: a study of 35 cases, *Dig Dis Sci* 47:2247–2253, 2002.

55. Bauer S, Joensuu H: Emerging agents for the treatment of advanced, imatinib-resistant gastrointestinal stromal tumors: current status and future directions, *Drugs* 75(12):1323–1334, 2015.

58. Miettinen M, Paal E, Lasota J, et al: Gastrointestinal glomus tumors: a clinicopathologic, immunohistochemical, and molecular genetic study of 32 cases, *Am J Surg Pathol* 26:301–311, 2002.

59. Wang ZB, Yuan J, Shi HY: Features of gastric glomus tumor: a clinicalpathologic, immunohistochemical, and molecular retrospective study, *Int J Clin Exp Pathol* 7(4):1438–1448, 2014.

61. Miettinen M, Majidi M, Lasota J: Pathology and diagnostic criteria of gastrointestinal stromal tumors (GISTs): a review, *Eur J Cancer* 38(Suppl 5):39–51, 2002.

74. An S, Jang J, Min K, et al: Granular cell tumor of the gastrointestinal tract: histologic and immunohistochemical analysis of 98 cases, *Hum Pathol* 46:813–819, 2015.

84. Hizawa K, Matsumoto T, Kouzuki T, et al: Cystic submucosal tumors in the gastrointestinal tract: endosonographic findings and endoscopic removal, *Endoscopy* 32:712–714, 2000.

87. Wegener M, Adamek R: Puncture of submucosal and extrinsic tumors: is there a clinical need? Puncture techniques and their accuracy, *Gastrointest Endosc Clin N Am* 5:615–623, 1995.

93. Demetri GD, Benjamin R, Blanke CD, et al: NCCN Task Force report: management of patients with gastrointestinal stromal tumor (GIST)— update of the NCCN clinical practice guidelines, *J Natl Compr Canc Netw* 5(Suppl 2):S1–S29, 2007.

95. Yasuda K, Cho E, Nakamima M, et al: Diagnosis of submucosal lesions of the upper gastrointestinal tract by endoscopic ultrasonography, *Gastrointest Endosc* 36:S17–S20, 1990.

96. Rösch T, Kapfer B, Will U, et al: Accuracy of endoscopic ultrasonography in upper gastrointestinal submucosal lesions: a prospective multicenter study, *Scand J Gastroenterol* 37:856–862, 2002.

105. Nickl N, Wackerbarth S, Gress F, et al: Management of hypoechoic intramural tumors: a decision tree analysis of EUS directed vs. surgical management, *Gastrointest Endosc* 51(4 Pt 2):AB176, 2000.

108. Kim MN, Kang SJ, Kim SG, et al: Prediction of risk of malignancy of gastrointestinal stromal tumors by endoscopic ultrasonography, *Gut Liver* 7:642–647, 2013.

109. Shah P, Gao F, Edmundowicz SA, et al: Predicting malignant potential of gastrointestinal stromal tumors using endoscopic ultrasound, *Dig Dis Sci* 54:1265–1269, 2009.

115. Catalano F, Rodella L, Lombardo F, et al: Endoscopic submucosal dissection in the treatment of gastric submucosal tumors: results from a retrospective cohort study, *Gastric Cancer* 16:563–570, 2013.

A complete reference list can be found online at ExpertConsult .com

32

Diagnosis and Treatment of Superficial Gastric Neoplasms

Satoru Nonaka, Ichiro Oda, and Yutaka Saito

INTRODUCTION

The incidence and mortality of gastric cancer have decreased in recent decades because of the reduction of *Helicobacter pylori* infection, development of endoscopic equipment, and refinement of endoscopic diagnostic and treatment techniques. However, it still remains among the most common malignancies, particularly in Asian countries. Although the prognosis of advanced gastric cancer is poor, the long-term outcome of early gastric cancer is favorable, so it is very important to endoscopically recognize cancers in the early phase. Therefore, endoscopists and gastroenterologists must have sufficient knowledge to provide a better quality of life and prognosis for patients with gastric cancer.

EPIDEMIOLOGY

Almost 1 million new cases of gastric cancer were estimated to have occurred in 2012 (952,000 cases, 6.8% of the total), making it the fifth most common malignancy in the world after cancers of the lung, breast, colorectum, and prostate.[1] More than 70% of cases occur in developing countries, and half the world total occurs in Eastern Asia. Age-standardized incidence rates are approximately twice as high in men as in women, ranging from 3.3 in Western Africa to 35.4 in Eastern Asia for men, and from 2.6 in Western Africa to 13.8 in Eastern Asia for women (Fig. 32.1).

Gastric cancer is the third leading cause of cancer death in both sexes worldwide (723,000 deaths, 8.8% of the total). The highest estimated mortality rates are in Eastern Asia (24 per 100,000 in men, 9.8 per 100,000 in women), with the lowest in Northern America (2.8 and 1.5, respectively). High mortality rates are also present in both sexes in Central and Eastern Europe, and in Central and South America.

Helicobacter pylori

In 1994, International Agency for Research on Cancer clarified *H. pylori* as a definite carcinogen of gastric cancer, and it is well known that most gastric cancer patients are positive for *H. pylori* infection.[2] *H. pylori* contributes to the development and progression of chronic gastritis that is present in most cases of gastric cancer, and it is associated with an increased cancer risk.[3] In fact, approximately 99% of Japanese gastric cancer patients are positive for *H. pylori*, and there is very low risk of gastric cancer in individuals that are negative for *H. pylori* infection.[4] The rates of incidence of and mortality from gastric cancer are still high in Japan, but there is a tendency to decrease both of these because of the recent reduction of *H. pylori* infection cases and the widespread use of eradication therapy for *H. pylori* (Fig. 32.2).[5] In addition, it has been reported that eradication therapy reduces the risk of gastric cancer as well as occurrence of metachronous gastric cancer after endoscopic resection.[6,7]

BACKGROUND OF DIAGNOSIS FOR EARLY GASTRIC CANCER

Treatment of gastric cancer remains a major clinical challenge. Survival of patients with early gastric cancer (EGC) is excellent, so early detection is essential for providing a more favorable

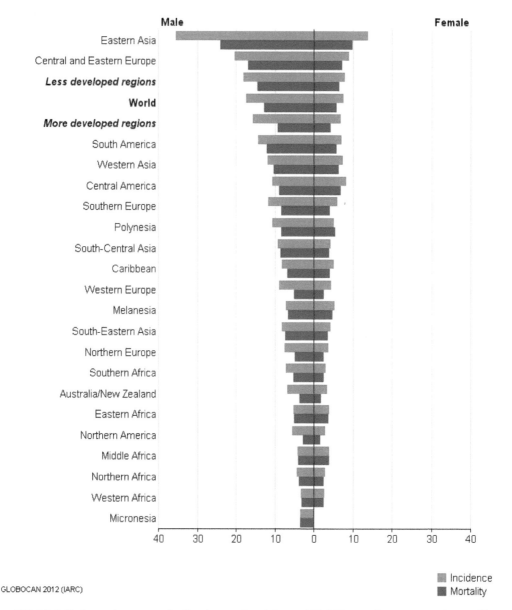

FIG 32.1 Estimated age-standardized rates (world) per 100,000 gastric cancer patients. (From International Agency for Research on Cancer [IARC]: GLOBOCAN 2012: Estimated cancer incidence, mortality and prevalence worldwide in 2012. Available at http://globocan.iarc.fr/Pages/fact_sheets_cancer.aspx. Accessed April 19, 2017.)

prognosis.[8–11] The 5-year disease-specific survival rate for surgical cases of intramucosal and submucosal invasive cancer is 99.3% and 96.7%, respectively.[11] It is also important for ensuring a better overall quality of life because endoscopic treatment provides a minimally invasive local resection for EGC with a negligible risk of lymph node metastasis, thereby preserving the patient's stomach.[12–14]

Japan has had a well-organized mass screening program for gastric cancer as an integral part of the public health service since the mid-1960s.[15] The Japanese mass screening program, however, most often utilizes gastrophotofluorography, which has comparatively poor resolution, and thus the sensitivity for EGC

has been quite low (39%) despite the sensitivity for advanced gastric cancer being high (92%).[16] Recent advances in endoscopy have had a substantial impact on improving early diagnosis, and EGC now accounts for approximately 50% of all gastric cancers treated at major medical facilities in Japan.[8,9] In fact, most cases (78%) of EGC at the National Cancer Center Hospital (NCCH) in Tokyo were recently detected by endoscopy.[17] A preponderance of those patients with EGC were asymptomatic, and therefore it is extremely important to motivate adults to undergo an endoscopy examination even if they are asymptomatic. It has been reported that the results of a community-based, case–control study by endoscopic screening suggest a 30% reduction in gastric

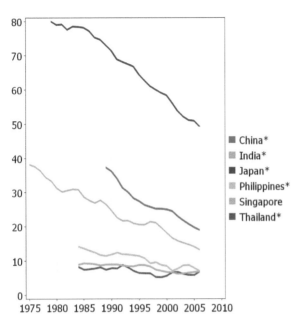

FIG 32.2 Trends in the incidence of stomach cancer in selected countries according to age-standardized rate (W) per 100,000 men. *, Regional data. (From International Agency for Research on Cancer [IARC]: GLOBOCAN 2012: Estimated cancer incidence, mortality and prevalence worldwide in 2012. Available at http://globocan.iarc.fr/Pages/fact_sheets_cancer.aspx. Accessed April 19, 2017.)

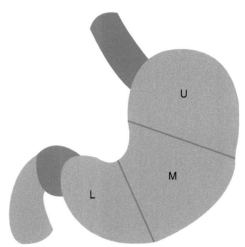

FIG 32.3 Three parts of the stomach. *U,* Upper third; *M,* middle third; *L,* lower third.

cancer mortality by endoscopic screening compared with no screening within 36 months before the date of diagnosis of gastric cancer.[18] Consequently, the guidelines for screening of upper gastrointestinal tract malignancies have been revised to allow the usage of endoscopy, which is expected to increase the early detection of gastric cancer.[19]

DESCRIPTION OF EGC

It is vital to describe tumors accurately using defined terminology to facilitate effective communications among endoscopists, surgeons, and pathologists.[20,21]

Tumor Location

The stomach is anatomically divided into three parts: the upper, middle, and lower thirds, as determined by lines connecting the trisected points on the lesser and greater curvatures (Fig. 32.3). The stomach's cross-sectional circumference is divided into four equal sections: the lesser and greater curvatures and the anterior and posterior walls.[20]

Macroscopic Type

Macroscopic types are defined as polypoid (0-I) and non-polypoid (0-II and 0-III). The polypoid (0-I) type is subdivided into protruded sessile (0-Is) and protruded pedunculated (0-Ip) subtypes. The non-polypoid type is subdivided into superficial elevated (0-IIa), flat (0-IIb), superficial depressed (0-IIc), and excavated (0-III) subtypes. A mixed type (e.g., 0-IIa+IIc, 0-IIc+IIa) is diagnosed whenever a lesion consists of at least two distinct macroscopic types and/or subtypes (Fig. 32.4).[20,21]

Tumor Invasion Depth

EGC is defined as cancer in which tumor invasion depth is confined to the mucosa or submucosa regardless of the presence of regional lymph node metastasis.[20] In Western countries, intramucosal cancer is commonly interpreted as high-grade dysplasia, particularly in relation to differentiated adenocarcinoma.

ENDOSCOPIC DIAGNOSIS OF EGC

EGC is usually characterized by only a slight change on the surface mucosa, particularly when the tumor invasion depth is intramucosal, so careful observation is paramount for detection.

Preparation

Optimal mucosal visualization is required for a thorough endoscopic examination. Mucosal flushing techniques have become standard practice in Japan to decrease foam and mucus that can obscure the field of view (Fig. 32.5).[22,23] Anti-foaming agents such as simethicone have been used since the 1950s, and more recent studies have shown that the addition of a mucolytic agent such as proteases further improves mucosal visualization. Flushing the entire stomach is time-consuming, but the early detection of EGC is difficult when large volumes of mucus and foam are present on the surface of the mucosa. Optical digital chromoendoscopy (e.g., narrow-band imaging [NBI, Olympus, Tokyo, Japan], etc.) and magnifying endoscopy are not helpful without this basic step. In addition, patients are routinely instructed to drink 100 mL of water containing 2 mL of simethicone and 20,000 units of Pronase (Sigma-Aldrich, St. Louis, MI) (a commercially available mixture of proteases) 10 minutes prior to endoscopy examination at NCCH to shorten flushing time.

Systematic Examination

A systematic recording routinely produces 30 to 40 endoscopic images of the whole stomach, including suspected lesions as well as normal-appearing areas (Fig. 32.6; Video 32.1). It is very important to maintain an adequate bend of the endoscope and to use the retroflexion view for the gastric body and cardia, as various angles and views are useful to detect the tiny abnormalities. Moreover, cloudiness of the lens also interferes with a careful observation, so one should use a lens cleaner just before

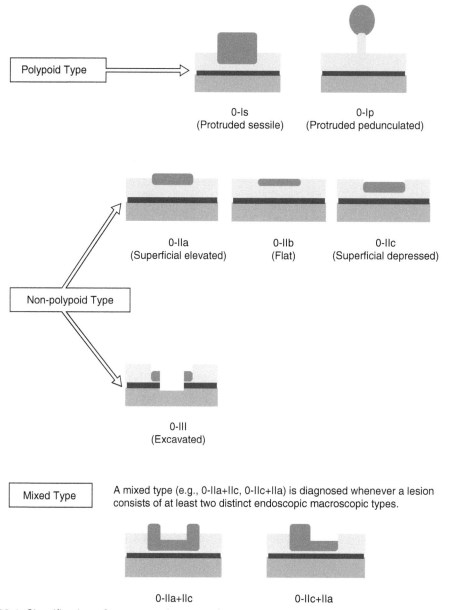

FIG 32.4 Classification of macroscopic types of early gastric cancer. (Modified from Endoscopic Classification Review Group: The Paris endoscopic classification of superficial neoplastic lesions: esophagus, stomach, and colon: November 30 to December 1, 2002. *Gastrointest Endosc* 58[6]:S3–S43, 2003.)

endoscopy. Some EGCs involve only a slight mucosal change that may be misdiagnosed as gastritis or erosions, so it is important to review the database of endoscopic images cautiously. Such endoscopic images are also useful for educational purposes and especially helpful for less experienced endoscopists. During endoscopy, adequate air insufflation is necessary, particularly to detect lesions located between folds (Fig. 32.7).

Identification and Diagnosis of EGC
Chromoendoscopy
Appropriate use of chromoendoscopy helps to highlight tissue appearance (Figs. 32.8–32.10).[24,25] In the stomach, 0.2% indigo-carmine dye solution is generally used as a topical contrast agent in Japan. It is essential to wash and remove any mucus on the

surface of the mucosa before using indigo-carmine dye, as lesions with a clear border cannot be easily visualized in the presence of mucus. Examination time is limited, however, so it is impractical to spray indigo-carmine dye throughout the stomach during every examination. Consequently, an abnormality suggesting possible EGC, such as a subtle red or pale color change or a slightly depressed or elevated change in the mucosa, should first be detected before spraying indigo-carmine dye (see Figs. 32.8–32.10). Other subtle changes that suggest possible EGC include a rough mucosal surface, an altered or missing vascular pattern, and loss of luster. The most important consideration is to identify the abnormal finding using white-light imaging before applying other modalities including chromoendoscopy, NBI, and magnifying endoscopy.

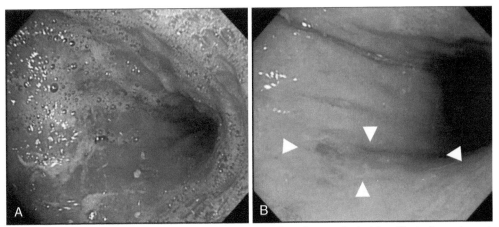

FIG 32.5 **A,** Mucus coating the gastric mucosa. **B,** Gastric neoplasia identified after adequate mucosal flushing *(arrowheads)*.

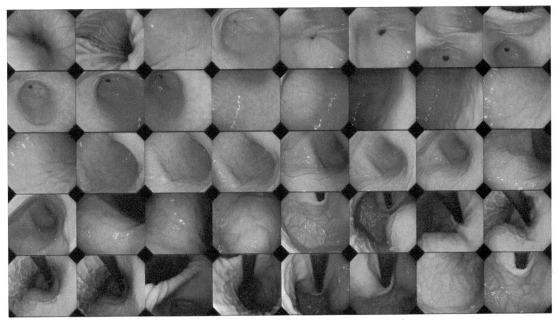

FIG 32.6 Systematic examination of the stomach.

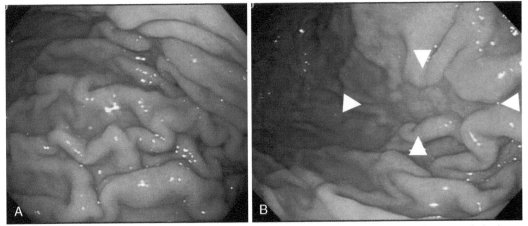

FIG 32.7 **A,** Gastric mucosa before insufflation. **B,** Adequate insufflation reveals a gastric lesion that was hidden in the folds *(arrowheads)*.

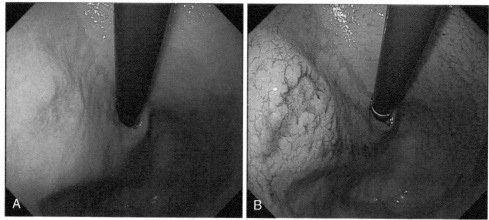

FIG 32.8 **A** and **B,** Examples of differentiated-type early gastric cancer. Reddish depressed lesions can be seen in the atrophic area.

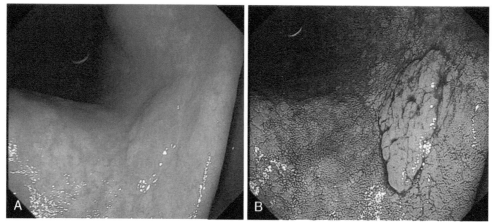

FIG 32.9 **A** and **B,** Examples of differentiated-type early gastric cancer. Note elevated lesions with reddish color in the atrophic area.

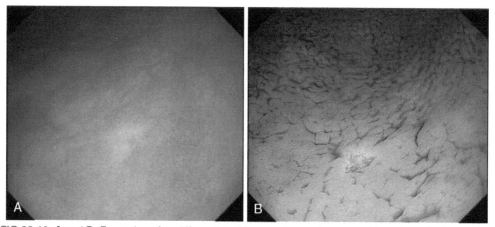

FIG 32.10 **A** and **B,** Examples of undifferentiated-type early gastric cancer. Note the pale depression in the near atrophic border.

Recent Advanced Techniques and Magnifying Endoscopy

Recent endoscopic imaging technology advances such as NBI, blue laser imaging, and iScan (Pentax Medical, Tokyo, Japan) with magnification have enabled endoscopists to observe microvascular (MV) and microsurface (MS) patterns.[26–29] In 2016, the magnifying endoscopy simple diagnostic algorithm for early gastric cancer (MESDA-G) was proposed by three Japanese institutions[30] (Fig. 32.11). If we detect a suspicious lesion, identification of a demarcation line (DL) between the lesion and the background mucosa is the first step in distinguishing EGC from a noncancerous lesion.[30] If a DL is absent, the diagnosis of a benign lesion may be made.[30] If a DL is present, the subsequent presence of an irregular MV pattern and an irregular MS pattern should be determined.[30] If irregular MV and/or MS patterns are present within the DL, the diagnosis of EGC can be made (Figs. 32.11 and 32.12).[30]

Histology

Histological type correlates with macroscopic appearance and tumor location (Table 32.1). Macroscopically, most undifferentiated-type EGCs consist of depressed lesions that are pale in color, whereas most differentiated-type EGCs are either depressed lesions that are red in color or elevated lesions that are either red or pale in color. The most frequent location also differs between the two histological types. Most differentiated-type EGCs are located in an atrophic area and most undifferentiated-type EGCs are located either in a non-atrophic area or near an atrophic border (see Figs. 32.8–32.10). As a result, the presence and extent of any atrophic change must be considered during endoscopic examination.

It is well known that there are many differences in histopathological diagnosis between Japan and Western countries. Since the Vienna classification was published in 2000, differences have been elucidated in the gastrointestinal tract between the East and West (Table 32.2).[31] It is generally thought to be divided

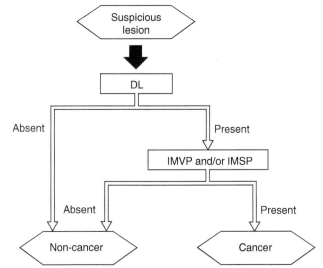

FIG 32.11 Magnifying endoscopy simple diagnostic algorithm for gastric cancer (MESDA-G). *DL,* Demarcation line; *IMVP,* irregular microvascular pattern; *IMSP,* irregular microsurface pattern.

TABLE 32.1 Correlations Between Histological Type and Endoscopic Finding of Early Gastric Cancer

Endoscopic Finding	HISTOLOGICAL TYPE	
	Differentiated (tub1, tub2, pap)	Undifferentiated (sig, por)
Macroscopic appearance	Depressed, red Elevated, red or pale	Depressed, pale
Location	Atrophic area	Non-atrophic area Near atrophic border

pap, Papillary adenocarcinoma; *por,* poorly differentiated adenocarcinoma; *sig,* signet ring cell carcinoma; *tub1,* well-differentiated tubular adenocarcinoma; *tub2,* moderately differentiated tubular adenocarcinoma.

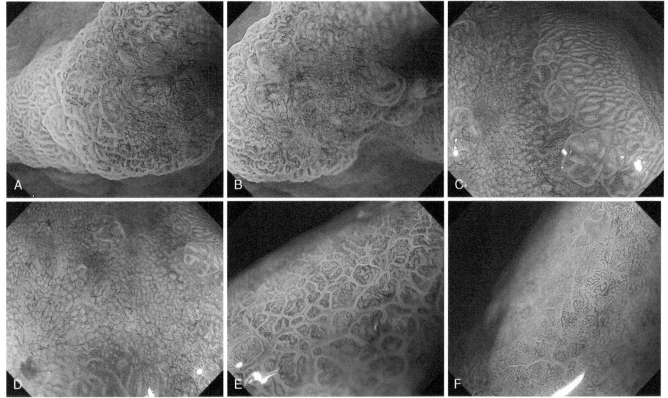

FIG 32.12 **A** to **F,** Irregular microvascular (MV) and surface (MS) pattern with demarcation line (DL).

TABLE 32.2 Vienna Classification of Gastrointestinal Epithelial Neoplasia

Category 1	Negative for neoplasia/dysplasia
Category 2	Indefinite for neoplasia/dysplasia
Category 3	Non-invasive low-grade neoplasia (low-grade adenoma/dysplasia)
Category 4	Non-invasive high-grade neoplasia: 4.1 High-grade adenoma/dysplasia 4.2 Non-invasive carcinoma (carcinoma in situ)[a] 4.3 Suspicion of invasive carcinoma
Category 5	Invasive neoplasia: 5.1 Intramucosal carcinoma[b] 5.2 Submucosal carcinoma or beyond

[a]Non-invasive indicates absence of evident invasion.
[b]Intramucosal indicates invasion into the lamina propria or muscularis mucosae.
From Schlemper RJ, Riddell RH, Kato Y, et al: The Vienna classification of gastrointestinal epithelial neoplasia. *Gut* 47(2):251–255, 2000.

TABLE 32.3 Correlations Between Macroscopic Type and Invasion Depth of Early Gastric Cancer

Macroscopic Type	INVASION DEPTH	
	Mucosal	Submucosal
0-I (n = 66)	43% (28)	57% (38)
0-IIa (n = 356)	71% (254)	29% (102)
0-IIb (n = 10)	80% (8)	20% (2)
0-IIc (n = 1488)	63% (931)	37% (557)
0-IIc+IIa (n = 19)	53% (10)	47% (9)
0-IIa+IIc (n = 132)	35% (46)	65% (86)
0-IIc+III (n = 15)	60% (9)	40% (6)
Total (n = 2086)	62% (1286)	38% (800)

into three categories, which include adenoma (low-grade dysplasia in the West), intramucosal adenocarcinoma (high-grade dysplasia in the West), and submucosal adenocarcinoma.

Targeted and Negative Biopsy

After detecting a lesion, we perform a biopsy for histological diagnosis. Random biopsies are not recommended, but a targeted biopsy is important for accurately diagnosing EGC. If we examine an EGC that has already been diagnosed histologically and is thought to be a candidate for endoscopic resection, negative biopsies taken from the surrounding area of the lesion are necessary to confirm the extent of malignant cells and prevent a positive margin for cancerous cells in the resected specimen histologically. A targeted biopsy from the lesion should only be performed if an abnormality that is suspicious of EGC is identified in the screening or surveillance endoscopy. After confirming the biopsy result, re-examination is usually conducted as a pre-treatment check, including negative biopsies taken from the surrounding area, to know a treatment plan with scope movement, angle, and distance between the scope and lesion. Because endoscopic diagnosis is subjective, there is always the possibility of misdiagnosis as well as the risk of performing an unnecessary biopsy.

ENDOSCOPIC STAGING OF INVASION DEPTH

Accurate endoscopic determination of invasion depth for gastric cancer is crucial for making a proper decision on treatment strategy. Endoscopic resection preserves the stomach, thus improving patient quality of life compared with surgery, and is accepted in many countries as a less invasive method for local resection of EGCs that have a negligible risk of lymph node metastasis.[32,33] Remarkable progress has been made in the development and refinement of endoscopic resection methods over the past 20 years. Techniques including endoscopic mucosal resection (EMR) and endoscopic submucosal dissection (ESD) have become the standard treatment method. At the same time, the indications for endoscopic resection have expanded.[34,35] Consequently, the number of EGC patients undergoing endoscopic resection is increasing, particularly in Asian countries.[36–43] Therefore, accurate differential endoscopic diagnosis between mucosal and submucosal invasion depths of EGC has become even more important for determining the indications for such procedures. Endoscopy

is the primary modality for diagnosing gastric cancer, but it can also be helpful in determining invasion depth. Direct visualization is somewhat subjective in nature, however, and there is a need for objective criteria.

A system for classifying macroscopic types of gastric cancer was first introduced in Japan, and correlations have subsequently been reported between macroscopic type and invasion depth of EGC.[20,21] Macroscopic classification is a relatively objective criterion, therefore, and its proper use is helpful in the determination of invasion depth.

Correlations Between Macroscopic Type and Invasion Depth

Table 32.3 indicates the correlations between macroscopic type and invasion depth for EGC previously reported in the Paris endoscopic classification of superficial neoplastic lesions.[21] In general, non-polypoid type without mixed type (0-IIa, 0-IIb, or 0-IIc) lesions have a lower risk of submucosal invasion compared with polypoid-type (0-I) and 0-IIa+IIc mixed type lesions. A description of the endoscopic estimation of invasion depth for EGC according to each macroscopic type is given in the following section.

Cases

A. 0-I type
   ✓ Tumor size correlates with depth of invasion, as lesions ≤ 2 cm usually indicate mucosal invasion (Fig. 32.13)
   ✓ Lesions > 3 cm have an even higher probability of submucosal or deeper invasion (Fig. 32.14)
   ✓ Lesions between 2 and 3 cm have an approximately 50% probability of submucosal invasion. Sessile subtype lesions have a somewhat higher risk of submucosal invasion compared with pedunculated subtype lesions

B. 0-IIa type
   ✓ Depth of invasion is usually mucosal, as tumor size does not correlate with invasion depth (Fig. 32.15)
   ✓ Lesions with a central depression or uneven surface are associated with submucosal invasion (Fig. 32.16)

C. 0-IIc type
   ✓ The following endoscopic findings suggest submucosal invasion:
      • Thickening of the gastric wall at the depression (see Fig. 32.16)

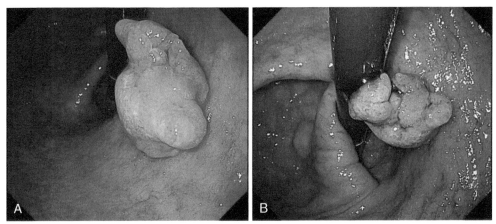

FIG 32.13 **A** and **B,** Example of a mucosal lesion. Endoscopic images reveal a polypoid-type (0-I) lesion 20 mm in size with subpedunculation on the lesser curvature of the upper gastric body.

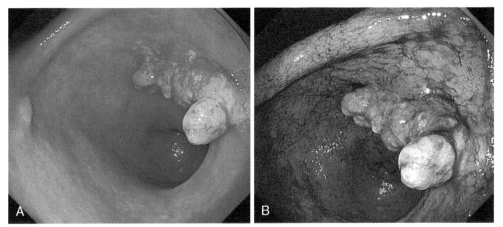

FIG 32.14 **A** and **B,** Example of a lesion with submucosal invasion. Endoscopic images reveal a polypoid-type (0-I) lesion 35 mm in size with a reddish color and erosion on the lessor curvature to posterior wall of the antrum.

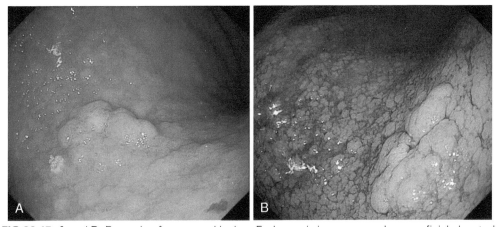

FIG 32.15 **A** and **B,** Example of a mucosal lesion. Endoscopic images reveal a superficial elevated-type (0-IIa) lesion 20 mm in size on the posterior wall of upper gastric body.

- Rigidity of the gastric wall at the depression (Figs. 32.16 and 32.17)
- Disappearance of mucosal surface pattern in the depression (Fig. 32.18)
- Nodule in the depression (uneven surface) (see Fig. 32.18)

- Intense redness of the depression (Fig. 32.19)
- Depression with submucosal tumor-like surrounding elevation (Fig. 32.20)
- Swelling of converging folds (Fig. 32.21)
- ✓ Lesions without any of the aforementioned findings are probably mucosal lesions (Fig. 32.22)

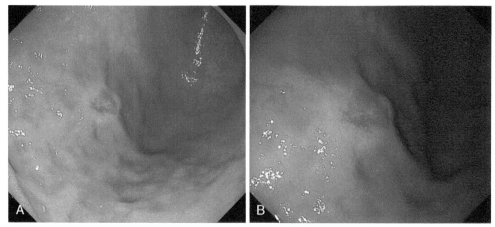

FIG 32.16 **A** and **B,** Example of a lesion with submucosal invasion. Endoscopic images reveal superficial elevated-type lesion with a central depression (0-IIa+IIc) 15 mm in size on the greater curvature of the middle gastric body. Lesion indicates thickening of the gastric wall and rigidity.

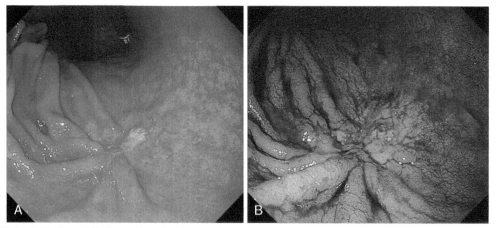

FIG 32.17 **A** and **B,** Example of a lesion with submucosal invasion. Endoscopic images reveal a superficial depressed type (0-IIc) lesion with an ulcer scar 30 mm in size on the anterior wall of the middle gastric body. There is wall thickening and rigidity in the center of the ulcer scar.

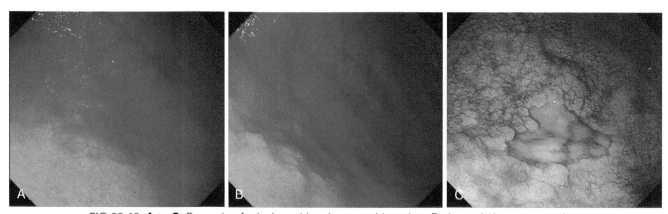

FIG 32.18 **A** to **C,** Example of a lesion with submucosal invasion. Endoscopic images reveal an intensely reddish superficial depressed type (0-IIc) lesion with nodular finding 15 mm in size on the greater curvature of the lower gastric body. Chromoendoscopy using indigo-carmine dye shows disappearance of the mucosal surface pattern in depression.

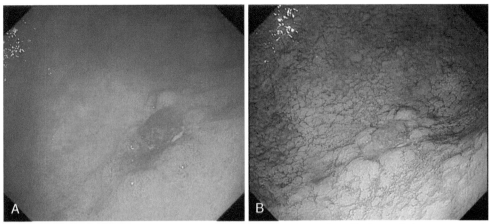

FIG 32.19 **A** and **B,** Example of a lesion with submucosal invasion. Endoscopic images reveal a remarkably reddish superficial elevated-type lesion with a central depression (0-IIa+IIc) 20 mm in size on the greater curvature of the middle gastric body. The tumor has a strongly reddish depression with surrounding elevation.

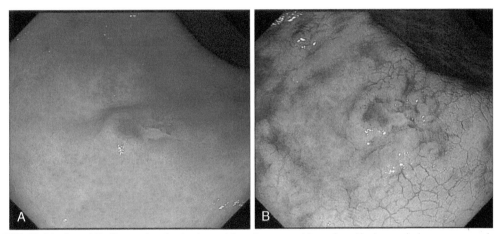

FIG 32.20 **A** and **B,** Example of a lesion with submucosal invasion. Endoscopic images reveal a superficial depressed type (0-IIc) lesion with surrounding elevation 15 mm in size on the greater curvature of the upper gastric body. The tumor has a submucosal tumor-like surrounding elevation on the oral side.

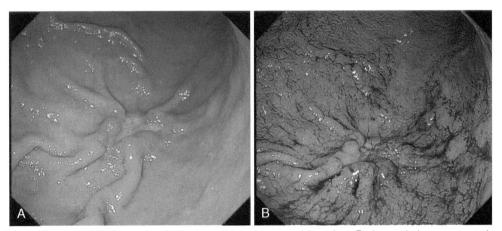

FIG 32.21 **A** and **B,** Example of a lesion with submucosal invasion. Endoscopic images reveal a superficial pale depressed type (0-IIc) lesion having fold convergences with swelling 30 mm in size on the greater curvature of the lower gastric body. The tumor has wall thickening and remarkable surrounding elevation with swelling fold convergences.

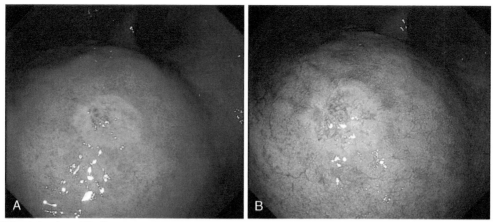

FIG 32.22 **A** and **B,** Example of a mucosal lesion. Endoscopic images reveal a superficial depressed type (0-IIc) lesion without any endoscopic findings that suggest submucosal invasion 10 mm in size on the anterior wall of the middle gastric body.

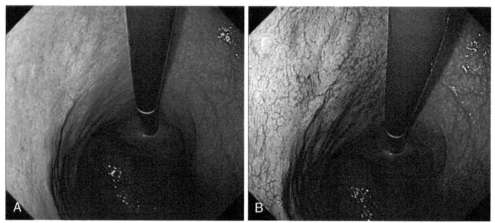

FIG 32.23 **A** and **B,** Example of a mucosal lesion. Endoscopic images reveal a superficial depressed-type (0-IIc) lesion with ulcer scar 30 mm in size on the posterior wall of the middle gastric body. There was no finding of submucosal invasion.

✓ Mucosal lesions are generally smaller than submucosal lesions

✓ For lesions with an ulcer, it is difficult to estimate invasion depth because fibrosis results in rigidity. Mucosal lesions with an ulcer do not usually have thickening of the gastric wall, submucosal tumor-like surrounding elevation, or a large nodule in the depression (Fig. 32.23). In contrast, submucosal lesions with an ulcer often have thickening of the gastric wall (see Fig. 32.21)

D. 0-IIa+IIc type

  ✓ Mixed types, particularly 0-IIa+IIc types, are generally associated with submucosal invasion (Fig. 32.24)

  ✓ When IIc components are clearly seen as less prominent, the lesion is often submucosal (Fig. 32.25)

Endoscopic Ultrasonography

Endoscopic ultrasonography (EUS) is one of the current modalities for determining invasion depth for EGC. In particular, EUS using a miniprobe (20 MHz) has demonstrated a high diagnostic accuracy for distinguishing between mucosal and submucosal lesions.[44–47] EUS accuracy is lower, however, for patients with larger lesions, undifferentiated-type lesions, lesions with concomitant ulceration, protruded lesions (type 0-I), and lesions

located in the upper third of the stomach.[48,49] In daily clinical practice the application of EUS for all EGCs is impractical, and therefore it should be reserved for selected cases in which tumor depth is difficult to determine. Although there are generally fewer EGC cases and more EUS examinations in Western countries, the convex method of EUS is not adequate to obtain a precise image of each layer and accurately diagnose tumor depth of the mucosa or submucosa.

When using a miniprobe, the normal gastric wall is visualized as the mucosa (combination of the first and second hypoechoic layers) and the submucosa (third hyperechoic layer). The muscularis propria is visualized as the fourth hypoechoic layer and the fifth hyperechoic layer is the serosa, including the subserosa (Fig. 32.26).[50] According to Yanai et al (1993), the thin layer between the second and third hyperechoic layers corresponds to the muscularis mucosae.[51] Invasion depth is diagnosed by the presence or absence of normal gastric wall architecture destruction (Figs. 32.27 and 32.28).

Depth Predictive Score

The Paris classification provides a relatively objective method for endoscopic diagnosis of EGC macroscopic types while simultaneously estimating invasion depth. Endoscopic prediction

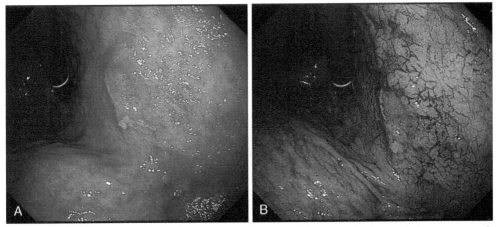

FIG 32.24 **A** and **B,** Example of a lesion with submucosal invasion. Endoscopic images reveal a mixed-type lesion with elevation and slight central depression (0-IIa+IIc) 20 mm in size on the lesser curvature of the middle gastric body. The whole area of the lesion shows elevation and hardness.

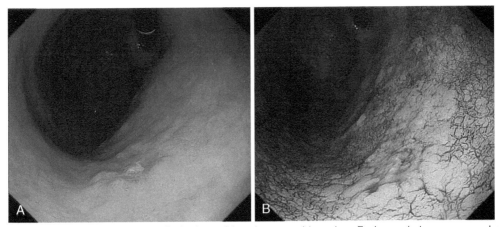

FIG 32.25 **A** and **B,** Example of a lesion with submucosal invasion. Endoscopic images reveal a mixed-type lesion with elevation and clear depression in the greater curvature side (0-IIa+IIc) 30 mm in size on the anterior wall of the middle gastric body. The depression area is seen as well-demarcated reddish change.

of invasion depth, however, is not always accurate, even with the proper use of macroscopic classification when supported by EUS, and thus further improvement in determining the depth of invasion is still necessary.[52,53] As a result, we have suggested a simple invasion depth predictive scoring system to more accurately and objectively estimate the invasion depth of EGC.[54] This concept is particularly expected to contribute to EGC diagnosis in Western countries.

SUMMARY OF DIAGNOSIS

Although endoscopic diagnosis and staging of EGC remain a clinical challenge, they are imperative for providing a better patient prognosis and quality of life. As a first step, it is important to motivate even asymptomatic individuals to undergo an endoscopy screening examination. Next, a fundamental understanding of EGC and proper endoscopic techniques such as adequate preparation, systematic examination, and the use of chromoendoscopy, optical image-enhanced endoscopy, and targeted biopsy are essential for early detection. Finally, accurate

endoscopic estimation of invasion depth for EGC is required for making proper decisions on treatment strategy.

BACKGROUND OF ENDOSCOPIC RESECTION FOR EGC

Endoscopic resection is widely accepted as an effective, minimally invasive treatment technique for EGC with a negligible risk of lymph node metastasis.[14,55] Endoscopic resection preserves the functional stomach and therefore improves patient quality of life compared with radical surgery. Remarkable progress has been made in the past decade in the field of endoscopic resection for gastric cancer, both in terms of expansion of the indications and in terms of improvements of the technique. The indications for endoscopic resection of EGC have been expanded based on an estimation of the risk of lymph node metastasis in cases of EGC from a large number of surgical cases.[32,33] The technique of endoscopic resection has been improved from EMR to ESD for R0 resection.[36–43] EMR procedures include inject and cut, strip biopsy, EMR with a cap-fitted endoscope, endoscopic aspiration mucosectomy, and EMR with a ligating device, etc., whereas ESD is a relatively new endoscopic resection method that facilitates en bloc resection. This section addresses the indications, results, some technical tips, and complications of ESD for EGC.

Indications of ESD for EGC

Endoscopic resection is generally indicated for EGC patients with a negligible risk of lymph node metastasis because it is a local resection without lymph node dissection. The estimated incidence of lymph node metastasis in mucosal and submucosal gastric cancer is approximately 3% and 20%, respectively.[32,33] If patients who have zero risk of lymph node metastases could be identified with certainty, endoscopic resection would be the ideal treatment method for these patients. However, it is not possible to exclude the presence of lymph node metastasis by computed tomography, positron emission tomography or EUS with certainty because lymph node metastases from EGC are often too small. As a result, the indication for endoscopic resection in patients with EGC is determined based on evaluation of clinicopathological findings that are considered to be associated with a negligible risk of lymph node metastasis. In the past, the accepted indications for endoscopic resection in cases of EGC were small intramucosal cancers measuring 2 cm or less in diameter, differentiated histopathological type, and absence of ulceration.[34] In an effort to expand the indications, Gotoda et al (2000) and Hirasawa et al (2009) reviewed surgical cases and identified other characteristics of EGC that were associated with a negligible risk of lymph node metastasis, as follows:[32,33]

Differentiated histopathological type, intramucosal cancer, greater than 2 cm in diameter, without ulceration

Differentiated histopathological type, intramucosal cancer, 3 cm or less in diameter, with ulceration

Undifferentiated histopathological type, intramucosal cancer, 2 cm or less in diameter, without ulceration

Differentiated histopathological type, 3 cm or less in diameter, minute submucosal (SM1) cancer

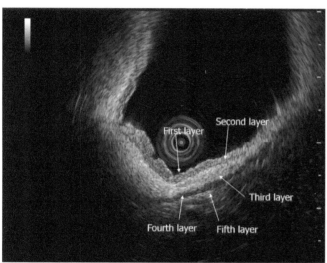

FIG 32.26 Endoscopic ultrasound features of a normal gastric wall. The first and second hypoechoic layers correspond to the mucosa, the third hyperechoic layer represents the submucosa, the fourth hypoechoic layer represents the muscularis propria, and the fifth hyperechoic layer represents the serosa, including the subserosa.

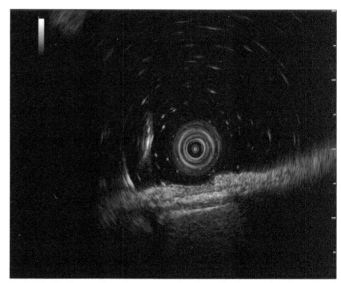

FIG 32.27 Example of a mucosal lesion. Endoscopic ultrasound reveals irregularity of the first layer and low echoic change of the second layer. The third layer is intact, and the thin, low echoic line that indicates the muscularis mucosae can be seen between the second and third layer.

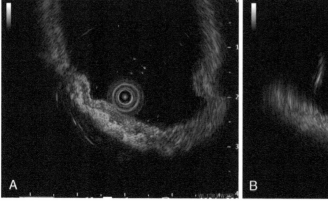
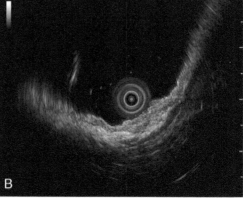

FIG 32.28 A and B, Example of a lesion with submucosal invasion. Endoscopic ultrasound reveals the thickness of the second layer and thin third layer, with the fourth layer intact.

Note that lymphovascular infiltration (ly(-), v(-)) should always be excluded, as this finding correlates with a greatly increased risk of lymph node metastases. The histopathological type is classified as either differentiated type or undifferentiated type. The former includes papillary adenocarcinoma and tubular adenocarcinoma (well and moderately differentiated), and the latter includes poorly differentiated adenocarcinoma, signet ring cell carcinoma, and mucinous adenocarcinoma.

Thus, these expanded indications now include larger lesions and lesions with ulceration. Such lesions were previously resected surgically owing to the difficulty in effectively using EMR techniques for resection in this context. As a result, ESD was developed to achieve en bloc resection even for larger and ulcerative lesions.

Clinical Results

ESD is associated with a very high rate of en bloc resections, regardless of the tumor location, tumor size, and the presence of ulceration. In our previously published case series, we achieved a very high rate (98%; 1008/1033 patients) of en bloc resections.[42] Similarly, other studies have also reported high rates of en bloc resection, ranging from 92.7% to 98.0%.[41,42,56–63] In addition, a meta-analysis revealed a higher rate of en bloc resection in patients undergoing ESD compared with those undergoing EMR.[64] After ESD, the curability is assessed based on the completeness of removal of the primary tumor and a zero possibility of lymph node metastasis. If the lesion was resected en bloc and is a ly(-), v(-) intramucosal cancer without ulceration, with negative resected margins, 2 cm or less in diameter, and shows differentiated histopathological type, it can be considered a curative resection. If a lesion was resected en bloc with negative margins, is ly(-), v(-), and fulfills one of the following criteria (Fig. 32.29):
1. > 2 cm in diameter, differentiated histopathological type, intramucosal, without ulceration, or
2. ≤ 3 cm in diameter, differentiated histopathological type, intramucosal, with ulceration, or
3. ≤ 2 cm in diameter, undifferentiated histopathological type, intramucosal, without ulceration, or
4. ≤ 3 cm in diameter, differentiated histopathological type, SM1 invasionthen the resection can be considered an "extended-indication" curative resection. As for the long-term outcomes of curative resection and extended-indication curative resection, there have been few published reports with median follow-up periods of more than 5 years.[65–69] The Japan Clinical Oncology Group (JCOG) carried out a clinical trial validating

gastric ESD for expanded indications, with the exception of those with undifferentiated type (previously mentioned lesions 1 and 2) (JCOG 0607), and the 5-year overall survival (OS) was 97.0% (95% confidence interval [CI]: 95.0%–98.2%).[70] The lower limit of the 95% CI for the 5-year OS was higher than the threshold 5-year OS (86.1%), and the primary endpoint was met. Therefore, ESD has become a standard treatment for EGC of expanded indications based on these results. Furthermore, a clinical trial assessing the validation of gastric ESD for expanded indications with undifferentiated-type (JCOG 1009/1010) has already finished enrollment and is now in the observation phase.[71] Moreover, a Japanese multicenter, prospective cohort study of endoscopic resection for EGC using a Web registry (J-WEB/EGC) is now ongoing, with approximately 10,000 patients in 41 institutions throughout Japan. It is hoped that the study will clarify long-term outcomes.[72]

Technical Tips Regarding ESD Performed for EGC
Basic Movement Is Dependent on ESD Device

A number of ESD devices have been developed that have just now become available for clinical use. These devices are divided into two major types: the IT-type knife and needle-type knife devices. The IT-type knife devices include the IT knife, IT knife 2, and IT knife nano (KD-611L, KD-611L, KD-612L; Olympus Medical Systems Corp., Tokyo, Japan), and the needle-type knife devices include the needle knife, hook knife, Dual Knife, (KD-1L-1, KD-620LR, KD-650 L; Olympus Medical Systems Corp., Tokyo, Japan), and FlushKnife BT (DK2618JB; Fujifilm Corp., Tokyo, Japan), among others. Importantly, these two different types of devices require completely different approaches. The IT-type knife has an insulated ceramic ball at the tip of the knife, which prevents gastric wall perforation. Therefore, we use the metallic blade between the tip and the sheath while using the IT-type knife for cutting. When using the IT-type knife, it must be pulled from the far side to the near side before the metallic blade can be used for cutting purposes. In contrast, ESD performed with a needle-type knife device requires an entirely different approach. As the tip of the knife is not insulated, the tip can be used for cutting purposes. Basically, the knife tip should be slid from the near side to the far side to avoid perforation. Pulling of a needle-type knife from the far side to the near side, as in the case of the IT-type knife, is associated with a high risk of perforation.

ESD Strategy

The ESD procedure consists of the following steps:
1. The lesion margin is identified and marked at a distance of approximately 3 to 5 mm outside the margin by argon plasma coagulation or with a needle-type knife
2. The mucosa is lifted by submucosal fluid injection followed by mucosal incision with the ESD knife
3. Submucosal dissection under the lesion is performed with the ESD knife

The set-up of high-frequency electrical surgical units (VIO300D; ERBE Corp., Tubingen, Germany and ESG-100; Olympus Medical Systems Corp., Tokyo, Japan) depends on the endoscopist's preference. The set-up of the gastric ESD used in our endoscopy unit is shown in Table 32.4.

When we use the IT-type knife as the main device for ESD, an initial incision is made at the far point (i.e., as shown on the TV monitor) with the needle-type knife, because a subsequent mucosal incision using the IT-type knife is then performed from

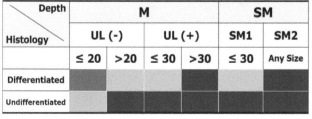

Depth	M				SM	
Histology	UL (-)		UL (+)		SM1	SM2
	≤ 20	>20	≤ 30	>30	≤ 30	Any Size
Differentiated						
Undifferentiated						

M, intramucosal; SM, submucosal; UL, ulcer finding; SM1, <500μm; SM2, ≥500μm

■ **Absolute Indication** ■ **Surgery**

■ **Expanded Indication**

FIG 32.29 Expanded pathological criteria for curative endoscopic resection of gastric cancer.

TABLE 32.4 Setup of High-Frequency Electrical Surgical Units in the Gastric Endoscopic Submucosal Dissection

	VIO300D		ESG100	
	Device	Setting	Device	Setting
Marking	APC	Forced APC 1.5 L/min 30 W	Needle Knife Dual Knife	Forced coag 1 20 W
First incision	Needle Knife Dual Knife	Endocut I E3-D2-I3	Needle Knife Dual Knife	Pulse cut slow 40 W
Mucosal incision	IT Knife 2 Dual Knife	Endocut I E3-D2-I3	IT Knife 2 Dual Knife	Pulse cut slow 40 W
Submucosal dissection	IT Knife 2 Dual Knife	Endocut I E3-D2-I3 Swift coag/ dry cut E5 50W	IT Knife 2 Dual Knife	Pulse cut slow 40 W Forced coag 2 50 W
Minor oozing	IT Knife 2 Dual Knife	Swift coag E5 50 W	IT Knife 2 Dual Knife	Forced coag 2 50 W
Major bleeding	Coagrasper (G)	Soft coag E5 80 W	Coagrasper (G)	Soft coag 80 W

the far side to the near side. When a lesion is located on the antrum, ESD is performed with a straight view, so that the initial incision is made at the distal side of the lesion, which corresponds to the far side on the TV monitor (Video 32.2). In contrast, the procedure is reversed for lesions located on the gastric body: the initial incision is made on the proximal side of the lesion, which corresponds to the far side on the TV monitor, because we use the retroflex view for lesions located on the gastric body. The mucosal incision is started from the point of the initial incision and pulled toward the near side. The IT-type knife should be placed in a tangential position parallel to the mucosa, and not in a vertical position, to provide for adequate depth of the mucosal incision. The final step is the actual submucosal dissection under the lesion. Submucosal dissection using the IT-type knife can also be performed from the near side on the TV monitor because it is easier to dissect lengthwise than widthwise using the IT-type knife. Therefore, we start the submucosal dissection from the distal outside to the proximal inside. We then proceed to make a depression at the near side, after which we dissect widthwise, hooking the IT-type knife on the edge of the depression. It is important to always move parallel to the gastric wall curvature to avoid perforation. Recently, we have reported the near-side approach method to more easily control bleeding and to shorten the procedure time for the lesion located on the gastric body, although the conventional method that is described earlier is the basic strategy (Video 32.3).[73]

In contrast, the procedure is reversed when the needle-type knife is used as the main device for ESD. The incision is started from the near side on the TV monitor, and then the knife tip is slid from the near side to the far side. Submucosal dissection using the needle-type knife is also performed from the near side to the far side (see Video 32.3). Thus, ESD requires a completely different approach, depending on which type of device is being used during the procedure.

Training for ESD

ESD requires a high level of technical expertise, and it may appear technically challenging to less experienced endoscopists. ESD trainees at the NCCH in Tokyo, Japan, follow a step-by-step process for learning ESD techniques. The first step entails acquiring a basic knowledge and understanding of EGC and ESD, in particular, the diagnosis of EGC and the indications for ESD. The next step for trainees is to observe expert endoscopists in action as they perform various ESD procedures. The third step involves trainees acquiring firsthand experience by assisting experts during actual ESDs. This is followed by the fourth step, in which ESD training is further refined using animal models. In the final step, it is important for trainees to start performing ESDs on lesions that are technically less challenging, including those that are located in the lower third of the stomach and those that are small in size and do not show ulcer fibrosis. Trainees perform their first 10 ESDs with direct hands-on support from highly qualified endoscopists, and then start to perform ESDs by themselves with mostly verbal guidance from expert endoscopists. As their ESD technique improves, trainees are gradually assigned to perform ESDs on lesions located in the middle and upper thirds of the stomach, and lesions that are larger in size. Based on our training program, the step-by-step training system at our center has been highly effective, with an en bloc resection rate of 100% and a low complication rate. As a result of this program, the point on the learning curve at which our trainees acquire the basic technical skills for successfully performing ESD in the lower third of the stomach is 30 cases.[74]

COMPLICATIONS

ESD is associated with a relatively high risk of complications. Bleeding and perforation are the two major complications. Endoscopists must be aware not only of the risk factors and the incidence of complications, but they must also know how to effectively manage complications.

Perforation

Most perforations occur during ESD, and the reported risk of perforation is in the range of 1.2% to 5.2% for gastric ESD.[42,43,58,61–63,75–80] In terms of delayed perforation occurring after the completion of gastric ESD, in one study such perforations occurred in six (0.5%) out of 1159 consecutive patients with 1329 EGCs treated by ESD.[81] The possible mechanisms for perforations induced by ESD are unanticipated injury of the muscularis propria caused by insufficient submucosal injection or miscalculation of the gastric wall curvature. To avoid perforation, adequate space in the submucosal layer between the muscularis propria and the mucosal layer is essential. To this end, a sufficient amount of submucosal injection solution must be injected. To lift the mucosa for the longer procedure period required by ESD, the effectiveness of sodium hyaluronate, glycerol, or a combination of sodium hyaluronate and glycerol has been reported previously.[41,82–84] The use of an injection solution mixed with indigo-carmine dye for submucosal injection is effective for better recognition of the gastric wall curve because it allows distinction of the (white) muscularis propria from the (blue) submucosal layer. The use of a transparent attachment to the scope to lift the mucosal layer is also useful for recognizing the gastric wall curve. If perforation is recognized during the procedure, endoscopic clipping can be performed (Fig. 32.30). In

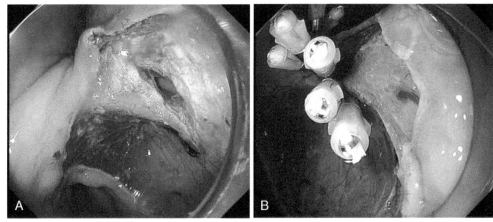

FIG 32.30 **A** and **B,** Endoscopic submucosal dissection (ESD) was performed for early gastric cancer located in the gastric angle, and perforation occurred during submucosal dissection. En bloc resection was immediately completed and perforation can be seen clearly with extra-wall yellow tissue. The endoscopic closure using endo-clips was successfully conducted and the patient had no symptoms after the ESD procedure.

the past, gastric perforations occurring during endoscopic resections of early cancers invariably necessitated emergency surgery, which effectively meant that all the benefits of endoscopic resection were lost. Endoscopic clips were originally developed for hemostatic purposes. Closure of a perforation using such clips after snare excision of a gastric leiomyoma was first reported by Binmoeller et al in 1993.[85] In 2006, endoscopic closure with endoscopic clips for endoscopic resection-related gastric perforations was reported to be effective in a series of consecutive cases.[75] In that study, 115 (98.3%) of 117 patients with gastric perforations were successfully treated conservatively by the use of endoscopic clips for closure of the perforations.

Bleeding

Bleeding complications associated with ESD can be subdivided into immediate (intraoperative) bleeding occurring during the procedure and delayed bleeding occurring after the procedure. Immediate bleeding is infrequent with EMR, but is quite common with ESD. Management of immediate bleeding plays a critical role in the successful completion of ESD. Electrocautery is used for hemostasis in cases of immediate bleeding occurring during ESD, because endoscopic clips interfere with the subsequent resection procedure.[86,87] Electrocautery is usually carried out using different devices depending on the degree of bleeding. Minor oozing can be controlled by electrocautery using a cutting device, such as the IT knife 2, Hook knife, Dual knife, and FlushKnife BT. It is also necessary to pre-coagulate to prevent bleeding using a cutting device when vessels are found during the procedure. Electrocautery using hemostatic forceps, such as the Coagrasper (G) (FD-410LR/FD-412LR; Olympus Medical Systems Corp.) or hot biopsy forceps (Radial Jaw; Boston Scientific Japan Corp, Tokyo, Japan), is suitable for arterial bleeding. The critical step for achieving adequate hemostasis is identification of the exact bleeding point using water flushing. Endoscopes equipped with water jet systems (GIF-Q260J; Olympus Medical Systems Corp.; EG-450RD5; Fujifilm Corp., Tokyo, Japan), which are useful for precisely determining the bleeding point, have recently become available for clinical use.

The reported incidence of delayed bleeding after ESD is in the range of 0% to 15.6%.[42,43,58,61–63,76–80,88,89] This wide range is partly due to differences in the definition of delayed bleeding among reported studies. If delayed bleeding were defined as bleeding requiring endoscopic treatment with any clinical symptoms of bleeding such as hematemesis and melena, the reported incidence is 3% to 8%.[42,62,63,76,78–80,88] All endoscopic treatment modalities can also be used individually or in combination for achieving hemostasis in cases of delayed bleeding after endoscopic resection. Different modalities are applied according to the time of onset of delayed bleeding. In cases with delayed bleeding occurring in the early phase after ESD, the artificial ulcer floor is still soft with little granulation tissue, so that endoscopic clips or electrocautery using hemostatic forceps can be applied to control the bleeding. In cases of delayed bleeding occurring in the later phase after ESD, the artificial ulcer floor is hard with granulation tissue, so the injection method is preferably used to control bleeding.

SUMMARY OF ENDOSCOPIC TREATMENT

Endoscopic resection is indicated for EGCs with a negligible risk of lymph node metastasis. ESD offers the advantage of achieving en bloc resection. Step-by-step training is important for training in ESD techniques. The technique employed for ESD depends on which type of device (IT-type knife or needle-type knife) is used during the procedure. ESD is associated with a relatively high risk of complications. Endoscopists must be aware of not only the incidence and risk factors for complications, but they must also know how to effectively manage these complications.

KEY REFERENCES

1. International Agency for Research on Cancer: The GLOBOCAN Project website. 2012. Estimated Cancer Incidence, Mortality and Prevalence Worldwide in 2012. Population fact sheets and cancer fact sheets. Available at http://globocan.iarc.fr/Default.aspx. (Accessed 17 April 2017).

2. International Agency for Research on Cancer: Schistosomes, liver flukes and Helicobacter pylori, *IARC Monogr Eval Carcinog Risks Hum* 61: 177–240, 1994.

3. Uemura N, Okamoto S, Yamamoto S, et al: Helicobacter pylori infection and the development of gastric cancer, *N Engl J Med* 345(11):784–789, 2001.

4. Matsuo T, Ito M, Takata S, et al: Low prevalence of Helicobacter pylori-negative gastric cancer among Japanese, *Helicobacter* 16(6): 415–419, 2011.

5. Asaka M, Kimura T, Kudo M, et al: Relationship of Helicobacter pylori to serum pepsinogens in an asymptomatic Japanese population, *Gastroenterology* 102(3):760–766, 1992.

6. Ford AC, Forman D, Hunt RH, et al: Helicobacter pylori eradication therapy to prevent gastric cancer in healthy asymptomatic infected individuals: systematic review and meta-analysis of randomised controlled trials, *BMJ* 348:g3174, 2014.

7. Fukase K, Kato M, Kikuchi S, et al: Effect of eradication of Helicobacter pylori on incidence of metachronous gastric carcinoma after endoscopic resection of early gastric cancer: an open-label, randomised controlled trial, *Lancet* 372(9636):392–397, 2008.

8. Nakamura K, Ueyama T, Yao T, et al: Pathology and prognosis of gastric carcinoma. Findings in 10,000 patients who underwent primary gastrectomy, *Cancer* 70:1030–1037, 1992.

14. Soetikno R, Kaltenbach T, Yeh R, et al: Endoscopic mucosal resection for early cancers of the upper gastrointestinal tract, *J Clin Oncol* 23:4490–4498, 2005.

18. Hamashima C, Ogoshi K, Okamoto M, et al: A community-based, case-control study evaluating mortality reduction from gastric cancer by endoscopic screening in Japan, *PLoS ONE* 8:e79088, 2013.

19. Hamashima C, Ogoshi K, Narisawa R, et al: Impact of endoscopic screening on mortality reduction from gastric cancer, *World J Gastroenterol* 21:2460–2466, 2015.

20. Japanese Gastric Cancer Association: Japanese classification of gastric carcinoma – 3rd English Edition, *Gastric Cancer* 14:101–112, 2011.

21. Participants in the Paris Workshop: The Paris endoscopic classification of superficial neoplastic lesions: esophagus, stomach, and colon, *Gastrointest Endosc* 58(6 Suppl):S3–S43, 2003.

27. Ezoe Y, Muto M, Uedo N, et al: Magnifying narrowband imaging is more accurate than conventional white-light imaging in diagnosis of gastric mucosal cancer, *Gastroenterology* 141:2017–2025, 2011.

30. Muto M, Yao K, Kaise M, et al: Magnifying endoscopy simple diagnostic algorithm for early gastric cancer (MESDA-G), *Dig Endosc* 28:379–393, 2016.

31. Schlemper RJ, Riddell RH, Kato Y, et al: The Vienna classification of gastrointestinal epithelial neoplasia, *Gut* 47:251–255, 2000.

32. Gotoda T, Yanagisawa A, Sasako M, et al: Incidence of lymph node metastasis from early gastric cancer: estimation with a large number of cases at two large centers, *Gastric Cancer* 3:219–225, 2000.

33. Hirasawa T, Gotoda T, Miyata S, et al: Incidence of lymph node metastasis and the feasibility of endoscopic resection for undifferentiated-type early gastric cancer, *Gastric Cancer* 12:148–152, 2009.

34. Japanese Gastric Cancer Association: Japanese gastric cancer treatment guidelines 2014 (ver. 4), *Gastric Cancer* 20:1–19, 2017.

35. Ono H, Yao K, Fujishiro M, et al: Guidelines for endoscopic submucosal dissection and endoscopic mucosal resection for early gastric cancer, *Dig Endosc* 28:3–15, 2016.

37. Inoue H, Takeshita K, Hori H, et al: Endoscopic mucosal resection with a cap-fitted panendoscope for esophagus, stomach, and colon mucosal lesions, *Gastrointest Endosc* 39:58–62, 1993.

40. Ono H, Kondo H, Gotoda T, et al: Endoscopic mucosal resection for treatment of early gastric cancer, *Gut* 48:225–229, 2001.

42. Oda I, Gotoda T, Hamanaka H, et al: Endoscopic submucosal dissection for early gastric cancer: technical feasibility, operation time and complications from a large consecutive series, *Dig Endosc* 17:54–58, 2005.

43. Oda I, Saito D, Tada M, et al: A multicenter retrospective study of endoscopic resection for early gastric cancer, *Gastric Cancer* 9:262–270, 2006.

69. Suzuki H, Oda I, Abe S, et al: High rate of 5-year survival among patients with early gastric cancer undergoing curative endoscopic submucosal dissection, *Gastric Cancer* 19:198–205, 2016.

70. Hasuike N, Ono H, Boku N, et al: A non-randomized confirmatory trial of an expanded indication for endoscopic submucosal dissection for intestinal-type gastric cancer (cT1a): the Japan Clinical Oncology Group study (JCOG0607). Gastrointestinal Endoscopy Group of Japan Clinical Oncology Group (JCOG-GIESG), *Gastric Cancer* 2017. Feb 21, [Epub ahead of print].

A complete reference list can be found online at ExpertConsult .com

33

Palliation of Gastric Outlet Obstruction

Emo E. van Halsema, Paul Fockens, and Jeanin E. van Hooft

MALIGNANT GASTRIC OUTLET OBSTRUCTION

Malignant gastric outlet obstruction (MGOO) is a syndrome caused by intestinal obstruction due to tumor growth in the pyloric region or duodenum (Fig. 33.1). Because of this mechanical obstruction, food and fluids accumulate in the stomach, which results in gastric distention. Patients with MGOO usually present with nausea and vomiting (85%), regurgitation (70%), abdominal pain (65%), and complaints of early satiety.[1,2] Western studies mainly report pancreatic cancer (51%–73%) as the underlying disease,[1,3–6] whereas gastric cancer (31%–69%) is the main cause of MGOO in Asian studies.[7–11] Other causes for MGOO are bile duct cancer, metastatic disease, duodenal cancer, gallbladder cancer, ampullary cancer, and lymphoma.[1,8,11] MGOO can be a clinical diagnosis when a patient with a known advanced gastroduodenal malignancy develops obstructive symptoms due to disease progression. However, at first presentation and when an intervention is considered, adequate imaging (i.e., contrast-enhanced computed tomography [CT] scan) is required to confirm tumor growth in the pyloric-duodenal region, to examine the location, extent, and resectability of the tumor, to look for signs of biliary obstruction, and to exclude a second intestinal obstruction distal to the duodenum. One should also be aware of benign causes of gastric outlet obstruction, such as motility disorders, pancreatic pseudocysts, ulcer-related complications, caustic ingestion, gallstone obstruction (Bouveret's syndrome), Crohn's disease, tuberculosis, or bezoars.[12–14] Endoscopy can therefore be of additional value in the diagnostic process to examine and sample the gastroduodenal area. Cytological or histological confirmation of malignancy is desirable before a definite surgical or endoscopic intervention is offered to the patient.

PALLIATIVE TREATMENT: SURGICAL BYPASS VERSUS ENDOSCOPIC STENT PLACEMENT

Patients with MGOO usually have advanced, unresectable disease with a poor prognosis. A mean survival of approximately 100 days (3.3 months) has been reported in a meta-analysis.[15] Palliative measures should therefore aim for comfort and resolution of obstructive symptoms. Traditionally, patients underwent surgical gastrojejunostomy to bypass the malignant obstruction. Nowadays, endoscopic self-expandable metal stent (SEMS) placement is also a valid treatment option for the palliation of MGOO. Three randomized controlled trials (RCTs) have been published that compared surgical gastrojejunostomy with SEMS placement (Table 33.1).[16–18] The largest and most recently published trial showed that a surgical gastrojejunostomy (open procedure in 16/18 patients) was superior to endoscopic SEMS placement with regard to long-term relief of symptoms, recurrent obstructive symptoms, and reinterventions.[16] There were no differences in health-related quality of life scores and overall survival.[16] The other two trials did not report significant differences in long-term outcomes between surgical gastrojejunostomy and SEMS placement, but the RCTs all showed clear benefits of SEMS placement in the short term: patients had a more rapid recovery of oral food intake and a shorter hospital stay.[16–18] SEMS placement also resulted in lower medical costs per patient.[16] Based on these results, the authors of the largest trial recommended SEMS placement only in patients who have a life expectancy of less than 2 months.[16] The better long-term outcomes of surgical gastrojejunostomy in comparison with SEMSs have also been confirmed by more recently published studies, including a meta-analysis.[15,19,20] So, because of the better short-term results (faster recovery of oral intake and shorter hospitalization), endoscopic SEMS placement is generally offered as a palliative intervention to patients in poor clinical condition who are unfit for surgery and have a short life expectancy of weeks to a few months.

THE ENDOSCOPIC PROCEDURE

Preparation and Materials

Endoscopic SEMS placement is generally performed as an outpatient procedure. Endoscopic gastroduodenal SEMS placement carries a high risk of aspiration because of the food and fluid accumulation in the stomach. Therefore, it is recommended

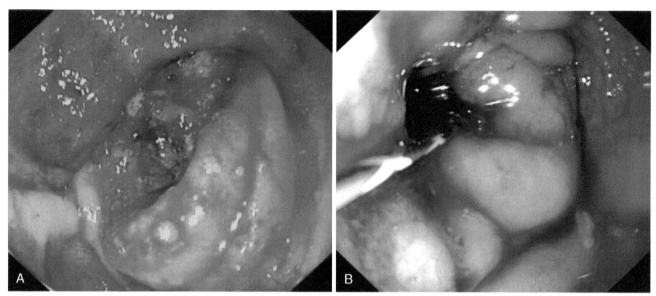

FIG 33.1 A, Endoscopic view of a duodenal carcinoma and a pancreatic carcinoma invading the duodenum with **B,** a guidewire advanced across the tumor, causing gastric outlet obstruction.

TABLE 33.1   Randomized Controlled Trials Comparing Surgical Gastrojejunostomy and Self-Expandable Metal Stent Placement

	Treatment	Technical Success	Clinical Success*	Complications	Recurrent Symptoms	Reinterventions	Hospital Stay	Median Survival
Jeurnink et al, 2010[16]	GJ N = 18	94%	83%	Wound infection: 2 Delayed gastric emptying: 2 Temporary paralytic ileus: 1 Urinary tract infection: 1	6%	11%	15 days	78 days
	SEMS N = 21	95%	86%	Stent migration: 1 Stent obstruction: 3 Delayed gastric emptying: 3 Bacterial infection: 1	24%	33%	7 days	56 days
Mehta et al, 2006[17]	GJ N = 13	100%	NR	Gastroparesis: 3 Hematemesis: 2 Port site infection: 1 Deep venous thrombosis: 1 Pneumonia: 1	NR	NR	11.4 days	NR
	SEMS N = 12	83%	NR	None	0%	NR	5.2 days	NR
Fiori et al, 2004[18]	GJ N = 9	100%	89%	Wound infection: 1 Anastomotic bleeding: 1 Delayed gastric emptying: 3	0%	11%	10 days	NR
	SEMS N = 9	100%	100%	Stent migration: 1 Stent obstruction: 1 Delayed gastric emptying: 1 Epigastric pain: 1	11%	0%	3.1 days	NR

*Defined as resolution of obstructive symptoms
GJ, gastrojejunostomy; *NR,* not reported; *SEMS,* self-expandable metal stent.

that the patient fast from solids for at least 12 hours before the procedure, instead of the regular 6–8 hours before upper gastrointestinal endoscopy. Depending on the patient's symptoms, gastric tube placement is indicated to empty the stomach before the endoscopic procedure. Intubation can be considered even when the aspiration risk is anticipated to be high. SEMS placement can be performed under conscious sedation (e.g., with midazolam or fentanyl) or deep sedation with propofol. In most cases of symptomatic MGOO, the tumor cannot be traversed with the endoscope. Therefore, fluoroscopic guidance is recommended

because it enables the endoscopist (1) to check whether cannulation through the tumor has been successful (intraluminally into to distal duodenum), (2) to get an impression of the length of the obstruction, and (3) to optimize the positioning and deployment of the SEMS using the radiopaque markers on the stent delivery system and using the visibility of the SEMS itself. A mono- or multilumen endoscopic retrograde cholangiopancreatography (ERCP) guiding catheter is used to advance a guidewire across the obstructing tumor into the distal duodenum and jejunum.

Cannulation

The technical success rate of gastroduodenal SEMS placement is high (90%–100%), but when technical failure occurs, it is mainly caused by the inability to pass the guidewire across the tumor.[21] This critical maneuver also carries a small (< 1%) risk for guidewire perforation.[21] Successful cannulation therefore starts with a good endoscopic position. Before gently advancing the guidewire, the endoscopist should carefully inspect the obstruction to get an impression of the lumen and the direction in which the guidewire should be advanced. Once the guidewire is past the obstruction, a catheter (either mono- or multilumen) can be advanced over the guidewire. The advantage of a multilumen guiding catheter is that a contrast agent can be injected through the open lumen without the need to first remove the guidewire. On the other hand, a monolumen catheter costs less, and should therefore be used in the case of easy access through the stricture with the guidewire. To choose the optimal stent size, the endoscopist estimates the length of the tumor using contrast injection to delineate the distal margins of the tumor or by pulling back an inflated balloon into the distal end of the stricture under fluoroscopic guidance. With the latter technique, an extraction balloon should be used to prevent any perforation that may occur due to accidentally inflating a dilation balloon inside the stricture. Interpretation of CT imaging before starting the endoscopic procedure can also help estimate the size of the tumor.

SEMS Deployment

The next step is to exchange the guiding catheter for the stent delivery system (Fig. 33.2). Nowadays, stent delivery systems are usually designed for through-the-scope (TTS) deployment, whereas some SEMS designs are delivered over a guidewire using fluoroscopy, also referred to as over-the-wire (OTW). TTS delivery systems require a working channel of at least 3.7 mm, necessitating the use of a therapeutic endoscope. With OTW delivery systems, the endoscopist can also reintroduce the

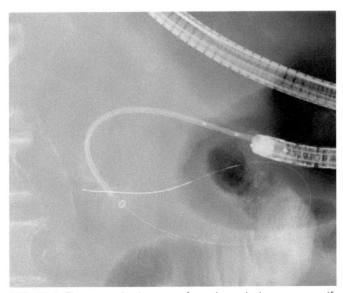

FIG 33.2 Fluoroscopic image of a through-the-scope self-expanding metal stent delivery system that is being advanced over the guidewire.

endoscope alongside the stent delivery system for an endoscopic view during SEMS deployment. Endoscopy allows visualization of the proximal end of the SEMS, which is usually indicated by a colored mark on the delivery system. So, together with an endoscopic view and fluoroscopic guidance, optimal positioning of the SEMS can be achieved. Once the endoscopist is satisfied with the position, the SEMS can be carefully deployed by pulling back the outer sheath that covers the SEMS. The endoscopist should be aware that SEMSs can shorten upon deployment. It is therefore important to read the instructions supplied by the manufacturer to understand what the radiopaque markers on the SEMS itself or on the stent delivery system indicate. Most stent delivery systems also allow for recapture and repositioning of the SEMS until a certain "point of no return" has been reached. Once the SEMS is fully deployed (Fig. 33.3), it takes 1–3 days to reach the maximum expansion diameter. Therefore, patients are instructed to carefully expand their diet from liquids to soft solids to solid food in the first 3 days after the procedure. In the palliative setting, patient comfort and personal dietary wishes should be respected as much as possible, but at the same time, patients should be instructed as to how to prevent food bolus obstruction of the SEMS. Some recommend a low-fiber diet and, when possible, that the SEMS is placed distal to the pylorus so that only digested stomach contents will pass through the SEMS. Others allow patients with a gastroduodenal SEMS to have a normal diet and prefer placing the proximal flare of the SEMS against the pylorus to prevent migration into the distal small bowel. Data are lacking to support either of these practices. Nevertheless, patients should be instructed to chew well, to avoid swallowing large pieces of food, and to have a glass of water present when eating. They should also be careful when eating (or avoid eating) solid foods that may easily obstruct the SEMS, such as mushrooms or meat or fish containing pieces of bone.

SELF-EXPANDABLE METAL STENTS

The endoscopist should be aware that there are different stent models available for the treatment of MGOO. The main problems encountered with the use of SEMSs are tumor growth through or over the stent mesh and stent migration, which causes the recurrence of obstruction symptoms. The current stents therefore all have features designed to reduce these risks. SEMSs generally consist of a wire mesh framework made of nitinol, an alloy of nickel and titanium. They usually have a cup- or funnel-shaped flare at the proximal side or at both ends. SEMSs can be uncovered or covered by a silicone or polytetrafluoroethylene membrane. The covering prevents tumor ingrowth, and thereby reduces the risk of recurrent obstruction. Covered stent models are either fully covered or partially covered. Partially covered stent designs have the advantage of preventing tumor ingrowth due to their partial covering, and they also reduce the risk of stent migration because the uncovered parts of the SEMS become embedded by the intestinal wall. Four RCTs have been published that compared the outcomes of uncovered and covered SEMSs for the treatment of MGOO (Table 33.2).[2,22–24] The authors of the largest and most recently published trial (2015) concluded that the partially covered SEMS used in their study was superior to the uncovered SEMS regarding stent patency and the reobstruction rate.[2] Another trial also reported significantly fewer reinterventions with the use of a partially covered SEMS because of a lower rate of reobstruction due to tumor in- or overgrowth.[23] The two other trials were included in a meta-analysis that compared the clinical

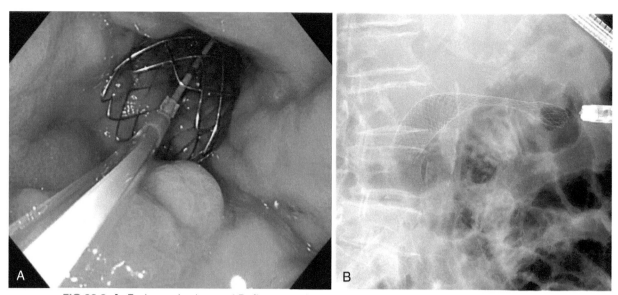

FIG 33.3 A, Endoscopic view and **B,** fluoroscopic image of a fully deployed self-expanding metal stent in the gastric antrum.

		Technical Success	Clinical Success*	Stent Dysfunction	Reinterventions	Stent Patency	Median Survival
	Stent						
Lee et al, 2015[2]	UCSEMS N = 51	96%	90%	Reobstruction: 38% Stent migration: 5%	16 wk: 39%	16 wk: 41%	NR
	PCSEMS N = 51	98%	96%	Reobstruction: 7% Stent migration: 10%	16 wk: 24%	16 wk: 69%	NR
Maetani et al, 2014[22]	UCSEMS N = 31	100%	94%	Reobstruction: 19% Stent migration: 3% Stent fracture: 6% Insufficient expansion: 0% Perforation: 0%	NR	Failed: 29%	93 d
	PCSEMS N = 31	100%	87%	Reobstruction: 0% Stent migration: 6% Stent fracture: 3% Insufficient expansion: 6% Perforation: 3%	NR	Failed: 16%	73 d
Shi et al, 2014[23]	UCSEMS N = 32	97%	94%	Reobstruction: 22% Stent migration: 0% Food impaction: 3%	23%	NR	Mean: 212 d
	PCSEMS N = 33	97%	94%	Reobstruction: 3% Stent migration: 6% Food impaction: 3%	9%	NR	Mean: 231 d
Kim et al, 2010[24]	UCSEMS N = 40	100%	90%	Reobstruction: 44% Stent migration: 8% Stent collapse: 0% Stent fracture: 0% Perforation: 0%	NR	Median: 13 wk	19 wk
	PCSEMS N = 40	100%	95%	Reobstruction: 3% Stent migration: 32% Stent collapse: 3% Stent fracture: 10% Perforation: 3%	NR	Median: 14 wk	26 wk

TABLE 33.2 Randomized Controlled Trials Comparing Uncovered and Covered Self-Expandable Metal Stents

*Relief of obstruction and/or improvement in gastric outlet obstruction scoring system (GOOSS) score after technically successful self-expanding metal stent placement
NR, not reported; *PCSEMS,* partially covered self-expandable metal stent; *UCSEMS,* uncovered self-expandable metal stent; *wk,* weeks.

outcomes of uncovered and covered SEMSs for the palliation of MGOO.[25] A total of 849 patients from nine comparative studies were analyzed, and showed no significant differences in stent patency, overall complications, and reintervention rates.[25] The only significant association was the higher migration rate and lower reobstruction rate seen with the use of covered SEMSs.[25]

PREDICTORS FOR STENT FAILURE

Clinical success of SEMS placement is usually defined as improvement in oral food intake or relief of obstructive symptoms in the first week after the procedure. In the literature, the clinical success rates range from 63%–99%.[1,6,26–28] Performance status and the presence of peritoneal carcinomatosis have been identified as important predictors for clinical failure after SEMS placement. A Karnofsky performance score of 50 or less and an Eastern Cooperative Oncology Group performance status of 3 or higher were independent predictors for clinical failure, with odds ratios ranging from 1.2–10.2.[7,11,29–31] The same applies to the presence of peritoneal carcinomatosis, with odds ratios ranging from 1.2–35.7.[7,9,20,29,30] One should realize that the aforementioned factors are only relative contraindications because clinical success rates of 69% and 88% have been reported in patients with a Karnofsky performance score of 50 or less or peritoneal disease, respectively.[9,11] Therefore gastroduodenal SEMS placement in patients with a poor performance status and/or peritoneal carcinomatosis should be considered on an individual basis. Other variables such as the site of obstruction, administration of chemotherapy, and the underlying malignancy showed inconsistent correlations with the clinical outcomes of SEMS placement.[5,7–9,11,20,31–36]

STENT PATENCY AND ADVERSE EVENTS

In the RCTs, stent dysfunction from any cause during follow-up was reported in 16%–59% of patients, depending on the type of SEMS (see Table 33.2).[2,22] Large prospective cohort studies have reported a median stent patency ranging from 73–91 days.[6,28] A pooled analysis of the prospective literature including almost 1300 patients reported that stent dysfunction occurred in 20% of patients treated with pyloric or duodenal SEMS placement.[21] Stent dysfunction mainly consists of reobstruction due to tumor growth (13%) and stent migration (4%).[21] The use of uncovered SEMSs is associated with reobstruction (15% vs. 5%), whereas covered SEMSs show an increased risk of stent migration (11% vs. 2%).[21] Other stent-related adverse events are relatively rare, and include: stent compression by tumor pressure (< 2%), insufficient stent expansion (< 1%), food occlusion (< 1%), and stent fracture (< 1%).[21] Recurrent obstructive symptoms caused by stent dysfunction can be treated with a second SEMS by stent-in-stent placement (in case of reobstruction; Video 33.1) or stent replacement (in case of migration). The outcomes of secondary SEMS placement for stent dysfunction are comparable to the outcomes of primary SEMS placement: in retrospective series, the technical and clinical success rates ranged from 98%–100% and 81%–92%, respectively.[37–40] Stent dysfunction after secondary SEMS placement was reported in 17%–34% of cases.[37–40]

Another non-negligible risk is the occurrence of intestinal perforation. This has been reported in approximately 1% of patients who underwent gastroduodenal SEMS placement.[21] Perforations can be procedure-related or can develop at any time after the procedure, and often result in surgical repair.[21] Gastrointestinal bleeding occurred in 4% of patients, although major bleeds were rare (< 1%).[21] Table 33.3 provides an overview of the adverse events reported in the prospective literature after pyloric or duodenal SEMS placement for MGOO.

BILIARY DRAINAGE

A point of discussion is whether or not duodenal SEMS placement should be preceded by biliary SEMS placement. After duodenal SEMS placement, endoscopic biliary access via ERCP through the SEMS will be technically challenging. When signs of biliary obstruction are already present, then biliary drainage is indicated before the duodenal SEMS procedure. It has been demonstrated in uncontrolled retrospective series that combined biliary and duodenal stenting is feasible and effective (Fig. 33.4).[51–55] So far, there is no convincing evidence to combine duodenal SEMS placement with preceding biliary SEMS placement when the patient does not have any clinical, biochemical, or radiological signs of a biliary outflow obstruction. An observational study retrospectively compared the occurrence of obstructive jaundice after duodenal covered SEMS placement in patients with (N = 53) or without (N = 53) a concomitant biliary SEMS.[56] In both groups, no cases of jaundice were reported after 90 days of follow-up, although the duodenal SEMS covered the major duodenal papilla in all patients.[56] Another retrospective comparative study also suggested that covered SEMS placement across the papilla did not increase the risk of reintervention.[57] When a patient develops obstructive jaundice or cholangitis after duodenal SEMS placement, biliary drainage can be achieved via the percutaneous transhepatic route. There are also reports of endoscopic biliary SEMS placement through the mesh of a duodenal SEMS.[58–60] The evidence of endoscopic ultrasound (EUS)-guided biliary drainage by choledochoduodenostomy or hepaticogastrostomy using a SEMS or a plastic stent is emerging, but randomized studies are still lacking.[60–64]

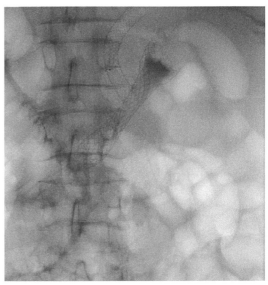

FIG 33.4 Fluoroscopic image with a duodenal self-expanding metal stent (SEMS) that bridges the major duodenal papilla with a biliary SEMS in situ.

TABLE 33.3 Adverse Events in Nonrandomized, Prospective Studies

	Patients (N)	Reobstruction*	Migration	Perforation	Bleeding	Other
UCSEMS						
Sasaki et al, 2016[41]	39	8%	0%	0%	0%	Aspiration: 10%
Tringali et al, 2014[1]	108	16%	2%	2%	5%[†]	Abdominal pain: 2% Other GI events: 16%
Van den Berg et al, 2013[27]	46	20%	4%	2%	0%	Stent compression: 4% Food impaction: 2% Motility disorder: 11% Pain: 2% Other GI events: 24%
Costamagna et al, 2012[6]	202	12%	1.5%	0.5%	1%[†] 2%[‡]	Abdominal pain: 3% Food impaction: 0.5% Vomiting: 0.5%
Dolz et al, 2011[32]	71	14%	0%	3%	7%[†]	Pain: 3% Insufficient expansion: 4%
Van Hooft et al, 2011[42]	52	21%	4%	0%	0%	Pain: 8% Motility dysfunction: 12%
Maetani et al, 2010[43]	53	13%	0%	2%	2%[‡]	Food impaction: 2% Stent fracture: 2% Insufficient expansion 4% Obstructive jaundice: 2%
Shaw et al, 2010[44]	70	4%	1%	0%	1%[†] 1%[‡]	Insufficient expansion: 1%
Havemann et al, 2009[26]	45	9%	7%	4%	0%	0%
Lee et al, 2009[28]	84	19%	0%	0%	0%	0%
Piesman et al, 2009[45]	43	9%	0%	5%	2%[‡]	Stent malposition: 2% Stent collapse: 2% Insufficient expansion: 5% Occlusion by jejunal wall: 2% Vomiting: 9% Other GI events: 7%
Van Hooft et al, 2009[46]	51	12%	2%	0%	4%[‡]	Motility dysfunction: 4% Intermittent pain: 4% Other GI events: 6%
PCSEMS						
Shi et al, 2013[47]	37	0%	0%	0%	41%[†] 3%[‡]	Food impaction: 5% Abdominal pain: 38%
Isayama et al, 2012[48]	50	10%	6%	2%	0%	Insufficient expansion: 2% Other GI events: 4%
Kim YW, et al, 2011[49]	50	8%	10%	0%	0%	Stent compression: 10%
Lee et al, 2009[28]	70	7%	17%	0%	0%	0%
Kim JH, et al, 2007[50]	213	8%	4%	0%	1%[†]	Stent collapse: 4% Food impaction: 2% Obstructive jaundice: 2%

*By tumor in- or overgrowth
[†]No intervention required
[‡]Major hemorrhage requiring intervention
GI, gastrointestinal; PCSEMS, partially covered self-expandable metal stents; UCSEMS, uncovered self-expandable metal stents.

NEW DEVELOPMENTS

Endoscopic bypass of the obstructed gastric outlet by an endoscopically created gastrojejunostomy is a developing area.[65–68] The aim of this minimally invasive technique is rapid relief of obstruction due to the endoscopic approach, as well as long-term intestinal patency conferred by the gastroenteric anastomosis that bypasses the obstructed duodenum. Two studies reported the use of magnets to create a pressure-induced fistula between the gastric wall and the jejunum.[68,69] After dilation of the duodenal stenosis, a magnet was placed distally from the tumor that was then joined with a magnet in the stomach. After 7 to 10 days, a SEMS with wide flanges was placed through the fistulous tract. Success rates of 87% (13/15) and 67% (12/18) were reported.[68,69] Stent migration was the main problem encountered, occurring in approximately 25% of patients.[68,69] One of the studies was prematurely terminated because of an intestinal perforation caused by the distal end of the stent.[68] A more recently published technique to create a gastrojejunal anastomosis is EUS-guided placement of a lumen-apposing metal stent (LAMS).[65–67] In this approach, the small bowel adjacent to the gastric wall is identified with EUS. To facilitate EUS visibility, one can use contrast injection, a water-inflated balloon, or a double-balloon tube to fill a segment of the small bowel with water. The small bowel loop is subsequently punctured with a fine-needle aspiration needle, and a guidewire is advanced through the needle into the distal jejunum. The puncture tract is either dilated or entered using the cautery tip of the LAMS delivery system. Under fluoroscopic guidance, the LAMS is placed through the gastrojejunal anastomosis to ensure luminal patency. In pilot studies, the technical and clinical success rates ranged from 90%–92% and 85%–100%, respectively.[65–67] No cases of stent migration were reported with the use of LAMSs. In one study, technical failure (2/20) was caused by dislocation of the jejunal loop, resulting in misplacement of the LAMS with direct visualization of the abdominal cavity through the LAMS.[65] Thus, endoscopic bypass seems to be a promising alternative to surgical gastrojejunostomy, although we need more experience with the technique and evaluation by RTCs to determine its role in the management of MGOO.

KEY REFERENCES

1. Tringali A, Didden P, Repici A, et al: Endoscopic treatment of malignant gastric and duodenal strictures: a prospective, multicenter study, *Gastrointest Endosc* 79:66–75, 2014.

2. Lee H, Min BH, Lee JH, et al: Covered metallic stents with an anti-migration design vs. uncovered stents for the palliation of malignant gastric outlet obstruction: a multicenter, randomized trial, *Am J Gastroenterol* 110:1440–1449, 2015.

5. Oh SY, Edwards A, Mandelson M, et al: Survival and clinical outcome after endoscopic duodenal stent placement for malignant gastric outlet obstruction: comparison of pancreatic cancer and nonpancreatic cancer, *Gastrointest Endosc* 82:460–468 e2, 2015.

6. Costamagna G, Tringali A, Spicak J, et al: Treatment of malignant gastroduodenal obstruction with a nitinol self-expanding metal stent: an international prospective multicentre registry, *Dig Liver Dis* 44:37–43, 2012.

7. Hori Y, Naitoh I, Ban T, et al: Stent under-expansion on the procedure day, a predictive factor for poor oral intake after metallic stenting for gastric outlet obstruction, *J Gastroenterol Hepatol* 30:1246–1251, 2015.

9. Lee JE, Lee K, Hong YS, et al: Impact of carcinomatosis on clinical outcomes after self-expandable metallic stent placement for malignant gastric outlet obstruction, *PLoS ONE* 10:e0140648, 2015.

11. Yamao K, Kitano M, Kayahara T, et al: Factors predicting through-the-scope gastroduodenal stenting outcomes in patients with gastric outlet obstruction: a large multicenter retrospective study in West Japan, *Gastrointest Endosc* 84(5):757–763.e6, 2016.

15. Nagaraja V, Eslick GD, Cox MR: Endoscopic stenting versus operative gastrojejunostomy for malignant gastric outlet obstruction-a systematic review and meta-analysis of randomized and non-randomized trials, *J Gastrointest Oncol* 5:92–98, 2014.

16. Jeurnink SM, Steyerberg EW, van Hooft JE, et al: Surgical gastrojejunostomy or endoscopic stent placement for the palliation of malignant gastric outlet obstruction (SUSTENT study): a multicenter randomized trial, *Gastrointest Endosc* 71:490–499, 2010.

20. Park CH, Park JC, Kim EH, et al: Impact of carcinomatosis and ascites status on long-term outcomes of palliative treatment for patients with gastric outlet obstruction caused by unresectable gastric cancer: stent placement versus palliative gastrojejunostomy, *Gastrointest Endosc* 81:321–332, 2015.

21. van Halsema EE, Rauws EA, Fockens P, et al: Self-expandable metal stents for malignant gastric outlet obstruction: a pooled analysis of prospective literature, *World J Gastroenterol* 21:12468–12481, 2015.

24. Kim CG, Choi IJ, Lee JY, et al: Covered versus uncovered self-expandable metallic stents for palliation of malignant pyloric obstruction in gastric cancer patients: a randomized, prospective study, *Gastrointest Endosc* 72:25–32, 2010.

25. Pan YM, Pan J, Guo LK, et al: Covered versus uncovered self-expandable metallic stents for palliation of malignant gastric outlet obstruction: a systematic review and meta-analysis, *BMC Gastroenterol* 14:170, 2014.

27. van den Berg MW, Haijtink S, Fockens P, et al: First data on the Evolution duodenal stent for palliation of malignant gastric outlet obstruction (DUOLUTION study): a prospective multicenter study, *Endoscopy* 45:174–181, 2013.

30. Jeon HH, Park CH, Park JC, et al: Carcinomatosis matters: clinical outcomes and prognostic factors for clinical success of stent placement in malignant gastric outlet obstruction, *Surg Endosc* 28:988–995, 2014.

35. Kim CG, Park SR, Choi IJ, et al: Effect of chemotherapy on the outcome of self-expandable metallic stents in gastric cancer patients with malignant outlet obstruction, *Endoscopy* 44:807–812, 2012.

37. Jin EH, Kim SG, Seo JY, et al: Clinical outcomes of re-stenting in patients with stent malfunction in malignant gastric outlet obstruction, *Surg Endosc* 30:1372–1379, 2016.

50. Kim JH, Song HY, Shin JH, et al: Metallic stent placement in the palliative treatment of malignant gastroduodenal obstructions: prospective evaluation of results and factors influencing outcome in 213 patients, *Gastrointest Endosc* 66:256–264, 2007.

54. Mutignani M, Tringali A, Shah SG, et al: Combined endoscopic stent insertion in malignant biliary and duodenal obstruction, *Endoscopy* 39:440–447, 2007.

56. Poincloux L, Goutorbe F, Rouquette O, et al: Biliary stenting is not a prerequisite to endoscopic placement of duodenal covered self-expandable metal stents, *Surg Endosc* 30:437–445, 2016.

57. Kim SY, Song HY, Kim JH, et al: Bridging across the ampulla of Vater with covered self-expanding metallic stents: is it contraindicated when treating malignant gastroduodenal obstruction?, *J Vasc Interv Radiol* 19:1607–1613, 2008.

60. Khashab MA, Valeshabad AK, Leung W, et al: Multicenter experience with performance of ERCP in patients with an indwelling duodenal stent, *Endoscopy* 46:252–255, 2014.

62. Ogura T, Chiba Y, Masuda D, et al: Comparison of the clinical impact of endoscopic ultrasound-guided choledochoduodenostomy and hepaticogastrostomy for bile duct obstruction with duodenal obstruction, *Endoscopy* 48:156–163, 2016.

64. Wang K, Zhu J, Xing L, et al: Assessment of efficacy and safety of EUS-guided biliary drainage: a systematic review, *Gastrointest Endosc* 83:1218–1227, 2016.

65. Itoi T, Ishii K, Ikeuchi N, et al: Prospective evaluation of endoscopic ultrasonography-guided double-balloon-occluded gastrojejunostomy bypass (EPASS) for malignant gastric outlet obstruction, *Gut* 65:193–195, 2016.

A complete reference list can be found online at ExpertConsult.com

34

Duodenal and Papillary Adenomas

Amir Klein and Michael J. Bourke

INTRODUCTION

Duodenal polyps are uncommon. They can be found in 0.3%–4.6% of patients undergoing upper gastrointestinal endoscopy, and are usually an incidental finding.[1-4] Adenomas account for approximately 7% of all duodenal polyps. They are most commonly found in the second part of the duodenum, and are usually solitary, flat, sessile lesions.[5-8] Duodenal adenomas can be classified as papillary adenomas (PAs) when primarily involving the papilla Vateri, or duodenal adenomas (DAs) when there is no involvement of the papilla. These adenomas can be further classified as sporadic papillary adenomas (SPAs) or sporadic duodenal adenomas (SDAs), i.e., those not associated with genetic polyposis syndromes, or as those related to familial adenomatous polyposis (FAP). It is estimated that 40% of duodenal adenomas are sporadic and 60% are related to FAP.[9]

Endoscopic resection (ER) of DA and PA is quickly becoming the treatment of choice for noninvasive lesions, even when they are very extensive.[10-14] Although no systematic comparative data exist, due to the lower risks of morbidity, mortality, and long-term digestive dysfunction, ER is considered preferable to surgery. ER in the duodenum requires a diverse range of endoscopic skills. These include proficiency in advanced endoscopic resection techniques, experience with pancreaticobiliary endoscopy, and the ability to identify and manage complications. These procedures should be performed by experienced endoscopists practicing in tertiary referral centers with access to surgical and interventional radiology support. A structured approach to lesion assessment, technical aspects of resection, and postresection surveillance is required.

EPIDEMIOLOGY AND NATURAL HISTORY

SDAs are rare, and most are discovered incidentally during esophagogastroduodenoscopy (EGD) performed for other indications.[3,15] In a similar fashion to colonic carcinogenesis, 30%–80% of SDAs demonstrate malignant progression through the adenoma-to-carcinoma pathway. In one study, 21% of lesions with low-grade dysplasia (LGD) showed progression to high-grade dysplasia (HGD), and the presence of HGD and a lesion size of more than 20 mm were independently associated with progression to adenocarcinoma.[16] In other studies, invasive adenocarcinomas were often found within small bowel adenomas, and residual adenomatous tissue was found adjacent to, or within, most carcinomas.[15,17] It is therefore recommended that all SDAs be removed.

SPAs are also uncommon, and have been reported to occur at a rate of 0.04%–0.12% in autopsy series.[18,19] Today, with the increasing performance of EGD and endoscopic retrograde cholangiopancreatography (ERCP), these adenomas are more frequently recognized at an asymptomatic stage. Similar to SDAs, SPAs appear to follow the adenoma-to-carcinoma paradigm, and should thus be removed.[20,21] However, SPAs are thought to progress to cancer more rapidly than nonpapillary duodenal adenomas.[22]

The molecular and genetic pathways of the adenoma-to-carcinoma sequence in SDA/SPA are less well established. In one study, approximately 75% of duodenal adenomas (both sporadic, FAP-related, and those involving the papilla) showed Wnt signaling pathway abnormalities.[23] KRAS mutations were found in 18% of SDAs, 9% of FAP-related adenomas, and 44% of SPAs.

No BRAF mutations were identified, and both p53 and DNA mismatch repair mutations were rare. In another study, the CpG island methylator phenotype (CIMP) was analyzed in ampullary and nonampullary SDAs.[24] Thirty-three percent of duodenal adenomas were CIMP+, and CIMP+ status was associated with advanced age, large lesions, villous histology, MLH1 methylation, and KRAS mutations. These results suggest that duodenal adenomas develop via similar mechanisms as colonic adenomas, and that CIMP+ duodenal adenomas may have a higher risk of developing malignancy.

SDAs are also considered surrogate markers for colonic neoplasia. Several retrospective case control studies have demonstrated a significantly higher risk of colonic neoplasia in patients with sporadic duodenal adenomas when compared with their matched controls (relative risk [RR] 2.5–7.8).[25,26] Thus, all patients with SDA/SPA should undergo colonoscopy at some point.

In contrast, patients with FAP have a much higher prevalence of DA or PA. Duodenal or papillary adenomas are found in more than 90% of patients with FAP, and 3%–10% will progress to malignancy over their lifetime.[27–30] In patients with FAP, duodenal adenomas are usually multiple, sessile, and located in the second and third parts of the duodenum.[31] The Spigelman staging system[32] is used to stratify disease burden and predict the risk of malignant transformation. The risk of duodenal cancer increases with age and with progressive adenoma stage.[29,33] DA may also occur in association with MYH-associated polyposis and Lynch syndrome.[34,35]

CLINICAL PRESENTATION

As previously mentioned, DAs are usually asymptomatic, and the majority are discovered incidentally during routine EGD performed for other indications. Rarely, very large lesions may present with gastrointestinal bleeding or obstructive features. PA may present with abdominal pain, recurrent pancreatitis, malaise, or anorexia. However, most noninvasive lesions are asymptomatic and are found incidentally during EGD or ERCP performed for other indications. Symptoms such as jaundice may result from invasive malignancy or intraductal extension, but may alternatively be caused by a concurrent benign condition such as common bile duct (CBD) stones.

INDICATIONS AND PATIENT SELECTION

ER should be considered for any noninvasive DAs/PAs, because it potentially offers significant advantages over operative management. Long-term cure rates can be expected in more than 90% of patients undergoing ER. Periprocedural complications are not uncommon (bleeding up to 25%, perforation up to 3%, recurrence up to 30%); however, they are usually not severe, and are managed successfully endoscopically or with conservative management without long-term sequelae.[12,36–40] In comparison, a conservative surgical procedure (transduodenal resection/ampullectomy) carries a morbidity rate of 20%–30%, a mortality rate of 0%–6%, and a residual disease rate of 13%–100%. The more radical pancreaticoduodenectomy has even higher rates of morbidity and mortality (25%–50% and 3%–9%, respectively).[41–46]

The patient's medical history, including his or her medication list, has to be thoroughly reviewed and the patient's comorbidities constantly factored into the therapeutic process. This is especially important because, compared with similar size adenomas in the colon, the risk for malignant transformation appears to be reduced, the time course more prolonged, and the ER procedure more technically challenging and associated with greater incidence of complications.[31]

To achieve endoscopic cure, the entire lesion must be accessible to resection, and the risk of submucosal invasive cancer (SMIC) and lymph node metastases (LNM) negligible. Lesions with LGD or HGD confined to the mucosa are considered suitable for ER.[47] Lesions with suspected SMIC or LNM require surgery to achieve cure, and are not suitable for ER. For PA, lymphovascular invasion and moderate or poor tumor differentiation confer additional risks for LNM.[48–50] T1 lesions (limited to the papilla vateri or sphincter of Oddi) harbor an appreciable rate of LNM (18%) and are best managed surgically.[48,51] Papillectomy may serve as the definitive staging tool and finally determine the need for additional therapy such as surgery. On the other hand, endoscopic cure of selected well-differentiated T1 papillary carcinomas has been demonstrated in small case series,[49] presenting a therapeutic alternative for patients unfit for surgical resection.

PA may contain an intraductal component or a lateral spreading component, or can involve the minor papilla. PA with intraductal extension limited to the papillary complex or extending 1 cm or less beyond the duodenal wall may be removed by ER. Lesions with more extensive intraductal involvement have higher failure rates with ER, and at present are best referred for surgical resection, although with expanding possibilities of cholangioscopy, such as intraductal radio frequency ablation (RFA), this may change in the future.[52–56] Lateral spreading lesions of the papilla (LSL-P) may be very large (in excess of 50–60 mm) and involve the entire duodenal circumference. Although uncommon, LSL-Ps may be cured endoscopically at rates comparable to lesions confined to the papilla, albeit with an elevated risk of bleeding.[47,57] Lesions involving the minor papilla are rare, hence data on resection and outcomes are limited.[57,58]

LESION ASSESSMENT AND STAGING

The lesion's size, the degree of circumferential involvement, and the relationship to the papilla should be carefully assessed. This may require use of a side-viewing duodenoscope. Chromoendoscopy or narrow-band imaging may be used to better delineate the lesion margin and histologic grade.[59] For DA, the presence of a depressed component (0-IIc of the Paris classifications), a type V Kudo pit-pattern, surface bleeding, fixation to the duodenal wall, or ulceration or a nonlifting sign raise concern for SMIC, and warrant consideration for surgical referral.[1] For PA, smooth, elevated lesions and an umbilicated appearance may be associated with a higher risk of SMIC.[47,60] According to Japanese data, ER of DA can be performed on lesions with a depressed element (Paris IIc, IIa + IIc) up to 10 mm in diameter and on nondepressed adenomas up to 50 mm in diameter, as the risk of SMIC in these groups is very low.[61] In expert hands, lesions up to 80 mm and even full circumference lesions without evidence of SMIC can be successfully removed by piecemeal endoscopic mucosal resection (EMR), albeit with higher risks of complications (mainly delayed bleeding).[39,62,63]

For FAP-related DA/PA, the neoplastic burden in the duodenum (as assessed by the Spigelman endoscopic and histologic classification system) is an additional factor in the selection of ER versus surgical management.[32] At present, it is not clear whether endoscopic intervention significantly alters the course of the disease or avoids the need for major surgery (Whipple resection) in patients with a significant duodenal polyp burden. However, it is current practice to endoscopically remove all large (> 1 cm) duodenal adenomas in patients with FAP unless there is suspicion of advanced histology and submucosal invasion (SMI).

The role of endoscopic ultrasound (EUS) in the assessment of DA has not been systematically evaluated, but its use is likely to be limited (similar to its use for large laterally spreading lesions in the colon), as advanced endoscopic imaging appears to be the most accurate means of predicting SMIC. However, for PA, especially lesions greater than 2 cm, preresection staging with EUS, magnetic resonance cholangiopancreatography, contrast-enhanced multidetector computed tomography (CT), and careful cholangiopancreatography (usually at the time of ampullectomy) are usually necessary. The presence of SMI or LNM, the extent of any intraductal component, and the presence of pancreatic duct anatomic variants (such as pancreas divisum) are assessed. No one test has emerged as the gold standard for T or N staging, and they are considered complementary. EUS provides superior T staging and comparable N staging to CT and magnetic resonance imaging.[64,65] Published accuracy rates vary from 55% to 90% in T staging and 50% to 80% in N staging.[66]

RESECTION PRINCIPLES AND TECHNIQUES

Duodenal Adenoma

- As most DAs are flat sessile lesions, ER is most commonly accomplished by standard EMR (Video 34.1).[31,67] Modifications to the standard technique, such as cap-assisted EMR and underwater EMR, have also been described.[68,69]
- En bloc EMR is considered for lesions up to 15–20 mm, whereas larger lesions require piecemeal EMR for complete and safe removal (Figs. 34.1 and 34.2).[1,13] Smaller piece sizes are required in the duodenum as compared with the colon, and safety should always be the primary concern.

- Endoscopic submucosal dissection has limited applicability in the resection of DA, due to an unacceptably high frequency of severe complications (mainly perforations, which occur in up to 25% of cases) during or following the procedure.[70,71]
- The submucosal injection solution is composed of a colloid solution (most commonly 0.9% saline, succinylated gelatin, or hydroxyl-ethyl-starch); diluted epinephrine, which may reduce intraprocedural bleeding; and an inert dye (indigo carmine or methylene blue), which delineates the submucosal layer from the underlying muscle layer. The submucosal injection should create a robust and sustained "cushion" between the mucosa and the muscularis propria, thus reducing the risk of deep tissue entrapment in the snare, transmural thermal injury, and perforation.[13,67,72]
- Microprocessor-controlled electrosurgical generators delivering alternating cycles of high-frequency short-pulse cutting with more prolonged coagulation current are most commonly used today. Tissue impedance is sensed via signals from the return electrode, adjusting power output accordingly to minimize the risk of deep tissue injury.
- CO_2 should be used routinely. Abundant data from colonoscopy, ERCP, and colonic EMR studies demonstrate that the use of CO_2 results in a significant reduction in postprocedural pain and admissions, without any adverse effects.[73,74]

Papillary Adenoma

- The standard technique for en bloc papillectomy has been described in detail (Video 34.2).[60] Briefly, the snare tip is anchored above the apex of the papilla at approximately the 12 to 1 o'clock position. The snare is then opened fully, and gently drawn down over the papilla as the endoscope is advanced. The snare is then closed slowly and fully while the tip is maintained impacted above the papilla. The mobility of the papilla relative to the duodenal wall is confirmed, and

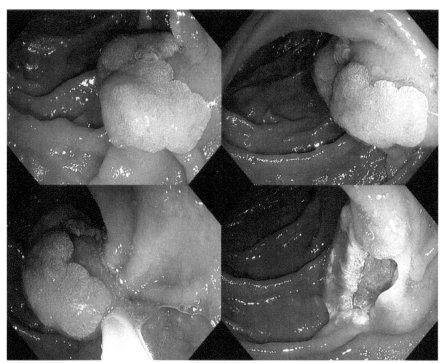

FIG 34.1 En bloc endoscopic mucosal resection of a 15-mm duodenal lateral spreading lesion.

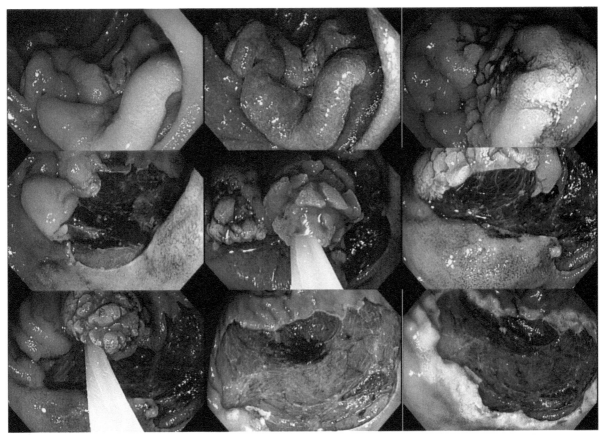

FIG 34.2 Piecemeal endoscopic mucosal resection of a 40-mm duodenal lateral spreading lesion.

the lesion is transected by continuous current application (we use Endocut Q effect 3 cut duration 1, cut interval 6; ERBE, Tübingen, Germany) (Fig. 34.3).

- En bloc papillectomy is associated with a lower rate of incomplete resection and residual disease.[37,75] Lesions limited to the papillary mound, or those with less than 10 mm extension to the duodenal wall and that are up to 20 mm in size, can usually be resected en bloc (Fig. 34.4).[37,38,60]
- Prior sphincterotomy should definitely be avoided because the papillary complex tends to retract following sphincterotomy, and this can seriously impede attempts at en bloc resection.
- For LSL-P, resection of the extrapapillary component follows the principles of EMR for DA.[14,31] Resection should preferably proceed along the duodenal folds, aiming to isolate the papilla for en bloc resection at the end (Video 34.3). Care should be taken to avoid overinjection or injection within the papillary mound, which may lead to a buried papilla between adjacent elevated mucosa ("canyon effect"), hindering adequate snare capture (Fig. 34.5).
- Pancreatic stent placement reduces the risk of postprocedure pancreatitis, and should be performed routinely.[76,77] The pancreatic orifice is usually identified as a slit-like opening in the 5 o'clock position within the base of the papillectomy site.
- Cholangitis following ampullectomy is uncommon, and routine postpapillectomy sphincterotomy or stenting is not mandatory.[57] However, for advanced resection requiring a longer procedure time, multiple submucosal injections, and extensive piecemeal resection, we often perform biliary stenting to avoid the small risk of papillary stenosis and cholangitis.[37,47,78]
- When intraductal extension is suspected, balloon trawls can be used to deliver distal disease for snare resection.[79] Alternatively, if the CBD is large enough, a fully covered self-extending metal stent (FCSEMS) can be placed and removed at scheduled surveillance. This will result in a CBD orifice of 10 mm in diameter, and easy access can be obtained to excise the residual tissue.

Postprocedure Care

ER of DA/PA is best scheduled during the morning to allow ample time for recovery and identification of adverse events. We routinely admit all patients for observation over a period of 24 hours. However, practice differs between centers, and in some, patients are discharged following an uncomplicated resection of DA/PA. If there is significant postprocedural pain, imaging from the case is carefully reviewed, and a CT scan with oral contrast ordered. Patients who are well may be discharged the following day. High-dose proton pump inhibitors (PPIs) are prescribed for 4 to 6 weeks, although there are no systematic data to support this practice. For PA, an abdominal film is obtained after 10 to 14 days to ensure pancreatic duct stent migration. A stent that has not migrated is removed endoscopically.

Surveillance endoscopy is performed at 4 to 6 months following the index procedure. If an FCSEMS was inserted during the index procedure, it is removed then. This can be successfully achieved in all cases in our experience, and complications related

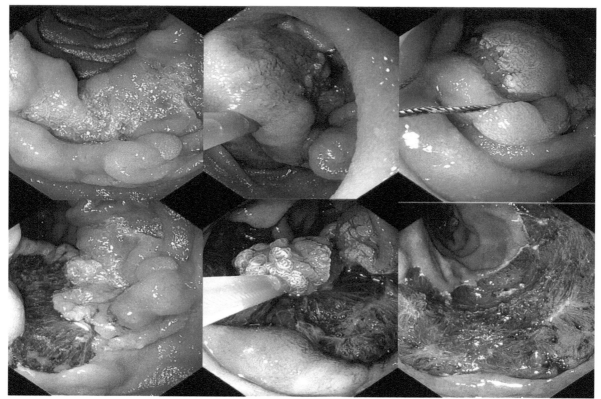

FIG 34.3 Piecemeal endoscopic mucosal resection of a 60-mm hemicircumferential duodenal lateral spreading lesion.

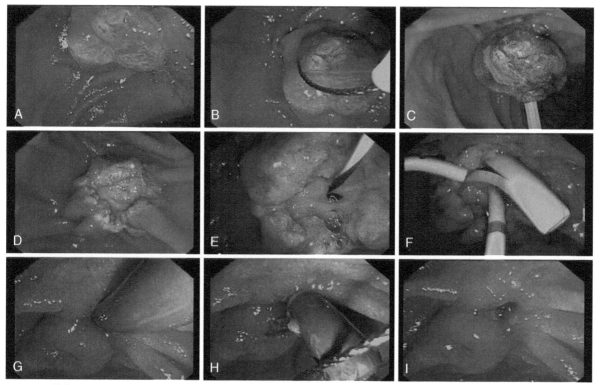

FIG 34.4 En bloc papillectomy of a 15-mm papillary adenoma. **A,** After careful interrogation, **B,** the snare is anchored at the 11 o'clock position and **C,** brought down over the papilla. **D,** Following transection, **E,** the pancreatic duct is cannulated. In this case, **F,** biliary stenting is also performed. **G–I,** During surveillance, the stents are removed, revealing a clean scar with no residual adenoma.

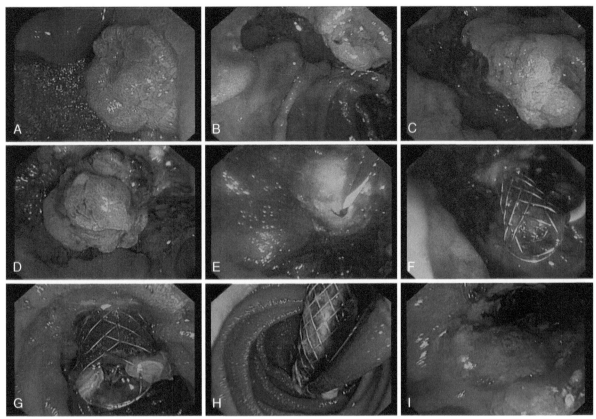

FIG 34.5 **A,** Endoscopic resection (ER) of lateral spreading lesions of the papilla. **B** and **C,** Piecemeal endoscopic mucosal resection of the lateral spreading component is performed, **D,** isolating the papilla for en bloc resection. **E** and **F,** ER is followed by pancreatic and biliary stenting. **G–I,** The stents are removed during surveillance.

to stent removal are rare.[80,81] The post-ER scar (and the distal CBD in PA cases) is carefully examined endoscopically for the presence of residual/recurrent neoplastic tissue, which can be managed by snare excision. If the tissue is especially adherent, then cold forceps avulsion followed by thermal ablative techniques (such as snare tip soft coagulation [STSC] or, more recently, RFA) can be used.

Adverse Events

Despite the advantages of ER for noninvasive DA/PA, the incidence of treatment-related adverse events is generally greater than for ER of similar-sized lesions elsewhere in the gastrointestinal tract. Contributing factors include a relatively thin, fixed duodenal wall, a rich vascular supply, and additional site-specific complications such as pancreatitis. Tables 34.1 and 34.2 summarize outcomes and adverse events of ER of PA and DA, respectively.

Bleeding is the most common adverse event following ER of DA/PA. Intraprocedural bleeding is common, varies greatly between studies due to heterogeneity in definition, and can usually be successfully managed endoscopically. We prefer STSC (Soft Coag effect 4, 80W, ERBE VIO 300 [ERBE, Tübingen, Germany]) as previously described for colonic EMR for nonpulsatile intraprocedural bleeding.[82] Pulsatile bleeding or bleeding unresponsive to STSC can be controlled with coagulation forceps using the same electrocautery settings. Endoscopic clip placement may be applied where other therapies fail, but caution should be exercised to avoid clipping muscle to muscle; because the duodenal wall

is relatively fixed, the muscle layer can be torn, and delayed perforation may ensue. We prefer to clip mucosa to mucosa.

Delayed bleeding occurs in 2%–18% and in 5%–26% of patients following ER of PA and DA, respectively, increasing up to 30% in patients with lesions greater than 30 mm in size,[7,8,12,14,52,70,75,78,83–89] with the most consistent risk factor being lesion size.[40,85,86] Patients without hemodynamic compromise or evidence of ongoing bleeding may be managed conservatively with inpatient observation, intravenous PPI, and fasting, as bleeding may be self-limiting. If endoscopic intervention is required, coagulation forceps are preferred after careful localization of the bleeding point. In cases with massive bleeding unresponsive to endoscopic therapy, angiographic embolization should be considered. ER in the duodenum is a very high bleeding risk procedure, and we generally advocate a more conservative approach to management of periprocedural anticoagulation and antiplatelet therapy than for procedures performed elsewhere in the gastrointestinal tract. An individualized approach in coordination with the cardiology/hematology team regarding bridging of necessary anticoagulation and withholding of antiplatelet therapy is advised.[90]

Perforations are reported in of 0%–3.6% of patients undergoing ER of PA/DA.[8,12,84–86,91,92] Early recognition and management are crucial. Endoscopic clip closure is feasible and suitable for injuries detected during the procedure. Small delayed perforations may respond to hypervigilant conservative management comprising intravenous antibiotics, bowel rest, and close clinical and

TABLE 34.1 **Endoscopic Resection of Papillary Adenomas: Outcomes and Adverse Events**

Reference	Study Type	Number of Patients	Mean Lesion Size (mm)	Technical Success	Bleeding	Perforation	Pancreatitis	Salvage Surgery	Follow-Up (mo)	Recurrence
Wiriyaporn et al, 2014	R	182	19.8	73.6%	12.6%	1.6%	3.8%	NR	22.7	15%
Napoleon et al, 2014	P (M)	79	16.3	87.3%	10%	3.6%	20%	n = 1	36	7.2%
Ismail et al, 2014	R	61	20	NR	18%	3.3%	9.8%	NR	14	25%
Laleman et al, 2013	R	91	NR	78%	12.1%	0%	15.4%	n = 13	32	18.3%
Patel et al, 2011	R	38	NR	81%	5%	0%	8%	NR	17	16%
Irani et al, 2009	R	102	24	84%	5%	2%	10%	n = 1	32	8%
Bohnacker et al, 2005	P	106	20	73%	13%	0%	6%	n = 15	40	15%
Catalano et al, 2004	R (M)	103	22.5	80%	2%	0%	5%	n = 10	36	10%
Cheng et al, 2004	R	55	15	74%	7%	2%	9%	n = 5	30	33%
Kahaleh et al, 2004	P	56	22	86%	4%	0%	7%			
Summary (range)			15–24	73%–93%	2%–18%	0%–3.6%	3.8%–20%	1–15	15–40	7.2%–33%

M, multicenter; *NR*, not reported; *P*, prospective; *R*, retrospective.

TABLE 34.2 **Endoscopic Resection of Nonpapillary Duodenal Adenomas: Outcomes and Adverse Events**

Reference	Study Type	Number of Patients	Mean Lesion Size (mm)	Technical Success	Bleeding	Perforation	Salvage Surgery	Follow-Up (mo)	Recurrence
Chemaly et al, 2008	R	37	19	97%	10%	n = 1	NR	15	3%
Alexander et al, 2009	R	21	27.6	78%	n = 1	0	NR	13	22%
Kedia et al, 2010	R	36	NR	78.6%	14%	0	NR	NR	NR
Kim et al, 2010	R	17	15.1	100%	n = 1	0	NR	29	0
Fanning et al, 2012	R	50	24.2	94%	12%	n = 1	n = 2	11	0
Basford et al, 2014	R	34	25	97%	n = 3	0	NR	NR	NR
Navaneethan et al, 2014	R	54	15.1	92.6%	n = 2	n = 1	n = 1	10.8	n = 1
Seo et al, 2014	R	45	9.1	91.1%	0	n = 3 (ESD)	NR	24.8	n = 1
Nonaka et al, 2015	R	121	12	NR	12%	2% (ESD)	n = 1	51	0
Singh et al, 2016	R	68	22	96%	12%	n = 2	n = 1	15	25%
Klein et al, 2016	R	106	25	96%	15%	n = 3	n = 2	22	14.4%
Summary (range)			9–28	60%–100%	0%–26%	0%–6%	NR	6–25	0%–22%

ESD, endoscopic submucosal dissection; *M*, multicenter; *NR*, not reported; *P*, prospective; *R*, retrospective.

radiological monitoring.[75] CT with oral contrast is the diagnostic procedure of choice, and if a large perforation is identified or an active leak persists, early surgical repair is indicated.[93,94] For ER of PA, FCSEMS are highly valuable for distal CBD or peri-ampullary injuries.[95]

Unique Site-Specific Complications

Pancreatitis complicates 4%–20% of ER procedures performed to treat PA.[52,57,75,96] Randomized and observational data support the routine placement of pancreatic stents,[77] and 5Fr stents are preferred over 3Fr stents.[97] We recommend deployment of the stent with the proximal tip below and not crossing the genu. Cholangitis is uncommon, and may be managed with intravenous antibiotics. ERCP and stent placement may be necessary. Papillary stenosis is an uncommon long-term complication occurring in 1%–2% of cases.[47,76,89] In our experience, most cases resolve following careful balloon dilation and/or serial stent placements. Duodenal luminal stenosis can occur after ER of lesions with extensive circumferential involvement.[63] In such cases, a preemptive dilation management strategy commencing 3 to 4 weeks after resection is appropriate.[59]

Endoscopic Outcomes

Outcomes of ER for DA and PA are reported mainly in retrospective case series, which are usually small and heterogeneous in terms of patient and lesion characteristics. Nevertheless, complete successful removal of DA/PA in a single session has been reported in 70% to 100% of cases, and long-term endoscopic cure of DA/PA can be expected in more than 80% of cases.[7,12,52,57,75,78,83–89,91,98]

Several studies reported on the number of EMR sessions required to achieve complete resection of DA. In these studies, 80% of adenomas were completely removed in a single EMR session, 17% in two sessions, and the remaining 3% in three sessions. A relationship between lesion size, percentage of luminal circumference involved, and EMR success has also been demonstrated,[8] with success rates of 94.7%, 45.5%, and 0% for lesions involving less than 25%, 25%–50%, and greater than 50% of the luminal circumference, respectively. In a recent report from a high-volume center, 87.5% of fully circumferential lesions, both with and without papillary involvement, were successfully removed in a single session.[63]

Recurrence of PA/DA following ER is not uncommon (0%–36% for DA and 0%–33% for PA),[12,13,52,57,70,75,78,85–89,98] and lesion size and piecemeal resection have been identified as risk factors for recurrence.[86,99] These relatively high recurrence rates highlight the need for a meticulous surveillance protocol, which includes initial endoscopic surveillance at 4 to 6 months with subsequent annual surveillance for 5 years to detect late recurrences.[75] For PA, endoscopic surveillance is performed with a side-viewing instrument. The mucosal papillectomy site is inspected, and cholangiography with balloon trawl is often performed as well. Treatment of recurrent/residual disease can be safely and effectively accomplished with a combination of snare resection (we recommend Forced Coag; effect 2, 30W, ERBE VIO 300 [ERBE, Tübingen, Germany]), cold forceps avulsion, and adjuvant thermal ablation. When significant thermal therapy is applied adjacent to the biliary or pancreatic orifice, a stent should be placed to mitigate the risk of pancreatitis, cholangitis, and early stricture formation.

CONCLUSION

ER for DA/PA is a highly effective, though complex, endoscopic procedure. Although no direct comparisons exist, modeling suggests comparable efficacy with superior morbidity, mortality, and cost profile compared with surgery.[100] The adverse event rate of ER for DA/PA is significant compared with other endoscopic therapies, and as such they should be performed by experienced advanced endoscopists practicing in tertiary referral centers. A careful, structured, multidisciplinary approach to patient and lesion assessment, endoscopic management, and surveillance is mandatory.

KEY REFERENCES

2. Culver EL, McIntyre AS: Sporadic duodenal polyps: Classification, investigation, and management, *Endoscopy* 43(2):144–155, 2011.
3. Jepsen JM, Persson M, Jakobsen NO, et al: Prospective study of prevalence and endoscopic and histopathologic characteristics of duodenal polyps in patients submitted to upper endoscopy, *Scand J Gastroenterol* 29:483–487, 1994.
8. Kedia P, Brensinger C, Ginsberg G: Endoscopic predictors of successful endoluminal eradication in sporadic duodenal adenomas and its acute complications, *Gastrointest Endosc* 72(6):1297–1301, 2010.
12. Chemaly M, Ponchon T, Napoleon B, et al: Endoscopic resection of sporadic duodenal adenomas: an efficient technique with a substantial risk of delayed bleeding, *Endoscopy* 40(10):806–810, 2008.
14. Fanning SB, Bourke MJ, Williams SJ, et al: Giant laterally spreading tumors of the duodenum: endoscopic resection outcomes, limitations, and caveats, *Gastrointest Endosc* 75(4):805–812, 2012.
15. Sellner F: Investigations on the significance of the adenoma-carcinoma sequence in the small bowel, *Cancer* 66:702–715, 1990.
16. Okada K, Fujisaki J, Kasuga A, et al: Sporadic nonampullary duodenal adenoma in the natural history of duodenal cancer: a study of follow-up surveillance, *Am J Gastroenterol* 106(2):357–364, 2011.
17. Perzin KH, Bridge MF: Adenomas of the small intestine: a clinicopathologic review of 51 cases and a study of their relationship to carcinoma, *Cancer* 48(3):799–819, 1981.
21. Spigelman AD, Talbot IC, Penna C, et al: Evidence for adenoma-carcinoma sequence in the duodenum of patients with familial adenomatous polyposis. The Leeds Castle Polyposis Group (Upper Gastrointestinal Committee), *J Clin Pathol* 47(8):709–710, 1994.
32. Spigelman AD, Williams CB, Talbot IC, et al: Upper gastrointestinal cancer in patients with familial adenomatous polyposis, *Lancet* 2(8666): 783–785, 1989.
47. Hopper AD, Bourke MJ, Williams SJ, Swan MP: Giant laterally spreading tumors of the papilla: endoscopic features, resection technique, and outcome (with videos), *Gastrointest Endosc* 71(6):967–975, 2010.
52. Bohnacker S, Seitz U, Nguyen D, et al: Endoscopic resection of benign tumors of the duodenal papilla without and with intraductal growth, *Gastrointest Endosc* 62(4):551–560, 2005.
55. Rustagi T, Irani S, Reddy DN, et al: Radiofrequency ablation for intraductal extension of ampullary neoplasms, *Gastrointest Endosc* 2016, [Epub ahead of print].
57. Irani S, Arai A, Ayub K, et al: Papillectomy for ampullary neoplasm: results of a single referral center over a 10-year period, *Gastrointest Endosc* 70(5):923–932, 2009.
65. Chen CH, Tseng LJ, Yang CC, et al: The accuracy of endoscopic ultrasound, endoscopic retrograde cholangiopancreatography, computed tomography, and transabdominal ultrasound in the detection and staging of primary ampullary tumors, *Hepatogastroenterology* 48(42):1750–1753, 2001.
75. Ridtitid W, Tan D, Schmidt SE, et al: Endoscopic papillectomy: risk factors for incomplete resection and recurrence during long-term follow-up, *Gastrointest Endosc* 79(2):289–296, 2014.
77. Harewood GC, Pochron NL, Gostout CJ: Prospective, randomized, controlled trial of prophylactic pancreatic stent placement for endoscopic snare excision of the duodenal ampulla, *Gastrointest Endosc* 62(3):367–370, 2005.
80. Devière J, Reddy DN, Püspök A, et al: Successful management of benign biliary strictures with fully covered self-expanding metal stents, *Gastroenterology* 147(2):385–395, 2014.
86. Klein A, Nayyar D, Bahin FF, et al: Endoscopic mucosal resection of large and giant lateral spreading lesions of the duodenum: success, adverse events, and long-term outcomes, *Gastrointest Endosc* 84(4): 688–696, 2016.
88. Napoleon B, Gincul R, Ponchon T, et al: Endoscopic papillectomy for early ampullary tumors: long-term results from a large multicenter prospective study, *Endoscopy* 46(2):127–134, 2014.
97. Afghani E, Akshintala VS, Khashab MA, et al: 5-Fr vs. 3-Fr pancreatic stents for the prevention of post-ERCP pancreatitis in high-risk patients: a systematic review and network meta-analysis, *Endoscopy* 46(7):573–580, 2014.

A complete reference list can be found online at ExpertConsult .com

35

Acute Colonic Pseudo-Obstruction

Robert J. Ponec and Michael B. Kimmey

INTRODUCTION

Acute colonic pseudo-obstruction (ACPO) is a disorder characterized by massive dilation of the colon in the absence of mechanical obstruction. This severe motility disturbance, also known as *Ogilvie's syndrome*,[1] usually develops in hospitalized patients, and is associated with various medical and surgical conditions. The tension on the colon wall resulting from the extreme dilation can lead to ischemic necrosis and perforation, especially in the cecum. The rate of spontaneous perforation has been reported to be 3% to 15%, with an attendant 40% to 50% mortality rate.[2–5] Despite the potential risk of perforation, approximately 75% of patients with ACPO recover over an average of 3 to 5 days when treated using a variety of conservative measures.[3,4] During the sometimes prolonged recovery phase, however, ACPO contributes greatly to patients' discomfort and immobilization, and prevents institution of enteral nutrition.

The risk of major complications/mortality and the morbidity of the long recovery led to a search for effective and safe therapies, not only to prevent ischemia and perforation but also to speed resolution. Very few controlled trials have evaluated the standard therapies used for ACPO. Nonetheless, conservative management strategies such as nasogastric (NG) suction and measures taken to correct precipitating factors have been the mainstay of treatment.

For the minority (approximately 25%) of patients who fail to respond to conservative therapy and for patients who have severe or prolonged colonic dilation risking perforation, more active interventions are instituted. In the past, surgical cecostomy and hemicolectomy were the main options for severe or refractory cases. Subsequently, colonoscopy and various radiologic procedures were reported to help decompress the colon.[5–11] Medications such as neostigmine have also been shown to be effective.[12] The

timing and combination of conservative and more active interventions must be individualized according to the severity of ACPO and the patient's comorbidities.

EPIDEMIOLOGY

ACPO is relatively uncommon. It can be triggered by various acute medical and surgical illnesses. Typically, rapid-onset abdominal distension begins within a few days of the start of the underlying illness.[2] Because ACPO is uncommon, one must look at reviews that examine several years of reported cases before one can draw conclusions about the epidemiology of the condition. Numerous case reports and reviews describe specific triggers. However, each proposed underlying condition seems to be associated with the development of ACPO in only a very small percentage of cases (Table 35.1). ACPO has been reported after various surgeries, including orthopedic, urologic, gynecologic, and neurologic surgeries, as well as organ transplants.[3,4,13–18] It is seen in obstetrics after vaginal deliveries and cesarean sections.[3,19] Trauma and burn patients sometimes develop ACPO.[3,4,20] Various medical illnesses are known to cause ACPO, including sepsis, respiratory failure, mechanical ventilation, renal failure, myocardial infarction, vascular emergencies, sickle cell crisis, and cancer.[3,4,21–25] Many medications can precipitate or worsen ACPO, especially narcotic analgesics and any medication that decreases peristalsis, such as tricyclic antidepressants or anticholinergic drugs.[5,8,26–28] Although the connection between any of these causes and ACPO is most likely through a disturbance in the autonomic innervation of the bowel, other variables, such as patient age, comorbidities, and factors such as immobility, medications, and electrolyte imbalances, are contributing factors.[2]

In one review of 351 ACPO cases from 1948 to 1980, 88% followed surgery, trauma, or acute medical illness.[3] The remaining

TABLE 35.1   Conditions Associated With Acute Colonic Pseudo-Obstruction

Surgical	Obstetric	Trauma	Medical Illness	Medication
Orthopedic	Normal delivery	Fractures	Sepsis	Narcotic analgesics
Urologic	Cesarean section	Burns	Neurologic disorders	Tricyclic antidepressants
Gynecologic			Cancer	Anesthetic agents
Abdominal			Chemotherapy	Antiparkinson drugs
Transplant			Radiation therapy	Anticholinergics
			Hypothyroidism	
			Myocardial infarction	
			Stroke	
			Respiratory failure, mechanical ventilation	
			Renal failure	
			Electrolyte imbalance (potassium, magnesium, calcium, phosphorus)	
			Viral infections (herpes, varicella zoster)	

12% were classified as idiopathic. This review reported a 15% perforation rate, with a 45% mortality in patients with colonic perforation. This high mortality was attributed in part to the fact that these patients already had serious underlying medical or surgical problems.

In another review of 400 patients from 1970–1985, 95% of the cases had identifiable underlying medical, surgical, or obstetric conditions[4]; this left only 5% to be categorized as idiopathic. ACPO usually developed within 5 days of onset of the underlying condition. The median patient age was approximately 60 years, and the male-to-female ratio was 1.5:1. The perforation rate was 20%, and mortality in patients with perforation was approximately 40%. Overall, mortality in the group was 15%. The mortality rate was affected by age, cecal diameter, length of dilation of colon, presence of ischemia in the bowel wall, and patient comorbidities. One important observation in this review was that patients with a cecal diameter of 8 to 25 cm usually had viable colon without significant ischemia. Thus, cecal size alone is not the only factor in the risk of perforation. Other variables, such as the acuity of the onset and the duration of distention, were also potentially important factors.

A more recent review by Ross et al (2016) of over 100,000 cases from 1998–2011 found a higher rate of ACPO incidence than previously reported (approximately 100/100,000 adult inpatients/year). They noted that, although the incidence rate has increased, the overall mortality has decreased. They found a 7.7 % overall mortality. There was, as expected, much higher mortality in those that failed medical therapy and needed endoscopy or surgery.[7]

PATHOGENESIS

In 1948, Ogilvie[1] first described massive colonic distention in two patients who exhibited onset of abdominal distention over a few weeks, rather than the more acute presentation that we currently refer to as Ogilvie's syndrome. Ironically, by today's criteria, neither patient would be categorized as having ACPO. Both patients were ultimately found to have widespread intra-abdominal malignancy with retroperitoneal involvement of nerve plexuses, leading Ogilvie to speculate that disruption of the autonomic innervation of the colon was the underlying cause of the disorder.[1]

Despite the wide variety of possible triggers for ACPO, the presentation is remarkably consistent. Generally, patients develop severe abdominal distention within 5 days of the onset of the medical or surgical insult. The intestinal dilation is usually most pronounced in the colon, especially proximal to the splenic flexure. On x-ray examination, the appearance is very similar to that of a patient who actually has an obstruction near the upper left colon/splenic flexure, leading to the term *pseudo-obstruction*. These facts led to the hypothesis that the final common pathway of the development of the disease is an acute cessation of effective colonic motility resulting from a disruption of the autonomic supply of the left side of the colon. One hypothesis was that excess sympathetic stimulation of the colon was inhibiting contraction. This hypothesis seemed to be supported by the observation that ACPO can occur in any sort of severe physical stress. In addition, epidural anesthesia to decrease sympathetic output has been reported to be beneficial for ACPO.[29] However, when guanethidine was used to block sympathetic tone, there was very little effect on colonic function in patients with ACPO.[30]

The leading current theory about the pathogenesis of ACPO is that a decrease in parasympathetic stimulation of the colon is more important than an excess of sympathetic input.[31] In the study of guanethidine mentioned previously, patients were first given guanethidine and then treated with neostigmine to block acetylcholinesterase. Patients had a prompt return of colonic function only after receiving the neostigmine, leading to the idea that a loss of parasympathetic tone is important in the development of ACPO. Some authors speculate that the parasympathetic deficiency is most pronounced in the left colon because of disruption of supply from the sacral plexus; this may explain why the left colon is contracted and aperistaltic in ACPO. Since these pioneering studies, the one medical treatment that has had the most consistent success in treatment of ACPO has been the use of neostigmine to cause a sudden increase in acetylcholine concentration at parasympathetic nerve synapses and an increase in colon peristalsis. However, there are other complex mechanisms that are thought to contribute to ACPO, including changes in nitric oxide release, stimulation of opioid receptors on the bowel wall, reflex inhibition of colonic motility caused by stretch-sensitive mechanoreceptors in the gut wall once severe dilation has occurred, etc.[32]

Other factors that likely contribute to the pathogenesis of ACPO are chronic underlying bowel motility disorders and constipation, patient immobility, electrolyte imbalance, medications such as narcotics, and mechanical ventilation. These other factors may worsen the autonomic imbalance, directly suppress muscular function of the colon, or simply increase the amount of gas that is entering the digestive tract, as occurs with mechanical ventilation. At least 50% of patients with ACPO have significant electrolyte abnormalities, especially low potassium, magnesium, and calcium.[4] Secretory diarrhea (with high potassium and low sodium concentration in the stool) can occur in ACPO. This is thought to be due to the effects of autonomic nervous system disturbance and colonic distension on the activity of the apical (BK) potassium channels in the colonic mucosa.[33]

The most feared complication of ACPO is colon perforation. When perforation occurs, it is usually in the right colon, especially the cecum. This relates to the high wall tension in the cecum leading to ischemic necrosis and wall disruption. The right side of the colon, which naturally has a thinner wall and a larger diameter than the left side, has the highest wall tension when the colon is distended. This occurrence is described well by Laplace's law: $T = P \times R/2d$, where T is wall tension, P is pressure in colon lumen, R is radius of the colon, and d is the thickness of the colonic wall. This equation helps explain how small changes in colonic radius in the setting of severe distention of the thin-walled cecum can lead to relatively large changes in wall tension and increase the risk of perforation.

Usually the perforation risk is not very high in patients with a cecal diameter of less than 12 cm. Nonetheless, studies have shown that patients with ACPO and a cecal diameter greater than 25 cm can recover without incident, and that this may also occur in patients with prior or chronic dilation. Other variables, such as elasticity of the muscle wall, adequacy of blood supply, and time course of distention, must be important as well in determining whether the colon remains viable. Some studies indicate an association between the duration of ACPO and perforation risk, and indicate that patients with persistence of distention for more than 5 days have higher perforation rates.[34]

CLINICAL FEATURES

ACPO is seen mainly in patients who are hospitalized for an acute medical, surgical, obstetric, or traumatic event. The condition progresses at a variable rate, usually over 2 to 7 days. The nearly universal symptom is progressive abdominal distention. The reported frequency of other symptoms is quite varied. Abdominal pain (10%–80%), nausea (10%–60%), vomiting (10%–60%), diarrhea (30%–40%), constipation (40%–50%), and respiratory compromise resulting from distention all have been reported.[3–5,8] Patients with ischemia and perforation are much more likely to have abdominal pain and fever.

Physical examination findings include a markedly distended abdomen that is usually tympanitic on percussion. Bowel sounds are often present. Although some tenderness has been noted (in 60% of patients in some reports), significant tenderness or guarding should raise suspicion for perforation.

Laboratory abnormalities include an elevated white blood cell count in up to 25% of patients without perforation and in almost 100% of patients with perforation.[4] Abnormalities are often seen in electrolytes such as potassium, calcium, magnesium, and phosphorus. Abnormal thyroid function is not caused by ACPO, but can occur concurrently, and is thought to contribute to colonic dysfunction. These various laboratory values should be checked in patients with ACPO and corrected, as needed.

Abdominal x-ray films show distention of the colon that is usually most pronounced in the cecum, as well as the ascending and transverse areas. In contrast to patients with severe obstipation, the colon is filled primarily with gas, not stool. There is often an apparent "cutoff" near the splenic flexure with a collapsed left colon. The location of the cutoff varies. In one review, the cutoff was at the splenic flexure in 56% of patients, at the hepatic flexure in 18%, and at the descending or sigmoid colon in 27%.[36] Although the small bowel usually exhibits less dilation in ACPO, one report indicated that 80% of patients had some small bowel dilation.[36] Air-fluid levels have been reported in 40% of patients. On x-ray, gas in the bowel wall and free intraperitoneal air are indicative of colonic ischemic necrosis and perforation, respectively. Radiographic studies like computed tomography (CT) scan or water-soluble contrast enema are often needed to rule out a true mechanical obstruction. As discussed in the treatment section, the use of water-soluble contrast material has been reported to have a therapeutic effect in some patients.[32,35] Abdominal CT scan with intravenous (IV) contrast has largely replaced contrast enemas in most centers for a number of reasons. In addition to being easier to perform, CT is safe and is often readily available. There is concern about perforation with contrast enema, as the study may put more pressure into an already distended colon. The CT accurately measures cecal diameter, which is important in determining risk of perforation. CT can detect thickening of the bowel wall and bowel wall gas as an indicator of ischemic necrosis and impending perforation.[36]

DIFFERENTIAL DIAGNOSIS

Two major considerations in the differential diagnosis of ACPO are mechanical bowel obstruction and toxic megacolon resulting from an enteric infection or inflammatory bowel disease (IBD). In addition, patients are sometimes first diagnosed with chronic colonic pseudo-obstruction when they are hospitalized for other reasons, making it important to establish early that the condition is truly acute and not chronic.

Mechanical colon obstruction from causes such as colon cancer, sigmoid volvulus, and diverticulitis must be confidently ruled out before considering specific therapies for ACPO. Often, the fact that patients with ACPO continue to have watery bowel movements is helpful to indicate that a complete obstruction is unlikely. In some cases, the presence of some gas in the rectum or throughout the entire colon, as seen on plain x-ray, also helps rule out obstruction. Nonetheless, these indicators are not totally reliable. Either CT scan, water-soluble contrast enema, or colonoscopy may be required to rule out mechanical obstruction.

Toxic megacolon resulting from infections such as *Clostridium difficile* should be considered in patients who have been exposed to antibiotics or prolonged care in a hospital or nursing facility, where they may have contracted the infection. Generally, such patients have severe diarrhea before the onset of the abdominal distention. Other colonic infections leading to toxic megacolon have been reported, particularly in immunosuppressed patients. In some cases, these patients have a presentation that is seemingly indistinguishable from classic ACPO. However, when the colonic distention is due to infection, patients usually have (1) an elevated white blood cell count; (2) more widespread thickening of the bowel wall on x-ray films (especially on CT); and (3) endoscopic evidence of severe colonic erythema, edema, ulceration, or pseudomembranes on flexible sigmoidoscopy or colonoscopy. Stool studies for enteric pathogens and *C. difficile* toxin are important in this setting.[37]

Similarly, toxic megacolon resulting from IBD can usually be differentiated from ACPO by a review of the patient's clinical history, laboratory results, x-ray films, and findings on endoscopy.[38] Patients with IBD should have had a history of diarrhea (often bloody) and abdominal cramps before the development of colonic distention. Blood test results usually show leukocytosis. Abdominal x-ray films/CT often show bowel wall edema. Sigmoidoscopy should show changes consistent with IBD.

Lastly, the presence of chronic pseudo-obstruction can often be excluded by a careful review of the patient's history, old records, and prior abdominal radiographs when available.

TREATMENT

Because ACPO is uncommon, there have been few randomized controlled trials to actually test the treatments that are currently considered the standard of care. Most data are from reviews, observational studies, and case presentations. Therapy is generally divided into conservative measures and active interventions. Because at least 75% of patients with ACPO experience resolution with a combination of conservative measures, these are generally tried first for at least 24 to 48 hours in most patients before more active interventions are considered.[39] Reported success from these measures ranges from 33% to 100%, and is usually approximately 75%.[20]

The following sections describe conservative therapy, medication therapy, colonoscopy, and surgical approaches for ACPO. These treatments are often combined (simultaneously or sequentially). Conservative measures are typically continued when more active interventions are added. The order and combination of these measures must be individualized to a patient's clinical presentation and course. For instance, a patient with a cecal diameter of over 12 cm and other high risk features may be better served by starting active therapy sooner, rather than waiting 24 to 48 hours while giving conservative measures. There have been a number of excellent reviews recently on the topic of treatment of ACPO.[32,39–50,50a] Fig. 35.1 outlines a proposed treatment algorithm for most patients with ACPO, modified from the American Society for Gastrointestinal Endoscopy (ASGE) practice guideline on treatment of this condition.[39] In the algorithm, a key point is that this is a treatment for acute colonic distention, not chronic pseudo-obstruction. First, ischemia and perforation need to be excluded. Then, mechanical obstruction from tumors or benign strictures (e.g., diverticulosis, sigmoid volvulus, etc.) is treated with endoscopic techniques or surgery, or at least ruled out with appropriate imaging. Finally, one starts down the path of the algorithm to treat ACPO only after all these other possibilities are convincingly ruled out.

Conservative Therapy

Conservative measures for treatment of ACPO include most, if not all, of the following, depending on individual circumstances.[26] The patient is made *nil per os* (NPO), and NG suction is used to prevent more gas from entering the gastrointestinal tract. At least initially, osmotic laxatives (especially fermentable ones like lactulose) should be avoided, as they can increase colonic distension and gas. Patients should be mobilized as much as possible. If the patient is bed-bound, the patient's position should be

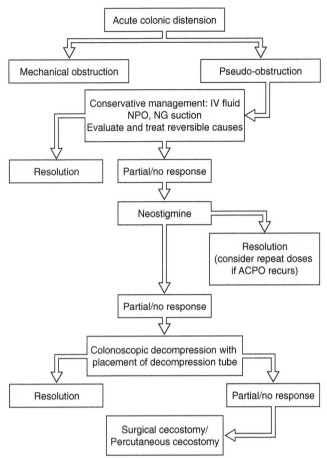

FIG 35.1 Suggested algorithm for the management of acute colonic pseudo-obstruction (ACPO). This algorithm has been adapted from the practice guideline published by the American Society for Gastrointestinal Endoscopy. *IV*, intravenous; *NG*, nasogastric; *NPO, nil per os*. (From Dominitz J, Baron T, Harrison M, et al: The role of endoscopy in the management of patients with known and suspected colonic obstruction and pseudo-obstruction. *Gastrointest Endoscopy* 71[4]:669–679, 2010.)

changed often from side to side and, when possible, into the prone and knee-to-chest position. A search for contributing factors should be made, with correction of as many as possible. One should withdraw medications that interfere with colonic motility, such as narcotic analgesics, anticholinergics, and calcium channel blockers. Laboratory tests should include complete blood count, comprehensive chemistry panel, and lactic acid level. If there is diarrhea, then stool should be sent for *C. difficile* toxin detection and for cultures. Electrolyte imbalance (especially potassium, calcium, magnesium, and phosphorus) should be corrected. Regular rectal examinations every 6 hours have been advocated as a way to encourage passage of colonic gas. Placement of a rectal tube is more often used for this purpose. Gentle tap water enemas are controversial, but are advocated by some authors as a way to liquefy remaining stool. A water-soluble contrast enema, which can liquefy stool, is commonly performed to exclude mechanical obstruction. Some authors have reported a stimulant effect on motility that sometimes speeds recovery.[35] The use of prophylactic antibiotics has not been studied, and is not common practice. If a patient has a fever or an elevated white blood cell count, broad-spectrum antibiotics can be considered while a careful evaluation is under way for signs of colonic ischemia, perforation, or other infections.

Conservative measures are continued for 24 to 48 hours before more active intervention is initiated. This recommendation is not based on controlled data, but rather on the observation that patients whose severe colon dilation (> 12 cm) persists for 4 to 5 days have a higher risk of ischemia and perforation.[4]

Although conservative therapy is generally successful, return of colon function in responders takes an average of 5 days. During this time, patients are contending with the consequences of ACPO, including distention, pain, prevention of enteral nutrition, compromised respiratory status, and delay in ambulation that can lead to other morbidities such as thromboembolism, atelectasis, and pneumonia. These facts have led to a search for a safe and effective treatment not only for patients who are refractory to conservative measures but also to provide a prompter resolution early in the course of the illness. Numerous active interventions have been reported to be useful for ACPO, including medications such as neostigmine,[12] colonoscopy with or without placement of a decompression tube,[51-55] diatrizoate meglumine (Gastrografin [Bracco Diagnostics Inc., Monroe Township, NJ]) enema,[35] radiologic procedures such as placement of a colonic decompression tube,[11] cecostomy (surgical, endoscopic, or radiologic), and surgical resection of part of the colon (mainly reserved for cases of perforation or significant ischemic necrosis).

Medical Therapy

Medications that stimulate colon motility have become the key part of active therapy. The most promising medication so far for treatment of ACPO is neostigmine, an inhibitor of acetylcholinesterase. Neostigmine causes a transient but significant increase in acetylcholine concentration, resulting in a pronounced increase in cholinergic stimulus throughout the body, including in the colon wall at the synapses between the gut wall nerves and the gut smooth muscle. The leading theory about the pathogenesis of ACPO is that there is an autonomic imbalance, with an increase in sympathetic tone and a decrease in the parasympathetic stimulus of the colon. Both these changes are thought to have a negative impact on colon motility. This theory led to studies of drugs that either decrease sympathetic tone or increase parasympathetic tone as a means to restore colon function.

In the 1960s, Neely and Catchpole (1971)[56] studied the effects of guanethidine (a sympathetic antagonist) and neostigmine (Prostigmin [Abbott Bioresearch Center, Worcester, MA], a cholinergic drug) on small bowel motility and found that these medications seemed to restore peristalsis. In 1992, Hutchinson and Griffiths[30] treated 11 ACPO patients first with guanethidine and then with neostigmine. They found that 8 of 11 patients had prompt return of bowel motility but only after the neostigmine infusion. In 1995, Stephenson and coworkers[14] presented results from a study showing that 11 of 12 ACPO patients treated with 2.5 mg of IV neostigmine had prompt resolution of their condition. These observations were confirmed by subsequent studies, including prompt clinical resolution in 75% of ACPO cases as presented by Turegano-Fuentes and coworkers[57] in 1997 and in 26 of 28 cases treated by Trevisani and colleagues,[58] whose results were published in 2000. Physiologic studies with neostigmine indicate that its indirect effect on muscarinic receptors in the bowel wall, which are presumably mediated through increased local acetylcholine concentrations, results in

increased colonic tone and increased coordinated colonic propulsion.[59]

Because ACPO often resolves with conservative therapy alone, controlled trials of neostigmine and other therapies are important. The first prospective randomized controlled trial on the use of IV neostigmine included 21 patients with ACPO (refractory to at least 24 hours of conservative measures and with a cecal diameter > 10 cm) who were randomly assigned to receive a 3-minute IV infusion of either 2.0 mg of neostigmine or saline administered by a physician blinded to the treatment allocation.[12] The endpoints included immediate passage of flatus and stool; the amount of decrease in the measured abdominal girth; and the change in the diameters of the cecum, ascending, and transverse colon on abdominal x-ray films obtained 3 hours later (Fig. 35.2). Of the 11 patients randomly assigned to neostigmine, 10 had prompt resolution with substantial responses in all the measured endpoints. The one nonresponder subsequently had a response when an open-label neostigmine dose was given 3 hours later. The median time to passage of flatus was 4 minutes (range 3–30 minutes). None of the patients given placebo responded, despite the continuation of conservative measures in all patients. Seven patients from the placebo group were subsequently treated with open-label neostigmine 3 hours later, and all had a prompt response. Since this publication, several uncontrolled studies and case reports have also reported similar results, with approximately 80% to 90% of patients usually showing a prompt response to the drug. Different doses have been used, ranging from 1 mg to 2.5 mg, either by slow IV push or by IV infusion for instance, over 30 minutes. A similar number of patients exhibited a sustained response after a single dose of neostigmine in these other studies as well, usually approximately 60% to 70%.[60-68] Some studies have shown success with repeated doses of the drug for patients with partial responses and recurrences, with the number of patients experiencing a sustained response increasing to the 80% to 90% range.[14] See Table 35.2 for a summary of the evidence for the use of neostigmine for ACPO.[32,48,69]

Factors that predict response to neostigmine have been examined. One retrospective review showed an 89% initial response and a 61% sustained response to a single dose of neostigmine. The authors found that narcotic medication use decreased not only the spontaneous resolution rate but also the response rate to neostigmine. Ambulatory patients had higher response rates as well. Interestingly, colon diameter and the duration of ACPO before treatment did not influence response rate.[63] Another prospective study enrolled 27 patients and found that electrolyte abnormalities and the use of antimotility drugs were associated with decreased response to neostigmine.[64]

Side effects of neostigmine include abdominal pain, nausea, vomiting, sweating, excess salivation, bronchospasm, and symptomatic bradycardia. Patients at risk for bradycardia, such as patients with preexisting bradyarrhythmias and patients receiving β-blockers, are at potentially higher risk of complications from neostigmine, as are patients with severe bronchospasm. Some caution in patient selection is needed. Nonetheless, neostigmine can be used in most patients with ACPO when proper monitoring and precautions are in place. Patients should be kept supine on a pad or bedpan for the first 30 minutes after neostigmine administration, and should be monitored by continuous electrocardiogram and frequent, intermittent blood pressure measurements. Transient bradycardia can occur but usually resolves quickly without treatment because of the short half-life of

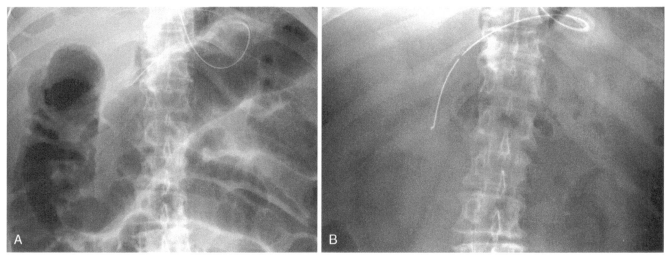

FIG 35.2 **A,** Dilated transverse colon and hepatic flexure in a patient with acute colonic pseudo-obstruction. A nasogastric tube is present in the stomach. **B,** Colonic gas is no longer present 3 hours after administration of neostigmine. The nasogastric tube remains in place. (From Ponec RJ, Saunders MD, Kimmey MB: Neostigmine for the treatment of acute colonic pseudo-obstruction. *N Engl J Med* 341[3]:137–141, 1999. Copyright © 1999 Massachusetts Medical Society. All rights reserved.)

TABLE 35.2   Studies on Intravenous Neostigmine for Acute Colonic Pseudo-Obstruction

Authors	# of Patients	Initial Success (%)	Long-Term Success (%) (Including Second Dose)
Prospective Randomized Controlled Trials			
Ponec et al, 1999	21	91	82
Amaro et al, 2000	20	94	89
van der Spoel et al, 2001	13	85	85
Fanaei et al, 2008	42	95	95
Uncontrolled Trials, Prospective and Retrospective			
Combination of studies 1992–2006	150	80% average response (range 64%–93%)	96% average response (range 31%–100%)

neostigmine. Atropine should be immediately available but should be given only if bradycardia is severe, prolonged, or associated with significant hypotension or persistent symptoms. Although neostigmine is partly cleared by plasma cholinesterase, approximately one-half of the clearance occurs in the kidneys; patients with renal failure have a prolonged half-life of neostigmine. In anephric patients, the elimination half-life is approximately 180 minutes, compared with 80 minutes in patients with normal renal function.[70]

Administration of glycopyrrolate, a selective anticholinergic agent, has been proposed as a way to decrease neostigmine side effects like bradycardia and bronchoconstriction. Because it has less effect on the bowel, glycopyrrolate might not interfere with the stimulatory effect of neostigmine in restoring colonic contraction. Although there has not been an organized study on this combined neostigmine/glycopyrrolate administration specifically in patients with ACPO, one controlled study in spinal cord injury patients showed that the combination was as effective as neostigmine alone in prompting colon evacuation. In addition, bradycardia and bronchoconstriction were not seen when the drugs were given together.[71] Because it seems to be rapidly effective in most patients with ACPO and has a low side effect profile

compared with other active therapies, such as colonoscopy or surgery, neostigmine appears early in the suggested treatment algorithm (see Fig. 35.1).[37,72,73] Although mainly studied in adult patients, there have been case reports of successful use in pediatric patients as well.[24,25,74] Most studies indicate that, as long as conservative measures are continued, the recurrence rate of ACPO after neostigmine is low.[12] Nonetheless, repeat doses can be tried in case of recurrence before resorting to more invasive techniques. Because the elimination half-life is 80 minutes, retreatment is not advisable at intervals less than every 3 hours.

Because there is the issue of recurrence of colonic distension after neostigmine, as well as after colonoscopic decompression, efforts have been made to reduce recurrence. One controlled study showed that, after successful decompression with either neostigmine or colonoscopy (with decompression tube placement), the administration of polyethylene glycol solution (PEG) twice daily (orally or per NG mixed with water) for 7 days reduced the recurrence rate for colonic distension (0/15 in PEG group vs. 5/15 in placebo group).[75]

Slower infusion of neostigmine has been proposed for ACPO. Neostigmine drip over 24 hours at 0.4 to 0.8 mg/hr has been shown to be very effective in critically ill intensive care unit patients with ileus and ACPO. Eleven out of thirteen patients in the neostigmine group recovered bowel motility and passed stools, whereas none of the eleven in the placebo group did. Interestingly, these authors did not observe the neostigmine side effects of bradycardia or bronchospasm.[76] Others have also shown success in treating patients who were refractory to bolus neostigmine by giving slow infusion of neostigmine at 0.4 mg/hr. There were few side effects.[77]

Although oral neostigmine is not recommended, a long-acting oral acetyl cholinesterase inhibitor, pyridostigmine, has been tested in patients with ACPO. Seven patients with refractory ACPO that recurred after neostigmine treatment and colonic decompression were given pyridostigmine 10–30 mg PO twice daily. All seven had successful resolution of ACPO.[78]

Other medical therapies have been reported, including prokinetic drugs such as metoclopramide,[79] erythromycin,[80,81] and cisapride.[82] Most of these reports have been anecdotal, involving only one or two patients. Published reports on the use of metoclopramide have been disappointing. Some reports have questioned the wisdom of applying a prokinetic such as metoclopramide out of concern that its main stimulus is on emptying the upper gut; this theoretically may deliver even more gas to the colon without adequate stimulus of the colon itself, and worsen the distention there. As the use of opioid medications has been associated with ACPO, and also with failure to respond to conservative and neostigmine therapy, there may theoretically be some benefit to the use of peripheral μ-opioid receptor blockers like methylnaltrexone. There are case reports of the successful use of methylnaltrexone in ACPO.[83,84] However, the results from studies on the use of this and other peripheral μ-opioid receptor antagonists like alvimopan have been quite mixed.[83,85,86] Additionally, case reports have described some success with 5-HT$_4$ receptor agonists like prucalopride and tegaserod, but more study is needed.[87,88]

Colonoscopy

Colonoscopy is useful in treating ACPO in many ways. First, it is used to suction extra gas and decompress the colon directly. Colonoscopy is also used to rule out mechanical obstruction and to check for signs of colonic mucosal ischemia and necrosis. Lastly, it can be used to place a guidewire into the proximal colon, over which a decompression tube can be placed. The reported rate of intubation proximal to the hepatic flexure in the setting of ACPO is at least 70%.[5]

Although there are no randomized controlled trials proving its efficacy, colonoscopic decompression has been central in the treatment of ACPO patients who fail conservative and pharmacologic measures. Its successful use was first reported in 1977 by Kukor and Dent.[6] Since then, numerous uncontrolled studies have reported initial clinical success with colonoscopy in approximately 70% of cases.[8,9,15] Nonetheless, a high recurrence rate of 40% may lead to the need for repeated colonoscopies (sometimes two or more additional procedures) to maintain the response.[5,8,51,89] Several authors have reported a lower recurrence rate if a decompression tube is left in place, especially if it is proximal to the hepatic flexure.[52] One institution compared the recurrence rate in patients who received colonoscopy with decompression tube placement with historical controls who received colonoscopy alone, and found recurrence rates of 0% versus 45%, respectively.[53] Some authors have criticized uncontrolled studies on colonoscopic decompression because they do not include control groups that receive conservative therapy alone (which may have differed over

time) and have a referral bias, in that they only involve patients who were specifically referred for the purpose of colonoscopic decompression.[5,54]

The potential benefits of colonoscopy with respect to diagnosis and therapy need to be weighed against the risks of the procedure. The risk of further inflating and stretching an already dilated and unprepared colon leads many to suggest that colonoscopy should not be used up front as a diagnostic tool, especially as there are safer diagnostic alternatives like CT scan.[48,49] As a therapeutic maneuver, colonoscopy has more acceptance, but is still considered a high risk procedure with uncertain outcome that often needs to be repeated due to recurrence of ACPO, clogging, or dislodgement of the decompression tube, if one is placed.[8] A summary of the expert consensus on several aspects of therapeutic colonoscopy for ACPO follows.[55] Colonoscopy in ACPO patients is technically difficult (performed in the unprepared colon of seriously ill patients) and carries an increased perforation risk of approximately 3%.[8,54] It should be performed only by expert endoscopists. A gentle tap water enema can be given first, but is usually not needed because the stool remaining in the colon is usually already liquefied. In addition, enemas may increase the risk of perforation in patients with ACPO. During colonoscopy, air insufflation must be kept to a minimum. Use of carbon dioxide is preferable because it can be absorbed. As each new dilated segment is entered with the colonoscope, it should be suctioned and decompressed. The mucosa should be washed periodically to examine for ischemic changes, including duskiness to frank cyanosis, mucosal hemorrhage, and ulceration. Cecal intubation is desirable but not critical. One should try to advance the colonoscope at least to the hepatic flexure. Fluoroscopy is useful for helping determine the position of the colonoscope tip and for placement of a decompression tube, and should be used regularly.

Traditionally, it has been recommended that, if mucosal ischemia is found, the colonoscope should be withdrawn, and the patient should be sent for urgent surgical resection, usually of the right colon, which is usually the area that is most severely affected. However, successful treatment with conservative measures and tube decompression has been reported even in patients with endoscopic evidence of ischemia without necrosis (e.g., deep ulceration, exudate, black mucosa).[90] Thus, colonoscopic decompression can still be tried as the primary therapy when the mucosal appearance noticeably improves promptly with decompression, or if the changes seen indicate that there is still intact colon wall (erythema, mucosal hemorrhage, and scant shallow ulceration only).

A tube for decompression should be placed at the initial colonoscopy, if possible. This can be a frustrating endeavor, and even with excellent technique and fluoroscopic guidance, there is a tendency for the decompression tube to migrate distally in the colon either during placement, when the guidewire is pulled back, or in the 24 hours after placement. Various techniques have been described. The most popular and most effective to date is the placement of a guidewire through the colonoscope when the colonoscope tip is in the cecum or at least proximal to the hepatic flexure. The colonoscope is withdrawn over the wire, and the wire is used to guide a decompression tube into position. Fluoroscopy should be used to confirm that the colonoscope is in a straight or a "question mark" configuration without looping prior to placement of the guidewire, and to assure that the guidewire remains in a nonlooped configuration during withdrawal of the colonoscope and subsequent passage of the decompression tube. A final position of the tube with the tip proximal to the splenic flexure can be satisfactory. Commercially available decompression kits use a 0.035-inch wire, an inner stiffening catheter, and outer drainage catheters that range from 7-Fr to 14-Fr in diameter. Other authors suggest using stiffer wires and larger tubes, such as a modified 18-Fr Levin or an NG tube. The tube is taped securely to the buttock, placed on low intermittent suction, and flushed with water (50–150 mL) at least every 6 hours to decrease clogging. Endoscopic treatment of ACPO was reviewed by Saunders in 2007,[43] and was also outlined in 2010 in the ASGE practice guideline.[39]

Daily abdominal x-ray films should be performed. The diameter of the cecum, ascending colon, and transverse colon should be tracked, and one should be vigilant for signs of pneumatosis and free intraperitoneal air. Although there is sometimes a dramatic decrease in colonic dilatation immediately after decompression, more commonly the colonic dilatation decreases gradually (Fig. 35.3). One study showed that the mean change in cecal diameter 4 hours and 1 day after colonoscopic decompression was only approximately 2 cm.[91] Thus, patience is advised, as long as the patient is clinically improving and the tube is in good position and flushes easily.

One report describes an alternative method for advancing a transanal decompression tube into the proximal colon using a steerable tricomponent coaxial catheter under fluoroscopic guidance.[11] Successful placement proximal to the hepatic flexure and decompression were seen in four consecutive patients. Percutaneous endoscopic cecostomy[92] can be performed in patients with refractory or recurring colonic distention, so long as there are no signs of ischemic necrosis. The technique is virtually identical to the placement of a percutaneous endoscopic gastrostomy. Acute and delayed complications, including perforation, abscess, and peritonitis, are reported to be an issue with percutaneous cecostomy.[32,48,93]

Surgery

Surgery is reserved for patients with ACPO who fail medical and colonoscopic therapy, or for patients with advanced ischemia or evidence of colonic perforation. Retrospective studies have shown that surgery is associated with higher morbidity and mortality than other therapies. This finding probably reflects the fact that the patients selected for surgery had more severe ACPO and more serious underlying conditions, although the extra morbidity of general anesthesia and an abdominal operation in such patients undoubtedly also has a significant impact.

For patients without peritoneal signs or evidence of perforation or severe ischemic bowel, tube cecostomy is advocated. Cecostomy has a high success rate in terms of decompression of the right colon.

For patients with peritoneal signs, a more extensive exploration is recommended, with the surgical findings guiding the type of intervention.[2] If, at surgery, a viable cecum is found, a tube cecostomy can still be performed. However, if there is significant ischemia or perforation, then colonic resection is advised, with the decision whether to do a primary anastomosis versus an ileostomy and mucous fistula depending on the patient's condition and the degree of peritoneal contamination.

In addition to the more traditional open surgical approach and placement of a Foley catheter or similar drain into the cecum, there are other variations on the technique. One is to perform

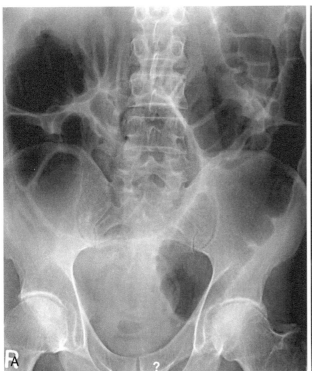
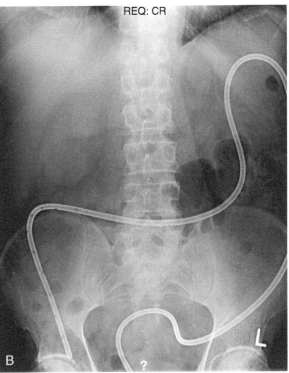

FIG 35.3 A, Plain abdominal radiograph from a patient with acute colonic pseudo-obstruction. **B,** Radiograph after colonoscopy and placement of a 14-Fr colonic decompression tube reveals a significant reduction in colonic gas. (From Nietsch H, Kimmey MB: Acute colonic pseudo-obstruction. In Waye J, Rex DK, Williams CB, editors: *Colonoscopy: principles and practice,* London, 2004, Blackwell Science, pp 596–602.)

laparoscopy first to check cecal viability, and then to use the laparoscope to help place a cecostomy tube. T-fasteners are used to hold the cecal wall up against the abdominal wall.[94]

Other methods of placing cecal tubes have been reported.[95] Radiologic methods have used fluoroscopy or CT scan to guide placement of T-fasteners and drainage tubes in the cecum.[10,96-98] Most authors argue that, given the availability and effectiveness of neostigmine and colonoscopy, surgery should be reserved for patients who have signs of perforation or peritonitis. Surgery for decompression in "refractory" cases should be infrequent.[32,48,99]

FUTURE TRENDS

The major challenge in assessing therapies for ACPO is that it is an uncommon condition that most often occurs in seriously ill hospitalized patients. It causes perforation in approximately 3% of patients, with up to 50% mortality if this occurs. Thus, prospective controlled studies designed to demonstrate a difference in hard endpoints such as perforation and death are not likely to be forthcoming. However, controlled trials that track intermediate endpoints such as colon diameter and clinical resolution of the distention are possible. Since the first randomized controlled trial was performed using neostigmine, there have been a number of other trials, mostly retrospective and uncontrolled, that confirmed that the initial and sustained success for neostigmine is approximately 80% to 90%, and that it is often useful in recurrences. In addition, there is evidence that PEG solutions are helpful in preventing recurrences after initial success with conservative measures, neostigmine, or colonoscopy.

Most cases of ACPO resolve with conservative therapy, but the time to resolution can be many days, making spontaneous resolution still a significantly morbid event. Emphasis should be placed on finding therapies that speed resolution safely and with minimal dependence on invasive procedures. A 2012 review concluded that neostigmine certainly speeds resolution of ACPO.[47]

Because ACPO can occur as the result of nearly any severe medical condition or any surgery, it is hard to imagine how to prevent it completely. Nonetheless, certain situations are especially associated with ACPO, such as severe trauma, major orthopedic procedures, and pelvic surgeries. Although this has not been systematically studied, it is logical to hypothesize that early, prophylactic application of some of the measures described in the sections on conservative and medication therapy might prevent some cases.

Medication is likely to be the biggest area of future research in ACPO. Although it already has a good track record, neostigmine has its limitations. It is relatively contraindicated in patients with certain cardiac and pulmonary conditions, and a significant minority of ACPO patients do not respond to it or experience recurrence after an initial response. As has been reviewed in this chapter, there may be ways to address these limitations. One is to infuse neostigmine more slowly, such as over 30 minutes, or even as a 24-hour infusion at 0.4–0.8 mg/hr. Another is to pretreat with glycopyrrolate, which has been shown to block the cardiac and respiratory side effects without much impact on neostigmine's effect on the bowel.[100] Whether this combination will be as successful as neostigmine alone remains to be proven. For recurrent or refractory ACPO, oral pyridostigmine or 24-hour infusion of neostigmine have both shown promise, but confirmatory studies are needed.

Safer prokinetic agents could be applied earlier and more liberally. These could include μ-opioid receptor antagonists and 5-HT$_4$ receptor agonists to restart bowel motility. These could be helpful as preventive treatment in high-risk patients (like certain surgical and trauma cases), in initial medical therapy, and also to prevent recurrences. So far, none of these "safer" agents have come anywhere close to the effectiveness of neostigmine, but hopefully there will be more research on them in the future.

Lastly, although colonoscopy already has a high success rate, improvements in minimally invasive endoscopic techniques would be of further benefit, such as better decompression tubes.

Nevertheless, it is important to remember that, despite all the research on new therapies, three out of four patients do resolve with standard conservative measures, as outlined in this chapter. For the one in four that does not respond, we are fortunate to have a treatment algorithm that works for most cases. Additionally, there is hope that, in the future, with more study and further improvements to this algorithm, ACPO will usually be corrected promptly, greatly decreasing its morbidity and mortality.

KEY REFERENCES

1. Ogilvie H: Large-intestine colic due to sympathetic deprivation: a new clinical syndrome, *BMJ* 2:671–673, 1948.
3. Nanni G, Garbini A, Luchetti P, et al: Ogilvie's syndrome (acute colonic pseudo-obstruction): review of literature (October 1948 to March 1980) and report of four additional cases, *Dis Colon Rectum* 25:157–166, 1982.
4. Vanek VW, Al-Salti M: Acute colonic pseudo-obstruction (Ogilvie's syndrome): an analysis of 400 cases, *Dis Colon Rectum* 29:203–210, 1986.
5. Jetmore AB, Timmcke AE, Gathright B, et al: Ogilvie's syndrome: colonoscopic decompression and analysis of predisposing factors, *Dis Colon Rectum* 35:1135–1142, 1992.
6. Kukor JS, Dent TL: Colonoscopic decompression of massive nonobstructive cecal dilation, *Arch Surg* 112:512–517, 1997.
8. Geller A, Petersen BT, Gostout CJ: Endoscopic decompression for acute colonic pseudo-obstruction, *Gastrointest Endosc* 44:144–150, 1996.
12. Ponec RJ, Saunders MD, Kimmey MB: Neostigmine for the treatment of acute colonic pseudo-obstruction, *N Engl J Med* 341:137–141, 1999.
14. Stephenson BM, Morgan AR, Salaman JR, et al: Ogilvie's syndrome: a new approach to an old problem, *Dis Colon Rectum* 38:424–427, 1995.
30. Hutchinson R, Griffiths C: Acute colonic pseudo-obstruction: a pharmacologic approach, *Ann R Coll Surg Engl* 74:364–367, 1992.
31. Stephenson BM, Morgan AR, Drake N, et al: Parasympathomimetic decompression of acute colonic pseudo-obstruction, *Lancet* 342:1181–1182, 1993.
32. DeGiorgio R, Knowles CH: Acute colonic pseudo-obstruction, *Br J Surg* 96:229–239, 2009.
39. Dominitz J, Baron T, Harrison M, et al: The role of endoscopy in the management of patients with known and suspected colonic obstruction and pseudo-obstruction, *Gastrointest Endoscopy* 71:669–679, 2010.
40. Saunders M, Kimmey M: Systematic review: acute colonic pseudo-obstruction, *Aliment Pharmacol Ther* 22:917–925, 2005.
43. Saunders M: Acute colonic pseudo-obstruction, *Gastrointest Endoscopy Clin N Am* 17:341–360, 2007.
48. Jain A, Vargas HD: Advances and challenges in the management of acute colonic pseudo-obstruction (Ogilvie syndrome), *Clin Colon Rectal Surg* 25:37–45, 2012.
55. Rex DK: Colonoscopy and acute colonic pseudo-obstruction, *Gastrointest Endosc Clin N Am* 7:499–508, 1997.
56. Neely J, Catchpole B: Ileus: the restoration of alimentary-tract motility by pharmacological means, *Br J Surg* 58:21–28, 1971.
57. Turegano-Fuentes F, Munoz-Jimenez F, Dell Valle-Hernandez E, et al: Early resolution of Ogilvie's syndrome with intravenous neostigmine: a simple, effective treatment, *Dis Colon Rectum* 40:1353–1357, 1997.

58. Trevisani GT, Hyman NH, Church JM: Neostigmine: safe and effective treatment for acute colonic pseudo-obstruction, *Dis Colon Rectum* 43:599–603, 2000.

63. Loftus CG, Harewood MD, Baron TH: Assessment of predictors of response to neostigmine for acute colonic pseudo-obstruction, *Am J Gastroenterol* 97:3118–3122, 2002.

65. Trevisani G, Hyman N, Church J: Neostigmine: safe and effective treatment for acute colonic pseudo-obstruction, *Dis Colon Rectum* 43:599–603, 2000.

69. Valle RG, Godoy FL: Neostigmine for acute colonic pseudo-obstruction: a meta-analysis, *Ann Med Surg* 3(3):60–64, 2014.

75. Sgouros S, Vlachogiannakos J, Vassiliadis K, et al: Effect of polyethylene glycol electrolyte balanced solution on patients with acute colonic pseudo obstruction after resolution of colonic dilation: a prospective, randomised, placebo controlled trial, *Gut* 55:638–642, 2006.

76. van der Spoel J, Oudemans-van Straaten H, Stoutenbeek C, et al: Neostigmine resolves critical illness-related colonic ileus in intensive care patients with multiple organ failure—a prospective, double-blind, placebo-controlled trial, *Intensive Care Med* 27:822–827, 2001.

A complete reference list can be found online at ExpertConsult .com

36

Colorectal Cancer Screening and Surveillance

Charles J. Kahi and Joseph C. Anderson

CHAPTER OUTLINE

INTRODUCTION

Colorectal cancer (CRC) is a global public health threat. The lifetime risks of an individual developing or dying from CRC are approximately 5% and 2.5%, respectively; worldwide, there are an estimated 1.4 million new cases and 700,000 deaths annually.[1] In the United States, approximately 135,000 new cases and 49,200 deaths were estimated to occur in 2016.[2]

The fundamental aim of screening for CRC is to decrease CRC risk, as well as mortality, which is related directly to disease stage at diagnosis. Patients with early-stage disease are usually asymptomatic and have high 5-year survival rates; therefore, the key to timely diagnosis is the identification of at-risk patients before symptoms occur. CRC is an eminently "screenable" cancer: the disease is common and generally has a long latency period, early detection can decrease mortality, effective screening methods are available, resources are available to provide screening and to provide diagnostic tests for those with positive screening results, screening is cost-effective, and screening modalities are accepted by patients and health care providers. Population-based studies show that screening can decrease the incidence of and mortality from CRC. In the United States, there has been a steady decline in the overall incidence of CRC in individuals 50 years or older since 1985, a trend that has been partly attributed to screening.[3,4] Beyond early detection, a unique attribute of CRC is that it is amenable to primary prevention (Fig. 36.1) via the detection and removal of precancerous polyps.

Several different strategies for CRC screening exist, each with advantages and limitations pertaining to effectiveness, risk, cost, and availability. Some countries, such as the United States, Germany, and Poland, have well-established colonoscopy-based screening programs, whereas others utilize fecal tests and sigmoidoscopy as "gateway" tests and refer patients with positive results to colonoscopy. Modern screening strategies emphasize the importance of prevention and risk stratification, grouping patients into average- and high-risk categories.[5] The final common pathway for all screening programs is colonoscopy; hence, the effectiveness of screening depends heavily on the availability of high-quality colonoscopy.

This chapter will provide an overview of CRC epidemiology and present screening and surveillance approaches for average-risk and high-risk individuals.

EPIDEMIOLOGY

Global Perspective

The incidence of CRC varies around the world, with the highest rates reported in industrialized Western countries. Conversely, the rates are lowest in India and Africa.[1] Migrant studies show relatively rapid rises in incidence in immigrant groups, usually matching host country rates within two generations. These observations highlight the importance of environmental, lifestyle, and dietary factors in the pathogenesis of CRC.

Demographic Factors

Age is the single most important risk factor for CRC. The incidence increases gradually with age, and increases exponentially after the age of 50 (Table 36.1).[2] Nearly 95% of cases are diagnosed after age 50, providing a strong rationale for the recommendation to start screening at 50 for most average-risk individuals. Although men have higher age-adjusted CRC incidence and mortality, the cumulative lifetime risk of CRC is similar for men and women (4.7% and 4.4%, respectively). Race and ethnicity are also important risk factors (Table 36.2). African Americans have the highest incidence and mortality rates among all racial groups in the United States,[2] but uncertainty remains regarding whether this is due primarily to biological differences, lifestyle factors, or disparities in access to health care. A family history of CRC

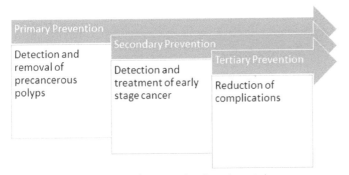

FIG 36.1 Levels of prevention in colorectal cancer.

TABLE 36.1   Probability (%) of Colorectal Cancer by Age and Sex

	Male	Female
< 49 yr	0.3 (1 in 300)	0.3 (1 in 318)
50–59 yr	0.7 (1 in 149)	0.5 (1 in 195)
60–69 yr	1.2 (1 in 82)	0.9 (1 in 117)
≥ 70 yr	3.7 (1 in 27)	3.4 (1 in 30)
Lifetime	4.7 (1 in 21)	4.4 (1 in 23)

Data from Siegel RL, Miller KD, Jemal A: Cancer statistics, 2016. *CA Cancer J Clin* 66(1):7–30, 2016.

TABLE 36.2   Incidence and Mortality of Colorectal Cancer by Race and Ethnicity

	INCIDENCE		MORTALITY	
Race	Male	Female	Male	Female
White	47.4	36.2	18.2	12.9
Black	60.3	44.1	27.6	18.2
Asian	39.0	29.2	13.0	9.4
American Indian	50.4	40.1	18.8	15.6
Hispanic	44.6	30.6	15.6	9.6

Rates are per 100,000 population and are age-adjusted to the 2000 United States standard population.
Data from Siegel RL, Miller KD, Jemal A: Cancer statistics, 2016. *CA Cancer J Clin* 66(1):7–30, 2016.

is present in approximately 20% of CRC cases.[6] A systematic review of lifetime risk associated with familial CRC found that the relative risk of CRC was 2.3 with an affected first-degree relative, 3.9 if the relative was diagnosed before age 45, and 4.2 if more than one relative was affected.[7] The effect of family history on risk of CRC decreases with age, and some analyses report that the risk is mildly increased if there is a second- or third-degree relative with CRC.[8] A family history of adenomatous polyps before the age of 60 has also been reported to increase CRC risk, but this may only be true if the index family member had advanced adenomas.[5]

Modifiable Risk Factors

It is estimated that two-thirds of the risk for CRC may be attributable to potentially modifiable environmental factors. There is considerable evidence linking cigarette smoking, obesity, metabolic syndrome, low levels of physical activity, and heavy alcohol consumption with increased CRC risk.[9] Diets that are high in fat and red meat and low in fiber have also been linked to CRC development. Conversely, there is strong evidence showing that individuals who use nonsteroidal antiinflammatory drugs (NSAIDs) and aspirin have a lower risk of developing colon adenomas and CRC. In addition, calcium supplementation and postmenopausal hormone replacement therapy have been associated with decreased CRC risk. It is important to emphasize that these medications are associated with adverse effects, and universal CRC chemoprevention is not recommended in lieu of screening in average-risk individuals. However, the United States Preventive Services Task Force (USPSTF) recently issued a Grade B recommendation to initiate low-dose aspirin use for the primary prevention of cardiovascular disease (CVD) and CRC in adults aged 50 to 59 years[10] who have a 10% or greater 10-year CVD risk, are not at increased bleeding risk, have at least a 10-year life expectancy, and are committed to taking low-dose aspirin daily for at least 10 years.

PATHOGENESIS

CRC is a heterogeneous disease with regards to tumor development, and each CRC is characterized by a unique molecular profile. Until recently, conventional adenomas were thought to be the only major CRC precursor, with the Fearon-Vogelstein model[11] describing a sequence of progressive molecular alterations leading from adenoma to carcinoma. It is currently recognized that there are three major pathways to colorectal carcinogenesis: the chromosomal instability (CIN) pathway, the microsatellite instability (MSI) pathway, and the serrated neoplasia pathway. It is important to know that these pathways are not mutually exclusive, but the understanding that there are three main pathways has changed the CRC pathogenesis paradigm and impacted approaches to screening and surveillance.

CIN accounts for approximately 60%–70% of all CRCs, and is initiated by mutation of the adenomatous polyposis coli (APC) gene. Subsequent mutations in KRAS and p53 are involved in the progression of an adenoma to advanced adenoma and cancer. CRCs arising along the CIN pathway are typically microsatellite stable and have low level of CpG island methylation. The CIN pathway is thought to take approximately 10 to 15 years from adenoma to CRC.

The MSI pathway is also adenoma-based, and approximately 15% of all CRCs demonstrate MSI. Some of these cancers arise from germline mutations in the mutation mismatch repair (MMR) genes (Lynch syndrome). The majority, however, are associated with epigenetic hypermethylation of the MLH1 MMR gene, which is also one of the molecular events in the serrated neoplasia pathway. Progression to cancer along the MSI pathway is accelerated compared to CIN, taking 3 to 5 years.

The serrated neoplasia pathway is increasingly recognized as an important contributor to CRC. The molecular hallmark is hypermethylation of the promoter CpG island, and the precursor lesion is the sessile serrated polyp (SSP), which can conceptually be thought of as an adenoma equivalent. Hypermethylation is an epigenetic phenomenon, as it alters gene expression without affecting the genetic sequence.[12–15] Tumors that exhibit hypermethylation can be classified as CpG island methylator phenotype (CIMP) high or low. The presence of CIMP is strongly linked with mutations in the oncogene *BRAF*, which have been observed even in diminutive serrated aberrant crypt foci.[16,17] MLH1 hypermethylation with subsequent microsatellite instability leads to

TABLE 36.3 Screening in Patients at Increased or High Risk for Colorectal Cancer

Persons at High Risk	Start Time	Recommended Strategy
FAP	Age 10–12 years	Annual sigmoidoscopy and counseling to consider genetic testing for APC mutations. Colectomy should be considered if FAP is confirmed by genetic testing.
Lynch syndrome	Age 20 to 25 years or 10 years before the youngest case in the immediate family	Colonoscopy every 1–2 years. Genetic counseling to consider testing for MMR mutations. Screening for extracolonic cancers.
Chronic ulcerative colitis or Crohn's colitis	8 years after the onset of pancolitis or 12–15 years after the onset of left-sided colitis	Colonoscopy every 1–2 years. Screening for dysplasia using chromoendoscopy with targeted biopsies, or random biopsies.
Persons at Increased Risk		
CRC or adenomatous polyps in a first-degree relative ≥ 60 years or in two second-degree relatives with CRC	Age 40 years	Intervals as per average-risk screening recommendations.
CRC or adenomatous polyps in a first-degree relative before 60 years or in two or more first-degree relatives at any age	Age 40 years, or 10 years before the youngest case in the family	Colonoscopy every 5 years.
Personal history of resected CRC		High-quality perioperative clearing, followed by colonoscopy 1 year after resection. If negative, repeat in 3 years. If 3-year examination is negative, repeat in 5 years and at 5-year intervals thereafter. Local surveillance can be considered for rectal cancer resected without total mesorectal excision.
One or two small tubular adenomas		Colonoscopy after 5–10 years.
Three to ten adenomas or one adenoma ≥ 1 cm or any adenoma with villous features or high-grade dysplasia		Colonoscopy after 3 years.
More than 10 adenomas		Colonoscopy after < 3 years.
Piecemeal resection of sessile adenoma		Colonoscopy after 2–6 months.

APC, adenomatous polyposis coli; *CRC*, colorectal cancer; *FAP*, familial adenomatous polyposis; *MMR*, mismatch repair gene.

the development of cytological dysplasia within the SSP and accelerates the progression to CIMP high CRC.[18,19] Available evidence suggests that the progression time for the serrated neoplasia pathway is comparable to that of the CIN pathway, although an aggressive course has been observed when MLH1 is inactivated.

SCREENING STRATEGIES: GENERAL APPROACH

As previously discussed, cancer screening is traditionally focused on the detection of early asymptomatic disease (secondary prevention). However, because most CRCs develop from precursor polyps, there is an opportunity for primary prevention via the detection and removal of polyps. The most recent US guidelines distinguish between tests designed for cancer detection and those designed for cancer prevention.[5] The "ideal" screening strategy has not been defined, as screening decisions often depend on resource availability, variation between and within countries, and patient and provider preference. The mainstay tests for early cancer detection are the fecal tests; these are most effective in programmatic approaches (the test is repeated at regular intervals, and there is high patient compliance) and when colonoscopy resources are available to investigate positive tests. The main modality for cancer prevention is colonoscopy because it alone can provide the benefit of polyp detection and polypectomy in one examination. In any context, it is critical that providers

recognize higher risk situations, as such patients require more intensive screening (Table 36.3). This includes patients with a personal history of CRC or adenomatous polyps, a personal history of inflammatory bowel disease (ulcerative colitis or Crohn's disease), a strong family history of CRC or polyps, or a known family history of a hereditary CRC syndrome such as familial adenomatous polyposis or Lynch syndrome. Average-risk patients, who contribute the largest proportion of CRC cases, can be offered the screening modalities and testing intervals discussed in subsequent sections (Table 36.4).

Several groups have issued CRC screening guidelines, with differing recommendations regarding preferred strategies (Table 36.5). In general, however, the guidelines agree that CRC screening is indicated starting at the age of 50 in average-risk individuals, and should be part of a programmatic structure that ensures that tests are repeated at recommended intervals and that positive tests are followed up appropriately.

SCREENING IN AVERAGE-RISK INDIVIDUALS

Stool-Based Colorectal Cancer Screening Tests

Randomized controlled trials (RCTs) have shown that, among patients who undergo screening with fecal occult blood testing (FOBT) compared to unscreened controls, cancers are discovered at an earlier stage, and mortality is reduced by 15% to 33%.[20–24] In the 30-year follow-up study of the Minnesota FOBT trial,

TABLE 36.4   Screening Modalities (ACS-MSTF-ACR Guidelines)

Test	Interval	Key Points
Tests for Early CRC Detection		
High-sensitivity gFOBT	Annual	2–3 samples at home Positive test requires colonoscopy
FIT	Annual	Needs to be programmatic Positive test requires colonoscopy
Stool DNA	Every 3 years	Collection more challenging (packaging, preservatives) Higher cost Positive test requires colonoscopy
Tests for CRC Prevention		
FSIG	Every 5 years	Bowel preparation More discomfort (no sedation) Limited protection Positive test requires colonoscopy
Colonoscopy	Every 10 years	Complete bowel prep Sedation is usually used Higher risk (bleeding, perforation); risks are rare and associated with polypectomy
DCBE	Every 5 years	Complete bowel preparation More discomfort (no sedation) Falling out of favor Option if incomplete colonoscopy and no CTC
CTC	Every 5 years	Complete bowel preparation Polyps ≥ 6 mm require colonoscopy Polyps < 5 mm not reported Extracolonic abnormalities

ACR, American College of Radiology; *ACS,* American Cancer Society; *CRC,* colorectal cancer; *CTC,* computed tomography colonoscopy; *DCBE,* double contrast barium enema; *FIT,* fecal immunochemical test; *FSIG,* flexible sigmoidoscopy; *gFOBT,* guaiac fecal occult blood test; *MSTF,* Multi-Society Task Force.
Modified from Levin B, Lieberman DA, McFarland B, et al: Screening and surveillance for the early detection of colorectal cancer and adenomatous polyps, 2008: a joint guideline from the American Cancer Society, the US Multi-Society Task Force on Colorectal Cancer, and the American College of Radiology. *CA Cancer J Clin* 58(3):130–160, 2008.

TABLE 36.5   Colorectal Cancer Screening Recommendations for Average-Risk Individuals

Guideline	Recommendation Highlights
USPSTF	Adults aged 50 to 75 years: Screen for CRC starting at age 50 years. Adults aged 76 to 85 years: The decision to screen for CRC is an individual one. Screening tests There are numerous screening tests to detect early-stage colorectal cancer, including stool-based tests (gFOBT, FIT, and FIT-DNA), direct visualization tests (flexible sigmoidoscopy, alone or combined with FIT; colonoscopy; and CT colonography), and serology tests (SEPT9 DNA test). The USPSTF found no head-to-head studies demonstrating that any of these screening strategies are more effective than others, although they have varying levels of evidence supporting their effectiveness, as well as different strengths and limitations. Starting and stopping ages The USPSTF concluded that the evidence best supports a starting age of 50 years for the general population. The age at which the balance of benefits and harms of CRC screening becomes less favorable varies based on a patient's life expectancy, health status, comorbid conditions, and prior screening status. The USPSTF does not recommend routine screening for CRC in adults 86 years and older. The USPSTF concludes with high certainty that the net benefit of screening for CRC is substantial. The USPSTF concludes with moderate certainty that the net benefit of screening for CRC in adults aged 76–85 years who have been previously screened is small. Adults who have never been screened are more likely to benefit. Screening is most appropriate for those healthy enough to undergo treatment and those without comorbid conditions that significantly limit their life expectancy.
ACS-MSTF-ACR	Make a distinction between tests for early CRC detection (fecal tests) and structural tests leading to CRC prevention, with a preference for tests with higher sensitivity that do not require frequent application. The health care provider should inform the patient about the benefits and drawbacks of each option to help decision making.
ACG	Preferred screening/prevention test: Colonoscopy Preferred screening/detection test for patients who decline cancer prevention tests: FIT African Americans: Offer screening starting at age 45.
NCCN	Preferred strategy: Colonoscopy every 10 years. Alternatives: Yearly gFOBT or FIT, or sigmoidoscopy every 5 years with or without annual stool testing.
Canadian Task Force on Preventive Health Care	Adults aged 50 to 74: Either gFOBT or FIT every 2 years or flexible sigmoidoscopy every 10 years. Adults aged ≥ 75: No screening. Colonoscopy not recommended for CRC screening.

ACG, American College of Gastroenterology; *ACR,* American College of Radiology; *ACS,* American Cancer Society; *CRC,* colorectal cancer; *FIT,* fecal immunochemical test; *gFOBT,* guaiac fecal occult blood test; *MSTF,* Multi-Society Task Force; *NCCN,* National Comprehensive Cancer Network; *USPSTF,* United States Preventive Services Task Force.

CRC mortality was reduced with annual screening (relative risk [RR] 0.68; 95% confidence interval [CI] 0.56–0.82) and biennial screening (RR 0.78; 95% CI, 0.65–0.93).[25] "Traditional" FOBT involves the use of an alpha-guaiaconic acid–impregnated card and a hydrogen peroxide developing solution.[26] The presence of heme results in a chemical reaction that causes the card to turn a bluish-green color. Three separate samples are needed to maximize sensitivity, and annual testing is recommended.

The newer fecal immunochemical test (FIT) involves the use of labeled antibodies on a card, which bind specifically to human hemoglobin. CRC screening by annual FIT testing has been recommended by the United States Multi-Society Task Force (USMSTF).[27] Erosions or stomach ulcerations due to chronic NSAID or aspirin use do not alter FIT performance because globin (as opposed to heme) is degraded in the small intestine. FITs are typically quantitative but can be designed to indicate a positive test depending upon a prespecified cutoff. A commonly used cutoff is 20 μg hemoglobin (Hgb)/g feces. In one study, at a cutoff of 20 μg Hgb/g feces, the specificity of FIT was 95%. In addition, the FIT had a much higher sensitivity than the FOBT (73.3% vs. 33.3%, respectively).[28] As the FIT uses only a single card and requires no special dietary restrictions, it may be associated with higher patient compliance than the FOBT.[29] Large observational studies examining results from programs using FIT-based screening demonstrated significant reductions in CRC mortality.[30,31]

The FIT has been shown to have a high sensitivity for CRC; approximately 80% in a large meta-analysis.[32] However, the sensitivity of FIT for advanced adenomas (23.8%) is lower than it is for CRC,[33] and test is relatively insensitive for SSPs because these lesions tend to be less vascular than conventional adenomas and thus less prone to bleeding.

Currently, there are four long-term trials comparing the FIT to colonoscopy-based screening (Table 36.6). It is anticipated that these trials will provide important outcome data, including CRC mortality and incidence. Interim results of the Spanish colonoscopy versus fecal immunochemical testing in colorectal-cancer screening (COLONPREV) trial have shown that, likely due to a higher participation rate, the FIT had similar CRC detection rates (30 CRCs; 0.1%) compared to colonoscopy (33 CRCs; 0.1%), whereas colonoscopy had higher rates of advanced adenoma detection than the FIT (1.9% vs. 0.9% respectively, $p < 0.001$). These findings demonstrate the magnitude of the impact that participation rates can have in large CRC screening programs.

A consensus statement for the FIT was recently published by the USMSTF on Colorectal Cancer.[26] The recommendations provided can be divided into several categories. With regards to the FIT performance, the USMSTF recommends:
- Screening using one sample collected annually
- Use of quantitative tests versus qualitative using a lower cutoff level (20 μg/g or lower)
- Patients should be told that they should not adjust their diet or medications during stool collection for the FIT
- The sample should be a spontaneously passed stool rather than one collected from a digital rectal exam in the office
- There should be no need to adjust handling of the sample based on temperature

The USMSTF also provides recommendations for standards to ensure the quality of a FIT screening program:
- ≥ 60% of those offered testing should complete the process
- < 5% should have samples that cannot be processed by the lab
- ≥ 80% of those with a positive FIT result should have a colonoscopy
- Adenoma detection rate (ADR) targets for colonoscopies done for positive FIT results should be ≥ 45% in men and ≥ 35% in women

The rationale for using fecal DNA (fDNA) for CRC screening is that tumor cells and DNA are shed in the feces of adults with these cancers.[34] An early study examined an fDNA test that was designed to detect CIN abnormalities (k-ras, APC, and p53), BAT-26 (a measure of MSI), and DIA (DNA Integrity Assay), a marker for dysfunctional apoptosis.[35] However, the sensitivity for CRC was low (51.6%).

Modifications to the fDNA test have included new markers such as the hypermethylated *vimentin* gene, as well as methods to neutralize the effect of bacterial enzymes.[36] A 2014 trial compared the fDNA test to the FIT in nearly 10,000 patients who had a complete screening colonoscopy (n = 9989).[37] The sensitivity for CRC was higher for the fDNA test that for the FIT (92.3% vs. 73.8%). Specifically, the fDNA test detected 60 of a total of 65 cancers, whereas the FIT detected 48. Both tests performed poorly with respect to the detection of advanced neoplastic lesions (fDNA sensitivity: 42.4%, FIT sensitivity: 23.8%); however, the fDNA test outperformed the FIT for the detection of serrated lesions, likely due to its hypermethylation assay.

Serological Biomarkers

Hypermethylated Septin 9 is a biomarker that has been shown to be present in a high percentage of CRC tissue specimens, as well as in the blood of patients with CRC. The use of a blood test to screen for CRC has several advantages, including no sedation requirement, no bowel preparation requirement, and

TABLE 36.6 Ongoing Screening Colonoscopy Randomized Controlled Trials

RCT	Setting	Comparison	Primary Outcome
ColonPrev NCT00906997	Spain	Screening colonoscopy versus biennial FIT	10-year CRC and incidence
NordICC NCT00883792	Sweden, Norway, the Netherlands, Poland	Screening colonoscopy versus no screening	15-year CRC and incidence
CONFIRM (VA CSP 577) NCT01239082	United States VA system	Screening colonoscopy versus annual FIT	10-year CRC mortality
SREESCO NCT02078804	Sweden	Screening colonoscopy versus 2 FIT rounds versus no screening	15-year CRC mortality

CRC, colorectal cancer; *FIT*, fecal immunochemical test; *RCT*, randomized controlled trial.

the lack of potential complications arising from the test. Recent studies (2015) have demonstrated that the sensitivity of the Septin 9 blood test for CRC ranges from 51% to 95.6%, and the specificity ranges from 80% to 98.9%.[38] However, the sensitivity for adenomas is much lower (10% in one study).[39] Thus, the septin 9 blood test is not currently recommended as a primary screening modality.

Tests for Structural Examination of the Colon

Sigmoidoscopy

The value of sigmoidoscopy for CRC screening is now supported by RCT evidence showing significant levels of protection against CRC (Table 36.7).[40–43] Sigmoidoscopy effectively protects against distal CRC and is an attractive option, given its cost-effectiveness and lower risk for harm than colonoscopy. The benefit of a one-time sigmoidoscopic examination to decrease the risk of CRC mortality extends beyond 10 years.[40] No RCTs comparing colonoscopy with sigmoidoscopy have been or are likely to be performed in the near future; however, indirect comparisons of results from observational studies suggest that there is a 40% to 60% lower CRC incidence and mortality risk after screening colonoscopy, although risk reduction was statistically significant for deaths from cancer of the proximal colon only.[44] The use of sigmoidoscopy in the United States has been declining, coincident with the rise of screening colonoscopy.

Colonoscopy

Colonoscopy has been increasingly used as a CRC screening modality in the United States since the 1990s. Colonoscopy allows direct visualization of the entire colon, it can interrupt the progression of precancerous polyps to cancer by polypectomy, and it allows clinicians to determine appropriate surveillance intervals based on the findings of the index examination. Other advantages include less frequent intervals between examinations and increasing acceptability and tolerability of modern sedation techniques. Average-risk patients with negative screening colonoscopy results have lower CRC incidence on long-term follow-up, extending beyond 10 years.[45,46] Screening colonoscopy was first endorsed by professional societies in 1997[47] and approved for Medicare beneficiaries in 2001. RCTs comparing colonoscopy to other modalities are now underway, but there is a large body of observational literature supporting the effectiveness of screening colonoscopy. A recent (2016) population-based German study showed that cancers detected by screening colonoscopy had a lower stage than those diagnosed by colonoscopy in patients with symptoms; the magnitude of stage shift was comparable to patients undergoing screening by the FOBT.[48] The National Polyp Study[49] reported a 76% reduction in the incidence of CRC in a cohort of patients with adenomas who underwent colonoscopy and polypectomy compared with a Surveillance, Epidemiology, and End Results reference group, and follow-up revealed a 53% reduction in CRC mortality after a median of nearly 16 years.[50] However, several studies published subsequent to the National Polyp Study have shown lower reduction in CRC incidence after colonoscopy and polypectomy. Important observations can be derived from recent studies. First, although colonoscopy can achieve significant overall levels of protection against CRC, it may not protect against proximal CRC to the same extent as it does against distal CRC (Table 36.8).[45,51–54] Second, and arguably more importantly, the issue of variable protection against CRC appears to be intricately linked to operator-dependent quality factors. The issue of optimal bowel preparation is largely addressable with the adoption and widespread use of split dosing, in which at least half of the preparation is given on the morning of the colonoscopy. Such regimens improve preparation quality, particularly in the right colon.[55] However, most of the limitations of colonoscopy can be accounted for by operator-dependent, and thus potentially reversible, factors. The ADR is now validated as a powerful surrogate marker of colonoscopy performance quality. In a large study based on data from the Polish CRC screening program, Kaminski et al (2010)[56] showed that the risk of interval CRC was 10-fold higher for patients who underwent colonoscopy by operators with an ADR less than 20% compared with those with an ADR 20% or higher. Corley et al (2014)[57] evaluated 314,872 colonoscopies performed by 136 gastroenterologists in the Kaiser Permanente Northern California system and ADRs ranging from 7.4% to 52.5%. Among patients of physicians with ADRs in the highest quintile, as compared with patients of physicians with ADRs in the lowest quintile, the adjusted hazard ratio for any interval cancer was 0.52 (95% CI, 0.39–0.69), for advanced-stage interval cancer, 0.43 (95% CI, 0.29–0.64), and for fatal interval cancer, 0.38 (95% CI, 0.22–0.65). Each 1% increase in the ADR was associated with a 3% decrease in the risk of cancer (hazard ratio, 0.97; 95% CI, 0.96–0.98). The specialty of the colonoscopy provider is associated with quality, with gastroenterologists outperforming other specialists. Variable quality also affects polypectomy. Pohl et al (2013)[58] performed biopsies on the margins of 346 polypectomy sites after apparently complete resection. The incomplete resection rate (as evidenced by residual microscopic neoplastic tissue) was 10% and ranged from 6.5% to 22.7% among different endoscopists. Larger polyp size and SSP histology were predictors of incomplete resection.

TABLE 36.7   Flexible Sigmoidoscopy Randomized Controlled Trials

Author (Year)	Setting	Primary Comparison	CRC Incidence (95% CI)	CRC Mortality (95% CI)
Atkin (2010) UK Trial	United Kingdom	Invitation for one-time screening between ages 55 and 64 versus no further contact	HR = 0.77 (0.70–0.84)	HR = 0.69 (0.59–0.82)
Segnan (2011) SCORE	Italy	Invitation for one-time screening between ages 55 and 64 versus no further contact	RR = 0.82 (0.69–0.96)	RR = 0.78 (0.56–1.08)
Schoen (2012) PLCO	United States	Screening between ages 55 and 74 and repeat screening in 3–5 years, versus usual care	RR = 0.79 (0.72–0.85)	RR = 0.74 (0.63–0.87)
Hoff (2014) NORCCAP	Norway	One-time screening with or without one-time screening FOBT, compared to no screening	HR = 0.80 (0.70–0.92)	HR = 0.73 (0.56–0.94)

Intention-to-treat (intention-to-screen) for all analyses
CI, confidence interval; *CRC,* colorectal cancer; *FOBT,* fecal occult blood testing; *HR,* hazard ratio; *RR,* relative risk.

TABLE 36.8   Association of Colonoscopy and Colorectal Cancer Incidence and Mortality

Author (Year)	Setting	Study Design	Primary Measurement	Overall CRC (95% CI)	Left-Sided CRC (95% CI)	Right-Sided CRC (95% CI)
Baxter (2009)	Ontario, Canada	Population-based, case-control	Exposure to colonoscopy between case patients who died of CRC and controls	OR = 0.63 (0.57–0.69)	OR = 0.33 (0.28–0.39)	OR = 0.99 (0.86–1.14)
Mulder (2010)	Netherlands	Population-based, case-control	Exposure to colonoscopy between case patients diagnosed with CRC and controls	OR = 0.56 (0.33–0.94)	OR = 0.36 (0.17–0.76)	OR = 0.98 (0.42–2.25)
Brenner (2010)	Saarland, Germany	Population-based, cross-sectional	Prevalence of advanced colorectal neoplasms according to previous colonoscopy history	PR = 0.52 (0.37–0.73)	PR = 0.33 (0.21–0.53)	PR = 1.05 (0.63–1.76)
Singh (2010)	Manitoba, Canada	Population-based, cohort	CRC mortality after colonoscopy compared to the general population	SMR = 0.71 (0.61–0.82)	SMR = 0.53 (0.42–0.67)	SMR = 0.94 (0.77–1.17)
Brenner (2011)	Rhine-Neckar, Germany	Population-based, case-control	Odds of CRC associated with previous colonoscopy	OR = 0.23 (0.19–0.27)	OR = 0.16 (0.12–0.20)	OR = 0.44 (0.35–0.55)
Baxter (2012)	United States	SEER-Medicare data, case-control	Exposure to colonoscopy between case patients who died of CRC and controls	OR = 0.40 (0.37–0.43)	OR = 0.24 (0.21–0.27)	OR = 0.58 (0.53–0.64)

CI, confidence interval; *CRC,* colorectal cancer; *OR,* odds ratio; *PR,* prevalence ratio; *SEER,* Surveillance, Epidemiology, and End Results; *SMR,* standardized mortality ratio.

It is estimated that more than 70% of interval CRC cases are attributed to missed lesions, with incomplete resection accounting for another 10% to 27%.[59] This means that the great majority of the variable effectiveness of colonoscopy is attributed to operator-dependent factors, which could potentially be overcome with educational and quality improvement initiatives. Quality monitoring and improvement are now an integral part of modern colonoscopy practice (Table 36.9).[60]

There has been considerable recent interest in the serrated neoplasia pathway, given its disproportionate contribution to interval CRC. Hyperplastic polyps (HPs) were long considered to be benign lesions with no clinical significance. However, these lesions are part of a larger heterogeneous group of lesions known as serrated polyps, and SSPs and traditional serrated adenomas (TSAs) are considered premalignant, similar to conventional adenomas. Distinguishing HPs from SSPs can be difficult, due to poor reproducibility among pathologists' readings, as well as overlap in morphological features, and the proportion of HPs that have been reclassified as SSPs after pathologic reassessment has ranged from 5.8% to 11.8%.[61–65] SSPs can be flat and more difficult to detect and resect completely than adenomas. Thus, it is not surprising that detection rates can vary among endoscopists[66,67] and centers.[68] There have been several small reports that demonstrate a long-term risk for CRC in patients with serrated polyps.[63,69,70] However, data from 2015 suggest that patients with large serrated polyps may have a similar risk for CRC as patients with advanced neoplasia in a follow-up period of approximately 10 years.[71] One large study from Norway observed that out of 23 large unresected serrated polyps, none progressed to malignancy.[71] These data suggest that large serrated lesions may represent surrogate markers for individuals at risk for CRC, rather than precursors. A 2016 large population-based study conducted in Denmark showed that patients with SSPs were three times more likely to develop CRC on follow-up, whereas the odd ratios for patients with dysplastic SSP and TSA were 4.76 and 4.84, respectively.[72] The USMSTF on Colorectal Cancer guidelines for colonoscopy surveillance after screening and polypectomy present recommendations for surveillance of individuals with SSP[73] that generally follow an approach similar to that recommended for conventional adenomas (Table 36.10).

However, it is important to recognize that these recommendations are based on low-quality data, and longitudinal follow-up studies are needed to better inform surveillance after SSP resection.

Computed Tomography Colonography

The 2008 USMSTF guidelines recommend computed tomography colonography (CTC) every 5 years as an acceptable CRC screening test.[74] The American College of Gastroenterology guidelines recommend that CTC replace double contrast barium enema as an alternative to their preferred screening test, conventional colonoscopy.[75] CTC has also been recently included as a CRC screening option by the recent USPSTF recommendations.[76]

CTC is a process that uses computed tomography (CT) to recreate the large bowel in two- or three-dimensional images. The CTC images, which are typically interpreted by a radiologist, are used to detect polyps in the large bowel that appear as protruding lesions into the lumen. The process involves the patient cleansing their large bowel with a purgative agent, similar to conventional colonoscopy. The bowel regimen also involves the intake of a tagging solution that contains barium sulfate to identify stool. The patient then undergoes a process similar to a CT, with air or CO_2 used to insufflate the large bowel through a tube inserted into the rectum. If polyps are detected during CTC, a referral must be made for a conventional colonoscopy. Absolute CTC contraindications include pregnancy and an allergy to iodinated contrast.

Potential advantages for CTC include the lack of a sedation requirement and good performance for large lesions (> 1 cm).[77,78] The American College of Radiology Imaging Network trial, which enrolled 2500 participants, demonstrated a high (90%) sensitivity for large (≥ 1 cm) polyps.[77] CTC also has a low complication rate of 0.03% or less.[79–81] One benefit of CTC as compared to conventional colonoscopy is increased patient compliance with screening. Compliance rates for screening were improved in military facilities where CTC was offered as an option.[82] The development of a noncathartic preparation regimen may offer the greatest advantage to CTC with regards to compliance. Studies have demonstrated sensitivities of nearly 80% for polyps of 6 mm or larger.[83,84] Another trial in which patients were invited for CTC versus conventional colonoscopy screening demonstrated

TABLE 36.9   Colonoscopy Quality Indicators

Preprocedure

1. Frequency with which colonoscopy is performed for an indication that is included in a published standard list of appropriate indications, and the indication is documented	Process	> 80%
2. Frequency with which informed consent is obtained, including specific discussions of risks associated with colonoscopy, and fully documented	Process	> 98%
3. Frequency with which colonoscopies follow recommended post-polypectomy and post–cancer resection surveillance intervals and 10-year intervals between screening colonoscopies in average-risk patients who have negative examination results and adequate bowel cleansing (priority indicator)	Process	≥ 90%
4. Frequency with which ulcerative colitis and Crohn's colitis surveillance is recommended within proper intervals	Process	≥ 90%

Intraprocedure

5. Frequency with which the procedure note documents the quality of preparation	Process	> 98%
6. Frequency with which bowel preparation is adequate to allow the use of recommended surveillance or screening intervals	Process	≥ 85% of outpatient exams
7. Frequency with which visualization of the cecum by notation of landmarks and photo documentation of landmarks is documented in every procedure (priority indicator) Cecal intubation rate with photography (all examinations) Cecal intubation rate with photography (screening)	Process	 ≥ 90% ≥ 95%
8. Frequency with which adenomas are detected in asymptomatic average-risk individuals (screening) (priority indicator) Adenoma detection rate for male/female population Adenoma detection rate for male patients Adenoma detection rate for female patients	Outcome	 ≥ 25% ≥ 30% ≥ 20%
9a. Frequency with which withdrawal time is measured	Process	> 98%
9b. Average withdrawal time in negative result screening colonoscopies	Process	≥ 6 min
10. Frequency with which biopsy specimens are obtained when colonoscopy is performed for an indication of chronic diarrhea	Process	> 98%
11. Frequency of recommended tissue sampling when colonoscopy is performed for surveillance in ulcerative colitis and Crohn's colitis	Process	> 98%
12. Frequency with which endoscopic removal of pedunculated polyps and sessile polyps < 2 cm is attempted before surgical referral	Outcome	> 98%

Postprocedure

13. Incidence of perforation by procedure type (all indications vs. colorectal cancer screening/polyp surveillance) and post-polypectomy bleeding Incidence of perforation—all examinations Incidence of perforation—screening Incidence of post-polypectomy bleeding	Outcome	 < 1 : 500 < 1 : 1000 < 1%
14. Frequency with which post-polypectomy bleeding is managed without surgery	Outcome	≥ 90%
15. Frequency with which appropriate recommendation for timing of repeat colonoscopy is documented and provided to the patient after histologic findings are reviewed.	Process	≥ 90%

From Rex DK, Schoenfeld PS, Cohen J, et al: Quality indicators for colonoscopy. *Am J Gastroenterol* 110(1):72–90, 2015.

that the rate of identifying advanced neoplasia by CTC was similar, largely due to a higher compliance in the CTC arm of the study.[85]

The potential downsides for CTC were outlined by the Centers for Medicare and Medicaid Services (CMS) in their denial of coverage for CRC screening.[86] Concerns raised included the low sensitivity and specificity for smaller polyps, high colonoscopy referral rate for abnormal findings (up to 30%),[87] and high rates of extracolonic findings.[77,87] There was also concern about the performance of CTC in older adults, including rates of colonoscopy referral.[77,78,87] Radiation exposure from initial CTC and the attendant follow-up studies is also an issue.

Denial of coverage for screening by CMS has limited the widespread use of CTC. In practice, CTC is currently mostly used to complete the large bowel evaluation in patients who have had an incomplete colonoscopy or cannot undergo colonoscopy. Overall, CTC performs well for cancers and large (> 1 cm) polyps, but concerns regarding smaller lesions (< 6 mm), radiation exposure, surveillance intervals, and extracolonic findings mean that further study is still needed. However, the noncathartic CTC may increase patient participation, and thus help reduce CRC incidence and mortality.

Colon Capsule Endoscopy

The colon capsule was first used 10 years ago, and has since been modified to include a wide-angle lens and the ability to take up to 35 images per second, increasing its sensitivity. A 2010 meta-analysis of 14 studies demonstrated that the sensitivity of the second-generation capsule is 86% and 87% for polyps of 6 mm or larger and 10 mm or larger, respectively.[88] Colon capsule endoscopy (CCE) has received approval by the Food and Drug

TABLE 36.10 Post-Polypectomy Surveillance Guidelines in Average-Risk Individuals

Baseline Finding	Recommended Interval (Years)
No polyps	10
Small rectal or sigmoid hyperplastic polyps	10
1–2 small tubular adenomas	5–10
3–10 tubular adenomas	3
> 10 adenomas	< 3
Villous adenoma or adenoma with high-grade dysplasia	3
Small SSP without dysplasia	5
SSP ≥ 10 mm, or SSP with dysplasia, or TSA	3
Serrated polyposis syndrome	1

"Small" = < 10 mm; *SSP*, sessile serrated polyp; *TSA*, traditional serrated adenoma

and Administration for use in individuals with incomplete colonoscopies. Thus, the role of CCE is to complete large bowel inspection of adults who have had an incomplete colonoscopy.[89] In a study of 75 patients with an incomplete colonoscopy, CCE visualized the proximal colon that was not seen in the colonoscopy exam in more than 90% of cases.[90] The effectiveness of CCE can be limited by poor bowel preparation. Thus, patients whose exams are limited by an inability to purge their colon may not be good candidates for CCE. This technology may be most useful for patients whose colonoscopy is limited by anatomical abnormalities related to tortuous or redundant large bowels. Current USMSTF, USPSTF, and American College of Gastroenterology Guidelines for CRC screening do not include CCE.[27,75,91] More data regarding performance characteristics will be needed to address the role of CCE in CRC screening.

SURVEILLANCE

Surveillance intervals should be based on evidence showing that interval examinations prevent interval CRC and decrease cancer-related mortality; however, guidelines are currently based on advanced adenomas as a surrogate marker. Key principles of current guidelines are the risk stratification of patients based on the findings at the baseline colonoscopy and the assumption that the baseline colonoscopy is of high quality and involved adequate bowel preparation (see Table 36.10). The USMSTF guidelines[73] identify two major risk groups based on the likelihood of developing advanced neoplasia during surveillance: low-risk adenomas (1–2 tubular adenomas < 10 mm) and high-risk adenomas (adenomas with villous histology, high-grade dysplasia, ≥ 10 mm, or three or more adenomas). Conversely, the British Society of Gastroenterology[92] stratifies patients into three groups: low risk (1–2 adenomas < 10 mm), intermediate risk (3–4 small adenomas or one ≥ 10 mm), and high risk (≥ 5 small adenomas or ≥ 3 with at least one ≥ 10 mm), and they recommend that the high-risk group undergo surveillance at 1 year because of concerns about missed lesions at baseline.

Patients with resected CRC represent a high-risk group requiring a more intensive approach. The USMSTF has published updated guidelines[93] that recommend, in addition to high-quality perioperative clearing colonoscopy, surveillance after 1 year, followed by colonoscopy at 3- and 5-year intervals.

ACKNOWLEDGMENT

The authors wish to acknowledge Dr. David Lieberman's contribution to this chapter in the previous edition of this textbook.

KEY REFERENCES

2. Siegel RL, Miller KD, Jemal A: Cancer statistics, 2016, *CA Cancer J Clin* 66:7–30, 2016.
5. Levin B, Lieberman DA, McFarland B, et al: Screening and surveillance for the early detection of colorectal cancer and adenomatous polyps, 2008: a joint guideline from the American Cancer Society, the US Multi-Society Task Force on Colorectal Cancer, and the American College of Radiology, *Gastroenterology* 134:1570–1595, 2008.
6. Lin JS, Piper M, Perdue LA, et al: Screening for colorectal cancer: a systematic review for the US Preventive Services Task Force: Evidence synthesis no. 135. AHRQ publication 14-05203-EF-1. Agency for Healthcare Research and Quality, Rockville, MD, 2016.
10. Bibbins-Domingo K, US Preventive Services Task Force: Aspirin use for the primary prevention of cardiovascular disease and colorectal cancer: U.S. Preventive Services Task Force Recommendation Statement, *Ann Intern Med* 164:836–845, 2016.
11. Vogelstein B, Fearon ER, Hamilton SR, et al: Genetic alterations during colorectal-tumor development, *N Engl J Med* 319:525–532, 1988.
19. Snover DC, Ahnen DJ, Burt RW, Odze RD: Serrated lesions of the colon and rectum and serrated polyposis. In Bozman F, Cameiro F, Hurban R, editors: *World Health Organization classification of tumours. Tumors of the Digestive System*, Lyon, France, 2010, International Agency for Research on Cancer (IARC) Press, pp 160–165.
25. Shaukat A, Mongin SJ, Geisser MS, et al: Long-term mortality after screening for colorectal cancer, *N Engl J Med* 369:1106–1114, 2013.
26. Robertson DJ, Lee JK, Boland CR, et al: Recommendations on fecal immunochemical testing to screen for colorectal neoplasia: a consensus statement by the US Multi-Society Task Force on Colorectal Cancer, *Gastroenterology* 152(5):1217–1237.e3, 2017.
32. Lee JK, Liles EG, Bent S, et al: Accuracy of fecal immunochemical tests for colorectal cancer: systematic review and meta-analysis, *Ann Intern Med* 160:171, 2014.
33. Imperiale TF, Ransohoff DF, Itzkowitz SH, et al: Multitarget stool DNA testing for colorectal-cancer screening, *N Engl J Med* 370:1287–1297, 2014.
44. Brenner H, Stock C, Hoffmeister M: Effect of screening sigmoidoscopy and screening colonoscopy on colorectal cancer incidence and mortality: systematic review and meta-analysis of randomised controlled trials and observational studies, *BMJ* 348:g2467, 2014.
45. Brenner H, Haug U, Arndt V, et al: Low risk of colorectal cancer and advanced adenomas more than 10 years after negative colonoscopy, *Gastroenterology* 138:870–876, 2010.
49. Winawer SJ, Zauber AG, Ho MN, et al: Prevention of colorectal cancer by colonoscopic polypectomy. The National Polyp Study Workgroup, *N Engl J Med* 329:1977–1981, 1993.
50. Zauber AG, Winawer SJ, O'Brien MJ, et al: Colonoscopic polypectomy and long-term prevention of colorectal-cancer deaths, *N Engl J Med* 366:687–696, 2012.
55. Kilgore TW, Abdinoor AA, Szary NM, et al: Bowel preparation with split-dose polyethylene glycol before colonoscopy: a meta-analysis of randomized controlled trials, *Gastrointest Endosc* 73:1240–1245, 2011.
56. Kaminski MF, Regula J, Kraszewska E, et al: Quality indicators for colonoscopy and the risk of interval cancer, *N Engl J Med* 362:1795–1803, 2010.
57. Corley DA, Levin TR, Doubeni CA: Adenoma detection rate and risk of colorectal cancer and death, *N Engl J Med* 370:2541, 2014.
58. Pohl H, Srivastava A, Bensen SP, et al: Incomplete polyp resection during colonoscopy-results of the complete adenoma resection (CARE) study, *Gastroenterology* 144:74–80.e1, 2013.

60. Rex DK, Schoenfeld PS, Cohen J, et al: Quality indicators for colonoscopy, *Gastrointest Endosc* 81:31–53, 2015.

66. Kahi CJ, Hewett DG, Norton DL, et al: Prevalence and variable detection of proximal colon serrated polyps during screening colonoscopy, *Clin Gastroenterol Hepatol* 9:42–46, 2011.

73. Lieberman DA, Rex DK, Winawer SJ, et al: Guidelines for colonoscopy surveillance after screening and polypectomy: a consensus update by the US Multi-Society Task Force on Colorectal Cancer, *Gastroenterology* 143:844–857, 2012.

74. Levin B, Lieberman DA, McFarland B, et al: Screening and surveillance for the early detection of colorectal cancer and adenomatous polyps, 2008: a joint guideline from the American Cancer Society, the US Multi-Society Task Force on Colorectal Cancer, and the American College of Radiology, *Gastroenterology* 134:1570–1595, 2008.

76. Lin JS, Piper MA, Perdue LA, et al: Screening for colorectal cancer: updated evidence report and systematic review for the US Preventive Services Task Force, *JAMA* 315:2576–2594, 2016.

78. Pickhardt PJ, Choi JR, Hwang I, et al: Computed tomographic virtual colonoscopy to screen for colorectal neoplasia in asymptomatic adults, *N Engl J Med* 349:2191–2200, 2003.

93. Kahi CJ, Boland CR, Dominitz JA, et al: Colonoscopy surveillance after colorectal cancer resection: recommendations of the US Multi-Society Task Force on Colorectal Cancer, *Gastroenterology* 150:758–768.e11, 2016.

A complete reference list can be found online at ExpertConsult .com

37

Colonoscopic Polypectomy, Mucosal Resection, and Submucosal Dissection

Heiko Pohl, Peter Draganov, Roy Soetikno, and Tonya Kaltenbach

CHAPTER OUTLINE

INTRODUCTION

Related to the central role of colonoscopy within colorectal cancer (CRC) screening and surveillance, most gastroenterologists spend the majority of their time in the colon looking for and removing neoplastic polyps in an effort to reduce the risk of CRC incidence and death.[1,2]

However, the benefit of colonoscopy in reducing CRC relies on the adequate detection and removal of polyps. Although the majority of CRC that are diagnosed following a colonoscopy are likely related to missing a lesion at the prior colonoscopy, incomplete resection has been considered to be a cause for these post-colonoscopy cancers in 10% to 30% of cases.[3] For colonoscopy to be effective, it is therefore not only important to minimize miss rates, but also to assure complete polyp resection.

Studies have shown that incomplete resection is frequent. In the Complete Adenoma Resection (CARE) study, 10% of all 5- to 20-mm neoplastic polyps were incompletely removed.[4] Perhaps more important, there was a broad variation across endoscopists from 6% to 23% incomplete resection rate. This underlines the need for improving quality of resection and agreeing on a standardized approach. This chapter will review safe and effective resection techniques of colonic lesions. Specifically, we will review what is needed to perform polyp resection, basic and advanced polypectomy, special techniques to improve efficacy and safety of resection, and discuss future directions.

DIFFERENTIAL DIAGNOSIS

Colonic lesions are classified as either epithelial or nonepithelial. Epithelial lesions include neoplastic adenomas (serrated, tubular, tubulovillous, villous), carcinomas, and nonneoplastic polyps (hyperplastic, juvenile, hamartoma, inflammatory). Occasionally, numerous lesions are encountered during colonoscopy of patients who have polyposis syndromes, including familial adenomatous polyposis (adenomas), Peutz-Jeghers syndrome (hamartomas), juvenile polyposis (juvenile polyps), or Cowden's syndrome (hamartomas). In addition, patients with hereditary non-polyposis CRC may harbor multiple advanced neoplastic lesions. Nonepithelial colonic lesions typically arise in the submucosa, muscularis propria, or serosal layers of the colonic wall and include lipomas, leiomyomas, carcinoids, lymphomas, and metastatic tumors. Indentations of the colonic wall by adjacent organs or endometrial implants on the serosa can also have the appearance of subepithelial lesions.

Careful endoscopic observation of the surface features of the lesion can often allow differentiation of epithelial from nonepithelial origin because nonepithelial lesions are usually covered by normal mucosa. Using currently available high-definition colonoscopes with image-enhanced capabilities, such as narrow-band imaging (NBI), it is increasingly possible to distinguish between nonneoplastic and neoplastic polyps, and to recognize superficial early adenocarcinoma.[5,6] Lesions that are amenable to endoscopic resection are typically mucosal lesions. Subepithelial lesions can sometimes be removed safely when they are located above the muscularis propria, as evidenced by their endoscopic appearance, response to submucosal saline injection, and, if needed, endoscopic ultrasound. Generally, biopsy should be performed if possible for lesions that are not amendable to endoscopic resection to ascertain their histology. These lesions should be endoscopically marked for surgical planning with submucosal tattoo and/or radiopaque clips.

CONSIDERATIONS BEFORE POLYP RESECTION

Indications and Contraindications

Treatment decisions must consider whether substantial risks exist and whether the patient's overall life expectancy is likely to be affected by the generally slow progression of colonic adenomas. The average transition time from non-advanced adenoma to cancer has been estimated to take more than 20 years,[7] so patients with advanced comorbid illnesses and limited life expectancy may not benefit from adenoma resection.

Colonoscopy is usually inappropriate in patients who are pregnant[8] or have fulminant colitis, suspected intestinal perforation, fresh intestinal anastomosis, a recent myocardial infarction, or stroke. With respect to antithrombotic management, polypectomy and mucosal resection are considered higher risk procedures and should generally not be performed in patients who have uncorrected bleeding disorders. High-quality bowel preparation is crucial for detection of subtle lesions and for resection of particularly large or difficult lesions when an elevated risk of perforation exists. Poor bowel preparation is also a contraindication for performance of complex polypectomy due to the risk of peritoneal contamination in the event of a perforation.

Management of Antithrombotic Agents

Polypectomy and mucosal resection are considered procedures at higher risk for bleeding.[9] Risks related to interrupting antithrombotic medications for polypectomy need to be balanced against the risks of significant bleeding during and after the procedure. Recommendations for the management of antithrombotic agents are provided in the recently updated American Society for Gastrointestinal Endoscopy (ASGE) guidelines.[9]

Anticoagulant Agents

Patients on warfarin at relatively low risk of thromboembolic complications can discontinue the medication 5 days before the procedure and resume it shortly after polypectomy. Patients on a novel oral anticoagulant should discontinue the medication between 1 and 6 days prior to surgery dependent on the half-life of the medication and the creatinine clearance.[9] High-risk patients, such as patients with atrial fibrillation and concomitant valvular disease, should be bridged with heparin or a heparin derivative (e.g., low-molecular-weight heparin). Warfarin generally can be resumed on the night of the procedure, with heparin resumed earlier at 2 to 6 hours after the procedure if necessary, based on the risk of thrombosis. Although there are no data on when to resume novel oral anticoagulants, these agents should probably be restarted 5 to 7 days after a large polyp resection with a higher bleeding risk to achieve a therapeutic level.[10]

Antiplatelet Agents

Whereas the risk of polypectomy bleeding is low for patients on acetylsalicylic acid (ASA) or nonsteroidal antiinflammatory drugs (NSAIDs), patients on thienopyridine (e.g., clopidogrel) have a high bleeding risk.[9] Therefore, patients on ASA/NSAIDs should continue these medications. Cessation may only be considered for patients at low risk for a thromboembolic event and who are undergoing a complex polypectomy (e.g., endoscopic mucosal resection [EMR] or endoscopic submucosal dissection [ESD]). Generally, when we believe that the risk of bleeding after endoscopic removal of a large or complex lesion is significant, we recommend that patients refrain from taking platelet inhibitors 7 days before the procedure and for approximately 7 days after it.

Thienopyridines should be stopped, or switched to ASA if the thromboembolic risk is high. Patients on double antiplatelet agents (ASA and clopidogrel) should stop the thienopyridine 5 to 7 days prior to the procedure, and ASA should be continued. Following drug-eluting coronary stent placement, an elective procedure should be deferred if possible up to 12 months, until ASA can be safely withheld.[9]

Antibiotic Prophylaxis for Endocarditis

The ASGE and the American Heart Association guidelines state that antibiotic prophylaxis solely to prevent infective endocarditis is no longer recommended before endoscopic procedures, including diagnostic colonoscopy and polypectomy.[11]

INSTRUMENTS AND EQUIPMENT

Dependent on the complexity of polypectomy, knowledge and familiarity with required equipment and accessories is essential for safe and effective polyp resection.

Colonoscope

The choice of colonoscope is dependent on personal preference. It needs to promote adequate position, visualization, and resection of the colonic lesion. The colonoscope should allow adequate flushing and be equipped with a water jet. Simethicone is often added to water to eliminate gas bubbles and improve visualization. Simethicone residue within the endoscope may be difficult to remove, and some manufacturers recommend the lowest dose of simethicone possible.[12]

CO$_2$ Insufflation

Insufflation should be done with CO_2. Its clinical utility as an insufflating gas for colonoscopy has been well established.[13] CO_2 is readily absorbed through the colonic mucosa. Because of the lower amount of retained gas in the colon, patients are more comfortable and less likely to have abdominal pain following the procedure. It is also nonflammable, and the risk of colonic perforation, which has been reported with air insufflation, should be zero. Finally, there have been rare case reports of fatal air embolism with other endoscopic interventions. Such risk does not exist when using CO_2 as the insufflating gas.

Snares

Both the endoscopist and the endoscopy assistant must be familiar with the type of snare used. These individuals must understand and have tactile knowledge of the opening and closing of the snare, the closing pressure required to produce optimal coagulation, and the relationship between the size of the tissue being strangulated and the amount of snare being closed. Various snares, each with a slightly different feature, are used for polypectomy and mucosal resection. The choice is based on personal preference, the size of the lesion, and the applied technique. Typically, small snares are used for small polyps, and larger snares for larger polyps. Stiffer snares are used for colonoscopic mucosal resection so that flat or depressed lesions and a healthy margin can be more easily captured in the snare.[14,15]

Injection Fluid

EMR and ESD generally require submucosal injection. Saline injection tends to be adequate for most cases of EMR. For more complex EMR cases and for all colorectal ESD, a solution that provides a longer-lasting submucosal cushion is highly recommended. At present in the United States, there is only one Food and Drug Administration–approved submucosal injectate (Eleview, Aries Pharmaceuticals, Inc., San Diego, CA). It contains a composition of polymer chains to provide a lasting cushion and methylene blue. Clinical studies are lacking, but preliminary data from animal model work appear promising.[16] Based on local availability the following solutions can be used off label:

- *Normal saline* can be used in the majority of cases of colonic EMR.
- Worldwide, *hyaluronic acid* (MucoUp, Seikagaku Corporation, Tokyo, Japan) is the most commonly used injection solution for colorectal ESD.
- *Sodium hyaluronate* (Healon, Abbott, Chicago, IL) dispensed as 10 mg/mL. 0.85-mL syringe is available in the US and is approved for intraocular injection during ophthalmic surgery. A typical dilution for ESD is one 0.85 mL syringe of hyaluronic acid mixed with 2.5 mL of normal saline and dye (indigo carmine or methylene blue) to desired color. Although this type of solution provides for excellent submucosal lift, the cost tends to be prohibitive for routine use.
- *Hydroxyethyl starch* (Hetastarch; available as Voluven, Fresenius Kabi Ltd., Runcorn, United Kingdom or Hespan, B. Braun Medical, Melsungen, Germany) dispensed as 500-mL bags. No dilution is necessary, dye can be added to the desired color, and the solution can be directly used for submucosal injection at the time of ESD. No data are available for the use in ESD, but a randomized controlled study showed that hydroxyethyl starch is superior to normal saline for EMR.[17]
- *Hypromellose* (Gonak, Akorn, Inc., Lake Forest, IL) is an ophthalmic solution used as artificial tears and is dispensed as a 15-mL vial. Typical dilution for ESD is to mix one 15-ml vial with 85 mL of normal saline. The use of hypromellose has been shown to be safe and effective in EMR, but data specifically pertaining to ESD are not available.[18]
- *Succinylated gelatin* (Gelufusine, B. Braun Medical) is a volume expander that is not available in the US. Its physical properties are similar to hydroxyethyl starch. It has been shown to reduce the number of resections during piecemeal mucosal resection and overall procedure time when compared with normal saline solution.[19]

Electrocautery

High-frequency electrical current is employed to facilitate cutting and to coagulate vessels at the resection margin. Electrical current is transformed to heat at high frequencies. The amount of heat that is produced in the tissue and determines cautery effects is dependent on the current density and tissue resistance. Current density is dependent on the contact (e.g., snare diameter); the smaller the contact area the higher the current density and the higher the heat. During polyp resection, the snare serves as the active electrode (high current density and heat), and the circuit is completed via a conducting grounding pad that is affixed to the patient's skin. Whereas current density is high at the snare, it is low at the grounding pad, and typically not noticed by the patient.[20]

Most electrocautery units allow three cautery modes: *cutting*, *coagulation*, or a *blend* of both. The *cutting* mode delivers a continuous sine-wave voltage pattern. When sufficient voltage is delivered with a resultant high current density, electrosurgical cutting ensues. This mode allows a swift cut through tissue without deep thermal tissue injury. The polyp base is desiccated based on the applied mechanical pressure of the snare loop onto the polyp base. This mode does not provide sufficient cautery time to seal blood vessels and bleeding is therefore a concern. In contrast, the *coagulation* mode provides less high-density current and therefore less heat. The tissue is coagulated while the snare is closed. This type of electrocautery snare resection may be considered a mechanical cut supported by coagulation. The concern is deep mural cautery injury. To minimize risk, cautery units provide a setting of cutting current alternating with coagulation current, also called *blended* mode. Realizing that heat production is dependent on tissue resistance, which is dependent on water content and changes during cautery, some cautery units provide a microprocessor-controlled current, which adjust the delivered energy to tissue resistance. This approach may optimize coagulation and cutting effects, and minimize risk.

Data on the optimal electrocautery mode are limited. A 2004 survey found that 46% of US endoscopists used blended and 46% coagulation mode.[21] Two retrospective studies suggest that coagulation may increase the risk of delayed bleeding and blended current of immediate bleeding.[22,23] Thus, the optimal electrocautery mode for polyp resection remains an important clinical question.

Argon Plasma Coagulation

Argon plasma coagulation (APC) is often used during EMR to cauterize residual polyp tissue and to ablate the resection margin.[24–27] APC produces electrically conducting argon plasma by guiding argon gas through a delivery catheter that also contains an electrode for delivery of high-frequency current. APC generally creates uniformly deep zones of desiccation, coagulation, and devitalization less than 3 mm in depth. Because the argon plasma conducts the current, APC can be applied without tissue contact.[20]

Other Instruments

Other instruments that are often used during polypectomy and mucosal resection include the standard sclerotherapy injection needle, endoclip, endoloop, and retrieval net.[28,29] Detailed examples of use of these instruments, which are important for colonoscopic resection, are described subsequently in the section on Techniques.

GENERAL APPROACH TO REMOVING A COLORECTAL POLYP

Independent of the type or complexity of resection, the following six components are common to all endoscopic resections of colonic lesions (Table 37.1). These include assessment of the lesion, decision whether to resect, position, resection, checking for completeness, retrieval and preparation of the specimen for interpretation.

Assessment of the Polyp

The macroscopic classification of adenomas and early colorectal neoplasms is crucial in the discussion of diagnosis and treatment

TABLE 37.1	**Components of Polyp Resection**	
Components of Resection	**Approach**	**Questions**
1. Assess the lesion		
Size	Use objective size reference	What tool for resection?
Morphology	Paris classification	Invasive cancer?
	LST	What portion to resect first?
Surface pattern	NICE (Kudo, Sano)	Invasive cancer?
Nonlifting sign	Submucosal injection	Invasive cancer?
2. Decide whether to resect	Weigh pros and cons	Sufficient skill, support, equipment?
3. Assume optimal position	Consider cap, retroflexion, overtube, gastroscope	Should be easy
4. Complete resection	Basic vs. advanced	How to assure curative resection?
5. Assure completeness of resection	Take time and use enhanced imaging	Did I achieve a healthy margin?
6. Retrieve and prepare the polyp	Suctioning, Roth net or with the scope, pin large specimen to orient lesion for pathologic sectioning and assessment	Is the deep margin free of cancer?

LST, Laterally spreading tumor; NICE, Narrow-Band Imaging International Colorectal Endoscopic.

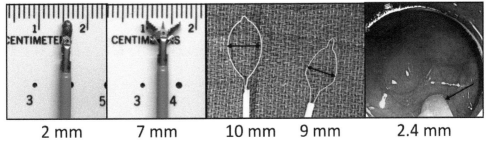

FIG 37.1 Examples of tools that can be used as a reference to estimate polyp size.

of early CRC. Typically, endoscopic resection can be considered for mucosal lesions. Submucosal lesions may require additional endosonographic evaluation. The following characteristics affect the decision whether to resect and what approach to choose.

Size

Several studies have shown variability in estimation of polyp size.[30–32] To minimize subjectivity, a reference tool may be used to estimate size. For instance, snares have predefined opening diameters and can serve as a reference (e.g., 10 mm) when positioned on or aside the polyp (Fig. 37.1). Furthermore, the snare catheter has a determined size (2.4 mm) and can also serve as a reference tool. Catheter tips could also be marked (mm/cm) to allow a more accurate assessment of size; however, this is cumbersome in clinical practice, and more applicable to studies. Because risk and surveillance management is based on size ranges, one may label polyps of 10 mm or less as diminutive (1–5 mm) and small (6–9 mm), estimate large (≥ 10 mm) by 5-mm increments up to 30 mm, and 10-mm increments for larger lesions. For very large lesions, the extent of the lesion circumference (25% increments) and across more than one fold should be noted, as these may affect difficulty of resection or risk of stenosis. To recognize the full extent of a lesion also requires clear visualization of the margin of the lesion. Digital or traditional chromoendoscopy typically help to contrast the lesion from the normal mucosa. A distal attachment cap is helpful to "spread out" the lesion slowly and inspect the margin. Submucosal injection with a contrast agent may further demarcate the lesion more clearly. Marking of the margin may be helpful in some cases before mucosal resection and submucosal dissections.

Morphology

Appearance is an important aspect to consider in preparation for resection. It provides information on the risk of prevalent cancer. In Western countries polyps have been broadly classified into pedunculated, sessile, and flat lesions. More recently, the Paris classification (2002), which is built on the well-established Japanese classification, has been promoted for worldwide use (Fig. 37.2).[33,34] The Paris classification broadly categorizes lesions into protuberant (Paris I) and flat lesions (Paris II). Protuberant lesions protrude more than 2.5 mm from the mucosa into the lumen. These include pedunculated (Ip), subpedunculated (Isp), and sessile (Is) lesions. Flat lesions are categorized as elevated lesions (but less than 2.5 mm height) (IIa), completely flat lesions that are leveled with the surrounding mucosa (IIb), and depressed lesions that are beneath the level of the surrounding mucosa (IIc). A polyp may also be elevated and have a depressed area, in which case it should be labeled IIa + c. Some snare catheters measure 2.5 mm in diameter and can therefore help to distinguish between Paris I and II.

More recently non-pedunculated lesions larger than 10 mm have been described as lateral spreading tumors (LSTs) (Fig. 37.3). The term refers more to the growth pattern rather than the endoscopic appearance. LSTs are categorized into LST-granular (LST-G), which have a carpeted nodular appearance, and into LST-nongranular (LST-NG), which may present with a flat surface or bulky appearance. This distinction is important, because LST-NG are more likely to contain invasive cancer. LST-NG are also more difficult to resect and may require en bloc resection to ensure cure. As with Paris, there could be a combination of both characteristics, which is called *mixed LST*.

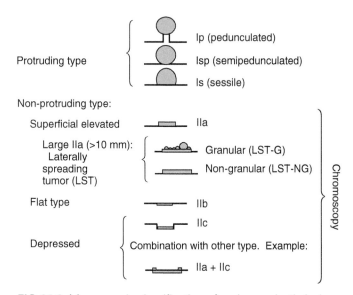

FIG 37.2 Macroscopic classification of early neoplastic lesions of the colon and rectum. This classification provides a more precise schematic description of early neoplastic lesions. In addition to the commonly described pedunculated and sessile lesions, the classification provides the appropriate descriptors for flat and depressed lesions. The classification is particularly useful for the endoscopist in deciding the treatment strategy of early colorectal carcinomas because the risk of submucosal invasion of these lesions corresponds to the endoscopic appearance and size. Image-enhanced endoscopy is useful to study the surface details and border of the non-protruding type. *LST-G,* Granular laterally spreading tumor; *LST-NG,* nongranular laterally spreading tumor; *LST,* laterally spreading tumor.

Surface Pattern

Since Kudo published his description of polyp surface pattern in 1996, several other classifications have been introduced.[35] The Kudo classification relies on chromoendoscopy and high-magnification imaging (100×) to visualize mucosal pit patterns, which can provide insights as to the pathology of the lesion. Pit patterns may reflect the tangential structure of the glands of the lesion. As the structural organization of the glands becomes disordered or even absent, as it does in invasive carcinoma, the pattern may become disorganized. The pit pattern may therefore provide clues about the presence and degree of neoplasia. According to Kudo, such assessment requires additional dye staining and high-magnification endoscopes. Dye-based enhancement typically includes diluted indigo carmine. Crystal violet, although not available for use in the United States, is also often applied in Japan when using high optical magnification (Fig. 37.4).

With the advancements in image-enhanced endoscopy, Kudo's principles have been applied to readily available high-resolution endoscopy and digital chromoendoscopy. Most commonly used are Sano and NBI International Colorectal Endoscopic (NICE) classifications, both using NBI. Sano classifies polyps into three categories (I, II, and IIIa and IIIb) based on presence, order, and regularity of capillary vessels.[36] The NICE classification uses polyp color, vessels, and surface pattern to categorize polyps into three types (Fig. 37.5).[37] A bland color, none or isolated lacy vessels, and a uniform pattern of spots (crypts) characterize hyperplastic

polyps (NICE Type 1). In contrast, adenomas have an overall brown appearance, and oval, tubular, or branched white structures surrounded by brown vessels (NICE Type 2). Invasive cancer is characterized by disrupted or absent vessels and an amorphous or absent surface pattern (NICE Type 3). Accurate recognition of polyp architecture and surface pattern is important when considering real-time optical polyp diagnosis as part of a resect-and-discard strategy, and when making a decision whether to attempt a polyp removal.

The application of a standard classification of colorectal lesions is the first step in stratifying which lesions are more likely to contain advanced pathology. Standard imaging, in some cases with image enhancement, is generally adequate to assess cancer depth.

Nonlifting Sign

Observation of the lesion during and after submucosal saline injection during mucosal resection is a simple but important method to assess the potential for deeply invasive carcinoma (Fig. 37.6).[38–40] Lesions may not lift because of desmoplastic reaction, invasion from the lesion itself, or submucosal fibrosis from prior multiple biopsy, cautery, tattoo injection, or ulceration. Several studies have reported the diagnostic operating characteristics of the nonlifting sign. The positive predictive value of the nonlifting sign is approximately 80%.[41] The correlate of the nonlifting sign when submucosal injection is not used is the inability to capture the lesion in the snare. Difficulties encountered during attempted snare resection should alert the endoscopist to the possibility of deep invasion.

Decision to Resect a Polyp

The decision on whether and how to resect a polyp is influenced by three main questions:
1. What is the malignant potential?
2. Do I have the skill to perform a complex resection?
3. Do I have technical assistance, the necessary equipment, and time to perform the resection?

Colonoscopic resection should be performed in patients for whom the removal of a polyp is likely to provide benefit. Endoscopic assessment for possible prevalent cancer and its depth of invasion are important in planning the resection. Lesions assessed to be noninvasive are most likely to benefit from endoscopic treatment. Lesions with minimal or moderate risk for submucosal invasion can be treated with endoscopy (see later), provided that the endoscopist believes that the lesion can be safely removed in its entirety and that the potential benefits of endoscopic treatment outweigh the risks. Patients whose lesions are strongly suggestive of invasive cancer should be referred to surgery after a confirmatory biopsy because endoscopic resection would expose them to unnecessary risks. Colonoscopic resection of neoplasms with deeply submucosal invasive cancer is generally difficult, has a high risk of bleeding, perforation, recurrence, and metastasis, and should be avoided.

A resection should only be performed if the endoscopist has the knowledge and expertise and supporting staff to complete the procedure. This is particularly relevant for removal of larger lesions by EMR or ESD. Rescheduling the patient may appear as a disservice to the patient. However, it may benefit the patient overall and improve outcome. The patient may be better served, when referred to a specialist, if the resection is not performed under time pressure, and if increased risks and alternatives are discussed with the patient prior to resection.

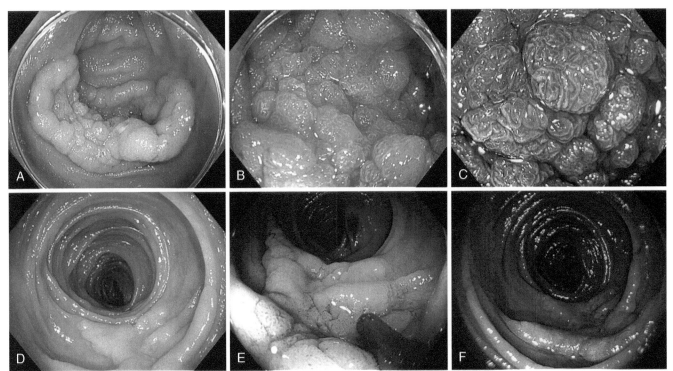

FIG 37.3 Non-polypoid lesions 10 mm or larger in diameter are referred to as laterally spreading tumors (LSTs). They have a low vertical axis and extend laterally along the luminal wall. LSTs are morphologically subclassified into granular type (LST-G) **(A–C)**, which have a nodular surface, and nongranular type (LST-NG), which have a smooth surface **(D–F)**. This macroscopic distinction is important to facilitate the endoscopic removal plan as it provides information about the risk of cancer or submucosal fibrosis to anticipate the technical ease or difficulty of the removal.

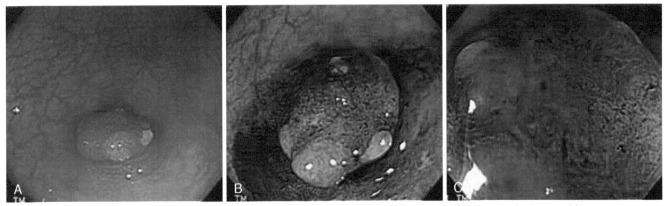

FIG 37.4 Close-up observation of the surface of lesions using magnification endoscopy with crystal violet chromoscopy can improve endoscopic assessment. **A,** A 7-mm superficial elevated lesion with depression. **B,** Crystal violet has been applied. **C,** On close examination using magnification endoscopy (100×), the pit pattern was consistent with a deeply submucosal invasive pattern. The patient underwent surgical resection where a deep submucosal invasive adenocarcinoma metastatic to local lymph nodes (2/7) was removed.

Colonoscope Position

An important aspect of endoscopist skill to perform endoscopic interventions is to achieve full control over the tip of the endoscope and assume an optimal position to complete the task. For polyp resection, this includes the "o'clock" position of the lesion and the distance of the lesion to the tip of the endoscope. Naturally, a 5 to 6 o'clock position is ideal with colonoscopes that

have the working channel opening in the same location. The key is not the position of the lesion, but the position of the lesion in reference to the endoscope. The endoscope-to-lesion distance is optimal if it allows full control over accessory equipment when engaging the polyp. As a general rule, closer is better. The optimal position is dependent on techniques and the tools, and affected by location of the lesion in the colon and with respect to a fold. For EMR and ESD, sufficient time should be

	Type 1	Type 2	Type 3
Color	Same or lighter than background	Browner relative to background	Brown to dark brown relative to background; sometimes patchy whiter areas
Vessel	None, or isolated lacy vessels coursing across the lesion	Brown vessels surrounding white structures	Has area(s) of disrupted or missing vessels
Surface Pattern	Dark or white spots of uniform size, or homogeneous absence of pattern	Oval, tubular or branched white structure surrounded by brown vessels	Amorphous or absent surface pattern
Most Likely Pathology	**Hyperplastic or Sessile Serrated Polyps (SSP)**	**Adenoma**	**Deep submucosal invasive cancer**
Examples	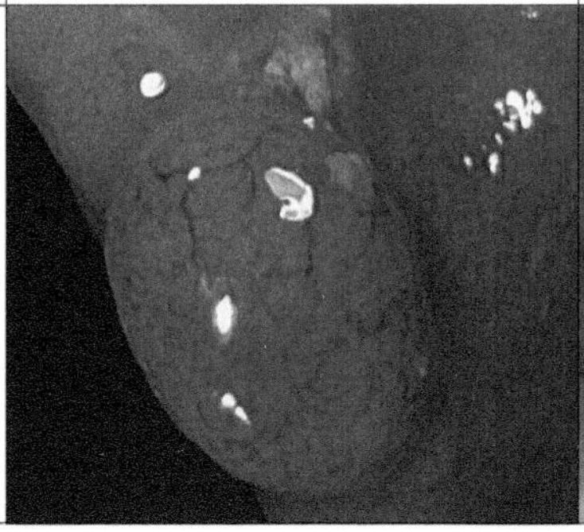	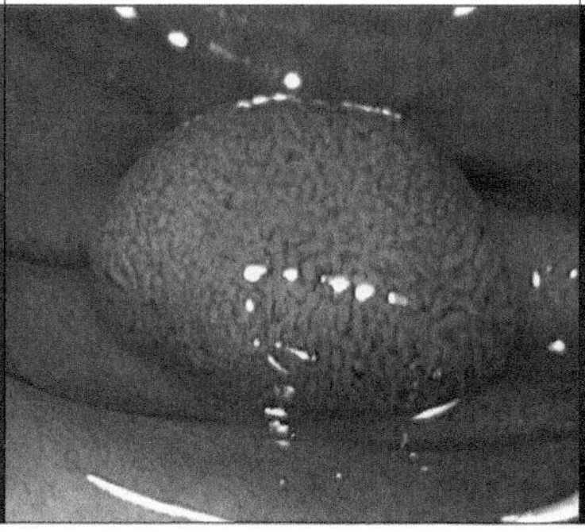	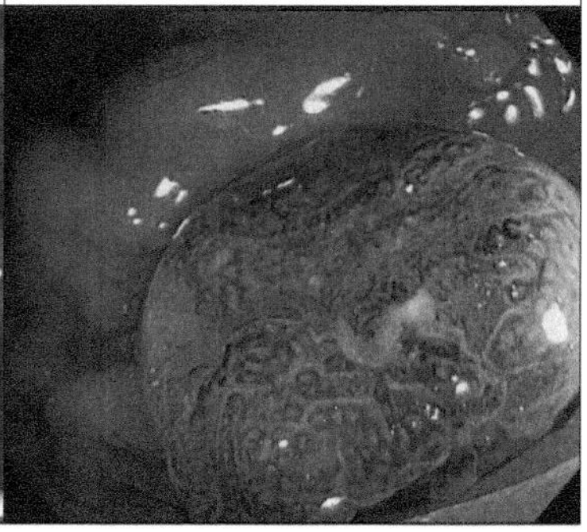

FIG 37.5 Narrow Band Imaging International Colorectal Endoscopic (NICE) Classification. Optical diagnosis of diminutive colorectal polyps by using the NICE classification. The use of confidence levels (high or low) in making an optical diagnosis is important in its implementation in clinical practice.

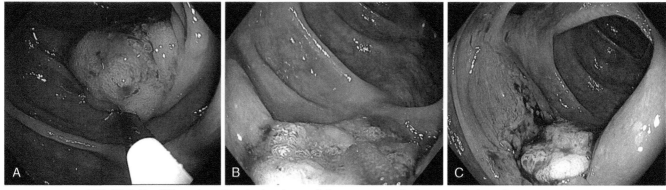

FIG 37.6 Nonlifting sign. The lesion has a full appearance that suggests invasive cancer, but prior pathology revealed only villous adenoma. **A–C,** Nonlifting sign. Injection of saline mixed with diluted indigo carmine into the submucosa beneath this lesion does not result in lifting of the lesion; instead, the lesion infolds as only the submucosa of the normal surrounding mucosa is expanded.

spent to assess the optimal position for resection, including the possibility of retroflection. If the location is difficult, alternative approaches should be considered. These include the use of an overtube (for proximal lesion location) and use of a gastroscope (easier retroflection in the rectum). A distal transparent cap that extents beyond the tip of the endoscope may ease resection of more complex lesions.[42] The cap allows stabilization of the mucosa and may improve position to lesions that are located on the proximal side of a fold.

Method of Resection

The type of resection is primarily defined by size and endoscopist preference. Different resection techniques are described later.

Completeness of Resection

Completeness of resection has received much attention over the past years. We realized that polyps are often incompletely resected, and that incomplete resection likely contributes to the risk of

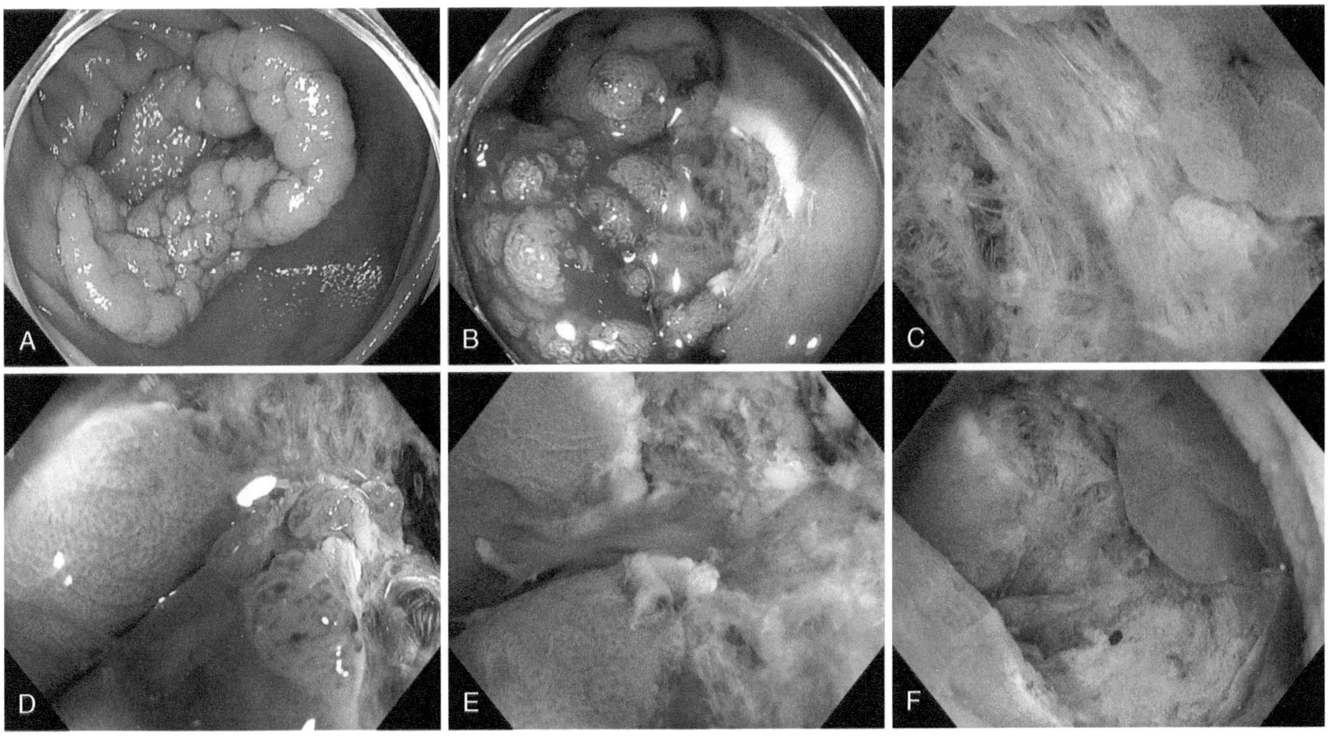

FIG 37.7 Inspect resection margins. **A,** Large cecal lateral spreading granular-type lesion. **B,** Inject and cut endoscopic mucosal resection is initiated from the periphery with clean margin. Further inspection shows **C,** no local residual, and **D,** local neoplastic residual, which is then **E,** removed using snare resection. **F,** Complete inspection of the margin defect shows no visible residual.

post-colonoscopy cancers, that is, those that occur after a complete colonoscopy.[3,4] Therefore, extra attention should be given to the polyp margin after resection. Although no study has formally examined the benefit, detailed inspection of the margin to assess for residual polyp tissue should be done. Although digital chromoendoscopy (e.g., NBI) may be used, the time spent to meticulously examine the resection margin is probably the most important aspect to assure completeness of resection. A distal cap may help to improve visualization of the margin. Residual polyp tissue should be removed (Fig. 37.7).

Retrieval and Preparation for Pathology

Each polyp should be retrieved for pathology examination. Retrieval options are based on the location, the size of the resected polyp, the type of the colonoscope (diameter of working channel), and the need for completing the remaining examination. Most polyps are sufficiently small to fit through the working channel. Larger polyps may be retrieved with a net or by suctioning them onto the orifice of the working channel and withdrawing them with the endoscope. Both options require reintroduction of the colonoscope to complete the examination. In some instances, one may decide to further cut a larger lesion into smaller pieces to allow suction through the working channel and avoid reintroducing the colonoscope.

In some countries, it is mandatory for the pathologist to provide information on the margins of the resected polyp.[43,44] However, there has been no study that clearly shows that polyp tissue at the margin of the resected polyp is predictive of incomplete resection. Moreover, cautery artifact and orientation of the specimen may impair adequate evaluation of margin involvement.

For larger lesions with signs of advanced neoplasia and early cancer, specimens should be prepared for optimal pathology assessment and to allow interpretation of a deep margin of an early cancer. For this purpose, specimens are pinned on a cork or on styrofoam before fixation in formalin. This will help the pathology assistant to cut and prepare specimens for optimal orientation. Mucosal or early submucosal cancers have a low risk of lymph node involvement. If the deep margins of such lesions are clear, surgery may be avoided. The risk and benefits of this decision, however, need to be discussed with the patient.

RESECTION TECHNIQUES

Basic Polypectomy

Definition

Basic polypectomy refers to resection of a polyp with one tool that does not require additional adjunctive means. Polyps that can be removed by basic resection technique are typically small, and because most polyps are small, the vast majority of polyps can be removed by this technique. Generally, all polyps should be removed by mechanical means. Two tools are available: biopsy forceps and resection snare. Both can be used with and without electrocautery, which is also known as cold and hot resection. The addition of electrocautery may reduce the immediate risk of bleeding and promote complete polyp removal by ablating residual polyp tissue. To date, there is little evidence to support the benefit of electrocautery resection for basic polypectomy.

The upper size limit that supports a basic resection technique (and that does not require submucosal injection) is unclear, and depends on local practice and individual preference. In a 2016

TABLE 37.2   Recommended Resection Method by Polyp Size

Polyp Size	Resection Method
1–2 mm	Cold forceps or cold snare
1–9 mm	Cold snare
≥ 10 mm	Hot snare with or without submucosal injection (consider cold snare if concerns about deep thermal injury)
≥ 15 mm	Submucosal injection/EMR
≤ 25 mm	Attempt en bloc EMR

EMR, Endoscopic mucosal resection.

study, hot snare resection was similarly effective in completely removing polyps up to 14 mm in size when compared to resection following submucosal injection. Whereas there was a nonsignificant trend favoring submucosal injection for polyps of 15 to 19 mm, submucosal injection showed a clear benefit for polyps 20 mm or larger.[45] These results reflect our current practice. Whereas most polyps up to 15 mm may be removed without submucosal injection, submucosal injection is used for larger polyps. Table 37.2 provides the suggested resection approach based on polyp size.

Resection Tools

Hot forceps resection has been commonly used in the past. However, it is often incomplete, and histopathology specimens may be difficult to interpret.[46,47] The greatest concern is the potential for deep tissue injury and increased risk of postpolypectomy syndrome, delayed bleeding, and perforation.[47] Therefore, hot biopsy forceps should not be used for basic polyp resection.

Cold forceps resection is the most commonly used means for resection for small diminutive polyps (≤ 4 mm) in the United States.[48] Despite its inefficiency for resection of larger lesions, it is still frequently used for large polyps.[49] Cold snare resection is frequently used for diminutive polyps, and hot snare resection has been the most common resection method for removal of polyps of 5 mm or greater.[48]

Head-to-head comparisons of cold forceps with cold snare resection have shown that both are equally effective for complete polyp removal for up to 3-mm polyps, whereas resection of larger polyps is more frequently complete when using a snare.[50–52] However, even with a snare, incomplete resection of diminutive and small polyps occurs.[51] A dedicated cold snare with a stiff wire may more frequently allow complete resection than a standard snare that is typically used for cold or hot snare resection. In one study dedicated cold snare resection of up to 10-mm polyps resulted in a lower incomplete resection rate of 9% compared to 21% when using a standard snare.[15] In clinical practice, however, most endoscopists currently use a hot snare for polyps that are 5 mm or larger.[48] It should be noted that there is no evidence that the addition of cautery promotes completeness of resection. The results of the CARE study, where all 5- to 20- mm polyps were removed by hot snare, still found an incomplete resection rate for 5- to 7-mm polyps of 6%,[4] very similar to results from cold snare studies. More recently, cold snares have been used for resection of larger polyps. Although it may lead to mild immediate bleeding (similar to taking mucosal biopsies), studies suggest that cold snare resection of polyps up

to 10 mm in size is at least as safe and effective as hot snare resection.[15,53–55] In one randomized study among patients who were on anticoagulants, the risk of immediate and delayed bleeding with cold snare resection was lower compared with hot snare resection (immediate bleeding: 6% vs. 23%; delayed bleeding: 0% vs. 14%).[54] Although mild bleeding after cold snare resection may occur, two other randomized studies have described no immediate bleeding event that required an intervention (e.g., clip placement).[53,56] The upper size limit for cold snare resection is yet unclear. Case series have reported feasibility of piecemeal removal of polyps larger than 20 mm in size.[57,58] In their 2017 guidelines the European Society of Gastrointestinal Endoscopy supports the resection of all sessile polyps larger than 10 mm with cold snare resection owing to its superior safety profile.[14] Cold snare resection of larger polyps (< 20 mm) can be considered if there is concern about deep thermal injury. Evidence for these recommendations is still lacking. It remains unclear if the increased need for piecemeal resection with larger polyp size will increase the risk for incomplete removal.

Cold Forceps Technique

A cold forceps may be used for resection of polyps that are more difficult to engage with a snare, either related to location or due to very small size (≤ 2 mm). The added benefit of using a forceps is immediate retrieval of the specimen with the forceps. The disadvantage is the possibility of not removing the entire polyp and the need for a repeat bite, which makes the resection via piecemeal resection and increases uncertainty for complete removal.[59] Using a large-capacity forceps does not seem to decrease the need for additional biopsies but may improve completeness of resection,[59,60] and even after visibly complete removal resection may still be incomplete in 20% of polyps of 6 mm or less.[59] Therefore, we consider it preferable to use a cold snare for all polyps of 3 mm or larger.

Cold Snare Technique

We suggest a cold snare as the primary resection tool for all diminutive polyps (Fig. 37.8). A cold snare can be safely used for polyps up to 10 mm in size. Some snares do not allow swift cold cutting through the base, and a dedicated cold snare may be preferable. Hot snare resection for polyps of 6 mm or larger remains an alternative. Polyps larger than 10 mm should be removed by hot snare given the lack of robust data for efficacy and safety of cold snare resection.

After sufficient insufflation and assuming an optimal position, the snare is opened and placed around the polyp head. The goal is to obtain a small healthy tissue margin around the polyp base to ensure complete resection. This is achieved by first carefully anchoring the snare tip at the proximal side of the polyp, approximately 1 to 2 mm away from the polyp base. The snare is then placed around the polyp base and the tip of the snare catheter gently anchored 1 to 2 mm distal to the polyp margin. The snare is slowly closed while maintaining gentle pressure of the catheter tip on the mucosa and suctioning some air. This gentle push allows engagement of a small healthy margin (Video 37.1). The removed polyp will remain at the resection spot and can now be easily accessed and retrieved through the working channel. Inspection of the margin follows the resection. Additional washing with the water jet may help to reduce mild bleeding, and also leads to mild submucosal lifting of the margin, which may then facilitate the ability to assess the margin. Residual polyp tissue can be removed with a cold snare or a forceps. There

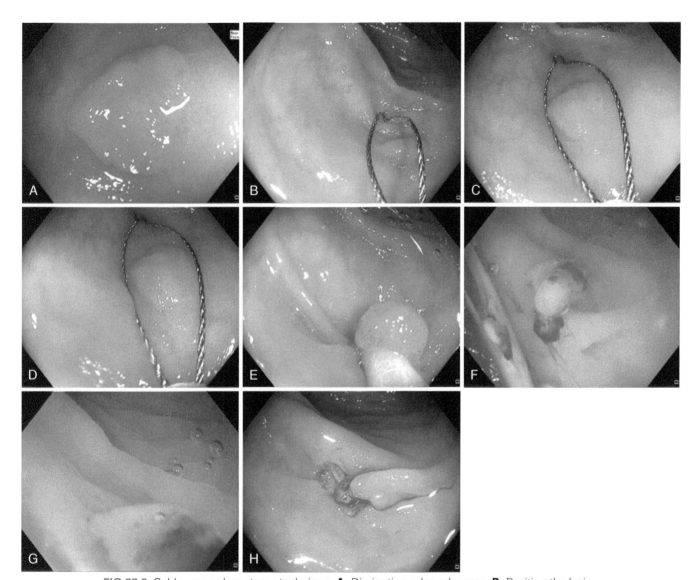

FIG 37.8 Cold snare polypectomy technique. **A,** Diminutive colon adenoma. **B,** Position the lesion at 5 o'clock in line with the colonoscope accessory channel. Engage the snare tip against the mucosa on the proximal side of the lesion, and open slowly. **C,** Open the snare until it has normal surrounding tissue and slightly move the endoscope distally as the snare is being opened according to the size of the lesion. **D,** While the snare is initially "closed" in a slow and steady manner, keep the endoscope tip deflection downward to apply gentle pressure against the mucosa (the ensnared polyp should not be lifted or tented during closure). **E,** Continue to maintain some tension on the snare catheter with gentle forward pressure during closure to avoid slipping of the snare upward, away from the submucosa and consequent shaving of the lesion. As the snare wire is closed, it will capture normal tissue. **F,** Once you have secured the normal tissue, then the lesion can be "cut." The snare "close" is slow and steady, the snare "cut" is faster. **G,** In the 5 o'clock position, the cut polyp typically remains in place for efficient retrieval. **H,** Minor post-cold snare oozing is expected and self-limiting.

have been no studies to show that a larger mucosal defect related to a healthy margin is associated with a higher risk of bleeding. Small flat lesions may be difficult to remove. Aspirating the lesion into the suctioning channel of the colonoscope for 5 seconds will create a pseudopolyp (suction pseudopolyp technique) and facilitates snare capture and resection.[61]

Hot Snare Technique

Resection with electrocautery snare is very similar to the cold snare technique, with the exception of the cutting maneuver.

The polyp is sufficiently exposed by insufflating air and brought into an optimal position. The polyp is then engaged by anchoring the catheter tip 1 to 2 mm distal to the polyp base. The snare is then closed while maintaining gentle pressure with the catheter tip onto the mucosa and suctioning some air. After tightly closing the snare around the polyp base, the entrapped polyp is now lifted or "tented" away from the colonic wall to avoid deep cautery tissue injury (Video 37.2). The polyp is then resected by applying electrocautery while fully closing the snare. The lift-and-cut technique represents the major difference compared with the gentle push-and-cut technique with cold snare resection. It is possible that lifting of the entrapped polyp may promote snare slippage away from the polyp base and therefore not include a healthy margin. Following the lift-and-cut resection, the margins should be carefully examined for residual polyp tissue.

Some endoscopists prefer to take the snare from the assistant and cut through the polyp base when applying electrocautery. This may be of benefit when performing resection of larger polyps to get a "feel" of the amount of entrapped polyp. This tactile feedback may be more relevant when applying forced coagulation, which can be understood as cautery-assisted mechanical cutting. In contrast, blended current applies a high energy and desiccates through tissue ("like a hot knife through butter") based on the pressure applied by the snare on the tissue. Here, the intermittent coagulation current "seals" any potentially bleeding vessels. The tactile feedback is therefore less present when applying this electrocautery mode. Overall, there have been no formal studies to show that any available setting should be preferred (Box 37.1).

Advanced Polyp Resection
Snare-Loop Polypectomy
Pedunculated and semipedunculated lesions (Paris Ip and Isp) may be resected by snare-loop polypectomy at the middle or upper stalk. Sessile lesions can be resected by a similar technique at the base. Large polyps (> 2 cm) or polyps with a thick stalk carry a higher risk of immediate or delayed bleeding. Prophylactic treatment to close off blood vessels in the stalk before resection prevents immediate or delayed bleeding (Fig. 37.9).[62–64]

One prophylactic method is the application of endoloops, which are detachable nylon loops that are applied to the base of the polyp stalk to strangulate the vessels supplying the polyp. Randomized trials have shown that prophylactic placement of an endoloop significantly reduced the rate of bleeding.[62,65] Another randomized trial of large pedunculated colon polyps showed significantly lower and less severe delayed bleeding among patients following prophylactic detachable snare placement and clip application to the residual stalk compared with patients who underwent prophylactic epinephrine injection alone.[64] However, placement of the endoloop in pedunculated polyps that have short stalks can be difficult. Massive bleeding can occur if the endoloop slips right after snare polypectomy.[66] In addition, the endoloop is made of nylon, which can be too floppy for ensnaring the polyp. In a more recent randomized trial (2014) among 195 patients with pedunculated polyps with a minimum stalk diameter of 5 mm, the bleeding rate was similar following prophylaxis with placement of an endoloop (5.7%) or clips (5.1%).[27] Although this study showed that prophylactic clipping was not inferior to using an endoloop, placement of clips for polyps with a large stalk may be difficult to achieve.

Because massive colonic bleeding can easily cause immediate loss of visualization, other prophylactic techniques may be more appropriate. Seitz et al (2003) used diluted epinephrine to inject to the base of the stalk before polypectomy.[67] Because the effect of epinephrine is transient, the site was then clipped. Other authors have reported safe use of endoclips before polypectomy (Fig. 37.10).[27] En bloc resection is a key component of precise pathologic staging in cases of polyps containing invasive cancer. A case series of giant pedunculated polyps described a greater than 80% volume reduction after 4 to 8 mL of 1:10,000 epinephrine injections into both the polyp head and the stalk. The dramatic volume reduction decreased the need for piecemeal

---

BOX 37.1   Rules of Endoscopic Resection

1. Remove in one piece if safely possible
2. Finish polyp resection in one session. A delayed resection will increase the risk of incomplete polyp removal
3. Obtain a healthy margin
4. Mechanical removal is superior to ablation
5. Avoid taking a biopsy if a patient will return for an EMR or ESD. High-quality endoscopic images are superior to biopsy for the referring endoscopist to assess the amenability of the lesion for endoscopic resection and plan for the appropriate resection procedure

EMR, endoscopic mucosal resection; *ESD,* endoscopic submucosal dissection.

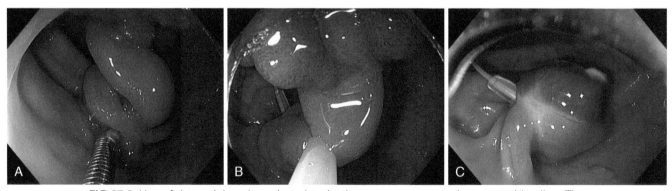

FIG 37.9 Use of the endoloop in pedunculated polyp to prevent postpolypectomy bleeding. The endoloop is used like a snare, except it can be detached after its deployment at the base of the polyp. **A,** The endoloop has been applied at the base of a large pedunculated lesion to ligate the feeding vessel. **B,** The polyp head has an ischemic purple appearance, and then an electrocautery snare has been placed above the loop with sufficient room to prevent the endoloop from slipping off after transection. The ideal way to snare a pedunculated polyp that has been looped is to tighten the snare as much as possible to make the snared plane smaller than the plane that has been looped. **C,** Resection site immediately after resection. A small blood vessel is visible. There was no bleeding after resection.

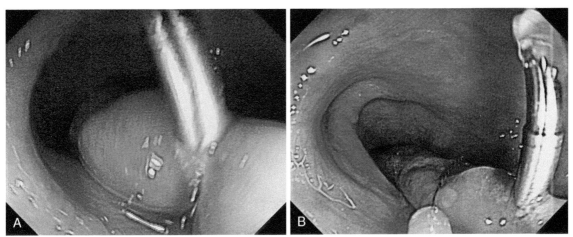

FIG 37.10 An alternative to endoloops for preventing postpolypectomy bleeding is the endoclip. **A,** A single endoclip has been applied at the lower part of a long polyp stalk. **B,** The polyp appeared dusky after the endoclip placement, indicating effective strangulation of the stalk. The snare was subsequently positioned above the clip, and electrocautery was applied. It is important to avoid touching the clip with the snare during electrocautery application.

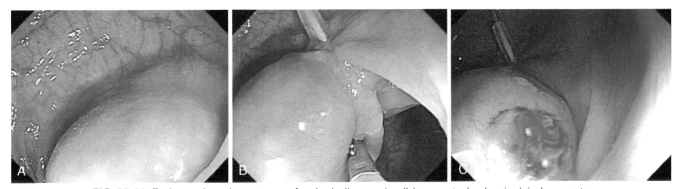

FIG 37.11 Endoscopic polypectomy of colonic lipoma (well known to be benign) is known to carry a high risk of perforation. The ligate and let go technique is safe and efficacious to treat colonic lipoma. **A,** Typical appearance of a colonic lipoma. Originally, the lesion was sessile (not shown), but by repositioning the patient to make it "hanging," the lesion became pedunculated because its weight had pulled it from its point of attachment. **B,** Ligation of the point of attachment using an endoloop caused the lesion to become ischemic. **C,** Biopsy on biopsy showed the naked fat, confirming the diagnosis. There was no residual on follow-up colonoscopy a few months later.

resection.[68] In addition to reducing bleeding, the prophylactic use of the endoloop or endoclip at the base of large pedunculated polyps to facilitate en bloc rather than piecemeal resection has been described. The loop-and-let-go technique may be useful for the treatment of large pedunculated lesions, especially colonic lipomas (Fig. 37.11).[69]

Endoscopic Mucosal Resection

Non-polypoid lesions can be difficult to capture with standard snare and polypectomy techniques, and it may be impossible to perform en bloc resection of large flat lesions using standard polypectomy techniques. Furthermore, the application of electrocautery may lead to a burn injury of the muscularis propria. A mucosal resection technique using submucosal injection can ameliorate these technical difficulties and risks. The indications of colonoscopic mucosal resection and submucosal dissection are presented in Box 37.2.

Various resection techniques have been described.[70] EMR refers to the inject-and-cut technique, which is most common. It was first described as the stripped biopsy method by Karita et al (1991).[71] The key aspects of submucosal injection are to inject a sufficient amount and to recognize the presence of the nonlifting sign. The ideal solution, which would form a substantial bulge and would not dissipate quickly, has not yet been defined. Physicians in the United States routinely use saline (Fig. 37.12).

Over the past decade, EMR has replaced surgical resection. It has been shown that it can achieve complete polyp removal in more 90% of lesions.[72,73] Considering the morbidity and potential mortality (albeit low) with surgical resection, and the required postsurgical care, EMR is more cost effective than surgical resection.[74] Therefore, endoscopic resection should be the first-line treatment for any colon polyp.

Submucosal injection lifts the polyp from the submucosal layer. The benefit is threefold. It creates a more protuberant

---

BOX 37.2 **Indications for Colonoscopic Mucosal Resection and Submucosal Dissection**

I. Requires a team to safely and efficaciously perform endoscopic mucosal resection (EMR) or submucosal dissection

II. The neoplasm does not have features of deep submucosal or deeper invasion

III. EMR: Lesion (non-polypoid or sessile) with mucosal neoplasia requiring resection at the submucosa to ensure cure. If the lesion is suspected to contain high-grade dysplasia or superficial submucosal invasion, EMR is indicated, provided that the lesion is within the scope of the EMR technique for en bloc removal

IV. Endoscopic submucosal dissection: Lesion requiring en bloc resection:
    1) Lesions for which en bloc resection with snare EMR is difficult to apply
      • Large nongranular lesion (laterally spreading tumor-nongranular) with slight depression
      • Lesions with suspected cancer and suggesting shallow submucosal invasion
      • Large depressed-type tumors
    2) Mucosal tumors with submucosal fibrosis
    3) Sporadic localized tumors in conditions of chronic inflammation such as ulcerative colitis
    4) Local residual or recurrent early carcinomas after endoscopic resection

IV. Pathologic evaluation provided proof of cure:
    A. Well-differentiated carcinoma (without poorly differentiated)
    B. Without lymphatic or vascular invasion
    C. Intramucosal cancer, regardless of size (limit of involvement in the United States)
    D. Minute submucosal invasion less than 1000 μm from the muscularis mucosa, or if the muscularis mucosa is absent, depth of measurement is performed from the surface of lesion
    E. Vertical and lateral margins are free of carcinoma

---

lesion, particularly of flat polyps, which can then be more easily engaged into a snare. It provides a safety cushion between the mucosal polyp and the muscularis propria when applying electrocautery by better distribution of current into the wide fluid cushion.[75] Last, the added contrast media generally demarcates the polyp margin from normal surrounding mucosa.

When should EMR instead of simple snare resection be used? A 2016 study suggests a possible benefit of submucosal injection for lesions 15 mm or larger, and clear benefit for lesions greater than 20 mm.[45] In practice, the size cutoff is determined by local practice and individual preference. Anecdotally, European endoscopists tend to inject smaller polyps than endoscopists from North America.

Once the decision is made to proceed with EMR, the resection needs to be planned. Can the lesion be removed in one piece (en bloc), or will it require piecemeal resection? If piecemeal, where should the resection start? Which snare is preferable?

En bloc resection: Resection in one piece is typically attempted for polyps up to 25 mm in size. It is associated with a lower risk of recurrence when compared to piecemeal resection.[76] The complication risk may be increased when attempting larger en bloc resection. The technique of en bloc resection is identical to hot snare resection following submucosal injection.

Piecemeal resection: The approach to piecemeal resection depends on the morphology, size, and location of the lesion. The following suggestions should be considered:

• The area of the polyp with the highest risk of cancer should be resected first. An LST-NG or mixed morphology has a higher risk of prevalent cancer than an LST-G.[77] Cancer is more commonly located in the protuberant portion (Paris Is) of the polyp. Retrieval of this specimen and preparation for pathology evaluation as detailed previously is mandatory to assess for possible deep invasion of cancer.

• Submucosal injection can help to improve visualization and positioning of the polyp. For instance, if a polyp is partially or completely located behind a fold, injection should start from the proximal margin of the lesion. This will lift the polyp toward the visual field of the colonoscope and ease resection.

• Submucosal injection may be applied liberally and may be used to "mold" the shape of the lifted lesion (dynamic injection; Fig. 37.13). By changing the needle catheter during injection (e.g., lifting), using subtle tip deflection into the lumen, gentle pull of the needle catheter back, and slight suctioning of the lumen, the shape of the submucosal cushion can be changed, which may improve positioning of the polyp and enhance engagement of the polyp into the snare.

The technical approach to EMR follows the principles of hot snare resection (Video 37.3). After the submucosal injection, the snare is positioned around the target area. A rim of normal mucosa is included. While maintaining gentle pressure of the snare onto the colonic wall, air is gently aspirated, and the snare closed. This combined maneuver of aspiration and closure promotes full engagement of the target tissue into the snare. Once the snare is closed, air is reinsufflated to visualize adequate entrapment of the polyp. The snare catheter is then moved back and forth (tucking) to ensure that no muscularis propria is enclosed in the snare. If the endoscopist is confident that snare closure is optimal, the snare is moved away from the wall and completely closed while applying electrocautery. After resection, the area should be flushed and carefully inspected for deep mural injury. A black or a yellow "bull's eye" at the resection base (or yellow "target sign" at the base of the resected polyp) may indicate perforation or impending perforation (serosal fat). Such a defect needs to be closed immediately. Once closure is ensured, resection can be continued. After the entire polyp is removed, the resection margin and the polyp base are carefully examined using white light and digital chromoendoscopy for any remaining polyp tissue.

Removing residual tissue islands may be challenging. The general principle holds that mechanical removal is superior to ablation. A dedicated stiff cold snare may engage small polyp islands more reliably. If this is not possible, residual tissue can be removed by avulsion. The tissue is grabbed with a forceps and pulled slowly and tangentially to obtain a larger tissue piece. Any bleeding that occurs with these cold resection techniques is typically mild and self-limited. If mechanical attempts to remove residual tissue fail, ablation should be applied. This can be done with APC. Alternatively, soft coagulation cautery may be safely applied through the snare tip.

Following visible complete resection, additional ablation of the resection margin may reduce risk of recurrence (see later). Retrieval of resection specimen can be accomplished with a net and withdrawal of the colonoscope. Specimens that indicate suspicion of prevalent cancer should be pinned to allow optimal preparation by the pathology lab for assessment of deep margin involvement.

Modified EMR Techniques

Underwater resection. Complete water immersion of the polyp may facilitate capture of the lesion with the snare and promote

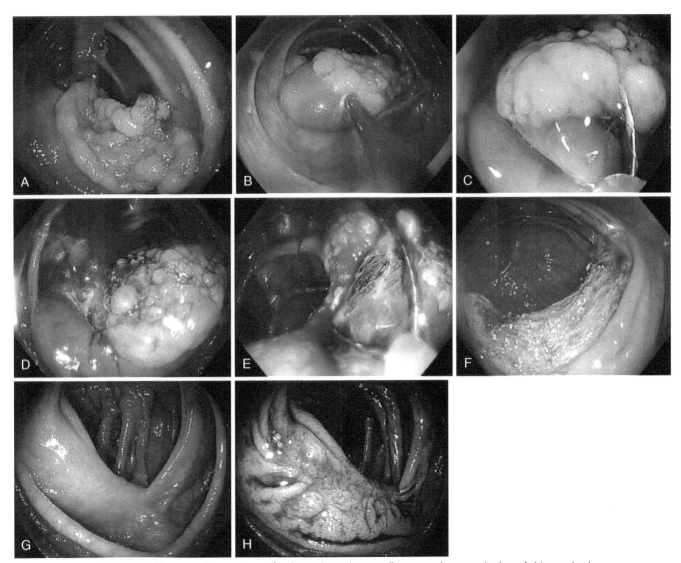

FIG 37.12 Piecemeal resection of a large lateral spreading granular type lesion. A biopsy had been performed to document that the lesion was a large villous adenoma, as was suspected from its endoscopic appearance. **A,** The lesion was located adjacent to the ileocecal valve. **B,** A large amount (40–50 mL) of saline mixed with a few drops of 0.2% indigo carmine was injected into the submucosa to lift the lesion. Efforts were made to inject so that the lesion does not tilt away from the colonoscope. **C,** The first piece was resected using a stiff snare at the edge of the lesion. By resecting the lateral margin first, the endoscopist developed an understanding of the depth of the lesion and the location of the submucosal plane. **D,** A small piece of the lesion had been resected. The visible bluish layer was the submucosa. **E,** Subsequent resections were performed without proceeding deeper than the submucosa. The remaining large piece of the lesion was snared. Note the position of the snare: parallel with the bowel wall. **F,** Appearance after piecemeal resection, which was completed approximately 40 minutes later. Argon plasma was applied to ensure complete eradication of the villous adenoma. **G** and **H,** The area of prior resection on follow-up 3 months later. There was no residual adenoma.

en bloc resection. Within the water-filled colon segment, the colonic wall is not expanded, and the muscularis propria tends not to involute into the lumen and become at risk for capture in the snare. Submucosal injection to create a safety cushion can therefore be deferred.

In a recent study, en bloc resection of 2- to 4-cm polyps was accomplished in 29 out of 53 lesions (55%). Outcomes were at least comparable to standard EMR with four complications, including one delayed bleeding event. Recurrence at first follow-up

was noted in 5% of patients. The drawback of this technique is impaired visualization in patients with suboptimal prep or with intraprocedural bleeding. However, these results encourage comparative studies.

Cold snare resection EMR. The upper size limit for cold resection of polyps has been increased to include LST lesions. The argument for cold snare resection is to lower the risk of delayed bleeding complications. Furthermore, complications related to cautery use, such as perforation or post-polypectomy syndrome,

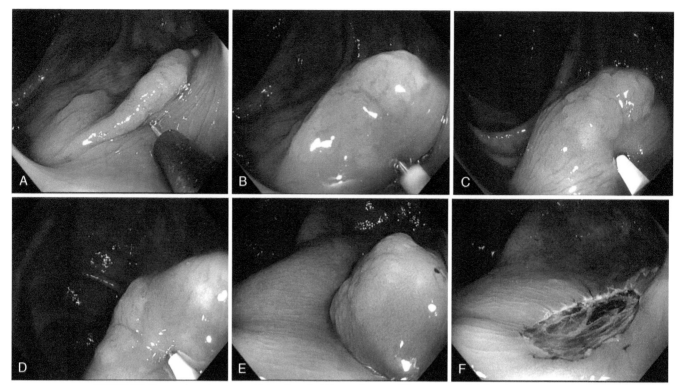

FIG 37.13 Dynamic submucosal injection. **A,** We evaluate a 15-mm superficially elevated serrated-appearing lesion under white light with diluted indigo carmine solution. In preparation for resection, we ensure optimal positioning of the targeted lesion to the 5–6 o'clock position and plan the path of injection. **B,** We place the needle catheter next to the lesion to then expose and insert the needle into the submucosa. **C,** We rapidly inject the mixture of saline and diluted indigo carmine into the submucosa with simultaneous adjustments of the needle catheter and endoscope tip to ultimately lift the lesion upward. **D,** As the injection proceeds to the right, the direction of the injection is slightly altered to the left and then upward again in order to guide the creation of the focal submcuosal bleb. **E,** During this process, we slightly suction the lumen in order to decrease wall tension, and then are able to place a snare around the lesion, and **F,** complete en bloc resection.

would not occur with this technique. Case series have shown that it is technically feasible and does not lead to increased intraprocedural bleeding complications.[57,58] Drawbacks may include impaired visualization from intraprocedural bleeding and smaller resection pieces. Both may increase the risk of recurrence.[78] Data on longer-term outcomes and recurrence are needed, and this approach is therefore considered experimental.

Submucosal resection with band ligation. This technique can be particularly useful for resection of submucosal lesions, such as carcinoid tumors in the rectum (Fig. 37.14).[79,80] After the endoscope is fitted with the ligation device, the target area is ligated, with or without prior deep submucosal injection. Standard polypectomy is performed below the rubber band. Small submucosal lesions may require prior markings at their periphery, achieved by brief bursts of cautery using the tip of a snare, because such lesions may be difficult to find after the ligation device has been fitted to the endoscope. Cap-assisted EMR has been popular and efficacious for resection of superficial early cancer in the esophagus and stomach, but in general it should not be used in the colon, as the thin muscularis propria of the colon can easily be suctioned into the cap, potentially leading to perforation.

Special Considerations

Location in the ileocecal (IC) valve. Position in the IC valve is not necessarily a contraindication for EMR. In a case series of 53 patients, LSTs could be successfully removed, and surgery avoided, in 43 patients (81%).[81] Recurrence was observed in 8 patients (20%), which could be managed endoscopically in all cases. Infiltration of the ileum and involvement of both IC valve lips were associated with failure of EMR. It should be pointed out that the published data are from a very experienced group and that technical success may not be generalizable. Furthermore, these results also point out that documentation of localization should be detailed and should state whether the superior and inferior lips, and the anterior and posterior angles of the IC valve, are involved.

Location in the appendiceal orifice. Extension of a lesion into the orifice of the appendix is only possible if the margin within the orifice is visible, which is in accordance with the principles of mucosal resection.

Location at the anorectal junction. Lesions involving the anal canal may be technically challenging because of impaired visibility (Fig. 37.15). Resection may be facilitated with the use of a cap (antegrade view) and the use of a gastroscope, which has greater

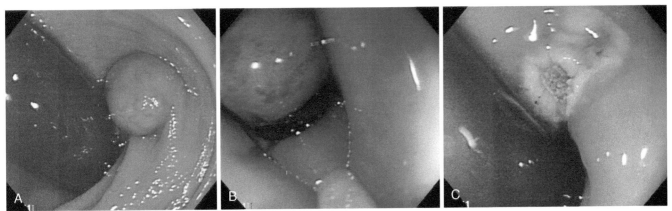

FIG 37.14 Endoscopic submucosal resection of a small carcinoid tumor in the rectum using a band ligation device. **A,** Lesion. **B,** After deep submucosal injection of saline and placement of a band using the ligation device, a snare is seen transecting the lesion as cautery is applied. **C,** Resection margin. The lesion was contained within the resected specimen with a clear margin (not shown). By cutting immediately below the band, a deeper resection can be performed.

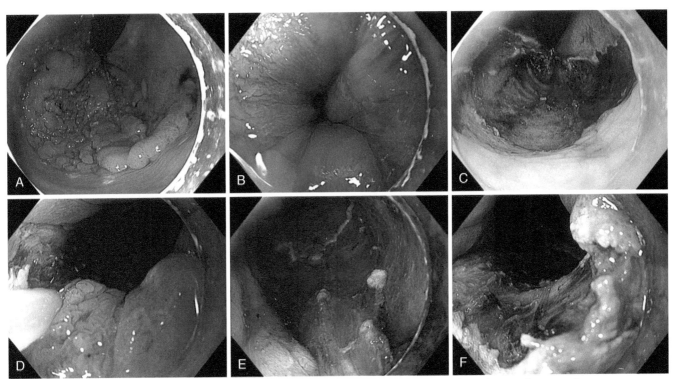

FIG 37.15 Distal rectal lesion involving the anal canal. **A,** A large 5-cm lateral spreading granular type lesion on the anterior wall of the distal rectum is seen in retroflexion, and **B,** extending into the anal canal. **C,** Piecemeal endoscopic mucosal resection is performed, and the mucosal defect can be seen. **D,** Inspection of the anal canal for residual neoplasia to target for resection requires the use of a cap. Position of the snare for resection of the neoplasia. **E** and **F,** Further inspection shows no further residual.

flexibility when resection is performed in retroflexion. Resection may include the squamous epithelium of the anal canal, which has a somatic sensory nerve supply and therefore requires anesthesia prior to resection. For such instances, a long-acting local anesthetic (e.g., bubivacaine) may be added to the submucosal injection fluid. Furthermore, rectal veins drain directly into the systemic system and not through the portal system with

its protective reticuloendothelial function. This may increase the risk of systemic bacteremia related to repeated submucosal injection and large-field resection, and antibiotic prophylaxis may be considered (although this has not been adopted into guidelines). Finally, hemorrhoidal plexus may be a concern for increased bleeding. However, the hemorrhoid vessels are located deep within the submucosa and are protected by the submucosal cushion. Injection should be placed just aside the hemorrhoidal columns to lower bleeding risk and ensure a safe submucosal lift between the polyp and the hemorrhoids. The Australian Colonic Endoscopic Resection (ACE) study group describes their standardized approach using local anesthetics and prophylactic antibiotics for lesions greater than 40 mm and within 5 cm of the dentate line.[82] Efficacy and safety was similar to resection of lesions in the proximal rectum.

Circumferential extension. No size limit for resection of LST lesions has been described. Polyps up to 16 cm in size have been excised by EMR. However, size appears to be less a limiting factor for mucosal resection than polyp morphology or location. Lesions that occupy the entire circumference are rare. In a case series, they represented approximately 1% of all LSTs larger than 20 mm, with the majority being located in the rectum or sigmoid colon.[83] Complete removal was accomplished of all 12 lesions in this series. Lumenal stenosis after resection is a concern, although symptomatic stricturing that required dilatation occurred in only two cases (17%). Recurrence after resection, which appears to be more frequent than seen with the average LST, could be successfully treated by repeated endoscopic resection.

Submucosal lesions. Endoscopic resection is also used increasingly to remove submucosal lesions, where the risk of metastasis is low.[70] In particular, rectal carcinoids up to 10 mm without any adverse features can be treated by endoscopic resection. A 2014 systematic review supports endoscopic resection of up to 16-mm rectal carcinoids followed by careful histological assessment.[84]

Endoscopic Submucosal Dissection

En bloc endoscopic resection of early gastric cancer was first described in 1988,[85] but it was not until 1999 that the first report of the use of a specialized knife was published in the Japanese literature[86] and soon after the term *ESD* was coined. Although the development of endoscopic therapy of early gastric cancer was the main driving force behind the evolution of ESD in the East, the first English language description of ESD was in the rectum.[87] Since then in the East, ESD has quickly gained popularity and has become a routinely used modality for the management of superficial lesions containing early cancer or high-grade dysplasia throughout the gastrointestinal tract.

The use of ESD over EMR in selected colonic lesions has been supported by two meta-analyses showing well-documented higher en bloc and curative resection rates, as well as decreased local recurrence.[88,89] An increased rate of adverse events with ESD mostly related to perforation and bleeding was shown in one of these meta-analyses,[89] but this was not confirmed by the other meta-analysis.[88] Importantly, the overwhelming majority of adverse events were successfully managed by endoscopic means. Nevertheless, ESD tends to be a lengthier procedure than EMR and requires extensive training. As a result, in the West expertise is not widely available.

At present, the majority of colonic lesions can be managed by EMR, but ESD expands the opportunity for patient cure and should be given strong consideration in the following circumstances[90]:

- LST-NG type. This recommendation is driven by the higher propensity of LST-NG for submucosal invasion. Even if malignant submucosal invasion is not present, LST-NGs tend to not lift well with submucosal injection due to submucosal fibrosis, which makes EMR technically difficult and complete resection frequently unsuccessful.

- Large LST-G type. ESD should be considered in LST-Gs measuring greater than 30 mm with large nodule(s) or large depressed areas due to the higher risk of submucosal invasion in these lesions.[91]
- Mucosal tumors with submucosal fibrosis, such as seen with post-EMR recurrences, lesions only partially removed by EMR, lesions that have been sampled with partial snare resection to obtain a large specimen for pathology, and tattoo placed under the lesion. Similarly, lesions in conditions of chronic inflammation, such as ulcerative colitis, tend to have a higher degree of submucosal fibrosis and may preferentially be approached by ESD.[92]
- Lesions with high suspicion for invasive cancer with invasion into the superficial submucosa (< 1000 μm). Assessment of invasion depth is typically based on the Kudo classification, and Kudo pattern Vi is consistent with superficial submucosal invasion whereas Kudo pattern Vn is seen with deep invasion. This differentiation can be very difficult if expertise in magnification endoscopy and chromoendoscopy with crystal violet is not available. The more practical NICE classification has been shown to have high sensitivity and specificity to detect deep submucosal invasion (NICE Type 3), precluding the use of ESD.[93] Patients with T1 lesions with less than 1000-μm submucosal invasion, well differentiation, and without lymphatic or vascular invasion have minimal risk of lymph node metastasis. Thus, patients can be informed about the risk of metastasis compared with the risk of surgery in making a decision regarding surgical resection.

ESD in the colorectum follows the same principles as ESD in the esophagus and stomach,[94] but as the technique has evolved a few technical considerations and variations have emerged.

- Mucosal markings around the lesion are typically not needed because lesion border tends to be easy to identify.
- A full circumferential incision is usually not done. The typical strategy of colorectal ESD is to perform a partial circumferential incision followed immediately by some submucosal dissection. This strategy is mostly driven by the very quick dissipation of the submucosal injectate. To further address this issue, the pocket-creation technique has been described. After creating an initial mucosal incision large enough to accommodate passage of the scope into the submucosal space, a large submucosal pocket is created undermining the lesion. This prevents leakage of injection solution and provides good tissue traction.[95]
- Change of patient position is frequently needed to provide some gravity-driven tissue retraction. Counter-traction is not easy to achieve, but the string and clip method appears to be more practical and may be considered in select cases.[96]
- A variety of bridging techniques have been described using a combination of components from ESD and EMR techniques. Multiple terms have been used in the past (circumferential incision EMR, circumferential submucosal incision EMR, EMR precutting, universal ESD), but the Japan Gastroenterological Endoscopy Society (JGES) guidelines streamlined the terminology and now two categories are recognized: precutting EMR and hybrid ESD[90]:
    - In precutting EMR, the tip of a standard snare or ESD knife is used to create a circumferential incision around the lesion. This is followed by application of snare for lesion removal without any submucosal dissection.
    - In hybrid ESD circumferential incision is performed and some degree of submucosal dissection is carried out prior

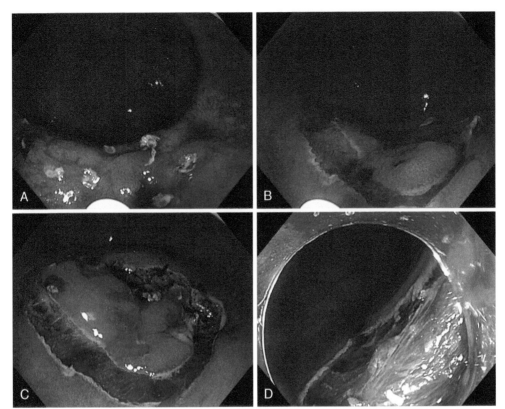

FIG 37.16 Hybrid endoscopic submucosal dissection. **A,** Non-polypoid flat dysplastic lesion is seen in a patient with ulcerative colitis. The periphery is marked. Severe submucosal fibrosis prevents both lifting and snare capture of the lesion, and **B,** hybrid endoscopic submucosal dissection (ESD) is pursued, with circumferential incision using a dual knife, and **C,** some submucosal dissection. **D,** The post-resection defect is seen.

to the application of the snare. Again, the tip of a snare or dedicated ESD knife can be used for the circumferential incision/submucosal dissection portion of the procedure (Fig. 37.16).

- Injection solution that provides a long-lasting submucosal cushion is required for ESD. This is preferred in the colon, where normal saline injection tends to dissipate rapidly. The available injection solutions options are discussed earlier in this chapter in the section on Instruments and Equipment.
- Specialized electrocautery equipment and in-depth knowledge of electrocautery principles are essential for successful ESD:
  - The use of an electrocautery unit providing modulated current capabilities is mandatory. The ASGE Technology Status Evaluation Report provides a detailed review of the technical characteristics and the available options in the United States.[20]
  - The exact settings of the electrosurgical generator (type of modulated current, power output, effect, duration, etc.) vary for different stages of the procedure (e.g., marking vs. circumferential incision vs. submucosal dissection), the type of instrument used, the lesion location (e.g., stomach vs. colon), and the different models of electrocautery generators. Some specific suggestions are summarized in a 2015 ASGE Technology Status Evaluation Report focusing on ESD.[29]
  - It should be emphasized that the recommended electrocautery settings differ greatly among experts performing an ESD. The main reason for this substantial variability is

that beside the factors listed earlier (stage of the procedure, type of instrument, and lesion location), other variables can significantly contribute to the final tissue effect. These include the surface area of the device electrode in contact with the tissue, the speed of movement of the electrode, the pressure applied with the electrode, the presence of coagulated tissue debris sticking to the electrode, the target tissue itself (fibrotic vs. high water content), and the grounding pad placement (pad should be placed on the patient flank rather than the lower extremity). Therefore, expert recommended settings will be a good starting point, but it is critical to note that the final tissue effect will significantly depend on a multitude of other factors, most importantly, the endoscopist's ESD technique. ESD has expanded our armamentarium to manage dysplastic and early cancerous lesions in the colon and is now routinely performed in the East. As ESD evolves, the anticipation is that increasing training opportunities, device innovations, and familiarity with the procedure will lead to full acceptance with expanding indications in the West.

TECHNIQUES TO IMPROVE EFFICACY AND SAFETY OF POLYPECTOMY

Prevention and Treatment of Recurrence

Because prior resection attempts increase the risk, one basic rule of EMR is to complete the resection in one setting. Of note, intraprocedural bleeding is a risk factor for recurrence. The reason

TABLE 37.3 **Factors Associated With Delayed Bleeding Following Endoscopic Resection of Large Non-Pedunculated Colorectal Polyps**

Study	Liaquat 2013[102]	Burgess 2014[78]	Albeniz 2016[101]	Zhang 2015[103]
Design	Retrospective	Prospective	Prospective	RCT*
Patients, n	463	1172	1274	348
Polyp size	≥ 20 mm	≥ 20 mm	≥ 20 mm	≥ 10 mm
Factors				
Proximal location†	**2.9** (1.3–6.9)	**3.7** (2.1–6.7)	**4.8** (2.4–9.7)	-
Size	**1.3** (1.1–1.7) (10-mm increments)	Not associated	**1.9** (1.0–3.7) (≥ 40 mm vs. < 40 mm)	-
Clip closure	**6.1** (2.0–18.6)‡	-	**3.6** (1.2–10.5)§	**1.1** vs. **6.7%**‖
Intraprocedural bleeding	-	**2.2** (1.2–4.0)	-	-
Cautery setting	-	**2.0** (1.0–4.0)¶	Not associated	-
ASA ≥ 3	-	Not associated	**1.9** (1.0–3.6)	-
Antiplatelet	-	Not associated#	**3.2** (1.2–8.5)**	-
Epinephrine	-	Not associated	Not associated	-

*Lesions were removed by endoscopic mucosal resection, endoscopic submucosal dissection (ESD), or hybrid ESD.
†Proximal to transverse colon.
‡Complete closure vs. no closure (historical controls).
§Complete closure vs. no closure; clip closure was selective at endoscopist discretion.
‖p = 0.012.
¶Microprocessor controlled vs. not microprocessor controlled.
#Any antiplatelet agent.
**Aspirin.
ASA, Aspirin; *RCT,* randomized controlled trial.

for this is very likely related to impaired visualization and missing residual polyp tissue.

Non-visible residual polyp at the resection margin has been considered the source for regrowth. Therefore, some endoscopists use ablation of the margin after visibly complete removal. A small randomized trial of using APC of the resection margin after resection in 21 patients showed a lower recurrence rate in the ablated patients (1/10 vs. 7/11).[97] However, this study was criticized for its small sample size and high incomplete resection rate in the control group (64%). In addition, the study was performed before high-definition endoscopes and digital chromoendoscopy were available. Recent preliminary results from the ACE group (2016) support ablation of the margin after resection. Among a total of 768 patients with polyps of 20 mm or larger, ablation of the margin using soft coagulation reduced the polyp recurrence rate from 20% to 6%.[98] In contrast, the same group showed that extending the resection to include a large, healthy margin did not appear to reduce the recurrence rate (12% in the standard group vs. 10% in the healthy margin group).[99] Despite these two seemingly opposing findings, the conclusion is twofold. First, ablation of the margin may be considered in routine practice. Second, even with dedicated attention to the margins, recurrence will occur in some patients. A possible reason for recurrence despite clearing the margins may be related to tissue bridges between the removed pieces that may serve as the nidus for regrowth.[100] Therefore, fewer pieces may lower the risk of recurrence; however, this has not been formally examined. Resection of recurrent lesions should follow the same principles of initial resection, that is, mechanical before ablation. However, in some instances, surgical removal is needed.

Reducing the Risk of Delayed Bleeding

Delayed bleeding is the most common serious complication related to EMR. Table 37.3 provides a summary of prior studies that examined potential risk factors. Size and proximal location, particularly in the ascending colon and cecum, have been consistently shown to be associated with increased risk of delayed bleeding.[78,101,102] Other factors that were found in some but not other studies include age 75 years or older, comorbidities (ASA ≥ 3), use of anticoagulation medication,[101] and use of electrocautery that is not microprocessor controlled.[78]

Two interventions have been examined to reduce the risk of delayed bleeding. First, the addition of epinephrine to the submucosal injectate does not appear to reduce the risk of delayed bleeding after EMR.[78] Second, closing the mucosal defect after resection with clips may reduce the risk of delayed bleeding.[101–103] A larger retrospective study by Liaquat et al (2013) showed a delayed bleeding rate of 2% if clip closure was performed compared with a 10% bleeding rate when the mucosal defect was not closed with clips.[102] These results are supported by a large prospective cohort study from Spain, where complete clip closure was associated with a reduced bleeding risk (whereas risk appeared to be increased if the defect was only partially closed).[101] Both studies are limited by their design (retrospective, uncontrolled). Selection bias is a potential problem, and obtained results may be affected by unmeasured confounders (for instance, lesions that were clipped might have been lower risk lesions). Therefore, the results cannot be generalized. A 2015 randomized trial from China might have overcome such limitations; however, smaller lesions (≥ 10 mm) were included, different resection methods applied (EMR, ESD, and hybrid ESD), and outcomes, particularly bleeding, not clearly defined.[103] The detected difference in delayed bleeding of 1.1% in the clip closure group compared with 6.7% in the control group therefore needs to be interpreted with caution. Although these studies suggest that clip closure may reduce the risk of delayed bleeding, convincing evidence for this approach is still lacking and it can therefore generally not be recommended. Aside from efficacy, cost-effectiveness analyses do not currently support general clip closure after EMR.[99,104] Clip closure may be considered for individual patients that are considered at higher risk of bleeding (proximal location and on anticoagulation). A large-scale multicenter, randomized trial is under way and will provide further guidance (ClinicalTrials.gov identifier: NCT01936948).

Marking the Polypectomy Site

The site of a lesion can be marked with ink (e.g., SPOT, GI Supply, Camp Hill, PA) injected into the submucosa or by placement of a single or multiple radiopaque clips (Fig. 37.17).[88,89] Both techniques are safe and simple to perform, although the endoclip may not be palpable and may not stay in place for a prolonged period. If marking is performed prior to endoscopic resection, it is important to inject the ink several centimeters away from the lesion because the injectate will result in submucosal fibrosis that can complicate resection.

Retrieving the Specimen

The benefits of mucosal resection or polypectomy can be assessed only by a properly prepared pathologic examination. The retrieval net is useful in recovering a specimen[90] from an en bloc resection of a flat or depressed lesion. Smaller pieces can be collected through the accessory channel. The net, snare, basket, and multipronged grasper are other accessories that can be useful for removal of large pedunculated polyps.

MANAGEMENT AND SURVEILLANCE AFTER POLYPECTOMY

Surveillance guidelines, for example, from the US Multi-Society Task Force on Colorectal Cancer, should be applied to determine the appropriate colonoscopy surveillance interval following polyp removal.[105] After piecemeal resection of large lesions, a repeat colonoscopy is typically performed within 3 to 6 months to assess for local recurrence.[106] The postmucosectomy scar site should be carefully examined; image-enhanced endoscopy techniques may be useful to show the presence of the innominate grooves across the scar and normal pit or microvessel patterns. Khashab et al (2009) reported a high predictive value for long-term eradication in cases where the postmucosectomy scar site showed both normal macroscopic and microscopic (biopsy) findings.[107] In cases with residual neoplasia, appropriate therapy with biopsy or repeat EMR is prudent, and another surveillance colonoscopy should be performed at 6 months. There is no clear guidance regarding a surveillance interval following a normal first follow-up examination. Even in the absence of biopsy-proven recurrence or residual adenoma at initial surveillance colonoscopy within 6 months, there is still a risk of recurrence at the following examination within the following year that may range between 4% and 10%.[72,108] Therefore, a second surveillance examination 1 year after the first seems appropriate. If negative, the surveillance interval may be extended to 3 years. Subsequent intervals may then follow based on findings and in accordance with the guidelines.[105]

The management of patients with polypoid lesions with invasive carcinoma is evolving. With increased ability to remove larger lesions, more patients are found to have T1 cancer within a removed polyp. The risk of recurrence is dependent on the risk of incomplete resection and lymph node metastasis.

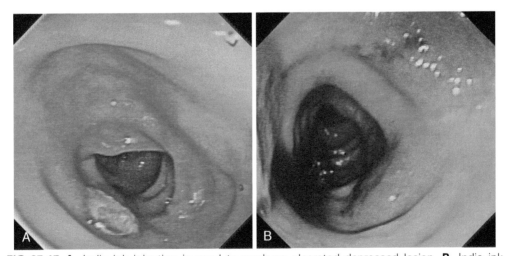

FIG 37.17 **A,** India ink injection is used to mark an ulcerated depressed lesion. **B,** India ink solution was injected submucosally at three separate points. The depressed lesion was later shown to be an adenocarcinoma invading deep into the submucosa. Locations of the tattoos (distal, proximal, same level of the lesion) must be documented precisely, especially in cases of flat and depressed lesions. These lesions are often not palpable by the surgeon. Sometimes an endoclip is used in addition to India ink to mark the site on radiographs taken immediately after colonoscopy; this can assist in surgical planning, particularly when laparoscopic resection is contemplated in cases in the left colon. In these cases, the clip, as seen in the abdominal x-ray, can provide the precise location of the lesion.

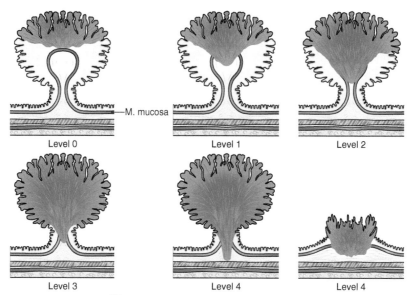

FIG 37.18 Haggitt et al (1985)[111] stratified the level of cancer submucosal invasion by the following criteria: *level 0*, carcinoma in situ (i.e., no extension below the muscularis mucosa); *level 1*, carcinoma invading through the muscularis mucosa but limited to the head of the polyp (i.e., above the junction between the adenoma and its stalk); *level 2*, carcinoma invading the level of the neck (i.e., the junction between adenoma and its stalk); *level 3*, carcinoma invading any part of the stalk; and *level 4*, carcinoma invading into the submucosa of the bowel wall below the stalk. In malignant sessile lesions, invasive carcinoma is considered as level 4.

Endoscopic resection has been shown to be safe and curative for low-risk T1 cancers, – those with only superficial submucosal invasion (≤ 1000 μm), absence of poor differentiation, tumor budding, or lymphovascular invasion[109–111] (Fig. 37.18). Risk of recurrence after resection of low-risk cancers is approximately 1%; however, it increases to 5% for cancers with high-risk histological features.[109,112,113] The risk of recurrence also appears to be greater for rectal cancers compared with other colon cancers.[112] Among patients with recurrence, however, the prognosis may be poor. Given the importance of complete resection to achieve cure, endoscopists need to have a high degree of suspicion for possible early invasive carcinoma. Image-enhanced techniques are therefore a mandatory asset for complex polyp removal. If early invasive cancer is suspected, and endoscopic resection is still considered, en bloc resection should be the goal as it improves the chance of complete removal. In these cases, ESD may be the preferred choice.

COMPLICATIONS

Complications of polypectomy and mucosal resection include bleeding, transmural burn, and perforation. Familiarity with the endoscopic findings, symptoms, and signs and treatment of complications is a prerequisite for performance of colonoscopic polypectomy and mucosal resection.

Postpolypectomy Bleeding

Postpolypectomy bleeding can occur during or after the procedure. The overall risk of severe bleeding related to polypectomy has been reported from large studies to be between 0.4% and 0.9%, or approximately 1 in 200 procedures.[114–118] The reported incidence varies according to the definition of bleeding, as well as the size

and type of lesions resected. It increases with polyp size and proximal polyp location. Delayed bleeding is the most common complication following EMR, occurring in 2% to 10% of patients, and several techniques may be applied to prevent risk of bleeding, as discussed earlier.

A variety of techniques are useful to treat active immediate or delayed bleeding. In cases with delayed bleeding, the bowel should be purged prior to performing the colonoscopy, although successful treatment of delayed postpolypectomy bleeding without prior bowel preparation has been reported and may be useful in more severe bleeding events.[119] These include application of a hemoclip or an endoloop, the use of APC, injection of dilute epinephrine, cauterization using monopolar or bipolar instruments, soft coagulation current, or use of a coagulation grasper (Coagrasper, Olympus, Center Valley, PA).[120,121] The selected method depends on the severity of bleeding and the bleeding lesion. For mild bleeding, our preferred technique is application of soft coagulation current.[122] More severe bleeding can be controlled with the coaggrasper or with a hemoclip (Fig. 37.19). If endoscopic treatment fails, selective angiogram with embolization or surgery is employed.

Postpolypectomy Syndrome

Postpolypectomy syndrome, also called transmural burn syndrome, is thought to occur when cautery injury causes full-thickness necrosis of the bowel wall. Patients typically present with fever, localized abdominal tenderness (often with rebound tenderness), and leukocytosis. Computed tomography may show local inflammatory changes that may mimic findings of diverticulitis. The onset of symptoms is commonly within a few hours of the polypectomy. It occurs in 0.1% to 0.5% of patients following a polypectomy.[114,115] Patients who are suspected to have

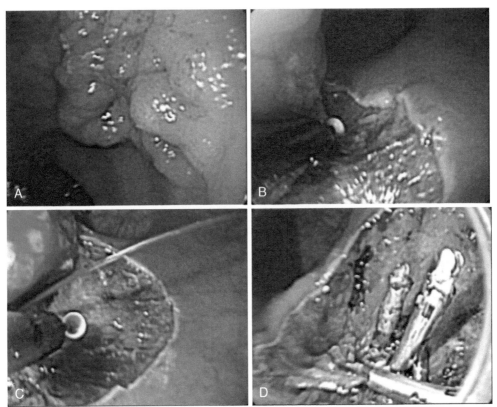

FIG 37.19 Immediate endoscopic submucosal dissection (ESD) bleeding. **A,** A large lateral spreading granular type rectal lesion. **B,** ESD technique is performed to remove the lesion. **C,** During submucosal dissection, arterial bleeding is encountered. **D,** Hemostasis is achieved using endoscopic clips, and the resection is complete.

postpolypectomy syndrome typically require admission with bowel rest and antibiotics, although successful outpatient treatment has been described.[123] Most patients recover uneventfully.

Perforation

Perforation can occur when the muscularis propria is included in the tissue grasped by a snare; this accident may happen, for example, when a large sessile polyp that is draped over a fold is grasped in its entirety. Perforation is rare with basic polypectomy, and occurs in up to 1% with EMR and 4% with ESD.[28,89,101,124,125] Techniques that may decrease the risk of capturing the muscularis propria have been summarized. A target sign at the base of the mucosal defect or the polyp following a resection is a sign of deep wall injury. A yellow defect target sign may represent serosal fat and indicates impending perforation. In the Australian cohort EMR of 911 large sessile polyps, a target sign was noted in 1.5% and an open perforation in 0.5%. All lesions were successfully closed with clips.[126] Other studies have similarly shown that the majority of perforations following a polyp removal can be closed with clips.[101,125,127]

FUTURE TRENDS

Basic polyp resection has seen a shift from hot to cold snare resection. Although early studies suggest that cold snare resection is at least as safe and effective as hot snare resection, future studies should provide more solid data from comparative effectiveness studies and identify the upper size limit for routine cold snare removal.

Advances in the technology and technique of colonoscopy have allowed us to manage increasingly complex colorectal lesions via endoscopy. Learning and using these new technologies and techniques may be demanding, but they enable us to perform endoscopic resections of larger, more complex lesions that previously would have required major abdominal surgery. Considering efficacy and cost, it is no longer justified to perform surgical resection of these lesions as the first treatment approach. At the same time, practice may vary. Regional or population-based studies may help to understand variations and whether additional training is required to provide effective and safe care. Particularly with respect to the resection of larger colorectal lesions, the following questions deserve attention:

- How can EMR reliably achieve complete resection?
- What technique provides the safest resection and minimal risk of bleeding?
- What is the optimal electrocautery setting for resection?
- How should antithrombotic agents be managed following removal of large polyps?
- When should ESD be used instead of EMR?

Studies are ongoing that will provide some answers to these questions and provide guidance to establishing a standardized efficacious and safe approach to resection of large colorectal lesions. Although resection of large lesions is technically feasible, resection may be tedious, is often incomplete at the initial session, requires extensive skill and experience, and the risk of complications is still substantial. These drawbacks call for a more elegant, safe, and reliable technique. Modified EMR and ESD techniques are attempts in that direction. New ideas and technological developments are needed to optimize our current techniques.

Finally, we recognize that resection of large lesions requires advanced endoscopy skills. Large polyp resection should be performed by endoscopists with sufficient experience and training in removing such lesions. Simplifications in the technology and techniques of resections would allow them to be used more widely and ultimately benefit more patients.

KEY REFERENCES

2. Corley DA, Jensen CD, Marks AR, et al: Adenoma detection rate and risk of colorectal cancer and death, *N Engl J Med* 370:1298–1306, 2014.

4. Pohl H, Srivastava A, Bensen SP, et al: Incomplete polyp resection during colonoscopy-results of the complete adenoma resection (CARE) study, *Gastroenterology* 144:74–80 e1, 2013.

5. ASGE Technology Committee, Abu Dayyeh BK, Thosani N, et al: ASGE Technology Committee systematic review and meta-analysis assessing the ASGE PIVI thresholds for adopting real-time endoscopic assessment of the histology of diminutive colorectal polyps, *Gastrointest Endosc* 81:502 e1–502 e16, 2015.

24. Moss A, Bourke MJ, Williams SJ, et al: Endoscopic mucosal resection outcomes and prediction of submucosal cancer from advanced colonic mucosal neoplasia, *Gastroenterology* 140:1909–1918, 2011.

28. ASGE Technology Committee, Hwang JH, Konda V, et al: Endoscopic mucosal resection, *Gastrointest Endosc* 82:215–226, 2015.

29. ASGE Technology Committee, Maple JT, Abu Dayyeh BK, et al: Endoscopic submucosal dissection, *Gastrointest Endosc* 81:1311–1325, 2015.

33. The Paris endoscopic classification of superficial neoplastic lesions: esophagus, stomach, and colon: November 30 to December 1, 2002, *Gastrointest Endosc* 58:S3–S43, 2003.

34. Co K, editor: *Japanese classification of colorectal carcinoma*, Kanehara, 1997.

35. Kudo S, Tamura S, Nakajima T, et al: Diagnosis of colorectal tumorous lesions by magnifying endoscopy, *Gastrointest Endosc* 44:8–14, 1996.

37. Hewett DG, Kaltenbach T, Sano Y, et al: Validation of a simple classification system for endoscopic diagnosis of small colorectal polyps using narrow-band imaging, *Gastroenterology* 143:599–607 e1, 2012.

72. Moss A, Williams SJ, Hourigan LF, et al: Long-term adenoma recurrence following wide-field endoscopic mucosal resection (WF-EMR) for advanced colonic mucosal neoplasia is infrequent: results and risk factors in 1000 cases from the Australian Colonic EMR (ACE) study, *Gut* 64:57–65, 2015.

73. Hassan C, Repici A, Sharma P, et al: Efficacy and safety of endoscopic resection of large colorectal polyps: a systematic review and meta-analysis, *Gut* 65:806–820, 2016.

74. Jayanna M, Burgess NG, Singh R, et al: Cost analysis of endoscopic mucosal resection vs surgery for large laterally spreading colorectal lesions, *Clin Gastroenterol Hepatol* 14:271–278 e1–e2, 2016.

78. Burgess NG, Metz AJ, Williams SJ, et al: Risk factors for intraprocedural and clinically significant delayed bleeding after wide-field endoscopic mucosal resection of large colonic lesions, *Clin Gastroenterol Hepatol* 12:651–661 e1–e3, 2014.

88. Wang J, Zhang XH, Ge J, et al: Endoscopic submucosal dissection vs endoscopic mucosal resection for colorectal tumors: a meta-analysis, *World J Gastroenterol* 20:8282–8287, 2014.

89. Fujiya M, Tanaka K, Dokoshi T, et al: Efficacy and adverse events of EMR and endoscopic submucosal dissection for the treatment of colon neoplasms: a meta-analysis of studies comparing EMR and endoscopic submucosal dissection, *Gastrointest Endosc* 81:583–595, 2015.

93. Hayashi N, Tanaka S, Hewett DG, et al: Endoscopic prediction of deep submucosal invasive carcinoma: validation of the Narrow-Band Imaging International Colorectal Endoscopic (NICE) classification, *Gastrointest Endosc* 78:625–632, 2013.

94. Draganov PV, Gotoda T, Chavalitdhamrong D, et al: Techniques of endoscopic submucosal dissection: application for the Western endoscopist?, *Gastrointest Endosc* 78:677–688, 2013.

102. Liaquat H, Rohn E, Rex DK: Prophylactic clip closure reduced the risk of delayed postpolypectomy hemorrhage: experience in 277 clipped large sessile or flat colorectal lesions and 247 control lesions, *Gastrointest Endosc* 77:401–407, 2013.

103. Zhang QS, Han B, Xu JH, et al: Clip closure of defect after endoscopic resection in patients with larger colorectal tumors decreased the adverse events, *Gastrointest Endosc* 82:904–909, 2015.

105. Lieberman DA, Rex DK, Winawer SJ, et al: Guidelines for colonoscopy surveillance after screening and polypectomy: a consensus update by the US Multi-Society Task Force on Colorectal Cancer, *Gastroenterology* 143:844–857, 2012.

113. Yoshii S, Nojima M, Nosho K, et al: Factors associated with risk for colorectal cancer recurrence after endoscopic resection of T1 tumors, *Clin Gastroenterol Hepatol* 12:292–302 e3, 2014.

118. Warren JL, Klabunde CN, Mariotto AB, et al: Adverse events after outpatient colonoscopy in the Medicare population, *Ann Intern Med* 150:849–857, W152, 2009.

126. Burgess NG, Bassan MS, McLeod D, et al: Deep mural injury and perforation after colonic endoscopic mucosal resection: a new classification and analysis of risk factors, *Gut* 2016. [Epub ahead of print].

127. Kim JS, Kim BW, Kim JI, et al: Endoscopic clip closure versus surgery for the treatment of iatrogenic colon perforations developed during diagnostic colonoscopy: a review of 115,285 patients, *Surg Endosc* 27:501–504, 2013.

A complete reference list can be found online at ExpertConsult .com

38

Endoscopic Diagnosis and Staging of Inflammatory Bowel Disease

Anna M. Buchner and Gary R. Lichtenstein

INTRODUCTION

Over the past several decades, endoscopy has become an integral tool for diagnosing inflammatory bowel disease (IBD), including ulcerative colitis (UC) and Crohn's disease (CD), and staging disease activity. Both CD and UC are characterized by the presence of intestinal inflammatory changes and ulcerations, which are detected during an endoscopic evaluation and confirmed by histopathology examination of specimens obtained during endoscopy. However, the endoscopic evaluation of IBD includes not only diagnosing the disease, assessing the disease's extent, and staging its activity, but also monitoring the responses to various medical therapies (with mucosal healing serving as a predictor of disease course) and managing the disease's complications. Several endoscopic scoring systems have been utilized for assessing and staging disease activity, thus allowing estimates of the prognosis and efficacy of medical treatment in IBD patients.[1-5]

Current endoscopic modalities utilize not only high-definition endoscopes, but can also apply wide-field techniques such as chromoendoscopy (both dye-based and electronic based techniques) and, in some centers, small-field technologies such as confocal laser endomicroscopy (CLE) and endocytoscopy (EC), which facilitates our ability to not only detect but also to further characterize mucosal abnormalities and image ongoing physiologic processes in vivo. These newer endoscopic imaging technologies may not only further improve detection and characterization of mucosal lesions, but also may have the potential to assess severity, disease extent, and response to treatment in patients with IBD.

Other endoscopic imaging tools, such as wireless video capsule endoscopy (VCE) and balloon-assisted enteroscopy, also include enhanced imaging of the small bowel (SB) in the setting of CD.

In this chapter, we review the most recent advances of endoscopic evaluation in the diagnosis and staging of IBD, and ultimately the role of endoscopy in the effective care of patients with IBD.

ENDOSCOPIC EVALUATION OF INFLAMMATORY BOWEL DISEASE

Diagnosing and Assessing Disease Presentation

Colonoscopy with endoscopic evaluation of the colon and distal ileum with biopsy is required in all patients who are clinically suspected of having IBD to effectively diagnose, stage disease activity and severity, and differentiate between UC and CD or other inflammatory entities such as ischemic colitis, infectious colitis, and diverticular-associated colitis. Based on various studies, colonoscopy with histopathology can accurately diagnose CD versus UC in 90% of patients.[4,6] Endoscopic features such as rectal sparing, the presence of skip lesions, terminal ileal involvement, fistulas, and strictures can be seen in CD (Figs. 38.1–38.3), whereas endoscopic features such as diffuse inflammatory changes with superficial ulcerations are suggestive of UC (Fig. 38.4). However, these endoscopic features are not specific to either CD or UC (Videos 38.1–38.3). Histopathology examination based on biopsies obtained from both normal-appearing mucosa and abnormal mucosa is an integral component of endoscopic evaluation in patients suspected to have IBD. Specific histologic features associated with chronic inflammation will permit differentiation of IBD from other colitides such as infectious colitis, segmental colitis associated with diverticulosis, and ischemic colitis. However, the diagnosis of CD based on endoscopic evaluation with histopathology assessment may still be challenging. Patients with a colonic presentation of IBD in whom the disease cannot be classified as UC or CD colitis are determined to have an unclassified type of IBD (IBD-U) (Fig. 38.5).[3,7]

Patients with CD may present with continuous rectal inflammation involving the whole rectum and extending more proximally without the presence of skip areas, deep ulcerations, and certain histologic features such as the presence of granulomas on histopathology examination.[8] In fact, some patients with CD may still have colonoscopy examinations with biopsies, which cannot

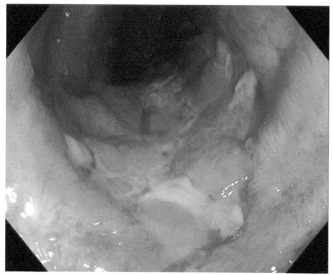

FIG 38.1 Cobblestoning mucosa in active Crohn's disease.

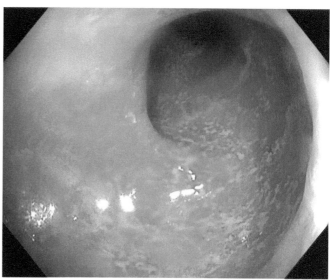

FIG 38.3 Crohn's colitis with aphthous ulcerations and white exudate.

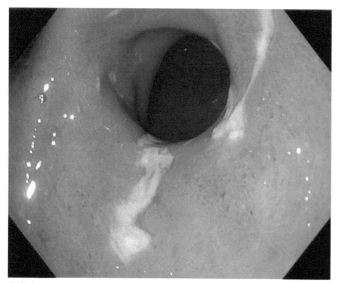

FIG 38.2 Multiple serpiginous ulcers in a patient with Crohn's disease.

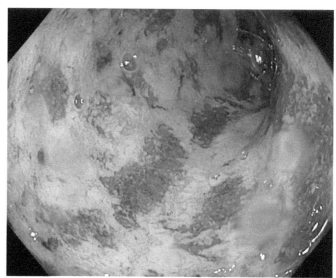

FIG 38.4 Ulcerative colitis with superficial ulceration, edema, and mucosal friability extending in a confluent manner starting from the rectum.

differentiate from that of UC. These patients with continuous inflammation beginning in the rectum and extending more proximally may be thus erroneously classified as having UC without further evaluation of the terminal ileum (TI). Thus, additional endoscopic evaluation of the TI during each colonoscopy examination is required to establish an appropriate diagnosis of IBD (Fig. 38.6). It may permit differentiation of UC from CD and further characterization of the subtypes of ileitis, specifically, CD ileitis and backwash ileitis. Backwash ileitis is typically a short segment of mildly inflamed mucosa of TI in the setting of existing colitis extending from the cecum without further progression to ulcerations, stenosis, and structuring.[3] Colonic pseudopolyps are usually seen in patients with UC, as the repeated cycle of ulceration and deposition of granulation tissue during the healing phase results in the development of inflammatory polyps (Fig. 38.7).

Diagnosing CD with SB involvement may be particularly challenging. The presence of SB involvement can be confirmed

in approximately 80% of patients with CD, including one-third of all cases with CD presenting with only isolated SB disease.[1] The most frequently encountered SB mucosal abnormalities suggestive of IBD include erosions, ulcers, erythema, villous blunting, and strictures, although they are not pathognomonic for CD as they can be seen in other conditions mimicking IBD. Table 38.1 summarizes frequent findings in IBD patients based on an endoscopic and histopathological evaluation.

VCE is another endoscopic tool that enables noninvasive visualization of the entire SB mucosa and is utilized in patients with suspected CD and established IBD, allowing the assessment of encountered SB mucosa abnormalities (see Figs. 14.4 and 17.5, as well as Videos 17.4 and 17.5).[9–12] Capsule endoscopy (CE) has been found to be more beneficial compared with push enteroscopy or radiologic imaging such as small bowel follow-through and computed tomography enterography in the

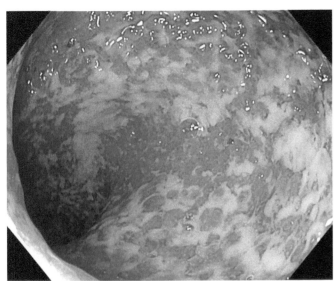

FIG 38.5 Colitis with superficial ulceration and edema. This appearance can be seen in both Crohn's colitis and ulcerative colitis.

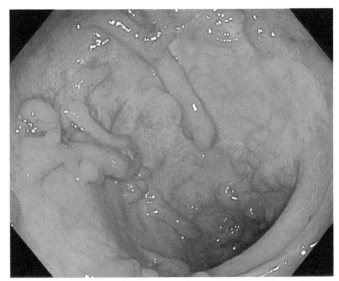

FIG 38.7 Pseudopolyps in a patient with ulcerative colitis.

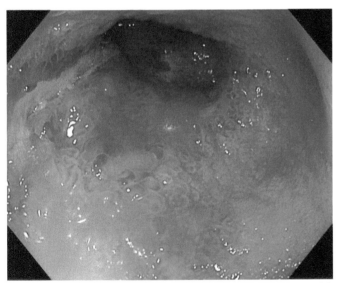

FIG 38.6 A patient with ileitis due to Crohn's disease with erythema, edema, and ulceration of the terminal ileum.

evaluation of patients with known CD.[13] The absence of typical capsule endoscopy features has a negative predictive value ranging from 96% to 100% based on available studies.[13–15]

VCE plays a role in re-evaluating patients with diagnosed UC when there is a question of a potential misclassification or potential misdiagnosis, as there are also certain conditions in which appearances can mimic CD-related changes, including nonsteroidal antiinflammatory drug (NSAID)-related injuries, ischemia, radiation enteritis, and drug-induced enteritis. Mehdi-zadeh et al (2008) confirmed that 15% of a total of 120 patients with UC were found to have CD based on the CE findings.[16]

Further SB visualization can be achieved with device-assisted enteroscopy such as single-balloon and double-balloon enteroscopy (DBE), as well as push enteroscopy.[17–19] The diagnostic yield of balloon-assisted enteroscopy has been reported to be

up to 59%.[17] Mensink et al (2010) demonstrated that DBE evaluation was deemed to change clinical management in 74% of patients with CD with SB involvement, as well as facilitate achievement of clinical remission in 88%.[19]

Based on a meta-analysis, the diagnostic yield of both VCE and DBE is comparable; however, VCE is still favored for the initial diagnostic approach as it is considered to be a non-invasive tool.[17,18]

In the pediatric population, upper endoscopy (esophagogas-troduodenoscopy [EGD]) is routinely performed when suspecting IBD, given the incidence of macroscopic involvement of the upper gastrointestinal tract reported to be as high as 30%, as well as the presence of microscopic changes seen in up to 60%.[20–22] This approach is supported by guidelines introduced by the European Crohn's and Colitis Organization (ECCO) recommending EGD for all pediatric patients suspected of having IBD, but it is not recommended routinely in adult populations.[20,21]

CD and UC can be classified based on endoscopic evaluation of disease location, maximal endoscopic involvement, and endoscopic presentation such as stricturing, penetrating versus nonstricturing, and nonpenetrating disease.[3,7,23] This classification is known as the revised Montreal classification and is highlighted in detail in Table 38.2.

The lack of clearly visible endoscopic features of inflammation may not always correlate with histopathology assessment. Therefore, obtaining biopsies during endoscopic evaluation from various segments of the colon, including those with a normal endoscopic appearance, is necessary for the true assessment of disease extent in patients with suspected IBD.[24]

Staging Disease Activity
Definition of Mucosal Healing
Mucosal healing (MH) refers to the endoscopic assessment of disease activity, and it has become increasingly important in the clinical management of patients with UC and CD. In addition, it has recently been used as an endpoint for clinical trials.[1,25] In general, there are no validated definitions of MH in the setting of IBD. MH has been typically recognized as a lack of ulcerations and erosions, and it has unequivocally been associated with better outcomes, including decreased hospitalization rates, sustained

TABLE 38.1 Frequent Endoscopic and Histopathology Findings in Ulcerative Colitis and Crohn's Disease

Disease	Colonoscopy With Ileoscopy	Esophagogastroduodenoscopy	Capsule Endoscopy	Histopathology
Ulcerative colitis	Rectum involved with continuous inflammatory changes and evident demarcation between normal and abnormal mucosa: Mucosal granularity, edema Friability and bleeding Pseudopolyps Backwash ileitis	Normal esophagus, stomach, and duodenum	Normal-appearing small bowel, with the exception of backwash ileitis	Disported crypt architecture Abscesses Goblet cells decrease Basal plasmacytosis Paneth cell metaplasia
Crohn's disease	Inflammatory changes either limited to the rectum, left colon, right colon, or diffuse May also extend to the ileum Segmental involvement; subtle and or serpingous ulcers Cobblestoning Further features that can be present or absent: Rectal sparing Aphtous ulcers Perianal ulcers Fistula Strictures	Inflammatory changes in the duodenum, edema, erythema, erosions, ulcers with thickened folds, friable mucosa Duodenal strictures Pyloric stricture	Mucosal abnormalities, erythema edema, erosions, ulcers	Distorted crypt architecture Occasional abscess Patchy distribution Non-caseating granulomas

TABLE 38.2 Revised Montreal Classification for Ulcerative Colitis and Crohn's Disease

Ulcerative Colitis (UC)	UC Definition	Endoscopic Involvement
E1	Proctitis	Rectum
E2	Left-sided colitis	Distal to splenic flexure
E3	Extensive colitis	Proximal to splenic flexure

Crohn's Disease (CD)	CD Location	CD Behavior
A1 ≤ 16 years	L1: Ileal	B1: non-stricturing, nonpenetrating
A2 = 17–40 years	L2: Colonic	B2: stricturing
A4 > 40 years	L3: Ileocolonic	B3: penetrating
	L4: isolated upper GI	+p: perianal disease is present

GI, gastrointestinal.
Adapted from ASGE Standards of Practice Committee, Shergill AK, Lightdale JR, et al: The role of endoscopy in inflammatory bowel disease. *Gastrointest Endosc* 81(5):1101–1121.e1–e13, 2015.

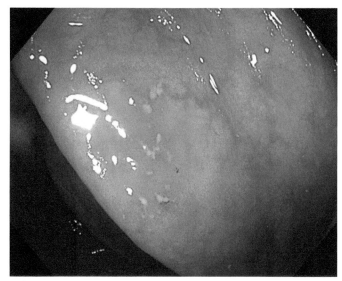

FIG 38.8 Mucosal healing with persistent colonic aphthous ulcers.

clinical remission, decreased need for corticosteroid use, decreased risk of colorectal cancer, and decreased rates of colectomy.[25–29]

In patients with UC, the absence of friability and erosions with the presence of a normal vascular pattern of the mucosa appears to represent an adequate definition of MH, as the presence of disease activity involves abnormality of the mucosa. This has been recognized by the International Organization of Inflammatory Bowel Disease (IOIBD) as "absence of friability, mucosal bleeding, erosions, and ulcers in all visualized segments are the required components of genuine endoscopic healing."[2] However, this definition has not been consistently accepted, as some studies

also include features of erythema and friability in the definition of MH.[30] On the other hand, diagnosing MH in CD may be particularly challenging given the transmural nature of the disease. Currently, in the setting of CD, MH has been recognized as the absence of any visible ulcers.[31] However, depending on the trial, the descriptive definition of MH in CD has also included an absence of inflammation, luminal narrowing, aphthous lesions, superficial and deep ulcerations, and nodules (Fig. 38.8).[32–34]

Endoscopic Scoring Systems in Ulcerative Colitis

A 2014 systematic review of the measurement of endoscopic healing in UC clinical trials revealed that currently utilized indices, such as the sigmoidoscopic component of the Mayo Clinic score

TABLE 38.3   Indices of Endoscopy-Based Disease Activity Used in Ulcerative Colitis: Mayo Endoscopic Score (1987) and UCEIS (2012)

Index	Study Design	Description	Applications	Level of Validation
Mayo Endoscopic Score (1987)	Prospective study	Four-grade scale: (1) Normal or inactive disease (2) Mild disease: erythema, decreased vascular pattern, mild friability (3) Moderate disease: marked erythema, absent vascular pattern, friability, erosions (4) Severe disease: spontaneous bleeding, ulcers	Numerous clinical trials	Not validated

UCEIS (2012)	Used in prospective studies	Grading system with a total score of 3–11 comprising three variable subscores;
		1. Vascular patterns: normal, patchy obliteration, obliterated
		2. Bleeding:
		  – None
		  – Mucosal
		  – Luminal:
		    – Mild
		    – Moderate to severe
		3. Erosions and ulcers:
		  – None
		  – Erosions
		  – Superficial ulcer
		  – Deep ulcer
			Recently developed	Validated

UCEIS, Ulcerative Colitis Endoscopic Index of Severity.
Data from Schroeder KW, Tremaine WJ, Ilstrup DM: Coated oral 5-aminosalicylic acid therapy for mildly to moderately active ulcerative colitis. A randomized study. *N Engl J Med* 317:1625–1629, 1987; Travis SP, Schnell D, Krzeski P, et al: Developing an instrument to assess the endoscopic severity of ulcerative colitis: the Ulcerative Colitis Endoscopic Index of Severity (UCEIS). *Gut* 61:535–542, 2012.

TABLE 38.4   Mayo Scoring System for Assessment of Ulcerative Colitis Activity

Stool frequency	0 = Normal 1 = 1–2 stools/day more than normal 2 = 3–4 stools/day more than normal 3 = > 4 stools/day more than normal
Rectal bleeding	0 = None 1 = Visible blood with stool less than half of the time 2 = Visible blood with stool half of the time or more 3 = Passing blood alone
Mucosal appearance at endoscopy	0 = Normal or inactive disease 1 = Mild disease (redness, decreased vascular pattern visible, friability) 2 = Moderate disease (marked erythema, no vascular pattern visible, friability, erosions) 3 = Severe disease (bleeding, ulceration)
Physician's global assessment of disease activity	0 (normal), 1 (mild), 2 (moderate), 3 (severe)

From Lewis JD, Shaokun C, Nessel L, et al: Use of the invasive components of the Mayo Score to assess clinical response in ulcerative colitis. *Inflamm Bowel Dis* 14(12):1660–1666, 2008.

and the Ulcerative Colitis Endoscopic Index of Severity (UCEIS), show the most promise as reliable evaluative tools of endoscopic disease activity in UC (Table 38.3).[35] The frequently used endoscopic component of the Mayo Clinic score, introduced by Schroeder et al in 1987, is based on an evaluation of vascular pattern, erythema, friability, erosions, and ulcerations.[36] The complete Mayo Scoring System (MCS) includes both endoscopic and clinical findings (Table 38.4).[36] Four variables of the MCS comprise stool frequency, rectal bleeding, physician's global assessment, and assessment of endoscopic severity seen in the rectosigmoid mucosa.[35] Complete response is defined as 0 for all defined variables. Partial response is defined as a substantial but incomplete improvement. The Mayo Endoscopic Score has been used in numerous trials and has been easy to apply in clinical practice, although interobserver agreement can vary. Some studies confirmed a high level of agreement (intraobserver: intraclass correlation coefficient [ICC]: 0.89; 95% confidence interval [CI]: 0.85–0.92), interobserver ICC: 0.79; 95% CI: 0.72–0.96), whereas others demonstrated only a fair or moderate agreement.[35,37] According to prior studies, the main limitation of using the Mayo score was assessment of mucosal friability. Subjective assessment of the mucosa lead to removal of friability in subsequent endoscopic scores and resulted in lack of validation.[38,39] However, in a systematic review by Samaan et al (2014), a variable of mucosal friability reported the highest agreement of over 90% among observers.[35] Feagan et al (2007) demonstrated that improvement in the Mayo score is clinically relevant, as it correlates with improvement in quality of life.[40] According to the Active Ulcerative Trials (ACT-1 and ACT-2) of infliximab, MH assessed by a Mayo Clinic score of 0 or 1 at week 8 (8 weeks after receiving infliximab) was associated with a significantly lower colectomy rate beyond 54 weeks.[41]

In addition, a new validated index, known as the UCEIS, has been introduced.[42] This index contains more detailed information on endoscopic assessment, such as vascular pattern, bleeding, and the presence of erosions/ulcerations, scored in the most severely affected part of the colon, and it additionally excludes friability from the analyzed parameters (Table 38.5). The UCEIS was originally developed as an 11-point score comprised of erosions/ulcers (1–4), vascular pattern (1–3) and bleeding (1–4). This scoring system has been simplified to an 8-point tool with parameters such as erosions/ulcers (0–2), vascular pattern (0–2),

TABLE 38.5   **The Ulcerative Colitis Endoscopic Index of Severity**

Descriptor (Score Most Severe Lesions)	Likert Scale Anchor Points	Definition
Vascular pattern	Normal (0)	Normal vascular pattern with arborization of capillaries clearly defined, or with blurring or patchy loss
	Patchy obliterations (1)	Patchy obliteration of vascular pattern
	Obliterated (2)	Complete obliteration of vascular pattern
Bleeding	None (0)	No visible blood
	Mucosal (1)	Some spots or streaks of coagulated blood on the surface of the mucosa ahead of the scope, which can be washed away
	Luminal mild (2)	Some free liquid blood in the lumen
	Luminal moderate or severe (3)	Frank blood in the lumen ahead of the endoscope or visible oozing from the mucosa after washing away intraluminal blood or visible oozing from a hemorrhagic mucosa
Erosions and ulcers	None (0)	Normal mucosa, no visible erosions or ulcers
	Erosions (1)	Very small (≤ 5 mm) defects in the mucosa white and yellow in color, with a flat edge
	Superficial ulcer (2)	Large (> 5 mm) defects in the mucosa, which are discrete fibrin-covered ulcers when compared with erosions, but remain superficial
	Deep ulcer (3)	Deeper excavated defects in the mucosa, with a slightly raised edge

Copyright Warner Chilcott Pharmaceuticals, although the index is freely available for use by investigators.
Adapted from Travis SPL, Schnell D, Krzeski P, et al: Developing an instrument to assess the endoscopic severity of ulcerative colitis: the Ulcerative Colitis Endoscopic Index of Severity (UCEIS). *Gut* 61:535–542, 2012.

TABLE 38.6   **Endoscopic Indices Used in Crohn's Disease**

Indices	Description	Summary
CDEIS	CDEIS evaluates: • Deep ulcerations: score 0 if absent or 12 if present • Superficial ulcerations: score 0 if absent or 6 if present • Length of ulcerated mucosa (0–10 cm): score 0–10 according to length in centimeters • Length of diseased mucosa (0–10 cm): score 0–10 according to length in centimeters • Grading (0–44) using the previous descriptive features such as ulceration's area of involvement, stenosis characteristics in colon and terminal ileum deep ulceration, superficial ulceration, and inflammation[1] – Complex (many variables and scores range from 0 to 44)	Detailed evaluation, assess global disease, partially validated, no validated definition of mucosal healing

SES-CD	Grading (0–56 points) using features such as size of the ulcers, degree of ulcerated surface, and presence of narrowing in the colon
	• Ulcers, inflammation, and narrowing
		Simplified version of the CDEIS, partially validated, high degree of correlation with the CDEIS for grading and responsiveness to changes
		  – Scores range from 0 to 60
		  – No validated definition of mucosal healing

CDEIS, Crohn's Disease Endoscopic Index of Severity; SES-CD, Simple Endoscopic Score for Crohn's Disease.
Data from Mary JY, Modigliani R: Development and validation of an endoscopic index of the severity for Crohn's disease: a prospective multicentre study. Groupe d'Etudes Therapeutiques des Affections Inflammatoires du Tube Digestif (GETAID). *Gut* 30:983–989, 1989; Daperno M, D'Haens G, Van Assche G, et al: Development and validation of a new, simplified endoscopic activity score for Crohn's disease: the SES-CD. *Gastrointest Endosc* 60:505–512, 2004.

and bleeding (1–4), and was found to have a satisfactory interobserver agreement (κ of 0.5).[42] The study has acknowledged the importance of using a standardized system of descriptive findings by observers for endoscopic severity evaluation, as well as the role of endoscopist experience and utilization of a centralized review of endoscopic video images.[42,43] All these factors may influence interobserver variations of disease activity endoscopic assessment. Feagan et al (2013) demonstrated excellent interobserver and intraobserver agreement of the UCEIS assessment among seven experienced central readers.[44] However, there are also some potential limitations of this index. The specific cutoffs corresponding to remission versus mild, moderate, and severe disease have not yet been fully characterized. In addition, Colombel et al (2016) confirmed that there is a high degree of correlation between findings from rectosigmoidoscopy versus colonoscopy in assessment of disease activity based on the UCEIS scores.[45] Nevertheless, the UCEIS index thus far represents the only validated endoscopic index for the evaluation of patients with UC and it is currently utilized in ongoing clinical studies.

Endoscopic Scoring Systems in CD

A 2014 systematic review of the measurement of endoscopic disease activity and MH in CD reviewed all available indices for CD and concluded that the Crohn's Disease Endoscopic Index of Severity (CDEIS) and the Simple Endoscopic Score for Crohn's Disease (SES-CD) are the most studied tools, although further validation for their broad use is still required[46] (Table 38.6).

The CDEIS, introduced in 1989 by Mary and Modigliani, is based on recognition of elementary features (no ulcerated lesions, ulcerations, and stenosis) associated with the pattern of their surface in five segments (rectum, sigmoid and left colon, transverse colon, and right colon and ileum).[32] Calculation of the CDEIS is very time consuming and requires significant training and experience, thus it is not broadly used. The calculated CDEIS score ranges from 0 to 44 and is illustrated in Table 38.6.[32] The CDEIS scores specific features such as the presence of deep ulcerations (12 if present), superficial ulceration (6 if present), the length of ulcerated mucosa ranging from 0 to 10 cm with scores of 0 to 10 according to the involved length, and finally the length of the diseased mucosa (0–10 cm). The numbers are added in each segment and divided by the number of segments evaluated. Additional points are given for an ulcerated stenosis, and a further 3 points are given for a nonulcerated stenosis. Based on subsequent studies, endoscopic remission (minor or no mucosal lesions) is defined as a CDEIS score less than or equal to 6, while complete endoscopic remission (mucosal healing; i.e., no lesions at all or scattered lesions) is defined as a CDEIS score of less than or equal to 3 or less than or equal to 4.[46–50] An endoscopic CDEIS response has been defined as a decrease from baseline of at least 3 points or 5 points or reduction of CDEIS by 50% or 75%.[46–50] Geboes et al (2005) defined the severity of the disease as mild, moderate, or severe based on CDEIS scores of below 5, between 5 and 15, and above 15, respectively.[51] Even though the CDEIS provides a complete and detailed examination of disease activity, the interobserver agreement for grading superficial and deep ulcerations is only reported to be fair, according to studies.[46] However, a 2016 study concluded that central reading of the CDEIS by four readers to evaluate CD severity had a very high level of intra-rater agreement (intra-observer ICC: 0.89; 95% CI: 0.86–0.93), although lower inter-rater agreement was seen (ICC: 0.71; 95% CI: 0.61–0.79).[52] The CDEIS has been used in trials on tumor necrosis factor (TNF) antagonists, thiopurines, and steroids.[25]

On the other hand, the simple endoscopic score for CD appears to be more practical and is based on four endoscopic variables to be scored 0–3 in the same five ileocolonic segments.[33] The SES-CD was demonstrated to have a high degree of correlation, with the CDEIS for grading of disease activity and responsiveness to changes in disease activity showing similar intraobserver and interobserver agreement.[33,46] Central reading of SES-CD by four experienced gastroenterologists was determined to have a high level of intra-rater and inter-rater reliability (intraobserver reliability ICC: 0.91; 95% CI: 0.87–0.94 and interobserver reliability ICC: 0.83; 95% CI: 0.75–0.89) based on data from a 2004 study.[33]

A CDEIS decrease of 6 points represents endoscopic response, according to some studies.[49] In a post-hoc analysis of data from the Study of Biologic and Immunomodulator Naive Patients in Crohn Disease (SONIC) trial, Ferrante et al (2013) concluded that endoscopic response (defined as a decrease from baseline in SES-CD or CDEIS of at least 50%) achieved at week 26 of treatment identified those most likely to be steroid free in clinical remission at week 50.[53] Further validation studies of indices are still needed, however.[35,46] Recent studies by Bouguen et al (2014)[54,55] evaluated the utility of MH as a treatment target in clinical practice settings. In individual settings of CD and UC, repeated endoscopic assessment of the disease within a minimum of 24 weeks, and treatment adjustments made based on that assessment, have improved the likelihood of achieving MH. However, further studies are needed to validate these observations. The practice of evaluating for MH after medication adjustment has been termed "treat to target."

Endoscopic evaluation of the intestinal mucosa also plays an important role in the postoperative management of patients with CD and allows the tailoring of medical therapy based upon the individual patient's disease behavior.[34,56] Staging of the severity

TABLE 38.7 **Rutgeert's Scale in Assessment of Postoperative Crohn's Disease (Endoscopic Recurrence Score)**	
Endoscopic remission	• i0: No lesions • i1: ≤ 5 aphthous lesions
Endoscopic recurrence	• i2: > 5 aphthous lesions with normal intervening mucosa • i3: diffuse aphthous ileitis with diffusely inflamed mucosa • i4: diffuse inflammation with large ulcers, nodules and/or narrowing

Data from Rutgeerts P, Geboes K, Vantrappen G, et al: Predictability of the postoperative course of Crohn's disease. *Gastroenterology* 99(4):956–963, 1990.

of endoscopic activity is assessed using Rutgeert's scores, which rank inflammation grossly from 0 to 4 in the neoterminal ileum where inflammatory changes after ileocolonic resection for CD typically recur.[34] The Rutgeert's score is based on an assessment of the number of aphthous lesions that are present, as well as the extent of ileitis and the presence of features such as ulcers, nodules, and narrowing (Table 38.7).[34] Based on this classification, patients with less severe endoscopic appearance and a score of 1 or less had a lower risk of clinical recurrence (8.6% at 8 years) after ileocecal resection, whereas 100% of patients with severe endoscopic changes and a Rutgeert's score of 4 had symptomatic recurrence by 4 years.[34] The endoscopic assessment of the neoterminal ileum between 6 and 12 months postsurgery is recognized to be helpful in risk-stratifying patients prior to initiating medical management, and can prevent symptomatic recurrence and the need for subsequent surgical interventions.[1,57] De Cruz et al (2015) utilized the Rutgeert's Postoperative Endoscopic Index in a randomized clinical trial aiming to identify the optimal strategy to prevent postoperative disease recurrence of CD.[58] The Postoperative Crohn's Endoscopic Recurrence (POCER) trial demonstrated that choosing treatment according to the clinical risk of recurrence and a postoperative colonoscopy at 6 months enabled clinicians to tailor therapy to the patient.[58] All patients with a high risk of recurrence in the study received postoperative anti-TNF or thiopurine therapy, and were randomly assigned to either an active group including a 6-month postoperative colonoscopy or a standard group with no 6-month postoperative colonoscopy. Selective immunosuppression, adjusted for early recurrence based on colonoscopy rather than routine use, lead to disease control in most patients.[58] This approach of personalized medicine with selective immunosuppression use, based on the endoscopic evaluation, adjusted for early recurrence rather than routine use, leads to disease control in most patients and is a viable strategy in high-risk patients.[58]

Crohn's Disease Small Bowel Endoscopic Scores

Scoring systems have been also utilized in SB assessment of CD by VCE.[59–61] The traditional threshold of more than three ulcers to diagnose CD has been proposed by Mow et al (2004), which yields a positive predictive value of only 50% lacks assessment of the distribution and severity, and has also not been formally validated.[59] The capsule endoscopy Crohn's disease activity index (CECDAI) was developed and subsequently validated with a scoring index, allowing the distinction between proximal and distal SB, as well as further evaluation of parameters such as inflammation, extent, and the presence of strictures.[60,61] The

Lewis score has been introduced and is comprised of a cumulative scoring system based on the features and distribution of villous edema, ulceration, and stenosis.[61] This scoring system has been converted into a software application that calculates the score automatically. The final score is calculated by adding the inflammatory score of the worst affected tertile to the scores of stenosis. The scoring system has been validated for reporting SB inflammatory activity with strong interobserver agreements in a practical clinical setting.[13,62] Cotter et al (2015)[12] confirmed strong interobserver agreements for determination of the Lewis score in a practical clinical setting, thus further validating this score for SB inflammatory activity. The Lewis score may show potential to be used for the diagnosis, staging, follow-up, and therapeutic assessment of CD with isolated SB involvement. Further validation studies assessing the clinical significance of inflammatory changes, as well as response to therapy, are still required.

There are no additional standardized scoring systems to evaluate SB lesions based on enteroscopy evaluation.

The Role of Endoscopy in Diagnosing and Staging Complications of IBD

Strictures

Strictures as complications of IBD occur in 25% of patients with CD and 10% with colonic IBD.[63] Endoscopic dilations have been demonstrated to be an effective and safe treatment for short strictures caused by CD, impacting substantially on the natural history of these patients (Fig. 38.9; also see Video 17.16).[63] Specifically, balloon dilation of strictures shorter than 4 cm and anastomotic stricture have been demonstrated to have better dilation outcomes. Endoscopic strictures in patients with UC require re-evaluation for SB disease to see if the disease is truly UC or CD. If UC is present, surgery is appropriate because a stricture can represent a colonic malignancy.[64] In a 2015 retrospective study of patients with IBD undergoing surgery for colonic strictures, 3.5% were found to have dysplasia or cancer.[64]

Perianal Fistulas

Endoscopic ultrasound has been used for the assessment of perianal fistulas and abscesses. A meta-analysis by Siddiqui et al (2012) on performances of magnetic resonance imaging (MRI) and endoanal ultrasound in CD patients demonstrated comparable sensitivities at detecting perianal fistulas, although the specificity for MRI was higher than that for endoanal ultrasound.[65] Both specificity values were still considered to be diagnostically poor; however, pelvic MRI has been recommended as the initial evaluation for perianal fistulas, according to ECCO guidelines.[57] Current American Society for Gastrointestinal Endoscopy (ASGE) guidelines suggest using endoscopic ultrasound for characterizing and managing fistulous perianal CD in conjunction with other imaging modalities.[3]

Role of the Latest Endoscopic Advances for Diagnosing and Staging Disease Activity in IBD

Over the last few decades, wide-field technologies with virtual chromoendoscopy (narrow-band imaging [NBI; Olympus, Tokyo, Japan], Fujinon intelligent color enhancement system [FICE; Fujinon, Saitama, Japan], iScan [Pentax Medical, Montvale, NJ]), and small-field technologies (such as CLE and EC) have been investigated to characterize detected mucosal abnormalities in patients with IBD. Virtual chromoendoscopy is known as the "push-button switch technique," and is based on capturing various wavelengths of reflected light through optical filters (NBI) or digital postprocessing of the endoscopic images (iScan, FICE). By enhancing altered mucosal surface and vascular patterns, virtual chromoendoscopy may image early signs of disease activity in a process known as *angiogenesis* within otherwise normal-appearing mucosa.[3] Neumann et al (2013) demonstrated that virtual chromoendoscopy with iScan has the potential to enhance assessment of disease severity and extent in mild or inactive IBD patients.[66] In their randomized controlled study of 78 patients with IBD, the endoscopic prediction of inflammatory extent and activity based on high-definition white light (HDWL) and virtual chromoendoscopy was made and compared with histological results.[66] Interestingly, the use of virtual chromoendoscopy did not significantly change the duration of the examination, but it significantly improved the characterization of mucosal inflammation and extent.[66] When compared with histological assessment, the overall agreement was 48% and 53% for HDWL assessment and 92% and 89% for virtual chromoendoscopy assessment, respectively.[66]

Further visualization of colonic mucosa with an image of ongoing physiologic processes in vivo can be achieved with small-field technologies such as CLE and EC.

EC (Olympus, Tokyo, Japan) allows microscopic imaging of the gastrointestinal mucosa after application of topical absorptive contrast with up to 1400-fold magnification. In a pilot study of IBD patients, Neuman et al (2013)[67] confirmed that EC could easily distinguish all inflammatory cells with a very high level of accuracy and demonstrated excellent 100% concordance

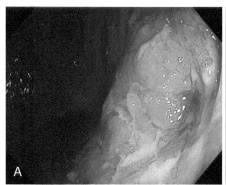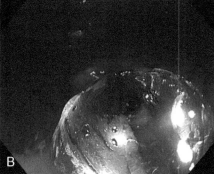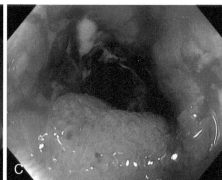

FIG 38.9 A, Ulcerated Crohn's stricture at the anastomosis. **B,** Balloon dilation of the stricture. **C,** Appearance of the stricture after dilation.

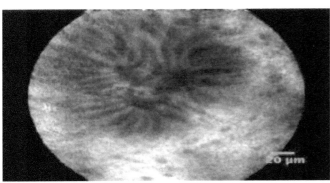

FIG 38.10 Confocal images of the colonic mucosa showing early inflammatory changes with increased colonic crypt tortuosity and fusion in a patient with Crohn's colitis.

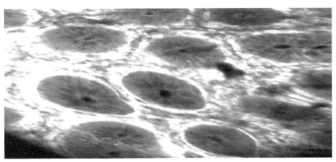

FIG 38.11 Confocal images of inflamed colonic mucosa with augmented vascularization and increased cellular infiltration in a patient with Crohn's colitis.

between EC and histopathology assessment for grading intestinal activity.

CLE can be performed using a Food and Drug Administration (FDA)-approved device: a standalone probe (herein termed *probe-based confocal laser endomicroscopy* [pCLE]) capable of passage through the accessory channel of most endoscopes (Cellvizio, Mauna Kea Technologies, Paris, France) and allowing 1000-fold magnification. Once the mucosal abnormality is detected during endoscopic evaluation, it can then be interrogated further by the confocal system for in vivo histology.[68] The CLE technique can also play a role in assessing and staging disease activity in addition to targeting biopsies to improve the early detection of neoplasia.[68,69]

Neumann et al (2012) proposed the Crohn's Disease Endomicroscopic Activity Score (CDEAS) to evaluate CD colitis activity in vivo based on typical inflammatory findings such as increased colonic crypt tortuosity, enlarged crypt lumen, microerosions, augmented vascularization, and increased cellular infiltration within the lamina propria (Figs. 38.10 and 38.11).[69] Quiescent CD colitis was also noted to have a significant increase in crypt and goblet cell numbers.[69] The inflammation activity of UC using CLE was also evaluated by Li et al (2010).[63] In their study, the endomicroscopy evaluation of crypt architecture and fluorescein leakage correlated well with traditional histology.[63]

Furthermore, CLE has also been studied to assess gastrointestinal barrier function. Using this technique, Kiesslich et al (2012) demonstrated that they could detect single-cell shedding and barrier loss in the TI of IBD patients and therefore predict relapse.[70] Specifically, CLE was used in detecting shedding epithelial cells and local barrier defects with fluorescein effluxing through the epithelium. Experiments on mice confirmed inward flow through some leakage-associated shedding events, which was increased when luminal osmolality was decreased. Interestingly, in IBD patients in clinical remission, this increased cell shedding with fluorescein leakage was associated with subsequent relapse within 12 months of endomicroscopic examination ($p < 0.001$).[70] The sensitivity, specificity, and accuracy of this grading system to predict a flare was 62.5% (95% CI: 40.8%–80.4%), 91.2% (95% CI: 75.2–97.7) and 79% (95% CI: 57.7–95.5), respectively.[70] This represents the truly great potential of the CLE system in staging disease activity and predicting disease course with a subsequent relapse. Similarly, Lim et al (2014) noted that CLE can detect epithelial damage and barrier loss in the duodenum of patients with CD and UC that is not apparent on conventional endoscopic evaluation.[71]

CLE has been also utilized for endoscopic molecular imaging, which has potential to enhance the detection of disease-specific targets and provide molecular-targeted therapies. The pilot study by Atreya et al (2014)[72] evaluated response to biological treatment with anti-TNF therapy. Topical antibody administration in 25 patients with CD led to the detection of intestinal membrane-bound TNF (mTNF)+ immune cells during CLE examination.[72] Patients with high numbers of mTNF+ cells had significantly higher short-term response rates (92%) at week 12 upon subsequent anti-TNF therapy compared with patients with low amounts of mTNF+ cells (15%).[72]

These results may facilitate early patient stratification in choosing therapeutic approaches. Endoscopic evaluation may also evolve beyond simply acting as a diagnostic tool into a prediction tool for molecular therapies in inflammation, guiding the treatment of patients, assessing the efficacy of biological treatment, and providing truly individualized therapy approaches.

SUMMARY

In summary, endoscopy is considered the gold standard technique for the diagnosis and staging of IBD and the evaluation of MH. Once IBD is diagnosed, frequent endoscopic assessment is associated with a higher rate of achieving MH.[73] Incremental changes in medication dosage or alteration of medications can occur. Frequent evaluation of the mucosa and optimization of therapy to achieve MH has been termed "treat-to-target."[74] Several studies have considered MH as an endpoint of significant importance, demonstrating that normalization of mucosa assessed by endoscopy and confirmed by histology ("deep remission") correlates with better clinical outcomes.[3,50,75]

Mucosal biopsy identifies persistent histologic disease activity, although the long-term clinical benefit of histological healing remains to be fully determined in spite of currently increasing evidence that supports achieving MH during therapy as a sign of adequate efficacy of treatment, reducing the need for hospitalization and surgical management, and impacting health-related quality of life in IBD patients.[26,76,77] The definition of MH has also been further defined in the setting of UC by the proposed guidelines, but needs to be further clarified in the setting of CD.[1] Current endoscopic tools (such as, for instance, the Mayo Endoscopic Score, CD Endoscopic Index of Severity, CDAI, etc.) utilized for assessment of disease were not initially created in accordance with the current mandate of the FDA, which requires the use of validated patient-reported outcomes (PROs). The current focus of the FDA is aimed at establishing and defining validated PROs in order to use this as a primary endpoint in clinical trials of IBD.[42] In the setting of IBD, PROs may provide an important complement to objective measures of intestinal inflammation otherwise obtained from endoscopic evaluation, and will serve as the ultimate endpoint in clinical trials. Currently, testing and refinement of proposed PRO measures in IBD are being investigated. Two interim PRO measures have been introduced.[50] In the setting of UC, a two-item PRO, including rectal bleeding and stool-frequency parameters of the MCS, has been used. In the setting of CD, a two-item PRO comprised of abdominal pain and stool frequency from the CDAI has been developed (PRO-2).[50]

Peyrin-Biroulet et al. (2016) proposed staging disease severity based on three domains, including impact of the disease on the patient (clinical symptoms, quality of life measured by PROs), measurable inflammatory burden based on endoscopic assessment and value of C-reactive protein, and disease course (including structural damage, history of surgical of intestinal resections, perianal disease, etc.).[74]

In the near future, a combination of symptomatic evaluation with defined PRO combined with endoscopic evaluation and staging severity of intestinal inflammation and assessing disease course may be particularly useful in staging disease severity in clinical practice as the main treat-to-target IBD-management strategy.

KEY REFERENCES

1. Annese V, Daperno M, Rutter MD, et al: European evidence based consensus for endoscopy in inflammatory bowel disease, *J Crohns Colitis* 7:982–1018, 2013.

2. D'Haens G, Sandborn WJ, Feagan BG, et al: A review of activity indices and efficacy end points for clinical trials of medical therapy in adults with ulcerative colitis, *Gastroenterology* 132:763–786, 2007.

4. Pera A, Bellando P, Caldera D, et al: Colonoscopy in inflammatory bowel disease. Diagnostic accuracy and proposal of an endoscopic score, *Gastroenterology* 92:181–185, 1987.

13. Dionisio PM, Gurudu SR, Leighton JA, et al: Capsule endoscopy has a significantly higher diagnostic yield in patients with suspected and established small-bowel Crohn's disease: a meta-analysis, *Am J Gastroenterol* 105:1240–1248, quiz 1249, 2010.

14. Jensen MD, Nathan T, Rafaelsen SR, et al: Diagnostic accuracy of capsule endoscopy for small bowel Crohn's disease is superior to that of MR enterography or CT enterography, *Clin Gastroenterol Hepatol* 9:124–129, 2011.

17. Manes G, Imbesi V, Ardizzone S, et al: Use of double-balloon enteroscopy in the management of patients with Crohn's disease: feasibility and diagnostic yield in a high-volume centre for inflammatory bowel disease, *Surg Endosc* 23:2790–2795, 2009.

18. Pasha SF, Leighton JA, Das A, et al: Double-balloon enteroscopy and capsule endoscopy have comparable diagnostic yield in small-bowel disease: a meta-analysis, *Clin Gastroenterol Hepatol* 6:671–676, 2008.

24. Floren CH, Benoni C, Willen R: Histologic and colonoscopic assessment of disease extension in ulcerative colitis, *Scand J Gastroenterol* 22:459–462, 1987.

25. Walsh A, Palmer R, Travis S: Mucosal healing as a target of therapy for colonic inflammatory bowel disease and methods to score disease activity, *Gastrointest Endosc Clin N Am* 24:367–378, 2014.

27. Rutgeerts P, Diamond RH, Bala M, et al: Scheduled maintenance treatment with infliximab is superior to episodic treatment for the healing of mucosal ulceration associated with Crohn's disease, *Gastrointest Endosc* 63:433–442, quiz 464, 2006.

29. Colombel JF, Rutgeerts P, Reinisch W, et al: Early mucosal healing with infliximab is associated with improved long-term clinical outcomes in ulcerative colitis, *Gastroenterology* 141:1194–1201, 2011.

31. D'Haens GR, Fedorak R, Lemann M, et al: Endpoints for clinical trials evaluating disease modification and structural damage in adults with Crohn's disease, *Inflamm Bowel Dis* 15:1599–1604, 2009.

32. Mary JY, Modigliani R: Development and validation of an endoscopic index of the severity for Crohn's disease: a prospective multicentre study. Groupe d'Etudes Therapeutiques des Affections Inflammatoires du Tube Digestif (GETAID), *Gut* 30:983–989, 1989.

33. Daperno M, D'Haens G, Van Assche G, et al: Development and validation of a new, simplified endoscopic activity score for Crohn's disease: the SES-CD, *Gastrointest Endosc* 60:505–512, 2004.

35. Samaan MA, Mosli MH, Sandborn WJ, et al: A systematic review of the measurement of endoscopic healing in ulcerative colitis clinical trials: recommendations and implications for future research, *Inflamm Bowel Dis* 20:1465–1471, 2014.

36. Schroeder KW, Tremaine WJ, Ilstrup DM: Coated oral 5-aminosalicylic acid therapy for mildly to moderately active ulcerative colitis. A randomized study, *N Engl J Med* 317:1625–1629, 1987.

38. D'Haens G, Feagan B, Colombel JF, et al: Challenges to the design, execution, and analysis of randomized controlled trials for inflammatory bowel disease, *Gastroenterology* 143:1461–1469, 2012.

40. Feagan BG, Reinisch W, Rutgeerts P, et al: The effects of infliximab therapy on health-related quality of life in ulcerative colitis patients, *Am J Gastroenterol* 102:794–802, 2007.

42. Travis SP, Schnell D, Krzeski P, et al: Developing an instrument to assess the endoscopic severity of ulcerative colitis: the Ulcerative Colitis Endoscopic Index of Severity (UCEIS), *Gut* 61:535–542, 2012.

44. Feagan BG, Sandborn WJ, D'Haens G, et al: The role of centralized reading of endoscopy in a randomized controlled trial of mesalamine for ulcerative colitis, *Gastroenterology* 145:149–157 e2, 2013.

45. Colombel JF, Ordas I, Ullman T, et al: Agreement between rectosigmoidoscopy and colonoscopy analyses of disease activity and healing in patients with ulcerative colitis, *Gastroenterology* 150:389–395 e3, 2016.

46. Khanna R, Bouguen G, Feagan BG, et al: A systematic review of measurement of endoscopic disease activity and mucosal healing in Crohn's disease: recommendations for clinical trial design, *Inflamm Bowel Dis* 20:1850–1861, 2014.

52. Khanna R, Zou G, D'Haens G, et al: Reliability among central readers in the evaluation of endoscopic findings from patients with Crohn's disease, *Gut* 65:1119–1125, 2016.

53. Ferrante M, Colombel JF, Sandborn WJ, et al: Validation of endoscopic activity scores in patients with Crohn's disease based on a post hoc analysis of data from SONIC, *Gastroenterology* 145:978–986 e5, 2013.

54. Bouguen G, Levesque BG, Pola S, et al: Feasibility of endoscopic assessment and treating to target to achieve mucosal healing in ulcerative colitis, *Inflamm Bowel Dis* 20:231–239, 2014.

62. Gralnek IM, Defranchis R, Seidman E, et al: Development of a capsule endoscopy scoring index for small bowel mucosal inflammatory change, *Aliment Pharmacol Ther* 27:146–154, 2008.

A complete reference list can be found online at ExpertConsult.com

39

Dysplasia Surveillance in Inflammatory Bowel Disease

Jimmy K. Limdi and Francis A. Farraye

INTRODUCTION

Patients with long-standing inflammatory bowel disease (IBD) are at an increased risk for development of colorectal cancer (CRC).[1,2] Risk factors for the development of CRC in ulcerative colitis (UC) or Crohn's colitis include young age of disease onset, longer duration of disease, greater extent of colonic involvement, coexistent primary sclerosing cholangitis (PSC), active endoscopic or histological inflammation, family history of CRC in a first-degree relative diagnosed before 50 years of age, a history of dysplasia, stricturing disease in UC, inflammatory ("pseudo") polyps, a shortened tubular colon, and possibly male gender.[3–9]

Of all the risk factors associated with the development of CRC in IBD, colitis-related dysplasia appears to confer the greatest risk, leading gastrointestinal (GI) societies to advocate colonoscopic surveillance to detect dysplasia in high-risk patients.[3–7,10,11] The goal of endoscopic surveillance is to reduce mortality and morbidity of CRC by either detecting and resecting dysplasia or detecting CRC at an earlier and potentially curable stage.[12,13] Surveillance strategies, until recently, relied on examination of the mucosa with targeted biopsies of visible lesions and random biopsy sampling, based on the prevailing notion that dysplasia is frequently not associated with visible mucosal abnormalities.[14] Meanwhile, advances in optical technology allowing for greater endoscopic identification of dysplasia and consensus that most dysplasia in patients with IBD is visible have led to a paradigm shift in our approach to surveillance and management of dysplasia.[12,15] This chapter will review the epidemiology of CRC in IBD, the evolution in our understanding of dysplasia, outline the most recent surveillance guidelines from scientific societies, and discuss the management of dysplasia and controversies therein.

EPIDEMIOLOGY OF CRC IN IBD

Colorectal cancer (CRC) in IBD, accounting for 1% to 2% of CRC cases in the general population, is responsible for 10% to 15% of all deaths in IBD patients.[16] Indeed, after genetic causes of CRC (such as familial adenomatous polyposis and Lynch syndrome), IBD ranks as the third highest risk factor for CRC, underpinning the need to better define associated risk factors and optimize surveillance strategies, thereby achieving meaningful reduction in IBD-CRC associated morbidity and mortality.[17]

The risk of CRC in IBD (and UC in particular) increases with time but risk estimates have been difficult to quantify, often limited by heterogeneity and methodology in the retrospective cohorts studied. A large meta-analysis in 2001 estimated a cumulative CRC risk of 2% at 10 years, 8% at 20 years and 18% after 30 years of colitis.[18] A 2012 population-based study from Copenhagen County, Denmark, demonstrated a decreasing incidence of CRC in IBD patients over the last few decades.[19] More recently (2015), a 40-year colonoscopic surveillance program from St. Mark's Hospital, UK, reported a cumulative incidence of developing CRC in IBD patients at 0.1% in the first decade since UC symptom onset, followed by 2.9%, 6.7%, and 10% by the second, third, and fourth decade, respectively.[20] The authors reported a significant decrease in the incidence of colectomy for dysplasia and a reduction in the incidence rate of advanced CRC and interval cancers over 4 decades of surveillance.[20] Population-based meta-analyses have shown an overall CRC incidence ratio of 1.7 in all IBD patients,[21] with patients with CD reported to have a 1.9-fold[22] and patients with UC having a 2.4-fold increase in lifetime CRC risk compared to the general population.[23] Thus, recent studies suggest a decrease in the risk of CRC in IBD, a temporal reduction that may be explained by more aggressive control of inflammation through medication, the greater uptake of surveillance colonoscopy allowing detection and resection of dysplastic lesions before the development of CRC, and appropriate timing of colectomy.[24,25]

RISK FACTORS FOR CRC IN IBD

Several risk factors are associated with the development of CRC in UC or Crohn's colitis as stated previously and include young

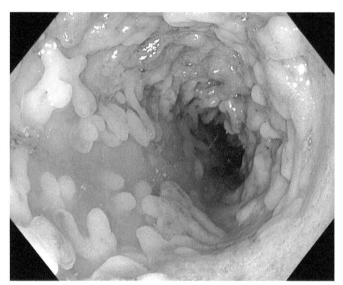

FIG 39.1 Pseudopolyps. (From Kakkar A, Farraye FA: Diagnosis and management of colorectal neoplasia in patients with inflammatory bowel disease. In Baumgart DC [Ed]: *Crohn's Disease and Ulcerative Colitis: Epidemiology and Immunobiology to a Rational Diagnostic and Therapeutic Approach.* New York, 2012, Springer, pp 701–712.)

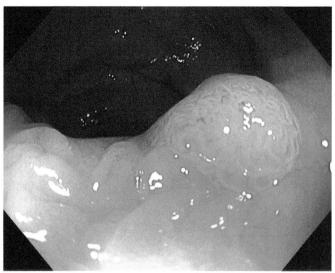

FIG 39.2 Polypoid dysplasia. (From Kakkar A, Farraye FA: Diagnosis and management of colorectal neoplasia in patients with inflammatory bowel disease. In Baumgart DC [Ed]: *Crohn's Disease and Ulcerative Colitis: Epidemiology and Immunobiology to a Rational Diagnostic and Therapeutic Approach.* New York, 2012, Springer, pp 701–712.)

age of disease onset, longer duration of disease, greater extent of colonic involvement, coexistent PSC, active endoscopic or histological inflammation, family history of CRC in a first-degree relative diagnosed before 50 years of age, a history of dysplasia, stricturing disease in UC, inflammatory ("pseudo") polyps, a shortened tubular colon, and male gender[3–9,26] (Fig. 39.1). Subtotal colitis or pancolitis confers the highest risk of developing CRC and patients with colonic CD disease involving more than one-third of the colon are also at increased risk of CRC.[27–29] The extent of colonic involvement should be based on both endoscopic and histological criteria and on whichever reveals more extensive disease.[3,5,30–32] Although patients with proctitis or distal proctosigmoiditis alone are not at increased risk compared with the general population, many patients with proctitis will develop more proximal disease over the course of their lifetime and a screening colonoscopy is recommended 8 years after the onset of symptoms even in patients with previously isolated proctitis to confirm extent of disease.[6,24,28,33] The relative risk (RR) of CRC rises with longer disease duration and is the rationale behind initiation of surveillance colonoscopy after 8 to 10 years of disease.[19,34] PSC confers a high risk for CRC. A meta-analysis of 11 trials reported a 4-fold increased risk of developing colonic neoplasia in patients with PSC and UC compared to those with UC alone.[35] Additionally, several clinical trials have demonstrated a persistently elevated risk of CRC in PSC despite undergoing orthotopic liver transplantation.[36–38] Thus, patients with IBD and PSC should undergo surveillance colonoscopy annually beginning at the time PSC is diagnosed.[3,5,6,10,31] Studies examining a link between early age of onset of IBD and CRC are conflicting and the American Gastroenterological Association (AGA) recommends that surveillance be based on duration of illness and not chronological age.[3]

The known risk factors for CRC in IBD are almost all non-modifiable with the possible exception of inflammation.[8,9,39] A positive association between the degree of microscopic inflam-

mation and advanced neoplasia has been noted in several studies.[8,9,39,40] Colonic strictures in UC (but not in CD), a shortened tubular colon, and multiple pseudopolyps also increase CRC risk, with the latter significantly limiting the ability to adequately survey the colon.[39–42] These clinically important associations must be considered when counselling patients about their risk of developing CRC and planning surveillance examinations.

Dysplasia

The detection of dysplasia is currently the best marker of CRC risk in IBD patients, the prevention of which is the ultimate goal of surveillance colonoscopy.[43–45] Biopsies taken at surveillance colonoscopy should be graded as "positive" for dysplasia, "negative" for dysplasia, or "indefinite" for dysplasia and further classified as low-grade dysplasia (LGD), high-grade dysplasia (HGD), or carcinoma.[46] Considerable interobserver variability exists amongst pathologists around interpretation of "low-grade" dysplasia and "indefinite for dysplasia" categories, mandating a second opinion from a specialist GI pathologist to confirm dysplasia when detected.[47] Older guidelines recommended that lesions be characterized as sporadic adenomas if found outside an area of known colitis or as dysplasia–associated lesion or mass (DALM) if detected within an area of colitis; however, this terminology has been abandoned and should no longer be used.[3–5,10,31,43,45,48,49] The terms "visible" and "invisible" should be used instead to describe dysplasia within clearly identified lesions or within random biopsy samples, respectively, with the addition of terms for ulceration and border of the lesion.[31,43] Visible dysplasia is further classified as polypoid (pedunculated or sessile) or nonpolypoid (superficial elevated, flat or depressed) in accordance with the Paris Classification[6,43,46] (Figs. 39.2 and 39.3). Accordingly, the term *endoscopically resectable* indicates that distinct margins of the lesion can be identified, the lesion appears completely excised on visual inspection after endoscopic resection,

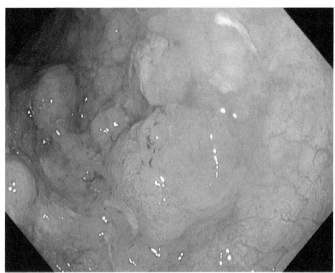

FIG 39.3 Nonpolypoid dysplasia. (From Kakkar A, Farraye FA: Diagnosis and management of colorectal neoplasia in patients with inflammatory bowel disease. In Baumgart DC [Ed]: *Crohn's Disease and Ulcerative Colitis: Epidemiology and Immunobiology to a Rational Diagnostic and Therapeutic Approach.* New York, 2012, Springer, pp 701–712.)

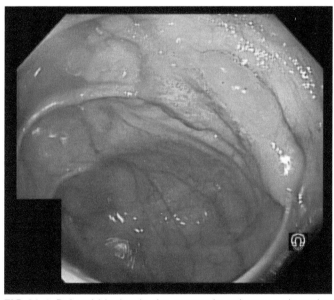

FIG 39.4 Polypoid lesion in the cecum in quiescent ulcerative colitis. (Courtesy Dr. Regi George, Pennine Acute Hospitals, Manchester, UK.)

histological assessment of the resected specimen is consistent with complete removal, and that biopsy specimens taken from mucosa immediately adjacent to the resection site are free of dysplasia on histological assessment (Fig. 39.4).[43]

Recognition that most dysplasia is endoscopically visible, bolstered by advanced imaging techniques facilitating dysplasia detection, has had a significant impact on modern dysplasia management and surveillance strategies.

Dysplasia Surveillance

The aim of endoscopic surveillance is the reduction of mortality and morbidity from CRC through detection and resection of dysplasia or by detecting CRC at earlier and potentially curable stages.[13] Endoscopic surveillance has been shown to reduce the risk of death from CRC in the IBD population and also to be cost-effective in various case-series, case-control studies and population-based cohort studies.[50–55] Thus, despite the lack of randomized controlled trials, the invasive nature of assessment, and utilization of societal resources, surveillance colonoscopy in IBD patients has been endorsed by multiple societies.[3–7,10,11] Most societies recommend that all patients with UC (including isolated proctitis) and Crohn's colitis should be offered screening colonoscopy approximately 8 to 10 years after onset of clinical symptoms to restage disease extent and evaluate features that may confer a higher risk for IBD–CRC.[3–7,10,11] In the absence of evidence from prospective studies, societies vary in their recommendations with surveillance intervals after a screening colonoscopy but universally agree and recommend annual screening for patients with the highest risk of IBD associated CRC.[3–7,10,11] Thus, patients with concomitant PSC, extensive colitis with active endoscopic or histological inflammation, a family history of CRC in a first-degree relative under the age of 50, a personal history of dysplasia, and stricturing disease (in UC patients) should be offered annual surveillance. Normal appearing mucosa appears to be associated with a lower risk of IBD associated colorectal neoplasia.[40] The British Society for Gastroenterology (BSG), European Crohn's and Colitis Organization (ECCO), National Institute for Health and Clinical Excellence (NICE), and Cancer Council of Australia (CCA) support a risk-stratification approach, increasing surveillance intervals to 5 years in lowest risk patients.[4,7,10] Societies in the United States do not currently recommend lengthening the surveillance interval to beyond 3 years.[3,5,6,43] Recommendations from the AGA guidelines are outlined in Box 39.1. The BSG guidelines incorporating risk factors and newer imaging techniques are outlined in Fig. 39.5.

The success of surveillance depends on several factors, of which the ability to detect dysplasia is probably most crucial. Surveillance traditionally performed by taking random colonic biopsies was based on the premise that dysplasia is frequently not associated with mucosal abnormalities.[12,14] To detect dysplasia with 90% probability, 33 serial colonic biopsies from four quadrant biopsy specimens need to be obtained every 10 cm from each anatomical segment of the colon, a practice endorsed by many GI societies.[3–5,55]

Evolution in endoscopic technology from standard definition (SD) colonoscopy using video chips to high-definition (HD) colonoscopy, and indeed evidence that most dysplasia is visible at standard white light colonoscopy, has challenged the practice of random biopsy sampling as the basis of surveillance assessment.[12,43]

The practice of random biopsies would sample less than 1% of total colonic mucosa, and one study suggested that up to 1266 random biopsies would be needed to detect one additional episode of dysplasia.[45,48] In a study in which UC patients underwent colonoscopy every 2 years, interval cancers were observed to develop between 10 and 28 months after dysplasia-free examination, reflecting poorly on the practice of random biopsies alone for dysplasia detection at surveillance.[56,57]

Surveillance strategies must take additional aspects such as resectability of dysplasia, anatomical features such as pseudopolyps, and a shortened tubular colon into consideration; these

BOX 39.1   AGA Surveillance Guidelines for CRC in Inflammatory Bowel Disease

- All patients, regardless of the extent of disease at initial diagnosis, should undergo a screening colonoscopy a maximum of 8 years after onset of symptoms, with multiple biopsy specimens obtained throughout the entire colon, to assess the true microscopic extent of inflammation.
- Patients with ulcerative proctitis or ulcerative proctosigmoiditis are not considered at increased risk for IBD-related CRC and thus may be managed on the basis of average-risk recommendations.
- Patients with extensive or left-sided colitis should begin surveillance within 1 to 2 years after the initial screening endoscopy.
- Patients with PSC should begin surveillance colonoscopy at the time of PSC diagnosis and then yearly.
- Patients with a history of CRC in a first-degree relative, ongoing active endoscopic or histologic inflammation, or anatomic abnormalities (shortened colon, multiple pseudopolyps, or stricture) may benefit from more frequent surveillance colonoscopy.
- Representative biopsy specimens from each anatomic section of the colon is recommended. Though no prospective trials have determined the optimal number of biopsies to take, one study has recommended a minimum of 33 biopsy specimens.
- Surveillance colonoscopy should ideally be performed when the patient is in remission.
- These recommendations apply to patients with Crohn's colitis who have disease involving at least one-third of their colon.

AGA, American Gastroenterological Association; *CRC*, colorectal cancer; *IBD*, inflammatory bowel disease; *PSC*, primary sclerosing cholangitis.
From Farraye FA, Odze RD, Iaden J, Itzkowitz SH: AGA technical review on the diagnosis and management of colorectal neoplasia in inflammatory bowel disease. *Gastroenterology* 138(2):746–774.e4, 2010.

may pose difficulties with dysplasia detection. Furthermore, colonic inflammation can make pathologic discrimination of dysplasia difficult; thus surveillance should ideally take place when the patient is in clinical remission. These factors merit careful consideration with patients when committing to a surveillance program. Evidence suggests that patients do not wish to consider colectomy until there is a relatively high certainty of cancer underpinning the importance of careful consideration and meticulous assessment, employing best available technology and technique to detect and resect dysplasia to avoid IBD-associated CRC and colectomy.[58]

New imaging techniques such as chromoendoscopy (CE), narrow band imaging (NBI), and confocal endomicroscopy have been developed as an adjunctive technique to detect more subtle mucosal abnormalities. Several studies have demonstrated a superior diagnostic yield and therapeutic advantage with CE when compared with standard random biopsy and white light technique for index screening of dysplasia in colitis,[59–63] supported by meta-analyses providing evidence that the use of CE with targeted biopsies is 8.9 times more likely to detect any dysplasia and 5.2 times more likely to detect nonpolypoid dysplasia than white light endoscopy (WLE) with random biopsy.[64,65] This evolution in knowledge has seen cautious translation in societal recommendations over the years. Although the American College of Gastroenterology's (ACG) 2010 guidelines considered it premature to endorse CE in low-risk patients,[5] the Crohn's and Colitis Foundation of America's (CCFA) 2004 and AGA's 2010 guidelines considered CE with targeted biopsies as a reasonable alternative to WLE for endoscopists experienced in this technique.[3,4] CE with targeted biopsies is endorsed by all recent European guidelines (ECCO, BSG, NICE) and recent American Society for Gastrointestinal Endoscopy (ASGE) guidance.[6,7,10] The recently published Surveillance for Colorectal Endoscopic Neoplasia Detection and Management in Inflammatory Bowel Disease Patients: International Consensus Recommendations (SCENIC) recommends CE over standard white light colonoscopy and suggest CE over HD colonoscopy for dysplasia surveillance in IBD, with meta-analysis demonstrating a significantly greater proportion of dysplasia detection at CE (RR 1.8, absolute risk increase 6%) than white light colonoscopy alone.[43] Furthermore, this strategy has also been shown to be cost-effective, especially with increasing surveillance intervals based on the risk of CRC.[66]

CE involves the use of topical contrast agents, either 0.1% methylene blue or 0.03% to 0.5% indigo carmine. Excellent bowel preparation is a prerequisite. Colonic mucosa is sprayed segmentally with contrast agent after cecal intubation and upon withdrawal, using a spray catheter or through the forward water-jet channel using an automated pump.[59–61,65–67] CE enhances mucosal irregularities and helps delineate the lesion morphology, size, and border to evaluate for endoscopic features of submucosal invasion (Figs. 39.6 and 39.7; Videos 39.1 and 39.2). Thus, endoscopically resectable lesions may be resected if feasible, or tattooed and referred to an endoscopist with expertise in endoscopic mucosal resection or dissection as appropriate. Targeted biopsies should be taken from lesions deemed endoscopically unresectable and lesions of uncertain significance. Furthermore, at least two histological staging biopsies from several colonic segments are recommended to determine histological extent and severity of disease, which, in turn, affects the risk of dysplasia.[6,7,10] Random biopsies are not recommended if CE is used for dysplasia surveillance.[6,7,10,11,31] Despite heightened sensitivity of CE in detecting dysplastic foci and other purported benefits, its universal adoption and acceptance has been met with by some scepticism.[44] The natural history of additional, smaller, flatter lesions identified at CE is poorly understood.[68] The rate of progression from indefinite and LGD to cancer appears to be low in some high-risk cohorts, even when considering variables such as PSC and previous advanced dysplasia.[69–72] Moreover, data from the Surveillance, Epidemiology and End results Medicare-linked database of patients over 67 years old showed that interval cancers 6 to 36 months after colonoscopy occurred in a much higher proportion of patients with IBD (15.1% with Crohn's disease and 15.8% with ulcerative colitis) than patients without IBD (5.8%), suggesting that clinically relevant areas of neoplasia may be missed with current colonoscopy surveillance.[57] Considering this, the SCENIC consensus acknowledges that its recommendation for CE over HD white light colonoscopy is conditional, being based on small observational studies.[43,73]

Since the publication of the SCENIC consensus paper in 2015, several studies have added to the body of evidence supporting CE as the preferred technique, with others expressing reservations regarding its universal adoption, through demonstration of its limitations and identifying gaps in our knowledge and understanding of the natural history of dysplasia.[20,74–78] Marion et al (2016) reported a follow-up evaluation of their 2008 study of patients in an IBD surveillance program.[74,79] Sixty-eight patients (from the original cohort of 115), with median disease duration of 21 years, were followed over a 5-year period, between 2005 and 2011. All patients underwent colonoscopy surveillance with random biopsy specimens, targeted WLE, and dye-spray CE. After a mean of three surveillance colonoscopies per patient, six

COLITIS SURVEILLANCE

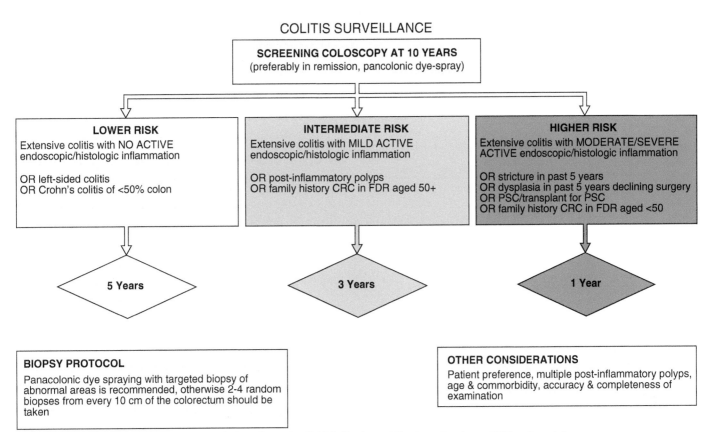

SCREENING COLOSCOPY AT 10 YEARS
(preferably in remission, pancolonic dye-spray)

LOWER RISK

Extensive colitis with NO ACTIVE endoscopic/histologic inflammation

OR left-sided colitis
OR Crohn's colitis of <50% colon

INTERMEDIATE RISK

Extensive colitis with MILD ACTIVE endoscopic/histologic inflammation

OR post-inflammatory polyps
OR family history CRC in FDR aged 50+

HIGHER RISK

Extensive colitis with MODERATE/SEVERE ACTIVE endoscopic/histologic inflammation

OR stricture in past 5 years
OR dysplasia in past 5 years declining surgery
OR PSC/transplant for PSC
OR family history CRC in FDR aged <50

5 Years

3 Years

1 Year

BIOPSY PROTOCOL

Panacolonic dye spraying with targeted biopsy of abnormal areas is recommended, otherwise 2-4 random biopses from every 10 cm of the colorectum should be taken

OTHER CONSIDERATIONS

Patient preference, multiple post-inflammatory polyps, age & commorbidity, accuracy & completeness of examination

FIG 39.5 Recommendations from the British Society of Gastroenterology. *CRC,* colorectal cancer; *FDR,* first-degree relative; *PSC,* primary sclerosing cholangitis. (From Cairns SR, Scholefield JH, Steele RJ, et al: Guidelines for colorectal cancer screening and surveillance in moderate and high risk groups [update from 2002]. *Gut* 59[5]:666–689, 2010.)

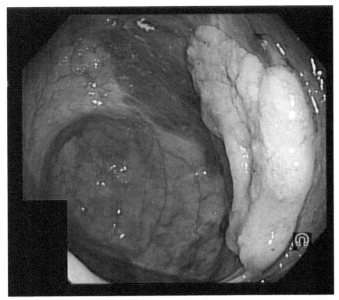

FIG 39.6 Cecal polypoid lesion in quiescent ulcerative colitis after indigo carmine dye spray. (Courtesy Dr. Regi George, Pennine Acute Hospitals, Manchester, UK.)

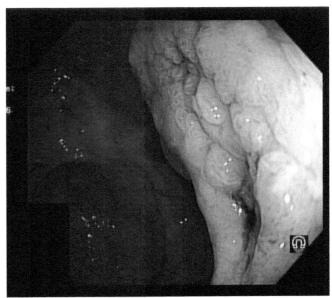

FIG 39.7 Cecal lesion in ulcerative colitis after dye spray. (Courtesy Dr. Regi George, Pennine Acute Hospitals, Manchester, UK.)

dysplastic lesions were detected by random biopsy technique, as compared with 11 and 27 dysplastic lesions seen at WLE and CE respectively.[74] CE demonstrated superiority to random biopsy specimens (odds ratio [OR] 5.4; 95% confidence interval [CI], 2.9–9.9) and targeted WLE (OR 2.4; 95% CI, 1.4–4.0). A negative result from CE assessment was the best indicator for a dysplasia-free outcome and a positive result was associated with earlier referral for colectomy (hazard ratio [HR] 12.1; 95% CI, 3.2–46.2). Notably, of the 10 patients with dysplasia referred for colectomy, no carcinomas were found.[74]

Gasia et al (2016), studied a cohort of 454 IBD patients undergoing surveillance assessments between 2011 and 2014.[75] Patients were examined using WLE, HD colonoscopy, virtual electronic, or dye spray CE. Just under one-third of patients underwent WLE or HD colonoscopy with random biopsy, and 14% had virtual CE with random biopsies. A smaller number of patients underwent dye-spray CE with random (n = 4) or targeted (n = 24) biopsies. Targeted biopsies identified more neoplastic lesions than random biopsies (19% vs. 8%). Four dysplastic lesions were seen at HD WLE. The investigators found no difference in yield between dye CE, virtual CE, and targeted WLE in the cohort of 454 patients studied. No dysplasia was identified, however, from random biopsy samples alone.[75] The futility of random biopsy has been demonstrated repeatedly and convincingly in several prospective studies.[45,48,56]

In a large Dutch multicenter study, Mooiweer et al (2015) studied the outcomes of adoption of CE from 440 colonoscopies in 401 patients compared with historical outcomes of 1802 colonoscopies in 772 patients with WLE.[78] No difference in dysplasia detection was noted in both groups (11% vs. 10%). An inherent limitation of the retrospective study was the lack of data for examination factors (including bowel prep and withdrawal time), but the remarkably stable neoplasia detection over a 10-year period in highly experienced hands suggests that CE is not superior to WLE.[78]

In contrast, another study from St. Mark's Hospital, London, reporting a 40-year experience with colonoscopic surveillance, found a recent increase in the incidence rate of dysplasia since the adoption of high-definition white light endoscopy (HD WLE) and CE for surveillance, but no decrease in the rate of colon cancer.[20] Although CE seemingly did not affect the outcome of CRC in IBD, there was a significant increase in the proportion of early-stage (Duke's A and B) versus late-stage (Duke's C & D) CRC in the most recent decade. HD WLE and CE were introduced at St. Mark's in 2006 and although patients were not randomized to CE between 2006 and 2012, the CRC incidence rate was 2.2/1,000 patient-years in patients receiving at least one CE versus 4.6 in those who had never received CE (p = 0.02).[20] Deepak et al (2016) from the Mayo Clinic reported an incremental diagnostic yield from CE.[76] In this retrospective study, IBD patients with colorectal dysplasia on WLE, endoscopic, and histologic findings (median disease duration 18 years) were compared among the index WLE, first, and subsequent CE.[76] Of 95 index cases, dysplasia was identified in 55 patients at index WLE. The first CE identified dysplastic lesions in 50 patients (34 new lesions not seen at index WLE), endoscopic resection was performed for 43 lesions, and 14 patients underwent surgery with two cases of CRC and three cases of HGD. From subsequent CE assessments, 34 lesions were identified in 20 patients. The data support CE as a surveillance procedure in high-risk patients.[76] Indeed, one of the arguments against "CE for all surveillance" is that the natural history of dysplastic lesions identified at CE remains

unknown. Choi et al (2016) identified four characteristics that were significantly associated with a later diagnosis of HGD or CRC.[20] Nonpolypoid lesion appearance, defined as Paris type 0-II (visible, slightly elevated, or depressed), type 0-III (excavated), or plaque-like, was the strongest factor (HR 8.6; 95% CI 3-24.8), but macroscopically invisible dysplasia (HR, 4.1; 95% CI, 1.3-13.4), lesion size of 1 cm or greater (HR, 3.8; 95% CI, 1.5-13.4), and previous history of indefinite dysplasia (HR, 2.8; 95% CI, 1.2-6.5) were also significant predictors. There was also strong positive correlation between the number of these risk factors present and a subsequent HGD or CRC diagnosis. The strongest risk factor, nonpolypoid dysplasia, was found at significantly greater frequency in those patients who underwent CE rather than white-light colonoscopy (15.8% vs. 7.8%, respectively), although exposure to CE did not lower the risk of HGD or CRC after Bonferroni correction for multiple testing.[20]

Successful delivery of dysplasia surveillance using CE, however, hinges on several factors, including appropriate training and expertise (endoscopist and nurses), lesion recognition, and interobserver variability amongst pathologists identifying and grading dysplasia, as well as operational barriers, such as the availability of dye and equipment and procedural time, which results in some hesitancy amongst gastroenterologists in adopting CE, and referral to "experts" for its provision in some instances.[43] The evidence favors CE for surveillance where suitable expertise is available and is backed by several scientific societies and international consensus opinion.[6,10,43] What constitutes "appropriately trained" for CE is currently debatable, as there is no standardized definitions or accreditation process. One study suggested that completion of 16 CE procedures may be adequate for dysplasia detection training using this modality, but this has not since been replicated.[73] A recent multicenter study from Spain has provided "real-world" experience in support of CE for IBD surveillance, challenging skepticism regarding the effectiveness of CE outside of a clinical trial setting and potential limitations posed by less experience with CE.[80] In a prospective study performed between 2012 and 2014, 350 patients with IBD on dysplasia surveillance were systematically evaluated using WLE (SD in 41.5% and HD in 58.5%) for each colonic segment, followed by CE with 0.4% indigo carmine. An incremental yield of 57.4% was noted with CE, comparable between SD and HD colonoscopy (51.5% vs. 52.3%; p = 0.30). A further interesting observation was a comparable dysplasia detection between expert and nonexpert colonoscopists (18.5% vs. 13.1%; p = 0.20) and no significant learning curve.[80] Endoscopic findings predictive of dysplasia were proximal colonic lesions, protruding morphology, loss of innominate lines, and a neoplastic Kudo pit pattern. Arguable limitations of the study include the potential for a "Hawthorne effect" (diligence with performance of colonoscopy in a prospective study) and an incremental yield from a "second look;" as there was also a small sample size, this study does provide proof of principle for the wider and realistic adoption of CE for dysplasia surveillance in high risk IBD patients and potentially in "nonexpert" hands.[80] Several excellent resources, however, are available for colonoscopists to enhance their skills.[43,65,81] Meanwhile, evolution in our knowledge of the natural history of dysplasia and the clinical implications of dysplasia found by CE through its wider adoption may close many gaps in our understanding of its real place in surveillance. Until then, the bulk of the evidence favors CE with targeted biopsy in individuals at high risk or those with previous dysplasia. In the remaining majority of patients undergoing surveillance

Summary of Recommendations for Surveillance and Management of Dysplasia in Patients With Inflammatory Bowel Disease

Detection of Dysplasia on Surveillance Colonoscopy

1. When performing surveillance with white light colonoscopy, high definition is recommended rather than standard definition (strong recommendations, low-quality evidence).
2. When performing surveillance with standard-definition colonoscopy, chromoendoscopy is recommended rather than white light colonoscopy (strong recommendation, moderate-quality evidence).
3. When performing surveillance with high-definition colonoscopy, chromoendoscopy is suggested rather than white light colonoscopy (conditional recommendation, low-quality evidence).
4. When performing surveillance with standard-definition colonoscopy, narrow band imaging is not suggested in place of white light colonoscopy (conditional recommendation, low-quality evidence).
5. When performing surveillance with high-definition colonoscopy, narrow band imaging is not suggested in place of white light colonoscopy (conditional recommendation, moderate-quality evidence).
6. When performing surveillance with image-enhanced high-definition colonoscopy, narrow band imaging is not suggested in place of chromoendoscopy (conditional recommendation, moderate-quality evidence)

Management of Dysplasia Discovered on Surveillance Colonoscopy

7. After complete removal of endoscopically resectable polypoid dysplastic lesions, surveillance colonoscopy is recommended rather than colectomy (strong recommendation, very low-quality evidence).
8. After complete removal of endoscopically resectable nonpolypoid dysplastic lesions, surveillance colonoscopy is suggested rather than colectomy (conditional recommendation, very low-quality evidence).
9. For patients with endoscopically invisible dysplasia (confirmed by a GI pathologist) referral is suggested to an endoscopist with expertise in IBD surveillance using chromoendoscopy with high-definition colonoscopy (conditional recommendation, very low-quality evidence).

GI, gastrointestinal; *IBD,* inflammatory bowel disease.
From Laine L, Kaltenbach T, Barkun A, et al: SCENIC international consensus statement on surveillance and management of dysplasia in inflammatory bowel disease. *Gastrointest Endosc* 81(3):489–501. e26, 2015.

colonoscopy, careful assessment with either HD WLE and random biopsies or CE with dye spray may be appropriate with no compelling mandate for one over the other at the present time. A summary of recommendations from the SCENIC consensus for surveillance and management of dysplasia in patients with IBD is outlined in Box 39.2.

OTHER ADVANCED IMAGING MODALITIES

Narrow Band Imaging

NBI, an optical CE technology that uses filters to enhance the contrast of the mucosa and vasculature, has not demonstrated an increased yield for dysplasia detection in randomized studies comparing NBI to either SD WLE or HD WLE.[82–85] Studies comparing NBI with CE have reported a numerically higher detection rate with CE but at meta-analysis the difference was not statistically significant.[84] A prospective, multicenter tandem surveillance study in patients with UC, comparing WLE with targeted and random biopsies to NBI, found no difference in

dysplasia detection rates.[86] The SCENIC consensus does not recommend NBI over dye spray CE.[43]

Confocal Laser Endomicroscopy

Confocal laser endomicroscopy (CLE) allows for "real-time" histology of lesions already detected at colonoscopy using intravenous administration of stains such as fluorescein. The endoscope integrates a confocal laser microscope into the distal tip of a conventional endoscope, or a CLE probe, which is passed through the working channel. After topical or intravenous application of a fluorescence agent, the CLE probe is applied to the mucosal surface. Fluorescein highlights the extracellular matrix allowing for in vivo evaluation.[87]

In a prospective trial with 161 UC patients randomized to combined CE and CLE or conventional WLE, neoplasia detection was 4.75-fold more with the combined approach ($p = 0.005$) requiring 50% fewer biopsies ($p = 0.008$) compared with conventional WLE.[88] A prospective study compared WLE with random and targeted biopsies (group I), CE with random and targeted biopsies (group II) and CLE with random and targeted biopsies (group III). No neoplasia was detected in group I; HGD was detected in two patients (4% detection rate) in group II; and in group III, HGD was detected in four patients (8% detection rate, $p = 0.05$).[89] Notably, all four lesions identified as neoplasia in the CLE group during the procedure were later confirmed at histology. The increased diagnostic yield of CLE with the need for fewer biopsies has been confirmed by other studies.[90,91] Despite encouraging data, the technique is currently limited by the increased length of time, being approximately 15 to 25 minutes more than WLE with target biopsy and CE with targeted biopsy, respectively;[89] a steep learning curve and cost (up to US $175,000 for the probe based system).[43,92–94]

Endocytoscopy

Endocytoscopy (EC) is a novel technique that allows highly magnified (up to 1400×) images of subcellular structures.[95] It uses either probe-based systems or EC-fitted endoscopes to obtain histology-equivalent images of the mucosa, following pretreatment with mucolytic agents and staining with dyes such as methylene blue and crystal violet.[95] A pilot study demonstrated that EC may accurately differentiate inflammatory cell populations in IBD, with prognostic implications, but no studies on dysplasia surveillance have been published to date.[96] The potential for EC to detect high-grade intraepithelial neoplasia in polyps, and to identify early dysplastic changes as part of the adenoma carcinoma sequence, shows promise for future applications in colitis-associated dysplasia.[97,98]

Molecular Imaging

The application of fluorescent substances (antibodies, nanoparticles, lectins, and peptides) acting as probes targeting molecular targets that play a role in GI disease is under study.[99,100] In a murine model, an enzymatically activated probe to detect cancer on a background of colitis, cancerous, and dysplastic cells showed a higher signal than inflamed tissue, confirmed at histology.[101] In a 2014 phase 1 study, patients with Crohn's disease with increased expression of membrane-bound tumor necrosis factor (TNF) as detected following the application of a fluorescent antibody to mTNF (probe), showed a higher response rate to anti-TNF therapy than patients with low mTNF expression.[102] This is an exciting advance with much promise for the potential for personalized management in the near future.[102]

Stool DNA Testing

The potential for stool DNA testing for genetic alterations that are part of the carcinogenesis cascade in IBD (e.g., BMP3 and mNDRG4) to improve colonoscopic yield is being studied.[103] In a 2016 study, using a Markov model to simulate the clinical course of chronic ulcerative colitis, analysis of stool DNA with CE for patients with positive results was noted to be more cost-effective than CE or WLE alone.[104] Cytobiology assays appear promising for detecting precancerous and cancerous lesions.[105] Likewise, molecular testing for alterations in mucosal antigens, cellular DNA content (e.g., p53 and APC gene mutations), and aneuploidy appear promising, although the predictive value of these changes is presently unclear.[105,106]

MANAGEMENT OF DYSPLASIA

The ability to accurately identify dysplasia and determine its potential resectability is key to further management.[43] CE and other image enhancing techniques have enhanced dysplasia detection and lesion delineation as described earlier. The SCENIC consensus recommends that lesion morphology be described as polypoid (pedunculated or sessile) or nonpolypoid (slightly elevated, flat, or depressed) and lesion borders classified as distinct or indistinct.[6,43,47] The presence of any overlying ulceration or features of submucosal invasion (such as depression or failure to lift with submucosal injection) may be indicative of underlying malignancy.[65]

A lesion detected at endoscopy should be identified as being within or outside an area of known colitis. Lesions in segments outside an area of known colitis should be treated as sporadic adenomas with standard post-polypectomy surveillance recommendations.[3,31,49,107] Lesions in an area of known colitis should be assessed for endoscopic resectability and completely resected, if possible, by an experienced endoscopist regardless of underlying colitis or grade of dysplasia. Inflammation, friability, and scarring can make such resection technically more difficult, in which case tattooing and photo documentation should be considered to aid subsequent surveillance or resection.[6,31,43] Colonic mucosa adjacent to the raised lesion should also be biopsied to evaluate for dysplasia. If complete resection is achieved, with dysplasia-free margins and no invisible dysplasia elsewhere in the colon, surveillance colonoscopy may be recommended rather than colectomy.[31,43] Societal recommendations with respect to surveillance after recommendations vary. Thus, ECCO recommends surveillance with CE at 3 months and then at least annually, whereas US Multi-Society guidelines suggest a close surveillance (< 12 months) for larger sessile lesions removed in piecemeal fashion or via endoscopic mucosal resection or endoscopic submucosal dissection, with longer surveillance intervals if the initial repeat colonoscopy result is negative.[31,49] Long-term follow-up studies of endoscopically resectable polypoid lesions are reassuring, demonstrating a low risk of developing dysplasia or carcinoma at follow-up,[108–112] with a 2014 meta-analysis also demonstrating a low risk of IBD-CRC following resection of polypoid dysplasia.[113] Patients diagnosed with dysplasia are themselves more likely to refuse or delay colectomy and prefer surveillance colonoscopy[43] and willing to accept an immediate colectomy only when the risk of synchronous CRC rises to above 73%.[58]

The management of nonpolypoid dysplastic lesions is more challenging. Two studies have demonstrated high cure rates after complete resection of circumscribed lateral spreading lesions and lesions with HGD.[114,115]

The SCENIC consensus supports surveillance colonoscopy after complete removal of endoscopically resectable nonpolypoid dysplastic lesions.[43] This recommendation is conditional, recognizing the higher CRC risk and greater endoscopic difficulty with resectability conferred by nonpolypoid lesions. Other guidelines recommend colectomy for nonpolypoid dysplastic lesions, considering such lesions generally not amenable to endoscopic resection.[3,7]

The management of endoscopically invisible dysplasia detected by random biopsies alone has also evolved considerably. Invisible dysplasia was defined by SCENIC as dysplasia identified on random (nontargeted) biopsies of colon mucosa without a visible lesion.[43] Data from St. Mark's Hospital using SD WLE indicates that 20% of patients with flat LGD detected by random biopsies had CRC at the time of immediate colectomy.[20] Ullman et al (2003) found synchronous advanced lesions, including flat HGD or CRC in 23% of patients undergoing colectomy for flat LGD detected on random biopsies using SD colonoscopes.[116] A systematic review of 20 studies and 477 patients with invisible LGD noted that 22% of patients with invisible LGD who had colectomy had CRC.[117] This rate of progression has been challenged by other studies.[118–120] Lim et al (2003) noted a 3% initial and 10% subsequent rate of progression from LGD to CRC in a ten-year period.[120] Extrapolation from data from previous studies should factor in recent recognition that most dysplasia is in fact visible, as well as evolution in endoscopic technology, which suggests that random biopsies showing invisible dysplasia in previous studies may have been taken from previously unrecognizable lesions, now visualized with modern endoscopic techniques.[12,43]

Studies from 2015 of CE or HD WLE have reported a 10% incidence of invisible dysplasia.[43] Until further evidence and our understanding of the natural history of dysplasia evolves and influences our practice through translation into more robust recommendations from GI Societies, the current consensus is as is outlined hereafter. The 2010 AGA guideline recommends colectomy for multifocal flat LGD.[3] The BSG also considers colectomy the best option for LGD but suggests CE if there is uncertainty with the diagnosis and regular surveillance for patients who decline colectomy.[10] The SCENIC consensus supports confirmation of dysplasia by a second GI pathologist and referral to an endoscopist with expertise in IBD surveillance and CE with HD to better inform subsequent decisions regarding surveillance versus colectomy.[43] If a visible dysplastic lesion is identified in the same region of the colon as the invisible dysplasia and the lesion can be resected endoscopically, it is suggested that such patients may remain in a surveillance program. If dysplasia is not found, individualized discussions involving the risks and benefits of surveillance versus colectomy are suggested.[43] Colectomy is the treatment of choice when HGD is confirmed by a second GI pathologist, or incompletely resected raised dysplasia is discovered.[3,10,43] In a review of 10 prospective surveillance trials from 1992, including 1225 patients, the prevalence of synchronous CRC in patients with flat HGD was 42%.[121] In the St. Mark's study of 600 patients in a surveillance program over 40 years, 45.5% of patients with flat nontargeted HGD detected on random biopsies using SD colonoscopes who underwent immediate colectomy had evidence of CRC in the colectomy specimen. Of those who deferred colectomy and continued surveillance, 25% later developed CRC.[20] The high rate of synchronous carcinomas,

TABLE 39.1 Society Guidelines for Detected Dysplasia

	Visible Dysplastic Lesion, Endoscopically Resectable With Negative Biopsies From Adjacent Mucosa	Visible Dysplastic Lesion, Endoscopically Unresectable, or Biopsies From Adjacent Mucosa With Dysplasia	Invisible High-Grade Dysplasia Detected by Random Biopsies	Invisible Low-Grade Dysplasia Detected by Random Biopsies
ECCO,[31] 2013	Surveillance at 3 months and then yearly, regardless of degree of dysplasia	Colectomy	Confirm by expert GI pathologist Rule out visible lesion with repeat chromoendoscopy surveillance Colectomy if confirmed	Confirm by expert GI pathologist Rule out visible lesion with chromoendoscopy surveillance Consider colectomy vs. intensified surveillance with random biopsies
CCA,[4] 2011	Surveillance	Colectomy	Confirm by expert GI pathologist Colectomy	Confirm by expert GI pathologist Multifocal: colectomy vs. intensified surveillance at 3–6 mo with chromoendoscopy, then annually Unifocal: consider surgery vs. surveillance at 6 mo then annually
BSG,[10] 2010	Surveillance	Colectomy	Not specifically mentioned	Confirm by expert GI pathologist Consider colectomy vs. intensified surveillance
ACG,[5] 2010	Surveillance	Colectomy	Confirm by expert GI pathologist Colectomy	Confirm by expert GI pathologist Colectomy vs. intensified surveillance
AGA,[3] 2010	Adenoma-like DALM; surveillance (6 mo)	Non-adenoma-like DALM; colectomy	Confirm by expert GI pathologist Colectomy	Confirm by expert GI pathologist Colectomy vs. intensified surveillance
ASGE,[6] 2015	Endoscopic surveillance at 1–6 and 12 months with biopsies of resection site	Repeat colonoscopy to check if endoscopically resectable. If unresectable, biopsy and tattoo. If dysplasia or cancer confirmed-proctocolectomy is recommended.	Confirm by expert GI pathologist and if confirmed recommend colectomy	Confirm by expert GI pathologist Repeat colonoscopy with surface chromoendoscopy by experienced colonoscopist. Obtain random biopsies in addition to targeted biopsies of lesions seen. Endoscopically invisible multifocal LGD recommend colectomy. For unifocal, flat, endoscopically invisible LGD decision should be individualized to offer colectomy vs. surveillance at 6 mo then annually.
CCFA,[3] 2005				Confirm by expert GI pathologist Multifocal or repetitive: colectomy Unifocal: colectomy; if patient opts for surveillance, then < 6-mo intervals recommended

ACG, American College of Gastroenterology; *AGA*, American Gastroenterological Society; *ASGE*, American Society for Gastrointestinal Endoscopy; *BSG*, British Society for Gastroenterology; *CCA*, Cancer Council of Australia; *CCFA*, Crohn's and Colitis Foundation of American; *DALM*, dysplasia-associated lesion or mass; *ECCO*, European Crohn's and Colitis Organization; *GI*, gastrointestinal; *LGD*, low-grade dysplasia.

when flat nontargeted HGD is found, is an indication for colectomy.[3] An endoscopically unresectable lesion or a lesion with dysplasia in the adjacent mucosa is an indication for colectomy.[6,31,43,65]

It is difficult to distinguish regeneration and repair from dysplasia in the presence of chronic active inflammation, frequently resulting in a pathologic finding that is "indefinite for dysplasia." Less is known about its significance in assessing CRC risk. In a study of 56 patients with biopsies indefinite for dysplasia, a 9% 5-year progression rate to HGD or CRC was observed.[116] Inflammation is possibly the only modifiable risk factor for CRC in IBD with a positive association between the degree of microscopic inflammation and advanced neoplasia.[8,9,39,40] Consequently, aggressive treatment of the underlying inflammation followed by endoscopic reevaluation, preferably with CE, is therefore recommended.[6,72] Furthermore, because the progression to CRC in patients with dysplasia is higher than without dysplasia, a further surveillance examination is advisable within 3 to 6 months.[3] A summary of societal guidelines for the management of dysplasia detected at endoscopic surveillance is shown in Table 39.1. The updated 2015 algorithm suggested by the ASGE for endoscopically visible lesions is shown in Fig. 39.8.

CONCLUSION

Colorectal cancer is a serious and potentially life-threatening complication of long-standing and extensive UC and colonic Crohn's disease. Of the myriad risk factors associated with the development of CRC in IBD, colitis-related dysplasia appears to confer the greatest risk. All patients with IBD should undergo

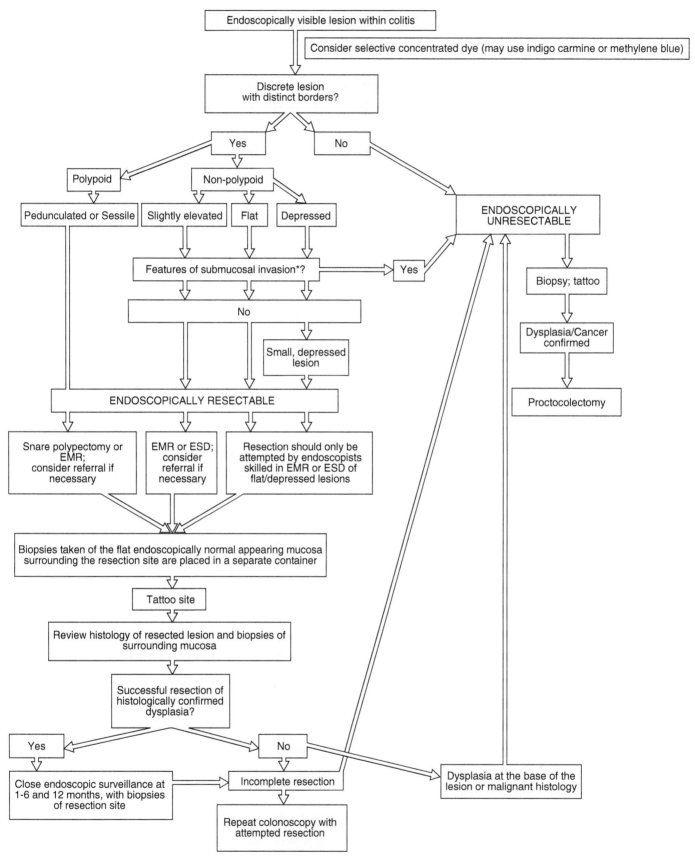

FIG 39.8 Recommended management of lesion detected during endoscopic surveillance. *Features of submucosal invasion include: depressions, failure to lift with attempted submucosal injection, or presence of overlying ulceration. *EMR*, endoscopic mucosal resection; *ESD*, endoscopic submucosal dissection. (From ASGE Standards of Practice Committee, Shergill AK, Lightdale JR, et al: The role of endoscopy in inflammatory bowel disease. *Gastrointest Endosc* 81[5]:1101–1121. e1–13, 2015.)

an initial surveillance colonoscopy 8 years after disease onset to assess the extent of colonic involvement, stratify risk of dysplasia, and determine surveillance interval. The goal of endoscopic surveillance is to reduce mortality and morbidity of CRC by either detecting and resecting dysplasia or detecting CRC at an earlier and potentially curable stage.

Understanding that most dysplasia is visible at colonoscopy, coupled with advances in optical technology, allowing for greater endoscopic resolution of dysplasia, has led to a paradigm shift in our approach to surveillance and management of dysplasia, with the bulk of evidence favoring CE or HD WLE at the very least for dysplasia detection. Adoption of CE as the gold standard of surveillance has been met with by skepticism, from conflicting data, operational barriers, and the need to understand the true impact of increasingly higher dysplasia detection on overall CRC mortality. The bulk of evidence, however, backed by recent consensus opinion, favors CE as a surveillance technique where appropriate expertise is available. Valid debate amongst experts notwithstanding, implementation of a risk stratification protocol that includes CE would be an effective approach, allowing earlier detection of dysplasia and colorectal neoplasia, determination of surveillance intervals with appropriate allocation of resources, and limiting morbidity from CRC, and indeed colonoscopy itself. Further prospective data are needed to define the true and long-term impact of dysplasia detection with modern techniques relating to IBD-CRC detection and survival. Meanwhile, the development of newer optical techniques and noninvasive methods for dysplasia detection has exciting implications for further research. The prospect of further intellectual effort invested in innovating and improving skills with established dysplasia detection techniques being rewarded through meaningful outcomes for our patients is now realistic.

KEY REFERENCES

3. Farraye FA, Odze RD, Eaden J, Itzkowitz SH: AGA technical review on the diagnosis and management of colorectal neoplasia in inflammatory bowel disease, *Gastroenterology* 138(2):746–774, 774 e1–e4, quiz e12–e13, 2010.

5. Kornbluth A, Sachar DB, Practice Parameters Committee of the American College of G: Ulcerative colitis practice guidelines in adults: American College Of Gastroenterology, Practice Parameters Committee, *Am J Gastroenterol* 105(3):501–523, quiz 524, 2010.

6. American Society for Gastrointestinal Endoscopy Standards of Practice Committee, Shergill AK, Lightdale JR, et al: The role of endoscopy in inflammatory bowel disease, *Gastrointest Endosc* 81(5):1101–1121 e1–e13, 2015.

7. Van Assche G, Dignass A, Bokemeyer B, et al: Second European evidence-based consensus on the diagnosis and management of ulcerative colitis part 3: special situations, *J Crohns Colitis* 7(1):1–33, 2013.

10. Cairns SR, Scholefield JH, Steele RJ, et al: Guidelines for colorectal cancer screening and surveillance in moderate and high risk groups (update from 2002), *Gut* 59(5):666–689, 2010.

12. Rutter MD, Saunders BP, Wilkinson KH, et al: Most dysplasia in ulcerative colitis is visible at colonoscopy, *Gastrointest Endosc* 60(3):334–339, 2004.

19. Jess T, Simonsen J, Jorgensen KT, et al: Decreasing risk of colorectal cancer in patients with inflammatory bowel disease over 30 years, *Gastroenterology* 143(2):375–381 e1, quiz e13–e14, 2012.

20. Choi CH, Rutter MD, Askari A, et al: Forty-year analysis of colonoscopic surveillance program for neoplasia in ulcerative colitis: an updated overview, *Am J Gastroenterol* 110(7):1022–1034, 2015.

21. Lutgens MW, van Oijen MG, van der Heijden GJ, et al: Declining risk of colorectal cancer in inflammatory bowel disease: an updated meta-analysis of population-based cohort studies, *Inflamm Bowel Dis* 19(4):789–799, 2013.

31. Annese V, Daperno M, Rutter MD, et al: European evidence based consensus for endoscopy in inflammatory bowel disease, *J Crohns Colitis* 7(12):982–1018, 2013.

34. Soetikno RM, Lin OS, Heidenreich PA, et al: Increased risk of colorectal neoplasia in patients with primary sclerosing cholangitis and ulcerative colitis: a meta-analysis, *Gastrointest Endosc* 56(1):48–54, 2001.

39. Rubin DT, Huo D, Kinnucan JA, et al: Inflammation is an independent risk factor for colonic neoplasia in patients with ulcerative colitis: a case-control study, *Clin Gastroenterol Hepatol* 11(12):1601–1608 e1–e4, 2013.

41. Rutter MD, Saunders BP, Wilkinson KH, et al: Cancer surveillance in longstanding ulcerative colitis: endoscopic appearances help predict cancer risk, *Gut* 53(12):1813–1816, 2004.

43. Laine L, Kaltenbach T, Barkun A, et al: SCENIC international consensus statement on surveillance and management of dysplasia in inflammatory bowel disease, *Gastroenterology* 148(3):639–651 e28, 2015.

44. Higgins PD: Miles to go on the SCENIC route: should chromoendoscopy become the standard of care in IBD surveillance?, *Am J Gastroenterol* 110(7):1035–1037, 2015.

47. Kaminski MF, Hassan C, Bisschops R, et al: Advanced imaging for detection and differentiation of colorectal neoplasia: European Society of Gastrointestinal Endoscopy (ESGE) Guideline, *Endoscopy* 46(5): 435–449, 2014.

54. Ananthakrishnan AN, Cagan A, Cai T, et al: Colonoscopy is associated with a reduced risk for colon cancer and mortality in patients with inflammatory bowel diseases, *Clin Gastroenterol Hepatol* 13(2):322–329 e1, 2015.

60. Rutter MD, Saunders BP, Schofield G, et al: Pancolonic indigo carmine dye spraying for the detection of dysplasia in ulcerative colitis, *Gut* 53(2):256–260, 2004.

64. Subramanian V, Mannath J, Ragunath K, Hawkey CJ: Meta-analysis: the diagnostic yield of chromoendoscopy for detecting dysplasia in patients with colonic inflammatory bowel disease, *Aliment Pharmacol Ther* 33(3):304–312, 2011.

65. Soetikno R, Subramanian V, Kaltenbach T, et al: The detection of nonpolypoid (flat and depressed) colorectal neoplasms in patients with inflammatory bowel disease, *Gastroenterology* 144(7):1349–1352, 52 e1–e6, 2013.

68. Marion JF, Sands BE: The SCENIC consensus statement on surveillance and management of dysplasia in inflammatory bowel disease: praise and words of caution, *Gastroenterology* 148(3):462–467, 2015.

74. Marion JF, Waye JD, Israel Y, et al: Chromoendoscopy is more effective than standard colonoscopy in detecting dysplasia during long-term surveillance of patients with colitis, *Clin Gastroenterol Hepatol* 14(5): 713–719, 2016.

75. Gasia MF, Ghosh S, Panaccione R, et al: Targeted biopsies identify larger proportions of patients with colonic neoplasia undergoing high-definition colonoscopy, dye chromoendoscopy, or electronic virtual chromoendoscopy, *Clin Gastroenterol Hepatol* 14(5):704–712 e4, 2016.

78. Mooiweer E, van der Meulen-de Jong AE, Ponsioen CY, et al: Chromoendoscopy for surveillance in inflammatory bowel disease does not increase neoplasia detection compared with conventional colonoscopy with random biopsies: results from a large retrospective study, *Am J Gastroenterol* 110(7):1014–1021, 2015.

81. Soetikno R, Sanduleanu S, Kaltenbach T: An atlas of the nonpolypoid colorectal neoplasms in inflammatory bowel disease, *Gastrointest Endosc Clin N Am* 24(3):483–520, 2014.

A complete reference list can be found online at ExpertConsult .com

40

Colonic Strictures

Andrew P. Copland and Andrew Y. Wang

INTRODUCTION

Colonic strictures are encountered with relative frequency in gastroenterology and colorectal surgery practices. The causes of these strictures are quite varied but the most common etiologies in adults include malignancy, diverticular disease,[1] ischemic injury,[2] inflammatory bowel disease (Crohn's disease),[1] surgical anastomoses, and radiation injury.[1] Less commonly, they can be seen in association with nonsteroidal antiinflammatory drug (NSAID)-induced injury,[3] pancreatitis,[4] endometriosis,[5] and as a complication of infections such as amebiasis.[6] A number of technical advances have made endoscopic management of these strictures possible. Endoscopic balloon dilation has been utilized since the 1980s,[7–9] whereas endoscopic placement of self-expanding metal stents (SEMS) has become increasingly utilized since the early 1990s.[10] Prior to any diagnostic or therapeutic endoscopy, patients with suspected colonic stricture or obstruction must be assessed with a careful physical examination and noninvasive radiographic imaging to exclude a surgical abdomen and the presence of luminal perforation.

INITIAL EVALUATION

Understanding the underlying etiology of a colonic stricture is critical to managing it appropriately. The diagnostic and therapeutic approach varies widely depending on whether a stricture is related to benign disease versus a malignancy. Inflammatory, ischemic, or anastomotic colon strictures can often be managed with endoscopic balloon dilation, but a malignant colonic stricture typically will not respond to conventional dilation therapy and will require either placement of a SEMS or surgical alternatives, such as diversion or resection.

In addition to identifying the etiology of a colonic stricture, it is also critical to define the location and morphology of the stricture. Fluoroscopic imaging (typically a barium enema or Gastrografin [Bracco Diagnostics Inc., Monroe Township, NJ] enema if a leak is suspected; Fig. 40.1A) or cross-sectional imaging (typically computed tomography scan [CT scan] with intravenous contrast in addition to oral or rectal contrast; see Fig. 40.1B) are important in confirming and delineating a colonic stricture. These radiographic imaging modalities are important to determine the number and location of colonic strictures, the degree and length of stricturing, and whether a perforation has already occurred. Additionally, cross-sectional imaging (typically a CT scan) enables assessment of the surrounding soft tissue, lymph nodes, and more distant organs, which can be critical in cases of mass lesions, as well as in inflammatory bowel disease, which can be further complicated by fistulas or abscesses.[11] Diagnostic endoscopy is also important in determining the etiology of a stricture as it can enable sampling for pathological diagnosis.

TECHNICAL CONSIDERATIONS FOR BALLOON DILATION

Dilating balloons are commercially available from various manufacturers. Balloon lengths range from 5.5 to 8 cm, and the dilating widths range from 6 to 20 mm, with various atmospheres of pressure being required to achieve a different balloon size depending on the balloon and manufacturer. Dilating balloon catheters come in gastroscope and colonoscope/enteroscope lengths and they can be purchased either with or without the ability to accommodate a guidewire. Most diagnostic gastroscopes (with a 2.8-mm accessory channel), and both pediatric and adult colonoscopes will accommodate these "through-the-scope" (TTS) catheters.

The commercially available dilating balloons can appear somewhat opaque when dilated in an insufflated lumen (particularly if they are filled with contrast for visualization under fluoroscopy). Replacing the air/CO_2 interface with water while pulling the dilated balloon snugly against the endoscope lens makes the balloon more transparent, allowing some visualization of the stricture lumen during dilation (Fig. 40.2, Video 40.1). When the lumen proximal to the stricture is endoscopically visible, fluoroscopy is not required. However, when visualization

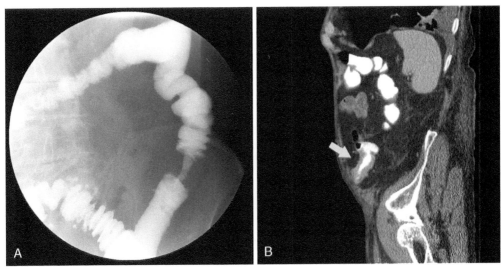

FIG 40.1 An "apple-core" lesion, which is pathognomonic for colonic adenocarcinoma, was found on **A,** a barium enema and **B,** on sagittal-views on a computed tomography (CT) scan. This left-sided colon stricture measured approximately 3 cm in length and would be ideal for stenting (as palliation or to assist in a single-stage surgical resection), as the proximal and distal colonic segments are straight and as this is a single stricture that is relatively short.

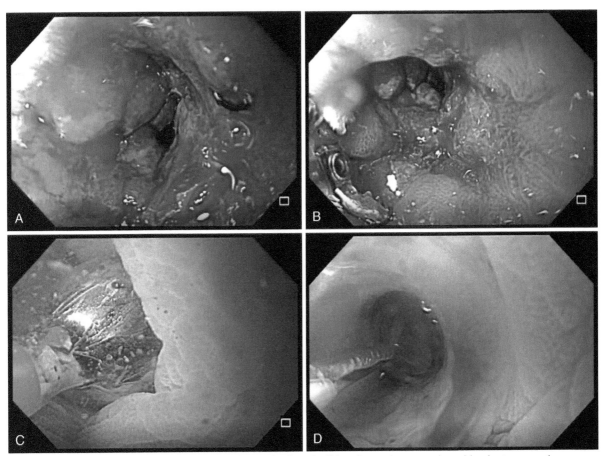

FIG 40.2 A patient with a history of colonic diverticulitis who underwent sigmoid colectomy and colostomy with subsequent takedown of the colostomy. **A,** She developed a tight stricture at the left-sided colorectal anastomosis that was erythematous and edematous. **B,** The stricture was approximately 3 mm in width (compared to opened biopsy forceps). **C,** A long 0.035-inch guidewire was passed across the stricture and a through-the-scope dilating balloon was used to dilate the stricture to 11 mm. **D,** Water was infused and the balloon was pulled close to the scope lens enabling visualization of the lumen of the stricture during dilation.

is poor due to tight, long, or angulated strictures, fluoroscopic guidance facilitates passage of a guidewire and then the dilating balloon catheter. Fluoroscopy is also valuable as contrast can be injected after dilation to ensure that contrast remains intraluminal and that there is no extravasation of contrast to suggest a bowel perforation.

For strictures that are tight, long (> 4 cm), or otherwise complex, a "ball-tipped" catheter can be used to inject contrast, navigate the stricture (given its atraumatic tip), and pass a guidewire. Additionally, dilation of strictures with significant inflammation, evidence of fistula, or an associated abscess should be avoided. Whereas most endoscopists likely have experience with TTS balloon dilation, there are no well-studied standard protocols for how to perform balloon dilation. In general, communication between the endoscopist and the assistant who is inflating the dilating balloon is critical, particularly as resistance to expansion of the balloon allows real-time assessment of the adequacy and risk of the dilation. Once a balloon size is reached that results in significant resistance to moving the balloon, most endoscopists adhere to the "rule of 3s," whereby dilation to three additional sizes provides treatment effect but also limits the risk of perforation (e.g., sequential dilation from 8 to 9 mm and then to 10 mm, etc.).[12]

Examination of a stricture can be done through the balloon or by deflation of the balloon in between sequential dilations. Evidence of a significant mucosal rent, or particularly of visible muscle fibers, should be a signal to cease further dilation. For a tight stricture, repeated dilations could be done in 2 to 4 weeks, with a reasonable eventual goal luminal diameter of 15 to 20 mm. If a stricture fails to respond or remain patent over two to three serial dilations, an alternative approach, such as surgical resection, should be strongly considered.

TECHNICAL CONSIDERATIONS FOR USE OF SEMS

Colonic SEMS have received United States Federal Drug Administration (FDA) 510(k) premarketing clearance "for palliative treatment of [colonic obstruction or] colonic strictures caused by malignant neoplasms, and to relieve large bowel obstruction prior to colectomy in patients with malignant strictures" (FDA 510(k): K113510, K061877). Furthermore, all commercially-available SEMS in the United States are uncovered, due to the high rate of migration associated with covered SEMS.[13] A comprehensive treatise on the use of colonic SEMS can be found in the American Society for Gastrointestinal Endoscopy Technical Review on "Role of self-expandable stents for patients with colon cancer."[13]

In general, uncovered SEMS in the United States come in discrete sizes that fall between 5.7 and 12 cm in length and with available body widths of 20, 22, and 25 mm (with variably flanged ends that are wider than the width of the stent body). Most commercially available uncovered SEMS in the United States are constrained on a 10-Fr catheter that can fit through the accessory channel of an adult colonoscope or through a therapeutic gastroscope, which allows for the stent to be placed using both endoscopic and fluoroscopic visualization.

In certain clinical situations, covered esophageal stents have also been used in an off-label manner to treat colonic strictures, particularly in cases of benign disease. Most covered esophageal stents come on a stiff introducer (ranging from 16-Fr to 24-Fr in size) that must be passed over a guidewire and cannot be passed through the scope channel or through severely angulated

areas (Video 40.2). These covered esophageal stents are constrained on shorter catheters, which usually limits their use to left-sided colonic strictures. There is one commercially available covered esophageal stent in the United States made by Taewoong Medical (Niti-S Esophageal TTS, Gyeonggi-do, South Korea) that comes on a 10.5-Fr flexible constraining catheter that can be deployed through the channel of a therapeutic gastroscope, which might enable successful covered metal stenting of difficult to reach or angulated colonic strictures (Video 40.3). We use covered esophageal stents to treat refractory or recurrent nonmalignant colonic strictures as an alternative to surgery; they may also be considered in patients with colonic obstruction with an uncertain diagnosis of malignancy.

We recommend using fluoroscopy whenever possible when attempting colonic stenting to help define the stricture and to adjunctively guide stent placement using the endoscope.[11] For left-sided colonic strictures, a therapeutic gastroscope is often the instrument of choice, but for right-sided strictures, a colonoscope may be required. Once the stricture has been reached, a long guidewire with a floppy tip (typically 0.035-inch guidewire for added stiffness) is passed across the stricture. We then suggest passage of a retrieval balloon of appropriate length across the stricture, which is then inflated to a large diameter (12–15 mm) and pulled back to define the proximal border of the stricture. An external marker (unbent paper clip affixed to the body) or an internal marker (endoclip or submucosal injection of a small amount of contrast) can then be placed to pinpoint the stricture for stenting. Deployment of TTS uncovered or covered metal stents follow similar principles and involve an assistant deploying the stent while the endoscopist pulls back on the restraining catheter until the stent is released.

MANAGEMENT OF BENIGN COLONIC STRICTURES

The published literature on the management of benign colonic strictures is largely focused on the inflammatory bowel disease population; in particular, on patients with Crohn's disease who will typically form strictures around the ileocecal valve and at surgical anastomoses (Fig. 40.3). The available data on management of strictures from other etiologies, such as diverticular disease, colonic ischemia, and radiation injury, are limited, and recommendations in the management of colonic strictures in these populations is largely extrapolated from patients with Crohn's disease or based on expert opinion.

The goal of endoscopic therapy for benign colonic strictures, in particular for stenotic surgical anastomoses, is to avoid the morbidity associated with surgical interventions in favor of less invasive therapy, sometimes coupled with medical therapy of any underlying disease. Endoscopic balloon dilation is the most often utilized tool. The technical success for strictures of the colon, including anastomotic strictures, is in excess of 86%.[14–18] In a retrospective study by Singh et al (2005),[16] a high technical success rate of 96.5% was reported following 29 dilations of 20 colon strictures with a long-term success rate of 76.5%. Similarly, Foster et al (2008)[17] reported a retrospective series of 24 patients with small and large bowel strictures who underwent a total of 71 dilations on 29 strictures. In this series, 92% of patients experienced symptomatic improvement.

However, long-term results are more tempered and suggest that nonmalignant colonic strictures often require subsequent interventions, including redilation and sometimes surgery. One large retrospective series spanning 22 years of experience found

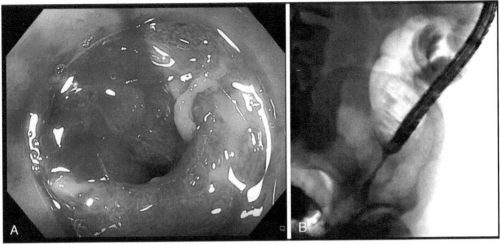

FIG 40.3 A 22-year-old man with long-standing ileal Crohn's disease presented with intermittent small bowel obstruction. **A,** Colonoscopy found an erythematous, ulcerated, stricture that was 3 to 4 mm in diameter. **B,** Injection of contrast via the colonoscope demonstrated a 5-cm-long, high-grade stricture consistent with fibrostenotic Crohn's disease that developed despite the patient having been on biologic therapy. Endoscopic balloon dilation to 10 mm resulted in temporary improvement in obstructive symptoms, but operative resection was eventually required for definitive management of this long fibrotic stricture.

that patients treated with balloon dilation required surgery in 13%, 26%, and 38% of cases at 1-, 3-, and 5-year follow-up, respectively.[18] Van Assche et al (2010)[19] described a retrospective series of 139 patients who underwent endoscopic dilation for short (< 5 cm) strictures and found that, whereas technical success rates were high (97%), 46% of patients required repeat dilation and 24% required a subsequent surgery over a median follow-up of 5.9 years. Another study in 2015 retrospectively reviewed a large series of 185 patients who underwent 462 endoscopic dilations over a mean follow-up of 3.9 years. They found that 36% of these patients required surgery.[20] The same group also demonstrated that patients with Crohn's who underwent surgery after dilation were more likely to require a stoma in their operative management (odds ratio [OR] 3.33, confidence interval [CI]: 1.14–9.78) and more likely to have a postoperative surgical site infection (OR 3.16, CI: 1.01–9.84). In aggregate, these data suggest that approximately 60% to 75% of patients with benign colonic strictures who undergo endoscopic dilation could avoid surgical intervention over a 5-year period.

It is important to know that balloon dilation for benign strictures, particularly in patients with Crohn's disease, is not without risk. Procedural complications can occur in approximately 5% of cases, with perforation occurring in 1.4% to 2.5% of cases and significant bleeding occurring in approximately 1% of cases.[18,19] Reassuringly, when compared to surgery, the rate of adverse events from endoscopic dilation in patients with Crohn's strictures is comparable to that associated with a planned surgical intervention.[21]

There are few validated clinical predictors for response to successful dilation of benign strictures. One important consideration is the complexity of the stricture. Patients with complex anastomoses or multiple strictures are less likely to have good treatment effect compared to those with a short, focal stricture in a straight colonic segment. A systematic review by Hassan et al (2007)[14] noted that the rate of long-term success was significantly higher for strictures less than 4 cm in length (OR

4.01). In the context of Crohn's disease, it is preferable to avoid dilation of an inflamed stricture given the transmural nature of Crohn's disease and the increased risk of perforation. In addition to conferring a higher risk of adverse events, the presence of ulcers within a stricture has also been noted to be a poor prognostic factor for dilation success, as has smoking.[15]

The available data on endoscopic therapy for other benign strictures, such those resulting from ischemic injury, diverticular disease, and radiation injury are limited. However, in general, we would recommend starting with graded endoscopic balloon dilation for treatment of nonmalignant colonic strictures prior to considering other alternatives.

One adjunctive therapy aimed at enhancing the effect of endoscopic dilation of benign strictures is steroid injection. East et al (2015)[22] demonstrated in a pilot study that, among 13 patients who underwent dilation, steroid injection was surprisingly associated with reduction in time to redilation. Conversely, a double-blind, randomized control trial of 29 pediatric patients with Crohn's strictures evaluated the use of intralesional steroid injection (triamcinolone 40 mg diluted in 5 mL of normal saline, which was injected deeply into the mucosa in 4 quadrants every 2 cm within the stricture) following balloon dilation (to a goal of 18 mm). These investigators demonstrated a statistically increased amount of time free from redilation ($p = 0.04$) and free of surgery in the steroid-treatment arm.[23]

SEMS should not be the first-line choice for management of benign colonic strictures, particularly as there are no FDA-approved covered colonic SEMS, and as uncovered colonic SEMS are typically not removable. However, for nonmalignant colonic strictures that are refractory or recurrent despite repeated attempts at endoscopic dilation, off-label use of fully covered SEMS is a consideration (see Videos 40.2 and 40.3). Caruso et al (2015)[24] reported on the use of fully covered SEMS for refractory anastomotic colorectal strictures and reported a 100% rate of technical and early clinical success in 16 patients with a median follow-up of 21 months. Prolonged clinical success was achieved in 9/16

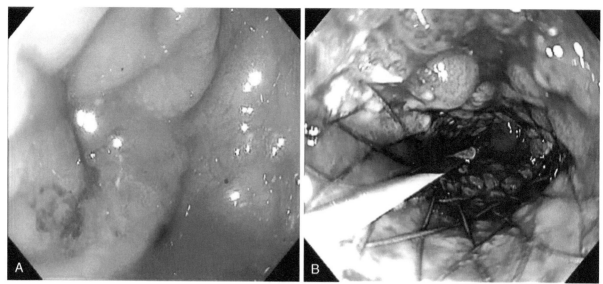

FIG 40.4 A patient with metastatic colon cancer presented with symptoms of obstruction. **A,** The colonic lumen was edematous and found to be completely obstructed. An uncovered self-expanding metal stent was deployed with immediate improvement in the luminal diameter. **B,** After stent deployment the obstructing tumor is more visible thorough the lattices of the stent. Please also refer to Video 40.4.

(56%) cases. There were no reported major complications, including perforation or bleeding. Stent migration occurred in 19% of cases, and larger median stent diameter was significantly associated with a more successful clinical outcome (26 mm vs. 20 mm, $p = 0.006$). Small et al (2008)[1] reported on a series of 23 patients with benign, obstructive, left colon strictures from 1999 to 2006 who had placement of uncovered or partially covered SEMS as a bridge to surgery. These investigators reported a high technical success rate of 95% in patients who had predominantly diverticular/inflammatory (16/23 patients) strictures. Major complications occurred in 38% of patients and included stent migration (n = 2), reobstruction (n = 4), and perforation (n = 2). Of the 19 patients who went on to have colectomy, 8 (42%) did not need a stoma after stenting.

Lastly, endosurgical techniques using a sphincterotome or a needle-knife to perform stricturoplasty have been described, which involves making careful radial incisions along the circumference of the stricture.[25–28] Whereas there is evidence that this may be a viable approach in select cases, such procedures should only be performed by interventional endoscopists with considerable experience and expertise and in settings with the appropriate radiological and surgical backup.

MANAGEMENT OF MALIGNANT COLONIC STRICTURES

The majority of malignant colonic strictures are caused by primary colorectal adenocarcinoma with the predominant lesion being found in the sigmoid or left colon.[29] Balloon dilation is not a useful therapeutic approach in the context of malignant colon strictures and management has focused on the appropriate use of SEMS and surgical intervention. SEMS can be used to treat patients with colonic strictures to (1) serve as palliation of obstructive symptoms in nonoperative candidates or (2) relieve acute obstruction as a bridge to surgery.

Palliative Stenting

SEMS are an important consideration for palliation among patients with incurable or inoperable malignant bowel obstruction (Fig. 40.4, Video 40.4). This approach can reduce rates of permanent ostomies, surgical morbidity, and length of hospital stays in this difficult-to-treat patient population.[30–32] In a retrospective series from 2011, Lee et al[33] noted a comparable success rate with palliative surgeries (100%) versus palliative SEMS placement (95.8%, $p = 0.12$). The SEMS group also had fewer early complications than the surgery group (15.5% vs. 32.9%, $p = 0.015$). The median duration of patency was shorter in the SEMS group (137 days) compared to the palliative surgery group (268 days, $p < 0.001$). However, after patients with SEMS occlusion were restented (required in 18 of the 30 patients), this extended the median patency duration to 229 days, resulting in comparable patency in both groups. Rates of major complications were not statistically different between the two groups (SEMS: 18.3% vs. surgery: 8.2%; $p = 0.074$). A randomized control study conducted in Australia enrolled 52 patients with a malignant, incurable, large-bowel obstruction (majority of patients from colorectal cancer) who were randomly assigned to surgical decompression or stent insertion. In this study of patients with advanced cancers and limited life expectancy (median survival of 5.2 months in the SEMS group and 5.5 months in the surgery group), stent use was found to be associated with several advantages including a quicker return to diet, decreased stoma rates, reduced postprocedural stay, and some quality-of-life benefits.[34]

As with any interventional procedure, a candid discussion regarding the risks and benefits of palliative SEMS placement is paramount and should be undertaken in the context of a patient's outlook, goals of care, and expected subsequent oncologic therapy. Some studies have suggested that, whereas short-term results, such as relief of obstruction, are quite good, there may be an increased rate of severe SEMS-related complication in the longer-term. A study by Fernandez-Esparrach et al[35] in 2010 described a prospective series of 47 patients in whom colorectal stenting for malignant obstruction was attempted. Eighty percent of these patients underwent stenting for palliative intent and median follow-up was 130 days. In this study, the long-term clinical failure rate was reported at 51% with major complications including stent migration (22%), recurrent obstruction (17%), perforation (7%), and tenesmus (5%). Stent migration was noted to occur between 6 and 56 days, whereas reobstruction was noted to occur between 67 and 332 days. One perforation in this study occurred 34 days after stent insertion, whereas the other two perforations occurred within the first 4 days following SEMS placement.

In our practice, we offer palliative uncovered SEMS placement to any patient with incurable cancer that presents with malignant colorectal obstruction without signs or evidence of perforation. Whereas a discussion between the endoscopist and the patient (which would ideally include the patient's family or support system) is of paramount importance given the potential risks associated with SEMS placement, we also make every effort to discuss the clinical situation with our surgical and medical oncology colleagues. Determination of which patients are deemed incurable and would benefit from palliative stenting might best be decided by multidisciplinary consultation or after discussion in a dedicated tumor board meeting. For example, given current treatment paradigms, oligometastatic colon cancer with isolated metastasis to the lung or liver may be amenable to chemotherapy and resection with some possibility of long-term remission or cure,[36] which might make palliative stenting (even for a temporary period) undesirable given the risks associated with the procedure. As current chemotherapy regimens can enable patients with advanced or metastatic colorectal cancer to have an expected survival often measured in years,[37] it is very important to inform patients regarding the potential long-term adverse events associated with colonic stenting, including bleeding and perforation. Finally, whereas we and others recommend SEMS placement as the preferred treatment for palliation of malignant colonic obstruction, prophylactic colonic stent placement is not recommended in patients who are not yet symptomatic.[11]

Stenting as a Bridge to Surgery

Patients with severe colonic obstruction are unable to undergo bowel preparation, which obviates a one-stage resection for left-sided colon cancers. However, preoperative colon preparation is not necessary in patients with obstruction from right-sided colon cancers. In addition to concerns regarding adequate colon preparation prior to surgery, patients who have colonic obstruction often have electrolyte disturbances and malnutrition due to progressive obstruction. As such, emergency surgery in the setting of a colon-cancer-related obstruction is associated with approximately 12% operative mortality, in addition to a significant rate of postsurgical complications.[38] Furthermore, postoperative mortality has also been shown to be higher in patients undergoing emergency surgery for colon cancer as compared to elective surgery.[32,38]

Retrospective and nonrandomized data have characterized SEMS placement as a useful way to avoid emergency surgery and bridge patients with colonic obstruction to an elective operation, thus reducing the need for a stoma and a staged-surgical procedure. Several pooled analyses have demonstrated rates of clinical success in excess of 91%.[30–32] In a prospective study of 182 patients from two large multinational registries by

Jimenez-Perez et al (2011),[39] the use of SEMS as a bridge to surgery in patients with malignant left-sided colorectal obstructions had a procedural success rate of 98% and a clinical success rate of 94%. The overall rate of adverse events was 7.8% (with 3% perforations, 1.2% stent migrations, 0.6% bleeding, and persistent colonic obstruction in 1.8%) and involved one death due to perforation. One hundred and fifty patients were able to undergo elective operations, and from this group only 9 patients (6%) required the creation of a stoma. Other series have suggested that SEMS placement as a bridge to surgery may decrease complication rates and shorten hospital stays.[32] Brehant et al (2009)[40] showed, in a series of 30 patients with mainly left-sided malignant colorectal obstructions treated with SEMS, that a diverting colostomy was able to be avoided in 77% of patients.

However, prospective randomized controlled trials (RCTs) have shown mixed outcomes regarding use of SEMS as a bridge to an elective or one-stage operation. In the first major RCT of SEMS as a bridge to elective surgery, Cheung et al (2009)[41] randomized 48 patients between 2002 and 2005 to either emergency open surgery or emergent SEMS placement with a subsequent one-stage laparoscopic procedure. The technical success rate was high at 83%, and the study noted no procedural complications associated with stenting. Furthermore, 67% of patients who underwent SEMS followed by laparoscopic surgery at a median of 10 days after stenting had a successful one-stage procedure, whereas only 38% of the patients who underwent emergency open surgery had a one-stage procedure. The SEMS group in this study had no permanent stomas. Other, larger studies have shown less encouraging results. Pirlet et al (2011)[42] published a French, multicenter, RCT that included 60 patients with malignant, left-sided, large bowel obstructions who were recruited between 2002 and 2006. Patients were randomized to either emergency surgery or SEMS placement with subsequent elective surgery. This study was ended early due to an increased rate of adverse events (two perforations during stenting procedures and an unexpectedly high rate of technical failures). This study demonstrated a low technical success rate of only 47% for SEMS placement and was not able to demonstrate a meaningful difference in their primary outcome of temporary or permanent stoma rates between treatment arms. Final analysis revealed no difference in secondary outcomes of mortality, morbidity, or length of hospital stay. In this trial, SEMS placement was attempted by radiologists in 13 patients and by gastroenterologists in 17 patients.

Another multicenter randomized trial by the Dutch Stent-In study group[43] enrolled 98 patients before it too was suspended after interim analysis showed no decisive clinical advantage of SEMS as a bridge to elective surgery versus emergency surgery for malignant bowel obstruction. Six of 47 patients in the SEMS arm experienced guidewire or SEMS-related perforation, and there was more postoperative anastomotic leakage in the SEMS arm (5/47 patients) compared to the emergency surgery arm (1/51 patients). Final analysis showed no difference between the treatment groups in 30-day mortality, overall mortality, and morbidity. Despite a goal of reducing need for stomas, over half of the patients in both groups required stomas during their clinical course. This was in part driven by an increased rate of anastomotic leak in the SEMS group requiring reoperation. This study from the Dutch Stent-In study group is also the only RCT to characterize quality-of-life outcomes for which there were no differences between the SEMS and surgery groups. In comparison to the French study,[42] SEMS were placed in this Dutch study only by experienced endoscopists who had placed more than 20 enteral stents, including at least ten colonic stents.[43]

Finally, a Cochrane analysis from 2011 examined five randomized trials comparing the use of SEMS versus emergency surgery in 207 patients with malignant colonic obstructions.[44] This pooled analysis again demonstrated a high rate of technical success for SEMS placement at 86%, and a rate of complications similar to that of emergency surgery. Successfully placed stents migrated out of place in only 2.1% of cases, and stent obstruction was relatively rare at 2.1% in the first 30 days. The overall 30-day mortality was similar among patients who underwent colonic stenting compared to those who had emergency surgery (2.3% for both groups); however, the total length of hospital stay was shorter in the colonic stenting group (11.5 days vs. 17.2 days).

Because of studies such as those presented, the European Society of Gastrointestinal Endoscopy (ESGE) Clinical Guideline on "Self-expandable metal stents for obstructing colonic and extracolonic cancer" recommends against use of colonic SEMS placement as a bridge to elective surgery.[11] However, it is our opinion that there is likely a select group of patients with malignant colonic obstruction who might benefit from SEMS placement as a bridge to either a more controlled elective operation or towards a single-stage procedure (for patients with left-sided obstruction). In particular, colorectal stenting as a bridge to surgery might offer a more favorable risk-benefit ratio in populations who require medical optimization prior to an operation, such as those with advanced age or complex medical comorbidities, including cardiopulmonary, renal, or metabolic disease.[11] The timing of subsequent elective surgery may also be an important variable in relieving obstructions in these subsets of patients. Prior studies have typically pursued elective surgery in fewer than 10 days after stent placement.[41-43] Given the lack of high-level evidence to support stenting (as a bridge to surgery) over emergency surgery for malignant colonic obstruction, the best outcomes are likely to be achieved if only those patients with favorable stricture location and morphology are offered preoperative stenting, and if these increased-risk procedures are performed by experienced endoscopists who also know when to abort a procedure if the odds of clinical success seem low once the stricture is endoscopically and fluoroscopically evaluated.

OTHER SEMS-RELATED ADVERSE EVENTS

The most serious SEMS-related adverse event is, of course, perforation, which can occur in the process of stenting (due to scope trauma or by guidewire or device passage) or after stent deployment. However, the most frequent SEMS-related adverse events include minor bleeding, abdominal pain, and stent migration.[32]

Whereas many studies have suggested that SEMS-related perforation occurs in less than 5% of cases, this complication does remain a prime concern among patients treated with SEMS.[30-32] A meta-analysis by Van Halsema et al[45] in 2014 pooled 4086 patients who underwent colorectal stent placement and demonstrated higher rates of perforation with a rate of 18.4% for benign strictures and a rate of 7.5% for malignant strictures. On subgroup analysis, patients who underwent dilation after stent placement had a significantly increased risk of perforation when compared to the nondilation group (20.4% vs. 0%, 95% CI: 6.5%–48.8%). This study also found that patients treated with a chemotherapy regimen containing the antiangiogenic

drug bevacizumab had an increased risk of perforation (12.5%, 95% CI: 6.4%–22.8%) as compared to patients who had no concomitant chemotherapy (9.0%, 95% CI: 7.2%–11.1%). Patients and referring physicians who request SEMS placement in the setting of large bowel obstruction from colorectal cancer should be aware of this issue, as some oncologists will not use bevacizumab in patients with SEMS for fear of a combined increased risk of hemorrhage and perforation. Furthermore, patients and referring surgical oncologists also need to be aware that a SEMS-related perforation in the setting of a resectable colorectal cancer might expose the peritoneum or retroperitoneum to cancer seeding, which may make a curable cancer incurable.

Stent migration is a relatively common event that can occur on average in 10% to 12% of cases.[30-32] Covered SEMS, which again are used in an off-label manner in the colon, are more prone to stent migration. Fortunately, SEMS migration can typically be managed endoscopically by removing the migrated stent with the goal of either placing a larger stent or a different type of stent that might be less prone to migration. Other alternatives to replacing a migrated SEMS include observation (particularly if the stricture has become more patent following stenting) or more definitive surgical intervention.

CONCLUSION

Colonic strictures present an interesting clinical and technical challenge to the gastrointestinal endoscopist. Endoscopic diagnosis and therapy can contribute meaningfully to the care of patients with benign and malignant strictures with a reasonable risk profile. Endoscopic dilation of benign strictures can help patients avoid the morbidity associated with operative resection. For patients with malignant strictures, endoscopic placement of SEMS can offer palliation of obstruction at the end of life or, in select patients, serve as a bridge to a safer, less morbid surgery. The role of the gastrointestinal endoscopist in the diagnosis and management of colonic strictures is sure to evolve as endoscopic techniques are refined and as new technologies and medical therapies are developed.

KEY REFERENCES

1. Small AJ, Young-Fadok TM, Baron TH: Expandable metal stent placement for benign colorectal obstruction: outcomes for 23 cases, *Surg Endosc* 22:454–462, 2008.
9. Whitworth PW, Richardson RL, Larson GM: Balloon dilatation of anastomotic strictures, *Arch Surg* 123:759–762, 1988.
11. van Hooft JE, van Halsema EE, Vanbiervliet G, et al: Self-expandable metal stents for obstructing colonic and extracolonic cancer: European Society of Gastrointestinal Endoscopy (ESGE) Clinical Guideline, *Endoscopy* 46:990–1053, 2014.
12. Shen B, Fazio VW, Remzi FH, et al: Endoscopic balloon dilation of ileal pouch strictures, *Am J Gastroenterol* 99:2340–2347, 2004.
13. Baron TH, Wong Kee Song LM, Repici A: Role of self-expandable stents for patients with colon cancer (with videos), *Gastrointest Endosc* 75:653–662, 2012.
14. Hassan C, Zullo A, De Francesco V, et al: Systematic review: endoscopic dilatation in Crohn's disease, *Aliment Pharmacol Ther* 26:1457–1464, 2007.
16. Singh VV, Draganov P, Valentine J: Efficacy and safety of endoscopic balloon dilation of symptomatic upper and lower gastrointestinal Crohn's disease strictures, *J Clin Gastroenterol* 39:284–290, 2005.
17. Foster EN, Quiros JA, Prindiville TP: Long-term follow-up of the endoscopic treatment of strictures in pediatric and adult patients with inflammatory bowel disease, *J Clin Gastroenterol* 42:880–885, 2008.

18. Gustavsson A, Magnuson A, Blomberg B, et al: Endoscopic dilation is an efficacious and safe treatment of intestinal strictures in Crohn's disease, *Aliment Pharmacol Ther* 36:151–158, 2012.

19. Van Assche G, Thienpont C, D'Hoore A, et al: Long-term outcome of endoscopic dilatation in patients with Crohn's disease is not affected by disease activity or medical therapy, *Gut* 59:320–324, 2010.

20. Lian L, Stocchi L, Shen B, et al: Prediction of need for surgery after endoscopic balloon dilation of ileocolic anastomotic stricture in patients with Crohn's disease, *Dis Colon Rectum* 58:423–430, 2015.

23. Di Nardo G, Oliva S, Passariello M, et al: Intralesional steroid injection after endoscopic balloon dilation in pediatric Crohn's disease with stricture: a prospective, randomized, double-blind, controlled trial, *Gastrointest Endosc* 72:1201–1208, 2010.

24. Caruso A, Conigliaro R, Manta R, et al: Fully covered self-expanding metal stents for refractory anastomotic colorectal strictures, *Surg Endosc* 29:1175–1178, 2015.

30. Sebastian S, Johnston S, Geoghegan T, et al: Pooled analysis of the efficacy and safety of self-expanding metal stenting in malignant colorectal obstruction, *Am J Gastroenterol* 99:2051–2057, 2004.

31. Khot UP, Lang AW, Murali K, et al: Systematic review of the efficacy and safety of colorectal stents, *Br J Surg* 89:1096–1102, 2002.

32. Watt AM, Faragher IG, Griffin TT, et al: Self-expanding metallic stents for relieving malignant colorectal obstruction: a systematic review, *Ann Surg* 246:24–30, 2007.

34. Young CJ, De-Loyde KJ, Young JM, et al: Improving quality of life for people with incurable large-bowel obstruction: randomized control trial of colonic stent insertion, *Dis Colon Rectum* 58:838–849, 2015.

35. Fernandez-Esparrach G, Bordas JM, Giraldez MD, et al: Severe complications limit long-term clinical success of self-expanding metal stents in patients with obstructive colorectal cancer, *Am J Gastroenterol* 105:1087–1093, 2010.

38. Biondo S, Marti-Rague J, Kreisler E, et al: A prospective study of outcomes of emergency and elective surgeries for complicated colonic cancer, *Am J Surg* 189:377–383, 2005.

39. Jimenez-Perez J, Casellas J, Garcia-Cano J, et al: Colonic stenting as a bridge to surgery in malignant large-bowel obstruction: a report from two large multinational registries, *Am J Gastroenterol* 106:2174–2180, 2011.

41. Cheung HY, Chung CC, Tsang WW, et al: Endolaparoscopic approach vs conventional open surgery in the treatment of obstructing left-sided colon cancer: a randomized controlled trial, *Arch Surg* 144:1127–1132, 2009.

42. Pirlet IA, Slim K, Kwiatkowski F, et al: Emergency preoperative stenting versus surgery for acute left-sided malignant colonic obstruction: a multicenter randomized controlled trial, *Surg Endosc* 25:1814–1821, 2011.

43. van Hooft JE, Bemelman WA, Oldenburg B, et al: Colonic stenting versus emergency surgery for acute left-sided malignant colonic obstruction: a multicentre randomised trial, *Lancet Oncol* 12:344–352, 2011.

44. Sagar J: Colorectal stents for the management of malignant colonic obstructions, *Cochrane Database Syst Rev* (11):CD007378, 2011.

45. van Halsema EE, van Hooft JE, Small AJ, et al: Perforation in colorectal stenting: a meta-analysis and a search for risk factors, *Gastrointest Endosc* 79:970–982 e7, quiz 83 e2, 83 e5, 2014.

A complete reference list can be found online at ExpertConsult .com

41

Infections of the Luminal Digestive Tract

C. Mel Wilcox and Christina Surawicz

INTRODUCTION

The diagnosis and management of luminal gastrointestinal (GI) tract infections has been an essential component of the practice of gastroenterology since the birth of the subspecialty. The emergence of endoscopy with mucosal biopsy as a safe and accurate diagnostic tool for patients with suspected infection has elevated the GI endoscopist to a key partner in the management team. The importance of the endoscopist may be best appreciated for patients who develop GI complications related to immune suppression, such as after organ transplantation, during chemotherapy, or with human immunodeficiency virus (HIV) infection. In these settings, infections are frequent, and the differential diagnosis and diagnostic approach to GI symptoms often differ from the normal host. This chapter provides an overview of GI infections from the endoscopist's perspective based on organ systems because the clinical presentation generally points to the site of gut involvement and dictates the diagnostic strategy. Several common themes are applicable to most GI infections:

1. The clinical presentation is dictated by the infecting pathogen.
2. The specific immunodeficiency state, its pathophysiology, and severity dictate the spectrum of complicating pathogens.
3. The severity and chronicity of infection for an immunosuppressed patient are dictated by the cause, duration, and type of immunodeficiency.
4. The endoscopic features of any GI infection are variable and overlapping, making definitive diagnosis by biopsy essential when other tests such as stool culture are negative. Biopsy of normal mucosa may be necessary in some situations.

EPIDEMIOLOGY

Immune Competent Patients

The frequency of luminal GI infections, spectrum of pathogens, severity of infection, and organ involvement are dictated by the combination of exposure, predilection (host factors), and organ-specific tropism of the infecting pathogen (Box 41.1). Most infections are transmitted by the fecal-oral route via contaminated food or water and are typically self-limited.[1] With the increase in international travel, geography plays an increasingly important role in the prevalence of some GI infections. Traveler's diarrhea, usually caused by enterotoxigenic *Escherichia coli*, is characteristically seen with travel to developing countries.[2] These travelers are at increased risk of other causes of diarrhea including invasive bacteria like *Campylobacter* and parasites like *E. histolytica*.

Pathogens are endemic in certain portions of the world and in specific regions within countries. For example, in the United States, histoplasmosis is endemic in the Midwest and Mississippi Valley. *Mycobacterium tuberculosis* (TB) is endemic in third world countries, and involvement of the GI tract is well recognized. Medications can also be an important risk factor. Antibiotics are the major risk factor for *C. difficile* infection (CDI). There is increasing evidence that acid suppressing medications increase the risk of most enteric infections, perhaps even CDI.[3]

Immune Suppressed Patients

For immunosuppressed patients, the incidence and severity of infection are often linked to the cause and degree of the immunodeficiency state. In addition, they are subject to opportunistic infections, defined as infection by a microorganism that does not typically cause disease. Patients undergoing solid organ

BOX 41.1   Factors Involved in the Prevalence and Type of Gastrointestinal Infections

Exposures	Geographic location
Immunodeficiency	Hospital setting
Transplant and type	Medication exposures
AIDS	
Cancer	

transplantation are at a heightened risk of infection early after transplantation because of profound medication-induced immunodeficiency.[4,5] It is also during this time that latent infections such as cytomegalovirus (CMV) and *Strongyloides* may become manifest. Over time, however, as drug-induced immunosuppression decreases as drugs are tapered, the incidence of infections decreases. Moreover, infections are more commonly observed after heart transplantation than liver transplantation because more potent and prolonged drug-induced immunosuppression is required to prevent cardiac rejection.

For patients infected with HIV, the incidence of GI infections increases markedly as immune function deteriorates, and the infection risk can be accurately stratified by the absolute CD4 lymphocyte count and HIV-1 RNA levels as higher HIV levels and lower CD4 lymphocyte counts correlate with the risk of opportunistic infections.[6–8]

Rarely, opportunistic infections have been observed in the apparently normal host, but in contrast to an immunodeficient patient, these infections are typically self-limited. Generally, the more severe the immunodeficiency state required for development of an opportunistic infection, the less likely the pathogen will be observed in the normal host. For example, until the advent of transplantation, CMV was a rare pathogen, and its identification in any patient suggests some type of immune dysfunction.[9,10] CMV is regarded as one of the most common opportunistic infections owing to the high prevalence of prior exposure to CMV, as reflected by seropositivity rates of more than 90% in developed countries,[11,12] and to the fact that CMV disease generally occurs from recrudescence of latent infection during periods of profound immunosuppression.

In summary, a careful history regarding potential exposure, cause and stage of immunodeficiency, if present, and specific epidemiologic factors germane to the clinical presentation will often help determine the potential causes of infection.

PATHOGENESIS

The pathogenic mechanisms of luminal GI infections include: (1) exposure to a pathogen, (2) reactivation of prior infection (recrudescence), (3) overgrowth of a commensal organism, and/or (4) local spread or dissemination. The specific organ involved with any infectious process, other than local spread, is dictated by the organ-specific tropism of the infecting pathogen. *Candida* and herpes simplex virus (HSV) almost exclusively infect squamous epithelium, whereas *Campylobacter jejuni* and *Shigella* species are colonic pathogens. Inherent to any discussion of pathogenesis is the issue of host-related factors. Numerous nonspecific and immune-based defense mechanisms both prevent and attenuate GI infections.[13] These defenses may be altered by disease, medications, organ dysfunction or organ absence (e.g.,

splenectomy), or as a part of the aging process. Saliva provides an effective physical barrier because of its physical properties. Moreover, immunoglobulins that are present in saliva and in intestinal secretions provide an important early line of defense. Gastric acid is a barrier to enteropathogens, and hypochlorhydria has been shown to be a risk factor for the development of cholera and other GI infections.[3,14] GI motility propels ingested pathogens through the gut and prevents stasis, which can lead to bacterial overgrowth. Inherent antibacterial proteins secreted by Paneth cells, termed *defensins,* seem to play a key role in the host response to bacterial infections of the gut.[15,16] The normal gut microbiota also plays a vital role in the prevention of infection such as CDI; its role in the prevention of other infections is unknown.

The mucosal immune system is composed of inflammatory cells, most notably T cells.[13,17] After exposure to a foreign antigen, these cells differentiate into helper or cytotoxic cells depending on whether the cells express the CD4 or CD8 receptor. The release of cytokines by these cells plays a crucial role in limiting infection but can also result in tissue damage. The critical role of the mucosal immune system in preventing and controlling infections is best shown by the array and severity of luminal GI infections that occur in AIDS, in which there is a progressive loss of CD4 lymphocytes from both the systemic circulation and the mucosal-based immune system.[18,19] Following HIV infection, there is a rapid, substantial and perhaps irreversible loss of mucosa associated lymphoid tissue based CD4 T-cells. Loss of these cells predisposes to small intestinal infections by opportunistic infections such as cryptosporidiosis and microsporidiosis. Likewise, lymphocyte dysfunction, either medication-induced or as part of an immunodeficiency state, predisposes to symptomatic primary infection or recrudescence (e.g., CMV).

In immune compromised patients, most viral GI infections considered here result from recrudescence of infection rather than recent exposure (primary infection). Normally, exposure to these infections occurs during childhood, and the systemic and mucosal-based immune systems keep these infections controlled. However, with immunodeficiency, disease may become overt. Conversely, *Candida* is a commensal organism of the oropharynx and esophagus and, although usually present in small numbers, overt *Candida* infection can be observed even in the normal host under certain conditions, such as antibiotic use; use of inhaled or ingested corticosteroids; antacid therapy or hypochlorhydria states; diabetes mellitus; alcoholism; malnutrition; old age; radiation therapy to the head, neck, and chest; and esophageal motility disturbances. Alterations in cellular immunity lead to Candidal colonization and superficial infection, whereas humoral immunity (granulocytes) prevents invasive disease and dissemination. Under conditions of absolute granulocytopenia or severely impaired granulocyte function, commensal bacteria, particularly gram-positive organisms, including *Streptococcus viridans,* Staphylococci, and other bacilli, may invade mucosa that has been damaged from gastric acid reflux disease, from radiation therapy, or from chemotherapy, leading to an active local infection and potential dissemination.[20]

GI infections may result secondarily from active disease in adjacent organs. Esophageal disease may be caused by contiguously infected mediastinal lymph nodes or pulmonary parenchymal infection[21] and by spread of infection via a draining fistula or obstructed lymphatics, resulting in tracheoesophageal fistula.[22] Widespread lymphohematogenous dissemination of opportunistic infections causes either diffuse or focal disease anywhere in the gut; this process is generally limited to only the most severely immunocompromised patients.[23,24]

Most intestinal infections result in tissue inflammation of varying degrees. Local upregulation of cytokines plays a central role in the local immune response to the pathogen but may also cause tissue injury. CMV esophagitis is associated with high mucosal concentrations of the proinflammatory cytokine tumor necrosis factor.[25] Toxin production, virulence factors, and the local microbiome will also determine the clinical expression and tissue damage caused by many GI infections, especially bacterial infections.[26,27]

Luminal digestive tract infections occur under specific epidemiologic conditions and in the appropriate host. The tissue-based immune system is crucial for preventing opportunistic infections; when this system is absent, infection with such pathogens may be chronic and potentially life-threatening. Exposure to the pathogen is important; however, concurrent predisposing factors that were elucidated previously, such as antibiotic or chemotherapy treatment, can play a pathogenic role in both the normal and the immunosuppressed host.

CLINICAL AND ENDOSCOPIC FEATURES

Numerous factors guide the approach to a patient with suspected GI infection. Given the breadth of potential etiologic pathogens, the diagnostic approach should be based on the character and chronicity of the symptoms, the organ system(s) involved, and the findings on physical examination.

Esophagus
Clinical Features
The most common cause of esophageal infection in both the normal host and the immunosuppressed patient is *Candida*, followed by the herpesviruses.[28] CMV occurs more commonly in patients with AIDS, whereas HSV is more often observed in the normal host and non–HIV-infected immunosuppressed patients.[29,30] Odynophagia is the characteristic symptom of esophageal infection, and infections resulting in esophageal ulceration almost uniformly cause odynophagia.[28–30] Although less common, dysphagia may be observed with esophageal infections, especially *Candida esophagitis*, or may represent esophageal obstruction or dysmotility from the infection or its sequelae (e.g., stricture). Odynophagia is almost uniformly present and is characteristically severe with CMV esophagitis. Chest pain, weight loss, and fever may be reported. The onset of symptoms is often more subacute than the acute presentation of HSV. A prior or coexistent diagnosis of CMV infection in other organs (e.g., retinitis or colitis) is frequent. Although rare in transplant patients, retinitis may be observed in approximately 15% of AIDS patients at the time of diagnosis of GI disease.[31] Bleeding is generally observed only when there is ulceration, and although generally mild, it can be severe if there is an associated coagulopathy. Pulmonary symptoms may predominate when there is fistula formation to the tracheobronchial tree or coexistent pulmonary involvement. Patients with AIDS often have multiple coexisting esophageal disorders, which further complicates management.[28,32]

Physical examination, particularly of the oropharynx, may be helpful in suggesting the diagnosis of esophageal infection. Approximately two-thirds of patients with AIDS and esophageal candidiasis have oral candidiasis (thrush).[33] In other immunocompromised patients, oropharyngeal candidiasis is also commonly associated with esophageal candidiasis.[28] Thrush may be absent, however, if antifungal therapy, such as nystatin, is currently administered. The presence of oropharyngeal candidiasis does not prove that *Candida* is the only cause of symptoms, and the absence of oropharyngeal candidiasis does not exclude *Candida esophagitis*. Patients with chronic mucocutaneous candidiasis may have fungal involvement of various mucous membranes, hair, nails, and skin and may have a history of adrenal or parathyroid dysfunction. Coexistent oropharyngeal ulceration is common in patients with HSV esophagitis but is infrequent in patients with CMV esophagitis or other systemic infections.[31,34]

After *Candida* species, herpesviruses are the most frequent infectious agents that cause esophagitis. After organ transplantation, HSV and CMV occur with equal frequency as causes of esophagitis,[28] whereas in patients with AIDS, HSV esophagitis is uncommon and far less frequent than CMV. In a study of 100 HIV-infected patients with esophageal ulcers, HSV was found in only nine (in four patients it was a copathogen with CMV).[30] HSV esophageal infection commonly manifests with the sudden onset of severe odynophagia, heartburn, or chest pain.[29,30] Autopsy studies suggest that esophageal symptoms may be absent. Herpes labialis (i.e., cold sores) and oropharyngeal ulcers may coexist, antedate, or develop during the esophageal infection, whereas skin infection is rare.[28] Numerous systemic manifestations, including low-grade fever or upper respiratory symptoms, may precede the onset of esophageal symptoms. In untreated immunocompetent persons, spontaneous resolution of HSV esophageal infection occurs within 2 weeks of the onset of symptoms. Rarely, bleeding is the initial presentation and may be observed in the absence of esophageal complaints.

The frequency of esophageal involvement with other pathogens is rare. Bacterial esophagitis has been observed in patients with severe neutropenia, usually patients with hematologic malignancies, but occasionally it is observed after bone marrow transplantation,[35] diabetic ketoacidosis,[36] steroid therapy, or in AIDS.[37,38] The presentation is similar to the presentation with other infectious agents.[39] Fungi other than *Candida* species and parasitic diseases have rarely been reported to involve the esophagus.[40–45]

The symptoms of esophageal TB depend on the degree and type of involvement.[22,46] Systemic symptoms of fever and weight loss are common. Pulmonary complaints often predominate because of a fistula to the trachea, bronchus, or pleural space. Dysphagia may be prominent with the formation of long strictures or traction diverticula resulting from the fibrotic response. Upper GI hemorrhage caused by esophageal ulcers or tuberculous arterioesophageal fistulas may rarely be the primary manifestation.[47] Other mycobacterial infections such as *Mycobacterium avium complex* (MAC) are rare.[48]

Barium radiography plays a minor role in the diagnosis of esophageal infection. In any patient, the presence of severe odynophagia limits the ability to drink barium, hampering the adequacy of the examination. Although specific barium esophagram findings may be more typical for certain disorders,[49] given the potential overlap, many of the findings are nonspecific, and endoscopy with biopsy is generally indicated. The wide spectrum of causes, coupled with the specific antimicrobial regimens that are required, necessitates a definitive diagnosis rather than empiric antimicrobial therapy except when Candida is highly expected. Nevertheless, a sinus tract or fistulous connection to the bronchial tree or mediastinum at the level of the hilum is highly suggestive of TB, although it may also be the result of malignancy. An esophageal neoplasm may be mimicked by an ulcerated

TABLE 41.1 Differential Diagnosis of Endoscopic Findings Based on Organ System and Pathogen

Finding	Esophagus	Stomach	Small Bowel	Colon
Plaque	*Candida* HSV	*Cryptococcus* MAC	MAC *Cryptococcus*	*Clostridium difficile* CMV
Inflammation*	HSV CMV	CMV *Cryptococcus* *Cryptosporidium*	*Cryptosporidium*	Bacteria CMV
Erosion or ulcer	Any infection	CMV TB Syphilis	CMV *Cryptosporidium* and *Cryptococcus*	Bacteria CMV *Histoplasma* Amebae *Strongyloides*
Stricture	CMV TB *Histoplasma* *Blastomyces*	*Cryptosporidium* TB	CMV TB	CMV TB
Mass	CMV TB	CMV	CMV	CMV *Histoplasma*

*Edema, subepithelial hemorrhage.
CMV, cytomegalovirus; *HSV*, herpes simplex virus; *MAC, Mycobacterium avium* complex; TB, *Mycobacterium tuberculosis.*

tuberculous granulomatous mass or CMV ulcer.[50,51] Chest radiography or computed tomography (CT) scan of the chest may support the diagnosis of TB, although a tissue diagnosis will be required.

Endoscopic Features

The characteristics of the esophageal lesions provide very important diagnostic clues. The location, size, and appearance of all endoscopic abnormalities should be documented because these features form the basis of the differential diagnosis and are useful for comparison on follow-up endoscopic examinations. The differential diagnosis of the lesion dictates how lesions should be sampled and what recommendations for diagnostic testing should be made on the biopsy or cytologic specimens (discussed later). Serologic testing plays no significant role in the diagnosis of acute infectious esophagitis. Endoscopic examination of the esophagus is the most sensitive and specific method for diagnosing esophageal candidiasis (Table 41.1).

The gross endoscopic appearance of *Candida esophagitis* is pathognomonic (Fig. 41.1) and may be graded according to published criteria.[52] A large, well-circumscribed ulceration should not be attributed to *Candida*. The endoscopic characteristics of HSV esophagitis reflect the pathologic changes. HSV esophagitis appears as discrete, usually small (< 1 cm), well-circumscribed, shallow ulcers; a diffuse erosive esophagitis; or, rarely, vesicles (Fig. 41.2).[28] Small, scattered lesions covered with exudate mimic esophageal candidiasis. Deep ulcers, as seen with CMV, are very rare. CMV esophagitis is characteristically associated with one or more ulcerations that can be quite striking in patients with AIDS. Nevertheless, as with other infections, variability has been reported with appearances ranging from multiple shallow ulcers, to solitary giant ulcers, to a diffuse superficial esophagitis (Fig. 41.3).[53] Although serologic testing is not helpful because of the high rate of prior exposure to CMV, the absence of CMV DNA or antigenemia in the blood would suggest an alternative diagnosis. Esophageal TB can manifest with a fistula to the tracheobronchial tree that is easily visualized endoscopically and rarely as an ulcer or mass lesion resembling a neoplasm. In normal hosts from

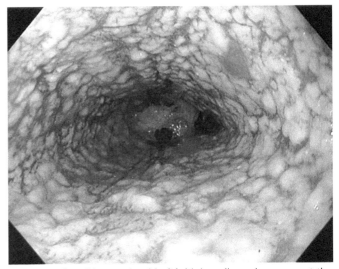

FIG 41.1 *Candida esophagitis.* Multiple yellow plaques coat the esophageal lumen. In several areas, the plaque has been removed, showing a normal-appearing underlying mucosa.

endemic areas in South America, *Trypanosoma cruzi* may involve the myenteric plexus of the esophagus, resulting in Chagas' disease and an appearance that is indistinguishable clinically, radiographically, manometrically, and endoscopically from idiopathic achalasia.[54] This diagnosis may be established by antibody testing. The endoscopic appearances of other rare infections have been described in case reports and resemble other infections.

Stomach
Clinical Features

Gastric infections are typically manifested by upper abdominal pain that is generally steady and may radiate to the back. Associated symptoms may include nausea with or without vomiting; vomiting may be prominent when mucosal infection is severe. Infrequently, nausea alone in the absence of abdominal pain may be observed. Fever and weight loss are variable. Diarrhea may be the prominent symptom if the infecting pathogen also involves the small bowel (e.g., *Cryptosporidium*). Bleeding, both occult and overt, is usually a marker of mucosal ulceration. However, because most gastric infections are superficial, severe bleeding is unusual unless there is an associated coagulopathy.

Worldwide, *Helicobacter pylori* is the most common gastric infection regardless of immune status. The prevalence of an infection has generally decreased in some parts of the world, particularly in the United States, although infection can approach 80% or more in selected populations.[55] The presence of *H. pylori* is also associated with hypochlorhydria (fasting gastric pH > 4) and the combination of *H. pylori* infection and HIV infection is more strongly associated with the prevalence of hypochlorhydria than either infection alone.[56,57] Because of the relative infrequency of gastric infections, understanding of the presentation and endoscopic findings of most of these infections is based on case reports or small series. With the exception of *H. pylori*, most infections of the stomach occur in the setting of an immunodeficiency state and include CMV; parasites and mycobacteria are uncommon.[58] In HIV-infected patients, there appears to be an inverse correlation between immune suppression as noted by CD4 lymphocyte count and the prevalence of active *H. pylori* infection.[57]

The primary symptom is dictated by the underlying cause. CMV gastric infection typically produces ulceration; abdominal pain with or without bleeding is the most frequent presentation. Mucosal infections that result in gastritis without ulceration, such as cryptosporidiosis, more commonly manifest with nausea without pain or may be asymptomatic. *H. pylori* infection of the stomach is generally considered an asymptomatic infection in most people regardless of immune status, but can be associated with dyspepsia and duodenal or gastric ulcer. Tuberculosis may cause antral narrowing with outlet obstruction, ulcer, or intramural abscess. Physical examination is generally unrevealing. Mild abdominal pain may be elicited on palpation of the epigastrium. Radiologic studies may suggest the presence of gastric infection. Although abnormalities can often be identified, the findings are typically nonspecific, and further investigation with endoscopy is often required. Barium findings of gastric infection may include fold thickening or ulceration, whereas the most common CT finding is wall thickening, usually diffuse, and focal lesions mimicking a mass lesion (Fig. 41.4). Neoplasms result in either focal or diffuse wall thickening depending upon etiology.

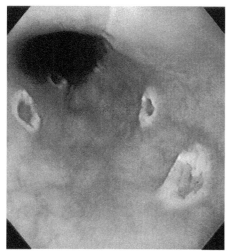

FIG 41.2 Herpes simplex virus esophagitis. There are multiple small ulcers, some of which have a "volcano" appearance typical for herpes simplex virus. The intervening mucosa is normal.

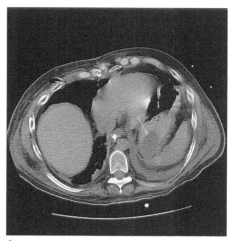

FIG 41.4 Gastric mucormycosis. Computed tomography (CT) scan shows a large hypodense area in the gastric wall *(arrow)*.

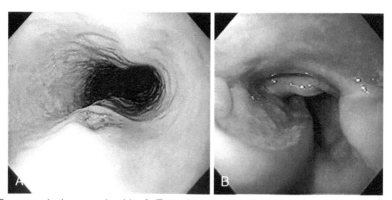

FIG 41.3 Cytomegalovirus esophagitis. **A,** Two ulcers in the mid-esophagus with normal surrounding mucosa. **B,** Large hemicircumferential ulcer in the mid-esophagus with heaped-up margins.

Endoscopic Features

Similar to all GI infections, the primary endoscopic abnormality is dictated by the infecting pathogen, and the severity of disease clinically and endoscopically depends on the presence and degree of immunodeficiency. *H. pylori* infection often results in no endoscopic findings or can be associated with a nodular (termed *chicken skin*) appearance due to the presence of lymphoid aggregates. *H. pylori* has also been associated with mucosa-associated lymphoid tumors which have a variable appearance, but typically ulcerated well circumscribed mass-like lesions or diffuse infiltration. CMV, the most common opportunistic gastric pathogen, generally manifests with a diffuse gastritis, characteristically with a hemorrhagic component (Fig. 41.5). Mucosal breaks are typical with focal or diffuse erosions or frank ulcerations (Fig. 41.6) that may be large, are usually well circumscribed, and may mimic a malignancy.[50] Ulcerations have also been described with other bacteria, fungi, and parasites.[59–62] The endoscopic features of gastric cryptosporidiosis and mycobacterial infection may appear as inflammation, polyps, or antral narrowing.[63–65]

In the normal host, gastric anisakiasis has been associated with ingestion of raw fish, and the *Anisakis* larvae may be visualized and removed at the time of endoscopy (Fig. 41.7).

Small Intestine
Clinical Features

The most common infections are viruses such as rotavirus and norovirus. The most common bacterial infection is enterotoxigenic *E. coli* (traveler's diarrhea), but epidemics of *Vibrio cholera* in endemic areas can have many affected patients with significant morbidity and mortality. Parasitic infections in the small bowel are mostly protozoa, with *Giardia lamblia* the most common, but include *Cryptosporidia, Cyclospora,* and *Cystoisospora.* The most common symptoms are diarrhea and abdominal pain. Diarrhea due to small intestinal pathogens is watery, and may be high volume when the organism impairs absorption or causes intestinal secretion like *Vibrio cholerae.* Diarrhea is not bloody as the organisms that infect the small bowel are generally not invasive or minimally so, with the exception of those bacteria that infect the ileo-colonic area, such as *Salmonella* and *Yersinia.* Associated symptoms include fever and crampy abdominal pain which is often periumbilical, and malaise. Dehydration and weight loss occur when the diarrhea is severe or chronic, and fat malabsorption may occur. Symptoms of fat malabsorption include greasy stools and symptoms of fat soluble vitamin deficiencies such as osteopenia/osteoporosis (vitamin D), night blindness (vitamin A), and easy bruisability (vitamin K). With these illnesses, physical exam is usually normal unless there is volume depletion. Diagnosis is usually made by stool culture when appropriate or ova and parasite (O&P) exam. With O&P exam, three specimens over several days will give the optimal yield. There is rarely a role for radiologic imaging or even endoscopy. If CT imaging is done, it may show small bowel wall thickening with invasive pathogens but this is a nonspecific finding and can be seen with inflammatory bowel disease (IBD) and other inflammatory diseases, or even small bowel malignancy like lymphoma.

The situation is different with immune suppressed individuals. With the exception of CMV, opportunistic small bowel infections are uncommon in transplant patients, but they are a hallmark

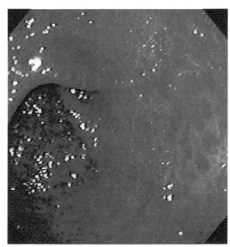

FIG 41.5 Cytomegalovirus gastritis. There is diffuse subepithelial hemorrhage, some of which is confluent in the gastric antrum. Several small erosions were also present in this patient.

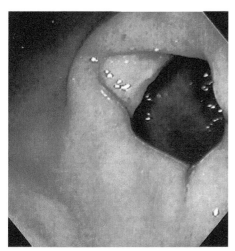

FIG 41.6 Pyloric channel ulcer resulting from cytomegalovirus. Hemicircumferential ulceration with a clean base in the pyloric channel. This lesion resembles a peptic ulcer.

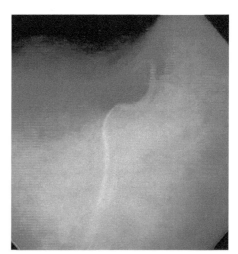

FIG 41.7 Anisakiasis. A well-circumscribed area of subepithelial hemorrhage is seen with a small worm emanating from the center of the hemorrhage. The worm was removed with biopsy forceps.

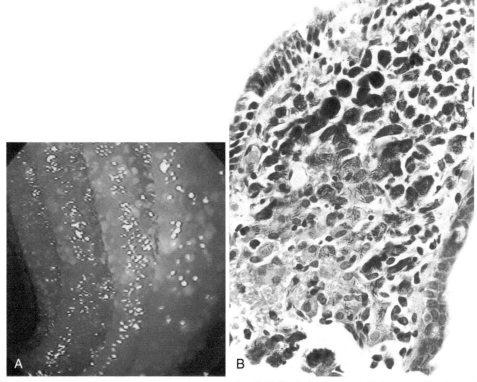

FIG 41.8 Duodenal *Mycobacterium avium* complex (MAC). **A,** Multiple well-circumscribed papular lesions typical for intestinal MAC. **B,** Acid-fast staining of mucosal biopsy specimens shows numerous mycobacteria filling the lamina propria.

of AIDS, where *Cryptosporidium* and *Microsporidia* are frequent pathogens, causing watery diarrhea, which is often severe. Less common is MAC, a pathogen principally restricted to patients with AIDS that is usually widely disseminated at the time of diagnosis[66] (Fig. 41.8). A localized proximal small bowel infection can occur with CMV, and distal ileitis has been reported with CMV, bacteria, mycobacteria, fungi, and parasites.[24,67–73]

Severe watery diarrhea causing dehydration is characteristic of intestinal cryptosporidiosis, whereas less severe diarrhea is observed with most other pathogens. Although crampy abdominal pain may be observed with any diarrheal disorder, more constant abdominal pain would be most typical for CMV enteritis and MAC.[66] Because CMV generally causes focal mucosal ulceration sparing the intervening mucosa, abdominal pain and overt bleeding can be observed in the absence of diarrhea. An acute abdomen can result from intestinal perforation due to CMV.[74]

Endoscopic Features

Most patients with small bowel infections will not need endoscopy, with the exception of those who are immune suppressed or those in whom a diagnosis of IBD is entertained. The endoscopic findings of small bowel infections vary from normal to widespread hemorrhage and ulceration. Focal erosions and ulcerations are typical for a viral infection with CMV, whereas minimal mucosal changes, if any, are common with parasitic diseases. Small bowel atrophy is associated with some of these infections and endoscopically mimics celiac sprue.[75] MAC infection has a characteristic appearance of small to confluent nodular lesions, often with a yellow color resembling Whipple's disease (see Fig. 41.8). Disseminated fungal infections can also manifest with small

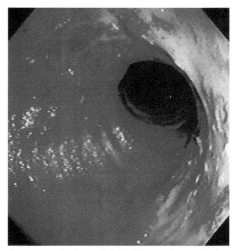

FIG 41.9 Cytomegalovirus ileitis. There is well-circumscribed hemicircumferential ulceration at the ileocolonic anastomosis after heart transplant and right hemicolectomy.

nodular lesions.[76] Rarely, obstructive symptoms may predominate if there is an obstructive process. Stricture and ulceration of the ileum is typical for TB and rare for CMV (Fig. 41.9); these are best characterized by radiographic rather than endoscopic examination.[77] Ileitis can also be observed with some bacterial infections, including *Yersinia* species and *Salmonella* species. The endoscopic and radiographic features of any severe ileitis may mimic Crohn's disease and underscores the importance of ileal examination with mucosal biopsy if colonoscopy is performed. Capsule endoscopy may also help characterize small bowel infections, although mucosal biopsy would require double-balloon enteroscopy.

Colon
Clinical Features

The most common symptoms are diarrhea and abdominal pain. In contrast to the large volume, watery diarrhea seen with small bowel pathogens, diarrhea due to colon pathogens tends to be smaller volume, can be bloody if the pathogen is invasive, and may be associated with tenesmus when there is rectal involvement, as is common with *Shigella* infection. Abdominal pain is most often left-sided unless there is right colon inflammation, as is seen with Shiga toxin *E. coli* (STEC). Other symptoms can include fever, malaise, and signs of volume depletion.[77] The physical examination is generally dictated by the infecting pathogen. With acute bacterial colitis, the patient may appear toxic and have significant abdominal tenderness suggesting an acute abdomen, and the pain may predominate over the diarrhea. The most common pathogens are, in order, *Campylobacter, Salmonella, Shigella* and STEC, both 0157:H7 strains and non-0157 strains. Rates of *C. difficile* infection have increased dramatically since the year 2000, and it should be considered in all acute diarrheal illnesses, not just as a consequence of antibiotics. CDI may complicate the illness in patients with IBD, especially in those with colonic involvement and with immune suppression. As the symptoms of IBD and CDI are the same, management can be challenging when CDI is adequately treated but the symptoms persist. Another challenge in management of IBD is the patient with ulcerative colitis (UC) who is severely ill and is refractory to immunomodulator therapy; in this situation, coinfection with CMV should be considered and endoscopy and biopsy can play an important role.[78] Less common bacterial pathogens are *Yersinia* (which has a predilection for the ileocolonic area and can thus mimic appendicitis and Crohn's disease), *Plesiomonas, Aeromonas* and noncholera *Vibrios*. Tuberculosis also has a predilection for the ileo colonic area.[79] The most common parasite to infect the colon is *E. histolytica*.

Evaluation. Recent American College of Gastroenterology guidelines (2016) on acute infectious diarrhea recommend microbiologic assessment of stool (i.e., stool culture for enteric pathogens) for immune competent individuals with dysentery (that is not travel related) and persistent diarrhea (14–30 days).[80] For travel-related diarrhea, empiric therapy was recommended, with the therapy depending on the severity of the illness. For diagnosis of CDI, most laboratories are moving to polymerase chain reaction (PCR) for detecting the toxin B gene in stools. Some still use enzyme-linked immunosorbent assay tests for toxin A and B.[81] Because PCR is very sensitive and 5% to 15% of individuals are carriers for *C. difficile*, only diarrheal stools should be tested. For diagnosis of TB, PCR of biopsy specimens is recommended as well as culture. For *Strongyloides*, serology and stool test combined give the best yield. In immune suppressed patients, the spectrum of pathogens includes the aforementioned, as well as opportunistic ones.

Depending on the clinical setting, CMV may be the most frequent opportunistic pathogen. Colonic CMV infection characteristically manifests as a chronic watery diarrhea; pain is often a prominent feature, and occult and overt bleeding may occur given the mucosal ulceration that is typical of colonic disease.[82]

When indicated, cross-sectional imaging may show colon wall thickening which is nonspecific. Cross-sectional imaging is reasonable to consider when there is severe abdominal pain and there are signs of toxicity. Colon wall thickening is nonspecific, and can be seen with invasive infections as well as ischemic colitis, and may be predominantly right-sided with STEC infection.[83]

Additional findings on CT may include small bowel thickening or lymphadenopathy.[84,85] Depending on the infectious cause, radiographic abnormalities may be either focal or diffuse. Barium enema examination, if indicated, should not be performed in patients with suspected colonic infection until all stool studies are collected.

Endoscopic Features

Colonoscopy can be very helpful in diagnosis of colitis, where the endoscopic findings can range from normal to severe pancolonic edema and ulceration. The colitis may be patchy, segmental, or diffuse. *Campylobacter, Shigella, Salmonella,* and *E. coli* 0157H7 infections may appear similar endoscopically with mucosal edema, subepithelial hemorrhage, erosions, and ulcers of varying size[86] (Figs. 41.10 and 41.11). Distal disease is typical for *Campylobacter* and *Shigella* infections, whereas infections with *Salmonella* and *Yersinia* preferentially involve the right colon and ileum.[86,87] *Salmonella typhi* infection results in lymphoid hyperplasia leading to ulceration at the site of Peyer's patches; this may explain its location in the bowel.[88]

In mild cases of *C. difficile* the colon may be normal, or there may be colitis in more severe cases. In the most severe form, pseudomembranous colitis, there are the classic appearing yellowish plaque-like membranes that are typically confluent (Fig. 41.12). However, pseudomembranes may be absent in patients with IBD and CDI, which may make the diagnosis more challenging. Subepithelial hemorrhage is characteristic of CMV infection, as is ulceration of variable distribution[89] (Fig. 41.13). An appearance of IBD, either UC or Crohn's disease, has been described with bacterial and CMV infections. Colorectal biopsy will usually make the distinction between infection and IBD[89] but cannot usually distinguish acute infection superimposed on chronic IBD. HSV can rarely involve the colon, but generally only the distal rectum and anus are involved, given the tropism of HSV for squamous mucosa. Amebic colitis may resemble a fulminant colitis or more commonly cause multiple ulcers that can be mistaken for Crohn's disease (Fig. 41.14).[90] The colonoscopic findings of cryptosporidiosis may be minimal edema or normal-appearing colon. TB may manifest with a mass lesion or serpiginous ulceration and nodularity.[91] Fungi have rarely been reported to involve the colon, with histoplasmosis noted to cause ulceration or mass lesions resembling carcinoma.[24,92] Helminthic and other pathogens of the colon have also been described (Fig. 41.15).[93,94]

PATHOLOGY

The pathologic features of GI infections depend on the infecting pathogen, and tissue tropism dictates the organ(s) of involvement.

Esophagus

The gross pathologic appearance of esophageal candidiasis ranges from a few white or yellow plaques on the mucosal surface to a dense, thick plaque coating the mucosa and encroaching on the esophageal lumen. Although potentially misinterpreted as "ulcer,"

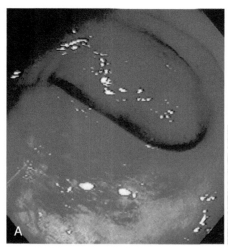
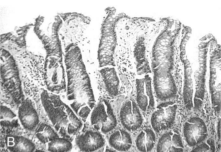

FIG 41.10 *Campylobacter* colitis. **A,** Focal area of subepithelial hemorrhage and erosion in the cecum. **B,** Hematoxylin and eosin staining of cecal biopsy specimens shows preserved architecture, mucosal edema, subepithelial hemorrhage, and acute inflammatory cells. These findings are typical for acute, self-limited colitis resulting from a bacterial infection.

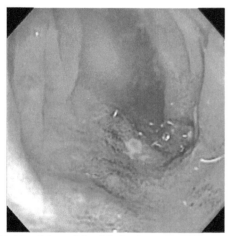

FIG 41.11 *Yersinia* colitis. Marked edema, hemorrhage and ulceration in the colon.

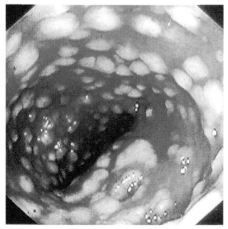

FIG 41.12 *Clostridium difficile* colitis. Typical yellow plaques are in the distal colon.

this plaque material is composed of desquamated squamous epithelial cells, admixed with fungal organisms, inflammatory cells, and bacteria.[51] True ulceration (granulation tissue) is rarely caused by *Candida* alone and has been documented most commonly in patients with profound granulocytopenia or when *Candida* is a coinfection with another cause of ulceration.[32] More deep-seated submucosal infections can occur with some fungi, and disseminated fungal infections can lead to ulceration.

Viral infection characteristically results in mucosal erosion and ulceration regardless of the site of infection. HSV infection is generally limited to squamous mucosa, where the earliest manifestation is a vesicle. As these vesicles enlarge and ulcerate, they coalesce to form larger, superficial lesions, which are typically focal, leaving the intervening mucosa normal. Microscopic examination of the squamous epithelial cells at the ulcer edge reveals multinucleation, ground-glass nuclei, and eosinophilic Cowdry's type A inclusion bodies that may take up half of the nuclear volume. With progression, these inclusion bodies may be surrounded by halos and may become more basophilic, filling, enlarging, and deforming the nucleus.

The histologic hallmark of CMV esophagitis is mucosal ulceration. Although variable, deep ulcers are very characteristic for disease in patients with AIDS, whereas in other immunocompromised patients, lesions tend to remain more superficial. Despite the depth of the lesions, perforation is rare. In contrast to HSV, the viral cytopathic effect of CMV is located in endothelial and mesenchymal cells in the granulation tissue of the ulcer base rather than in squamous cells. Inclusions are large (cytomegalic) and often have an eosinophilic appearance that may be located either in the nucleus or in the cytoplasm.[95] The inclusions can assume an atypical appearance, especially in patients with AIDS[96]; immunohistochemical stains play a valuable role in selected patients to confirm the presence of CMV, and they often highlight more infected cells than are appreciated by routine hematoxylin and eosin staining.[97] CMV may coexist with HSV or *Candida* or other pathogens in patients with AIDS. The gross pathologic appearance of bacterial esophagitis depends on the etiologic pathogen and ranges from diffuse, shallow ulcerations

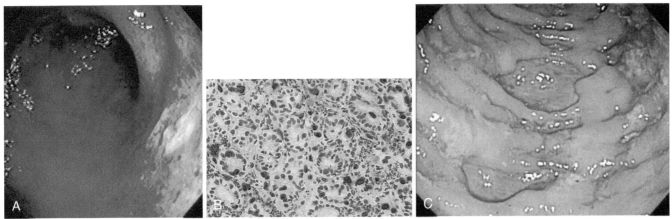

FIG 41.13 Cytomegalovirus (CMV) colitis. **A,** Diffuse subepithelial hemorrhage typical for CMV infection. **B,** Immunohistochemical stain for CMV antigens highlights the numerous infected cells. **C,** Large, well-circumscribed ulcerations potentially suggesting Crohn's disease.

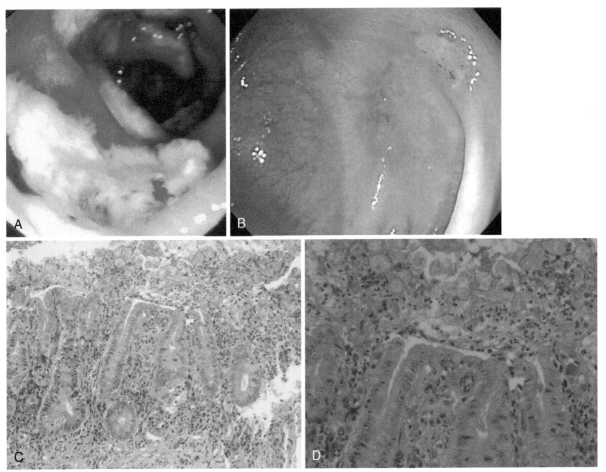

FIG 41.14 Amebic colitis. **A,** Patchy erosions and ulcer are suggestive of inflammatory bowel disease. **B,** Well circumscribed ulcer. **C,** Acute colitis with overlying inflammatory exudate which **D,** on close-up shows the typical amoebic structures. (**A,** Courtesy John L. Meisel, MD.)

to ulcers associated with erythema, plaques, pseudomembranes, nodules, or hemorrhage.

Microscopic examination reveals pseudomembranes and bacterial invasion that may be superficial and limited to squamous epithelium or may be invasive and transmural with infiltration of blood vessels (i.e., phlegmonous esophagitis). Esophageal

actinomycosis is characterized by ulceration and sinuses leading from abscess cavities with sulfur granules and filamentous gram-positive branching bacteria seen on tissue biopsy specimens.[40] In the one reported case, *B. henselae* esophagitis resulted in multiple nodules resulting from a lobulated proliferation of capillary vessels lined by plump endothelial cells.[38]

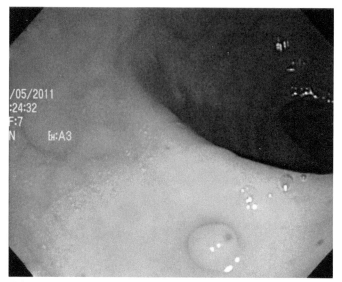

FIG 41.15 *Schistosomiasis* of the colon. Solitary nodule in the descending colon.

Stomach

Bacterial infection of the stomach is generally limited to *H. pylori* infection, which has the characteristic chronic active gastritis often with lymphoid aggregates.[98] These bacteria may be highlighted accurately by additional staining methods, including immunohistochemical stains. Phlegmonous gastritis, whose pathogenesis is not well understood, may involve gram-positive and gram-negative bacilli.[99]

Small Bowel

Small bowel biopsy is helpful to detect parasites like *Giardia*, *Cryptosporidia*, *Cystoisospora*, and *Strongyloides*. When the lamina propria is filled with macrophages, a periodic acid–Schiff (PAS) stain will be positive in MAC infection, differentiating it from Whipple's disease. Rare findings include lymphoma or other obscure infections. Biopsy of normal appearing mucosa is indicated when looking for infections or a cause of chronic diarrhea.

Colon

The main role of colorectal biopsy for the diagnosis of colitis is to distinguish infection from IBD. In the former, normal colonic architecture is usual, inflammation is predominantly acute, and there are no basal lymphoid aggregates. In UC, the inflammation is diffuse and limited to the mucosa. The hallmark is distorted crypt architecture, with acute and chronic inflammation and basal inflammation with plasma cells and lymphoid aggregates. In Crohn's disease, inflammation is typically patchy, but can be transmural. Granulomas can be found in up to 20% of biopsies, and can be found in biopsies of normal mucosa. However, granulomas are not specific for Crohn's disease, and can be seen with tuberculosis (they are typically more numerous though may not be caseating), *Yersinia*, schistosomiasis (surrounding the organism) and rarely in syphilis. Colorectal biopsy may also show ulcers with ameba on the surface (see Fig. 41.14).

Colorectal biopsy is also helpful to diagnose a CMV superinfection complicating IBD, especially UC, if typical inclusions are seen, but should be supplemented with another technique such

as culture or PCR testing. Biopsy cannot distinguish a bacterial infection superimposed on chronic IBD.

Special Stains

Although generally an excellent stain, hematoxylin and eosin staining may not identify all pathogens. Various pathogen-specific stains are available to aid in the identification of nearly all common GI infections (with the exception of non-herpesviruses). These stains highlight infecting pathogens and make identification easier. Immunohistochemical stains for viral antigens are very helpful when examining for herpesviruses.[100] Because a battery of stains is not routinely performed on all biopsy specimens, communication with the pathologist is essential to ensure appropriate pathologic evaluation.[101] Intestinal TB and MAC may be hard to distinguish because both may have granulomas present in ulcer tissue, with mycobacteria identifiable by mycobacterial staining. MAC, in contrast to TB, may not result in well-formed granulomas. Staining for MAC with PAS stain characteristically yields an abundance of organisms (see Fig. 41.8B), whereas tuberculous bacilli may be few in number, even in patients with AIDS.

DIFFERENTIAL DIAGNOSIS

Diagnostic considerations are determined by the clinical presentation, risk group, severity of immunodeficiency, and specific endoscopic findings. Although overlap is broad, some endoscopic abnormalities are typical for a specific pathogen and may be organ-specific (see Table 41.1). In the esophagus, CMV esophagitis and the idiopathic esophageal ulcer of AIDS are difficult to differentiate.[31,102] These two processes generally result in one or more large ulcers. Pill-induced esophagitis must be excluded by history because the pathologic findings of esophageal biopsy specimens are similar. Likewise, distal esophageal ulcer may suggest gastroesophageal reflux disease, and the histopathologic features cannot distinguish this from idiopathic esophageal ulcer. The clinical history is different, however, and the endoscopic appearance helps suggest gastroesophageal reflux. Small esophageal ulcers can be observed in the acute phase of HIV infection, which can mimic viral or pill-induced esophagitis.[103] Esophageal strictures can result from opportunistic infections.[104] The history coupled with mucosal biopsy helps differentiate infection from gastroesophageal reflux disease.

The appearance of the small bowel is similar in many infections and can be normal. The cause of bacterial colitis, with the exception of *C. difficile*, can rarely be differentiated by presentation or endoscopic appearance alone, although some infections may favor a proximal or distal location. In this setting, stool culture and blood culture may be diagnostic. In an immunosuppressed patient with chronic diarrhea, one or more colonic ulcers associated with subepithelial hemorrhage are highly suggestive for CMV, but this appearance can result from other disorders as well.[89,105]

Description of Techniques

No specific techniques are generally required for the endoscopic evaluation of GI infection. Based on the suspected cause clinically, endoscopically, and pathologically, additional stains may be required, necessitating close collaboration with the pathologist to diagnose these infections accurately. Because most infections can be diagnosed on tissue biopsy alone, multiple biopsy specimens of endoscopic abnormalities should be obtained to increase

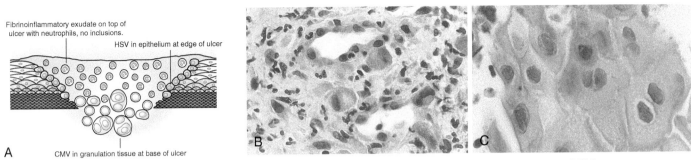

FIG 41.16 **A,** Location of viral cytopathic effect in mucosal ulceration. Herpes simplex virus (HSV) can be found at the ulcer edge, whereas cytomegalovirus (CMV) is located in granulation tissue deep in the ulcer bed. **B,** Large cells with intranuclear inclusions typical for CMV. **C,** Multinucleated cells in squamous tissue typical for HSV. (From Lazenby AJ: Gastroenterologist/pathologist partnership. *Tech Gastrointest Endosc* 4[2]:95–100, 2002.)

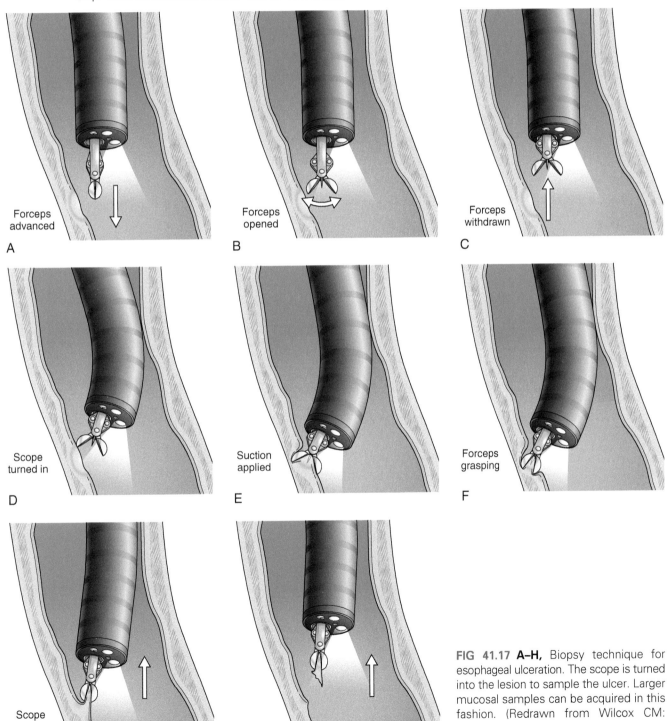

FIG 41.17 **A–H,** Biopsy technique for esophageal ulceration. The scope is turned into the lesion to sample the ulcer. Larger mucosal samples can be acquired in this fashion. (Redrawn from Wilcox CM: Approach to esophageal disease in AIDS: a primer for the endoscopist. *Tech Gastrointest Endosc* 4[2]:59–65, 2002.)

diagnostic yield. Even when the mucosa appears normal, multiple biopsy specimens should be taken when infection is suspected. During endoscopy, mucosal lesions can be brushed and submitted for cytologic evaluation, or biopsy specimens can be obtained for histologic diagnosis. Esophageal brushings with cytologic evaluation may be diagnostically helpful in certain diseases, such as those resulting from *Candida* and HSV, but are not helpful for diagnosis of CMV disease.

Viral culture of biopsy specimens may increase the diagnostic yield, although false-positive and false-negative results occur, and viral cultures are less sensitive than multiple biopsy specimens. Use of shell vial techniques improves the turnaround time for CMV culture to 48 hours. Bacterial culture of colonic biopsy specimens has been found in some series to enhance the diagnostic yield but is not typically done. Cytologic brushings and endoscopic mucosal biopsy specimens should be taken from the ulcer edge when HSV disease is suspected because the viral cytopathic effect is best identified in epithelial cells rather than in granulation tissue in the ulcer bed.[106] In contrast, a biopsy specimen of the ulcer base must be obtained when viral infection is suspected with CMV (Fig. 41.16). Multiple biopsy specimens (up to 10) may be required to establish the diagnosis in patients with AIDS and should be taken from the base of the ulcer.[107] Overall, mucosal biopsy for histologic diagnosis is the preferred method to distinguish the cause of ulcer.[108] Culture of an aliquot of stool obtained at colonoscopy and bacterial culture of mucosal biopsy specimens may increase the diagnostic yield.[109]

As mentioned previously, many histologic stains are available to identify pathogens. Immunohistochemical staining on biopsy samples using specific monoclonal antibodies to viruses such as HSV and CMV helps confirm the diagnosis when the viral cytopathic effect is difficult to appreciate. We generally rely on histology for the diagnosis of viral GI infections and use brushings and viral culture selectively. A technique first described for gastric biopsies, whereby the forceps are tilted into the lesion and the tissue is avulsed, is especially useful for taking samples from esophageal lesions (Fig. 41.17). Lastly, as noted previously, communication with the pathologist is essential so that appropriate attention can be drawn to specific pathogens and so that special stains can be performed.

KEY REFERENCES

1. DuPont HL: Persistent diarrhea. A clinical review, *JAMA* 315: 2712–2723, 2016.
2. Steffen R, Hill DR, DuPont HL: Traveler's diarrhea: a clinical review, *JAMA* 313:71–80, 2015.
3. Bavishi C, DuPont HL: Systematic review: the use of proton pump inhibitors and increased susceptibility to enteric infection, *Aliment Pharmacol Ther* 34:1269–1281, 2011.
4. Fishman JA: Infection in solid-organ transplant recipients, *N Engl J Med* 357:2601–2614, 2007.
7. Wilcox CM, Saag MS: Gastrointestinal complications of HIV infection: changing priorities in the HAART era, *Gut* 57:861–870, 2008.
8. Xiao J, Gao G, Li Y, et al: Spectrums of opportunistic infections and malignancies in HIV-infected patients in tertiary care hospital, China, *PLoS ONE* 8:e75915, 2013.
10. Lancini D, Faddy HM, Flower R, et al: Cytomegalovirus disease in immunocompetent adults, *Med J Aust* 201:578–580, 2014.
28. Baehr PH, McDonald GB: Esophageal infections: risk factors, presentation, diagnosis, and treatment, *Gastroenterology* 106:509–532, 1994.
29. Wang HW, Kuo CJ, Lin WR, et al: Clinical characteristics and manifestation of herpes esophagitis, *Medicine (Baltimore)* 95:e3187, 2016.
30. Wilcox CM, Schwartz DA, Clark WS: Esophageal ulceration in human immunodeficiency virus infection: causes, diagnosis, and management, *Ann Intern Med* 123:143–149, 1995.
32. Wilcox CM: Evaluation of a technique to evaluate the underlying mucosa in patients with AIDS and severe *Candida* esophagitis, *Gastrointest Endosc* 42:360–363, 1995.
49. Levine MS, Rubesin SE, Laufer I: Barium esophagography: a study for all seasons, *Clin Gastroenterol Hepatol* 6:11–25, 2008.
52. Wilcox CM, Schwartz DA: Endoscopic-pathologic correlates of *Candida* esophagitis in acquired immunodeficiency syndrome, *Dig Dis Sci* 41:1337–1345, 1996.
53. Wilcox CM, Straub RA, Schwartz DA: Prospective endoscopic characterization of cytomegalovirus esophagitis in patients with AIDS, *Gastrointest Endosc* 40:481–484, 1994.
55. Eusebi LH, Zagari RM, Bazzoli F: Epidemiology of Helicobacter pylori infection, *Helicobacter* 19:1–4, 2014.
56. Nevin DT, Morgan CJ, Graham DY, et al: *Helicobacter pylori* gastritis in HIV-infected patients: a review, *Helicobacter* 19:323–329, 2014.
77. Dickinson B, Surawicz CM: Infectious diarrhea: an overview, *Curr Gastroenterol Rep* 16:399, 2014.
78. Lee HS, Park SH, Kim SH, et al: Risk factors and clinical outcomes associated with cytomegalovirus colitis in patients with acute severe ulcerative colitis, *Inflamm Bowel Dis* 22:912–918, 2016.
80. Riddle MS, DuPont HL, Connor BA: ACG clinical guideline: diagnosis, treatment, and prevention of acute diarrheal infections in adults, *Am J Gastroenterol* 111:602–622, 2016.
82. Blanshard C, Francis N, Gazzard BG: Investigation of chronic diarrhoea in acquired immunodeficiency syndrome: a prospective study of 155 patients, *Gut* 39:824–832, 1996.
89. Wilcox CM, Chalasani N, Lazenby A, et al: Cytomegalovirus colitis in acquired immunodeficiency syndrome: a clinical and endoscopic study, *Gastrointest Endosc* 48:39–43, 1998.
100. Abreu MT, Harpaz N: Diagnosis of colitis: making the initial diagnosis, *Clin Gastroenterol Hepatol* 5:295–301, 2007.
102. Wilcox CM, Schwartz DA: Endoscopic characterization of idiopathic esophageal ulceration associated with human immunodeficiency virus infection, *J Clin Gastroenterol* 16:251–256, 1993.
107. Wilcox CM, Straub RF, Schwartz DA: A prospective evaluation of biopsy number for the diagnosis of viral esophagitis in patients with HIV infection and esophageal ulcer, *Gastrointest Endosc* 44:587–593, 1996.
108. Wilcox CM, Rodgers W, Lazenby A: Prospective comparison of brush cytology, viral culture, and histology for the diagnosis of ulcerative esophagitis in AIDS, *Clin Gastroenterol Hepatol* 2:564–567, 2004.

A complete reference list can be found online at ExpertConsult .com

42

Techniques in Enteral Access

Stephen A. McClave

INTRODUCTION

Using the gut to provide nutritional therapy by the enteral route plays a pivotal role in patient outcome in the critical care setting. Failure to use the gut for nutrition results in the gut becoming a proinflammatory organ, and results in increasing oxidative stress and higher risk of complications.[1] Early enteral access and utilization of the gut in contrast, promote or support the mass of gut-associated lymphoid tissue (GALT), as well as mucosal-associated lymphoid tissue (MALT) at distant sites like the liver, lungs, and kidney.[2] This process accounts for the "nonnutritional benefits" of nutritional therapy, contributing to an appropriate immune response, downregulation of inflammation, and a reduction in the rate of long-term complications. The sicker the patient, the greater the need to maintain gut integrity. Enteral nutrition support becomes a therapeutic tool or pharmacologic agent capable of changing outcome by reducing nosocomial infection, multiple organ failure, and hospital length of stay.[3,4] Recent literature confirms that aggressive enteral tube feeding decreases the rate of complications when compared to "standard therapy," which is defined as patients who are allowed to advance to either an oral diet on their own as tolerated or parenteral nutrition (PN).[5,6]

However, obtaining enteral access early in the course of a critically ill patient may be difficult. Patients in this setting are at the height of the hypermetabolic response, often requiring high doses of narcotic analgesia and sedation; thus, they are prone to ileus, gastroparesis, and high gastric residual volumes. Transporting these patients to the radiology suite for placement of feeding tubes is difficult, as they are unstable. Such transport leads to delays in getting tubes placed and has been shown to increase the risk of complications (such as aspiration, hemody-

namic instability, and new cardiac dysrhythmias).[7,8] Bedside techniques to place feeding tubes are essentially blinded, which carries some additive risk. Although bedside techniques may be sufficient in a large number of patients in the critical care setting, the success rate for bedside placement decreases as disease severity increases, and there is greater need to place the tube lower in the gastrointestinal (GI) tract.

In long-term acute care and in the chronic management of patients recovering from stroke and neurologic injury, percutaneous endoscopic techniques provide a more reliable semi-permanent enteral access, affording a number of options in a variety of patients. Insertion of a feeding tube distal to the stomach and into the small bowel has been shown to reduce the incidence of regurgitation and aspiration.[9,10] In a 2016 meta-analysis performed in preparation for societal guidelines, small bowel feeding was shown to significantly reduce the incidence of aspiration pneumonia when compared with gastric feeding.[11] In patients with severe gastroparesis, percutaneous endoscopic techniques may provide a gastrostomy tube for decompression and a direct jejunostomy tube for continued enteral feeding. In patients with recurrent flares of chronic pancreatitis, placement of an endoscopic jejunostomy tube may provide therapeutic options which preserve nutritional status, decrease dependance on narcotic analgesia, and reduce the number of hospitalizations per year. In patients with dysphagia resulting from neurologic injury, these percutaneous endoscopic feeding tubes are easily removable should the patient recover function and resume adequate volitional oral intake.

The role of the endoscopist in these settings is critical. One must have the skills to place the tube at the appropriate level in the GI tract, and most techniques can be performed at the bedside in the intensive care unit (ICU) without transport to the radiology suite. The endoscopist has the expertise in gut physiology, thereby allowing for adequate monitoring of enteral nutrition therapy and distinguishing tolerance of feeds from intolerance. Endoscopists have the capabilities to provide simple techniques by which to manage complications. In the absence of such expertise for enteral access, the use of PN increases significantly, a change in management strategy that may negatively impact patient outcome.

HOW TO ESTABLISH AN ENDOSCOPY SERVICE FOR ENTERAL ACCESS

Several important steps should be taken to set up an effective endoscopic enteral "tube service." The nutrition literature is so strong regarding the beneficial effects of enteral feeding in the critical care setting that multidisciplinary nutrition teams are under significant pressure to get tubes in early and get feeds started quickly. The endoscopist should establish rapport with the multidisciplinary nutrition team and provide a timely response to consults for request for enteral access. This can be facilitated by flexibility with potential time slots in the endoscopy schedule to make room for add-on cases for enteral access. It is important to provide same-day service when a request for access is placed to deliver the best patient care. In general, it helps treat a request for enteral access for a patient in the ICU as one would respond to a request to evaluate a patient with GI bleeding.

The two most important endoscopes needed to outfit an endoscopic enteral tube service are a pediatric colonoscope and a small-caliber gastroscope with an insertion tube outer diameter

less than 6 mm. A pediatric colonoscope is usually the best choice for endoscopic nasoenteric tube (ENET), percutaneous endoscopic gastrojejunostomy (PEGJ), and direct percutaneous endoscopic jejunostomy (DPEJ) because of its length and relative stiffness. Although a push enteroscope is an adequate substitute for the pediatric colonoscope, the greater flexibility of the small bowel enteroscope promotes looping or curling in the stomach. The small-caliber gastroscope has the advantage that it can be passed via the transnasal route at the bedside with no sedation, making it an ideal choice in cases requiring ENET placement. The small-caliber endoscope can also be passed through a mature percutaneous endoscopic gastrostomy (PEG) tract ostomy for placement of a one-piece PEGJ. When a 28-Fr PEG is in place, this same endoscope may be passed through the PEG itself for purposes of conversion to a two-piece PEGJ. The endoscopist is encouraged to learn one technique well for each of the four procedures (ENET, PEG, PEGJ, and DPEJ), and then later experiment with many other techniques to find his or her personal favorite. When choosing an enteral access technique, priority should be placed on ones that allow "untethered" endoscopy to place a wire. Techniques which require dragging a wire down through the GI tract, or even worse, dragging the feeding tube itself, are less successful, more frustrating for the operator, and more likely to be displaced (Fig. 42.1).

Fluoroscopy is valuable early in the learning curve, but all these techniques may be performed easily at the bedside or in the endoscopy suite without fluoroscopy. The ability to come to the ICU and place these tubes endoscopically without fluoroscopy avoids the need to transport the patient out of the ICU, increases

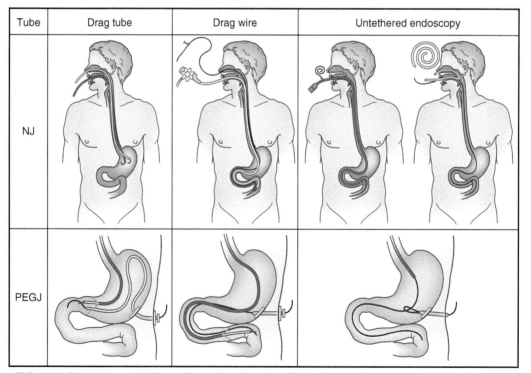

FIG 42.1 Prioritizing techniques for enteral access. Dragging a tube into place increases the chance for proximal displacement when the scope is withdrawn. Dragging a wire is better, but torsion on the wire still impedes endoscopy. "Untethered" endoscopy techniques allow placement of a wire and then delivery of the tube over that wire directly into the small bowel without the need to drag either into place using the endoscope. *NJ*, nasojejunal; *PEGJ*, percutaneous endoscopic gastrojejunostomy.

flexibility in scheduling, and avoids the cost and exposure to radiation involved with fluoroscopy. Having appropriate ancillary devices such as wires, biopsy forceps, and snares that are long enough (such that they can be passed out through the colonoscope and still have a workable length beyond the tip of the scope) and having key accessories such as a hemoclip (to secure the distal tube tip to the intestinal mucosa) or bandage clips (to secure the proximal end of the tube to the skin), all improve the efficiency and success rate for these procedures. It is important to maximize lubrication when working with feeding tubes, both by activating the hydrophilic lubricant on the inner surface of the tube by water infusion, and by applying a vegetable spray or surgical lubricant to the outer surface.

ENDOSCOPIC NASOENTERIC TUBES

Endoscopic nasoenteric tubes (ENET) placement is most commonly required in the critical care setting. Severity of critical illness, complications of sepsis and multiple organ failure, and therapeutic strategies such as placement on mechanical ventilation are all factors indicating the need for early enteral access. Establishing enteral access and initiating enteral feeds is considered part of the basic resuscitation of these patients. ENET placement deep into the jejunum is specifically reserved for those critically ill patients who demonstrate intolerance to initial nasogastric feeding (due to poor gastric emptying, ileus, regurgitation, or aspiration) and those who are at high risk for aspiration. Several techniques have been described for ENET placement.

Over-the-Guidewire Technique

The over-the-guidewire technique may be more difficult technically than other ENET procedures because of the oronasal transfer and wire exchanges (removing the endoscope from the wire and placing the feeding tube over the wire) (Fig. 42.2). However, this technique is the one ENET procedure that most reliably places the feeding tube at or below the ligament of Treitz. Before performing an endoscopy, the oronasal transfer tube is placed through one nostril, brought out of the mouth, and then clamped to the side using a hemostat. The pediatric colonoscope is passed through the mouth, down the esophagus and stomach, and into the small bowel. As the endoscopist traverses the duodenum, it is important to pay attention to landmarks of the duodenal bulb, and the C-loop. The long, straight segment immediately after the duodenal C-loop is the distal duodenum leading up to the ligament of Treitz. The ligament of Treitz is the first turn after this long segment. Paying attention to these landmarks helps assure the endoscopist as to the location of the tip of the endoscope within the GI tract. Passing the endoscope one to two loops below the ligament of Treitz helps anchor the tip of the wire during subsequent wire exchanges (see Fig. 42.2A). Once the endoscope has been passed as deep as possible, the wire is extended out from the end of the endoscope until it meets gentle resistance.

The first wire exchange involves removing the endoscope off the wire without displacing the tip. The key point to this aspect of the procedure is that the endoscopist places one hand on the endoscope as he or she removes it from the mouth and the other hand on the wire as it is passing into the operating channel of the endoscope at the other end (see Fig. 42.2B). An assistant may support the weight of the scope, keeping it from bowing in the middle during the wire exchange. As the endoscopist pushes the wire out the end of the tube with one hand, and withdraws

the scope with the other, a "keyhole technique" should be used. To keep the folds of the small bowel from passing off the end of the endoscope too quickly, a rolling motion should be used where the scope is withdrawn 5 cm and then pushed back in 2 to 3 cm (the same technique used to keyhole the pylorus in order to visualize the duodenal bulb as the scope is withdrawn from the small bowel on esophagogastroduodenoscopy). As a result, the bowel will come off the end of the scope in measured fashion 1–2 folds at a time (see Fig. 42.2C). The point at which the colonoscope has been withdrawn off the wire, the tip of the wire is protruding from the patient's mouth. The oronasal transfer of the wire, if done incorrectly, will cause a loop to form in the mouth and/or displacement of the tip of the wire from the small bowel back into the stomach. The tip of the wire is placed through the oronasal transfer tube, passing the excess wire out of the end of the transfer tube protruding from the nose (see Fig. 42.2D). Before the final loop protruding from the mouth is withdrawn or eliminated, the index finger is passed through the mouth, pinning the wire against the posterior wall of the oropharynx (see Fig. 42.2F). While firmly holding the wire against the posterior pharyngeal wall, traction is placed on the end of the wire protruding from the nose, completely eliminating the loop protruding through the mouth (see Fig. 42.2E). With the wire now protruding from the nose, the second and final wire exchange is made. This latter wire exchange may be accomplished using one of two different techniques. One technique involves carefully passing the feeding tube over the wire in a manner similar to the first wire exchange (see Fig. 42.2G). Again, the endoscopist is careful to place one hand at the nose as he or she inserts the tube, with the other hand at the opposite end of the feeding tube where the wire is being withdrawn. The rate of the tube passing down into the nose should match exactly centimeter for centimeter the rate of the wire being withdrawn at the other end, to avoid deflecting the tip of the wire (see Fig. 42.2G). An alternative technique for this second wire exchange involves pinning the end of the wire to a bed rail or bedside table establishing a "point in space" (see Fig. 42.2H). Assistants help keep the wire straight and level while the endoscopist slides the feeding tube over the fixed wire into final position.

Drag and Pull Technique

This technique is facilitated by placing one or two extra guidewires (for a total of 2 or 3) through the nasoenteric tube prior to placement. Two to three centimeters of the soft tip of one wire should protrude out through the distal end of the tube. This assembly is then passed down through the nose into the stomach, followed by passage of the endoscope alongside the tube, down through the mouth, and into the stomach. Once in the stomach, a long biopsy forceps is used to grab the soft tip of the wire protruding from the feeding tube. The endoscope holding the wire is then passed into the small bowel, hopefully down to or beyond the ligament of Treitz (Fig. 42.3A).

From the point of deepest insertion, the endoscope is then slowly withdrawn back toward the stomach as the biopsy forceps holding the wire is advanced, holding the tip of the wire in place in the small bowel. Once the endoscope is positioned back into the stomach, the feeding tube is advanced over the wire down to its tip, which is still being held by the biopsy forceps (see Fig. 42.3B). Only at this point are the biopsy forceps opened and the wire is released. The biopsy forceps are then withdrawn back into the endoscope and the endoscope is slowly withdrawn back out through the esophagus and mouth. The keys to success for

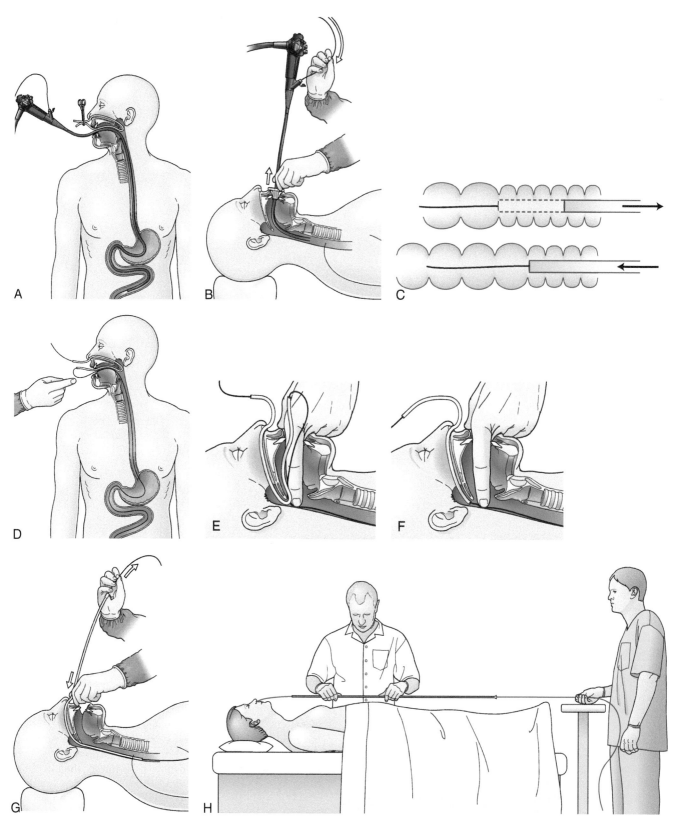

FIG 42.2 Over-the-guidewire endoscopic nasoenteric tube (ENET) technique. **A,** The pediatric colonoscope is passed down below the ligament of Treitz and the wire extended out beyond the end of the scope. **B,** In the initial wire transfer, the scope is withdrawn out from the mouth at the same rate the guidewire is passed down through the operating channel, to prevent displacement of the wire tip from its position in the small bowel. **C,** The keyhole technique is used for withdrawing the endoscope off the guidewire. With the bowel pleated on the end of the endoscope, the endoscope is withdrawn 5–6 cm. By quickly pushing the endoscope back in 2–3 cm, the bowel comes off the end of the endoscope 1–2 folds at a time. **D,** With the wire protruding out through the mouth, the tip of the wire is then passed through the oronasal transfer tube. **E** and **F,** The index finger is then used to pin the wire against the posterior pharyngeal wall while traction is placed on the wire protruding out through the nose, pulling on the wire until the wire is straight and tension is felt against the finger in the posterior pharynx. **G,** In one technique for the final wire transfer, the feeding tube is passed over the wire down through the nares at the exact same rate that the wire is withdrawn out from the distal end of the feeding tube, again to avoid displacing the wire tip. **H,** In an alternative technique for the final wire transfer, an assistant pins the wire to a "point in space" (using a bedside table), and the tube is then slid over the fixed wire into final position.

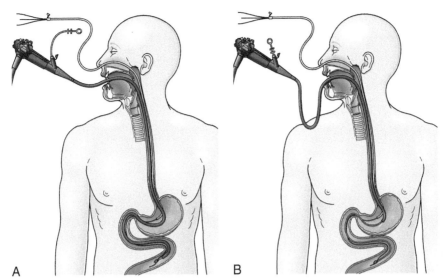

FIG 42.3 Drag and pull endoscopic nasoenteric tube (ENET) technique. **A,** The feeding tube is stiffened with three guidewires and then passed into the stomach, where one of the three guidewires is passed out beyond the end of the feeding tube. This one wire is grabbed with biopsy forceps and the pediatric colonoscope drags the wire down below the ligament of Treitz. **B,** As the endoscope is withdrawn back into the stomach, the biopsy forceps are pushed out to hold the wire in position below the ligament of Treitz. With the endoscope still positioned in the stomach, the feeding tube is advanced over the wire until it meets the biopsy forceps at the distal end. The endoscope is then withdrawn out through the mouth before all the guidewires are removed.

this procedure are a pair of biopsy forceps that are long enough (≥ 240 cm), and the stiffening of the feeding tube with extra guidewires (which facilitates removal of the endoscope without displacing the tube back into the stomach) (see Fig. 42.3B).

Transnasal Technique

Availability of a small-caliber gastroscope affords the endoscopist the opportunity for a simple technique for ENET placement. The key to success with this technique is the placement of a biopsy forceps or a Savary guidewire down through the operating channel, which serves to stiffen the instrument and increase the ease with which it may be passed through the bowel. Transnasal passage of the endoscope is tolerated well by the patient and sedation is not usually required. After intubating the esophagus and stomach, the endoscope is passed as far as possible, usually to the third or fourth portion of the duodenum. At this point, the stiffening device is withdrawn and a guidewire is placed down through the operating channel out as far as possible until meeting gentle resistance (Fig. 42.4). Using the wire exchange system described in the over-the-guidewire technique, the small-caliber gastroscope is then withdrawn off the wire. Obviously, no oropharyngeal transfer of the wire is required, and the feeding tube may be immediately passed directly over the wire. Wire exchanges are somewhat more tenuous and difficult with this procedure because the wire is usually not passed as deep into the small bowel as in the over-the-guidewire technique described earlier, and the tip may be displaced more easily back into the stomach.

Alternate Options

In a simpler version of the previously mentioned drag and pull technique, a knotted suture line is attached to the distal end of the feeding tube, and then the tube is passed through the nares down into the stomach. The endoscopist passes the endoscope alongside the tube through the mouth, down into the stomach, grabbing the knotted suture with biopsy forceps (Fig. 42.5A). It can be surprisingly difficult and frustrating to drag the tip of the feeding tube through the pylorus and down into the duodenum. The success of this sometimes awkward procedure is improved by using a knotted suture line instead of a loop or single strand on the tip of the tube (see Fig. 42.5B), by adding a second guidewire to stiffen the tube to prevent displacement upon withdrawal of the endoscope, and by keeping the biopsy forceps 1 to 2 cm away from the tip of the endoscope to enhance visualization (see Fig. 42.5A).

Another alternate technique utilizes adding one or two extra guidewires (for a total of two or three) to the feeding tube to increase stiffness, and then passing the tube through the nares down into the esophagus and stomach. The endoscope is passed through the mouth alongside the tube down into the stomach, and the tip of the stiffened tube is simply pushed or nudged using open biopsy forceps through the pylorus into the duodenal bulb (see Fig. 42.5C). Continuing to watch endoscopically from the stomach, the endoscopist pushes the stiffened feeding tube from the outside proximal end in an effort to pass the distal tip around the C-loop and into the third and fourth portion of the duodenum (see Fig. 42.5C).

The most reliable of the three alternate methods uses an 8-Fr nasoenteric tube, which is passed through the operating channel of the endoscope after it has been passed through the esophagus and stomach into the small bowel. This procedure's success is enhanced by using a large channel therapeutic endoscope and a small-bore (8-Fr) nasoenteric tube which has a removable proximal feeding cap. Because the endoscope is passed through

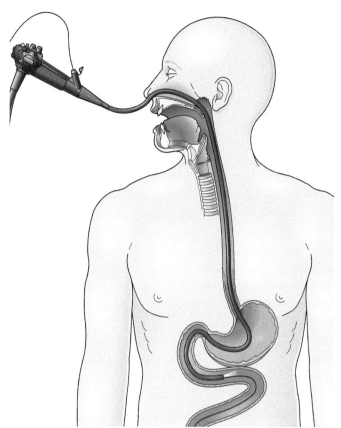

FIG 42.4 Transnasal endoscopic nasoenteric tube (ENET) technique. After first placing biopsy forceps down through the operating channel to stiffen the endoscope, a small-caliber (< 6-mm diameter) gastroscope is passed through the nares down into the stomach and beyond the pylorus. A guidewire is passed through the operating channel out beyond the end of the endoscope, and then the endoscope is subsequently withdrawn. The final feeding tube is passed over the wire.

the mouth, it does require placement of an oronasal transfer tube and the subsequent transfer of the tube from the mouth out through the nose (see Fig. 42.5D), using the method described in the over-the-guidewire technique.

Securing Tube With Nasal Bridle

For any case in which the time and expense of endoscopic placement of a nasoenteric tube is required, consideration should be given to securing the tube with a nasal bridle. Although this technique may seem barbaric and somewhat punitive to the patient, selection of the proper tube for the nasal bridle results in a degree of discomfort that is no different than the presence of the nasoenteric tube alone. The timing of the nasal bridle placement is important, and should be done initially before endoscopy is performed (before the patient is agitated from the passage of the endoscope). Two separate but similar techniques may be used to establish a nasal bridle. In one technique, two 5-Fr neonatal feeding tubes are used (Fig. 42.6A). The first tube is passed through one of the nares and brought out through the mouth, while the second is passed through the other nares and likewise brought out through the mouth. The two ends protruding from the mouth are then secured together by a single suture, or are simply tied together by hand using a square knot. Traction

is placed on one end protruding from the nares, pulling the nasal bridle into place (pulling the knotted juncture out through the nares such that one of the tubes passes into the nares around the nasal septum and out the other nares) (see Fig. 42.6A). An alternate technique uses a commercial device with two flexible rubber sticks, each with a magnet at one end (see Fig. 42.6B). A cloth ribbon is attached to the opposite end of one of the sticks. Each stick is passed through a separate nares, allowing the magnetic tips to click together in the posterior hypopharynx. Traction is applied to one of the sticks to pull the cloth ribbon into final position in one nares, around the nasal septum, and then out the other nares (see Fig. 42.6B). The oronasal transfer tube is then placed and the rest of the ENET procedure commences thereafter. At the completion of the ENET placement, the feeding tube is taped to the 5-Fr nasal bridle tube (beginning 1 cm below the nose and wrapping the tape downward over the feeding tube and bridle until the bridle is completely covered; see Fig. 42.6A), or clipped to the cloth ribbon (see Fig. 42.6B).

PERCUTANEOUS ENDOSCOPIC GASTROSTOMY

Placement of a percutaneous endoscopic gastrostomy (PEG) tube provides a more reliable and semi-permanent enteral access compared to the ENET, and should be considered in any patient requiring specialized nutrition therapy for greater than 4 weeks' duration. Because an incision is made, those patients who are not already on antibiotics do need a single dose for antibiotic prophylaxis (a third-generation cephalosporin is appropriate) at the time of the initial procedure. Identifying landmarks with an indelible marker, such as the midline and the costal margins, provides good orientation during the procedure and avoids the possibility of lacerating the left lobe of the liver with placement too close to the costal margin. Antiplatelet or anticoagulant therapy is not a contraindication to these percutaneous techniques. Aspirin does not have to be stopped prior to the procedure. Patients on warfarin (Coumadin, Bristol-Myers Squibb Company, Princeton, NJ) may be switched to low molecular weight heparin (Lovenox, sanofi-aventis US LLC, Bridgewater, NJ) 1 week prior to the procedure (holding the dose on the morning of the procedure). If patients on clopidogrel (Plavix, Bristol-Myers Squibb) cannot be switched to aspirin alone 5 days before the procedure, the procedure may still be performed with caution (adding epinephrine to the anesthetic used for the initial skin incision to promote vasoconstriction, avoiding large superficial blood vessels in the skin or gastric mucosa, and setting the external bolster somewhat more firmly against the abdominal wall to achieve compression).

In the past, the traditional location for PEG placement has been in the left upper quadrant in the vortex formed by the midline and the left costal margin (Fig. 42.7A). Relocating the site of routine PEG placement down lower close to the umbilicus and even to the right of the midline should be considered for two good reasons. First, as shown on computerized tomography (CT) scan (see Fig. 42.7B), the area of greatest interface between the stomach and anterior wall that provides the shortest, most direct passage into the stomach, is located at this site. The traditional site in the left upper quadrant creates a tract that is longer and more tangential as it enters the stomach. However, even more importantly, this lower position on the abdomen places the PEG in the antrum, which facilitates conversion of the PEG to a PEGJ should the patient develop intolerance to gastric feeding later on. Site selection is further enhanced by

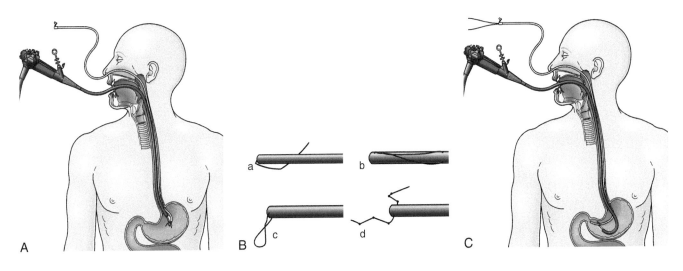

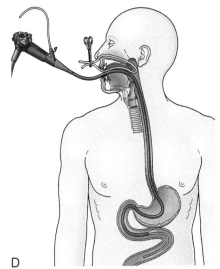

FIG 42.5 Additional endoscopic nasoenteric tube (ENET) options. **A,** One option involves two knotted sutures, attached to the distal end of the feeding tube, which is then passed through the nares down into the stomach. Biopsy forceps passed through the gastroscope grab the knotted suture and drag the tube down below the pylorus into the distal duodenum. **B,** This figure shows how the knotted suture is superior to a single or double suture line (which may adhere with gastric juices and mucous to the feeding tube) and a loop of suture (which may become tangled and twisted). **C,** A second option involves two or three guidewires passed through the feeding tube, which is subsequently passed through the nares down into the stomach. The endoscope is passed through the mouth down into the stomach where biopsy forceps are used to push or shove the stiffened feeding tube through the pylorus. The tube can then be advanced further down into the distal duodenum by pushing from the outside. **D,** Another option involves the passage of an 8-Fr feeding tube through the operating channel of a therapeutic gastroscope, which has been passed to the distal duodenum or proximal jejunum. After advancing the feeding tube out beyond the end of the endoscope, the endoscope is withdrawn out from the mouth and the tube is transferred via a larger oronasal transfer tube out through the nose.

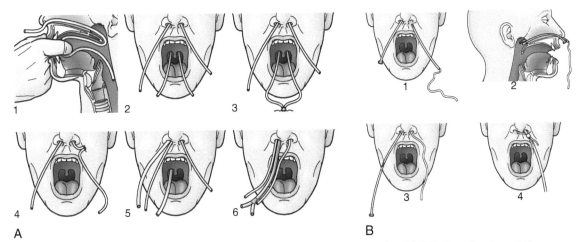

FIG 42.6 Bridle technique for securing endoscopic nasoenteric tube (ENET) **A,** using two 5-Fr neonatal feeding tubes or **B,** a commercial device using two flexible sticks with magnetic ends. The numbers identify the sequential steps in each procedure.

instilling 500 mL of air through the nasogastric tube into the stomach and obtaining an abdominal film in the hour prior to PEG placement. Putting a coin in the umbilicus serves as an obvious landmark on the abdominal film, the position of which can be compared to the costal margins. The position of the air

bubble with respect to the coin and the costal margins help select the specific PEG site. (see Fig. 42.7C).

Palpating the stomach and obtaining translumination through the abdominal wall is a valuable reassurance for proper PEG site selection. If there is any question (especially in cases of obesity),

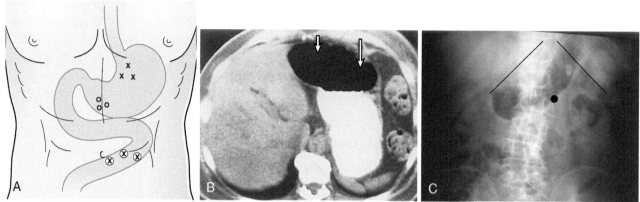

FIG 42.7 Steps to localize percutaneous endoscopic gastrostomy (PEG), percutaneous endoscopic gastrojejunostomy (PEGJ), and direct percutaneous endoscopic jejunostomy (DPEJ) sites. **A,** The traditional PEG site is marked by the *x* in the left upper quadrant. Better placement is above the umbilicus, close to the midline, or slightly to the patient's right of midline position *(circles)*. The PEG is in the gastric antrum, which is ideal should the patient require conversion later to a PEGJ. *X with circles* show the tremendous variability in the site for DPEJ placement, which can occur anywhere from the left costal margin down to the left iliac crest. **B,** Computerized tomography (CT) scan shows that the PEG site slightly above or to the patient's right of the umbilicus coincides with the area with the most direct, perpendicular, and shortest tract into the gastric antrum *(short arrow)*. Traditional sites in the left upper quadrant have a longer, more tangential tract into the midbody or even lower fundus *(long arrow)*. **C,** Placing a coin in the umbilicus *(dark circle)* and injecting 500 mL of air through a nasogastric tube before PEG placement helps identify the gastric antrum, easing selection of the PEG site.

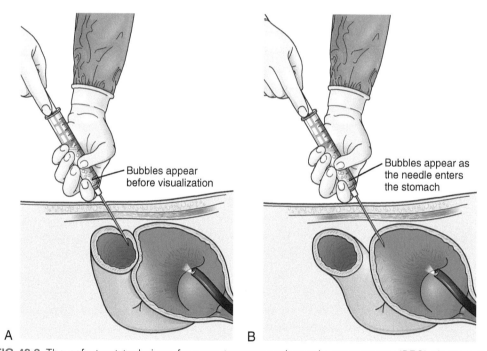

FIG 42.8 The safe tract technique for percutaneous endoscopic gastrostomy (PEG) placement helps **A,** avoid inadvertent tracking through an adjacent loop of bowel before **B,** passage into the stomach.

a safe tract technique may be utilized to assure that no intervening loop of bowel exists between the stomach and the anterior abdominal wall (Fig. 42.8). Using a 22-gauge spinal needle and a syringe with 1 to 2 mL of saline, the needle is passed through the abdominal wall at the proposed PEG site. If bubbles appear in the saline just as the needle passes into the lumen of the stomach (as seen by endoscopy), there is some reassurance that the tract is appropriate. If bubbles appear before the needle passes into the stomach, there may be an intervening loop of bowel present (see Fig. 42.8). The length of the skin incision should be adequate just to accommodate the diameter of the feeding tube.

Ponsky Pull and Sachs-Vine Push Technique

For PEG placement, the Ponsky pull and Sachs-Vine push techniques are virtually indistinguishable, provide no real advantage over the other, and may be selected based on personal preference of the operator. Once the PEG site is selected, the skin is anesthetized, a small incision is made, and the initial trocar is passed into the stomach. In the Sachs-Vine push technique, a single-stranded wire is passed through the trocar in the stomach and secured by a snare passed through the endoscope. With the Ponsky pull technique, a blue double-stranded wire loop is passed through the trocar and grabbed by the snare (Fig. 42.9A).

The wire passed by either technique is then brought out through the mouth. In the Sachs-Vine push technique, a long 2- to 3-foot plastic pointed leader is fused to the proximal end of the feeding tube, facilitating passage over the single-stranded guidewire. This assembly is pushed down the wire, through the esophagus, and out through the gastric and abdominal wall (see Fig. 42.9B). In contrast, the Ponsky pull technique involves a loop on the end of the feeding tube which is affixed to the double-stranded blue loop of wire protruding from the patient's mouth. Attaching the two wire loops is made easier by remembering the phrase "blue through," which describes the blue double-stranded wire being passed first through the silver loop on the end of the feeding tube (see Fig. 42.9B). Once the knot between the wire loops is secured, the feeding tube is then pulled down through the esophagus into the stomach and out through the abdominal wall into the final position (see Fig. 42.9C).

As a general rule when setting the external bumper, a close fit causes fewer subsequent complications than a tight fit, which can later lead to pressure necrosis and buried bumper syndrome. A quick and easy procedure to facilitate setting adequate tension between the bumpers involves following the PEG tube down through the esophagus by snaring the endoscope to the internal bolster (Fig. 42.10A). As shown in the top of Fig. 42.10A, snaring one-third of the internal bolster makes it easy to release the bolster once the endoscope is led down into the stomach. As the tube is pushed or pulled down through the esophagus and stomach, the endoscope is brought down easily with it into position into the stomach. Once the snare is released, the external bolster may be set with the internal bolster under direct endoscopic visualization (see Fig. 42.10B). Drawing a figure and marking the exact number on the tube for the position of the external bolster is a valuable aid for nursing care and may be placed on the chart for reference at any time (see Fig. 42.10B).

Russell Introducer Technique

In patients with a large exophytic oropharyngeal or esophageal carcinoma, the Russell introducer technique should be considered to reduce the likelihood for tumor implantation of the PEG site. This is a technique commonly used by radiologists, but is easily performed by the endoscopist. Localization of the PEG site, position of the endoscope, and passage of the initial trocar are identical to the previous two techniques. With the trocar in place, a single-stranded guidewire is passed into the stomach and then held firmly by a snare protruding from the endoscope (Fig. 42.11A). Continuing to hold the wire throughout the procedure maintains a "safety line" of access to the gastric lumen.

The stomach has to first be secured to the anterior wall by T-fasteners (see Fig. 42.11A). Although a variety of commercial models of these fasteners exist, the design for deployment is

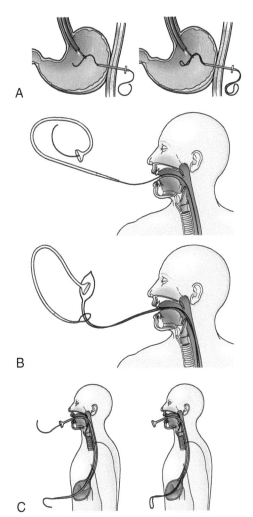

FIG 42.9 Comparison of the Sachs-Vine push versus the Ponsky pull technique for percutaneous endoscopic gastrostomy (PEG) placement. **A,** In the Sachs-Vine technique, a single wire is passed through the trocar and grabbed with the snare, whereas a wire loop is passed through the trocar in the Ponsky pull technique. **B,** A long, 2-foot plastic leader attached directly to the feeding tube allows the entire ensemble to passed or pushed over the wire in the Sachs-Vine push technique, whereas the blue wire loop can be attached to a wire loop on the end of the feeding tube in the Ponsky pull technique, allowing the tube to be pulled into position. **C,** In the Sachs-Vine technique, the tube attached to the plastic leader is pushed through the esophagus and out through the gastric wall, whereas in the Ponsky pull technique, the wire loop pulls the feeding tube down through the esophagus and out through the gastric wall.

similar. As shown in Fig. 42.11A, this particular technique involves a narrow-gauge introducer trocar in which the T-fastener is placed in a distal slot. A 22-gauge spinal needle is helpful as a sounding device to determine the appropriate tract for each T-fastener. After making a nick in the skin with a scalpel blade, the device is passed through the abdominal wall. The T-fastener is deployed in the stomach by a central canula. After removing the small trocar and canula for the T-fastener, a cotton roller ball and two metal fastening devices are cinched down until there is mild tension on the outer abdominal wall against the T-fastener on

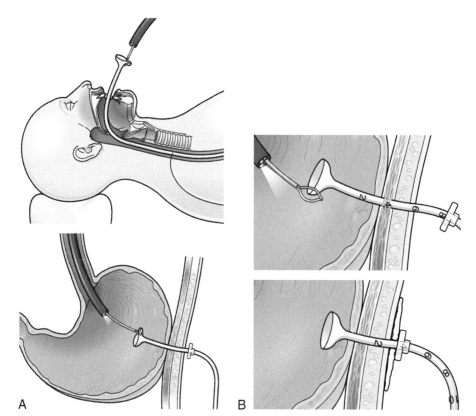

FIG 42.10 Following the percutaneous endoscopic gastrostomy (PEG) tube down into place and positioning the external bolster for appropriate tension. **A,** Just before the feeding tube is pushed or pulled down through the oropharynx and esophagus, a snare passed through the endoscope is snared to the internal bolster of the feeding tube, securing the endoscope to the tube. The endoscope is then pulled down through the oropharynx and esophagus as the PEG is brought down into position. **B,** Once in the stomach, the snare is released and the bumper is positioned gently up against the gastric wall. The external bumper is positioned with a single layer of gauze underneath. A final figure indicating the appropriate number on the feeding tube for position of the external bolster may be drawn and recorded on the patient's chart.

the inside of the stomach. Crimping the two metal fasteners holds the T-fastener in place. Anywhere from two to four T-fasteners should be placed circumferentially around the trocar before proceeding further (see Fig. 42.11A).

With the stomach affixed to the anterior wall by the T-fasteners, the tract over the wire is dilated by Seldinger-type dilators of increasing size. Three to five dilators are passed over the wire, with the snare holding the wire on the inside of the stomach (see Fig. 42.11B). Once the tract has been fully dilated, a peel-away sheet overlying a larger bore canula is passed over the wire and into the stomach (see Fig. 42.11B, bottom).

Most of the Russell introducer kits do not come with an external bolster and are instead designed or anticipated to be sutured to the skin. A simple homemade external bolster may be created by a short segment from any small Salem sump, Foley catheter, or other larger gauge feeding tube, and placed over the feeding tube prior to passage into the stomach (see Fig. 42.11C). Once the external bolster is in place, the feeding tube may be placed over the wire through the peel-away sheet into the stomach. The internal balloon is then inflated, the peel-away sheet is removed, and the external bolster is then placed into position (see Fig. 42.11C).

PERCUTANEOUS ENDOSCOPIC GASTROJEJUNOSTOMY

For patients with documented intolerance to gastric feeding with nausea, vomiting, high gastric residual volumes, or evidence of gastroparesis, the percutaneous endoscopic gastrojejunostomy (PEGJ) provides an easy, although somewhat less reliable, long-term access to the small bowel. The success of this procedure is related to a number of factors. Localization of the PEG in the antrum is most important. The PEG should be cut down to approximately 10 cm in length to afford a maximum length of the jejunal tube for passage into the small bowel. If the PEGJ is performed at the time of initial PEG placement, then antibiotic prophylaxis should be used. A site just to the right and above the umbilicitus is the best site for placement into the antrum (see Fig. 42.7). A pediatric colonoscope is important to try to get one to two loops below the ligament of Treitz. Long biopsy forceps of greater than 350 cm in length are important to have a sufficient working length beyond the tip of the colonoscope (the accessory device must be twice the length of the scope plus 20 to 30 cm extra for a "working length"). The endoscopist should not use a snare to place wires in this procedure, as it can be

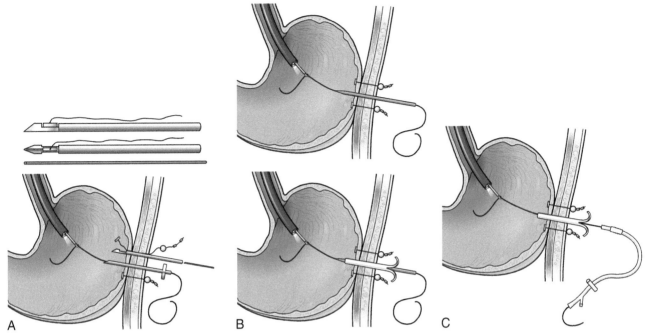

FIG 42.11 The Russell introducer percutaneous endoscopic gastrostomy (PEG) technique. **A,** After initial placement of the trocar and passage of a single stranded wire, the wire is held with some tension against external traction by a snare passed through the endoscope within the stomach. T-fasteners are then passed to secure the stomach up against the anterior abdominal wall. The top of this figure shows how the T-fasteners (with attached suture) are released by the canula device. **B,** Once the stomach is secured to the anterior abdominal wall, the tract is dilated over the guidewire by three Seldinger dilators of increasing size. After the last dilation, a peel-away sheath over the final dilator is passed into position and the dilator is removed. **C,** After first preloading an external bumper on the feeding tube, the feeding tube is passed over the wire through the peel-away sheath into the stomach where the internal bolster is inflated, the peel-away sheath is removed, and the external bolster is positioned down against the skin.

difficult to extract the snare from the tip of the wire once it is positioned in the small bowel.

One of the most important elements in the success of this procedure is the function of an air retention valve (Fig. 42.12). Although a number of commercial models are available (see Fig. 42.12A), a homemade air valve can be made from the cap of the feeding tube (creating a hole with a pair of scissors) (see Fig. 42.12B). The air valve allows passage of a wire or a snare through the PEG into the stomach without losing air insufflation. Failure to use or create an air valve significantly prolongs the procedure and can make visualization very difficult when passing the endoscope from the stomach into the small bowel.

Through-the-Snare Technique

This technique is the most reliable way to successfully place a PEGJ tube into the proximal jejunum at or below the ligament of Treitz. After cutting the PEG down to 10 cm, an air retention valve is fashioned and the snare is passed through the hole in the air valve positioned in the PEG into the stomach. The snare is opened, allowing the pediatric colonoscope to be passed down through the esophagus and stomach, through the snare, and on into the small bowel. Once the endoscope has been passed into the small bowel, the snare is closed once to make sure the endoscope has passed through the snare. The air valve may be backed out of the PEG at this point to decompress the stomach

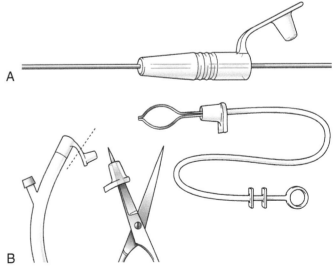

FIG 42.12 Commercial and homemade air valves. **A,** The top figure shows a commercial air valve passed over the guidewire, which is used most often during percutaneous endoscopic gastrojejunostomy (PEGJ) conversions. **B,** A homemade air valve may be created by cutting off the valve plug on a feeding tube, coring the valve out with a pair of scissors, and then passing a snare or wire through the valve.

and prevent looping or curling of the endoscope. The endoscope is passed, hopefully, one to two loops beyond the ligament of Treitz. At its deepest penetration, a guidewire is passed out further into the jejunum until gentle resistance is met. The key to success of this technique is the selection of a very long 480-cm standard guidewire. The wire that comes with PEG and PEGJ kits is usually substantially shorter than this (Fig. 42.13A). Using proper wire exchange techniques, the endoscope is withdrawn back to the proximal stomach above the level of the snare, keeping the tip of the wire in position in the small bowel (see Fig. 42.13B). Once the endoscope has been brought back to approximately 45 cm (from the incisors), the air valve is placed back into the PEG to insufflate the stomach and confirm position of the endoscope above the snare (see Fig. 42.13B). The snare is then closed on the wire and a loop of the wire is pulled out through the PEG to the outside (see Fig. 42.13C). The endoscopist separates the loop with his fingers, and has an assistant pull on the proximal wire extending out from the proximal operating channel of the endoscope. The movement of one side of the loop helps identify that end of the wire coming from the endoscope (see Fig. 42.13C). This end of the wire is then pulled out through the PEG, resulting in a straightened single-strand guidewire passing through the PEG and down into the small bowel (see Fig. 42.13D). The jejunal tube is then passed over the wire (using good wire exchange technique) into position in the small bowel. Having an assistant provide a point in space above the abdomen secures or fixes the guidewire, facilitating passage of the jejunal tube into final position.

Over-the-Guidewire Technique

Although this technique appears to be more simplified than the through-the-snare technique, it may be slightly more frustrating for getting proper placement of the jejunal tube well down into the small bowel. For this technique, an air retention valve is placed over a wire, and then the wire is passed through the PEG into the stomach. After passing the endoscope through the esophagus into the stomach, biopsy forceps are used to grasp the wire and walk it on down into the small bowel. The key to the success of this procedure is again using biopsy forceps that are greater than 350 cm in length, to afford a sufficient working length out beyond the end of the colonoscope. The colonoscope is hopefully passed down to a level at or below the ligament of Treitz (Fig. 42.14A). While still holding the wire in place at its distal tip, the biopsy forceps are slowly advanced as the endoscope is withdrawn back into the proximal stomach. The jejunal tube is then passed over the wire all the way down until it strikes the biopsy forceps still holding the tip of the wire in the small bowel (see Fig. 42.14B). Only at this point are the biopsy forceps opened, releasing the wire. The biopsy forceps are withdrawn back into the endoscope. It is important for the endoscopist to realize that if shorter biopsy forceps are used, the jejunal tube may strike the forceps holding the end of the wire while there is still a significant length of jejunal tube remaining outside the PEG. Although it is appropriate to open the biopsy forceps and release the wire at this point, the added length of the jejunal tube outside the PEG as the jejunal tube is pushed down and seated into position in the PEG often forms a loop in the stomach and the procedure has to be repeated.

Trans-PEG Gastroscopy Technique

This technique may be performed with a small-caliber gastroscope, but is only feasible if the patient's original PEG is 28-Fr in diameter. The technique can be performed through a PEG tube of smaller diameter, but a bronchoscope or ureteroscope may need to be substituted. The key to success with any of these small endoscopes is to stiffen the instrument by placing a biopsy forceps or a stiff guidewire down through the operating channel. Failure to do so will cause excessive looping or curling in the stomach and possible inability to transcend the pylorus. In this simple technique, the endoscope is passed through the PEG, down through the pylorus, and through the third and fourth portion of the duodenum. It is difficult to get beyond the ligament of Treitz with this endoscope alone, but passing the wire out through the end of the endoscope once it is positioned in the distal duodenum may allow passage of the wire into the proximal jejunum below the ligament of Treitz. The endoscope is then withdrawn and the jejunal tube is placed over the guidewire (Fig. 42.15).

If enough time has lapsed so a mature tract has already formed, a one-piece PEGJ can be placed through the existing PEG tract (Fig. 42.16). The original PEG should be removed in an atraumatic fashion. A small-caliber (< 6 mm) gastroscope is inserted through the PEG site and driven down below the ligament of Treitz. The soft-tipped end of the guidewire is fed through the scope and advanced as far as possible beyond the end of the endoscope, stopping when slight pressure is felt (see Fig. 42.16A). The scope is withdrawn, leaving the guidewire in place using the combination cm-by-cm and keyhole techniques described previously. The gastroscope is then reinserted through the nares or the mouth, passed down the esophagus, and positioned in the stomach to observe the position of the guidewire throughout the rest of the procedure. A one-piece PEGJ tube is fed over the wire, passing down into the small bowel while visualizing the wire and tube from the stomach to make sure a loop does not form in the process (see Fig. 42.16B). Once the tube has been passed far enough over the wire, the internal balloon bolster is inflated, the external bolster set, and the guidewire withdrawn. The key to success on this technique involves a long enough standard 0.035 wire (< 350 cm), thorough lubrication of the wire with silicone, and passage of the endoscope into the stomach the second time to watch out for looping of the wire or the tube.

Securing the PEGJ

The most frustrating aspect of the PEGJ procedure is that the jejunal tube frequently migrates back into the stomach. Two techniques may help prevent this. One is to use a rotatable endoscopic clip to clip a suture affixed to the distal end of the feeding tube to the intestinal mucosa. Although this is easy to perform, the clip may only hold the suture reliably in place for 7 to 10 days. A second technique is shown in Fig. 42.17, in which an anchor is created with a 1 cm segment from some other piece of tubing. A Salem sump, Foley catheter, or some other feeding tube may be used to create the 1-cm anchor. A 20-cm length of suture is affixed to the distal end of the feeding tube and then secured to the anchor. The anchor is placed over the guidewire ahead of the jejunal feeding tube in the final step of the PEGJ procedure, as the jejunal tube is passed over the wire into position in the small bowel (see Fig. 42.17).

It is important, at the completion of the PEGJ procedure by any of these methods, that the operator confirms the proper position endoscopically. If the jejunal tube forms a loop up toward the gastroesophageal junction, the procedure may need to be repeated to achieve deeper positioning into the small bowel (Fig. 42.18). The natural action of this loop is to displace the tube

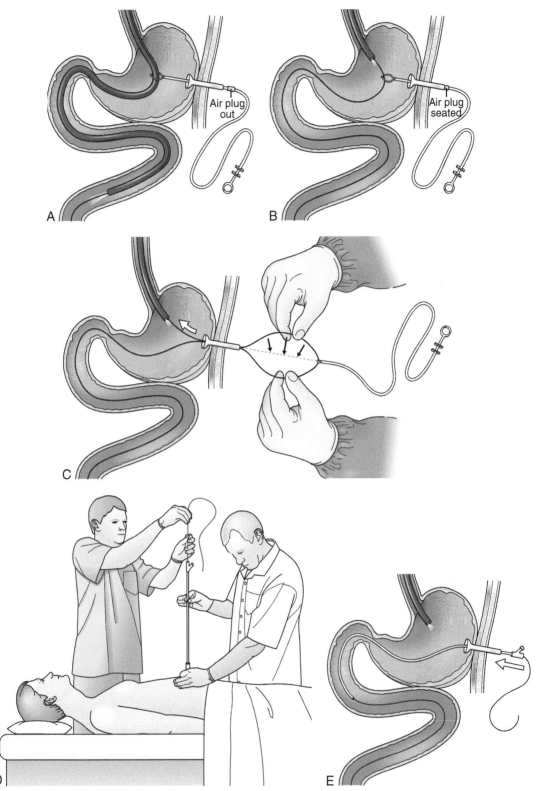

FIG 42.13 Through-the-snare percutaneous endoscopic gastrojejunostomy (PEGJ) technique. **A,** After initial placement of the percutaneous endoscopic gastrostomy (PEG), the PEG tube is cut down short to approximately 10 cm, and then a snare placed through a homemade or commercial air valve is passed into the stomach. A pediatric colonoscope is passed into the stomach, through the snare, and then down into the small bowel below the ligament of Treitz (after which the wire is extended beyond the end of the scope). **B,** Using careful wire transfer technique, the endoscope is withdrawn back to the proximal stomach, keeping the tip of the wire in place below the ligament of Treitz. The air plug may be seated to allow visualization of the snare within the stomach. **C,** The snare is then closed on the wire, which is pulled out through the PEG. While the assistant holds the wire loop coming out from the PEG, the operator pulls on the wire extruding from the operating channel of the scope, to indicate which side of the wire loop represents the proximal end of the wire. That loop is then pulled out through the PEG. **D,** An assistant provides a "point in space" to secure or fix the guidewire as the operator passes the jejunal tube down through the PEG. **E,** The jejunal extension tube is passed down into final position, with the tip located well below the ligament of Treitz.

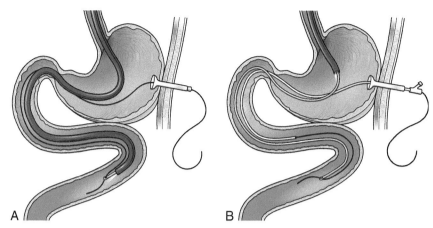

FIG 42.14 Over-the-guidewire percutaneous endoscopic gastrojejunostomy (PEGJ) technique. **A,** A single stranded guidewire passed through a valve (which is seated in the percutaneous endoscopic gastrostomy [PEG]) is grasped by biopsy forceps (passed down through a pediatric colonoscope). The endoscope holding the wire (via biopsy forceps) is passed down into the small bowel below the ligament of Treitz. **B,** The endoscope is then withdrawn back into the stomach as the biopsy forceps are pushed outward through the end of the scope, holding the wire in place below the ligament of Treitz. Once the scope has been withdrawn back into the proximal stomach, the jejunal extension tube is passed over the wire until the distal end strikes the biopsy forceps at the end of the wire.

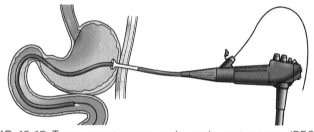

FIG 42.15 Trans-percutaneous endoscopic gastrostomy (PEG) gastroscope percutaneous endoscopic gastrojejunostomy (PEGJ) technique. After first stiffening the small-caliber 5.5-mm gastroscope with a biopsy forceps, the endoscope is passed through the PEG down to the distal duodenum and proximal jejunum. After removing the biopsy forceps, a single-stranded guidewire is passed out through the end of the endoscope hopefully beyond the ligament of Treitz. After the scope is withdrawn, the jejunal extension tube is passed over the wire.

upward toward the fundus, out from the small bowel. Proper positioning instead should have the appearance that the jejunal tube passes from the PEG directly toward the pylorus and down into the small bowel (see Figs. 42.13E and 42.16B).

DIRECT PERCUTANEOUS ENDOSCOPIC JEJUNOSTOMY

Although direct percutaneous endoscopic jejunostomy (DPEJ) may be the most technically demanding procedure for enteral access, it provides the most reliable semi-permanent access for the patient who has had difficulty with gastroparesis, nausea, vomiting, or previous intolerance to gastric feeding. Antibiotic prophylaxis is required for the DPEJ technique. Recommendations for the management of antiplatelet or anticoagulant therapy are similar to PEG placement. Although the DPEJ technique is very

similar to the Ponsky pull technique for PEG, a number of important differences exist. First, a much larger area of the abdomen from the costal margins bilaterally down to the iliac crests on both sides may need to be prepped because translumination may occur at more unusual sites anywhere over the abdomen. If the patient has had previous partial gastrectomy and rerouting of the GI tract, the DPEJ may end up being placed significantly to the right of the midline. The DPEJ is a two-person procedure, requiring an assistant at the level of the skin and a skilled endoscopist with the scope. The endoscopist should anticipate taking much longer time (anywhere from 5 to 30 minutes) to transluminate and to finger palpate the site. It is most appropriate to use a 22-gauge spinal needle as a sounding needle in attempts to intubate the small bowel. Again, the endoscopist should anticipate many more needle sticks with the spinal gauge needle compared to the PEG technique. The Ponsky pull technique is best suited for DPEG. The plastic leader on the Sachs-Vine push technique is not long enough to reach the small bowel site. Most importantly, a tube should be selected with a small internal bolster. A large balloon bolster may cause partial obstruction of the small bowel. A 14-16-Fr pediatric PEG tube with a flat or small mushroom internal bolster is ideal for this procedure. In passing the endoscope through the stomach and into the small bowel, it is important to pay attention to landmarks so that the endoscopist knows when the tip of the endoscope is below the ligament of Treitz. In a patient with Billroth II anatomy, it is important to document the efferent limb for DPEJ placement. The pediatric colonoscope is the instrument of choice in patients with intact anatomy or a "virgin abdomen." A more flexible gastroscope may be better suited for the patient with a partial gastrectomy and a Billroth II reanastomosis. In patients with an intact stomach, the colonoscope may need to be passed its entire length into the small bowel and withdrawn back to the proximal duodenum several times before a site can be identified by transillumination and finger palpation. Site selection is facilitated by searching for a site immediately beyond the ligament of Treitz,

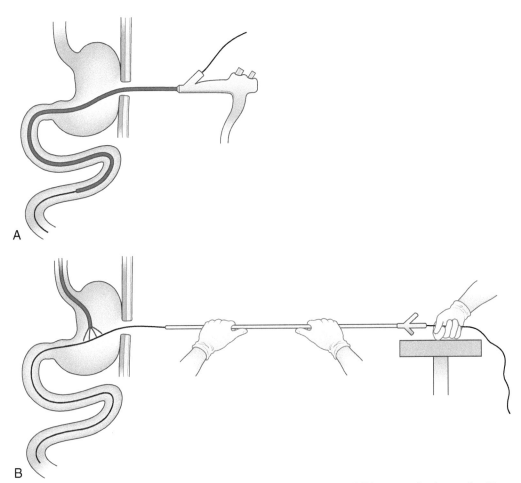

FIG 42.16 Placement of a one-piece PEGJ through a mature PEG tract. **A,** A small-caliber (< 6 mm) gastroscope is passed through the PEG stoma down below the ligament of Treitz, and the guidewire is passed further still down the jejunum. The endoscope is withdrawn off the wire. **B,** The same endoscope is passed down from the mouth or nares to the stomach to watch out for looping of the wire as the tube is passed over the wire into final position.

and subsequently passing into each successive length of bowel (moving distally) if unsuccessful.

At the beginning of the procedure, the assistant at the skin should have the anesthetic needle and syringe in one hand and the sounding needle in the other hand. As he or she visualizes an area of transillumination, a quick brief injection of the local anesthetic is followed by a quick abrupt puncture with the sounding needle. Care should be taken not to pass the sounding needle more proximally into the shaft of the endoscope. The endoscopist should place a snare through the instrument and out into the lumen, anticipating passage of the sounding needle into lumen of the small bowel (Fig. 42.19A). Once the small bowel is intubated, the sounding needle is grasped firmly with the snare and held in place by the endoscopist. The assistant at the skin then takes the trocar and passes alongside the sounding needle in the same axis to achieve intubation in the small bowel (see Fig. 42.19B). Glucagon may be given intravenously at this point to maintain a hypotonic bowel. Once the trocar is passed into the lumen of the small bowel, the snare is released from the sounding needle and repositioned on the trocar. The sounding needle is withdrawn and removed. Still holding the bowel in place with the snare affixed to the trocar, the double-stranded wire loop is passed through the trocar into the small bowel, and

the snare is slipped off the trocar, grabbing the wire loop within the lumen of the small bowel (see Fig. 42.19C). The wire is then fed through the trocar as the endoscopist removes the wire out through the stomach, esophagus, and the patient's mouth. Only at this point (see Fig. 42.19D) is further local anesthesia applied in the area of the wire, and an incision is made with the scalpel.

With the blue wire loop protruding out from the patient's mouth, the DPEJ tube is pulled down into position using the Ponsky pull technique. In comparison to the PEG (where passage of the endoscope post placement is optional), it is imperative to follow the internal bolster with the endoscope down through the stomach and small bowel into final position. The bolster has a tendency to pop down from one segment of bowel to the next. It is very difficult to confirm final position of the DPEJ by "blinded feel" alone, by measuring the distances (using the calibrated markings on the tube) between the skin and the internal bolster, or by palpating the internal bolster transabdominally with tension on the tube. Securing the end of the endoscope to the internal bolster with a snare (such as described earlier for the PEG procedure) will help facilitate this process.

Should the PEGJ tube need to be replaced because of deterioration, splitting, or shortening of the tube, an atraumatic technique should be utilized to protect the stomal tract and maintain wire

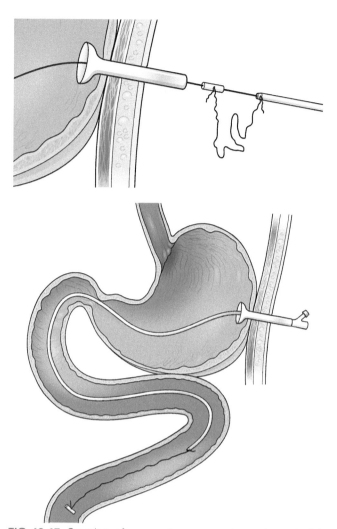

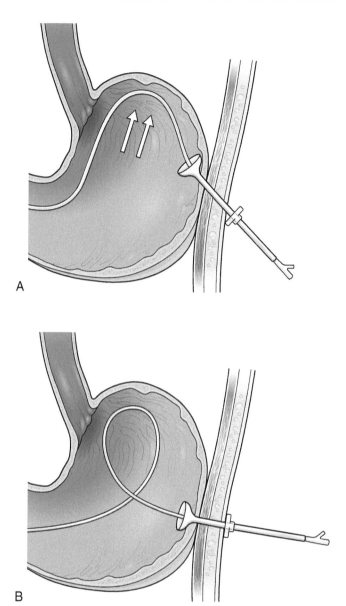

FIG 42.17 Creation of a percutaneous endoscopic gastrojejunostomy (PEGJ) anchor. A single 1-cm section of tubing is created from any tube that is roughly the same diameter as the feeding tube, which is then attached to the distal end of the feeding tube via a 20-cm silk suture. The anchor segment is preloaded on the guidewire ahead of the feeding tube and then passed down into position in the distal duodenum and proximal jejunum. After removal of the wire, the anchor will hopefully pass distally and help hold the distal tip of the jejunal extension tube in place.

FIG 42.18 Poor positioning of the jejunal extension tube after percutaneous endoscopic gastrojejunostomy (PEGJ) conversion. Poor placement is demonstrated by **A,** which shows that although the tip of the jejunal tube is well down past the stomach, the tube passes toward the gastroesophageal junction first before looping and then passing down to the pylorus. If the tube is left in this position after placement, this loop will serve to displace the tip of the jejunal tube back into the stomach. **B,** shows the jejunal extension tube looped back upon itself in the stomach following placement. Failure to correct this would also promote displacement of the tip back into the stomach.

access with the gut lumen (Fig. 42.20). The blue double-stranded wire loop is passed through the DPEJ (after cutting it down to 3 to 4 cm in length). The wire loop is grabbed by the snare (see Fig. 42.20A), which is then pulled back into the DPEJ tube (see Fig. 42.20B). A scalpel incision is made along the length of the tube (1 cm long), the snare is pulled out through the incision, and the snare wire loop is opened (see Fig. 42.20C). A "luggage tag" connection is made between the blue double-stranded wire loop and the snare wire. As the DPEJ tube stump is brought back into the bowel and out of the mouth, the blue wire loop is pulled back with it, facilitating replacement with the new DPEJ tube (see Fig. 42.20D).

POSTPROCEDURE CARE

Patient management and care of the enteral access site post placement is essentially the same for all the percutaneous

techniques. Patients are generally held nil per os (NPO) for 3 to 4 hours following initial placement, after which feeds may be initiated. Starting at a lower infusion rate of 25 mL/hr, feeds may be advanced as tolerated quickly every 6 to 12 hours such that goal infusion rate is obtained within 24 to 48 hours. For the first 7 to 10 days, a mild cleansing agent should be used once per day to clean the access site. Use of hydrogen peroxide washes or scented soaps, which contain an alcohol base, should be avoided

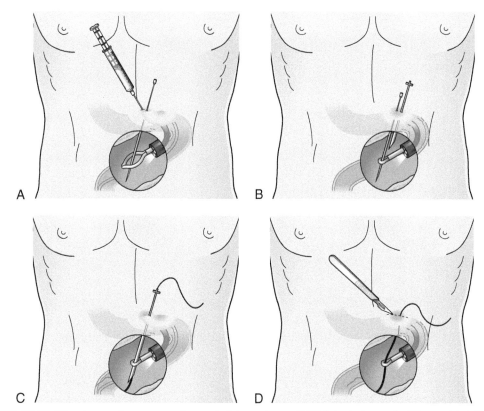

FIG 42.19 Direct percutaneous endoscopic jejunostomy (DPEJ) technique. **A,** After quick initial skin anesthesia, a 22-gauge sounding needle is passed into the small bowel and grasped with a snare passed through the operating channel of the endoscope positioned in the small bowel. **B,** While holding the sounding needle in place with the snare, the trocar is passed at the same angle into the small bowel. The snare is opened, the sounding needle is withdrawn, and the snare is transferred to the trocar. **C,** A double-stranded guidewire is then passed through the trocar, the snare is opened enough to fall back onto the wire, and then the trocar is removed. **D,** Only after the wire has been grabbed firmly by the snare should the skin incision be made over the guidewire. Once the double-stranded wire loop has been withdrawn out through the mouth, the final placement is made using the Ponsky Pull technique.

because they have a drying, desiccating effect on the tissue. Bandage dressings should be changed daily over this initial period. Four days after initial placement, the external bolster should be moved back to allow 0.5 to 1 centimeter of play between the skin and bolster. After 7 to 10 days, the frequency of dressing changes may be decreased.

ENET Complications

The most common complication of the ENET procedure is postinsertion displacement. Tubes placed intentionally in the small bowel may be displaced back into the stomach in 3.7% to 7.0% of cases.[12] Inadvertent removal of the nasoenteric tube completely occurs in 21% to 41% of patients.[13,14] Surprisingly, inadvertent removal does not always occur in a setting with the typical profile of the patient with altered mental status. Most cases of inadvertent removal involve patients with normal mental status, occurring as a result of routine nursing duties (arising from bed, transport out of the unit, physical therapy) when there has been failure to secure the tube by proper methods.[13] Securing the distal end of the nasoenteric feeding tube by using a clip (securing a suture on the tip of the tube to the intestinal mucosa) will not prevent displacement of the tube manually by the patient.

Securing the proximal end with a nasal bridle or some kind of bandage-clipping device (securing the proximal end to the skin) is needed. Displacement of nasoenteric tubes upon initial placement occurs in 0.3% to 15% of cases (mean 3% to 4%), but this is related more to blinded, bedside techniques using aspirate pH and auscultatory methods.[12,14,15] In these cases, pneumothorax, bronchopleural fistula, and even empyema (resulting from infusion of formula into the lung) may occur.[12] These latter complications do not usually occur as a result of endoscopic placement.

Additional minor complications include epistaxis, persistent gagging, knotting, breaking and kinking of the tube, or occlusion of the tube from clogging of the formula. Clogged feeding tubes are best treated with a pancreatin (Viokase) tablet crushed in warm water with bicarbonate, placed in a 10-mL syringe, and used as an irrigating solution. This has been shown in formal testing to be superior to a variety of soft drinks and papain (or meat tenderizer).[16] If the clot fails to clear with this irrigating solution alone, an endoscopic retrograde cholangiopancreatography (ERCP) catheter should be placed down through the tube to the level of the clot and infusion of the irrigating solution should be delivered directly at the site of the clot. If the clogged

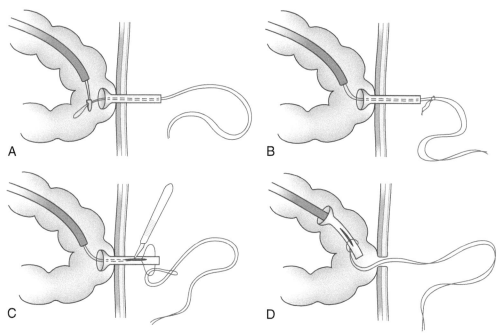

FIG 42.20 Atraumatic replacement of a DPEJ. **A,** The blue double-stranded wire loop is passed through the DPEJ (after cutting it down to 3–4 cm in length) and grabbed by the snare. **B,** The closed snare is then pulled back into the DPEJ tube. **C,** A scalpel incision is made along the length of the DPEJ tube (1 cm long), and the snare is pulled out through the incision. The snare wire loop is opened and a "luggage tag" connection is made between the blue double-stranded wire loop and the snare wire. **D,** As the DPEJ tube stump is brought back into the bowel and out the mouth, the blue wire loop is pulled back with it, facilitating replacement with the new DPEJ tube.

tube persists, further efforts to clear the clot may be accomplished by a mechanical declogging device such as an endoscopy brush or spiral-shaped mechanical declogger that can actually be rotated or screwed through the obstruction.

Sinusitis is a complication of prolonged nasoenteric tube placement, and should be a consideration in patients with such tubes who develop an unexplained fever. The incidence of sinusitis based on opacification of sinuses on radiograph or CT scan tends to be overreported at approximately 25%, whereas needle puncture and culture of effluent from the sinuses more accurately places the incidence at approximately 11.4%.[17] Esophageal stricture is a theoretical complication of long-standing nasoenteric tubes, but the incidence is not clear and is probably underreported. A long-standing nasal bridle, in place for greater than 1 to 2 months' duration, may erode through the nasal septum.

PEG Complications

Reports from the literature of overall complications related to PEG placement indicate that this minimally invasive procedure has low morbidity and negligible mortality.[18,19] Two large series published 15 to 20 years ago showed that the incidence of minor complications ranged from 4.9% to 13%, with major complications ranging from 1.3% to 3%.[18,19] Mortality in these two large series was only 0.2% to 1.0%.[18,19] Two other large series (2001) duplicated these results, showing that the rate of minor complications ranged from 10.3% to 10.7%, with major complications ranging from 1.0% to 2.4%.[20,21] There was no mortality in these more recent series. Minor complications described in these reports include peristomal wound infections, tube disintegration, clogging,

leakage, prolonged ileus, late inadvertent extubation, subcostal neuralgia, laceration of the left lobe of the liver, and delayed closure following removal. Major complications reported include aspiration, peritonitis, early premature removal, tumor implantation at the PEG site, buried bumper syndrome, gastrocolocutaneous fistula, necrotizing fasciitis, and hemorrhage.[18–21]

A benign pneumoperitoneum occurs in up to 40% of cases following routine PEG placement.[22] In the absence of peritoneal signs (e.g., rebound tenderness), this finding is innocuous and does not preclude feeding within 4 hours of tube placement. Pneumoperitoneum may or may not be accompanied by a large, air-filled, distended stomach, which can easily be decompressed by uncapping the newly placed PEG tube.[23] Prolonged ileus following PEG placement was described in 1% of patients in one large series.[21]

The incidence of aspiration following PEG placement is difficult to determine because of varying definitions (witnessed aspiration event vs. new infiltrate on chest radiograph vs. aspiration of gastric contents labeled with a radioisotope or fluoroscopic colorimetric microspheres). The risk of aspiration immediately related to the procedure of PEG placement itself has been reported to be less than 1% of cases,[18,24] and is thought to be related to oversedation, overinflation of the stomach, and performing the procedure in the supine position. Aspiration as a long-term complication of PEG placement has been reported in up to 18% of cases.[25] In one small prospective study, patients randomized to PEG placement had lower gastroesophageal reflux (as measured by 24-hour pH monitoring) compared to patients randomized to nasogastric feeding.[26] Risk for aspiration long term is related to patient age (older than 70 years), reduced level of consciousness, history of neuromuscular disease, delayed gastric emptying, endotracheal intubation, trauma to the abdomen or pelvis, bolus versus continuous feeds, and nursing care.[27,28] Risk for aspiration increases fourfold when patients are moved from the ICU (low patient-to-nurse ratio) out to the medical or surgical floor (high ratio).[27] These studies reporting aspiration post-PEG placement do not usually differentiate aspiration of contaminated oropharyngeal secretions from regurgitation and aspiration of contaminated gastric contents. Three studies would suggest that the aspiration of contaminated oropharyngeal secretions is at least an equivalent if not greater factor in colonizing the trachea and upper-respiratory tree than aspiration of bacteria-laden gastric contents.[29–31] Poor oral health has been well defined as an additional risk factor for aspiration in patients on tube feeding.[32]

Buried bumper syndrome is an underreported complication ranging from ulceration underneath the internal bolster to total erosion of the PEG tube out through the gastric and abdominal wall. It most often occurs as a result of excessive tension between the external and internal bolster, but additional predisposing factors include smaller, stiffer internal bolsters (made from silicone compared to polyurethane), presence of malnutrition or poor wound healing, or a significant weight gain in response to feeding.[24] Buried bumper syndrome may present simply as increased leakage around the PEG, infection at the PEG site, immobility of the catheter, resistance to infusion, or abdominal pain occurring with infusion of formula.[23,24,33,34] A wide variety of techniques are described in the literature to manage this complication. Usually the PEG tube has to be removed either by pulling it back into the stomach and out through the mouth or pulling it out through the abdominal wall. In patients where the PEG tube has not been used from several weeks to months, the internal bolster may be completely buried within the gastric and abdominal wall. In this situation, a needle-knife thermocoagulation catheter may be required to cut down to the bolster to facilitate removal.[33]

Gastrocolocutaneous fistulas may occur because of inadvertent puncture of an overlying loop of bowel at the time of initial placement, or as a delayed complication occurring because of migration or erosion of the tube over time into the colon.[24,35] Insufficient translumination, inadequate gastric insufflation at the time of initial placement, or previous abdominal surgery in which a loop of bowel may be tacked down by scar tissue are all risk factors increasing the likelihood for this complication.[23,24] Gastrocolocutaneous fistula may present acutely with peritonitis, infection, fasciitis, or obstruction to flow from infusion of the formula. More often it occurs chronically, presenting after several months with either stool appearing around the PEG tube or as insidious diarrhea in which the stool has the appearance of formula identical to that infused into the PEG. Frequently, this complication is not identified until the tube is removed and stool appears at the ostomy site. This complication is managed by first documenting the complication with radiographic contrast studies. Surprisingly, it is managed fairly easily by simply removing the PEG, placing a bandage over the defect, and allowing the site to heal. Operative takedown is only required if the fistula fails to close.[23,24]

PEG site infection is one of the most common complications of PEG placement. Risk for developing PEG site infection is related to patient factors (e.g., diabetes, obesity, malnutrition, or chronic use of steroids), factors involving technique (pull or push type PEGs vs. introducer PEGs, small incisions, and lack

of antibiotic prophylaxis), and nursing care (excessive traction on the bolsters). The incidence of wound infection around the PEG site ranges from 5.4% to 17.0%,[25,36,37] but the majority (more than 70%) are minor in degree.[38] Antibiotic prophylaxis at the time of initial placement is an important measure to reduce the incidence of this complication. In an older study, a single dose of antibiotic prophylaxis at the time of placement reduced the incidence of PEG site infection from 32% down to 7% ($p < 0.05$).[39] In a more recent (1999) study, a single dose of one or two antibiotics at the time of placement reduced the incidence of PEG site infection significantly from 13.2% to 0.5% compared to controls receiving no antibiotic prophylaxis ($p < 0.01$).[38] Patients already on concurrent antibiotics do not need additional prophylaxis at the time of PEG placement.[40] If infection develops around the PEG site, usually intravenous antibiotics and local wound care are sufficient to correct the complication. Surgical incision and drainage are rarely required. Actual peritonitis occurs less frequently in 0.4% to 1.5% of cases,[18,24,35,41] and is differentiated from simple PEG site infection by the development of peritoneal signs and rebound tenderness. Again, prompt broad-spectrum intravenous antibiotics are usually sufficient. But in the presence of peritonitis, contrast studies should be performed to rule out the presence of a leak. If there is leakage into the peritoneum, then surgical intervention is required.[24]

Hemorrhage is a rare complication involving less than 2.5% of cases.[24,35] A variety of etiologic factors may contribute to this complication, including direct puncture of a blood vessel or traumatic tearing of the esophagus or stomach upon initial placement, concomitant peptic ulcer disease, development of gastric ulcer underneath the internal bolster, or erosion of the posterior gastric wall opposite from the internal bolster of the PEG tube.[24,35] Management involves urgent endoscopy to document the source and appropriate steps to achieve hemostasis.

Leakage around the PEG site is reported in only 1% to 2% of cases,[21,41] but this probably represents underreporting of the incidence of this complication. Etiologic factors include corrosive agents (vitamin C ascorbic acid infused with formula, increased gastric acid arising from stop orders for prescribed acid-reducing agents, and continued hydrogen peroxide washes of the site following initial placement), cutaneous fungal infection around the site, development of granulation tissue, side-torsion on the tube creating ulceration on one wall of the tract, absence of an external bolster (allowing to-and-fro motion of the PEG tube through the tract), buried bumper syndrome, and PEG site infection. Management again depends on defining the exacerbating factors, which can usually be ascertained by careful examination of the PEG site. Initial physical exam should rule out PEG site infection, confirm there is no fixation of the tube (suggesting buried bumper syndrome), and make sure there is no ulceration of the tract indicating side-torsion. The patient's list of medications should be reviewed, a proton pump inhibitor should be added if this agent has not been ordered, ascorbic acid should be stopped, and consideration should be given to providing an antifungal cream or zinc oxide to the site. Side-torsion creating ulceration in the tract may require stabilization of the PEG tube with a vertical clamp (which prevents side-to-side motion). Granulation tissue around the PEG site may be treated with silver nitrate sticks. Options for those cases where there is no external bolster include replacing the PEG tube with a commercial replacement PEG set that contains an external bolster, or creating a homemade external bolster from the funneled end of a Foley catheter. PEG site infection should be treated, as should existence of the buried bumper syndrome according to previously described methods. The tract may be damaged to the point that diverting the stream of infused formula down into the small bowel (by converting the PEG to a PEGJ) or completely removing the PEG tube and placing a nasoenteric aspirate/feed tube to allow the site to heal may be required in more severe cases.

Accidental extubation of the PEG tube occurs in anywhere from 1.6% to 4.4% of cases, half of which occur prematurely prior to complete maturation of the PEG site.[20,25,35,37,42] Normally the PEG site should mature over 7 to 10 days, at which point the gastric wall becomes fused to the anterior abdominal wall. Maturation of the PEG tract may be delayed up to 4 weeks in the presence of chronic steroid use, malnutrition, or ascites. Management is surprisingly simple, as long as no peritonitis is present.[35] The patient may be brought back down to the endoscopy suite immediately, and a new PEG may be placed through the same site on the abdominal wall (although there is no need to pass through the same site on the gastric wall). The placement of the trocar should be done quickly to avoid prolonged insufflation and a large pneumoperitoneum. If this strategy is unsuccessful, a nasogastric (NG) tube can be placed for decompression, a broad-spectrum antibiotic should be started, and the PEG may be replaced later within 7 to 10 days. Only if peritonitis develops is surgical intervention required.[35] Once the PEG tract is mature, simple bedside replacement with a PEG tube (or endoscopic placement if the site closes down) may be sufficient.

Less common complications of PEG placement include tumor implantation at the PEG site, development of a broncoesophageal fistula, migration of the internal balloon bolster causing gastric outlet obstruction at the level of the pylorus, reversible apnea, subcostal neuralgia, and development of a gastroileocutaneous fistula.[20,43–47]

PEGJ AND DPEJ COMPLICATIONS

For obvious reasons, patients requiring placement of a PEGJ are at risk for all the complications previously described for placement of a routine PEG tube. The most common additional problem encountered with PEGJ tubes is inadvertent migration of the jejunal tube from the small bowel back into the stomach, which occurs in 27% to 42% of cases.[48–50] A number of factors contribute to this complication, including a large dilated atonic stomach, failure to cut the PEG tube down to a shortened length, insufficient length of the jejunal tube, placement of the initial PEG high in the stomach, surgical PEG placement (in which the PEG tube is tunneled in a direction that points toward the gastroesophageal junction), as well as recurrent nausea and vomiting. Steps that can be taken at the time of initial placement to reduce this complication include positioning the PEG tube immediately above and to the right of the umbilicus so that the entrance is in the gastric antrum, cutting the PEG tube down to approximately 10 cm in length, selecting a jejunal tube with the greatest length, and making sure that there is no loop in the stomach as the jejunal tube passes from the PEG to the pylorus. As mentioned earlier in the section on technique of PEGJ placement, securing the distal end to the intestinal mucosa with a clip or placement of an anchor device may help hold the jejunal tube in place for a brief period.

Complications arising from DPEJ placement differ very little from those encountered by routine PEG placement. Of note is the fact that a jejunocolocutaneous fistula may occur. Intermittent small bowel obstruction may occur when a larger balloon-type internal bolster is selected for the procedure. Volvulus leading to necrotic bowel has been described with DPEG.[51]

CONCLUSION

Multidisciplinary nutrition teams across the country are pressured to obtain early enteral access, as the weight of the literature shows that early use of the gut and maintenance of gut integrity significantly improves patient outcome. These teams rely on a skilled endoscopist to obtain enteral access, monitor enteral tube feeding, and help troubleshoot problems when the issue of intolerance arises. When a short-term nasoenteric feeding is required, or more long-term percutaneous access is needed, a variety of techniques exist for almost any patient situation. Under each category of access, the endoscopist should learn one main technique well, and then experiment enough with other techniques to know which one suits him or her best. Proper choice of instrument, correct accessory devices, and selection of the appropriate technique for the individual patient needs should optimize the chances for success and minimize the risk of complications when performing endoscopic procedures to obtain enteral access.

KEY REFERENCES

1. McClave SA, Heyland DK: The physiologic response and associated clinical benefits from provision of early enteral nutrition, *Nutr Clin Pract* 24:305–315, 2009.
2. Jabbar A, Chang WK, Dryden GW, McClave SA: Gut immunology and the differential response to feeding and starvation, *Nutr Clin Pract* 18:461–482, 2003.
3. McClave SA, Martindale RG, Rice TW, Heyland DK: Feeding the critically ill patient, *Crit Care Med* 42(12):2600–2610, 2014.
4. Patel C, Omer E, Diamond SJ, McClave SA: Can nutritional assessment tools predict response to nutritional therapy? *Curr Gastroenterol Rep* 18:15–19, 2016.
5. McClave SA, DiBaise JK, Mullin G, Martindale RG: ACG clinical guideline: nutrition therapy in the adult hospitalized patient, *Am J Gastroenterol* 111(3):315–334, 2016.
6. Lewis SJ, Andersen HK, Thomas S: Early enteral nutrition within 24 h of intestinal surgery versus later commencement of feeding: a systematic review and meta-analysis, *J Gastrointest Surg* 13(3):569–575, 2009.
9. Heyland DK, Drover JW, MacDonald S, et al: Effect of postpyloric feeding on gastroesophageal regurgitation and pulmonary microaspiration: results of a randomized controlled trial, *Crit Care Med* 29:1495–1501, 2001.
11. McClave SA, Taylor BE, Martindale RG, et al: Guidelines for the provision and assessment of nutrition support therapy in the adult critically ill patient: Society of Critical Care Medicine (SCCM) and American Society for Parenteral and Enteral Nutrition (A.S.P.E.N.), *JPEN J Parenter Enteral Nutr* 40(2):159–211, 2016.
12. Levy H: Nasogastric and nasoenteric feeding tubes, *Gastrointest Endosc Clin N Am* 8:529–550, 1998.
13. McClave SA, Sexton LK, Spain DA, et al: Enteral tube feeding in the intensive care unit: factors impeding adequate delivery, *Crit Care Med* 27(7):1252–1256, 1999.
18. Larson DE, Burton DD, Schroeder KW, et al: Percutaneous endoscopic gastrostomy: indications, success, complications, and mortality in 314 consecutive patients, *Gastroenterology* 93:48–52, 1987.
19. Grant JP: Percutaneous endoscopic gastrostomy, *Ann Surg* 217:168–174, 1993.
20. Rimon E: The safety and feasibility of percutaneous endoscopic gastrostomy placement by a single physician, *Endoscopy* 33(3):241–244, 2001.

21. Lin HS, Ibrahim HZ, Kheng JW, et al: Percutaneous endoscopic gastrostomy: strategies for prevention and management of complications, *Laryngoscope* 111(10):1847–1852, 2001.
23. Baskin WN: Enteral access techniques, *Gastroenterologist* 4:S40, 1996.
24. Safidi BY, Marks JM, Ponsky JL: Percutaneous endoscopy gastrostomy, *Gastrointest Endosc Clin N Am* 8:551–558, 1998.
28. McClave SA, DeMeo MT, DeLegge MH, et al: North American summit on aspiration in the critically ill patient: consensus statement, *JPEN J Parenter Enteral Nutr* 26(Suppl 6):S80–S85, 2002.
29. Pingleton SK, Hinthorn DR, Liu C: Enteral nutrition in patients receiving mechanical ventilation. Multiple sources of tracheal colonization include the stomach, *Am J Med* 80(5):827–832, 1986.
30. Torres A, el-Ebiary M, Gonzalez J, et al: Gastric and pharyngeal flora in nosocomial pneumonia acquired during mechanical ventilation, *Am Rev Respir Dis* 148(2):352–357, 1993.
31. Bonten MJ, Gaillard CA, van Tiel FH, et al: The stomach is not a source for colonization of the upper respiratory tract and pneumonia in ICU patients, *Chest* 105(3):878–884, 1994.
35. Schapiro GD, Edmundowicz SA: Complications of percutaneous endoscopic gastrostomy, *Gastrointest Endosc Clin N Am* 6:409–422, 1996.
36. Lockett MA, Templeton ML, Byrne TK, Norcross ED: Percutaneous endoscopic gastrostomy complications in a tertiary-care center, *Am Surg* 68(2):117–120, 2002.
37. Dwyer KM, Watts DD, Thurber JS, et al: Percutaneous endoscopic gastrostomy: the preferred method of elective feeding tube placement in trauma patients, *J Trauma* 52(1):26–32, 2002.
39. Jain NK, Larson DE, Schroeder KW, et al: Antibiotic prophylaxis for percutaneous endoscopic gastrostomy, *Ann Intern Med* 107:824–828, 1987.
42. Galat SA, Gerig KD, Porter JA, Slezak FA: Management of premature removal of the percutaneous endoscopic gastrostomy, *Am Surg* 56:733–736, 1990.

A complete reference list can be found online at ExpertConsult.com

43

Endoscopic Techniques for Weight Loss

Daniel Blero and Jacques Devière

CHAPTER OUTLINE

INTRODUCTION

Obesity is the pandemic of the 21st century and is associated with considerable morbidity and mortality.[1] Management of obesity depends on body mass index (BMI) and the presence of comorbidities, including heart disease, diabetes, hypertension, dyslipidemia, osteoarthritis, and sleep apnea.[2] Approximately 1.6 billion adults are overweight; at least 400 million adults are obese. The World Health Organization projected that by 2015, approximately 2.3 billion adults would be overweight, and more than 700 million would be obese. Previously considered a problem only in high-income countries, the number of overweight and obese individuals is now dramatically increasing in low- and middle-income countries, particularly in urban settings.[3]

At the present time, surgery is the only effective therapy for morbid obesity, defined as a BMI of 40 kg/m^2 or more, or as a BMI of 35 kg/m^2 or more in the presence of comorbidities.[4] Bariatric surgery has been shown to be effective in the long-term and significantly reduces the risk of mortality associated with morbid obesity. In the United States, the indications for bariatric surgery increased by 80% during the period 1998–2004.[5]

Bariatric surgery induces and maintains satisfactory weight loss while decreasing comorbidities in the overweight patient.[6] Efficacy varies with the type of procedure, which can be divided into restrictive (lap band, sleeve gastrectomy), malabsorptive (biliopancreatic diversion), or a combination of both (gastric bypass). Although very effective, laparoscopic and surgical bariatric procedures have complication rates of 3% to 20% and mortality rates of 1%.[7] Cardiopulmonary events and anastomotic leaks are the major sources of severe morbidities.

The demand for less invasive therapy for obesity led to the development of endoscopic technologies, potentially characterized by less invasiveness and fewer complications. Endoluminal surgery, performed entirely through a natural orifice, offers this potential for a less invasive weight loss procedure, possibly performed on an ambulatory basis, and might find its place in the current armamentarium for morbid obesity treatment, extending indications for treatment to patients with severe comorbidities and

older age and even to non–morbidly obese patients. We review the various endoluminal techniques that are either in routine use or in clinical evaluation and address the role of endoscopy in management of weight regain occurring after bariatric surgery.

ENDOSCOPIC OPTIONS FOR ENDOLUMINAL PRIMARY TREATMENT OF OBESITY

Similar to surgical procedures, the different options for endoluminal treatment of obesity can be divided between restrictive and malabsorptive procedures (Table 43.1).

Restrictive Procedures
Intragastric Balloons
The use of a fluid-filled intragastric balloon to induce weight loss in obese patients was first described in 1982.[8] Since then, numerous intragastric balloons have been in use worldwide, and several have been withdrawn from the market. The BioEnterics Intragastric Balloon (BIB; Allergan, Irvine, CA) or ORBERA (Apollo Endosurgery, Austin, TX) has a spherical shape and larger capacity than earlier models and has been the most extensively used device. Among the more recently improved minimally invasive procedures, the intragastric balloon has been one temporary nonsurgical option that can promote weight loss in obese patients by partially filling their stomach and inducing a sense of early satiety.[9,10] One of the major drawbacks of balloon implantation is weight regain after balloon removal. Two early studies help clinicians better understand what can be expected from balloon implantation.

In the first study, Mathus-Vliegen and Tytgat (2005)[11] included patients who had participated in a randomized controlled trial (RCT) comparing a balloon with a sham for a 3-month period in an additional trial which involved 9 months of balloon treatment and follow-up for 1 year after removal. The authors excluded 8 patients who had not met the weight loss goal during the first 3 months (5 patients) or who did not tolerate the balloon (3 patients). Although there was no difference between the sham and balloon during the first 3 months, after 1 year of balloon

TABLE 43.1 Available Bariatric Endotherapy Technology

Endoscopic Procedures	Mechanism	Human Applications	Limitations
Intragastric balloon	Restrictive	Prospective crossover study; > 2000 cases reported	Patient tolerance Limited effect (6 mo)
Endoluminal vertical gastroplasty	Restrictive	One prospective study (64 patients)	Long-term efficacy Depth of suture
Transoral gastroplasty	Restrictive	Multiple human studies (> 150 patients), multicentric RCT completed unpublished	Long-term outcomes Complications
Endoscopic sleeve gastroplasty	Restrictive	Large postmarketing studies (> 200 patients), no prospective evaluation with ITT analysis	Long-term outcomes Patients selection biases
Endoluminal suturing device	Restrictive	Limited human study (11 patients) Universal triangulation platform Use of stitches; transmural stitching	Long-term efficacy
POSE	Restrictive	Two prospective studies (n = 161 patients)	Long-term efficacy Intraprocedural drop out of patients
Aspiration therapy	Malabsorptive	11 + 25 patients treated	Adherence to protocol Parietal complications
DJBS	Malabsorptive	12 patients investigated	Patient tolerance Long-term safety and efficacy Reversibility Liver abscesses
Gastroduodenojejunal bypass sleeve	Restrictive & malabsorptive	13 patients investigated	Tolerance at the level of the cuff inserted at the cardia Long-term efficacy

DJBS, duodenojejunal bypass sleeve.

treatment, a mean weight loss of 21.3 kg (17.1%) was achieved in all patients; 12.6 kg (9.9%) was maintained at the end of the second balloon-free year. Overall, 47% of patients sustained a 10% weight loss at the end of 2 years of follow-up. Although this study did not show an independent benefit of balloon treatment beyond diet, exercise, and behavioral therapy in the first treatment, balloon treatment for 1 year, in the patients who tolerated the treatment, resulted in substantial weight loss, a significant part of which was maintained during the first year after removal of the balloon.[11]

The second study looked at the long-term outcome after treatment with an intragastric balloon for 6 months, with no structured weight maintenance program after balloon removal. After BIB placement, 100 consecutive morbidly obese individuals were prospectively followed; 97 patients completed the final follow-up at a mean of 4.8 years. After 6 months, 63% of patients had more than 10% baseline weight loss, whereas there were only 28% at final follow-up. At that time, 35 patients had undergone bariatric surgery, and 34 patients had no significant weight change from baseline.[12]

Finally, a 2015 systematic review and meta-analysis performed by the American Society for Gastrointestinal Endoscopy (ASGE) Bariatric Endoscopy Task Force demonstrated that an intragastric balloon results in 25.4% of excess weight loss (EWL) and 11.3% of total weight loss 1 year after balloon insertion (6 months after balloon removal).[13] The main side effects consisted in upper gastrointestinal (GI) complaints (abdominal pain and nausea), which were responsible for early removal in approximately 7.5% of patients. Serious adverse events are rare, including 0.1% with GI perforation and 1.4% with balloon migration.[13]

Different technical modifications of the fluid-filled balloons have been brought to potentially improve its efficacy, tolerance, or safety profile. Currently, however, none of these have been

proven to be superior.[14] The Spatz adjustable Balloon system (Spatz FGIA, Inc., New York, NY) has an extractable inflation tube for adjustment after initial filling either in case of intolerance or decreased efficacy. It has been associated with specific complications related to catheter impaction requiring surgical extraction. However, it is approved for 1 year implantation and, in a case-controlled study that required adjustment in 22.5% of patients, had an efficacy similar to 2 consecutive BIBs left for the same period, with a similar tolerance and safety profile (Video 43.1).[15] The ReShape Duo (ReShape, San Clemente, CA) is the second intragastric balloon approved by the Food and Drug Administration (FDA). It consists of two separately attached filled balloons (450 mL each). In the REDUCE pivotal FDA trial (a prospective, randomized controlled pivotal trial of a dual intragastric balloon for the treatment of obesity), which enrolled 326 patients,[16] patients treated with Duo achieved significantly more weight loss than those with diet and exercise alone (27.9% vs. 11.3% EWL). Gastric ulcerations at removal were reported in 10% of cases. In Europe, the high cost of this device limits its clinical use.

Air/gas-filled balloons have been proposed as an alternative to classic fluid-filled balloons. The Heliosphere BAG balloon (Helioscopie, Vienne, France) was reported as having a similar efficacy to the BIB, with possibly less discomfort.[17] However, a high rate of spontaneous deflation, the absence of a marker allowing early identification of a possible rupture, and technical difficulties in its positioning have limited its routine use.

Other gas-filled balloons can be swallowed without the need for endoscopy but still require endoscopy for removal (Obalon Therapeutics, Carlsbad, CA), and some are even designed to be swallowed as a pill and inflated in the stomach, and contain a resorbable valve, which would allow spontaneous deflation and uneventful migration (Allurion Technologies, Inc., Wellesley,

MA). However, the clinical data available with these techniques are currently insufficient to make any recommendation on their use.[18,19]

In summary, balloon implantation may be helpful for long-term weight loss in select patients. It is a potential option for patients who are unwilling to undergo bariatric surgery or who are not suitable candidates for bariatric surgery. Balloon implantation could also be used as a temporary measure in superobese patients to induce weight loss and decrease the risk of complications associated with further bariatric surgery.[20]

Suturing/Stapling Procedures

Another group of endoscopic procedures aims to offer a long-lasting reduction of gastric volume and decrease the distensibility of the stomach by suturing or stapling techniques. This endoluminal transoral restrictive surgery includes several techniques, the first one (EndoCinch) being performed with a device initially designed for treatment of gastroesophageal reflux disease (GERD).

Endoluminal vertical gastroplasty. The EndoCinch suturing system (C.R. Bard, Murray Hill, NJ) was initially designed for endoscopic treatment of GERD. This system allows the placement of a series of stitches in the lower esophagus to create a pleat at the level of the lower sphincter. Although associated with encouraging early results, use of the EndoCinch for the treatment of GERD has been called into question because of the lack of retention of plications in the long term.[21]

The device was then used to restrict the gastric cavity. The technique utilizes the deployment of seven sutures in a continuous and cross-linked fashion from the proximal fundus to the distal body. Again, despite initial encouraging results,[22] the latest development of the device (RESTORe Suturing system [Bard/Davol, Warwick, RI]), theoretically capable of full-thickness tissue apposition, found that sutures were not durable over time, leading to a lack of effectiveness.[23]

Transoral gastroplasty. Transoral gastroplasty (TOGa System; Satiety, Inc., Palo Alto, CA) used the first endoscopic stapling device to create a full-thickness plication in the proximal stomach with a strictly endoluminal approach.

The system consisted of the TOGa Sleeve Stapler, a flexible 18-mm diameter shaft device, which rides over a guidewire for introduction, and accommodates a standard endoscope up to 8.6 mm in diameter. It created full-thickness plications of the anterior and posterior walls of the stomach, which are acquired using vacuum pots located parallel to the staple line (Fig. 43.1).

Two successive human pilot series[24,25] reported a mean EWL of 16%, 23%, and 25% at 1, 3, and 6 months, respectively, with the first design of the instrument, and 19%, 34%, and 46% at 1, 3, and 6 months, respectively, after some technical modifications. No severe adverse events were reported. A 1-year follow-up on a larger multicenter European study involving 53 patients has confirmed these data, with an EWL at 12 months of 39% in morbidly obese patients.[26] Although the technique was performed under general anesthesia, recovery was very fast, and the procedure could be performed within 30 to 45 minutes on an outpatient basis, suggesting that this technique might become an interesting first step for bariatric treatment strategy. A multicenter randomized sham-controlled study was performed in 11 centers comparing the active and sham procedure (2:1 ratio) in a series of more than 300 patients. This RCT showed significant but modest differences between the two groups, with two severe complications. The FDA required additional data. Due to a shortage of financing, the company closed and sold its assets. Interestingly, the company

that acquired these assets refused to provide the clinical data for publication of this RCT.

Endoscopic Sleeve Gastroplasty

The Overstitch device (Apollo Endosurgery, Austin, TX) is an FDA-approved suturing device able to place full-thickness stitches across the gastric wall. Placement of multiple stitches from the antrum to the fundus is performed to reproduce a kind of restriction comparable to a sleeve gastrectomy. The first study published reported a mean percentage EWL of 54% and 21 kg of total weight loss at 1-year postprocedure in 22 patients out of 25 (3 dropped out).[27] During the follow-up, 1 patient underwent an additional intervention due to the loosening of the stitches. Interestingly, no major side effects were noted. A more recent study (2016) reported on 91 patients with a BMI above 30 treated in an open-access environment.[28] The authors reported a total body weight loss (TBWL) of 17.6% at 12 months, with a 76% follow-up rate and improvement of comorbidities. Only 1 severe complication (perigastric leak) occurred and was managed conservatively. Further data are needed to determine the long-term benefits of this technique.

Primary obesity surgery endoluminal. Using their Incisionless Operating Platform (USGI Medical, San Clemente, CA), the primary obesity surgery endoluminal (POSE) procedure places anchoring structures across the gastric wall, introducing an area of transmural plications within the corpus and the fundus, up to the gastroesophageal junction. Lopez-Nava et al (2015)[29] enrolled 147 patients in a prospective study over 1 year, with a highly controlled behavioral and nutritional follow-up. Thirty-one patients were lost to follow-up. In the 119 remaining patients, a mean of 44% EWL (15 kg of total weight loss) was observed without any serious adverse event.[29] A sham-controlled trial involving 332 patients (ESSENTIAL) has also been conducted. Results indicated 4.9% TBWL in the treatment arm and 1.38% in controls. The mean percent change in TBWL was 3.6 times greater in the active treatment group. The response rates were 41.6% for the active arm and 22% in the sham arm. However, the study did not reach its primary endpoint, which was defined as 5% TBWL at 12 months.[30]

Endoluminal suturing device. More recently, Huberty et al (2016) reported the use of a new triangulation platform and endoscopic stitchers (Endo tools SA[ETT], Gosselies, Belgium), with which they could perform multiple double transmural plicatures along the greater curvature of the stomach to create a restrictive gastroplasty (Videos 43.2 and 43.3). No severe adverse events were recorded for the first 11 obese patients treated. The percentage of EWL was 41% at 6 months.[31] Again, broader experience and long-term technical and clinical outcomes will be necessary.

Articulating circular endoscopic (ACE) stapling procedure. The ACE stapling device (Boston Scientific, Marlborough, MA) is a rotatable device allowing eight plications at the level of the fundus, reducing the proximal gastric volume. In a pilot study, the investigators also added two plications at the level of the antrum. At 1 year of follow-up, plications persisted and the median EWL was 34.9%.[32]

Malabsorptive Procedures

Aspiration Therapy

This procedure is based on a well-known endoscopic tool adapted for the purpose of inducing weight loss. It requires the implantation of a 30-Fr gastrostomy tube, called an *A-tube*, in obese

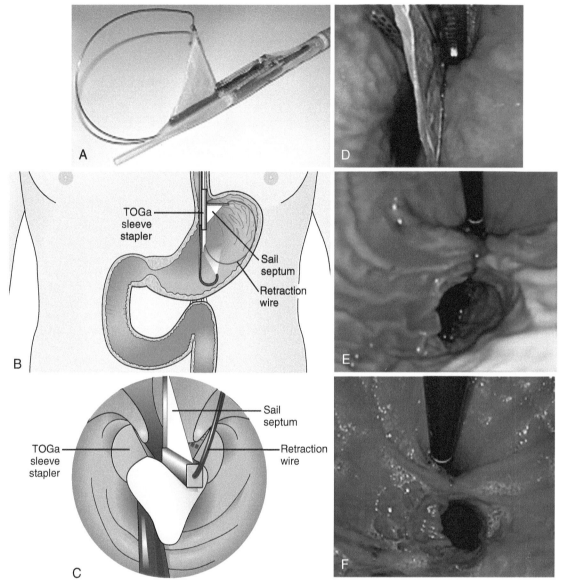

FIG 43.1 **A** to **F,** Transoral gastroplasty procedure.

patients. The patient uses it 20 minutes after ingestion, to aspire 30% of each meal. The system is called the Aspire Assist (Aspire Bariatrics, King of Prussia, PA). There are two studies published. In the latest and largest one, including 22 out of 25 patients, mean EWL was 40.8% and TBWL was 14.8% after 6 months of use. Three patients dropped out because of time constraints (the system involves the evacuation of food three times daily). No nutritional deficiencies were reported.[33] A pivotal multicenter randomized study is ongoing in the United States.

Duodenojejunal Bypass Liner or EndoBarrier Device

The bypass technique has to be considered in line with the development of metabolic surgery and, particularly, with the clinical observation that bypassing the proximal bowel improves type 2 diabetes and induces weight loss, a feature that partly explains the greater improvement of diabetes observed in patients undergoing a laparoscopic Roux-en-Y gastric bypass (RYGB) for weight loss compared with a purely restrictive procedure.[34]

The first strictly endoluminal device used to bypass the proximal small intestine is the duodenojejunal bypass liner, also called the EndoBarrier (GI Dynamics, Watertown, MA). It is composed of a self-expanding implant that is placed in the duodenum and has antimigration features. It is attached to a 60-cm plastic sleeve that extends into the proximal jejunum and works by creating a physical barrier between food that has been ingested and the intestinal wall and biliopancreatic secretions (Fig. 43.2). The device is left in place for a maximum of 3 to 6 months and is removed with a dedicated and relatively easy system.

Three RCTs including 174 patients (90 received the EndoBarrier and 84 were the control arm) have been scrutinized by the ASGE Bariatric Endoscopy Task Force. This analysis demonstrated no statistical difference in terms of weight loss (%EWL) at 12 months after EndoBarrier insertion. On the other hand, this meta-analysis found a persistent effect 12 months after implantation on glycated hemoglobin, which had dropped by 1% (93 patients, 52 treated and 41 controls). More importantly, they

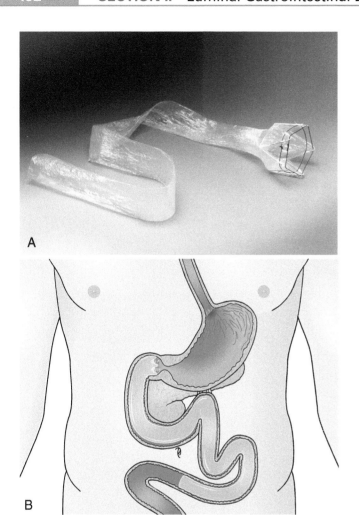

FIG 43.2 A, Duodenojejunal sleeve. **B,** Schematic representation of the sleeve in place in the proximal jejunum. (**A,** Used with permission of GI Dynamics, Inc., Lexington, MA.)

also reported that the rate of early retrieval for intolerance of the device was as high as 18%.[35] In 2016, authors from Denmark found a modest effect of the EndoBarrier on weight loss, but did not find any glycemic improvement.[36] Finally, a 2015 report of liver abscesses (4 out of 325 patients) complicating the insertion of the EndoBarrier in the pivotal RCT in the United States precluded the actual development of the device.[37]

Gastroduodenojejunal Bypass Sleeve

The gastroduodenojejunal bypass sleeve is another implantable device, potentially mimicking more closely RYGB (Valentx Inc., Carpinteria, CA). A plastic cuff with a 120-cm long sleeve is implanted endoscopically and laparoscopically at the level of the cardia. It reproduces not only the restrictive component of the surgical RYGB in its proximal part but also the malabsorptive component by ensuring that food has no contact with the bile and chyme coming from the papilla. This device was prospectively implanted in 12 patients. Early removal was necessary in 2 of them secondary to intolerance. Among the 10 remaining patients, the cuff partially detached from the cardia in 4. This detachment was presumed to explain a lower weight loss in that group of patients. Finally, the percentage of EWL at 1 year in the study was 36%. Interestingly, all comorbidities improved during the 12 months of the trial.[38]

Other Procedures
Electrical Stimulation

Gastric electric stimulation can induce food intake reduction and gastroparesis, as well as modulate appetite-regulatory hormones. The Tantalusmeal activated device (MetaCure USA Inc., Orangeburg, NY) consists of 3 pairs of electrodes connected to a pulse generator that only delivers stimulation when eating starts. In a pilot study of 11 patients, an absolute weight loss of 5.3 kg and an improvement of diabetes control was reported after 6 months.[39]

Injections: Botulinum Toxin

Injection of botulinum toxin A (BoTox) into the gastric wall induces local and temporary paralysis of the muscle, which inhibits

TABLE 43.2 **Available Intragastric Balloons**			
Balloon Type	**Fluid or Air Filled**	**Particularities**	**Weight Loss**
Orbera (Apollo Endosurgery, Austin, TX)	Fluid	Spherical silicone balloon Largest experience	Median % of Excess Weight Loss at six months ~25%[13]
Spatz Adjustable Balloon System (Spatz FGIA, New York, NY)	Fluid	Spherical balloon connected to a catheter for adjustment.	Median % of Excess Weight Loss at 12 months ~45.7% Increased early intolerance (21/73)[50]
ReShape Duo Integrated Dual Balloon System (ReShape Medical, San Clemente, CA)	Fluid	Two independent balloon linked by a flexible tube	Median % of Excess Weight Loss at 6 months ~25%[16]
Elipse (Allurion Technologies, Wellesley, MA)	Fluid	Swallowable balloon, naturally excreted uneventfully	Loss of 2.4 kg at 6 weeks in 8 patients[18]
Obalon Gastric Balloon (Obalon Therapeutics, Carlsbad, CA)	Air	Swallowable balloon, 1–3 balloons could be inserted. Must be retrieved	Loss of 5 kg at 12 weeks in 17 patients[19] Spontaneous deflation
Heliosphere BAG (Helioscopie, Vienne, France)	Air	Spherical polyurethane and silicone balloon inserted under conscious sedation	Median % of Excess Weight Loss at 6 months ~24%[51] Spontaneous deflation

From Imaz I, Martinez-Cervell C, Garcia-Alvarez EE, et al: Safety and effectiveness of the intragastric balloon for obesity: a meta-analysis. *Obes Surg* 18(7):841–846, 2008.

the release of acetylcholine at the neuromuscular junction. This can delay gastric emptying and also modulate local hormonal secretions. In an RCT, prolonged gastric emptying and significant weight loss (11.0 kg +/− 1.0 vs. 5.7 kg +/− 1.1) were reported 8 weeks after treatment, and a meta-analysis further confirmed the efficacy of this treatment. However, its high cost and the need to be repeated every 3 to 6 months limits its applicability.[40,41]

Table 43.1 summarizes current techniques of bariatric endotherapy for which clinical data are available. Further data are likely to become available, and the role of endotherapy in the management of obese patients undergoing bariatric surgery is likely to increase, rendering necessary the integration of endotherapy into the armamentarium of the multidisciplinary treatment of these patients.

Table 43.2 summarizes the different types of balloons evaluated in terms of particularities and their EWL effects.

CONCLUSION

The role of endoscopy is expected to continue to evolve in the development of novel options for primary bariatric therapy, where endoscopy, in the setting of a multidisciplinary approach, is likely to represent a classic alternative within the upcoming years. Minimal thresholds have been defined for a technique to potentially be incorporated in clinical practice. They include an EWL of at least 25% at 12 months in patients with a BMI over 35. Obviously, not every technique will reach these thresholds, but if some do, and given the fact that a transoral approach has the major advantage of not compromising further surgery in the setting of a chronic, life-long disease, it is probable that primary endoscopic bariatric therapy will become part of the armamentarium for managing obese patients. In this case, it could become of particular interest as a first interventional therapy.

KEY REFERENCES

3. Glenny AM, O'Meara S, Melville A, et al: The treatment and prevention of obesity: a systematic review of the literature, *Int J Obes Relat Metab Disord* 21:715–737, 1997.

7. Rosenthal RJ, Szomstein S, Kennedy CI, et al: Laparoscopic surgery for morbid obesity: 1,001 consecutive bariatric operations performed at The Bariatric Institute, Cleveland Clinic Florida, *Obes Surg* 16:119–124, 2006.

8. Nieben OG, Harboe H: Intragastric balloon as an artificial bezoar for treatment of obesity, *Lancet* 1:198–199, 1982.

10. Genco A, Bruni T, Doldi SB, et al: Bioenterics intragastric balloon: the Italian experience with 2515 patients, *Obes Surg* 15:1161–1164, 2005.

11. Mathus-Vliegen EM, Tytgat GN: Intragastric balloon for treatment-resistant obesity: safety, tolerance, and efficacy of 1-year balloon treatment followed by a 1-year balloon-free follow-up, *Gastrointest Endosc* 61:19–27, 2005.

12. Dastis NS, François E, Deviere J, et al: Intragastric balloon for weight loss: results in 100 individuals followed for at least 2.5 years, *Endoscopy* 41:575–580, 2009.

21. Schwartz MP, Wellink H, Gooszen HG, et al: Endoscopic gastroplication for the treatment of gastroesophageal reflux disease: a randomized sham controlled trial, *Gut* 56:20–28, 2007.

26. Familiari P, Costamanga G, Blero D, et al: Transoral gastroplasty for morbid obesity: a multicentre trial with a 1-year outcome, *Gastrointest Endosc* 74:1248–1258, 2011.

27. Lopez-Nava G, Galvao M, Bautista-Castaño I, et al: Endoscopic sleeve gastroplasty with 1-year follow-up: factors predictive of success, *Endosc Int Open* 4:E222–E227, 2016.

29. Lopez-Nava G, Bautista-Castaño I, Jimenez A, et al: The primary obesity surgery endoluminal (POSE) procedure: one year patient weight loss and safety outcomes, *Surg Obes Relat Dis* 11:861–865, 2015.

30. Sullivan S, Swain JM, Woodman G, et al: Randomized sham-controlled trial evaluating efficacy and safety of endoscopic gastric plication for primary obesity: the ESSENTIAL trial, *Obesity (Silver Spring)* 25:294–301, 2017.

31. Huberty V, Ibrahim M, Hiernaux M, et al: Safety and feasibility of an endoluminal-suturing device for endoscopic gastric reduction (with video), *Gastrointest Endosc* 85(4):833–837, 2017.

39. Sanmiguel CP, Conklin JL, Cunneen SA, et al: Gastric electrical stimulation with the TANTALUS system in obese T2D patients: effect on weight and glycemic control, *J Diabetes Sci Technol* 3:964–970, 2009.

41. Bang CS, Baik GH, Shin IS, et al: Effect of intragastric injection of Botulinum Toxin A for the treatment of obesity: a metaanalysis and metaregression, *Gastrointest Endosc* 81:1141–1149, 2015.

A complete reference list can be found online at ExpertConsult .com

44

Management of Post-Bariatric Complications

Allison R. Schulman, Marvin Ryou, and Christopher C. Thompson

INTRODUCTION

Obesity is a global epidemic, and has resulted in a substantial increase in the number of bariatric procedures performed worldwide.[1-4] As the field of bariatric surgery continues to grow with the increasing prevalence of obesity, a greater number of patients are referred for endoscopic evaluation after bariatric surgery. Despite improvement in the performance of bariatric surgery over the past decade, complications from the procedures are not uncommon. The type of complications and overall risk of adverse outcomes vary according to baseline patient characteristics, the duration of time since the operation, and the type of bariatric surgery performed.

A basic understanding of the anatomic changes and potential complications associated with bariatric procedures is essential for optimal assessment and appropriate treatment. A substantial number of these complications necessitate endoscopic interventions for accurate diagnosis and effective, minimally invasive management. This chapter will review the major complications, early and late, associated with the most commonly performed bariatric surgeries, and the endoscopic diagnosis and management of these complications.

ROUX-EN-Y GASTRIC BYPASS (RYGB)

The RYGB has traditionally been the most common bariatric surgery procedure performed worldwide.[1] The surgery involves the creation of a small gastric pouch and an anastomosis to a Roux limb of the jejunum (Fig. 44.1A). The expected endoscopic findings following RYGB are therefore a normal esophagus and gastroesophageal junction leading into to a gastric pouch, typically 30 mL in volume at the time of bypass surgery. The gastrojejunal

anastomosis (GJA) is typically sized 10 to 12 mm, beyond which the efferent Roux limb is found, typically 75 to 150 cm in length. The jejunojejunal anastomosis leads to the common limb and the pancreaticobiliary limb (including duodenum and ampulla); however, intubation of the latter, for endoscopic retrograde cholangiopancreatography (ERCP) or assessment of the gastric remnant, is often technically challenging.

Although this altered anatomy leads to weight loss through a variety of mechanisms, there are several complications associated with this procedure, some of which are related to the altered anatomy, and others of which are specific to the surgical technique or approach (i.e., laparoscopic vs. open).

Marginal Ulcerations

Marginal ulceration at the site of the GJA is not uncommon, and has been reported in up to 16% of patients after gastric bypass surgery (Fig. 44.2A).[5-9] The clinical presentation can range from being asymptomatic to having severe pain and obstructive symptoms or gastrointestinal bleeding, and, rarely, can present as perforation.

The mechanisms underlying the development of marginal ulceration have not been fully elucidated, and the etiology of this complication is likely multifactorial. There is substantial evidence that acidity plays a major role in the disease pathophysiology. Several potential inciting factors have been implicated including ischemia from the surgical creation of an anastomosis, foreign body materials (including staples or nonabsorbable sutures), gastrogastric fistula (GGF) which lead to excessive acid exposure from gastric remnant, nonsteroidal antiinflammatory drugs (NSAIDs), immunosuppressive agents, smoking, and gastric pouch orientation or size.[6,9-14] The relationship between *Helicobacter pylori* (*H. pylori*) infection and the development of marginal

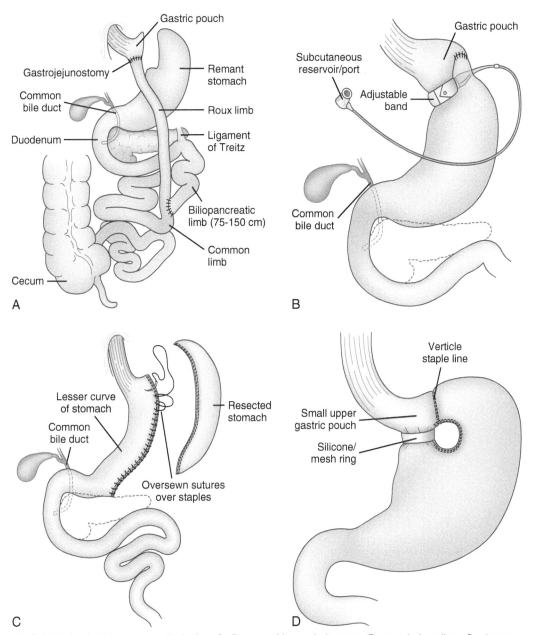

FIG 44.1 Bariatric surgeries including **A,** Roux-en-Y gastric bypass, **B,** gastric banding, **C,** sleeve gastrectomy, and **D,** vertical banded gastroplasty.

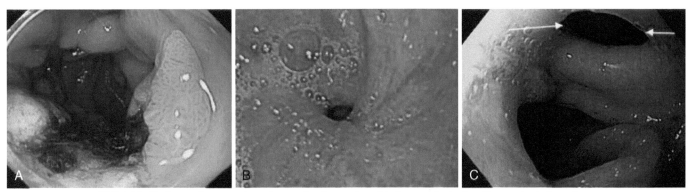

FIG 44.2 Endoscopic examples of complications of gastric bypass including **A,** marginal ulceration, **B,** stenosis of the gastrojejunal anastomosis, and **C,** gastrogastric fistula *(arrows)*.

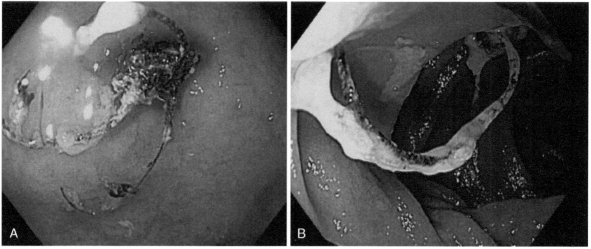

FIG 44.3 Suture material found in **A,** the gastric pouch and **B,** gastrojejunal anastomosis.

ulceration is controversial; however, a 2017 nationwide analysis suggests a strong association.[15-21]

During endoscopic evaluation, the gastric pouch should be closely inspected for a GGF. Endoscopic removal of foreign material, such as nonabsorbable suture or staples, should also be performed at the time of ulcer diagnosis[22] (Fig. 44.3). Pouch biopsies for *H. pylori* are less reliable, as most of the stomach where *H. pylori* resides is inaccessible.

The majority of patients with marginal ulcerations respond to medical therapy including high-dose proton pump inhibitor (PPI) therapy. PPI administration should be in soluble or open capsule form to enhance absorption, as recent evidence (2016) suggests it significantly decreases time to ulcer healing.[23] The addition of liquid sucralfate has also been advocated, in addition to smoking cessation and indefinite discontinuation of NSAIDs.

Endoscopic suturing techniques to oversew the ulcer have been described, with small case series demonstrating technical feasibility and efficacy.[24] Surgical revision of the gastrojejunostomy with truncal vagotomy has traditionally been performed in the small percentage of patients who do not improve. Reoperation, however, carries significant morbidity and a 7.7% recurrence rate.[25]

Stomal Stenosis

Stricture of the GJA, also known as *stomal stenosis*, has been reported in up to one-fifth of patients undergoing RYGB, although the majority of studies report an incidence of less than 10%[8,26-33] (see Fig. 44.2B). Strictures can occur weeks to years after surgery. This complication is more common in patients undergoing laparoscopic RYGB, possibly due to the use of small-diameter circular staplers during the construction of the gastrojejunostomy. Tension or ischemia at the site of anastomosis, in addition to ulceration or anastomotic leak, may also contribute.[34-36]

Stomal stenosis often leads to symptoms of progressive dysphagia, nausea, vomiting, and inability to tolerate oral intake. Endoscopic visualization is the first diagnostic tool.[37] Although there is no clear definition for stomal stenosis, diagnosis is typically made when a patient is symptomatic and passage of a standard upper endoscope through the GJA is met with resistance.

Endoscopic balloon dilation of the stricture is used almost exclusively to treat this complication (Fig. 44.4). Serial dilation

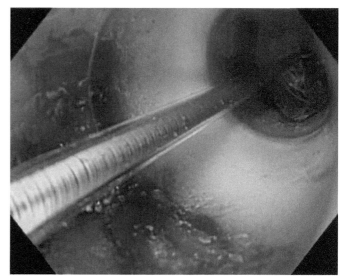

FIG 44.4 Endoscopic balloon dilation of stenosis of the gastrojejunal anastomosis.

using a through-the-scope balloon catheter should be performed with the goal of symptom resolution and target a stomal diameter of 8 to 12 mm, and rarely exceed 15 mm, as overzealous dilation may result in perforation or weight regain. The initial balloon size should be based on the estimated diameter of the anastomotic stricture, with effective dilation resulting in partial disruption of the GJA. A co-existent marginal ulceration may increase the risk of perforation, and dilation should be avoided or performed very carefully in this cohort of patients.

The majority of strictures can be effectively dilated in one or two sessions, with a 1- to 3-week interval between sessions. Other endoscopic interventions have also been reported with some success, including placement of a lumen-apposing metal stent (LAMS), needle-knife electroincision of the anastomosis, or steroid injection.[38-40] Surgical revision is required in a small percentage of patients who are refractory to endoscopic management, or in whom coexistent marginal ulceration precludes optimal treatment.[41]

Leaks

One of the most serious complications of bariatric surgery is postoperative leak, which occur at multiple points along any staple line, and typically within days to weeks following the operation. The incidence ranges from 0.1% to 5.6%, and revision surgery predisposes to increased risk of occurrence.[42–44] The most common presenting findings are tachycardia, leukocytosis, and elevated inflammatory markers, but can also present as hemodynamic instability or sepsis.[45]

Identification of the location of the leak is critical, as that will dictate appropriate management. Leaks occurring at the pouch or GJA can be managed with endoscopic placement of self-expandable metal stents. To prevent both incomplete closure as well as stent migration or mucosal hypertrophy leading to increased difficulty of stent extraction, it has been proposed that the optimal time for stent removal is between 6 to 8 weeks.[46] Leaks at other sites may not be amenable to stenting, and other modalities have had variable results. Chronic leaks with a walled-off cavity should be treated like walled-off pancreatic necrosis. Surgical exploration is often required in patients who are unstable.

Gastrogastric Fistula

A GGF is an abnormal communication between the gastric pouch and the excluded stomach, or gastric remnant (see Fig. 44.2C). In the era of nondivided gastric bypass, GGFs were one of the most common complications, occurring in upward of half of all patients. With the advent of the divided RYGB, in which the gastrointestinal stapler simultaneously places rows of staples and transects the tissue between the rows, the incidence of GGF has declined to less than 6%.[47–49] Marginal ulceration, gastric leak, and foreign body erosion have all been additional postulated mechanisms for the development of this complication.[47–49]

The most common presenting symptom is weight regain or inability to lose weight, although pain, nausea, reflux, and emesis are often reported.[39,50] Endoscopy and upper gastrointestinal series should be performed to make the diagnosis, although GGFs can often be seen on abdominal computed tomography scan with oral contrast. On endoscopic evaluation, careful examination of the pouch should be performed, as GGF are often small and can be overlooked.

If present, maximum medical therapy should be instituted, with over one-third of patients experiencing symptom resolution. If the GGF is associated with a marginal ulcer, an initial conservative approach consisting of high-dose PPI therapy and liquid sucralfate may be sufficient to allow for fistula closure. NSAID use and smoking should be strictly avoided.

In a patient with persistent symptoms that are clearly attributable to the fistula, closure is indicated. Traditionally, procedural intervention has been accomplished via a surgical approach. However, endoscopic suturing symptoms should be considered, and these are especially effective when the fistula is less than 1 cm.[51,52] Use of over-the-scope clips have been described in small case series, but should be used with caution, as these may interfere with subsequent surgical intervention if it is required.[53–55]

Gastrointestinal Bleeding

Gastrointestinal bleeding following RYGB is often seen at the gastrojejunal anastomosis (Fig. 44.5). Hematemesis is the most common clinical presentation in early postoperative bleeds. Endoscopic management can be challenging because of the higher risk of perforation at the newly created surgical anastomosis. Carbon dioxide should be utilized instead of air insufflation, and the use of nonthermal devices such as clips is preferred for hemostasis.

Beyond the early postoperative period, endoscopic therapy can be achieved by standard hemostatic interventions such as injection of vasoconstrictors, thermal therapy, or mechanical modalities. Discontinuation of NSAIDs and smoking are advised. Balloon-assisted enteroscopy is often required to access the jejunojejunal anastomosis and enable retrograde examination of the bypassed stomach and duodenum.

Cholelithiasis and Choledocholithiasis

The development of cholelithiasis is not uncommon following RYGB, and is estimated to occur in 28% to 71% of patients within 6 months following surgery, with up to 40% of these patients becoming symptomatic.[56] Rapid weight loss has been shown to contribute to the formation of gallstones by increasing the cholesterol saturation in the bile and the gallbladder mucin concentration.[56–61]

Choledocholithiasis after RYGB can be particularly challenging to treat via ERCP due to the relative inaccessibility of the duodenum (Fig. 44.6). Use of a balloon-assisted enteroscope, pediatric

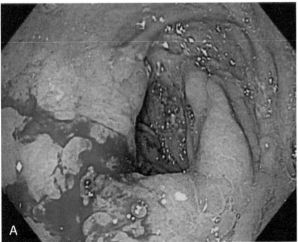
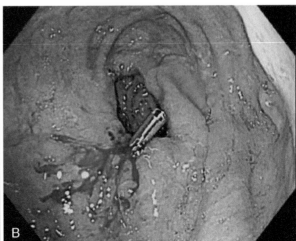

FIG 44.5 **A,** Bleeding marginal ulceration **B,** followed by endoscopic therapy.

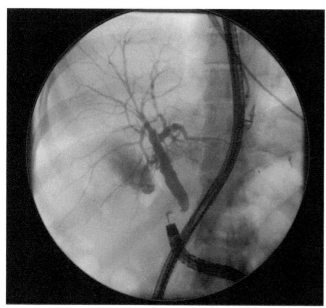

FIG 44.6 Use of balloon-assisted enteroscopy to perform endoscopic retrograde cholangiopancreatography in a Roux-en-Y gastric bypass patient.

colonoscope, spiral overtube, or duodenoscope back-loaded onto a guidewire is often required. If a GGF is present, the scope can pass directly through the remnant stomach and into the duodenum. Dilation of the GGF may be performed if it is too small for scope passage, although subsequent closure is a concern. Placement of a prophylactic gastrostomy tube into the bypassed stomach, or endoscopic ultrasound (EUS)-directed gastrostomy, has also been described.[62] An alternative emerging procedure is the EUS-directed transgastric ERCP (EDGE) procedure that allows direct access through placement of a LAMS between the pouch and the gastric remnant,[63,64] although persistent GGF formation remains a theoretical concern.

Dumping Syndrome

Early and late dumping syndrome occurs not uncommonly in patients who have undergone gastric bypass surgery when large quantities of simple carbohydrates are ingested. Early dumping typically occurs within 15 minutes of ingestion and has been attributed to rapid fluid shifts from the plasma into the bowel from hyperosmolality of the food. Late dumping occurs hours after eating and results from hyperglycemia and the subsequent insulin response leading to hypoglycemia. When hypoglycemia is severe, treatment with a low carbohydrate diet and an alpha-glucosidase inhibitor may be effective. Furthermore, restoration of gastric restriction using an endoscopic approach to reduce the aperture of the GJA has also demonstrated to be effective in management of this condition.[65] Symptoms of early and late dumping syndrome are shown in Box 44.1.

Failure to Lose Weight or Weight Regain

RYGB is associated with 15% to 35% failure, defined as inability to achieve significant weight loss or excessive weight regain after initial adequate weight loss.[66–70] Whereas this may be due to progressive dietary noncompliance, anatomic changes may also predispose to weight regain. Dilation of the GJA, development of a GGF, and enlargement of the gastric pouch also play a significant role in weight regain, with the size of the GJA correlating linearly with the degree of weight regain.[71]

Endoscopic suturing, plication devices, and thermal therapy including argon plasma coagulation have been used to tighten the stoma and reduce pouch volume, with suturing demonstrating sustained weight loss at 3 years and level I evidence in a randomized controlled trial[72] (Fig. 44.7). These endoscopic therapies offer a less invasive option for management of post-bypass weight regain, with minimal morbidity.

LAPAROSCOPIC ADJUSTABLE GASTRIC BANDING

Adjustable gastric banding is a restrictive procedure. Insertion of an adjustable, prosthetic band over the cardia of the stomach leads to formation of a gastric pouch with roughly 15 mL capacity (see Fig. 44.1B). The gastric band consists of a silicone ring connected to an infusion port, the latter of which remains in the subcutaneous tissue and can be easily accessed for saline injections to increase the degree of restriction. This type of procedure has the lowest peri-operative complication rate and mortality among all bariatric procedures; however, disadvantages include the presence of a foreign body.

Band-Related Complications

Band erosion is a severe complication of adjustable banding procedures and occurs in less than 10% of patients. Band erosion may occur early within weeks, or can be seen months and even years after operation.[73,74] Early erosions are usually secondary to undetected gastric perforations during surgery or early infection, whereas late erosions may be the consequence of gastric wall ischemia from an excessively tight band.

Clinical manifestations of this complication can range from weight gain to nausea and vomiting to life-threatening sepsis or massive hemorrhage, depending on the location of the erosion. Diagnosis can be made endoscopically, and depending on what portion of the band is visible, removal may be accomplished at the time of the procedure. Caution must be exercised if endoscopic removal of a gastric band is considered, especially when the penetration through the gastric wall is incomplete, as this endoscopic removal carries a high risk of gastric perforation.

Esophageal-Related Complications

Reflux esophagitis are not uncommon following banding procedures, and typically require acid suppression therapy and

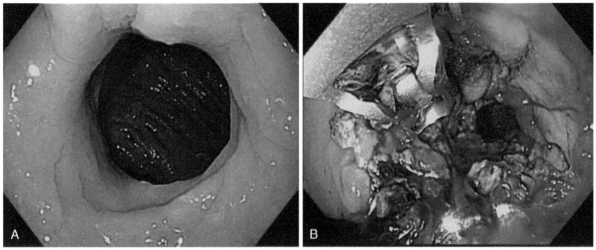

FIG 44.7 **A,** Dilated gastrojejunal anastomosis **B,** followed by endoscopic revision.

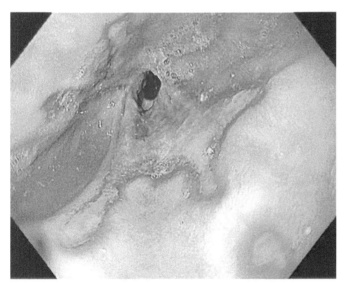

FIG 44.8 Severe esophagitis following laparoscopic adjustable banding.

deflation of the band[75,76] (Fig. 44.8). Surgical revision is considered in patients who are unresponsive to maximum medical therapy.

Esophageal dilation proximal to the band can also occur if the band is excessively inflated. Symptoms include reflux, epigastric discomfort, and inability to tolerate oral intake. Typically, treatment involves deflation of the band and diet modification, but worsening esophageal dilation and inadequate weight loss mandate replacement of the band in a new location or conversion to an alternative bariatric procedure.

SLEEVE GASTRECTOMY

Laparoscopic sleeve gastrectomy is a restrictive procedure in which a large portion of the greater curvature of the stomach is removed, with preservation of the pylorus and maintenance of physiological food passage (see Fig. 44.1C). Laparoscopic sleeve gastrectomy is increasingly being performed worldwide, and is now the most commonly performed bariatric surgery in the United States.

Stenosis

Stenosis following sleeve gastrectomy occurs in up to 4% of patients. The site of stenosis is typically at the incisura angularis, and may be the result of over-sewing the staple line or using a bougie that is too small. Symptoms of obstruction can occur depending on the severity of the narrowing.

This diagnosis is typically made by upper endoscopy or with fluoroscopy using an upper gastrointestinal series, but can often be missed by upper endoscopy, as often there is no physical resistance to gastroscope passage. Successful balloon dilation of both the pylorus and incisura starting with a 20-mm hydrostatic balloon, followed by pneumatic balloon dilation from 30 mm to 40 mm at increasing pressures every 2 to 4 weeks, has been demonstrated to be safe and with high efficacy rates, with a small case series demonstrating 94% patients with resolution of symptoms.[77] This new method may offer a less invasive alternative to surgical revision.

Anastomotic Leaks

Gastric leaks have been reported in up to 5.3% of patients, and usually occur along the superior aspect of the staple line just below the gastroesophageal junction. Leaks can be the result of inadequate healing of the gastric tissue from poor blood supply and oxygenation, or from heat generated from cautery during dissection of the greater curvature. This complication is one of the most serious. Endoscopic approaches have proven successful, and offer a less invasive first-line therapy to reoperation for many patients. If the leak occurs within 6 weeks, stent placement followed by dilation of the pylorus to treat distal obstruction should be performed. Leaks that occur more than 6 weeks following surgery require management similar to an endoscopic necrosectomy whereby pigtail stents are placed and tissue débrided. Endoscopic septotomy has also been described and used to facilitate healing of refractory leaks. This procedure is performed by incision and enlargement of the fistulous tract, thereby allowing direct communication with the gastric lumen and promoting internal drainage.[78]

VERTICAL BANDED GASTROPLASTY

Vertical banded gastroplasty (VBG) involves the creation of a small proximal gastric pouch of less than 50 mL lined by a vertical staple line and a tight prosthetic mesh that is sutured to itself but not the stomach (see Fig. 44.1D). This is a purely restrictive procedure and has the benefit of providing an outlet diameter that should remain constant.[48] Although this type of procedure has largely been replaced by other procedures, familiarity with the complications and the role of endoscopic management is still important.

Staple Line Dehiscence

Staple line dehiscence can result in a fistula to the fundus, often leading to failure to lose weight or weight regain following the procedure. It is found in as many as half of all patients on routine postoperative endoscopy, but has also been described following blunt abdominal trauma. Endoscopy is helpful in diagnosing and evaluating the disruption, and endoscopic suturing systems may ultimately prove to be effective in treatment of this condition.

Band Erosion

Band erosion develops in approximately 1% to 2% of patients with VBG, with clinical symptoms of weight regain and abdominal pain. Erosion of the mesh band is a late complication of this procedure, and can be removed via an endoscopic approach, but may ultimately require reoperation or conversion to RYGB.

Obstruction/Pouch Dilation

Obstruction from stomal stenosis can occur and be managed by endoscopic balloon dilation, although results are often short-lived and revision may be necessary when symptoms persist. Pouch dilation can occur as a consequence of stomal obstruction, band erosion, or staple line dehiscence. Endoscopy is the modality of choice for diagnosis.

CONCLUSION

Obesity is one of the most rapidly emerging health problems worldwide. Although bariatric surgery is effective in achieving weight loss and resolution of comorbidities, complications are not uncommon. A basic understanding of the anatomic changes and potential complications associated with bariatric procedures is essential for optimal assessment and appropriate management.

KEY REFERENCES

1. Buchwald H, Oien DM: Metabolic/bariatric surgery worldwide 2011, *Obes Surg* 23:427–436, 2013.
2. Buchwald H, Avidor Y, Braunwald E, et al: Bariatric surgery: a systematic review and meta-analysis, *JAMA* 292:1724–1737, 2004.
3. Arterburn DE, Olsen MK, Smith VA, et al: Association between bariatric surgery and long-term survival, *JAMA* 313:62, 2015.
10. Azagury DE, Abu Dayyeh BK, Greenwalt IT, et al: Marginal ulceration after Roux-en-Y gastric bypass surgery: characteristics, risk factors, treatment, and outcomes, *Endoscopy* 43:950–954, 2011.
12. Coblijn UK, Lagarde SM, de Castro SMM, et al: Symptomatic marginal ulcer disease after Roux-en-Y gastric bypass: incidence, risk factors and management, *Obes Surg* 25:805–811, 2015.
18. Lin Y-S, Chen M-J, Shih S-C, et al: Management of *Helicobacter pylori* infection after gastric surgery, *World J Gastroenterol* 20:5274, 2014.
21. Schulman AR, Abougergi M, Thompson CC: H. Pylori as a predictor of marginal ulceration: a nationwide analysis, *Obesity (Silver Spring)* 25(3):522–526, 2017.
22. Ryou M, Mogabgab O, Lautz DB, et al: Endoscopic foreign body removal for treatment of chronic abdominal pain in patients after Roux-en-Y gastric bypass, *Surg Obes Relat Dis* 6:526–531, 2010.
23. Schulman AR, Chan WW, Devery A, et al: Opened proton pump inhibitor capsules reduce time to healing compared with intact capsules for marginal ulceration following Roux-en-Y gastric bypass, *Clin Gastroenterol Hepatol* 15(4):494–500, 2017.
24. Jirapinyo P, Watson RR, Thompson CC: Use of a novel endoscopic suturing device to treat recalcitrant marginal ulceration (with video), *Gastrointest Endosc* 76:435–439, 2012.
28. Peifer KJ, Shiels AJ, Azar R, et al: Successful endoscopic management of gastrojejunal anastomotic strictures after Roux-en-Y gastric bypass, *Gastrointest Endosc* 66:248–252, 2007.
35. Fisher BL, Atkinson JD, Cottam D: Incidence of gastroenterostomy stenosis in laparoscopic Roux-en-Y gastric bypass using 21- or 25-mm circular stapler: a randomized prospective blinded study, *Surg Obes Relat Dis* 3:176–179, 2007.
37. Goitein D, Papasavas PK, Gagné D, et al: Gastrojejunal strictures following laparoscopic Roux-en-Y gastric bypass for morbid obesity, *Surg Endosc* 19:628–632, 2005.
39. Lee JK, Van Dam J, Morton JM, et al: Endoscopy is accurate, safe, and effective in the assessment and management of complications following gastric bypass surgery, *Am J Gastroenterol* 104:575–582, 2009.
43. Almahmeed T, Gonzalez R, Nelson LG, et al: Morbidity of anastomotic leaks in patients undergoing Roux-en-Y gastric bypass, *Arch Surg* 142: 954, 2007.
46. Merrifield BF, Lautz D, Thompson CC: Endoscopic repair of gastric leaks after Roux-en-Y gastric bypass: a less invasive approach, *Gastrointest Endosc* 63:710–714, 2006.
48. Stanczyk M, Deveney C, Traxler S, et al: Gastro-gastric fistula in the era of divided Roux-en-Y gastric bypass: strategies for prevention, diagnosis, and management, *Obes Surg* 16:359–364, 2006.
50. Huang CS, Forse RA, Jacobson BC, et al: Endoscopic findings and their clinical correlations in patients with symptoms after gastric bypass surgery, *Gastrointest Endosc* 58:859–866, 2003.
51. Fernandez-Esparrach G, Lautz DB, Thompson CC: Endoscopic repair of gastrogastric fistula after Roux-en-Y gastric bypass: a less-invasive approach, *Surg Obes Relat Dis* 6:282–288, 2010.
54. Flicker MS, Lautz DB, Thompson CC: Endoscopic management of gastrogastric fistulae does not increase complications at bariatric revision surgery, *J Gastrointest Surg* 15:1736–1742, 2011.
62. Thompson CC, Ryou MK, Kumar N, et al: Single-session EUS-guided transgastric ERCP in the gastric bypass patient, *Gastrointest Endosc* 80:517, 2014.
65. Fernández-Esparrach G, Lautz DB, Thompson CC: Peroral endoscopic anastomotic reduction improves intractable dumping syndrome in Roux-en-Y gastric bypass patients, *Surg Obes Relat Dis* 6:36–40, 2010.
71. Abu Dayyeh BK, Lautz DB, Thompson CC: Gastrojejunal stoma diameter predicts weight regain after Roux-en-Y gastric bypass, *Clin Gastroenterol Hepatol* 9:228–233, 2011.
72. Kumar N, Thompson CC: Transoral outlet reduction for weight regain after gastric bypass: long-term follow-up, *Gastrointest Endosc* 83:776–779, 2016.
77. Abidi W, Thompson CC: Systematic treatment of sleeve gastrectomy stenosis with hydrostatic and pneumatic balloon dilatation is safe and effective, *Gastroenterology* 150:S828–S829, 2016.

A complete reference list can be found online at ExpertConsult .com

45

Intramural and Transmural Endoscopy

Lyz Bezerra Silva and Ricardo Zorron

INTRODUCTION

Natural orifice transluminal endoscopic surgery (NOTES) is an evolving concept, combining minimally invasive surgery with flexible endoscopy, potentially representing a major paradigm shift to scarless surgery. Recently, NOTES went from few experimental reports to clinical series and multicentric studies.[1,2] Since the early concept, from pioneers such as Kalloo and Kantsevoy[3] in the United States, and Rao and Reddy[4] in India, NOTES has emerged as a promising new alternative to open and laparoscopic surgery for abdominal access. Potential benefits include decreasing surgical incision complications, such as incisional hernias, adhesions, intestinal obstruction, scars, and wound infection, together with better aesthetics. This evolution led to the first successful series of clinical applications in the literature for transvaginal (TV) and transgastric (TG) NOTES.[5]

Intramural surgery is an exciting new technical possibility, allowing for unimagined therapy for submucosal tumors, access for endoscopic techniques, and submucosal myotomy for achalasia. New tools and evolution of these techniques are changing the way many problems in gastroenterology are resolved. This chapter reviews early procedures and current clinical applications of intramural and transmural endoscopy.

INTRAMURAL ENDOSCOPY TECHNIQUES

Techniques for Creation of a Submucosal Working Space
Submucosal Endoscopy With Mucosal Safety Valve Technique
The submucosal endoscopy with mucosal flap (SEMF) technique may offer safe access to the peritoneal cavity for NOTES surgery.

The submucosal space functions as a tunneled portal and the free overlying mucosa as a protective sealant flap, minimizing contamination of the extraluminal peritoneal cavity.

In the original SEMF technique, balloon dissection combined with high-pressure carbon dioxide (CO_2) is used to dissect the submucosa.[6] A submucosal injection of saline is used to identify the submucosal tissue plane, then bursts of CO_2 are injected to create a gas-filled submucosal bleb, followed by injection of hydroxypropyl methylcellulose, which prevents gas escape. A mucosal incision is made with a needle-knife at one margin of the bleb/fluid cushion to allow entry below the mucosa. Balloon dissection can be performed to transform the submucosa into an intramural free space. Blunt dissection with grasping forceps can also be used (Fig. 45.1).

Chemically Assisted Submucosal Dissection Technique
Aiming to minimize mechanical trauma to the mucosal flap, mesna was discovered as a useful adjuvant to the blunt dissection, acting by chemically softening the submucosa. In this technique, mesna solution is injected into the saline submucosal bleb before initiating balloon dissection.[6]

Peroral Endoscopic Myotomy
Achalasia is an esophageal motility disorder for which treatment, until recently, was restricted to pharmacotherapy, balloon dilatation, botulinum toxin injection, and surgical intervention (e.g., Heller myotomy) with the aim to reduce lower esophageal sphincter pressure. Conservative treatment has limited efficacy, frequently needing repeated procedures, whereas surgical treatment requires additional fundoplication to prevent gastroesophageal reflux. Due to this, novel technologies have been explored to treat this pathology. Peroral endoscopic myotomy (POEM)

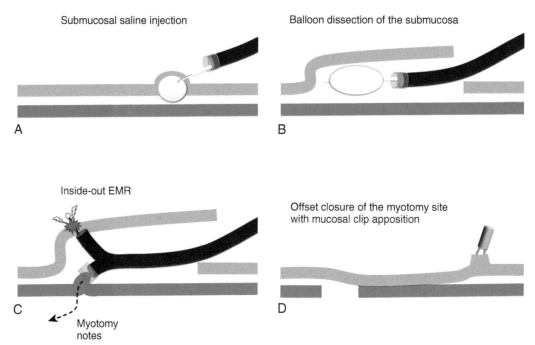

Submucosal saline injection

Balloon dissection of the submucosa

Inside-out EMR

Offset closure of the myotomy site
with mucosal clip apposition

A

B

C

D

Myotomy
notes

FIG 45.1 Submucosal flap construction. **A,** A small submucosal saline bleb is made to identify the submucosal tissue plane. **B,** After pretreatment of the submucosa with high-pressure carbon dioxide (CO_2) or mesna, balloon dissection is performed to create an open space within the submucosal tissue plane. **C,** The submucosal space is used as a working space for interventions such as inside-out submucosal endoscopy with mucosal resection, intramural myotomy, and offset access for natural orifice transluminal endoscopic surgery (NOTES) procedures. **D,** The muscular defect after myotomy is sealed with an overlying mucosal flap, and the submucosal tunnel is closed with mucosal clip apposition. *EMR,* endoscopy with mucosal resection.

is a novel procedure, first performed in humans by Inoue et al (2010),[7] that has been established as safe, minimally invasive, and with expected long-lasting symptom control.

The technique involves four major consecutive steps: esophageal mucosal incision and entry into the submucosal space; creation of a submucosal tunnel; incision of the esophageal muscles (myotomy); and closure of the mucosal incision. It can also be used in patients with recurrence after other treatments have been performed.

Technique

The procedure is carried out with the patient under general anesthesia, with positive pressure ventilation, using higher pressures than those generated by endoscopic CO_2 insufflation. A submucosal injection is administered at the level of the mid esophagus, 13 cm proximal to the gastroesophageal junction (GEJ), followed by injection of saline with 0.3% indigo carmine. A 2-cm longitudinal mucosal incision is made on the mucosal surface to create an entry to the submucosal space. A long submucosal tunnel is then created, of approximately half the circumference of the tubular esophagus. Dissection of the circular muscle bundle is subsequently initiated. When the tip of the endoscope reaches the stomach region, the submucosal space becomes wider, and muscle layer cutting is continued for approximately 2 cm distal to the GEJ. Complete division of the circular muscle bundle is confirmed by endoscopic appearance. The mucosal entry is closed with hemostatic clips.[7]

Results

In a series of 500 cases of patients who underwent POEM for achalasia, Inoue et al (2015) describe significant reductions in symptom scores and lower esophageal sphincter pressures.[8] Gastroesophageal reflux was noted in 16.8% of patients at 2 months and 21.3% at 3-year follow-up. Median total length of the endoscopic myotomy was 14 cm in the esophagus and 3 cm in the stomach. Median procedure time was 90 minutes (range: 70.8–119 minutes). Procedure-related adverse events were observed in 16 patients (3.2%). In all cases the POEM procedures were accomplished successfully, including those with adverse events. The overall success rate at 2 months, 1–2 years, and 3 years was 91.3%, 91%, and 88.5%, respectively.[8]

A meta-analysis evaluating studies using POEM for achalasia, comprising 1045 patients, concluded that there was no difference between POEM and laparoscopic Heller myotomy in reduction in Eckhart's score, postoperative pain and analgesic requirements, length of hospital stay, adverse events, and gastroesophageal reflux. Operative time was significantly lower for POEM. In the review, POEM was effective for achalasia, with similar outcomes as surgical myotomy.[9]

After several published series, POEM can be offered to almost all achalasia patients, with a low complication rate. According to Inoue et al, sigmoid esophagus, dilated esophagus, and long duration of symptoms do not appear to be a barrier to successful treatment with POEM.[8]

TRANSGASTRIC ENDOSCOPIC SURGERY

TG NOTES was the first natural orifice access proposed by researchers, mainly because of familiarity of gastroenterologists and surgeons with upper flexible endoscopy, and the availability of endoscopic sets. TG procedures have the potential of completely avoiding incision complications, and may produce less pain.

Technique of Transgastric Surgery

The patient is sedated with general anesthesia and placed in a Lloyd-Davies position. Pneumoperitoneum can be achieved using a Veress needle, followed by insertion of an umbilical laparoscopic optic, which allows peritoneoscopy to evaluate the feasibility of the procedure, safe transluminal entrance of the endoscope to the abdominal cavity, and facilitates closure of the gastric wound after the procedure.

The access technique starts by perorally passing a flexible endoscope into the stomach. The gastric contents are aspirated before advancement into the peritoneal cavity, and lavage with dilute chlorhexidine can be performed. Use of an esophageal overtube can protect against esophageal trauma due to instrumentation. The site of the gastric puncture is selected by laparoscopic guidance, with two relatively avascular areas in the stomach considered adequate for the approach: the proximal body, midway between the lesser and greater curvatures of the stomach, and a similar site in the distal antrum.[4] The gastric fundal region is avoided because of danger of damaging short gastric vessels and the spleen. A perforation of the wall is created by needle knife at the chosen site. The needle is withdrawn and an endoscopic balloon dilator is passed over the hole and positioned across the gastrotomy. The balloon is dilated completely and the endoscope is progressed into the peritoneal cavity.

Specimens can be extracted without special bags, and when the specimen diameter exceeds the diameter of the esophagus, open conversion by umbilical access and extraction is the solution.

An issue of the TG approach is reliable gastrotomy closure, as postoperative leaks for TG abdominal surgery cannot be tolerated. Tissue apposition and clipping have been widely used since early reports, but the endoscopic clipping devices were developed for control of gastrointestinal bleeding and are therefore unreliable for NOTES closure.

The use of endoscopic clips for closure was reported in most experimental studies and in the first casuistic of Rao and Reddy.[4] Differently from a gastric incision or an iatrogenic perforation, the gastrotomy created by the balloon dilation technique closes spontaneously after removal of the endoscope. Multiple clips can be applied to approximate and close the wound, starting from the periphery and moving to the center. However, most clips approximate only mucosa, and this can be an issue for further applications. Similar techniques have been used to close the gastric defects following endoscopic mucosal and submucosal resections.

In the laparoscopic closure, another 3-mm trocar can be inserted to aid in gastrotomy closure, using single-hand suture, by inserting a needle-holder through this trocar and a laparoscope through the umbilical trocar. This closure is also monitored by the endoscope, which is withdrawn and kept in the gastric lumen while the bytes are taken.[1]

There are now several novel full-thickness closure devices, such as T-Tag tissue anchors (Olympus Corporation of the Americas, Center Valley, PA), the flexible linear stapling device (Power Medical Interventions, Langhorne, PA), the G-Prox (USGI, San Clemente, CA), the Eagle Claw (Olympus), the OverStitch (Apollo Endosurgery, Austin, TX), and the OTSC (Over The Scope Clip, Germany). Studies are under way to evaluate the efficacy of these new methods. Apollo Overstitch is currently the most reliable method of closing gastric defects, and there are growing applications in endoscopic sleeve gastroplasty for primary endoscopic therapy for obesity[10] (Fig. 45.2).

TG Cholecystectomy

Usually, one 3- or 5-mm trocar is placed at the umbilicus for guiding the endoscope's safe TG exit, and later, for retracting the gallbladder fundus. Dissection can be performed either endoscopically or laparoscopically. In the series by Dallemagne et al (2009), the umbilical trocar was also used to allow entry of a laparoscopic clip applier.[11]

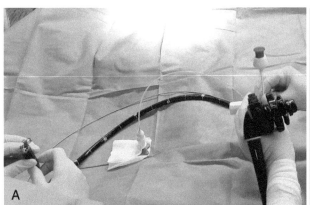 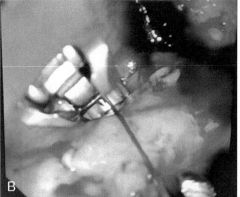

FIG 45.2 A, The Apollo Overstitch suturing device is currently used to close gastric and esophageal defects, fix gastroesophageal stents, and perform primary endoscopic therapy for obesity. Assembly of the Apollo Overstich to the double-channel endoscope outside the patient. **B,** Internal view of endoscopic sleeve gastroplication (ESG) for morbid obesity. Six to nine sutures are placed in the greater curvature of the stomach for gastric reduction. The motility and emptying of the stomach are delayed, therefore producing restriction and feelings of satiety.

TG Appendectomy

TG appendectomies are performed initially using a 3- or 5-mm umbilical trocar to guide peritoneal access by the endoscope. The same trocar can later be used for retracting the appendix. All the steps are usually performed without any other extra trocars until the extraction of the specimen. At that point, a 5-mm right pararectal trocar can be inserted to aid in gastrotomy closure.

Clinical Transgastric Endoscopic Surgical Results

TG access was inspired by the initial description of Seifert et al (2000), who performed TG debridement of necrotizing pancreatitis using flexible endoscopy.[12] To date, there are only a few reports of clinical TG surgery for cholecystectomy, appendectomy, and cancer staging, with good results in a small number of cases.[1,4,13-19]

In the largest prospective multicenter database available in the literature, 362 patients were prospectively documented, including TG and TV cases, of which there were 29 TG cholecystectomies and 14 TG appendectomies.[1] The operative time for NOTES cholecystectomy did not differ significantly between TV (96.1 min) and TG access (110.93 min). In comparison to TV appendectomy, TG appendectomy had significant longer operative time (60.5 vs. 135.5 min). The main challenges were retroflection of the endoscope, generating difficulty in orientation and restricted dissection possibilities, and gastric opening and closure. In one TG cholecystectomy case, the retrieval specimen was too large (a 2.4-cm gallstone) and could not be extracted through the oropharynx, requiring removal through an umbilical incision. In two cases where no overtube was used, large specimens also caused esophageal hematoma and laceration, and longer operative times.

Complications were recorded in 32 patients in general (8.84%). In one case of TG cholecystectomy, the patient was readmitted on the 5th postoperative day due to diffuse abdominal pain and distention. Laparoscopy was performed and diffuse peritonitis caused by *Streptococcus faecalis* was found, but without gastric fistula. Abdominal fluid aspiration and washing with saline solution was performed, with good postoperative course. In one patient, the passage of a large calculi with an inflamed gallbladder led to perforation of the proximal esophagus requiring a thoracic operation and longer intensive care unit admission.

A longer learning curve for TG surgery is expected. The lack of instruments to perform adequate dissection and retraction, the need for retroflection and for flexible endoscopy skills, and the small size of the esophageal lumen contribute to longer operative times and complications than TV NOTES.

Large-specimen retrievals are not suitable for TG surgery, as the esophagus allows only a maximal instrumental (or specimen) diameter of approximately 2 cm. TV NOTES has less potential for complications such as fistula and peritonitis than other transluminal accesses. Potential disadvantages of NOTES surgery are the necessary use of antibiotics, possible trauma to the oropharynx, and risk of infection and morbidity of gastric, vaginal, and colonic access, still with longer operative times.

Currently, after all this clinical experience, TG abdominal surgery is limited to pancreatic endoscopy for debridement, pseudocyst drainage, and oncologic biopsies. Advanced flexible NOTES TG surgery is still waiting for technology to allow safe and effective applications.

TRANSVAGINAL ENDOSCOPIC SURGERY

TV access has been established in gynecology for many years and is increasingly used in abdominal surgery. In 1813 the German surgeon C. Langenbeck performed the first TV hysterectomy.[20] In 1901 the Russian physician Dimitri von Ott published the first report about the so-called ventroscopy,[21] access to the abdominal cavity by colpotomy without using optics. Decker designed his "Culdoscope" and performed diagnostic culdoscopy.[22]

In 2007, Tsin et al published a review of 100 culdolaparoscopic cases, referred to by the authors as "mini-laparoscopy assisted natural orifice surgery" (MANOS).[23] Multiple procedures were reported: appendectomy, cholecystectomy, salpingo-oophorectomy, myomectomy, ovarian cystectomy, and culdolaparoscopy during vaginal hysterectomy. In 2007, Zorron et al published the first cases of flexible NOTES TV cholecystectomy,[24] (Video 45.1) and soon other groups added more clinical experience.[25-29]

Transvaginal Access Technique

In the majority of procedures, the patient is placed in the lithotomy position, and vaginal preparation is carried out with povidone-iodine or chlorhexidine gluconate solution. TV access can be obtained under laparoscopic view of the cul-de-sac or directly by colpotomy without guidance from a laparoscope. A speculum is inserted into the vagina to expose the posterior fornix and visualize the cervix, and its posterior lip is retracted to facilitate visualization of the cervicovaginal junction. A small incision is made in the posterior fornix, usually under visualization from a laparoscopic camera in the abdomen. The safest area to access the abdomen is known as the *triangle of safety*: after visualization of the cervix and posterior fornix, a clock located at the base of the cervix is envisioned, with the superior two corners of the triangle being the 4 o'clock and 8 o'clock positions.[30] Insufflation is commonly performed with a Veress needle placed in the umbilicus or abdominal wall. Alternatively, TV insufflation of the peritoneal cavity can be achieved either with a Veress needle placed in the posterior cul-de-sac, transuterine, or through a transvaginally placed port. If a flexible endoscope is used, insufflation can be established through one of the working channels. A wide variety of different ports and systems are currently used for TV NOTES. For colpotomy closure, absorbable suture in either an interrupted or running fashion using the directly visualized TV technique is recommended.

In a prospective multicenter study, the German Registry for Natural Orifice Endoscopic Surgery, a total of 551 patients were reported.[2] Cholecystectomies were the main procedure (85.3%), appendectomies were performed in 7.3%, and six patients received bariatric operations. All NOTES operations were performed transvaginally, with the hybrid technique (with an additional transumbilical trocar) being used in 99.3%. Rigid endoscopes were used in most cases for TV access. One appendectomy for chronic appendicitis was performed using the pure NOTES technique, with a flexible endoscope and no transabdominal trocars. The overall complication rate was low (2.9%), occurring only in cholecystectomies.[2]

In the International Multicenter Trial on Clinical Natural Orifice Surgery, two access methods were described.[1] Some centers performed abdominal insufflation by means of a Veress needle in the abdomen, and others achieved good results by directly accessing the cavity through a direct-view vaginal access. Different techniques for TV cholecystectomy were described. A total NOTES dual scope method used two endoscopes through the vaginal

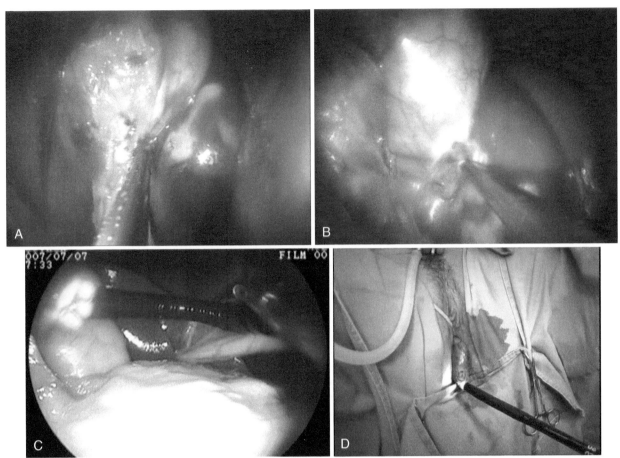

FIG 45.3 A, Transvaginal flexible cholecystectomy, dissection of gallbladder from the liver bed. **B,** Flexible endoscopic dissection of Calot's triangle by natural orifice transluminal endoscopic surgery (NOTES) transvaginal flexible cholecystectomy. **C,** Transvaginal introduction of two endoscopes (one gastroscope, one colonoscope) to perform total NOTES cholecystectomy. **D,** Transvaginal extraction of the specimen.

incision, with no use of laparoscopic instruments or camera (Fig. 45.3). A hybrid NOTES technique used the laparoscopy for safer access, visualization, and dissection, allowing a shorter operative time. Finally, TV trocars can also be used combined with mini laparoscopy instruments through the umbilicus. The complication rate for TV surgery was 6.9%. Mean intraabdominal CO_2 pressure did not show significant differences between the types of access and surgeries performed. Visualization of the cavity was mostly described to be of very good quality. When an abdominal trocar was inserted, insufflation through that trocar or Veress needle was preferred.[1]

In the series by Federlein et al (2010), satisfaction of patients with the result of the operation was high, and most would recommend TV access to others.[31] This painless access often requires very few postoperative analgesia. Dyspareunia has been mentioned as a possible complication of the TV approach, but it has not been recorded as a complication in most clinical series so far. On the contrary, TV access is used for diagnostic investigation of infertility, which in turn may be associated with sexual disturbance. The fornix of the vagina has very low sensible innervation. In our experience and from other authors, there is no detection of disturbance of sexuality in operated patients. The possibility of adhesion formation after incision of the posterior vault has thus far not been investigated.

Comparative studies on TV versus laparoscopic cholecystectomy have shown some advantages for the former.[32] In certain centers, TV cholecystectomy is no longer considered an experimental technique and may be routinely offered as a scarless option for cholecystectomy in female patients.

TRANSRECTAL NOTES AND TAMIS TOTAL MESORECTAL EXCISION

Transanal NOTES surgery has been the subject of a few recent experimental studies, suggesting that this access route can be an attractive option for treating colonic and abdominal diseases.[33–35] Technical obstacles for colonic access include risk of infection and leaks, safe entrance into the abdominal cavity, and reliable colonic closure, which all hinder transcolonic clinical applications.

Intrarectal surgery seems to add the advantages of transanally endoscopic microsurgery (TEM) together with transanal extraction of the specimen (natural orifice specimen extraction, or NOSE[35]), and can be performed either with flexible or with rigid instruments. We can imagine that in a few years, most colorectal surgery will be performed predominantly through natural orifices using single ports, endoscopes, transluminal devices, and even one-arm robotics and miniature robots, and cameras. It will be potentially possible to reach resections of any part of the colon as new technology becomes available.

Compared with TG access to the abdominal cavity, the transanal route offers potential advantages, by eliminating the need to retroflect the scope and other instruments in the upper abdomen. NOSE via TV and, more recently, transrectal access has been increasingly used to avoid larger incisions in laparoscopic surgery for large-organ extraction. NOTES TV sigmoidectomy, assisted by mini laparoscopy, was described by Lacy et al (2008), denominating the technique as MA-NOS in a patient with sigmoid cancer,[36] and Burghardt et al (2008) described the first case of NOTES TV right colectomy.[37]

Human Transanal Down-to-Up TME

The term *down-to-up total mesorectal excision* (TME) was coined in 2009 to describe the technique of cephalad progression of mesorectal dissection in transanal resections for rectal cancer.[38] Contrary to laparoscopic TME, this procedure allows easy identification of the distal limits of the tumor and promotes an excellent clearance of the distal resection margin. Our group published oncologic down-to-up TME (or transanal minimal invasive surgery TME [TAMIS-TME]) using a flexible colonoscope to enter the presacral plane and dissect the mesorectum (Fig. 45.4).

The current standard of care in the treatment of rectal cancer implies high ligation of the inferior mesenteric artery and total mesorectal resection with en bloc lymphadenectomy. The precise TME plane of dissection, described by Heald in the early 1980s, resulted in a better oncologic anatomical specimen without cell spillage, improving results and reducing the indication of abdomino-perineal resections.[39,40] From our experience with down-to-up TME, an adequate dissection with preservation of the mesorectal envelope can be achieved by flexible or rigid technique. Transanal NOTES TME is performed in the same anatomical plane but in the opposite direction (from anal to rectosigmoid junction), beginning the dissection by gaining access to the presacral plane between the presacral fascia and the mesorectum. The progression of the cephalad dissection is improved by the retropneumoperitoneum inside this avascular plane.

The history and progress of transrectal NOTES is undoubtedly due to the pioneer efforts of Gerhard Buess, who in the early 1980s described TEM, which is still the standard therapy for most low-rectal benign lesions.[41]

Down-to-Up Transanal NOTES TME Using a Single-Port Platform

Down-to-up TME using rigid intrarectal laparoscopy and a single-port device implies initial low circular full-thickness access to the anatomic plane of presacral space, evolving the dissection cephalad and circumferentially.[38] The patient is placed in the Lloyd-Davies position, receiving a single dose of intravenous antibiotic prophylaxis. Transabdominal laparoscopic high ligation and left-colon mobilization can be performed at the beginning or after the mesorectal resection. When the procedure is started with the laparoscopic step, care must be taken to not dissect the upper rectum and posterior mesorectum, due to the risk of gas leakage when performing transanal TME. The rectal lumen is disinfected with iodopovidone solution, and a disposable single-port access device is inserted transanally. It has three channels for instrumentation, and one or two additional channels for CO_2 insufflation. A laparoscopic camera and instruments are inserted through the port to act intraluminally. The inferior limits of the tumor are identified, and the lower resection limit is chosen at the desired line of anastomosis. A purse-string suture is transanally performed at an adequate distance from the tumor margin. This unique characteristic of the down-to-up technique allows for adequate visualization of the tumor margin and resection line, which is different from laparoscopic TME. The

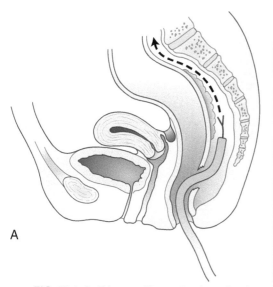

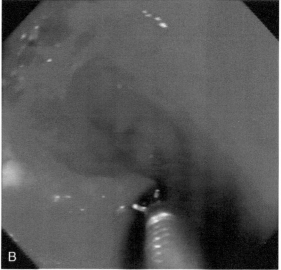

FIG 45.4 A, Diagram illustrating introduction of the endoscope in the presacral space for flexible natural orifice transluminal endoscopic surgery (NOTES) Down-to-Up total mesorectal excision (TME). The endoscope is inserted directly in the presacral space, 2–3 cm above the dentate line, allowing flexible dissection in the anatomic oncologic plane from below. **B,** Endoscopic view of flexible Down-to-Up TME for rectal cancer in a patient using a standard colonoscope. Total mesorectal resection is progressively accomplished using endoscopic monopolar scissors inside the ideal oncologic plane of dissection.

full-thickness circular incision reaches the plane between the presacral fascia and rectal fascia posteriorly, and the posterior wall of the vagina anteriorly, with cephalad progression. Transanal extraction of the specimen and section of the proximal colon is achieved. A transverse coloplasty can be performed in the proximal colon to improve functional results and hand-sewn or stapled coloanal anastomosis is performed.

Flexible Down-to-Up NOTES TME

Perirectal NOTES access with flexible TME using a standard colonoscope implies an initial low posterior perforation to the anatomic plane between the presacral fascia and the fascia propria, evolving the dissection proximally and circumferentially.[35] Preparation of the patient is as described previously. The necessary equipment is a single-channel videocolonoscope and a laparoscopic set. An anoscope is transanally inserted, and the rectum lumen is closed by a circumferential purse-string suture above the limit of rectal section, and the distal rectum is disinfected. The anal verge is identified, and a small posterior incision is performed exactly at the planned line of rectal resection, using monopolar cautery under direct view. The access orifice is tested by digital exploration, and the colonoscope is inserted directly in the perirectal retroperitoneal space. Total mesorectal resection is progressively accomplished using endoscopic monopolar scissors in the oncologic plane between the presacral fascia and the mesorectal fascia (see Fig. 45.4), with posterior and anterior cephalad progression, finally reaching the peritoneal cavity. To provide high vascular ligation, a laparoscopic camera is inserted through the umbilicus, allowing high ligature of inferior mesenteric artery at the level of aorta insertion, using a standard three-trocar technique, and also mobilizing the splenic flexure. The specimen is grasped and transanally extracted, followed by transanal stapled anastomosis. Proximal loop ileostomy is performed in most cases to protect the low anastomosis.

The use of the transanal approach for TME is evolving. There is growing experience worldwide and published casuistic work with consistent oncologic results, with dedicated teams that incorporated the technique as a surgical solution for difficult lower tumors. Other centers have incorporated transanal TME as the standard therapy for middle- and low-rectal cancers. In the future, with the availability of long-term oncologic and functional results, it will be possible to evaluate the standard use of the technique as the primary indication for most rectal cancers with surgical indication.

INTRAGASTRIC SINGLE-PORT SURGERY

An alternative method for transmural access of the stomach, intragastric single-port surgery (IGS) can be performed and allows for excellent exposition of difficult intragastric tumors, and to perform intragastric surgery when endoscopic therapy is limited.

Intragastric Single-Port Resection of Large Benign Tumors

Most benign intragastric tumors are treated endoscopically. In cases of tumors larger than 3 cm necessitating full-thickness resection involving a large gastric defect, IGS allows for safe and controlled resection even in difficult locations such as paraesophageal, using gastrointestinal laparoscopic staplers, coagulation, and sutures, without the need to previously enter the abdominal cavity laparoscopically.[42]

The technique involves the exteriorization of the gastric wall through the skin, fixation of the stomach to the skin, gastrotomy, and IGS (Fig. 45.5A–C). The tumor or bleeding lesion is localized, and successive intragastric stapling is performed to resect the lesion. In the case of gastric gastrointestinal stromal tumors, the resection can be performed intragastrically when more than 50% of the tumor is intragastric. When the tumor is exofitic to the abdominal cavity, a formal laparoscopic resection is indicated. Other indications are performing endoscopic retrograde cholangiopancreatography (ERCP) in altered anatomy after Roux-en-Y gastric bypass (RYGB), resection of recurrent Dieulafoy bleeding lesions (Video 45.2), and intragastric revision of pancreato-gastro anastomosis.

Transgastric ERCP in Excluded Stomach for Altered Anatomy After Roux-en-Y Gastric Bypass

The incidence of gallstone disease is increased after RYGB, mainly in the first postoperative year, due to the rapid weight loss. Management of choledocholithiasis in these patients can be challenging due to difficulty in accessing the common bile duct (CBD) as a result of surgically altered anatomy of the stomach and duodenum.[43] A combination of laparoscopy and endoscopy can be used to perform a TG ERCP along with laparoscopic cholecystectomy.

Access can be achieved by a 1-cm incision in the anterior wall of the remnant stomach and placement of a 15- to 18-mm trocar in the left abdomen, through which a side-view duodenoscope is passed, with the help of the surgeon, reaching the duodenum.[44-46] The procedure is then performed as a conventional ERCP.[47] In cases where this is technically difficult, an alternate technique can access the CBD via the jejunum, facilitated by a double-balloon enteroscope. This approach has a successful biliary cannulation rate of up to 60%.[48]

Falcão et al (2012) analyzed 20 patients submitted for TG laparoscopic ERCP, with papillotomy success in 100% of the cases without any serious complications. In a few cases the cystic duct was partially opened and a guidewire inserted that was exteriorized in the duodenal papilla, working as a guide for biliary catheterization.[47,49]

An innovative procedure can be performed using a single-port device inserted directly inside the excluded stomach, after its exteriorization through the abdominal wall (IGS). This method comprises the following technical steps: (1) insertion of the single port in one incision in the left upper abdomen; (2) adhesiolysis, cholecystectomy when indicated, localization and grasping of the excluded stomach; (3) removal of the single-port device; (4) exteriorization and fixation of the stomach to the skin; (5) gastrotomy and insertion of the single-port device, this time in an intragastric position; (6) progression of the endoscope through the single port, and ERCP and endoscopic papillotomy (see Fig. 45.5D). In our clinical series, ERCP was possible in all patients, and it is currently our standard technique for this common problem.

EXPECTATIONS OF NATURAL ORIFICE SURGERY

NOTES appears to be evolving as a feasible, safe, and reasonable option for transabdominal surgery, with the potential to avoid incision-related complications. Preliminary results of clinical experience have demonstrated acceptable complication rates in main international centers, low postoperative stay, and good cosmetic and pain requirement results. More important than

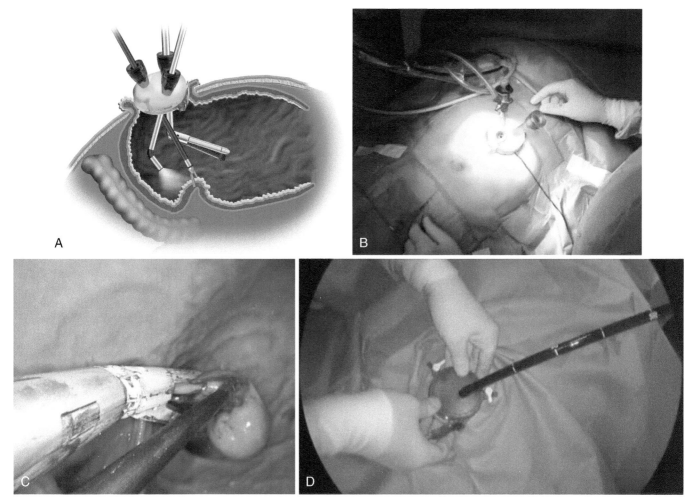

FIG 45.5 A, Schematic illustration of intragastric single-port surgery (IGS). The gastric wall is extracted and fixed to the skin. After this, an opening is made in the antrum to allow the introduction of a single-port device in an intragastric position. **B,** External view of IGS positioning for resection of a gastric gastrointestinal stromal tumor (GIST). **C,** Intraoperative view of IGS resection of a gastric GIST. Staplers and laparoscopic instruments can easily be introduced to perform full-thickness extraction of intramural tumors. **D,** Transgastric IGS-ERCP in excluded stomach for altered anatomy after Roux-en Y gastric bypass. The single port is intraabdominally inserted, then the excluded stomach is localized and exteriorized through the abdominal wall, and fixed to the skin. The endoscope is inserted percutaneously into the stomach and ERCP easily performed.

this, and perhaps crucial to indicate longevity for transluminal surgery, is the ability of surgeons and endoscopists to replace complex surgical procedures with simple endoscopic ones, and the identification of novel therapeutic targets.[50] Consistent advantages of natural orifice surgery over existing procedures are not evident yet, and future prospective clinical trials may be addressed to recognize the role of NOTES in surgery.

KEY REFERENCES

1. Zorron R, Palanivelu C, Galvao Neto MP, et al: International multicenter trial on clinical natural orifice surgery–NOTES IMTN study: preliminary results of 362 patients, *Surg Innov* 17(2):142–158, 2010.
2. Lehmann KS, Ritz JP, Wibmer A, et al: The German registry for natural orifice translumenal endoscopic surgery: report of the first 551 patients, *Ann Surg* 252(2):263–270, 2010.
3. Kalloo AN, Singh VK, Jagannath SB, et al: Flexible transgastric peritoneoscopy: a novel approach to diagnostic and therapeutic interventions in the peritoneal cavity, *Gastrointest Endosc* 60(1):114–117, 2004.
4. Rao GV, Reddy DN, Banerjee R: NOTES: human experience, *Gastrointest Endosc Clin N Am* 18(2):361–370, x, 2008.
5. Chukwumah C, Zorron R, Marks JM, Ponsky JL: Current status of natural orifice translumenal endoscopic surgery (NOTES), *Curr Probl Surg* 47(8):630–668, 2010.
6. Sumiyama K, Tajiri H, Gostout CJ: Submucosal endoscopy with mucosal flap safety valve (SEMF) technique: a safe access method into the peritoneal cavity and mediastinum, *Minim Invasive Ther Allied Technol* 17(6):365–369, 2008.
8. Inoue H, Sato H, Ikeda H, et al: Per-oral endoscopic myotomy: a series of 500 patients, *J Am Coll Surg* 221(2):256–264, 2015.
9. Talukdar R, Inoue H, Nageshwar Reddy D: Efficacy of peroral endoscopic myotomy (POEM) in the treatment of achalasia: a systematic review and meta-analysis, *Surg Endosc* 29(11):3030–3046, 2015.
10. Lopez-Nava G, Galvao M, Bautista-Castano I, et al: Endoscopic sleeve gastroplasty with 1-year follow-up: factors predictive of success, *Endosc Int Open* 4(2):E222–E227, 2016.

11. Dallemagne B, Perretta S, Allemann P, et al: Transgastric hybrid cholecystectomy, *Br J Surg* 96(10):1162–1166, 2009.

12. Seifert H, Wehrmann T, Schmitt T, et al: Retroperitoneal endoscopic debridement for infected peripancreatic necrosis, *Lancet* 356(9230): 653–655, 2000.

20. Sutton C: The history of vaginal hysterectomy. In Sheth SJ, editor: *Vaginal hysterectomy*, London, 2002, Martin Dunitz, p 3.

24. Zorron R, Filgueiras M, Maggioni LC, et al: NOTES transvaginal cholecystectomy: report of the first case, *Surg Innov* 14(4):279–283, 2007.

25. Marescaux J, Dallemagne B, Perretta S, et al: Report of transluminal cholecystectomy in a human being, *Arch Surg* 142:823–826, 2007.

30. Roberts KE, Solomon D, Bell RL, Duffy AJ: "Triangle of safety"— anatomic considerations in transvaginal natural orifice surgery, *Surg Endosc* 27(8):2963–2965, 2013.

31. Federlein M, Borchert D, Muller V, et al: Transvaginal video-assisted cholecystectomy in clinical practice, *Surg Endosc* 24(10):2444–2452, 2010.

35. Zorron R: Natural orifice surgery and single port access applied to colorectal surgery: the new era of intrarectal surgery? *G Chir* 32(3): 97–103, 2011.

36. Lacy AM, Delgado S, Rojas OA, et al: MA-NOS radical sigmoidectomy: report of a transvaginal resection in the human, *Surg Endosc* 22(7): 1717–1723, 2008.

37. Burghardt J, Federlein M, Muller V, et al: [Minimal invasive transvaginal right hemicolectomy: report of the first complex NOS (natural orifice surgery) bowels operation using a hybrid approach], *Zentralbl Chir* 133(6):574–576, 2008.

38. Zorron R, Phillips HN, Wynn G, et al: "Down-to-Up" transanal NOTES total mesorectal excision for rectal cancer: Preliminary series of 9 patients, *J Minim Access Surg* 10(3):144–150, 2014.

42. Zorron R, Bothe C, Holtmann M, Junghans T: Intragastrische (IGS) Single-Port Chirurgiie bei grossen gutartigen Magentumoren, *Zeitschrift Gastroenterol* 53(08):2014. KC096.

47. Falcao M, Campos JM, Galvao Neto M, et al: Transgastric endoscopic retrograde cholangiopancreatography for the management of biliary tract disease after Roux-en-Y gastric bypass treatment for obesity, *Obes Surg* 22(6):872–876, 2012.

48. Chu YC, Yang CC, Yeh YH, et al: Double-balloon enteroscopy application in biliary tract disease-its therapeutic and diagnostic functions, *Gastrointest Endosc* 68(3):585–591, 2008.

49. Falcão M, Campos JM, Galvão Neto M, et al: Colangiopancreatografía retrógrada endoscópica en pacientes con asa en Y-de-Roux, *Revista Chilena Cirugía* 64:238–244, 2012.

50. Pasricha PJ, Krummel TM: NOTES and other emerging trends in gastrointestinal endoscopy and surgery: the change that we need and the change that is real, *Am J Gastroenterol* 104:2384–2386, 2009.

A complete reference list can be found online at ExpertConsult .com

46

Endoscopic Full-Thickness Resection of Subepithelial Lesions of the GI Tract

Jennifer Maranki and Stavros N. Stavropoulos

INTRODUCTION

Over the past 15 years, the role of endoscopy in the removal of large and subepithelial lesions has expanded greatly. Whereas expertise in endoscopic submucosal dissection (ESD) has been long established in Asia, the technique has become more widely available in the West. With expanding indications, including the removal of muscularis propria (MP)-originating subepithelial tumors (SETs), the need for a safe and effective method for performing endoscopic full-thickness resection (EFTR) is critical. Suzuki et al (2001) reported on the use of EFTR and endoscopic complete defect closure in one duodenal and two rectal carcinoids, the first English-language report of the technique.[1] Lesions were suctioned and ligated within the cap of the devices, and in the duodenal case, laparoscopic assistance was required for microperforation closure.[1] Since then, a variety of techniques have been reported including those that are laparoscopy-assisted, device-assisted, and those that employ a free-hand approach.[2–4]

INDICATIONS AND CONTRAINDICATIONS FOR EFTR

Indications for EFTR are dependent on whether the lesion is in the upper or lower gastrointestinal (GI) tract. The most frequent indication for EFTR is SETs of 5 cm or less in diameter arising from or involving the MP based on endoscopic ultrasound (EUS) or computed tomography (CT) imaging.[5] These lesions are often gastrointestinal stromal tumors (GISTs), and National Comprehensive Cancer Network (NCCN) guidelines recommend removal of known or suspected GISTs that are symptomatic, have high-risk EUS features (including an irregular border, ulceration, cystic spaces, heterogeneity, and echogenic foci), or are greater than or equal to 2 cm in size.[6] Pathologic features that indicate a higher risk of metastasis or recurrence include mitotic index and Ki-67 status.[7,8] Another indication is recurrence of mucosal lesions following endoscopic mucosal resection (EMR) or ESD at a surgical resection site.[5] Any SET that is symptomatic should also be resected.[9]

Contraindications for EFTR can be divided into patient- and tumor-related factors. Patient-related contraindications include the presence of high surgical risk due to severe comorbidities, including bleeding or coagulation disorders, and severe cardiopulmonary disease; pregnancy; inability to tolerate anesthesia; and anatomic issues that would preclude passage of the EFTR or suturing device. Tumor-related factors that are contraindications are the presence of a large extramural component; tumors with a high risk of lymph node spread or evidence of systemic spread; and features suggestive of aggressive behavior.[5,9] Notably, carcinomas should be resected with a pre-closure method of EFTR to prevent contamination of the peritoneal cavity with malignant cells.[10–12]

EFTR OF SUBEPITHELIAL TUMORS ARISING FROM THE MUSCULARIS PROPRIA

EFTR allows for minimally invasive, "scarless," organ-preserving, en bloc resection of tumors ranging from 2 to 5 cm. Tumors less than 2 cm are rarely symptomatic and carry low risk of malignant transformation, whereas tumors greater than 5 cm in diameter typically have higher malignant potential[13] and are often difficult to extract from the mouth or the anus, making surgical resection a better option.

The most commonly encountered neoplastic SET is a GIST, and management decisions are based on size and mitotic rate. Whereas tissue acquisition via EUS-guided fine-needle aspiration or fine-needle biopsy is ideal, these techniques fail to obtain adequate histology in up to 40% of SETS.[14–16] Furthermore, assessment of mitotic index, a very important factor for risk assessment of GISTs,[13] frequently cannot be performed. NCCN consensus guidelines for known or suspected GISTs recommend resection for all lesions that are symptomatic, have high-risk EUS features (including irregular border, cystic spaces, ulceration, echogenic foci, and heterogeneity), or are greater than or equal to 2 cm in size.[7] Long-term annual surveillance is recommended for low risk GISTs less than 2 cm in size. This management plan is also utilized for other, indeterminate lesions or rare mesenchymal tumors for which there is a paucity of data to develop an evidence-based algorithm. As a result, a cumbersome, lifelong surveillance plan is undertaken, contributing not only to health care costs but also to substantial anxiety on the part of the patient.

Frequently, these lesions are located in anatomic areas such as the gastroesophageal junction, pre-pyloric antrum, cardia, and esophagus where organ-preserving tumorectomy via standard surgical approaches is difficult or impossible, and thus require more extensive organ resection. Because of these circumstances, a technique that achieves minimally invasive, organ-preserving, complete resection of such lesions via natural orifices following the tenets of natural orifice transluminal endoscopic surgery (NOTES), preserving the natural anatomy and minimizing morbidity, is highly desirable.

There are several reasons why endoscopic resection of these tumors is favorable. Based on tumor biology, these lesions are rarely aggressive and, unlike epithelial malignancies, carry minimal risk of lymph node involvement. Furthermore, unlike cancer resections, they do not require a large margin of uninvolved tissue for resection because they have a low chance of local recurrence even in cases of R1 (microscopic margin positive) surgical resection.[17] Additionally, these lesions in the wall of the GI tract typically grow into the lumen of the GI tract, making them easily identifiable and often amenable to enucleation without the need for resection of uninvolved tissue.

EARLIER EFTR TECHNIQUES

Although there is some overlap in terminology, the preponderance of recent literature utilizes the term EFTR to denote free-hand "pure NOTES" full-thickness resection of lesions with ESD-like technique and accessories. Later efforts incorporated a combined laparoscopic and endoscopic approach. A variety of techniques have been reported, with the role of endoscopy ranging from lesion and margin identification to almost complete endoscopic resection with laparoscopic defect closure.[18,19] The main drawback of these approaches is that they are more invasive and time-consuming than a purely endoscopic approach.

Device-assisted EFTR (DA-EFTR) utilizes devices to ensure serosal apposition prior to resection. DA-EFTR has been reported by means of tissue apposition devices that were designed for endoscopic anti-reflux procedures. Initially, the NDO Plicator device, which is no longer available, was used and, more recently, the GERDX device (G-SURG, Seeon-Seebruck, Germany) (Fig. 46.1), or over-the-scope nitinol clips (OTSCs) (Ovesco, Cary, NC) either via their original device designed for tissue apposition or a more recent adaptation by the same company (FTR device, Ovesco) specifically designed for DA-EFTR[9] have been used.

Potential advantages of DA-EFTR techniques include that they are easier and faster than free-hand EFTR and that pre-closure of the defect eliminates escape of luminal contents, which should decrease the risk of infection and potentially allow resection of epithelial malignancies without fear of disseminating malignant cells to the peritoneal or thoracic cavities. However, with current technology, DA-EFTR has significant limitations. The GERDX device is restricted to lesions less than 35 mm with a largely intraluminal growth pattern because of the progressive difficulty in placing full-thickness sutures as tumor size increases.[9,20] The GERDX device utilizes the placement of transmural resorbable sutures with serosa-to-serosa apposition underneath the SET followed by lesion resection. The OTSC method, even with the larger FTR device, is limited to epithelial lesions of less than 3 to 4 cm and subepithelial lesions less than 2 cm with intraluminal growth pattern only that are able to be suctioned completely into the device cap with subsequent clip deployment. Additionally, both the GERDX and OTSC devices are bulky and limited by the ability to advance the endoscope with the device to the area of interest, thereby making certain locations inaccessible to them. For example, the Ovesco FTR device, due to its very large size (outer diameter of 21 mm), is approved in Europe only for colonic lesions, although it has been used sporadically for selected upper gastrointestinal lesions by experts with significant experience.[21]

"Free-hand" EFTR represents an offshoot of ESD-based techniques utilizing the same knives but taking the plane of dissection deep to the submucosa, along the surface of the MP for submucosally located SETs (what has been termed endoscopic submucosal excavation [ESE]), or, for MP-based SETs, taking the dissection INTO the MP (termed variably endoscopic muscularis dissection, endoscopic enucleation, or endoscopic muscularis excavation [EME], the term we will use in this review). Initial attempts at endoscopic resection of MP-based SETs employed the ESE or EME technique (for SETs arising from the submucosa or MP, respectively) to resect small subepithelial lesions in the range of 2 to 3 cm in size with intraluminal growth. The lesions are excavated en bloc using ESD techniques maintaining a plane of resection along the inner circular muscle or the surface of the MP, avoiding perforation or full-thickness resection. Complete resection rates range from 65% to 100%, with relatively low rates of perforation (0% to 13%) that can be managed endoscopically with minimal morbidity, as well as a favorable overall adverse event profile.[22–32]

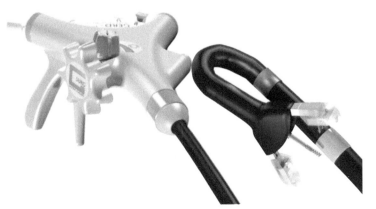

FIG 46.1 GERDX. (Image courtesy G-SURG GmbH, Seeon-Seebruck, Germany.)

These techniques are limited to lesions with purely intraluminal growth (no tumor component extending beyond the MP towards the peritoneal or thoracic cavities), as is also the case with the DA-EFTR technique. Additionally, for MP-based lesions, as full thickness resection is not undertaken, EME may leave tumor cells in the MP or serosa.

Two main techniques, EFTR and submucosal tunnel endoscopic resection (STER), have been developed to address these disadvantages of EME. They represent pure NOTES techniques that can achieve complete full-thickness resection of MP-based tumors independent of growth pattern using ESD techniques and tools. Both techniques arose within a climate of renewed interest in NOTES in the form of juxtaluminal, short-range NOTES procedures, referred to as *New NOTES* procedures. This renewed interest was sparked by the remarkable success of Per Oral Endoscopic Myotomy (POEM), the prototypical New NOTES procedure that has been credited as the first successful NOTES intervention.[33] Although EFTR is widely applicable in any location of the GI tract, STER is limited to locations where a submucosal tunnel can be successfully created (esophagus, distal stomach or rectum). In this chapter, we will focus on the EFTR technique, because the STER technique is better addressed as an offshoot of tunnel-based interventions such as POEM. The EFTR technique involves full-thickness removal of a SET by creating an intentional perforation, with subsequent endoscopic closure using endoscopic suturing[34] or clips and endoloop techniques consisting of the use of several endoclips, with subsequent placement of the endoloop to fix and tighten the clips together.[35,36]

EFTR, using a free-hand approach with ESD techniques and tools, was first reported in 2011 by two Chinese groups.[4,37] Wang and colleagues reported EFTR of 66 nonintracavitary stromal lesions less than or equal to 3.5 cm in size, and compared their experience to 43 patients with similar tumors who underwent laparoscopic surgery. Median operating times and hospital costs were lower in the endoscopic group, both techniques achieved R0 resection in all cases, and postoperative complications were significantly higher in the endoscopic group, which correlated with tumor size (14% vs. 26%).[37] That same year, Zhou and colleagues reported on EFTR of 26 gastric submucosal lesions arising from the MP (16/26 GISTs), with size ranging from 1.2 to 4.5 cm. Complete resection was achieved in all cases, and there were no instances of significant adverse events or complications.[4]

DESCRIPTION OF EFTR TECHNIQUE

In accordance with NOTES protocols, as a breach of the GI lumen is expected, prophylactic antibiotics should be administered, and the target organ must be meticulously irrigated and cleaned of all debris. Furthermore, optimally, the patient should be positioned to ensure that the area of resection is non-dependent to avoid extraluminal escape of significant amounts of luminal secretions, irrigation fluid, and blood once a full-thickness defect is present and prior to its closure. Following the procedure, patients should take nothing by mouth (NPO) for at least 24 hours, and radiographic imaging to test for leaks must be performed prior to the initiation of a liquid diet. If there are any concerns regarding how secure a closure has been achieved (which is not usually the case if effective suturing is possible, but may be the case when endoclips/endoloop techniques are used), nasogastric suction should be applied and possibly more prolonged NPO status.

The critical steps of the EFTR procedure are as follows (Figs. 46.2 and 46.3):

1. Using a solution of blue dye (methylene blue or indigo carmine) and saline, or other standard solutions used in ESD and EMR, submucosal injection is performed along the margin of the tumor.
2. Using an ESD knife, circumferential margination of the tumor is undertaken. The type of knife used is operator-dependent, but the most commonly used ones include the ERBE T-type Hybrid Knife (ERBE USA, Marietta, GA), the IT2 Knife (Olympus America), and the Hook Knife (Olympus America). For a complete listing of ESD knives and accessories, refer to the American Society for Gastrointestinal Endoscopy (ASGE) ESD Technology Status Evaluation Report.[38] Margination is complete when fully circumferential mucosal and submucosal dissection has been achieved.
3. Resection of the MP is performed, with special attention to the avoidance of tumor capsule disruption, as damage to the capsule may result in dispersal of tumor cells. Tumors that are deep in the MP may be adherent to the serosa, which requires resection of the MP and serosa. For certain more superficial MP-based tumors it may be possible to preserve the serosa. In this deep dissection, a knife with an insulated tip is often preferred to prevent injury to adjacent organs. Key aspects of the technique are to avoid overinsufflation and to be able to detect and treat tension capnoperitoneum, which can be vented by placing an angiocath or Veress needle in the right or left upper quadrant.
4. In the final stages of the resection, care is taken to avoid pushing the tumor into the peritoneum through the defect. Some operators use a double-channel endoscope with a grasper to secure the tumor during the final incision. Alternatively, a snare is used to make the final cut, which enables capture of the tumor immediately on completion of the final incision.
5. Several devices may be used for closure of the full-thickness defect. Closure devices include the combination of endoclips and endoloops,[19] OTSCs (Ovesco),[39] and an endoscopic suturing device (Overstitch, Apollo Endosurgery, Austin, TX).[34] A unique approach to closure is the omental patch technique, which involves suctioning a patch of omentum through the defect and securing it with endoclips onto the defect to "plug" the defect and achieve secure closure.[40]

EFTR OUTCOMES

Several case series using EFTR, mainly from China, have reported on the safety and efficacy for treatment of SETs, and are summarized in Table 46.1. Most lesions are between 15 and 30 mm in diameter, and are SETs in the upper GI tract, most of which are GISTs, followed by leiomyomas and smaller numbers of other mesenchymal tumors, such as glomus tumors and schwannomas. Procedure times range from 40 to 105 minutes, and en bloc resection is achieved in nearly 100%. Most common adverse events include localized peritonitis, pneumoperitoneum, abdominal distension or pain, fever, nausea and vomiting, and posterior pharyngeal pain likely due to minor trauma during peroral extraction of the larger tumors.[4,36,39,41–44] Of those with documented follow-up, none had evidence of recurrence. In a series of 48 patients from our center at Winthrop University, the only Western free-hand EFTR series to date, similar results using free-hand EFTR were achieved.[33,45]

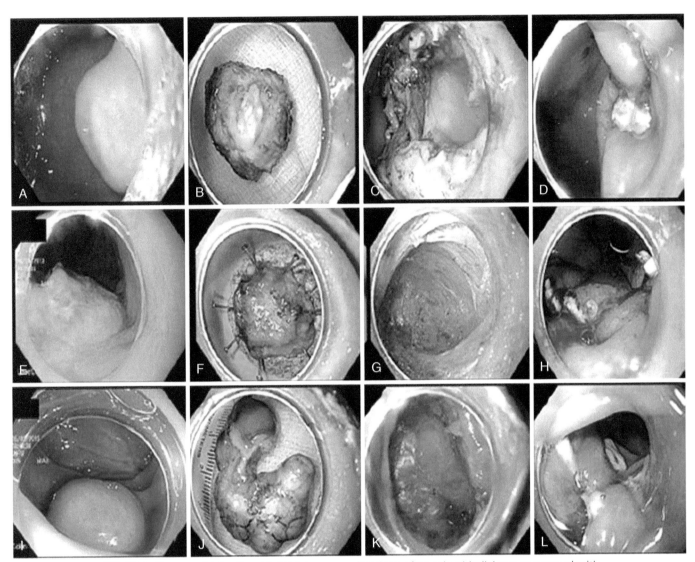

FIG 46.2 Closure of intentional full-thickness perforations after subepithelial tumor removal with endoscopic suturing device. **A,** Endoscopic image of gastric muscularis propria based subepithelial tumor. **B,** 2.5 cm schwannoma. **C,** Resection crater showing transmural fat. **D,** Endoscopic sutured closure of defect. **E,** Endoscopic image of rectal carcinoma superficially extending to muscularis propria. **F,** 1.3 cm rectal low-grade adenocarcinoma. **G,** Resection crater showing perirectal fat, circular muscle layer, and longitudinal muscle layers. **H,** Endoscopic sutured defect closure. **I,** Endoscopic image of sigmoid muscularis propria based subepithelial tumor. **J,** 3 cm leiomyosarcoma. **K,** Resection crater demonstrating peritoneal fat. **L,** Endoscopic sutured closure of defect. (From Stavropoulos SN, Modayil R, Friedel D: Current applications of endoscopic suturing. *World J Gastrointest Endosc* 2015;7[8]:777–789.)

In comparing EFTR to laparoscopic-assisted resection of small SETs, few series have been reported.[46] Wang et al (2016) reported on 68 total patients who underwent EFTR or laparoscopic resection. EFTR was associated with fewer complications and favorable en bloc resection.[47]

A study by Tan et al (2016) compared outcomes of EFTR versus STER for the removal of gastric GISTs in 52 patients. No differences were found in tumor size, en bloc resection rate, operation time or complications, hospital stay, or cost.[48]

There is a paucity of data on the use of EFTR techniques for treatment of lesions located beyond the esophagus and stomach.

Pure EFTR is rarely applied to substantial duodenal lesions due to the technical difficulty in closing large defects in the duodenum and the high risk of leaks and bleeding complications that are difficult to treat, often resulting in significant morbidity. Abe and colleagues in 2012 reported on laparoscopy-assisted EFTR of a duodenal carcinoid.[49] More recently, Schmidt et al (2015)[21] reported on EFTR of four duodenal lesions (two non-lifting adenomas and two carcinoids) using the FTR device. Mean resection size was 28.3 mm (range 22–40 mm). There were two cases of minor bleeding and no perforations, and R0 resection was achieved in 3 of 4 cases.[21]

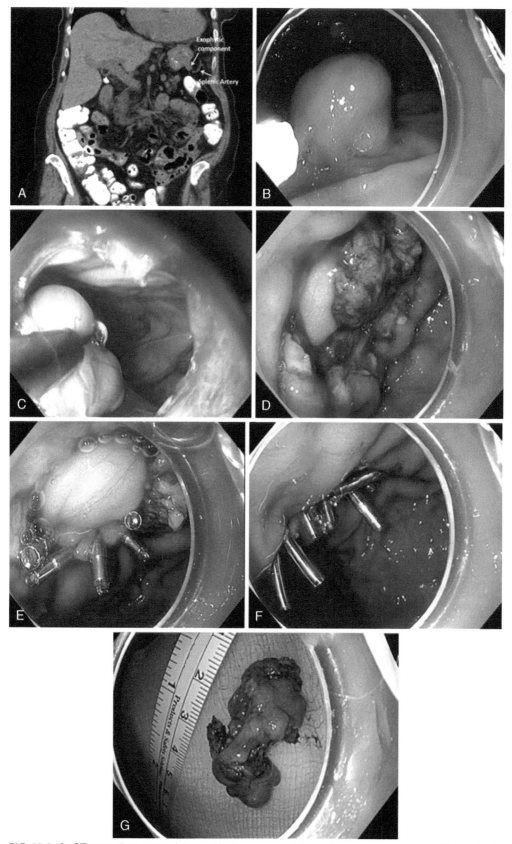

FIG 46.3 A, CT scan demonstrating exophytic portion of the subepithelial tumor abutting splenic artery. **B,** Endoscopic view of the endophytic portion along greater curvature of stomach. **C,** Extraluminal portion of the tumor retracted with the endoscopic submucosal dissection knife to show omental fat and intraperitoneal organs, seen through the full-thickness defect. **D,** Resection crater with omental fat. **E,** Omental fat clipped to the resection rim to seal the full-thickness defect. **F,** Two-layer closure with endoclips to approximate mucosa **G,** "Dumbbell" shaped tumor 4 × 2.5 cm with exophytic and endophytic lobulated components. Pathology: GIST (0 mitoses/50 hpf). (From Stavropoulos SN, Modayil R, Friedel D, Brathwaite CE: Endoscopic full-thickness resection for GI stromal tumors. *Gastrointest Endosc* 2014;80[2]:334–335.)

TABLE 46.1 Selected Series of EFTR Cases

Study	Year	Number of Cases	Lesion Location	Mean Tumor Size (cm)	Success Rate of en Bloc Resection (%)	Pathologic Diagnosis	Adverse Events
Zhou, et al[4]	2011	26	Gastric	2.8	100	16 GIST, 6 leiomyomata, 3 glomus tumors, 1 schwannoma	None
Wang, et al[37]	2011	31	Gastric	1.5	97	31 GIST	9 localized peritonitis
Xu, et al[3]	2013	19	Colonic	1.8	84	9 leiomyomata, 4 GISTs, 2 schwannomata, 2 fibromatoses, 1 granuloma, 1 hamartoma	2 localized peritonitis, 1 bleeding
Ye, et al[36]	2014	51	Gastric	2.4	98	30 GISTs, 21 leiomyomata	None
Huang, et al[41]	2014	35	Gastric	2.8	100	25 GISTs, 7 leiomyomata, 2 nerve tumors	5 pneumoperitoneum
Feng, et al[43]	2014	48	Gastric	1.6	100	43 GISTs, 4 leiomyomata, 1 schwannoma	5 abdominal distensions
Yang, et al[42]	2015	41	Gastric	1.6	100	33 GIST, 4 leiomyomata, 1 NET, 1 schwannoma, 1 pancreatic rest, 1 hyaline degeneration	2 abdominal pain, 1 fever, 1 dysuria, 1 nausea/vomiting, 1 pharyngeal pain, 1 upper abdominal tenderness
Guo, et al[39]	2015	23	Gastric	1.2	100	19 GISTs, 4 leiomyomata	2 localized peritonitis
Wu, et al[46]	2015	50	Gastric	3.4	100	50 GISTs	None
Shi, et al[44]	2016	68	Gastric	2.6	100	68 GISTs	1 Mallory Weiss syndrome, 1 delayed bleed
Wang, et al[47]	2016	35	Gastric	1.3	100	35 GISTs	4 intraoperative bleeding
Tan, et al[48]	2016	32	Gastric	1.5	97	32 GISTs	4 abdominal pain and fever, 1 delayed bleed
Schmidt, et al[12]	2016	106	Colonic	1.7	89	80 adenoma, 13 T1 carcinoma, 13 SETs	2 minor bleeds, 3 perforations (1 delayed)

EFTR has been used in the colon, with closure of the defect using clips. In a case series of 16 patients, two required laparoscopic assistance for defect closure, and two developed peritonitis.[3] DA-EFTR with the Ovesco FTR device may be an appropriate technique to remove epithelial lesions, such as advanced adenomas or intramucosal carcinomas, in the colon because pre-closure of the defect eliminates risk of extraluminal contamination (an important concern in the colon) and escape of malignant cells (which is a concern in epithelial neoplasms, unlike SETs). Even though these lesions are limited to the mucosa and thus amenable to EMR or ESD, DA-EFTR may facilitate resection of challenging lesions such as previously manipulated "non-lifting" lesions or lesions in difficult locations, such as near the appendiceal orifice. Salerno et al (2016) reported a case of EFTR using the FTR device to removal a 16-mm submucosal lesion of the right colon. Complete removal was achieved with no complications; pathology revealed a large B-cell lymphoma.[50] A large multicenter series from Germany reported application of DA-EFTR with the Ovesco FTR to 180 such lesions in the colon.[12] Outcomes were modest, and only lesions less than 3 cm were included. Complete R0 resection was only achieved in 78%. Full-thickness resection including MP was also only achieved in 78%. Significant adverse events, including events requiring emergency surgery (2 perforations [1 delayed], 1 appendicitis), occurred in 1.6%. Ten percent had residual/recurrent tumor even at limited 3-month follow-up. Seven percent required surgery within this 3-month interval. Hopefully, with continued device improvements, outcomes will improve.

In conclusion, in the hands of expert operators, EFTR appears to provide high rates of complete resection of SETs of 4 cm or less, with favorable procedural times and adverse event profile. EFTR provides advantages over laparoscopy-assisted procedures by allowing for optimum organ-sparing resection with minimal invasiveness. For lesions of 4 to 5 cm in size, a combined approach with laparoscopy may be preferred, as it provides an effective method for tumor extraction. For lesions larger than 5 cm, given the increased risk for aggressive behavior and challenges in manipulating and endoscopically extracting such large lesions, including risk of rupture due to central necrosis in larger tumors, traditional surgery is recommended. It should be emphasized that, due to the skills required for secure closure, avoidance of severe bleeding, and control of insufflation, EFTR should be attempted by operators with ESD mastery, under institutional review board protocol at least initially, and with surgical backup.[33]

SUMMARY

Current data indicate that EFTR in the hands of endoscopic resection experts represents a safe and effective pure NOTES approach for en bloc resection of SETs less than 5 cm in size, mainly located in the esophagus and stomach. Complete resection is achieved at high rates, with an acceptable adverse event profile. However, it should be emphasized that techniques for EFTR require a high degree of expertise, with mastery of ESD and submucosal tunneling techniques. Further improvements in closure devices such as the Overstitch system or other suturing devices in development, improvements in DA-EFTR devices such as the GERDX and FTR device systems, and the advent of novel devices, including robotic or lumen stabilization platforms currently under development (e.g., Lumen-R, Boston Scientific,

Marlborough, MA or DiLumen, Lumendi, Westport, CT), will likely push the field of EFTR forward and make it more widely accessible to advanced endoscopists beyond the current small group of resection experts.

KEY REFERENCES

1. Suzuki H, Ikeda K: Endoscopic mucosal resection and full thickness resection with complete defect closure for early gastrointestinal malignancies, *Endoscopy* 33(5):437–439, 2001.
3. Xu M, Wang XY, Zhou PH, et al: Endoscopic full-thickness resection of colonic submucosal tumors originating from the muscularis propria: an evolving therapeutic strategy, *Endoscopy* 45(9):770–773, 2013.
4. Zhou PH, Yao LQ, Qin XY, et al: Endoscopic full-thickness resection without laparoscopic assistance for gastric submucosal tumors originated from the muscularis propria, *Surg Endosc* 25(9):2926–2931, 2011.
5. Cai M, Zhou P, Lourenço LC, et al: Endoscopic full-thickness resection (EFTR) for gastrointestinal subepithelial tumors, *Gastrointest Endosc Clin N Am* 26(2):283–295, 2016.
7. von Mehren M, Randall RL, Benjamin RS, et al: Soft tissue sarcoma, version 2.2016, NCCN Clinical Practice Guidelines in Oncology, *J Natl Compr Canc Netw* 14(6):758–786, 2016.
9. Bauder M, Schmidt A, Caca K: Non-exposure, device-assisted endoscopic full-thickness resection, *Gastrointest Endosc Clin N Am* 26(2):297–312, 2016.
11. Goto O, Takeuchi H, Kitagawa Y, et al: Endoscopic submucosal dissection (ESD) and related techniques as precursors of "new notes" resection methods for gastric neoplasms, *Gastrointest Endosc Clin N Am* 26(2):313–322, 2016.
20. Schmidt A, Bauder M, Riecken B, et al: Endoscopic full-thickness resection of gastric subepithelial tumors: a single-center series, *Endoscopy* 47(2):154–158, 2015.
24. Lee IL, Lin PY, Tung SY, et al: Endoscopic submucosal dissection for the treatment of intraluminal gastric subepithelial tumors originating from the muscularis propria layer, *Endoscopy* 38(10):1024–1028, 2006.
25. Hwang JC, Kim JH, Shin SJ, et al: Endoscopic resection for the treatment of gastric subepithelial tumors originated from the muscularis propria layer, *Hepatogastroenterology* 56(94-95):1281–1286, 2009.
26. Probst A, Golger D, Arnholdt H, et al: Endoscopic submucosal dissection of early cancers, flat adenomas, and submucosal tumors in the gastrointestinal tract, *Clin Gastroenterol Hepatol* 7(2):149–155, 2009.
27. Shi Q, Zhong YS, Yao LQ, et al: Endoscopic submucosal dissection for treatment of esophageal submucosal tumors originating from the muscularis propria layer, *Gastrointest Endosc* 74(6):1194–1200, 2011.
30. Zhang Y, Ye LP, Zhou XB, et al: Safety and efficacy of endoscopic excavation for gastric subepithelial tumors originating from the muscularis propria layer: results from a large study in China, *J Clin Gastroenterol* 47(8):689–694, 2013.
31. Liu BR, Song JT, Qu B, et al: Endoscopic muscularis dissection for upper gastrointestinal subepithelial tumors originating from the muscularis propria, *Surg Endosc* 26(11):3141–3148, 2012.
33. Modayil R, Stavropoulos SN: A Western perspective on "New NOTES" from POEM to full-thickness resection and beyond, *Gastrointest Endosc Clin N Am* 26(2):413–432, 2016.
34. Stavropoulos SN, Modayil R, Friedel D: Current applications of endoscopic suturing, *World J Gastrointest Endosc* 7(8):777–789, 2015.
35. Zhang Y, Wang X, Xiong G, et al: Complete defect closure of gastric submucosal tumors with purse-string sutures, *Surg Endosc* 28(6):1844–1851, 2014.
36. Ye LP, Yu Z, Mao XL, et al: Endoscopic full-thickness resection with defect closure using clips and an endoloop for gastric subepithelial tumors arising from the muscularis propria, *Surg Endosc* 28(6):1978–1983, 2014.
39. Guo J, Liu Z, Sun S, et al: Endoscopic full-thickness resection with defect closure using an over-the-scope clip for gastric subepithelial tumors originating from the muscularis propria, *Surg Endosc* 29(11):3356–3362, 2015.
40. Stavropoulos SN, Modayil R, Friedel D, et al: Endoscopic full-thickness resection for GI stromal tumors, *Gastrointest Endosc* 80(2):334–335, 2014.
42. Yang F, Wang S, Sun S, et al: Factors associated with endoscopic full-thickness resection of gastric submucosal tumors, *Surg Endosc* 29(12):3588–3593, 2015.
46. Wu CR, Huang LY, Guo J, et al: Clinical control study of endoscopic full-thickness resection and laparoscopic surgery in the treatment of gastric tumors arising from the muscularis propria, *Chin Med J* 128(11):1455–1459, 2015.
47. Wang H, Feng X, Ye S, et al: A comparison of the efficacy and safety of endoscopic full-thickness resection and laparoscopic-assisted surgery for small gastrointestinal stromal tumors, *Surg Endosc* 30(8):3357–3361, 2016.
48. Tan Y, Tang X, Guo T, et al: Comparison between submucosal tunneling endoscopic resection and endoscopic full-thickness resection for gastric stromal tumors originating from the muscularis propria layer, *Surg Endosc* 2016. [Epub ahead of print].
50. Salerno R, Gherardi G, Paternò E, et al: Endoscopic full-thickness resection of a submucosal right colon lesion, *Endoscopy* 48(S 01):E376–E377, 2016.

A complete reference list can be found online at ExpertConsult.com

47

Extraintestinal Endosonography

Amit P. Desai and Frank G. Gress

INTRODUCTION

The use of endoscopic ultrasound (EUS) has grown over the last 30 years, and it is now a well-established diagnostic method for the assessment of a range of gastrointestinal (GI) disorders, including the evaluation and staging of many types of endoluminal cancers. This chapter discusses EUS applications relating to extraintestinal structures, organs, and lesions. The objectives of this chapter are to review the utility of EUS for evaluating the mediastinum in both benign and malignant disease processes, including the detection of mediastinal lymph node metastases in lung cancer. Mass lesions in the paragastric and retroperitoneal organs (excluding the bile duct, gallbladder, and pancreas) are reviewed, including detection of lesions of the adrenal gland, liver, and kidneys. Ascites and pleural fluid are examined along with unusual extraintestinal lesions.

LUNG CANCER

Lung cancer is the leading cause of cancer death in the United States in men and women, and has an overall 5-year survival rate of 15%.[1,2] Treatment decisions are based on the location and extent of the tumor. The presence of extrapulmonary metastasis is crucial because patients without mediastinal involvement are potential candidates for resection. The distinction between non–small-cell lung cancer (NSCLC), which accounts for 80% of tumors, and small-cell lung cancer (SCLC), which accounts for 20% of tumors, is important because of the more aggressive nature of SCLC. SCLC is usually classified as limited or extensive disease, although the criteria for these two categories remain controversial.[3–5] Although the TNM (primary tumor, regional nodes, metastases) staging system traditionally has not been used in staging SCLC, studies have suggested using the 7th

edition of the TNM classification scheme for clinical trials and registry information, to guide future management.[6–10] The forthcoming 8th edition of the TNM classification system has proposed changes to the T classification scheme, highlighting tumor size as a key feature.[11] Metastatic disease is detected in 80% of SCLC cases at the time of diagnosis and tends to spread quickly so that surgery is considered less often in SCLC compared with NSCLC. Although highly responsive to radiotherapy and chemotherapy, SCLC usually recurs within 2 years.

In comparison, half of NSCLC cases are localized or locally advanced and can be treated by surgery, the cornerstone of therapy for NSCLC, or with adjuvant therapy with or without resection.[12–14] NSCLC, which includes adenocarcinoma, squamous cell cancer, and large-cell cancer, was previously staged using the 2002 International Staging System.[14–16] Recently, NSCLC, has been staged using the 7th edition until December 31, 2017 (Box 47.1) and subsequently will be staged using the future 8th edition.[11] This section focuses on EUS applications in the diagnosis and staging of NSCLC, although much of what is covered can be applied to SCLC.

Staging and Staging Modalities

Mediastinal lymph node metastases are present in nearly half of all patients with NSCLC. Accurate staging of NSCLC is crucial in determining treatment options because the detection of mediastinal lymph node metastasis preoperatively has therapeutic implications. In the absence of distant metastasis, the documentation of mediastinal metastasis is probably the most common deterrent to cure.[17–28]

The TNM staging system used for lung cancer (see Box 47.1) designates metastasis to ipsilateral peribronchial or ipsilateral hilar lymph nodes, or both, and intrapulmonary nodes including involvement by direct extension of primary tumor as N1 disease;

BOX 47.1   International Staging System for Lung Cancer, 2007

Primary Tumor (T)

Tx: Primary tumor cannot be assessed

T0: No evidence of primary tumor

Tis: Carcinoma in situ

T1: Tumor < 3 cm without bronchoscopic evidence of invasion more proximal than the lobar bronchus (not the main bronchus unless superficial tumor of any size with invasion limited to the bronchial wall, which may extend proximal to the main bronchus)

     T1a: Tumor < 2 cm in size

     T1b: Tumor > 2 cm but < 3 cm in size

T2: Tumor > 3 cm but <7 cm, or any size with any of the following:

     Involves the main bronchus (at least 2 cm distal to the carina)

     Invades visceral pleura

     Associated with atelectasis or obstructive pneumonitis that extends to the hilar region but does not involve the entire lung:

     T2a: Tumor > 3 cm but <5 cm

     T2b: Tumor > 5 cm but <7 cm

T3: Tumor > 7 cm or directly invades any of the following:

     Chest wall, diaphragm, mediastinal pleura, or parietal pericardium or tumor in the main bronchus < 2 cm distal to the carina (without involvement of the carina)

     Atelectasis or obstructive pneumonitis of the entire lung

     Separate tumor nodules in the same lobe

T4: Tumor of any size that invades any of the following:

     Mediastinum, heart, great vessels, trachea, esophagus, vertebral body, or carina

     Separate tumor nodules in a different ipsilateral lobe

Nodal Involvement (N)

Nx: Regional lymph nodes cannot be assessed

N0: No regional lymph nodes metastasis

N1: Metastasis to ipsilateral peribronchial or ipsilateral hilar lymph nodes, or both, and intrapulmonary nodes including involvement by direct extension of primary tumor

N2: Metastasis to ipsilateral mediastinal or subcarinal lymph nodes, or both

N3: Metastasis to contralateral mediastinal, contralateral hilar, ipsilateral or contralateral scalene, or supraclavicular lymph nodes

Metastasis (M)

Mx: Distant metastasis cannot be assessed

M0: No distant metastasis

M1: Distant metastasis present

M1a: Separate tumor nodules in a contralateral lobe; tumor with pleural nodules or malignancy pleural or pericardial effusion

M1b: Distant metastasis

Stage Grouping

Occult carcinoma: TxN0M0

Stage 0: TisN0M0

Stage IA: T1a-bN0M0

Stage IB: T2aN0M0

Stage IIA: T1N1M0, T2bN0M0

Stage IIB: T2bN1M0, T3N0M0

Stage IIIA: T1N2M0, T2N2M0, T3N1-2M0, T4N0-1M0

Stage IIIB: T4 N2M0, Any TN3M0

Stage IV: Any T any N M1-b

Adapted from Goldstraw P, Crowley J, Chansky K, et al: The IASLC Lung Cancer Staging Project: proposals for the revision of the TNM stage groupings in the forthcoming (seventh) edition of the TNM classification of malignant tumours. *J Thorac Oncol* 2(8):706–714, 2007.

---

metastasis to ipsilateral mediastinal or subcarinal lymph nodes, or both, as N2; and metastasis to contralateral mediastinal, contralateral hilar, ipsilateral or contralateral scalene, or supraclavicular lymph nodes as N3. Although N2 disease is potentially resectable, most patients with N2 disease receive multimodality treatment (Table 47.1 and Fig. 47.1; see Box 47.1).[14-16,28,29]

Various techniques are currently available to diagnose and stage lung cancer, including x-rays, computed tomography (CT), magnetic resonance imaging (MRI), positron emission tomography (PET), endobronchial ultrasound (EBUS), and EUS. CT scan of the chest is the current standard by which mediastinal lymphadenopathy is detected. Generally, lymph nodes larger than or equal to 1 cm on chest CT scan are considered abnormal. A review of previously published studies reveals an accuracy of CT staging of the mediastinum of 52% to 88%.[30-40] This variation has been attributed to the wide range of correlation of lymph node size to the presence of malignant involvement. Although the general trend is increased risk for metastasis correlating with increasing lymph node size, lymph node size is not an accurate criterion for assessing risk. Problems associated with size as a criterion include the inability to differentiate inflammatory or reactive lymph nodes from malignant involvement. In one study, 37% of mediastinal lymph nodes that ranged in size from 2 to 4 cm were benign,[40] and 40% of enlarged nodes in another series were not cancerous.[41] Similarly, normal-sized lymph nodes can contain foci of cancer. McKenna et al (1985)[42] found no correlation between the presence of mediastinal nodal metastases

and nodal size. Metastases may be found in 21% of normal-sized nodes.[43]

MRI may be slightly superior to CT in the detection of mediastinal disease,[44] and PET has been shown to be superior to CT for staging for the mediastinum.[45,46] PET does not rely on an arbitrary cutoff of size to diagnose malignant nodes but detects the increased glycolytic rate in metabolically active tumors. In a meta-analysis, PET had a sensitivity of 79% and a specificity of 91% compared with CT, which had sensitivity and specificity of 60% and 77%, respectively, for the detection of mediastinal disease.[45] In another meta-analysis by Toloza et al (2003),[46] the performance characteristics of CT, PET, and EUS for staging the mediastinum in NSCLC were compared. PET was more accurate than CT or EUS for detecting mediastinal metastases, with a sensitivity of 84% and a specificity of 89% for PET compared with CT (sensitivity 57% and specificity 82%) and EUS (sensitivity 78% and specificity 71%). However, PET is limited for small lesions (≤ 1 cm), has false-negative results in tumors with low metabolic activity, and has false-positive results in benign lesions such as granulomatous disease. Although PET has a relatively high sensitivity, because of the importance and implications of staging, specificity is still too low, and pathologic staging is still generally sought.[47-49]

Fritscher-Ravens et al (2003)[50] performed a prospective comparison of CT, PET, and EUS for the detection of metastatic lymph nodes metastases in patients with lung cancer being considered for operative resection. After bronchoscopic evaluation,

TABLE 47.1 Lymph Node Map Definitions

Nodal Station	Anatomic Landmarks
N2 Nodes: All N2 Nodes Lie Within the Mediastinal Pleural Envelope	
1. Highest mediastinal nodes	Nodes lying above the horizontal line at the upper rim of the brachiocephalic (left innominate) vein where it ascends to the left, crossing in front of the trachea at its midline
2. Upper paratracheal nodes	Nodes lying above the horizontal line drawn tangential to the upper margin of the aortic arch and below the inferior boundary of the No. 1 nodes
3. Prevascular and retrotracheal nodes	Prevascular and retrotracheal nodes may be designated 3A and 3B; midline nodes are considered to be ipsilateral
4. Lower paratracheal nodes	Lower paratracheal nodes on the right lie to the right of the midline of the trachea between a horizontal line drawn tangential to the upper margin of the aortic arch and a line extending across the right main bronchus at the upper margin of the upper lobe bronchus and contained within the mediastinal pleural envelope; lower paratracheal nodes on the left lie to the left of the midline of the trachea between a horizontal line drawn tangential to the upper margin of the aortic arch and line extending across the left main bronchus at the level of the upper margin of the left upper lobe bronchus, medial to the ligamentum arteriosum and contained within the mediastinal pleural envelope
	Researchers may wish to designate the lower paratracheal nodes as No. 4s (superior) and No. 4i (inferior) subsets for study purposes; No. 4s nodes may be defined by a horizontal line extending across the trachea and drawn tangential to the cephalic border of the azygos vein; No. 4i nodes may be defined by the lower boundary of No. 4s and the lower boundary of No. 4, as described previously
5. Subaortic (aortopulmonary window)	Subaortic nodes are lateral to the ligamentum arteriosum or the aorta or left pulmonary artery and proximal to the first branch of the left pulmonary artery, and lie within the mediastinal pleural envelope
6. Paraaortic nodes (ascending aorta or phrenic)	Nodes lying anterior and lateral to ascending aorta and the aortic arch or the innominate artery, beneath the line tangential to the upper margin of the aortic arch
7. Subcarinal nodes	Nodes lying caudal to the carina of the trachea but not associated with the lower lobe bronchi or arteries within the lung
8. Paraesophageal nodes (below carina)	Nodes lying adjacent to the wall of the esophagus and to the right or left of the midline, excluding subcarinal nodes
9. Pulmonary ligament nodes	Nodes lying within the pulmonary ligament, including nodes in the posterior wall and lower part of the inferior pulmonary vein
N1 Nodes: All N1 Nodes Lie Distal to the Mediastinal Pleural Reflection and Within the Visceral Pleura	
10. Hilar nodes	Proximal lobar nodes, distal to the mediastinal pleural reflection and the nodes adjacent to the bronchus intermedius on the right; radiographically, hilar shadow may be created by enlargement of both hilar and interlobar nodes
11. Interlobar nodes	Nodes lying between the lobar bronchi
12. Lobar nodes	Nodes adjacent to the distal lobar bronchi
13. Segmental nodes	Nodes adjacent to the segmental bronchi
14. Subsegmental nodes	Nodes around the subsegmental bronchi

From Mountain CF, Dresler CM: Regional lymph node classification for lung cancer staging. *Chest* 111(6):1718–1723, 1997.

CT, PET, and EUS were performed to evaluate potential mediastinal involvement with bronchoscopic biopsy and cytology-proven ($n = 25$) or radiologically suspected ($n = 8$) lung cancer before surgery. Surgical histology was used as the gold standard and revealed NSCLC in 30 patients, neuroendocrine tumor in 1 patient, and benign disease in 2 patients. With respect to the correct prediction of mediastinal lymph node stage, the sensitivities of CT, PET, and EUS were 57%, 73%, and 94%; specificities were 74%, 83%, and 71%; and accuracies were 67%, 79%, and 82%, respectively. Results of PET could be improved when combined with CT (sensitivity 81%, specificity 94%, and accuracy 88%). The specificity of EUS (71%) was improved to 100% by fine-needle aspiration (FNA) cytology. Furthermore, Redondo et al (2015) performed a comparative study for evaluation of mediastinal lymphadenopathy, directly comparing PET-CT with EUS-FNA. Endosonographers were blinded to PET-CT results. With tissue being the gold standard, the sensitivity and specificity of EUS-FNA was 91.3% and 100%, respectively, compared with 75% and 25%, respectively, for PET-CT.[51] Overall, across both comparative studies, no single imaging method alone was conclusive in evaluating potential mediastinal involvement.

Whenever enlarged lymph nodes are seen in the mediastinum on chest CT scan, standard practice is to perform a lymph node biopsy for more accurate staging. The traditional methods for performing a lymph node biopsy are via CT or bronchoscopy, or both. Bronchoscopy with FNA is commonly used to evaluate suspicious paratracheal, hilar, and subcarinal lymph nodes seen on CT.[52–55] The role of bronchoscopy in the diagnosis and staging of NSCLC is well established and has a sensitivity of approximately 60%.[56–62] Bronchoscopy, however, is unable to access the aortopulmonary window or the inferior mediastinal nodes. CT-guided biopsy of the mediastinum is limited by overlying vascular and bony structures. When the lymph node status is not determined with CT or bronchoscopy or both, historically, mediastinoscopy, and in some cases limited thoracotomy, were performed to clarify the disease stage.[39,63–65] However, these procedures are significantly more invasive.[66] The advent of EUS and EBUS has made it possible to minimally invasively image the mediastinum with precise

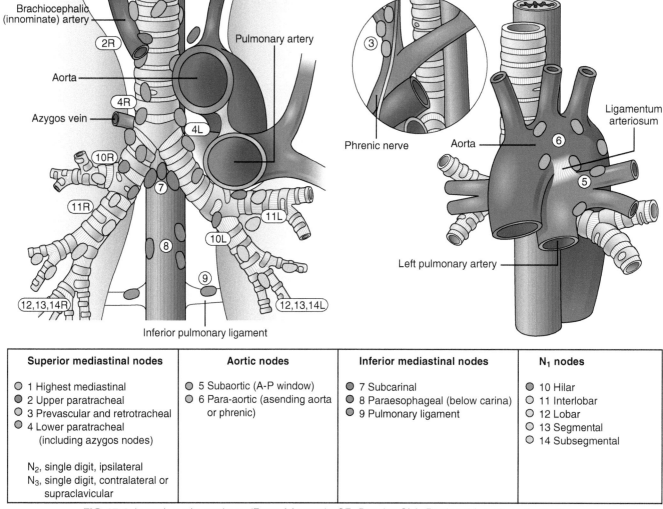

FIG 47.1 Lymph node stations. (From Mountain CF, Dresler CM: Regional lymph node stations for lung cancer staging. *Chest* 111:1718–1723, 1997.)

Superior mediastinal nodes	Aortic nodes	Inferior mediastinal nodes	N₁ nodes

○ 1 Highest mediastinal
● 2 Upper paratracheal
○ 3 Prevascular and retrotracheal
○ 4 Lower paratracheal
   (including azygos nodes)
 	
N₂, single digit, ipsilateral
N₃, single digit, contralateral or
   supraclavicular
	● 5 Subaortic (A-P window)
	○ 6 Para-aortic (asending aorta
	   or phrenic)
		● 7 Subcarinal
		● 8 Paraesophageal (below carina)
		● 9 Pulmonary ligament
			● 10 Hilar
			○ 11 Interlobar
			○ 12 Lobar
			○ 13 Segmental
			○ 14 Subsegmental

resolution, allowing for an accurate and safe method for staging lung cancer.[67–81]

Endoscopic Ultrasound and Endobronchial Ultrasound

EUS-guided FNA can sample suspicious posterior mediastinal lymph nodes, including aortopulmonary window, subcarinal, and inferior (below carina) paraesophageal nodes. Tracheal air artifact generally precludes reliable assessment of the anterior mediastinum lesions, pretracheal nodes, and upper paratracheal nodes; however, the advent of EBUS technology seems to be minimizing this limitation.

Sampling of suspicious lymph nodes is essential except in N1 nodes. EUS is best at accurately detecting mediastinal lymph node metastasis in the aortopulmonary window (station 5), subcarinal (station 7), and paraesophageal (station 8) regions (see Fig. 47.1). Several prospective studies evaluated the accuracy of EUS, EUS-guided FNA, and chest CT scan in detecting and staging mediastinal lymph node metastasis in patients with NSCLC based on correlation with surgical staging.[71,74] Gress et al (1997)[74] reported a study consisting of patients with NSCLC and enlarged mediastinal lymph nodes (> 1 cm) seen on chest CT scan. EUS criteria used to differentiate benign from malignant

lymph nodes resulted in an accuracy of 84% compared with 49% for CT. The sensitivity (64%) and specificity (35%) of CT scan was compared to the sensitivity (93%) and specificity (100%) of EUS-guided FNA of lymph nodes. A 2008 meta-analysis of 76 studies (44 EUS, 32 EUS-FNA) evaluating mediastinal lymph nodes reported a sensitivity of 84.7% (EUS on criteria alone) and 88% (EUS-FNA), and specificity of 84.6% (EUS on criteria alone) and 96.4% (EUS-FNA).[82] The authors conclude that EUS-FNA should be the diagnostic test of choice in evaluating mediastinal lymphadenopathy, however recognizing the limitation of EUS in the anterior mediastinum.

In an attempt to view the anterior mediastinum, EBUS-guided transbronchial needle aspiration (TBNA) was developed. A systematic review of EBUS-TBNA showed that it was a safe and effective modality to aid in the staging of NSCLC with a sensitivity ranging from 85% to 100%.[70] Eapen et al (2013) performed a prospective study on 1317 patients undergoing EBUS staging with a 1.4% complication rate, with transbronchial lung biopsy being the only major risk factor.[83] In an early, large-scale study, Wallace et al (2008)[71] compared the use of TBNA, EUS-FNA, and EBUS-TBNA using pathologic confirmation of malignancy or benign disease as the diagnostic standard. This group found

EBUS-FNA to be more sensitive, with a higher negative predictive value than TBNA. More importantly, they found the combination of EBUS-FNA with EUS-FNA to have a sensitivity of 93%, a positive predictive value of 100%, and a negative predictive value of 97%. A recent meta-analysis in 2013 by Zhang et al evaluating eight studies further confirmed the conclusion that combined technique was more sensitive and specific than either alone.[84] Given the combined high sensitivity and specificity of EUS-FNA and EBUS-FNA, many investigators have been seeking to perform a complete "medical mediastinoscopy," with the hope of avoiding the more traditional, invasive staging, including mediastinoscopy, of NSCLC before operative intervention.

Endoscopic Ultrasound Technique for Imaging the Mediastinum

After informed consent is obtained, the patient is placed in the left lateral decubitus position. After sedation, the echoendoscope is passed to the gastroesophageal (GE) junction in a manner similar to the passage of a duodenoscope. Many endosonographers first perform staging with a radial scanning echoendoscope and then switch to a dedicated biopsy echoendoscope or a curved linear array echoendoscope if FNA is to be performed.

When imaging the mediastinum, a thorough understanding of mediastinal anatomy relative to the esophagus is essential to perform a complete examination. Scanning should begin distally below the GE junction while withdrawing the scope proximally because this limits scanning artifacts. It is useful to press the transducer with its balloon partially inflated against the gut wall to minimize air artifacts and to anchor the transducer. In addition, the suction port is depressed to maintain optimal imaging by minimizing intraluminal air.

As the endosonographer withdraws the radial scanning echoendoscope, the aorta should be maintained in the 5 o'clock to 6 o'clock position in the ultrasound (US) field, which generally allows proper orientation of the paraesophageal structures. The aorta is easily recognized as a circular anechoic structure, approximately 1.5 to 2 cm in diameter, with a relatively bright border resulting from back wall enhancement (a normal artifact seen in vessels). As the echoendoscope is withdrawn into the distal esophagus, the aorta, spine, left lobe of the liver, inferior vena cava, and heart can be seen. The spine is also easily identified in the 7 o'clock position next to the aorta and has irregular echo features with artifacts produced by poor penetration of echoes through bony structures. The left lobe of the liver appears at the 6 o'clock to 12-o'clock position, and often the hepatic veins and inferior vena cava can be seen as they course through the liver. Slightly more proximally, the beating of the heart is appreciated as the left atrium comes into view at the 12 o'clock position. The mitral valve leaflets can be seen as the valve opens from the left atrium into the left ventricle, and the pulmonary veins can be seen entering the left atrium. The left pulmonary artery arches posteriorly to the left of the ascending aorta and tends to be easier to view than the right pulmonary artery, which can be seen just below the carina. The left ventricle, right atrium, and right ventricle lie deep to the left atrium; it can be more difficult to visualize these structures completely. As the aorta moves toward the left, the spine and azygos vein are seen posteriorly. The aortic outflow tract can be appreciated as the endoscope is withdrawn further. The spine continues to be a useful landmark because it consistently appears as a hyperechoic structure located posteriorly throughout the chest. Careful inspection of this area may reveal the thoracic duct adjacent to the aorta and spine.

The right lung appears as hyperechoic rings emanating from the 9 o'clock position, whereas the left lung appears at the 2 o'clock position. In the midesophagus, the right and left bronchi are easily demarcated by the hyperechoic rings (echogenic air) seen at the 11 o'clock and 1 o'clock positions. The two bronchi join to form the trachea normally at 27–28 cm from the incisors. The azygos vein can be seen coming into position to the right of the aorta and moves anterior to the spine and toward the right lung. As the endoscope is withdrawn further, the azygos vein can be seen to move forward and extend anteriorly into the superior vena cava. The ascending aorta can be difficult to trace because this structure runs deep to the hilar structures (pulmonary vessels), and because of air within the bronchi and trachea, the ascending aorta is often not fully imaged. In the proximal esophagus, the aortic arch is identified on the left and moves rightward and anteriorly across the screen. In the cervical esophagus, above the level of the aortic arch, the carotid vessels and, occasionally, the thyroid gland can be seen (Figs. 47.2 to 47.4).

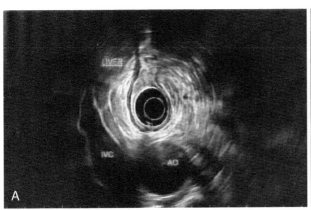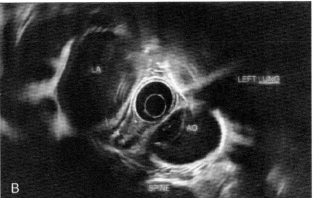

FIG 47.2 A, Radial imaging at the distal esophagus showing the liver, inferior vena cava (IVC), and aorta (AO). The spine lies immediately deep to the aorta. **B,** Imaging slightly higher in the distal esophagus showing the right lower lobe of the lung (RLL), left lung (LL), aorta (AO), spine (SP), and a portion of the left atrium (LA).

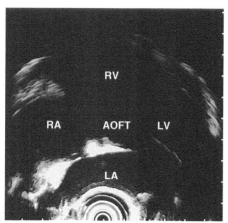

FIG 47.3 Radial endoscopic ultrasound (EUS) from the distal esophagus. The left atrium (LA), right atrium (RA), right ventricle (RV), and left ventricle (LV) can be seen. The leaflets of the mitral valve and the base of the aortic outflow tract (AOFT) are also visible.

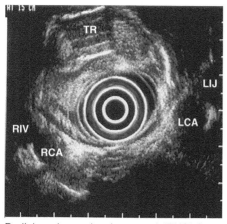

FIG 47.4 Radial endoscopic ultrasound (EUS) from the most proximal aspect of the esophagus. The left common carotid artery (LCA), left internal jugular vein (LIJ), right internal jugular vein (RIV), and right common carotid artery (RCA) are seen. In addition, the thyroid gland is seen on either side of the trachea (TR). *AOFT*, aortic outflow tract.

Evaluation of the mediastinum using linear EUS requires rotation of the echoendoscope every few centimeters for a thorough evaluation. As in radial EUS, vascular structures provide the major landmarks for orientation, and the home base structure is the descending aorta, which is first located approximately 35 cm from the incisors. The echoendoscope is rotated initially clockwise (right) bringing structures anterior to the esophagus into view and then counterclockwise (left) bringing posterior structures into view. The left atrium is found by rotating the shaft of the scope 180 degrees in the distal esophagus to midesophagus until a large, echolucent structure is seen within which the mitral valve leaflets are located. By tipping the scope upward and with slight withdrawal, the subcarinal lymph node station is located immediately beneath the endoscope at approximately 27 cm between the left atrium and right pulmonary artery. The aortopulmonary window is located by following the descending aorta cephalad to the arch and pushing the endoscope in again approximately 2 cm. The endoscope is turned 90 degrees clockwise and tipped up slightly until a cross-sectional view of the aortic arch and the more distally located left pulmonary artery are seen. The area between these structures is known as the *AP window*. Another potentially important area for FNA of lymph nodes is the celiac axis. This area is located by finding the abdominal aorta at the level of the GE junction and the takeoff of the celiac artery with the superior mesenteric artery just distal to this (Figs. 47.5 to 47.8).

TECHNIQUES FOR STAGING NON–SMALL-CELL LUNG CANCER WITH ENDOSCOPIC ULTRASOUND

In experienced hands and with careful planning, EUS of the mediastinum can be performed quickly, regardless of the type of EUS technology used. Prophylactic antibiotics are not administered unless recommended by the American Heart Association or the American Society of Gastrointestinal Endoscopy because EUS-guided FNA of mediastinal lesions is not associated with significant bacteremia. However, prophylactic quinolone antibiotics are recommended for FNA of cystic mediastinal lesions, which is similar to the recommendations for pancreatic cystic lesions and perirectal lesions.[85–92] The instrument is advanced into the stomach, and the celiac axis is imaged. The probe is slowly withdrawn to the GE junction and then cephalad using radial scanning images generally obtained with 7.5-MHz frequencies at each 1-cm interval while keeping the aorta at the 5 o'clock

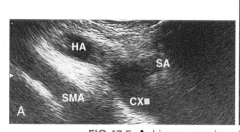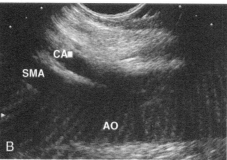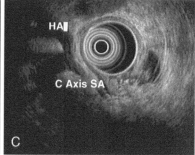

FIG 47.5 **A,** Linear array imaging of the celiac axis is depicted showing the takeoff of the superior mesenteric artery (SMA) and celiac axis (CX) along with the hepatic artery (HA) and splenic artery (SA) branches. **B,** More typical linear images as seen from the proximal stomach. **C,** Radial imaging showing the CX. *AO,* Aorta.

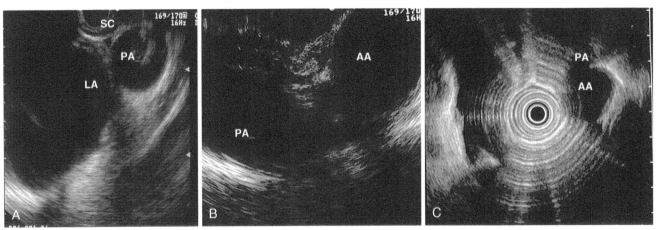

FIG 47.6 A, Curved linear array view through the midesophagus of the subcarinal (SC) region. The left atrium (LA) is next to the right pulmonary artery (PA) with the ascending aorta lying deep to these structures. **B,** Linear array view through the midesophagus of the aortic arch (AA) and the pulmonary artery (PA)–the "AP window." **C,** Radial imaging of the area of the AP window.

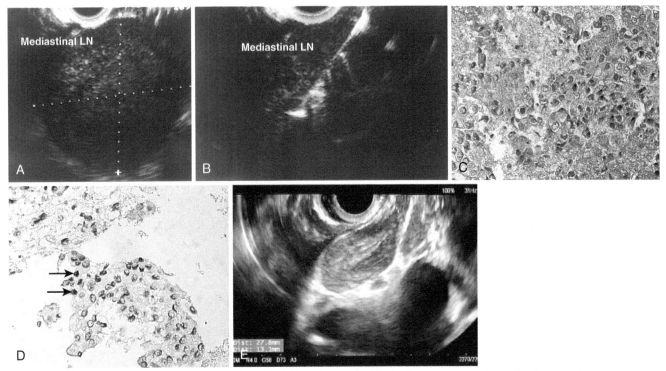

FIG 47.7 A, Mediastinal lymph node (LN) as imaged with the linear array endoscopic ultrasound (EUS) system. **B,** The fine-needle aspiration (FNA) needle is seen exiting the scope; the tip of the needle is seen to be in the center of the LN. **C,** High-power magnification of hematoxylin and eosin stain on cell block reveals metastatic adenocarcinoma. **D,** High-power magnification of immunoperoxidase stain on cell block. Tumor nuclei *(arrows)* are positive for TTF1 antibody consistent with non–small-cell lung carcinoma. **E,** Mediastinal lymph node as imaged with the linear array EUS system in a patient with prior history of Hodgkin's lymphoma.

or 6 o'clock position, as described earlier. All mediastinal lymph nodes seen are "mapped" by location according to the American Thoracic Society classification scheme (see Box 47.1, Table 47.1, Fig. 47.1, and Video 47.1).[14–16]

An objective determination is made as to whether the mediastinal lymphadenopathy detected by EUS is consistent with benign or malignant status according to previously reported

studies using the same criteria.[86,93–99] EUS criteria used to diagnose malignant lymph nodes are round shape, sharp distinct borders, hypoechoic texture, and a short-axis diameter greater than 5 mm. Each of these parameters should be present for a lymph node to be considered as potentially malignant; however, FNA has significantly improved the sensitivity and specificity of detection of malignant lymph nodes.[74,80,81,86,99,100]

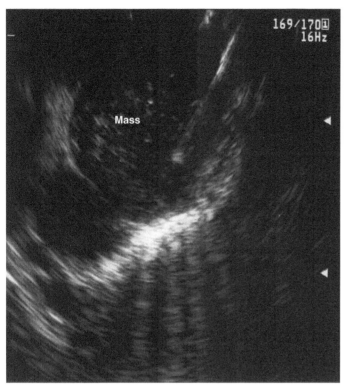

FIG 47.8 Linear endoscopic ultrasound (EUS) reveals a hypoechoic mass within the mediastinum. EUS-guided fine-needle aspiration (FNA) was performed and revealed metastatic non–small-cell lung cancer (cytology favored a large-cell neuroendocrine-type lesion).

The liver and left adrenal gland are carefully inspected, and any ascites or pleural fluid that is unexpectedly detected is inspected. If suspicious lymphadenopathy or other suspicious findings are seen that may represent metastatic disease, the linear echoendoscope is introduced (if not already in use), and EUS-guided FNA is performed. Many centers have successfully used only linear technology for diagnostic imaging and for obtaining needle aspiration cytologic samples, and this may become the modality of choice after gaining more experience with the technique.

TECHNIQUE FOR PERFORMING ENDOSCOPIC ULTRASOUND-GUIDED FINE-NEEDLE ASPIRATION

Mediastinal Lymph Nodes

At the present time, several EUS catheter–FNA needle systems are available with various needle lengths (up to 14 cm) and gauges (19–25-gauge) available. We routinely perform EUS-guided FNA on all posterior mediastinal lymph nodes that are suspicious for malignant involvement by clinical suspicion or EUS criteria, or both. Many patients have more than one suspicious lymph node or finding. In our patients, we sample only the most suspicious lymph node or finding that would have the greatest impact on the clinical staging (i.e., contralateral or subcarinal).

The EUS-guided FNA technique was initially developed for use with the linear array instrument and has been described elsewhere.[94–96,101,102] The unique viewing angle of the linear array transducer allows for observation of the needle as it exits the

biopsy channel and enables direction of the needle tip into the target lesion. A similar technique using a radial scanning echoendoscope has been reported; however, serious complications have been described via this technique, and it is not recommended.[93,102]

EUS-guided FNA involves the insertion of the FNA catheter device through the accessory channel of the echoendoscope followed by deployment of the needle under EUS guidance into the lymph node to be sampled. The handle mechanism is secured to the accessory port, and if the instrument has an elevator, the elevator should be fully released into the down position to allow easy passage of the needle. The elevator can be used during the biopsy to direct the needle gently into the lesion. Doppler is used to identify surrounding vascular structures. The FNA needle is slowly advanced toward the target lesion. With certain needles, it helps if the stylet is withdrawn a few millimeters (2–3 mm), and the needle and the stylet are then directed into the target. When the needle has entered the lesion, the stylet is advanced (to clear the needle) and then removed. The endosonographer or assistant applies suction to the catheter system using a 5-mL or 10-mL Luer-Lok syringe. Suction is followed by in-and-out movements of the catheter after firmly locking the needle–catheter system to the appropriate depth so that the needle is not advanced beyond a desired depth. Typically, we make 7 to 10 gradual in-and-out movements within the lesion. Before removing the needle, the negative pressure is released slowly, the needle is removed from the lesion, and subsequently the needle system is unscrewed from the echoendoscope. It has been suggested to perform EUS-guided FNA of lymph nodes without the use of suction, as suction may result in a bloody sample that may be more difficult for the cytopathologist to examine.[99]

We recommend having a cytopathologist or cytotechnologist present during the EUS-guided FNA portion to improve the efficiency of the technique and potentially obtain preliminary cytology findings. If a cytopathologist or cytotechnologist is unavailable, two to three passes should be performed for lymph nodes (or liver metastases) and five to six passes should be performed for masses (similar to pancreatic masses) to ensure adequate cellularity in more than 90% of cases.[99,103] However, this approach is associated with a 10% reduction in definitive cytologic diagnoses, increased time and risk, and the potential need for additional needles.[103]

The FNA sample obtained is prepared for review using Diff-Quik stain (HARLECO; EMD Chemicals, Inc., Gibbstown, NJ) applied to the slide containing the deposited specimen or fixed with ethanol. Additional passes are made until a positive cytology or adequate tissue sample is obtained. When lymphoma is suspected, additional material is collected if possible and placed in a preservative solution for subsequent flow cytometry and immunocytochemistry as indicated.[104,105] If an infection is suspected, a culture media can be used.

Other Malignant Mediastinal Disease

The most important indication for mediastinal imaging is the detection or staging (or both) of lung cancer. However, there are other indications for mediastinal EUS. There are several reports of EUS-guided FNA in the cytologic diagnosis and staging of mediastinal metastases from various extrathoracic malignancies. These include metastatic pancreatic, esophageal, gastric, colon, laryngeal, germ cell, renal cell, breast, and ovarian cancers.[75,76,78–79,106–109]

Devereaux et al (2002)[109] retrospectively reviewed a large, single-center experience with EUS-guided FNA for the diagnosis

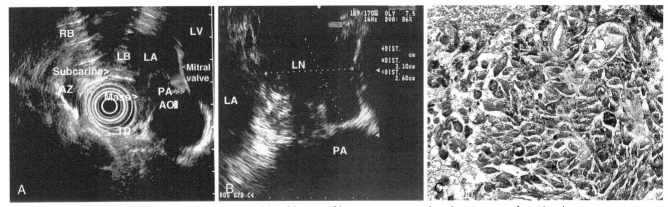

FIG 47.9 A 71-year-old woman with a history of breast cancer and melanoma was found to have mediastinal lymphadenopathy on chest computed tomography (CT). **A,** Radial endoscopic ultrasound (EUS) revealed a subcarinal 3.1- × 2.6-cm necrotic-appearing lymph node versus mass. **B,** Linear array imaging depicting fine-needle aspiration (FNA) of this lesion. **C,** High-power magnification of hematoxylin and eosin stain on cell block shows metastatic pigmented melanoma. *AO,* aorta; *AZ,* azygos vein; *LA,* left atrium; *LB,* left bronchi; *LN,* lymph node; *LV,* left ventricle; *PA,* pulmonary artery; *RB,* right bronchi; *TD,* thoracic duct.

of mediastinal mass or lymphadenopathy in the absence of known pulmonary malignancy. In this report, 49 patients were analyzed; a malignant process was diagnosed in 22 of 49 (45%), and a benign process was found in 24 of 49 (49%). These included four patients with previously undiagnosed lung cancer, whereas metastatic breast carcinoma was the most frequent (6 of 22 [27%]) lesion. EUS-guided FNA was diagnostic in 46 of 49 (94%) patients. Eloubeidi et al (2012) analyzed 116 patients with mediastinal lymphadenopathy of unclear etiology and found EUS-FNA sensitivity, specificity, and accuracy to reach almost 100% when on-site cytopathologist and special immunohistochemical stains were administered. Diagnoses ranged from lymphoma to solid-organ non-lung malignancies metastatic to the mediastinum.[110] This is consistent with recent studies that also support the use of EUS-FNA with flow cytometry for the diagnosis of mediastinal lymphoma.[111–113] In a multicenter study of 62 patients, Catalano et al (2002) found EUS-FNA to be diagnostic in 90% of cases, classified as benign, infectious, malignant pulmonary, and malignant mediastinal.[106] Panelli et al (2001) determined over a 5-year period that 2.5% (n = 33) of upper EUS examinations involved evaluation for mediastinal lymphadenopathy.[114] EUS-FNA was performed in 25 of 33, of which 22 (67%) were determined to be malignant.

Overall, the authors for these studies suggest that EUS-guided FNA can be a useful and minimally invasive technique for the cytodiagnosis of extrathoracic cancers that are metastatic to the mediastinum (Fig. 47.9).[115]

Nonmalignant Mediastinal Disease

Although commonly present in patients with suspected or known pulmonary malignancy, mediastinal lymph nodes are also present in patients with benign diseases such as histoplasmosis, sarcoidosis, and tuberculosis.[109,116–118] In addition, benign cystic structures such as congenital foregut cysts account for approximately 20% of mediastinal masses.[92]

Savides et al (1995)[117] described 11 patients with dysphagia who had a midesophageal submucosal mass or stricture. EUS findings consisted of large, matted posterior mediastinal lymph nodes in all patients. The diagnosis of histoplasmosis was

supported by the EUS finding of lymph node calcifications and response to treatment in seven of these patients without a malignancy in 20.5 months follow-up.

Sarcoidosis is a systemic granulomatous disease with a predilection for the lung and mediastinal lymph nodes. Historically, a transbronchial biopsy is carried out, which has a diagnostic yield of 40% with one biopsy and 90% when four biopsy specimens are obtained.[119] If the transbronchial approach is unsuccessful, more invasive diagnostic procedures such as mediastinoscopy or lung biopsy may be used. EUS has been reported to be an accurate and simple less invasive method for the diagnosis of sarcoidosis.[105,106,118–120] In two larger studies, Michael and colleagues[120] and Jamil and colleagues[121] reported a sensitivity greater than 80% in diagnosis sarcoidosis in patients with mediastinal lymphadenopathy, but failed to identify specific EUS characteristics (size, shape, echogenicity, or homogenicity) for sarcodosis. The authors conclude that FNA is a vital part of the evaluation. A study reporting the results of EUS-guided FNA evaluation in 19 patients with suspected sarcoidosis revealed enlarged mediastinal lymph nodes (mean size 2.4 cm) located subcarinally (n = 15), in the aortopulmonary window (n = 12), and in the lower posterior mediastinum (n = 5).[106] The nodes were described as isoechoic or hypoechoic, with "atypical" vessels in five cases. The aspirate obtained using EUS-guided FNA was adequate in all patients. Cytology showed epithelioid cell granuloma formation, and cultures for mycobacteria were negative in all of the patients except one, in whom the final diagnosis was tuberculosis. The specificity and sensitivity of EUS-guided FNA in the diagnosis of sarcoidosis were 94% and 100%. Furthermore, given sarcoidosis is a systemic disease, there is potential for EUS-guided FNA in the cytologic diagnosis of intraabdominal and pancreatic sarcoidosis, which is beyond the scope of this chapter (Figs. 47.10 and 47.11).[119,120,123,124]

Tuberculosis must be on the differential in the evaluation of benign mediastinal lymphadenopathy. One study[124a] found 2 patients with tuberculosis in 101 patients without a history of cancer who had EUS-guided FNA of mediastinal lymph nodes. This study highlights the need for acid-fast staining and culture to exclude tuberculosis in cases of noncaseating granulomas.

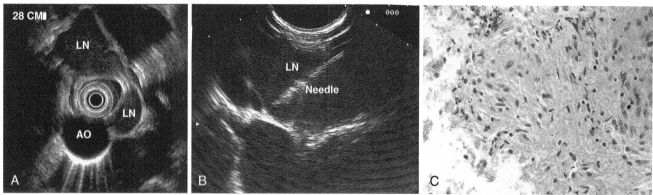

FIG 47.10 **A,** Radial imaging of large hypoechoic, oblong, and teardrop-shaped mediastinal lymph nodes (measuring up to 3.7 cm × 3.4 cm) in a patient with fever and elevated angiotensin-converting enzyme level. **B,** Fine-needle aspiration (FNA) performed with linear array echoendoscope. **C,** High-power magnification of hematoxylin and eosin stain on cell block reveals a noncaseating epithelioid granuloma consistent with sarcoidosis. Special stains (acid-fast bacilli, Gomori methenamine silver) to rule out tuberculosis and fungal infections were negative. *AO,* aorta; *LN,* lymph node.

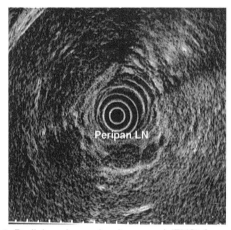

FIG 47.11 Radial endoscopic ultrasound (EUS) from the body of the stomach in a patient with a history of sarcoidosis with peripancreatic lymphadenopathy that increased in size on serial transabdominal imaging. EUS revealed several hypoechoic lymph nodes. Fine-needle aspiration (FNA) yielded tissue with prominent granulomatous inflammation thought to represent abdominal sarcoidosis. *LN,* lymph node.

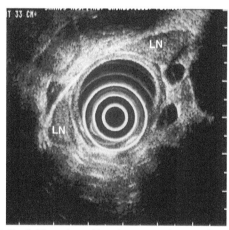

FIG 47.12 Radial imaging of benign-appearing mediastinal lymph nodes (LN).

Approximately 4% of regional lymph nodes of carcinomas have noncaseating epithelioid granulomas. Therefore a presumptive diagnosis of sarcoidosis or another granulomatous disease should be made only after careful exclusion of malignancy and close follow-up.[125] Detectable mediastinal lymph nodes may also be present in normal subjects and are often found in patients undergoing EUS examinations for various indications, which may be indicative of prior histoplasmosis or other pulmonary infections (Fig. 47.12).[117,126] Given the difficulty in differentiating benign from malignant disease, Janssen et al (2007) tested the use of elastography to aid in the evaluation of lymph nodes in the posterior mediastinum. A total of 50 patients underwent EUS biopsies and each lymph node was characterized by their elastography patterns. Two expert reviewers analyzed the elastography patterns. The accuracy was 81.8% and 87.9% to detect benign lymph nodes, 84.6% and 86.4% to detect malignant lymph nodes for two expert reviewers. The interobserver agreement kappa was 0.84. The authors present elastography as a complement to guide biopsies, as the results still remain inferior to EUS-guided biopsies.[127]

EUS is often useful in distinguishing cystic lesions from solid lesions in the mediastinum, whereas chest CT scan can have limited utility in providing this distinction.[90,128-133] The features used to classify cysts were as follows: benign simple cysts appear as anechoic or hypoechoic smooth, spherical structures with well-defined thin walls; esophageal duplication cysts are adherent to the esophagus, whereas cysts originating from the airways are designated as bronchogenic cysts. Cysts that do not fall into either category are termed *nonspecific duplication cysts.* A layered wall structure supports the diagnosis of duplication cyst but is not mandatory. Simple cysts include mesothelial cysts, lymphogenous cysts, and thoracic duct cysts. Simple cysts do not have a layered wall and do not have a connection to the airways or esophagus and are termed *nonspecific simple cysts.* When solid tissue is seen within the fluid, the cysts are considered complex (e.g., benign cystic teratoma, thymic cyst), and the diagnosis of a benign simple cyst is excluded.

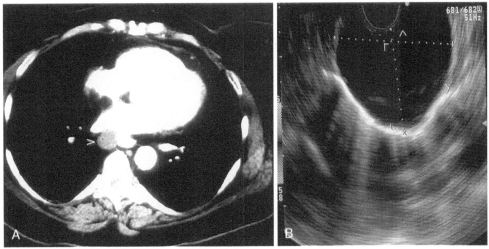

FIG 47.13 A, Chest computed tomography (CT) shows an ill-defined soft tissue density adjacent to the midesophagus. **B,** Linear array imaging of this lesion reveals a paraesophageal duplication cyst.

Posterior mediastinal cysts are usually benign; therefore obvious cysts should not be aspirated given the risks of mediastinitis (Fig. 47.13). FNA should be considered for hypoechoic lesions (when a cyst cannot be clearly distinguished from a solid tumor), but prophylactic antibiotics should be administered. Alternatively, an MRI or CT should be performed to confirm that there is a cyst. If FNA of a posterior mediastinal cyst is performed, intent should be for full drainage and a course of antibiotics.[134]

Adrenal and Renal Lesions

EUS can provide early excellent images of the left adrenal gland. The right adrenal gland is also accessible by EUS, and its routine evaluation may be feasible, although it is more difficult to visualize than the left adrenal gland and the procedure is not routinely performed.[135] The left adrenal gland is more difficult to view than the right gland when imaging with transabdominal US.[136–138]

When imaging the left adrenal gland, the echoendoscope is advanced into the proximal stomach, and the aorta is identified just below the GE junction. The splenic vein is imaged by advancing the transducer forward with a clockwise rotation. Following the splenic vein laterally, the splenic hilum is found by further clockwise rotation and slight withdrawal. The left kidney is imaged by advancing the scope from the splenic hilum with a slight counterclockwise rotation. The left adrenal gland lies just below the splenic vein, between the left kidney (superior and medial to the kidney) and the aorta. In a study by Chang et al (1996),[138] the average long-axis dimension of the adrenal gland was 2.5 cm and the short-axis dimension was 0.8 cm. The adrenal gland as imaged on EUS is homogeneous and hypoechoic with two basic morphologic types: seagull shape and elliptical shape. Occasionally, the adrenal gland can appear as both shapes in the same patient with a slight change in the orientation of the EUS probe tip.[138] In some patients, the central region of the gland may appear more echogenic than the peripheral region (Fig. 47.14).

Incidental benign adrenal lesions are commonly found on CT scans performed for various indications. Unless unequivocally benign, biopsy of these lesions should be performed in certain scenarios. CT scans performed in the staging work-up of lung cancer reveal that more than 16% of patients have adrenal masses

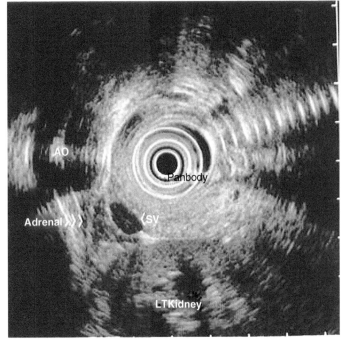

FIG 47.14 Radial imaging from the body of the stomach showing the left adrenal gland, aorta (AO), splenic vein (SV), left (LT) kidney, and body of the pancreas (Panbody).

on screening examination.[138–143] Metastasis to the adrenal glands as the cause of isolated mass lesions occurs in 32% to 93% of cases of NSCLC, as determined by FNA cytology.[141,144] In autopsy series of NSCLC, adrenal metastases are found in 59% of cases.[145,146]

EUS-guided FNA may provide an alternative to percutaneous aspiration technology in the evaluation of adrenal lesions. Chang et al (1995)[147] reported the identification of the left adrenal gland in 97% of 31 consecutive patients undergoing EUS for known pulmonary or GI malignancies, including one patient with a history of T1N0 lung cancer who was found to have metastatic disease with EUS-guided FNA. A more recent case series (2008) also suggests that the right adrenal gland may be more accessible by EUS-guided FNA than previously believed.[135] Given the clinical impact of an adrenal metastasis, routine assessment of the left and possibly right adrenal glands in patients with lung cancer is recommended during the EUS evaluation.[147] A meta-analysis identified 17 studies evaluating 416 patients undergoing EUS-FNA of adrenal lesions. Only one complication was identified, adrenal hemorrhage, which required a brief hospital stay, demonstrating the relative safety of the procedure.[148]

EUS of the right and left kidneys is possible because of the immediate approximation between the GI lumen and the kidneys. The right kidney can be imaged by placing the transducer in the second portion of the duodenum and rotating laterally. The left kidney can be imaged from the body of the stomach, posterior to the spleen, as described previously. The left kidney is often easier to show than the right kidney. The kidneys have a hyperechoic central medulla, a hypoechoic outer cortex, and a thin echogenic capsule (Fig. 47.15).

Approximately 85% of renal masses detected on CT are renal cell carcinomas, and 15% of CT-detected renal masses are benign lesions.[149,150] Biopsy of malignant-appearing masses that are resectable should not be routinely performed. Biopsy of a solitary renal mass is generally accepted in cases with a known primary extrarenal malignancy when the presence of a metastasis would alter management.[149,151] Biopsy specimens of renal masses have traditionally been obtained under either transabdominal US or CT guidance.[149,152] A few case reports exist showing the possibility of making a diagnosis of renal cell carcinoma using EUS-guided FNA[149,153]; however, further experience is required before the establishment of EUS-guided FNA as a modality for performing renal biopsy.

Ascites and Pleural Fluid

The identification of malignant pleural effusion or malignant ascites is diagnostic of advanced disease in various malignancies. EUS seems to be more sensitive than CT in the detection of small amounts of ascites and pleural fluid. Drainage of pleural fluid or ascites at the time of EUS is possible and can be helpful if positive for malignancy. The technique of EUS-guided FNA of ascites or pleural fluid is similar to the technique applied to other lesions. Seeding of malignant cells into the fluid through the GI tract is a concern. The site of needle penetration in the GI lumen must not be involved with tumor (Fig. 47.16).

Chang et al (1995)[147] reported the utility of EUS for the detection of ascites and EUS-guided FNA in 571 consecutive patients who underwent upper EUS for various indications.[154]

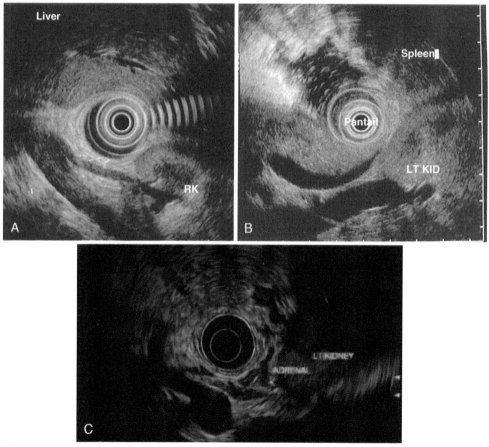

FIG 47.15 A, Radial imaging from the duodenum shows excellent images of the right kidney in this patient with malrotation of the right kidney (RK). The liver is seen in the upper portion of the image. **B,** Radial imaging from the body of the stomach shows the left (LT) kidney, spleen, body and tail of the pancreas (closest to the transducer) and above the splenic vein. The left renal vein is seen exiting the kidney. **C,** Radial imaging from the body of the stomach shows the LT kidney and adrenal gland.

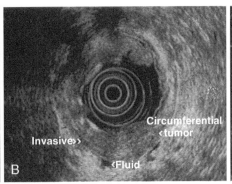
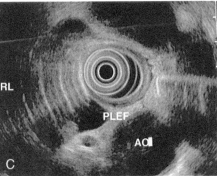

FIG 47.16 A, Radial imaging of trace ascites in a patient with pancreatic cancer. The pancreatic mass is seen below the ascites. **B,** Ascites in a patient with linitis plastica. **C,** Pleural effusion (PLEF) seen adjacent to the right lung (RL). *AO,* aorta.

EUS detected ascites in 85 (15%) patients, whereas CT-detected ascites in 14 (18%) of the 79 patients who underwent CT scanning before EUS. Of 85 patients, 31 underwent EUS-guided FNA paracentesis, and malignant ascites was diagnosed in 5 of these patients. Dewitt et al (2007) performed a retrospective study evaluating 60 patients undergoing EUS-FNA of ascites. Malignancy was revealed in 18 (30%) patients. Negative cytology did not exclude disease, as 3 (5%) patients ultimately were diagnosed with metastatic disease. Two patients experienced self-limited fever as a complication, suggesting the safety of EUS-FNA. The authors did find that EUS more readily identified ascites than CT, transabdominal US or MRI.[155]

Liver Lesions

EUS provides very good imaging of the left lobe of the liver and a significant portion of the right lobe of the liver. The left lobe and hilum of the liver are examined from the gastric body and fundus. The tip of the echoendoscope is placed in the gastric antrum; then, slowly withdrawing the echoendoscope, the tip is deflected up and rightward. When the liver comes into view, the instrument is rotated to evaluate portions of the liver. The right lobe of the liver is best imaged from the duodenum but can also be seen from the antrum. Liver lesions near the second or third portion of the duodenum, peripheral lesions near the dome of the diaphragm, and lesions in the inferior portion of the right lobe of the liver can be difficult to visualize (see Figs. 47.2 and 47.15).[156]

CT-guided and US-guided FNA of liver lesions have been reported to have sensitivities of 83% to 93% for the detection of malignant disease.[138,140–143] However, although rarely, percutaneous FNA of the liver has been associated with tumor seeding, intrahepatic hematoma, and hemorrhage.[157–161] Nguyen et al (1999)[156] postulated that EUS-guided FNA has the possible advantage over the percutaneous route due to shorter insertion length of the needle if the liver lesion is deep to the skin surface. With EUS-guided FNA, there is continuous visualization of the needle tip, which helps minimize risk for bleeding when the procedure is performed in conjunction with color flow and Doppler US.

Early experience suggests that EUS-guided FNA is comparable to CT-guided FNA in terms of safety and diagnostic utility for hepatic lesions.[156,162–166] Nguyen et al (1999)[156] conducted a prospective study in which 574 consecutive patients with a history or suspicion of GI or pulmonary tumor who were undergoing upper EUS examinations underwent EUS evaluation of the liver. They found small focal liver lesions that were undetected with conventional CT. Of these patients, 15 (2.6%) were found to have focal liver lesions (5 right lobe, 9 left lobe) and underwent EUS-guided FNA. The median largest diameter of the liver lesions was 1.1 cm (range 0.8–5.2 cm), and the mean number of passes per lesion was 2.0 (range 1–5 passes). Of the 15 liver lesions sampled via EUS-guided FNA, 14 were malignant and 1 was benign. Before EUS, recent CT depicted liver lesions in only 3 of 14 (21%) patients. In seven patients, the initial diagnosis of cancer was made by means of EUS-guided FNA of the liver. There were no immediate or late complications.

tenBerge et al (2002)[166] reported a multicenter study of 167 cases of EUS-guided FNA of the liver. Complications were reported in six (4%) cases, including death in one patient with an occluding biliary stent and biliary sepsis, bleeding (one case), fever (two cases), and pain (two cases). In 23 of 26 patients, EUS-guided FNA helped diagnose malignancy after a non-diagnostic percutaneous FNA. EUS was able to localize an unrecognized primary tumor in 17 of 33 (52%) cases after CT showed only liver metastases. This study highlights the fact that adequate biliary drainage is recommended in the setting of cholangitis before or coincident with the FNA procedure.

Dewitt et al (2003) performed a large single-center study to evaluate the clinical impact of benign and malignant solid liver lesions. The sensitivity for EUS-FNA for malignancy was 94% and malignancy was identified in 41% of patients who had negative prior CT or US. They reported a zero-complication rate.[167] EUS-guided FNA of liver lesions seems to be safe and effective and may become a more useful diagnostic method for liver lesions.

Miscellaneous

The close proximity of the intestinal tract to abdominal organs raises the possibility of EUS-guided FNA of idiopathic abdominal masses. Catalano et al (2002)[168] retrospectively evaluated the diagnostic accuracy of EUS-guided FNA of abdominal masses of unknown cause and its impact on subsequent evaluation. From five tertiary referral centers, 34 patients with idiopathic abdominal masses underwent EUS-guided FNA after evaluation including CT or transabdominal US, or both. CT showed an intraabdominal mass in all patients. Four patients had a history of intraabdominal cancer (two cervical, one ovarian, one colon), but these cancers were considered to be in remission. A final diagnosis for the mass lesions was established in all patients by various methods, including EUS-guided FNA, surgery, autopsy, or long-term follow-up. Abdominal masses were classified into three categories: infectious, benign or inflammatory, and malignant. EUS-guided FNA established a tissue diagnosis in 29 of 34 (85%) patients: infectious, 80% including abscess and infected pseudocyst; benign or inflammatory, 67% including hematoma or postsurgical inflammatory mass, leiomyoma, and sarcoidosis; and malignant, 91% including sarcoma, lymphoma, hepatoma, adenocarcinoma of unknown primary, ovarian cancer, transitional bladder carcinoma, uterine or cervical cancer, recurrent colon cancer, neuroendocrine tumor, paraganglionoma, metastatic lung cancer, and prostate cancer. EUS-guided FNA was instrumental in directing subsequent evaluation in 29 (85%) patients and therapy in 26 (77%). The number of fine needle passes needed for adequate tissue sampling was lower for nonmalignant (2.2–3.2 passes) versus malignant diseases (4.6 passes). A perirectal abscess developed in one patient and was treated successfully with antibiotics.

Cases using EUS-guided FNA to diagnose a schwannoma of the mediastinum[169] and a retroperitoneal neurilemoma have been described.[170] In addition, studies by Erickson and Tretjak (2000)[171] and Anand et al (2007)[172] have helped show that EUS-guided FNA is an effective method with a high sensitivity and specificity for diagnosing and altering patient management of nonpancreatic lesions adjacent to the GI tract.

Accessory spleen may be a potential cause of misinterpretation on EUS. Barawi et al (2003)[173] described the EUS features of accessory spleen in 10 (8 accessory spleen, 2 lobulated spleen) patients. The mean size of these lesions was 2.7 × 3.1 cm. Nine accessory spleens were round, and one was oval. All were located inferolateral to the pancreatic tail and medial to the spleen. All these lesions had a sharp and regular outer margin and homogeneous echo texture; four were hypoechoic and six were hyperechoic. CT scan may be helpful in confirming the presence of lobulated spleen and accessory spleen (Fig. 47.17).

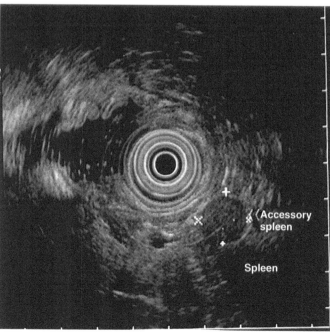

FIG 47.17 Radial imaging from the stomach of an accessory spleen.

One series described EUS-guided FNA of splenic lesions that were considered to be too small or dangerous for sampling with other modaliites.[174] In this series, a positive diagnosis was made in 10 of 12 patients (83%) for lesions ranging in size from 0.8 to 4.2 cm (median 1.4 cm). Bacteriology was positive for *Staphylococcus aureus* and *Serratia* in one patient each and for *Mycobacterium tuberculosis* in two patients. Diagnoses included lymphoma, sarcoidosis, abscesses, tuberculosis, metastatic colon cancer, and infarction (in one patient). One patient experienced pain after the procedure, but no hematoma was shown on subsequent US examination. Since this study, other studies have been performed supporting the possibility that EUS-guided FNA of splenic masses is feasible and safe.[175,176]

Complications

EUS-guided FNA is a relatively safe procedure compared with CT-guided FNA, bronchoscopy with transbronchial FNA, mediastinoscopy, or open or exploratory procedures. Generally, when complications occur, these are usually mild and self-limited. In reports and more recent prospective studies that have addressed complications of EUS-guided FNA, rare complications included endoscope-induced perforations, febrile episodes (after FNA of pancreatic cystic lesions), hemorrhage, pancreatitis, and pneumoperitoneum; false-positive diagnoses have been described.[177] As alluded to previously, the role of prophylactic antibiotics for EUS-guided FNA is unclear. The general practice has been to administer antibiotics to any patient undergoing FNA of cystic pancreatic or perirectal lesions. Barawi et al (2001)[85] studied 108 consecutive EUS-guided FNA cases that did not show bacteremia at 30 and 60 minutes after the procedure. However, the study by Van de Mierop et al (1999)[92] revealed a 19% incidence of bacteremia with EUS-guided FNA of solid lesions.

CONCLUSION

Over the last two decades, EUS has played an increasingly important role as an accurate and safe method for staging patients with NSCLC. EUS is now integrated into the evaluation of non-GI pathology, especially in the assessment of mediastinal pathology. EUS-guided FNA should be considered in patients in whom a previous attempt at lymph node FNA was unsuccessful using CT or bronchoscopy. Depending on the local expertise, EUS may be considered the primary procedure for biopsy of lesions arising from the posterior mediastinum, especially at levels 5 (aortopulmonic), 7 (subcarinal), or 8 (periesophageal) because these are most readily accessed by EUS. EBUS may also be considered where available to evaluate lesions in the anterior mediastinum traditionally not visualized well with EUS alone. This consideration is of particular relevance for staging of NSCLC, in which contralateral mediastinal lymph node metastases preclude curative resection. Identification of ipsilateral mediastinal lymph node involvement may be helpful for identifying patients who could benefit from neoadjuvant therapy. Mediastinoscopy, thoracoscopy, or partial thoracotomy could be reserved for patients with enlarged anterior lymph nodes or patients with suspicious nodes not successfully sampled by CT, bronchoscopy, EBUS, or EUS. EUS-guided FNA has been shown to be a highly accurate modality for evaluating unknown mediastinal masses or lymph nodes including lymphoma, sarcoidosis, and histoplasmosis.

In patients with otherwise operable lung cancer, EUS-guided FNA may be a viable alternative to percutaneous aspiration biopsy of a left adrenal mass. EUS can detect small focal liver lesions and small pockets of ascites or pleural fluid not detected by CT. Findings of EUS-guided FNA can confirm a cytologic diagnosis of metastasis and establish a definitive M stage that may change clinical management. EUS-guided FNA of renal masses may be a safe means of confirming the presence or absence of malignancy and may preclude the need for CT-guided studies. EUS-guided FNA provides minimally invasive tissue sampling and may obviate the need for exploratory laparotomy in cases of abdominal masses of undetermined origin.

KEY REFERENCES

2. Travis WD, Lubin J, Ries L, et al: United States lung carcinoma incidence trends: declining for most histologic types among males, increasing among females, *Cancer* 77:2464–2470, 1996.

6. Goldstraw P, Crowley J, Chansky K, et al: The IASLC Lung Cancer Staging Project: proposals for the revision of the TNM stage groupings in the forthcoming (seventh) edition of the TNM classification of malignant tumours, *J Thorac Oncol* 2:603–612, 2007.

8. Postmus PE, Brambilla E, Chansky K, et al: The IASLC Lung Cancer Staging Project: proposals for revision of the M descriptors in the forthcoming (seventh) edition of the TNM classification of malignant tumours, *J Thorac Oncol* 2:686–693, 2007.

9. Groome PA, Bolejack V, Crowley JJ, et al: The IASLC Lung Cancer Staging Project: validation of the proposals for revision of the T, N, and M descriptors and consequent stage groupings in the forthcoming (seventh) edition of the TNM classification of malignant tumours, *J Thorac Oncol* 2:694–705, 2007.

11. Goldstraw P, Chansky K, Crowley J, et al: The IASLC Lung Cancer Staging Project: proposals for revision of the TNM stage groupings in the forthcoming (eighth) edition of the TNM classification for lung cancer, *J Thorac Oncol* 11(1):39–51, 2016.

20. Martini N, Baines MS, McCormick PM, et al: Surgical treatment in non-small cell carcinoma of the lung: the Memorial Sloan-Kettering experience. In Hoogstraten B, Addis BJ, Hansen HH, et al, editors: *Treatment of lung tumors*, Heidelberg, 1987, Springer-Verlag, pp 111–132.

29. Glazer GM, Gross BH, Quint LE, et al: Normal mediastinal lymph nodes: number and size according to American Thoracic Society mapping, *AJR Am J Roentgenol* 144:261–265, 1985.

47. Flickling W, Wallace MB: EUS in lung cancer, *Gastrointest Endosc* 56:S18–S21, 2002.

50. Fritscher-Ravens A, Bohuslavizki KH, Brandt L, et al: Mediastinal lymph node involvement in potentially resectable lung cancer: comparison of CT, positron emission tomography, and endoscopic ultrasonography with and without fine-needle aspiration, *Chest* 123:442–451, 2003.

65. Merav AD: The role of mediastinoscopy and anterior mediastinotomy in determining operability of lung cancer: a review of published questions and answers, *Cancer Invest* 9:439–442, 1991.

68. Sugimachi K, Ohno S, Fujishima H, et al: Endoscopic ultrasonographic detection of carcinomatous invasion of lymph nodes in the thoracic esophagus, *Surgery* 107:366–371, 1990.

69. Schuder G, Isringhaus H, Kubale B, et al: Endoscopic ultrasonography of the mediastinum in the diagnosis of bronchial carcinoma, *Thorac Cardiovasc Surg* 39:299–303, 1991.

70. Varela-Lema L, Fernández-Villar A, Ruano-Ravina A: Effectiveness and safety of endobronchial ultrasound-transbronchial needle aspiration: a systematic review, *Eur Respir J* 33:1156–1164, 2009.

74. Gress FG, Savides TJ, Sandler A, et al: Endoscopic ultrasonography, fine-needle aspiration biopsy guided by endoscopic ultrasonography, and computed tomography in the preoperative staging of non-small-cell lung cancer: a comparison study, *Ann Intern Med* 127(8 Pt 1): 604–612, 1997.

76. Janssen J, Johanns W, Luis W, et al: Clinical value of endoscopic ultrasound-guided transesophageal fine needle puncture of mediastinal lesions, *Dtsch Med Wochenschr* 123:1402–1409, 1998.

84. Zhang R, Ying K, Shi L, et al: Combined endobronchial and endoscopic ultrasound-guided fine needle aspiration for mediastinal lymph node staging of lung cancer: a meta-analysis, *Eur J Cancer* 49(8):1860–1867, 2013.

91. Levy MJ, Norton ID, Wiersema MJ, et al: Prospective risk assessment of bacteremia and other infectious complications in patients undergoing EUS-guided FNA, *Gastrointest Endosc* 57:672–678, 2003.

95. Rex DK, Tarver RD, Wiersema MJ, et al: Endoscopic transesophageal fine needle aspiration of mediastinal masses, *Gastrointest Endosc* 37: 465–468, 1991.

99. Wallace MB, Kennedy T, Durkalski V, et al: Randomized controlled trial of EUS-guided fine needle aspiration techniques for the detection of malignant lymphadenopathy, *Gastrointest Endosc* 54:441–447, 2001.

102. Gress FG, Hawes RH, Savides TJ, et al: Endoscopic ultrasound guided fine needle aspiration biopsy utilizing linear array and radial scanning endosonography: results from a large single center experience, *Gastrointest Endosc* 45:243–250, 1997.

108. Hahn M, Faigel DO: Frequency of mediastinal lymph node metastases in patients undergoing EUS evaluation of pancreaticobiliary masses, *Gastrointest Endosc* 54:331–335, 2001.

155. DeWitt J, LeBlanc J, McHenry L, et al: Endoscopic ultrasound guided fine-needle aspiration of ascites, *Clin Gastroenterol Hepatol* 5(5): 609–615, 2007.

167. DeWitt J, LeBlanc J, McHenry L, et al: Endoscopic ultrasound–guided fine needle aspiration cytology of solid liver lesions: a large single-center experience, *Am J Gastroenterol* 98(9):1976–1981, 2003.

168. Catalano MF, Sial S, Chak A, et al: EUS-guided fine needle aspiration of idiopathic abdominal masses, *Gastrointest Endosc* 55:854–858, 2002.

177. Early DS, Acosta RD, Chandrasekhara V, et al: Adverse events associated with EUS and EUS with FNA, *Gastrointest Endosc* 77:839–843, 2013.

A complete reference list can be found online at ExpertConsult .com

SECTION III

Pancreaticobiliary Disorders

General Considerations and Techniques
Preparation for Pancreaticobiliary Endoscopy
Cholangiography and Pancreatography
Difficult Cannulation and Sphincterotomy
Endoscopic Ultrasound and Fine-Needle Aspiration for Pancreatic and Biliary Disorders
Endoscopic Ultrasound–Guided Access and Drainage of the Pancreaticobiliary Ductal Systems

Benign Biliary Disorders
Gallstone Disease: Choledocholithiasis, Cholecystitis, and Gallstone Pancreatitis
Postoperative Biliary Strictures and Leaks
Infections of the Biliary Tract
Sphincter of Oddi Disorders

Benign Pancreatic Disorders
Recurrent Acute Pancreatitis
Pancreatic Fluid Collections and Leaks
Chronic Pancreatitis

Neoplastic Pancreaticobiliary Disorders
The Indeterminate Biliary Stricture
Pancreatic Cystic Lesions
Evaluation and Staging of Pancreaticobiliary Malignancy
Palliation of Malignant Pancreaticobiliary Obstruction

48

Preparation for Pancreaticobiliary Endoscopy

Saurabh Chawla, Vikesh K. Singh, and Field F. Willingham

CHAPTER OUTLINE

INTRODUCTION

Pancreaticobiliary endoscopy focuses on the diagnosis and therapy of conditions involving the pancreas and biliary tree, and distinguishes itself from luminal endoscopy by a greater use of side-viewing endoscopes and echoendoscopes and the use of fluoroscopy. As discussed in Chapter 1, endoscopic retrograde cholangiopancreatography (ERCP) was first performed in the early 1970s, and endoscopic ultrasound (EUS) was introduced in 1980 for transluminal evaluation of the pancreas. During those early years, both ERCP and EUS were primarily diagnostic modalities and lacked therapeutic capabilities. Since then, pancreaticobiliary endoscopy has grown rapidly within the field of gastroenterology, with the development of new endoscopic devices, improvements in endoscopic imaging, and innovation in endoscopic techniques. Concurrent advancements in noninvasive imaging with increased resolution of computerized tomography (CT) scans and the advent of magnetic resonance cholangiopancreatography (MRCP) have redefined the role of pancreaticobiliary endoscopy. In addition, as will be discussed later in this chapter, the therapeutic potential of EUS is increasingly being recognized, and innovative therapeutic procedures using combined EUS and ERCP techniques are being developed.

Though pancreaticobiliary endoscopy may utilize different equipment and devices relative to luminal endoscopy, the fundamentals of patient preparation, reporting, documentation, and risk management overlap and remain applicable to these patients. This chapter will highlight some of the specific preparations that may be required for patients undergoing pancreaticobiliary procedures.

PATIENT-RELATED PREPARATION

Preprocedure Visit

Pancreaticobiliary diseases may range from relatively straightforward uncomplicated disorders such as choledocholithiasis or postoperative cystic duct leaks to more complex and challenging diseases such as primary sclerosing cholangitis, chronic pancreatitis, and disconnected pancreatic duct syndromes. In some cases, the availability of complementary diagnostic imaging (such as MRCP) and therapeutic procedures (interventional radiology, surgery) may impact management.

Therefore prior to performing pancreaticobiliary endoscopy, the indication for which the patient is referred must be carefully reviewed. This may or may not involve a clinic visit and physical examination. Typically, a comprehensive review of the laboratory and imaging data is required. For all patients, a frank discussion regarding the risks, benefits, and alternatives to the procedure must precede any endoscopic procedure. Clinic visits are more helpful for patients who will require multiple procedures and postprocedure admission to prepare them for periprocedural management. This provides an opportunity to establish a relationship and to prepare the patient for the sequence of events involved in their care.

Increasingly, endoscopists meet a patient for the first time in the preprocedure area on the day of endoscopy (open-access endoscopy).[1] Open-access endoscopy has gained popularity due to the increasing number of patients referred for screening colonoscopy who do not require a specialist visit prior to the procedure. With the increasing demand for endoscopic procedures, open-access endoscopy is also practiced in busy pancreaticobiliary endoscopy units. The basic tenets of open-access endoscopy include appropriateness of referral, patient acceptance and preparedness for endoscopy, informed consent, diagnostic yield of the endoscopy, and assurance that appropriate follow-up will be adhered to. For pancreaticobiliary endoscopy, it is important to review these requests on an individual basis. In such cases, the endoscopist should review the pertinent patient data prior to meeting the patient and allow time for a discussion, as stated earlier. Patient dissatisfaction and communication lapses are the leading cause of medicolegal claims, and may be much more common than true malpractice or medical negligence.[2]

Most pancreaticobiliary endoscopy is now performed under anesthesiology supervision. Preprocedure consultation may also be useful for patients with comorbidities to allow a preprocedure anesthesia evaluation that enables the anesthesiology team to complete their assessment of the patient and obtain any additional testing, such as an electrocardiogram or cardiac evaluation. This process may decrease procedural cancellations on the day of the endoscopy and can facilitate flow in the endoscopy unit.

Informed Consent

Consent is a voluntary agreement by a person with functional capacity for decision making, allowing a procedure to be performed on himself or herself. It is based on the principles of self-determination and autonomy, and requires that the provider or provider's representative provides the patient with substantive information necessary to make a reasoned decision.[3] In most circumstances, informed consent is also a requisite legal document, and failure to properly obtain informed consent can constitute medical battery and negligence.

It is especially important for pancreaticobiliary endoscopists to understand the concept of informed consent, as these procedures are frequently complex and may be associated with a higher rate of more serious adverse effects than other endoscopic procedures. Informed consent should be obtained after a detailed discussion of the nature of the proposed procedure, indication, and benefits, as well as potential risks and complications. Whenever possible, it is recommended that information in the form of non-technically worded handouts, fliers, or informational videos be shared with patients in advance of the procedure, giving them ample time to comprehend the planned procedure and allay their concerns.[4] A preprocedure visit or a well-documented preprocedure phone call can sometimes be utilized to help improve understanding of the procedure, and may allow time if there are additional concerns.

The consequences of not undergoing the procedure and the presence of alternatives to the procedure may also be very relevant to the discussion. Sometimes unanticipated procedures are needed in addition to the planned procedure, e.g., adding an unplanned EUS-guided rendezvous during a planned ERCP. Therefore some centers may require that these additional procedures be included as a part of the informed consent process. As a patient may withdraw consent at any time until the start of the procedure, it may be best if the consent is obtained on the day of the procedure. Often, the consent has a window of coverage within which the procedure must occur, or the consent will need to be repeated.

It is also recommended that a physician performing or participating in the procedure obtains the informed consent, thereby providing another opportunity to address any questions. Inadequacies in the informed consent process may impact patient-physician relationships, and are also one of leading components of legal claims and lawsuits against pancreaticobiliary endoscopists.[5]

Interdisciplinary Communication

In the area of pancreaticobiliary endoscopy, healthy and direct relationships with specialists in other disciplines are critical. Patients referred for pancreaticobiliary endoscopy often have complex neoplastic or inflammatory diseases and significant comorbidities. Very often, care is multispecialty, with patients frequently also receiving care from surgeons, oncologists, radiation oncologists, and/or interventional radiologists. Participation in multidisciplinary tumor boards with radiologists, medical and surgical oncologists, and pathologists is often helpful for outlining management plans for complex cases. Referral for pre-anesthesia evaluation for patients with significant comorbidities is frequently of benefit. Discussion with interventional radiologists and surgeons about the best approach for the management of the condition and complications, should they occur, is often of benefit if the presentation could be managed in several ways. Such collaboration may improve patient care and outcomes.[6] This is aptly illustrated in a 2014 single center study, where establishment of a multidisciplinary pancreatic cyst clinic led to a change in management of 30% of patients after a collaborative review of imaging features, cyst fluid analysis, cytology, and patient preference by gastroenterologists, pancreatic surgeons, radiologists, and cytopathologists.[7]

PROVIDER-RELATED PREPARATION

Provider Competence

Competence is the minimal level of skill, knowledge, and expertise required to safely and proficiently perform a procedure. Given the significant complications that may be associated with pancreaticobiliary endoscopy, it is very important that the endoscopist is competent and has the necessary skill set to perform the planned procedure. With the rapid pace of advancement, competence in pancreaticobiliary endoscopy requires not only adequate training but also an adequate case volume after training to maintain proficiency.

In 1996, a threshold of 100 ERCPs with 20 sphincterotomies was first proposed as a threshold for adequate training in ERCPs prior to independent practice. This threshold was soon challenged, and a more recent systematic review (2015) has suggested that 160–400 ERCPs may be required to achieve competency.[8] Similar numbers have also been proposed for EUS training.[9,10]

The increased scope and complexity of pancreaticobiliary endoscopy has led to a fourth year of advanced endoscopy training to achieve proficiency and certification in pancreaticobiliary endoscopy. It is, however, important to recognize that the number of procedures remains a surrogate for provider competence. Prospective multicenter studies on advanced endoscopy trainees have suggested that emphasis should be shifted to well-defined and validated competency thresholds for ERCPs and EUS rather than numbers alone.[11,12] It is important to recognize that, even if a provider is competent in performing the more common endoscopic procedures like stone extraction, stent placement, or fine needle aspiration, they may not have enough experience in the more complex procedures such as pancreatic necrosectomy or EUS-guided rendezvous. It has been demonstrated that high-volume endoscopists and centers have better outcomes than facilities where pancreaticobiliary endoscopy is performed less frequently (< 50 ERCP/year per endoscopist or < 87–200 ERCP/

year per center).[13,14] However, at this time, no guideline recommendations for case volume per endoscopist or center performing pancreaticobiliary endoscopy for maintenance of skills exist.

Another very important aspect of this field is the acquisition and safe adoption of new techniques and technology as they are introduced. The American Society of Gastrointestinal Endoscopy has published guidelines for the clinical application of these techniques that can be used by hospitals and practices for credentialing and granting privileges.[15] These guidelines recommend that emerging technologies can be stratified according to their complexity and general applicability. Training in minor new skills that are an extension of or advancement in a currently performed procedure or technique may be achieved by reading, viewing video recordings of the technique, or attending short courses. Training in major new skills that involve new techniques or procedures with a high level of complexity, interpretative requirements, and/or a new type of technology may require formal hands-on training under supervision, followed by documentation of competency.

Achieving competency in newer technologies depends on the individual endoscopist's skill set and prior training and the complexity of new technology. Therefore it is important for the endoscopist to adequately plan for the procedure prior to scheduling and to recognize if certain interventions or maneuvers are outside their skill set. In such cases, depending on the resources available, the provider may ask for supervision from a more experienced endoscopist or refer the patient to a center where such expertise is available. Representatives from industry may often provide assistance with training in the use of a particular accessory or endoscope, may provide case support, and may assist with materials and demonstration. This would not necessarily supplant training requirements for certain procedures that are high risk and represent a larger departure from procedures currently performed by the endoscopist.

ENDOSCOPY UNIT–RELATED PREPARATION

Endoscopy Unit Design

Ideally, the endoscopy suite for the performance of pancreaticobiliary endoscopic procedures should be 300 square feet or larger.[16] This is because pancreaticobiliary endoscopy requires additional equipment that may not be used for general endoscopy. This equipment may include EUS processors, electrohydraulic lasers, fixed table fluoroscopy, or portable C-arms. Frequently, these procedures also require anesthesiology support, and the presence of anesthesiology equipment, ventilators, and personnel requires additional space considerations. Equipment required for the procedures should be positioned to enable visualization, provider movement, and image transmission, all with the ultimate goal of facilitating a good procedural outcome for the patient.

Endoscopists are at increased risk for musculoskeletal injuries due to repetitive movements and possibly abnormal posture, and surveys of endoscopists have suggested musculoskeletal injury rates between 29% and 89%.[17] This risk may be greater in pancreaticobiliary endoscopists due to the longer duration of the procedures, thumb movement on the elevator of endoscopes, and the use of lead aprons, which leads to added strain to the neck and shoulders.[18] Therefore the endoscopy unit should be ergonomically designed and equipped to allow the endoscopist to stand on an antifatigue cushioned floor mat in a neutral position with video monitors positioned at eye level to minimize musculoskeletal stress and the risk of mechanical injuries.[17] Split

lead aprons are helpful in distributing the weight over the hips and less on the neck/lower back, and should be used if available.

A usual format that is followed is to center the room around the patient table and fluoroscopy equipment, such that adequate space is available at the head end for patient monitoring and anesthesia equipment, and for the endoscopist and the assistant to stand unencumbered on the side with access to control panels, monitors, and endoscopy devices. To achieve this, most high volume centers have dedicated pancreaticobiliary endoscopy procedure rooms with fixed table-mounted fluoroscopy equipment, boom- or wall-mounted video monitors, and storage for specialized endoscopic devices to efficiently and ergonomically perform these procedures. In lower-volume centers, where such dedicated fluoroscopy-enabled rooms are not present, portable C-arms may be brought in for performance of ERCPs. In such cases, it is important to remember the aforementioned principles and to position equipment prior to the start of the procedure, not only to allow for unobstructed and efficient conduct of the procedure but also to ensure that there is no impediment to accessing the patient or changing the position of the patient for resuscitation, should the need arise.

Pancreaticobiliary endoscopy requires frequent use of radiation, and may therefore expose the patient and endoscopy staff to the risk of radiation injury. Although most studies report that radiation exposure to providers and patients is well below the safety limits, the pancreaticobiliary endoscopy suite should be shielded to prevent radiation exposure outside the suite, and should have indicators for active fluoroscopy use. To mitigate the risk of radiation to endoscopy personnel, wraparound lead aprons, thyroid shields, and leaded eyeglasses should be provided and their use encouraged.[19] The endoscopy personnel should use dosimeters, and monthly evaluation of radiation exposure should be performed to keep track of cumulative radiation exposure for the endoscopy staff. Whereas some institutions require that nonradiologists undergo formal credentialing in the use of fluoroscopy, even if not mandatory, the pancreaticobiliary endoscopist and the endoscopy staff should at least have access to radiation safety information and be aware of the "ALARA" (as low as reasonably achievable) principle to decrease avoidable fluoroscopy use and radiation exposure.[18,20]

Staff Training

Endoscopy practice is most commonly performed with support from nonphysician staff in the endoscopy unit. This staff may involve nurses, endoscopy technicians, nursing aids, anesthesia personnel, and administrative staff. Whereas adequate criteria have been set for physician training and maintenance of competence, most endoscopy staff undergo on-the-job training, and training certification is largely voluntary. Organizations such as the Society of Gastrointestinal Nurses and Associates offer training and certification courses for nurses and associates, as well as ongoing education through various local, regional, and national conferences, to provide a forum for staff exposure to new developments and techniques in endoscopy.

Another means of providing continuing staff training involves hands-on product demonstrations in the endoscopy unit to familiarize the staff with the use of available equipment, a process that is commonly referred to as an *in-service*. This may be applicable not only to new devices but also to periodic updates on equipment that is infrequently used (e.g., a mechanical lithotriptor) or complex devices (e.g., electrosurgical generators). This may be facilitated by including industry representatives and training with the devices on animal explants or inanimate models. Such efforts are valuable in ensuring staff competency, facilitating the adoption of new technology, and eventually contributing to patient safety.[21]

Preprocedure Checklist

Since their introduction, surgical safety checklists have been shown to decrease complications, length of hospital stay, and mortality, and are now used in most operating rooms.[22] These checklists were initially introduced for preprocedure verification of the patient, site of surgery, and antibiotic prophylaxis, as well as postprocedure sponge counts; however, an ancillary benefit involved increased communication within the operating room, further increasing efficiency and minimizing errors. Variations on these checklists are now used in most procedures outside the operating room, including endoscopy.[23]

As an extension of these checklists, the endoscopist can discuss the planned endoscopic procedure, and the anticipated devices and accessories can be pulled in advance. This helps team members prepare for the procedure, gives team members a chance to ask for guidance on the use of devices they may not be comfortable with, and ensures that all the required equipment is present prior to the start of the procedure. Doing a huddle and performing preprocedure verification of accessories may occasionally mean the difference between the success and failure of complex therapeutic pancreaticobiliary endoscopy procedures.

Postprocedure Care

Increasingly complex therapeutic pancreaticobiliary endoscopic procedures are being performed on outpatients. Although the paradigm for most outpatient endoscopic procedures is early discharge after recovery from sedation, patients undergoing pancreaticobiliary endoscopy may require more prolonged postprocedure observation and aggressive postprocedure hydration, and occasionally have intraprocedural events or persistence of pain that may trigger further testing, procedures, or unplanned admissions.[24]

Frequently, complex pancreaticobiliary procedures are scheduled with a planned postprocedure admission. Therefore the unit should recognize that these patients may require close monitoring, and a protocol for postprocedure care should be developed by the physicians in conjunction with the postprocedure team and unit managers. Doing this allows the staff to assist with and facilitate the care of patients who may have unanticipated outcomes, and will ideally allow the busy outpatient endoscopy unit to run smoothly, without needing to divert staff or resources to attend to these patients.

CONCLUSION

The field of pancreaticobiliary endoscopy continues to advance at a rapid pace. New developments such as interventional EUS, management of peripancreatic fluid collections, pancreatic necrosectomies, and submucosal endoscopic procedures such as endoscopic submucosal dissection and peroral endoscopic myotomy are permitting more advanced care to be performed in a minimally invasive manner. As these novel technologies and approaches are adopted, it is important that patients be advised of the options and alternatives in their treatment. At times, the higher procedural risk of a surgery must be weighed against a higher chance of recurrence if an endoscopic resection is not

complete. The necessity of interspecialty communication and collaboration has grown with the proliferation of treatment paradigms.

In what settings is an endoscopic procedure preferable to a minimally invasive surgery? What are the risks of repeated endoscopic procedures, compared to the morbidity of a single definitive procedure? In complex cases or gray areas, it is generally best to involve stakeholders prior to the procedure, allowing surgery, interventional radiology, and/or oncology to weigh in, as this increases the odds of obtaining the best outcome for the patient. Preparation for advanced endoscopic procedures becomes more important as higher risk procedures, novel procedures, and innovative approaches are implemented. Ultimately, attending to the details before and after the procedure increases the chance of a successful endoscopy and an excellent outcome for the patient.

KEY REFERENCES

1. Chandrasekhara V, Eloubeidi MA, Bruining DH, et al: Open-access endoscopy, *Gastrointest Endosc* 81(6):1326–1329, 2015.
2. Cotton PB, Saxton JW, Finkelstein MM: Avoiding medicolegal complications, *Gastrointest Endosc Clin N Am* 17(1):197–207, ix, 2007.
3. Zuckerman MJ, Shen B, Harrison ME, 3rd, et al: Informed consent for GI endoscopy, *Gastrointest Endosc* 66(2):213–218, 2007.
4. Everett SM, Griffiths H, Nandasoma U, et al: Guideline for obtaining valid consent for gastrointestinal endoscopy procedures, *Gut* 65(10): 1585–1601, 2016.
5. Cotton PB: Analysis of 59 ERCP lawsuits; mainly about indications, *Gastrointest Endosc* 63(3):378–382, quiz 464, 2006.
6. Petty JK, Vetto JT: Beyond doughnuts: tumor board recommendations influence patient care, *J Cancer Educ* 17(2):97–100, 2002.
7. Lennon AM, Manos LL, Hruban RH, et al: Role of a multidisciplinary clinic in the management of patients with pancreatic cysts: a single-center cohort study, *Ann Surg Oncol* 21(11):3668–3674, 2014.
8. Shahidi N, Ou G, Telford J, Enns R: When trainees reach competency in performing ERCP: a systematic review, *Gastrointest Endosc* 81(6): 1337–1342, 2015.
9. Arya N, Sahai AV, Paquin SC: Credentialing for endoscopic ultrasound: a proposal for Canadian guidelines, *Endosc Ultrasound* 5(1):4–7, 2016.
10. Eisen GM, Dominitz JA, Faigel DO, et al: Guidelines for credentialing and granting privileges for endoscopic ultrasound, *Gastrointest Endosc* 54(6):811–814, 2001.
11. Wani S, Hall M, Keswani RN, et al: Variation in aptitude of trainees in endoscopic ultrasonography, based on cumulative sum analysis, *Clin Gastroenterol Hepatol* 13(7):1318–1325, e1312, 2015.
12. Wani S, Hall M, Wang AY, et al: Variation in learning curves and competence for ERCP among advanced endoscopy trainees by using cumulative sum analysis, *Gastrointest Endosc* 83(4):711–719, e711, 2016.
13. Cote GA, Imler TD, Xu H, et al: Lower provider volume is associated with higher failure rates for endoscopic retrograde cholangiopancreatography, *Med Care* 51(12):1040–1047, 2013.
14. Kalaitzakis E, Toth E: Hospital volume status is related to technical failure and all-cause mortality following ERCP for benign disease, *Dig Dis Sci* 60(6):1793–1800, 2015.
15. ASGE Guidelines for clinical application. Methods of privileging for new technology in gastrointestinal endoscopy. American Society for Gastrointestinal Endoscopy, *Gastrointest Endosc* 50(6):899–900, 1999.
16. Mulder CJ, Jacobs MA, Leicester RJ, et al: Guidelines for designing a digestive disease endoscopy unit: report of the World Endoscopy Organization, *Dig Endosc* 25(4):365–375, 2013.
17. Harvin G: Review of musculoskeletal injuries and prevention in the endoscopy practitioner, *J Clin Gastroenterol* 48(7):590–594, 2014.
18. Pedrosa MC, Farraye FA, Shergill AK, et al: Minimizing occupational hazards in endoscopy: personal protective equipment, radiation safety, and ergonomics, *Gastrointest Endosc* 72(2):227–235, 2010.

19. Seo D, Kim KH, Kim JS, et al: Evaluation of radiation doses in patient and medical staff during endoscopic retrograde cholangiopancreatography procedures, *Radiat Prot Dosimetry* 168(4):516–522, 2016.
20. Alzimami K, Sulieman A, Paroutoglou G, et al: Optimisation of radiation exposure to gastroenterologists and patients during therapeutic ERCP, *Gastroenterol Res Pract* 2013:587574, 2013.
21. Kaul V, Faigel D: The role of industry representatives in the endoscopy unit. 2015. American Society for Gastrointestinal Endoscopy. Available at https://www.asge.org. Accessed 8 February 2017.
22. Pugel AE, Simianu VV, Flum DR, Patchen Dellinger E: Use of the surgical safety checklist to improve communication and reduce complications, *J Infect Public Health* 8(3):219–225, 2015.
23. Matharoo M, Thomas-Gibson S, Haycock A, Sevdalis N: Implementation of an endoscopy safety checklist, *Frontline Gastroenterol* 5(4):260–265, 2014.
24. Cote GA, Lynch S, Easler JJ, et al: Development and validation of a prediction model for admission after endoscopic retrograde cholangiopancreatography, *Clin Gastroenterol Hepatol* 13(13):2323–2332, e2321–2329, 2015.

A complete reference list can be found online at ExpertConsult.com

49

Cholangiography and Pancreatography

Jeffrey J. Easler, Evan L. Fogel, and Stuart Sherman

CHAPTER OUTLINE

INTRODUCTION

Endoscopic cannulation of the major papilla with imaging of the biliary tree and the pancreatic ductal system (endoscopic retrograde cholangiopancreatography [ERCP]) was first successfully accomplished with an end-viewing duodenoscope and reported in 1968.[1] Subsequent development of side-viewing endoscopes with a catheter-deflecting elevator greatly advanced the technique. Diagnostic studies were supplemented by the first endoscopic sphincterotomies in the early 1970s.[2,3] Overall, these developments expanded the field of endoscopy and permitted the performance of less invasive diagnostic and therapeutic maneuvers in the pancreaticobiliary ductal system(s), which were previously limited to open surgical and percutaneous techniques.

In recent years, the refinement and proliferation of magnetic resonance imaging (MRI) and endoscopic ultrasound (EUS) techniques have changed the practice of ERCP. Now that quality diagnostic studies are readily available to the pancreaticobiliary endoscopist, ERCP has evolved from a stand-alone diagnostic procedure into an almost exclusively therapeutic endeavor. Although diagnostic indications for ERCP have now been displaced by the aforementioned less invasive, lower risk imaging modalities, the need for mastery of the radiographic findings of ERCP remains. Expert level execution and interpretation of

diagnostic ERCP is a crucial component for skillful, efficient deployment of therapeutic interventions. Diagnostic ERCP findings also complement (and, in a few scenarios, are superior to) noninvasive imaging modalities for establishing or excluding pathology (e.g., pancreatic ductal leaks and fistulae).

This chapter reviews the indications for ERCP, techniques involved in its performance, and frequently encountered normal and pathologic diagnostic findings.

INDICATIONS AND CONTRAINDICATIONS FOR ERCP

Imaging of the pancreaticobiliary ductal system without anticipated therapy is appropriate in a narrow set of clinical circumstances. Patients requiring ductal imaging who are unable to undergo MRI/magnetic resonance cholangiopancreatography (MRCP) (e.g., those with implantable devices and/or a large body habitus) may require diagnostic ERCP as a first diagnostic test for ductography. However, conditions that indicate ERCP as purely a diagnostic modality are usually exceptional (e.g., cholestasis without dilated ducts, suspicion of early sclerosing cholangitis, confirmation of pancreatic fistula after nondiagnostic imaging if clinical suspicion persists), and it should only be performed in a setting of at least moderate pretest suspicion. In certain settings, such as clinical diagnosis of acute cholangitis with shock or sepsis, therapeutic ERCP is considered lifesaving, and need not be preceded by cross-sectional imaging. Overall, ERCP is indicated in clinical settings in which there is significant suspicion of pathology and a clear intention for therapeutics. A general list of indications is shown in Table 49.1.

Most contraindications to ERCP are relative, and the degree of risk must be balanced against the potential benefit.[4–6] In patients with necrotizing pancreatitis and low clinical suspicion for ductal stones, ERCP is relatively contraindicated, as pancreatography may result in bacterial contamination of the pancreatic bed and undrained fluid collections. Other relative contraindications include unstable cardiopulmonary disease or severe coagulopathy. Patients with comorbid life-threatening conditions can have endoscopic retrograde cholangiography (ERC) performed in the intensive care unit (with or without fluoroscopy) if deemed medically necessary. ERCP with manometry and/or sphincterotomy is now generally not indicated in patients with type III sphincter of Oddi dysfunction, given the negative results of a 2014 high-quality, randomized study.[7]

ENDOSCOPIC EQUIPMENT

ERCP is performed using side-viewing instruments with video chip processors that provide high-quality images. Digital video systems (over fiberoptic) are now the standard, as they offer the advantage of television monitor viewing by all persons in the endoscopy suite, real-time teaching capabilities, and seamless coordination between the endoscopist and the ERCP team. Endoscopes have a working length of 120 cm and are generally categorized as diagnostic (11-mm distal diameter) or therapeutic (13.7-mm distal diameter). Some newer-generation endoscopes combine a large working channel diameter (up to 4.2 mm) with a standard 11-mm insertion tube diameter (Fig. 49.1). A pediatric duodenoscope with an outer diameter of less than 7.5 mm is available (Olympus America Inc., Center Valley, PA). Most ERCP examinations should now be performed with CO_2 insufflation. Data suggest that CO_2 insufflation reduces postprocedure abdominal distention and pain, and likely expedites recovery.[8]

Current-generation endoscopes are capable of undergoing submersion disinfection. After cleaning, endoscopes should be hung in vertical position to facilitate drying. However, in the setting of growing concern over carbapenem-resistant Enterobacteriaceae infections linked to contaminated duodenoscopes even after "standard" reprocessing procedures, enhanced techniques for disinfection and surveillance are now recommended.[9] Special attention should be given to the elevator mechanism during disinfection. Surveillance cultures of the duodenoscope instrument channel and its distal components are also recommended, with reprocessing of duodenoscopes if cultures are positive.[10]

TABLE 49.1	Indications for Endoscopic Retrograde Cholangiopancreatography	
Category	**Biliary**	**Pancreatic**
Diagnosis/ confirmation of suspected disorder	Obstructive jaundice/ cholestasis Ascending cholangitis Symptomatic choledocholithiasis Biliary lesion seen on other imaging test Biliary leak/fistula	Recurrent pancreatitis Main duct or mixed IPMN Chronic pancreatitis Pancreatic leak/fistula
Endoscopic therapy	Sphincterotomy Biliary drainage (stent) Bile duct stricture therapy	Sphincterotomy Pancreatic drainage Transpapillary therapy for pseudocysts Pancreatic duct stones/strictures Pancreatic leak/fistula
Endoscopic tissue and fluid sampling	Biopsy, brush cytology, fine needle aspiration, bile collection	Biopsy, brush cytology, pancreatic juice collection
Preoperative ductal mapping	Malignant and benign bile duct strictures	Chronic pancreatitis
Manometry	Sphincter of Oddi dysfunction	Idiopathic pancreatitis

IPMN, intraductal papillary mucinous neoplasm.

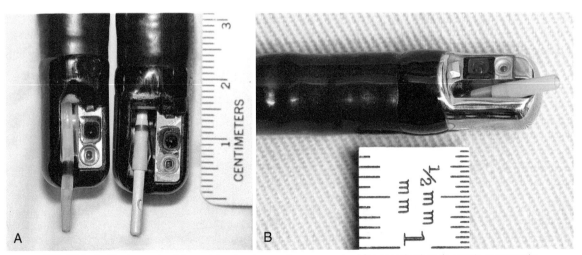

FIG 49.1 A, Photograph of two side-viewing endoscopes used for standard endoscopic retrograde cholangiography (ERC). Biopsy channel diameters range from 3.2–4.5 mm to accommodate a wide variety of accessories needed in diagnostic and therapeutic biliary studies. **B,** Newer-generation Olympus pediatric video duodenoscope for use in children weighing less than 10 kg.

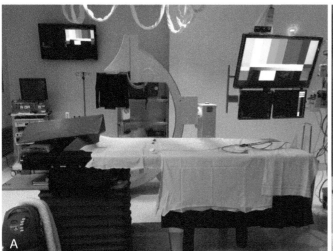
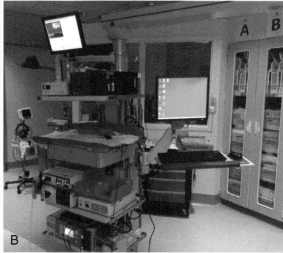

FIG 49.2 **A,** C-arm and table fluoroscopy unit. Table capable of tilt and cradle, C-arm tilt, and rotation offers viewing in multiple angles. Note lead apron drape from image intensifier and multiple high-resolution monitors. **B,** Tower with video recorder, video processor, and electrocautery unit. Note closet for storage of endoscopic accessories in the background.

Digital Imaging and Radiation Safety

Endoscopists at high-volume centers often have dedicated suites for ERCP. However, many physicians in the community and/or at lower-volume centers must coordinate procedures with a radiology department and use general purpose or angiographic units. Manufacturers now market dedicated fluoroscopy units for ERCP. Flat tables with a fixed overhead carriage have limited versatility. Consequently, the preferred x-ray table configuration includes the ability to tilt the patient's head up and down 30 degrees and has a C-arm carriage, which allows axial, cranial, caudal, vertical, and horizontal movements, to create image vectors from multiple angles (Fig. 49.2). Because the patient is usually positioned prone with the head at the foot of the table, having the ability to reverse the viewing image in both the vertical and the horizontal axes is helpful. In the past, endoscopists used older-generation x-ray units, including portable C-arm units with limited image resolution. This practice is no longer acceptable because high-quality fluoroscopy and quality images are key to accurate diagnosis and management. High-quality ERCP imaging requires resolution equivalent to that for neuroradiology (brain blood vessels). Resolution of greater than 2.5 line pairs per millimeter is strongly recommended for both fluoroscopy and final images (Fig. 49.3). This resolution is best accomplished with image intensifiers that have smaller diameters (6–9 inches).

Radiation safety standards should be followed.[11] Monitoring levels of personal exposure, selecting the highest-quality equipment, using radiation shielding, and undergoing formal training in techniques to limit exposure are recommended to limit cumulative radiation dosage to the patient and the ERCP team (Box 49.1). Collimating to the area of interest rather than magnifying is good practice. Use of newer-generation pulse fluoroscopy gives intermittent viewing, which, although slightly jerky, is often adequate for the majority of maneuvers during a case and with a fraction of the radiation exposure. Appropriate lead aprons, lead glasses, and thyroid shields are recommended (Fig. 49.4).

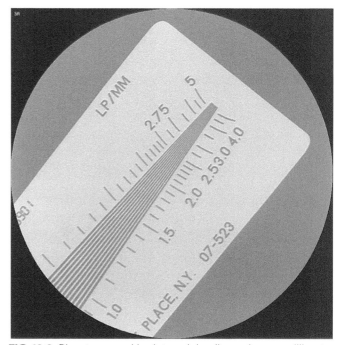

FIG 49.3 Phantom used in determining line pairs per millimeter resolution during fluoroscopy or image acquisition. Greater than 2.5-line pair resolution is recommended for optimal endoscopic retrograde cholangiopancreatography (ERCP) imaging. (Courtesy of Joe Edmiston, Indiana University Medical Center.)

ENDOSCOPIC TECHNIQUE

Upper Gastrointestinal Endoscopy

Initially, a brief endoscopic examination of the esophagus, stomach, duodenum, and major duodenal papilla is performed with the duodenoscope. Whereas views of the lumen are limited,

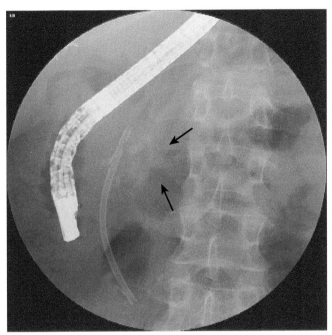

FIG 49.5 Plain x-ray film of right upper quadrant showing post–shock wave lithotripsy pancreatic calcifications (arrows) and residual biliary stent. This film serves as a background view for all subsequent contrast agent injections.

BOX 49.1   Strategies to Limit Personal Radiation Exposure During ERCP

Personal Shielding Protection

Full (wrap) coverage body aprons
Leaded glasses
Thyroid shield
Regular, systematic inspection of personal shielding for defects

Fluoroscopy Equipment

Under-couch x-ray tube preferred to over-couch and mobile C-arms
Leaded drapes, shielding between operator and collector
High-quality, digital systems

Operator Behavior

Use of collimation rather than magnification for enhanced images
Pulsed rather than continuous fluoroscopy
Use of "last image hold" over radiograph for reference
Use of endoscopic rather than fluoroscopic cues for appropriate ERCP maneuvers (e.g., exchange of endoscopic accessories within the duodenoscope channel)

Staff Monitoring and Education

Dual dosimeter monitoring with regular operator feedback
Displays with cumulative fluoroscopy time and radiation exposure
Structured training on fluoroscopy equipment and radiation safety

ERCP, endoscopic retrograde cholangiopancreatography.

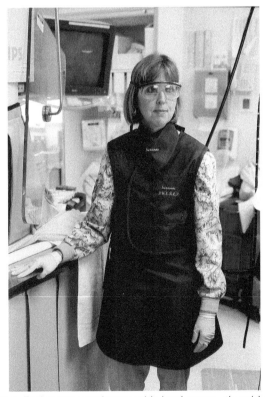

FIG 49.4 Endoscopy assistant with lead apron, thyroid shield, and lead glasses for optimal radiation safety.

a physician who is familiar with the endoscopic dynamics of operating a duodenoscope can often perform an adequate clinical examination of the patient's anatomy.

One should first attempt to exit the stomach with minimal residual intragastric air, as this permits *en face* papilla views and

facilitates optimal fluoroscopic images. Encountering obstruction (malignant or benign) of the gastric outlet or otherwise should prompt the physician to consider switching to an end-viewing endoscope to assess the need for endoscopic dilation or any further maneuvers to complete the case.

Other findings, such as varices, external compression of the gut wall, or edema of the medial wall of the duodenum, help quantify or localize disease processes. The major papilla is usually located on the medial aspect of the mid-descending duodenum, but may reside anywhere from the duodenal bulb to the transverse duodenum. Care should be taken to look for major papilla abnormalities (e.g., tumor, edema, enlarged orifice from stone or mucin passage), as they may also have diagnostic value and import for planning your approach. The location of orifices should be noted. A brief examination of the minor papilla may be helpful if initial pancreatography via the major papilla fails and pancreatic access is intended.

If the major papilla is not initially evident, gentle lifting of folds, greater air distention, and use of glucagon to inhibit peristalsis will likely expose the structure. If duodenal diverticula are present, the major papilla is most often on the diverticular rim, but the papilla is within the diverticulum *per se* in approximately 5% to 10% of cases.

Selective Cannulation of the Desired Duct

Prior to attempting cannulation, fluoroscopic inspection of the field of interest should be performed to take note of the initial duodenoscope position, stents, calcifications, masses, extraluminal air, and residual contrast material from prior radiographic studies (Fig. 49.5). A still image should be indexed to document any findings and serve as a baseline for comparative purposes, if there is any question of complications during the case (e.g., retroperitoneal air associated with perforation) (Fig. 49.6). The choice of initial cannulation tool is a personal preference (similar

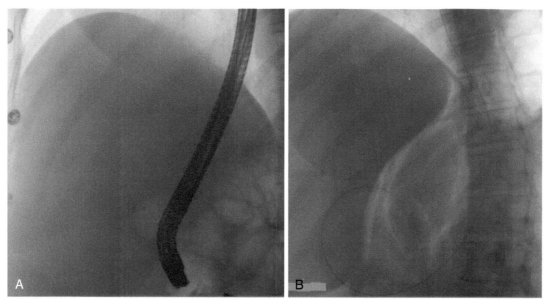

FIG 49.6 A, Preprocedure radiograph. **B,** Postprocedure radiograph demonstrating retroperitoneal air and an air nephrogram suggestive of retroperitoneal perforation secondary to sphincterotomy.

to choosing a tennis racket or golf club). One may begin with a simple single-lumen 5-Fr polyethylene catheter or an extraction balloon in the setting of prior sphincterotomy. If the orifice appears small, or cannulation of the minor papilla is desired, a catheter with a highly tapered tip (to 3-Fr) or a sphincterotome is desirable. However, if sphincterotomy is anticipated, a sphincterotome is the most cost-effective tool, and is now the standard for most biliary endoscopists as they approach a native papilla. Two-lumen or three-lumen accessories are most advantageous, as they have dedicated channels for independent deployment of a guidewire and injection of contrast medium. A guidewire may be used at any point to aid cannulation or maintain intraductal stability.

For the purposes of cannulation, orientation of the catheter tip toward the 11 o'clock to 12 o'clock position (Fig. 49.7) is ideal to access the bile duct, and orientation of the catheter toward the 1 o'clock to 4 o'clock position is ideal for pancreatic duct entry. However, the biliary orifice location may vary from 10 o'clock to 2 o'clock, depending on patient anatomy. Pancreatic cannulation is often easier than biliary cannulation, as the vector for cannulation is often *en face*.

Cannulation may initially be attempted either by gently threading the guidewire 1 to 2 cm into the desired channel (wire-guided cannulation) or by gentle impaction of the catheter tip in the papillary orifice. Growing evidence supports initiating cannulation by threading or "feathering" the guidewire for access (wire-guided cannulation). Meta-analysis–level data suggest that this technique facilitates cannulation and is associated with lower rates of post-ERCP pancreatitis.[12] However, wire-guided cannulation must be performed carefully, as unintended passage of the guidewire into the pancreatic duct is common during biliary cannulation, and is associated with pancreatitis. Wire-induced pancreatic duct perforation through a side branch (often at the genu) can occur if the guidewire is advanced beyond 2 cm without contrast agent injection to confirm position[13] (Fig. 49.8). Deep cannulation (> 1 cm penetration of the catheter into the duct) should then follow for a more secure intraductal position. This

allows contrast agent injection, fluid aspiration, patient position changes, and endoscope position changes without loss of access to the duct.

For biliary cannulation, 0.025- or 0.035-inch diameter wires are preferred. An 0.021- or 0.018-inch guidewire may be desired for pancreatic access, especially if access through the minor papilla is anticipated. Soft-tipped wires have the advantage of inducing less tissue trauma (e.g., fewer submucosal or other extraductal dissections). Torsion with advancement of an angled wire with a hydrophilic tip may facilitate access across angulated ductal anatomy. Ultimately, the specific devices used are much less important than the experience and skill of the endoscopist and the ERCP team members (Fig. 49.9).

If the cannulation is not optimal for the desired duct, an advantage of a sphincterotome is the ability to orient further by "bowing" the instrument. Decompressing air from the stomach and/or transitioning to a long position (advancing the duodenoscope such that the shaft is along the greater curvature) may also achieve the necessary angles. In patients with a prominent major papilla (protruding well into the duodenal lumen), the path of the biliary lumen is nearly always stair-stepped. Cannulation is initially cephalad, then more perpendicular into the wall, and then more cephalad again. The cannulation is partially accomplished by pulling the endoscope more cephalad, lowering the elevator, and moving the viewing lens very close to the papilla. Gentle guidewire manipulations and more perpendicular catheter orientation are required.

When difficult anatomy, pathology (e.g., ventral duct obstruction), or pancreas divisum prevents performance of pancreatography from the major papilla, pancreatography can be accomplished via the minor papilla, with a reported rate of success of greater than 90%, regardless of divisum anatomy.[14,15] This technique allows for pancreatography of the dorsal and ventral pancreatic ducts (through antegrade filling) in most patients, and may be an effective approach for endotherapy.[14]

The minor papilla is a slightly raised structure that can display frond-like mucosa. However, it often lacks a clear os. Usually, the minor papilla is located 2 to 3 cm proximal and slightly anterior and to the visual right of the major papilla; however, its location may vary along the duodenal wall. A gradual push of intravenous (IV) secretin (0.2 μg/kg body weight; 16 μg in most patients) over 60 seconds will frequently stimulate the flow of pancreatic juice into the duodenum and facilitate orifice identification. If the orifice is not detectable, methylene blue can be sprayed on the duodenal wall to facilitate visualization of the (relative clear) focal excretion of pancreatic juice. The minor papilla is best approached with an initial *en face* view facilitated by a long or semi-long duodenoscope position. Cannulation usually follows a slightly posterior and horizontal to mildly cephalad path.

Cannulation of the minor papilla can be achieved with a standard sphinctertome or with straight cannula accessories. However, due to the diminutive size of the os and the paraduodenal dorsal pancreatic duct, use of small-caliber tip accessories (3- or 4-Fr) and guidewires (0.018- or 0.021-inch) to facilitate deep cannulation with graded dilation of the os is preferred by experts.

If cannulation of the biliary tree is mandatory and initial attempts fail, several options exist. Attempting cannulation alongside a pancreatic duct guidewire or stent has a significant rate of reported success.[16] Precut entry is also a reasonable next maneuver, and should ideally be performed after placement of a pancreatic stent. Literature now suggests that, if deployed early during a difficult cannulation by those with experience with the technique, precut needle knife access does not elevate the risk of complications.[17–19] Endosonographic rendezvous and drainage techniques may be deployed in expert hands. However, the endoscopist at this juncture must take inventory of his or her skill set and balance a decision for aggressive, advanced access techniques against transfer to a facility with high-level expertise, as the literature reports that subsequent success rates approach 95% in the setting of transfer to an expert center.[20,21] When cannulation fails in the setting of biliary obstruction, one may also consider percutaneous drainage.

Contrast Medium and Image Acquisition

Standard ionic contrast medium (e.g., diatrizoate meglumine) at a 25% to 30% concentration is often called *half-strength*, and is most commonly used for cholangiography. Half-strength contrast medium permits adequate visualization of small ducts (2–6 mm in diameter) and allows filling defects (stones) to be seen in capacious, dilated ducts. However, biliary stricture detail, peripheral intrahepatic ducts, and pancreatic ducts are better defined with "full-strength" contrast medium (50%–60% concentration). Nonionic and lower osmolality contrast agents, which are more expensive, offer no safety advantage.[22] Many manufacturers have abandoned marketing of inexpensive ionic agents, making the use of nonionic agents necessary. Also of note, whereas a degree of absorption of contrast media has been reported, use of contrast media within the pancreaticobiliary system does not appear to elicit a clinical reaction, even in patients with a declared allergy to IV contrast media. Consequently, routine or even targeted prophylaxis for contrast media reaction is not recommended prior to ERCP.[23]

We prefer using 10- to 20-mL syringes for injection of contrast to decrease the need for frequent exchange of syringes (and the consequent potential to introduce air bubbles). The catheter should be preflushed with contrast prior to cannulation to avoid unnecessary injection of air from within the catheter lumen.

With each syringe exchange, one should aspirate back to remove any air bubbles from the Luer connector and flush to ensure that the contrast medium extends to the catheter tip. Contrast agent injection is performed with continuous fluoroscopic monitoring.

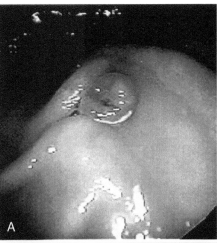
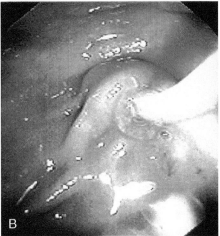
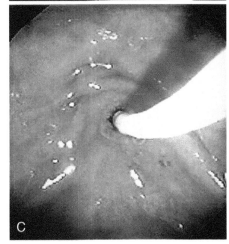

FIG 49.7 **A,** Endoscopic view of 5-Fr catheter oriented toward the 11 o'clock position of the major papilla. **B,** The bile duct is entered, and bile aspiration is confirmed by the yellow color in the catheter lumen. **C,** The catheter is oriented more toward the 3 o'clock position to enter the pancreas. *Continued*

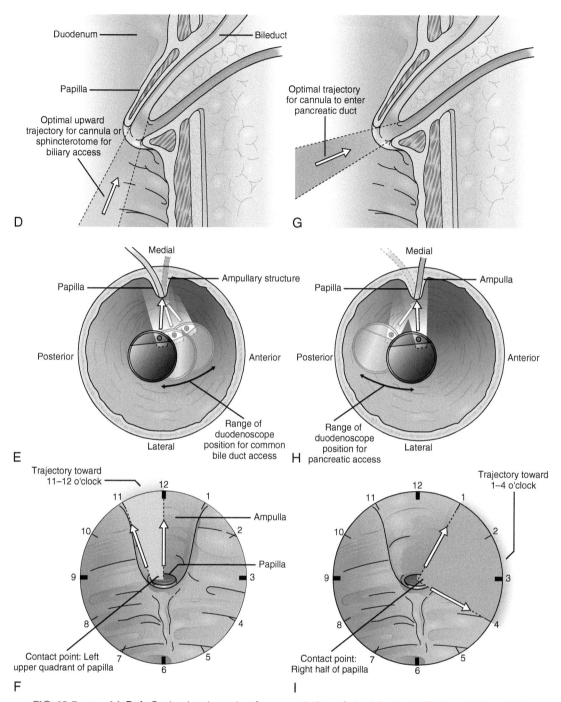

FIG 49.7, cont'd D–I, Optimal trajectories for cannulation of the bile duct (**D, E,** and **F**) and the pancreatic duct (**G, H,** and **I**), as projected in transverse (**E** and **H**), coronal (**D** and **G**), and sagittal (**F** and **I**) sections.

CHOLANGIOGRAM TECHNIQUE AND IMAGE INTERPRETATION

The density of contrast medium is greater than bile, and it flows along the most dependent route. The left lobe (lowest) fills quickest with the patient prone (Fig. 49.10A), the right lobe anterior segments fill next, and the right lobe posterior segments fill last (and may remain unfilled unless adequate volume and injection force are applied) (see Fig. 49.10B). However, injection

through a stone extraction balloon over a guidewire, inflated to prevent distal contrast flow targeting proximal portions of the biliary tree, allows for greater precision and control of contrast introduction.

The extent of ductal filling should be considered in advance of ERCP, and should be based on clinical history, preprocedure imaging, and intentions for therapy. In settings of tight biliary strictures, contrast medium filling upstream should be limited until catheter access above the stricture is achieved (Fig. 49.11).

In patients with diseases with a high potential for residual contrast in undrained segments following cholangiography, limited filling of the biliary tree is of greatest importance. Such clinical scenarios include diseases with complex biliary strictures involving multiple segments (e.g., perihilar cholangiocarcinoma and intrahepatic primary sclerosing cholangitis [PSC]). To facilitate this approach, a preprocedure reference MRCP or high-quality computed tomography (CT) scan provides a critical "road map" for planning biliary opacification and access during ERCP. High-resolution fluoroscopy is also ideal to delineate fine detail and small ductal structures. A technique utilizing air/CO_2 insufflation via an intraductal catheter, rather than contrast for cholangiography during stent exchanges and placement, may be suitable in patients with complex hilar strictures. Although there are reported cases of fatal air embolism with direct air insufflation of the biliary tree during cholangioscopy, case series suggest that this event is rare. The use of CO_2 may decrease this risk, and is weighed

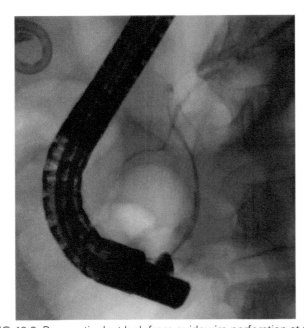

FIG 49.8 Pancreatic duct leak from guidewire perforation at the genu of the pancreas. This was successfully managed with a bridging pancreatic duct stent.

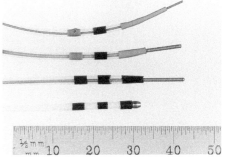

FIG 49.9 A well-equipped biliary diagnostic unit contains a wide variety of guidewires with varying characteristics, different sizes (0.018-inch, 0.025-inch, and 0.035-inch diameter), variable hydrophilic tips, and some groomable wires whose tip shape can be changed. Also shown are 5-Fr catheters with variable tip tapers or metal tips (bottom).

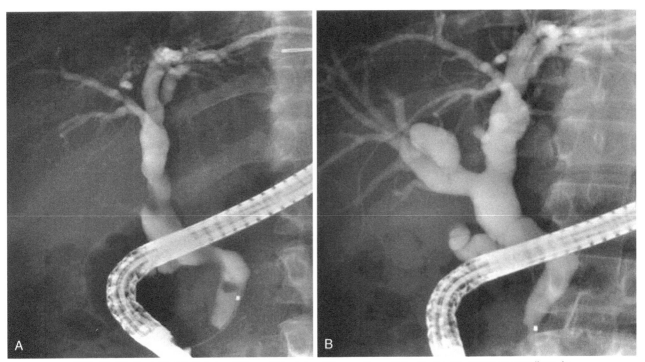

FIG 49.10 **A,** Initial left lobe filling. This lobe fills preferentially because contrast medium is heavier than bile and flows down into the dependent left lobe with the patient prone. This could be mistaken for complete biliary filling. **B,** When the patient is tilted head-down 20 degrees and more volume is added, the right lobe can be viewed. Wire access and balloon occlusion of the right hepatic duct may facilitate right system cholangiogram as well.

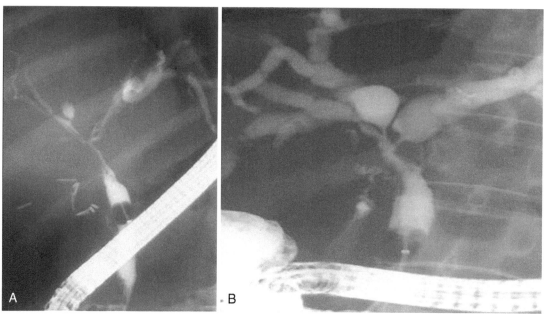

FIG 49.11 A, Cholangiocarcinoma involving the hepatic hilum. Only a limited amount of contrast medium is injected above the strictures to avoid contamination. More contrast medium should be injected only after the guidewire is advanced above the stricture. If additional upstream information is needed, magnetic resonance cholangiopancreatography (MRCP) or computed tomography (CT) scan is recommended. **B,** Excessive intrahepatic filling above hilar stricture. Unless subsequent bilateral drainage is achieved, the patient is at higher risk of postprocedure cholangitis.

against an advantageous decrease in the risk of cholangitis, which is a much more common sequela of ERCP when performed for complex hilar biliary strictures.[24–27] Finally, stent exchanges alongside or through (snare-over-the-wire technique) previously placed stents (before stent removal) ensure segmental wire access without the need for contrast injections (Video 49.1).

Multiple early views of the bile duct during filling are recommended to identify potential small filling defects (stones) that may be washed upstream (and then no longer be visible) or masked by dense contrast concentration in a dilated duct (Figs. 49.12 and 49.13). A "complete" cholangiogram requires filling of the peripheral intrahepatic radicles. The left lobe is more dependent in the prone position, and fills preferentially. Right lobe filling may require tilting the patient's head down 15 to 20 degrees on the fluoroscopy table, administering a more forceful injection using a balloon occlusion catheter, employing selective right lobe cannulation, or turning the patient to the supine position. Positioning the C-arm in the left posterior oblique position is ideal for collecting images at the bifurcation, as it diminishes two-dimensional overlap of primary and secondary segmental branches (Video 49.2). Placing the duodenoscope in a long position is effective for inspecting portions of the middle bile duct often obscured by the superimposed instrument shaft (Fig. 49.14; see also Video 49.2). Table 49.2 provides a list of common technical problems and clinical challenges encountered during cholangiopancreatography, with suggested steps for troubleshooting.

Features of a Normal Cholangiogram

A normal cholangiogram is shown in Fig. 49.15. Although controversial, there is evidence that indicates that the biliary tree does not dilate significantly after cholecystectomy in the absence of obstructing pathology.[28,29] The diameter of the common hepatic and common bile duct on ERCP is commonly 2 to 3 mm greater than is seen on CT or ultrasound. This difference is accounted for by filling (or overfilling) the ductal system with extra fluid (contrast medium) under greater pressure than physiologic secretory pressure.[30] Many centers accept 10 mm as the upper limit of the normal diameter of the common bile duct in adults. The cystic duct typically joins the common duct approximately halfway from the hilum to the papilla, but the location of this junction may vary. The intrahepatic radicles have a leafless tree-like branch pattern with marked variation in distribution. An aberrant, low-insertion, right hepatic duct, which connects to right posterior hepatic segments, is seen in 5% of patients (Figs. 49.16 and 49.17). These may be transected during laparoscopic cholecystectomy and give rise to problematic bile leaks from the disconnected segmental branch. Because the transected duct does not fill on ERCP, MRCP may be more diagnostic.[31] Numerous other nonpathologic anatomic variants have also been reported (at a frequency of 20%–30% in MRI series), and should therefore often be encountered by the discerning biliary endoscopist.[32,33] A detailed review of anatomic variants of biliary anatomy requires discussion well beyond the scope of this chapter (Fig. 49.18).

Biliary Stones and Acute Pancreatitis

Relative consensus now exists regarding the role of endoscopic cholangiography for suspected choledocholithiasis and acute pancreatitis. Gallstone pancreatitis is a common outcome of small stone (< 5 mm diameter) passage (see Fig. 49.13). In this latter setting, more than 80% of patients spontaneously pass the

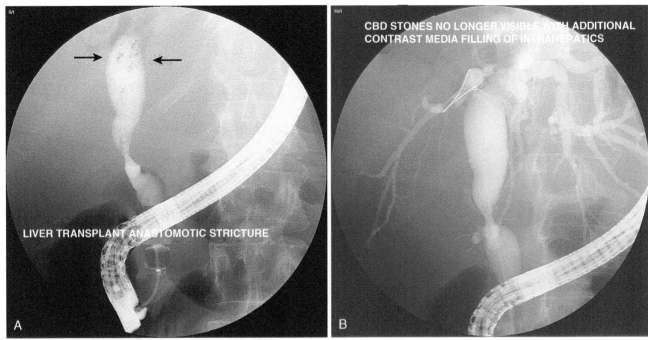

FIG 49.12 A, Patients with suspected common bile duct (CBD) stones (especially patients with dilated ducts) should have multiple early-filling biliary films taken to observe stones *(arrows)* **B,** before the stones are potentially washed upstream or masked by dense contrast material. The patient has had a liver transplant with duct-to-duct anastomosis. There is stricture at the anastomosis.

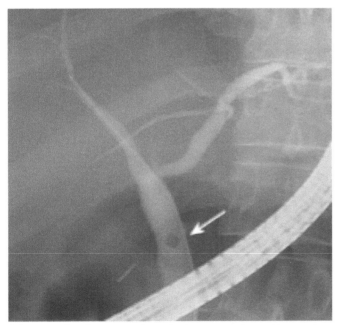

FIG 49.13 Small common hepatic duct stone *(arrow)* in a patient after cholecystectomy.

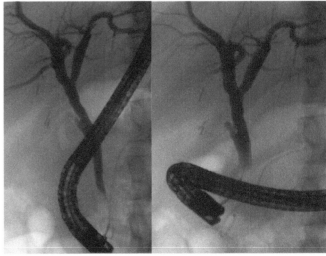

FIG 49.14 Transition of the duodenoscope from a short to a long position. This maneuver reveals the middle portion of the bile duct that was obscured by the overlying duodenoscope insertion tube.

stones from the bile duct into the duodenum. Consequently, selective use of ERC is recommended. Guidelines support an approach that targets patients who present with predictors for a retained common bile duct stone based on biochemical and radiographic testing. These indicators include: persistent or worsening cholestasis, dilated extrahepatic bile ducts, or clinical cholangitis.[34] Use of these predictors for decision making also applies in the setting of gallstone pancreatitis. This stems from meta-analysis–level data that confirm therapeutic ERCP to be beneficial in the setting of acute pancreatitis only in patients with high-level suspicion for choledocholithiasis (e.g. cholangitis or jaundice). Benefit does not correlate directly with the severity of pancreatitis.[35,36]

Whereas noninvasive imaging such as MRCP is helpful, it adds expense and should be reserved for patients who are at

TABLE 49.2   **Common General Problems and Challenges Encountered During Endoscopic Retrograde Cholangiography**

Cholangiographic Challenge or Clinical Suspicion	Potential Steps to Solve Problem
Obese patient	Increase kilo voltage Take extra exposures (a few are likely to be adequate) Review still images before deciding on therapy (i.e., do not rely only on fluoroscopy view)
Patient moves frequently	Take multiple exposures (one is likely to be clear) Increase kilo voltage to shorten exposure time
Terminal (preampullary) CBD not well seen	If patient has cholangitis with risk of sepsis if greater filling is performed, pass stone retrieval balloon to mid-CBD, inflate balloon, and inject contrast agent downstream of balloon (need appropriate "below the balloon" injection port). Tilt head up 5–20 degrees. If moderate amount of contrast agent already upstream in intrahepatic ducts, place catheter tip 1 cm above sphincter. Aspirate nonopacified bile until upstream contrast agent flows back into terminal CBD.
Patient has typical postcholecystectomy pain, but ERCP (or MRCP) is normal	Perform manometry Do not initiate ERCP if ducts are not dilated by noninvasive imaging and liver serum chemistries are normal
Cannot find papilla	Check fluoroscopy to ensure endoscope tip is in descending duodenum. Be sure of surgical anatomy (Roux-en-Y gastrojejunostomy?). Bile present—follow trail. Gently lift folds in candidate area. Find minor papilla, and search left and inferior. Give cholecystokinin or secretin to stimulate fluid flow.
Left and right hepatic ductal systems overlap at hilum, not well-defined	Fixed fluoroscopy table, roll patient to slight left posterior oblique position; use C-arm rotation to separate systems
Bile leak expected	Obtain multiple early images to locate leak site precisely before leak site contrast agent obscures view Limit injection to small amount of spilled contrast agent
Air bubbles introduced	Observe where bubbles went and where collected; if distal CBD, tilt head down and aspirate bubbles, bile, and contrast agent from terminal duct Consider tilting head up and observing bubble passage into intrahepatic ducts
Contrast agent or air in duodenum or stomach detracts from image quality	Aspirate all contrast agent and air from duodenum before imaging; do this routinely when injecting contrast agent
Endoscope repeatedly covers area of interest	Use C-arm (or patient positioning) to change angle Move the endoscope from short (lesser curve) to long (greater curve) position Place catheter upstream to hilum, slowly back endoscope into the stomach, aspirating air and spilled contrast agent as if a nasobiliary tube had been placed
Pyloric or duodenal narrowing precludes duodenoscope passage	Pass a stiff guidewire (Amplatz Super Stiff, Boston Scientific or SavaryWire) and catheter in to the transverse duodenum. Pass duodenoscope over the wire, paying attention to fluoroscopic alignment more than endocscopic view. Advance large (15–18 mm) balloon catheter over guidewire into transverse duodenum. Inflate extraction balloon and, with traction on the balloon catheter and duodenoscope reduction, advance duodenoscope beyond the stricture.

CBD, common bile duct; *ERCP,* endoscopic retrograde cholangiopancreatography; *MRCP,* magnetic resonance cholangiopancreatography.

high risk for adverse events linked to anesthesia, patients with altered foregut anatomy (post–bariatric surgery), and patients with moderate to low probability of ductal stones.[34] Patients with a very high or high probability for a retained bile duct stone should proceed directly to ERC. Patients with an intermediate probability for a retained bile duct stone should have a preceding MRCP or EUS, or should be considered for cholecystectomy with intraoperative cholangiogram if the gallbladder is in situ. A larger ductal stone in a patient following cholecystectomy is shown in Fig. 49.19A. Intrahepatic stones (with or without extrahepatic stones) are common in Asian populations, and may be associated with recurrent pyogenic cholangitis.[37] Fig. 49.19B shows right segmental branches with large fusiform stones. A stone impacted in the cystic duct may compress the common hepatic or common bile duct and cause obstructive jaundice (Mirizzi's syndrome). Cholangiogram may demonstrate only a common bile duct stricture in this scenario. Cross-sectional

imaging or cholangioscopy may be necessary to confirm the diagnosis. Table 49.3 reviews problems encountered in biliary stone cases and ways to troubleshoot them.

Biliary Strictures

Biliary strictures are abnormal narrowings of the ductal system resulting from compression (e.g., chronic pancreatitis), scar formation (e.g., postoperative), autoimmune disease (autoimmune cholangiopathy, PSC), or neoplasm (e.g., cholangiocarcinoma, pancreatic duct adenocarcinoma, metastases).[38,39] These typically manifest clinically with cholestasis, obstructive jaundice, or cholangitis. The etiology of the stricture is usually evident from the history (e.g., recent biliary surgery, risk factors for chronic pancreatitis, or elderly patients with weight loss) and preprocedure cross-sectional imaging (e.g., pancreatic or perihilar mass). Table 49.4 reviews problems encountered during cholangiography for bile duct strictures. Fig. 49.20 shows a smooth, tapered, long

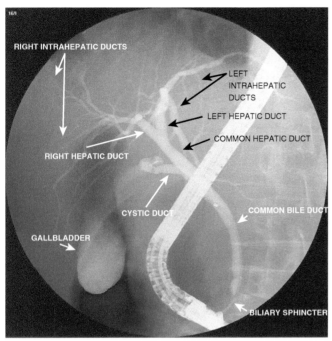

FIG 49.15 Normal cholangiogram with ductal segments labeled. Colon gas overlaps the gallbladder, making viewing suboptimal.

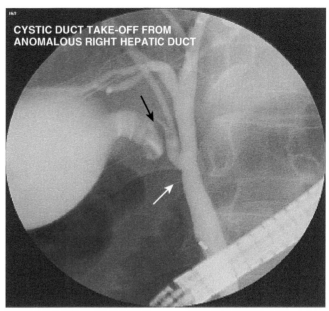

FIG 49.17 Aberrant posterior segmental hepatic branch arising from mid-extrahepatic duct *(white arrow)*. The cystic duct take-off *(black arrow)* is from the aberrant right hepatic duct.

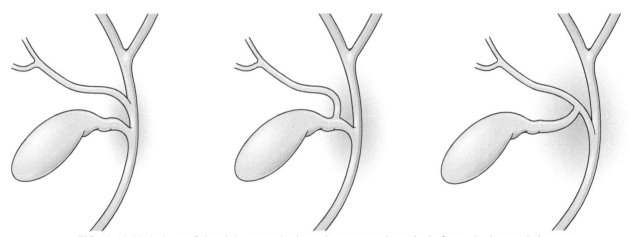

FIG 49.16 Variations of the right posterior hepatic segment branch. *Left,* cystic duct and aberrant right hepatic duct are adjacent to each other, but both are attached to the main extrahepatic duct. *Center,* aberrant right branch arises from cystic duct. *Right,* cystic duct arises from aberrant right branch.

TABLE 49.3 Challenges for Optimal Viewing of Stones

Cholangiographic Challenge or Clinical Suspicion	Potential Steps to Solve Problem
Probable bile duct stones (most are in terminal CBD at beginning of examination)	Inject contrast agent with catheter tip in sphincter segment (not deeply cannulated) Inject contrast agent slowly Take film exposures early after only 1–2 cm of duct filled and again at each 1–2 cm further filling With patient prone, tilt table head up 5–20 degrees to keep contrast agent near papilla
Gallbladder stones	Take multiple early-filling gallbladder films If overfilled, advance guidewire and catheter into gallbladder and aspirate excess contrast agent Take delayed films supine in 4–24 hr
Probable sludge seen in terminal CBD on early films	Stop contrast agent injection; aspirate bile through a "see-through" (non-opaque) catheter and confirm granular material
Cholangitis manifesting with purulent bile (with or without sepsis)	Aspirate bile from CBD (send for culture) and replace aspirated bile (e.g., 30 mL with less than 1/3 volume [10 mL] of contrast media); limit intrahepatic filling; do definitive intrahepatic duct and stone evaluation later when cholangitis is resolved

CBD, common bile duct.

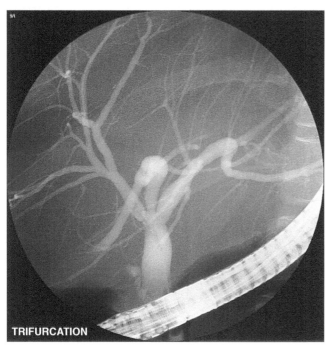

FIG 49.18 Trifurcation of intrahepatic ducts at the hilum.

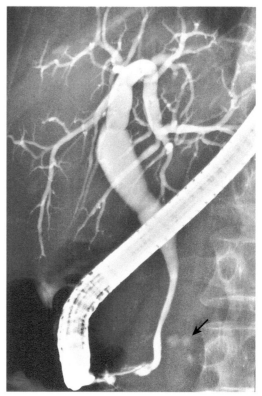

FIG 49. 20 Endoscopic retrograde cholangiography (ERC) showing long, smooth, tapered stricture within the pancreas with mild upstream dilation (the right lobe has not yet filled). Calcified stones *(arrow)* are seen in the head of the pancreas.

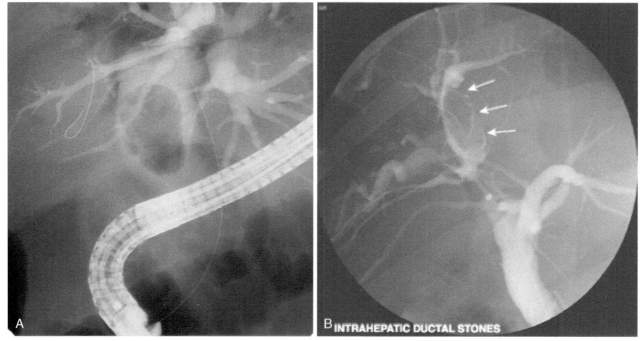

FIG 49.19 **A,** Large common bile duct stone. **B,** Large intrahepatic stones *(arrows).* Small common bile duct stones were also present. The gallbladder had been removed 5 years previously. These stones are much more common in Asian populations.

TABLE 49.4   Challenges in Detection and Optimal Viewing of Strictures

Cholangiographic Challenge or Clinical Suspicion	Potential Steps to Solve Problem
Hilar stricture	Take multiple early-filling views with varying degrees of angulation; especially obtain Y confluence view with left and right main hepatic ducts separated Fill only a tiny amount of duct upstream initially, and pass guidewire upstream before filling more; avoid thorough upstream filling (rely on MRCP or CT if that information is clinically needed) unless a guidewire and catheter have already been passed upstream and full stent drainage is certain
Common bile or common hepatic duct stricture with obviously dilated upstream ducts (per CT or MRI); need definition of upper rim of stricture	Inject more contrast agent with greater force (unless purulent bile) Advance catheter into right duct Consider aspirating bile from near hilum to "empty" right lobe to make space for contrast agent If prior sphincterotomy, use balloon occlusion Tilt head down 5–20 degrees
Probable sclerosing cholangitis setting or other intrahepatic stricturing; contrast agent preferentially enters gallbladder	Limit gallbladder filling in primary sclerosing cholangitis, because post-ERCP cholecystitis may occur; inflate balloon catheter above cystic duct take-off and inject upstream; after more aggressive intrahepatic filling, patient should remain on broad-spectrum antibiotics for 5–7 days
Sphincter segment appears narrow	This is usually a normal finding; dilated duct upstream or abnormal liver serum chemistries present suggests pathology Measure length of segment: > 12 mm suggests scar or tumor narrowing; correlate with normal or abnormal appearance of papilla; brush cytology, manometry, sphincterotomy with viewing inside ampulla, or endoscopic ultrasound may be needed to clarify
Is postsphincterotomy biliary orifice adequate?	Do manometry, pull-through stone retrieval balloon; size with hydrostatic balloon

CT, computed tomography; *ERCP,* endoscopic retrograde cholangiopancreatography; *MRCP,* magnetic resonance cholangiopancreatography; *MRI,* magnetic resonance imaging.

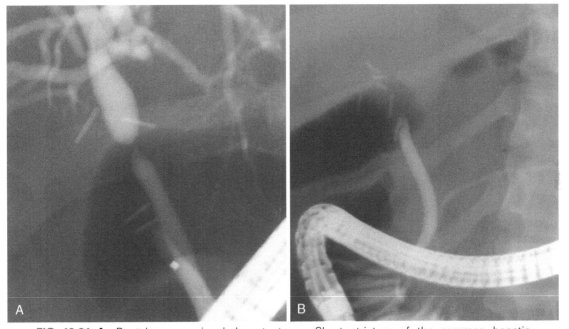

FIG 49.21 A, Post–laparoscopic cholecystectomy. Short stricture of the common hepatic duct is seen, with upstream dilation. The stricture occurred near clips, and is probably due to a thermal injury. **B,** Unintentional clip transection of the common bile duct at the cystic duct junction, which occurred at open cholecystectomy in a patient with prior upper abdominal radiation for lymphoma.

narrowing of the bile duct within the head of the pancreas in a patient with calcific chronic pancreatitis. Laparoscopic cholecystectomy is associated with thermal or mechanical injury, which results in stricture formation in 0.25% to 0.5% of patients.[40,41] Fig. 49.21A shows a typical postlaparoscopy stricture. Injuries during open cholecystectomy occur less frequently. Duct transections (see Fig. 49.21B) and duct resections are the most serious injuries.

Orthotopic liver transplant with duct-to-duct anastomosis results in pathologic narrowing at the anastomosis in 15% of patients (Fig. 49.22).[42] PSC is characterized by multifocal extrahepatic and/or intrahepatic strictures (Fig. 49.23).[39] The gallbladder and cystic duct are spared in this disease.

The goals of ERC in suspected PSC are to (1) treat dominant strictures, (2) guide sampling for diagnosis of cholangiocarcinoma,

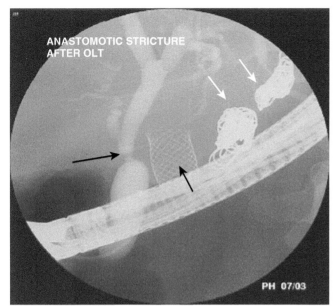

FIG 49.22 Orthotopic liver transplant (OLT) with duct-to-duct anastomosis. Narrowing of the anastomosis is seen just 10 days postoperatively *(long black arrow)*. Note endovascular metal stent (transjugular intrahepatic portosystemic shunt) used to treat prior variceal bleeding *(short black arrow)* and endovascular coils in the duodenal arcade from bleeding duodenal ulcers *(white arrows)*.

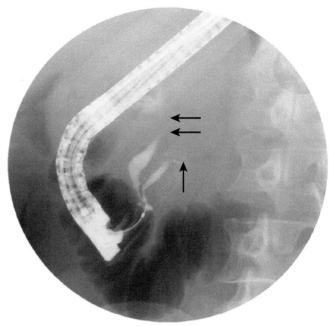

FIG 49.24 Typical double-duct sign of pancreatic cancer. *Double arrows* indicate common bile duct narrowing. *Single arrow* indicates pancreatic duct obstruction. This sign may also be seen in chronic pancreatitis.

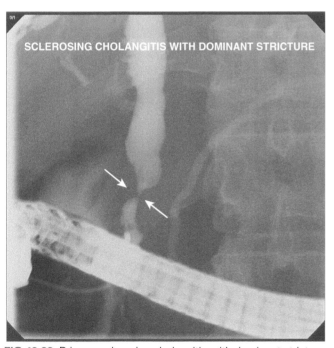

FIG 49.23 Primary sclerosing cholangitis with dominant stricture. All diagnostic studies were benign.

and (3) establish the diagnosis. However, with high-quality MRI/MRCP, performance of a "diagnostic" ERC for the sole purpose of establishing a diagnosis of PSC is no longer considered the standard of care.[43] The focus of ERCP in patients with PSC is endoscopic therapy and tissue sampling, given that the risk for bacterial cholangitis can range from 2% to 8%, despite antibiotic prophylaxis.[44,45] Cholangiocarcinoma is of particular concern in this population, as the lifetime risk is 20% and approaches 40% in patients with advanced cases who go on to transplantation. Overall, the role ERC plays in routine screening and surveillance is an area of controversy.[39,46] Pancreatic ductal adenocarcinoma is the most common stricture of malignant origin encountered on ERC. Cancer of the pancreatic head often presents with the classic double-duct sign (Fig. 49.24). Although this sign is present in patients with chronic pancreatitis, the presence of jaundice creates a clinical scenario with a high pretest suspicion for ampullary and/or peri-ampullary malignancy.[47]

Tissue sampling should be done on strictures that have any clinical suspicion for neoplasia. Brush cytology is the easiest to obtain, but detects cancer when present in only 30% to 50% of cases. Additional sampling with a second brush, forceps, endoluminal needles, and/or fluorescence in situ hybridization increases the diagnostic sensitivity by approximately 10%.[48,49] Single operatory digital cholangioscopy site-directed biopsies and EUS fine-needle aspiration (FNA) (for distal bile duct strictures) have incremental value, in that they increase sensitivity for neoplasia to 85% and 81%, respectively.[50,51]

Beyond radiographic findings of upstream bile duct dilation, elevated basal sphincter pressure (> 40 mm Hg, as evaluated by manometry), and biochemical liver function test abnormalities, stenosis at the major papilla can also be assessed via dedicated cholangiography of the distal bile duct. Sphincter stenosis can occur de novo or as a late complication of prior biliary sphincterotomy. Discrete, abrupt, short segment narrowing of the intraduodenal bile duct segment is often observed. Following sphincterotomy, the true diameter of the biliary sphincter may be difficult to judge, and may best be assessed with the assistance of a hydrostatic balloon inflated with contrast across the sphincter segment, sized to the upstream bile duct (Fig. 49.25).

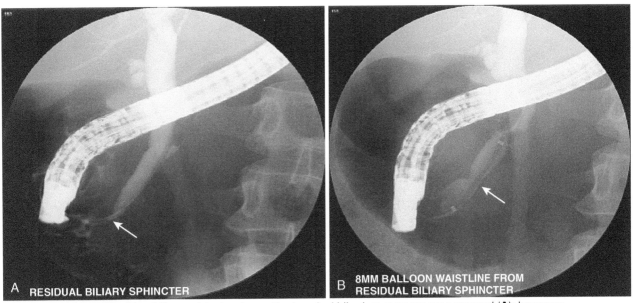

FIG 49.25 After biliary sphincterotomy, the terminal bile duct may appear narrowed (**A**); however, true sphincter size is probably best determined by inflation of a hydrostatic balloon within the sphincter segment, observing the residual waistline (**B**).

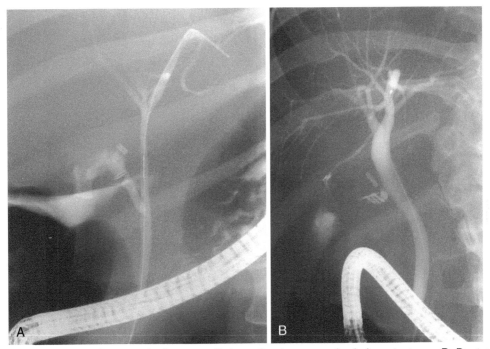

FIG 49.26 A, Leak from cystic duct seen 2 days after laparoscopic cholecystectomy. **B,** Duct of Luschka leak seen 7 days after laparoscopic cholecystectomy. These ducts are in close proximity to the gallbladder bed, and are exposed with free dissection of the gallbladder.

Biliary Leaks

Biliary leaks result from surgery complications or trauma (penetrating or nonpenetrating), or can be induced at the time of ERCP.[38] Laparoscopic cholecystectomy is most often associated with leaks from the cystic duct or the duct of Luschka (Fig. 49.26). Bile leaks typically cause right upper quadrant pain, fever, mildly abnormal serum liver chemistries, and leukocytosis. A typical duct of Luschka leak is seen in Fig. 49.26B, with the leak occurring from a small intrahepatic duct. A subhepatic contrast collection from

a cystic duct leak occurring after laparoscopic cholecystectomy is seen in Fig. 49.26A. A retrograde cholangiography–based grading system for the severity of biliary leaks after surgery has been reported. Based on the radiographic identification of a leak either before (high-grade) or after (low-grade) opacification of intrahepatic biliary radicals, this system may have practical applications for therapeutic decision making. A cohort study at a single center reported that more than 90% of patients with low-grade leaks and without additional, significant biliary pathology (e.g., bile duct stricture) were successfully managed

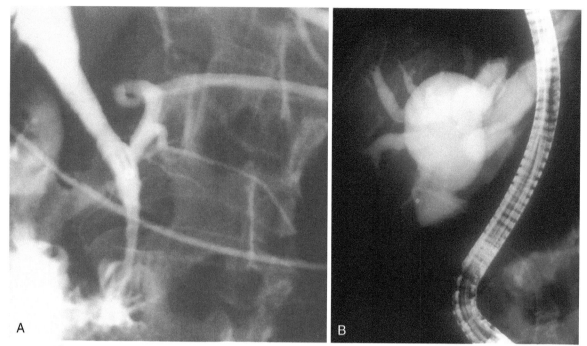

FIG 49.27 A, Anomalous pancreaticobiliary ductal junction with pancreatic duct joining the bile duct well outside the duodenal wall. Note the long common channel of at least 15 mm in length. **B,** Type I choledochal cyst.

with biliary sphincterotomy alone.[52] In a separate retrospective study evaluating clinical factors associated with failure of the first endoscopic intervention for management of bile leaks after cholecystectomy, high-grade leak was found to be a statistically significant predictor on multivariate analysis (odds ratio [OR] 26.8, $p < 0.001$).[53]

Anomalous Pancreaticobiliary Ductal Union

Anomalous pancreaticobiliary ductal union occurs in approximately 2% of people of Asian descent, but only 0.2% of Caucasian populations.[54,55] In this condition, the pancreaticobiliary junction occurs outside the duodenal wall, and simultaneous biductal filling occurs from major papilla injection through a common channel greater than 15 mm in length (Fig. 49.27A). Approximately one-third of these patients have an associated choledochal cyst (see Fig. 49.27B). Patients with an anomalous pancreaticobiliary junction are considered to be at high risk for gallbladder and bile duct cancer.[56]

PANCREATOGRAM TECHNIQUE AND IMAGE INTERPRETATION

Adjusting the C-arm for an anteroposterior (rather than a left posterior oblique) view to obtain images of the midline (head/genu of the pancreas) and left abdomen (body and tail) is optimal for acquisition of fluoroscopic and radiographic images of the pancreatic duct.

Safe imaging of the pancreatic ductal system necessitates the careful use of smaller volumes of contrast than are used to image the biliary system. This difference is crucial, as overfilling can occur with small volumes of contrast agent, and is an established risk factor for post-ERCP pancreatitis.[5] An approach of "feathering" contrast injections through gentle taps of pressure on the syringe is part of this subtle contrast injection technique. Overfilling is

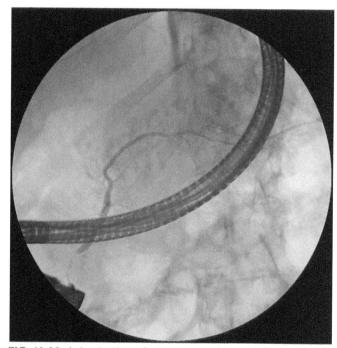

FIG 49.28 Acinarization of the pancreatic body from vigorous injection of contrast material.

best recognized as *acinarization*, which is the consequence of pressurized, densely opacified tertiary/quaternary and smaller pancreatic ductal structures. This appears as halos of fluffy radiographic structures along the pancreatic duct and its side branches (Fig. 49.28). Impaction of the catheter into a side branch, variant ductal anatomy, or injection downstream or upstream from a stricture/stone can cause segmental acinarization.

Caution is also advised in the setting of pancreatic fluid collections if formal drainage or surgery is not planned. Aggressive filling and consequent contamination of undrained cysts that follow pancreatitis (e.g., pseudocysts and walled-off necrosis) create a risk of infection. Antibiotic prophylaxis should be administered if this occurs.

FEATURES OF A NORMAL PANCREATOGRAM

The goal of endoscopic retrograde pancreatography (ERP) is to collect contrast-enhanced radiographic images of the shape, caliber, course, and pattern of distribution of the main pancreatic duct (and in some cases its side branches) to guide therapy. Some diagnostic limitations of ERP are that it offers little information regarding the parenchyma, rarely provides dimensions for communicating cystic structures (in the setting of careful injection technique), and provides very limited information regarding the overall dimensions of the gland itself. The structures that comprise the first-order pancreatic ductal system include: the main (ventral) pancreatic duct of Wirsung extending through the head and genu, the (dorsal) accessory duct of Santorini in the head of the pancreas, and the dorsal pancreatic duct in the body and tail of the pancreas.

The main pancreatic duct is smooth and tapers in diameter from the head to the tail (Fig. 49.29). Its course of filling on anteroposterior images begins by ascending on the left of the spine (head, genu) and progresses in a horizontal-oblique fashion over (body) and to the right (body, tail) of the lower thoracic or upper lumbar spine.[57] Focal nonpathologic indentations are sometimes noted at the genu near the approximate junction

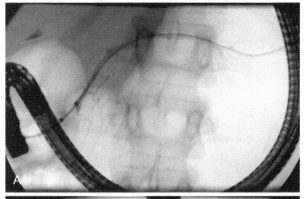

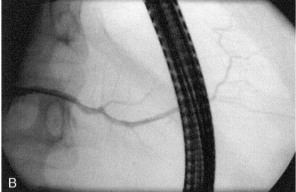

FIG 49.29 A and **B,** Normal dorsal duct pancreatogram of head (**A**) and body and tail (**B**) regions.

with the accessory duct, and in the body near the superior mesenteric vasculature.[58] Numerous postmortem and endoscopic studies have reported the length and diameter of the pancreatic duct. Postmortem values tend to be slightly higher than endoscopic values.[57] This may be due to the fact that, with age, the adult duct caliber appears to increase slightly, whereas the length is stable. The average length of a normal gland is approximately 17 cm, ranging from 9 to 24 cm. When the main duct is less than 9 cm in length, obstruction or atrophy should be suspected. The caliber of the pancreatic duct is most variable within the head of the gland. The normal diameter in the head is 3 to 4 mm (may range up to 6 mm), in the body 2 to 3 mm (up to 5 mm), and in the tail 1 to 2 mm (up to 3 mm).[57]

Visualization of side branches during pancreatography depends largely on technique and the force of contrast agent injection. Adequate visualization of side branches is by no means a routine maneuver in ERP, and it is often risky and irrelevant, as endoscopic therapeutic maneuvers are limited to the main pancreatic duct. Side branches are highly variable and asymmetric in the pancreatic head. However, they are regular and symmetric throughout the body and tail. A postmortem study reported a mean of 56 first-order branch ducts (range: 52–66).[59] Far fewer branches tend to be seen even with the most forceful pancreatogram.

Normal ductal anatomy can vary greatly between individuals. A single large, inferiorly directed "uncinate" branch is seen in 55% to 62% of pancreatograms.[58,60] The accessory pancreatic duct (duct of Santorini) is also reported to have significant variability. This duct fills in only 43% of ventral endoscopic pancreatogram series, yet it communicates with the main pancreatic duct in approximately 90% of postmortem specimens.[61] The diameter, course, and patency for drainage through the minor papilla also varies greatly. Comparative pancreatogram series describe its patency to be 40% to 70% in general ERCP studies (without necessarily involving a targeted cannulation through the minor papilla). However, its patency is 17% to 21% in patients either being evaluated for biliary pancreatitis and/or ultimately presenting with post-ERCP pancreatitis, implying that when patent, the accessory duct may augment decompression of the main pancreatic duct and prevent pancreatitis.[62,63]

ANATOMIC VARIANTS OF THE PANCREATIC DUCT

The pancreatic ductal system is subject to abnormal formation during embryogenesis (Fig. 49.30). The most important clinical variants develop between the sixth and eighth week of embryogenesis. The mechanism of their formation relates to either malrotation or malfusion of the ventral and dorsal embryonic pancreatic anlage and/or their respective ductal structures.

Failure of normal rotation and migration yields an annular pancreas, in which a portion of the ventral pancreatic anlage remains behind along the path of migration during organogenesis (Figs. 49.30 and 49.31). This band of incompletely migrated duct and parenchyma forms a partial or complete ring around the second portion of the duodenum, just proximal to the major papilla. Symptomatic variants can cause partial duodenal obstruction at any point during the lifetime of the patient. Annular pancreas may also cause episodic pancreatitis, but its association with other abnormalities makes interpretation of the exact etiology uncertain. For instance, approximately one-third of cases are associated with pancreas divisum.[64]

Pancreas divisum is the most common congenital variant (Fig. 49.32; see also Fig. 49.30). It occurs as a result of incomplete

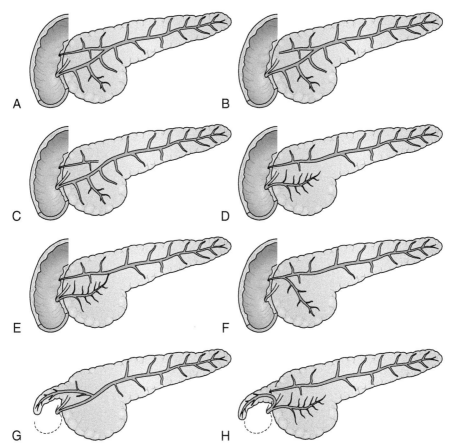

FIG 49.30 Variations in dorsal and ventral duct migration and fusion. **A,** Normal. **B,** Normal with imperforate minor papilla. **C,** Normal with disjunction of the accessory duct. **D,** Pancreas divisum. **E,** Incomplete pancreas divisum. **F,** Pancreas divisum with no ventral duct. **G,** Annular pancreas with normal fusion of ventral and dorsal ducts. **H,** Annular pancreas with associated pancreas divisum.

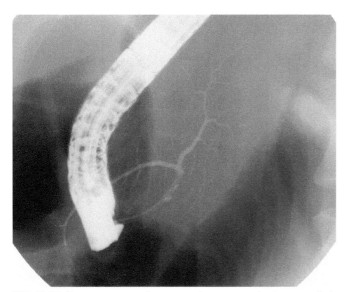

FIG 49.31 Pancreatogram demonstrating pancreatic duct morphology consistent with annular pancreas.

fusion of the ventral and dorsal ducts after migration of the ventral anlage. Pancreas divisum is found in 7% of people in autopsy series. Approximately 15% to 20% of cases are "incompletely" divided, which is characterized by a persistent, tiny communication through side branches of the dorsal and ventral systems.[65]

Ductography via the major papilla in patients with pancreas divisum can reveal a normal, small diameter or a nonexistent (30%) ventral pancreatic duct. A "Christmas tree" pattern along the ventral duct of Wirsung with side branches that progressively diminish in size is often identified with ventral ductography. Dorsal ductography is also necessary to differentiate pancreas divisum from "pseudodivisum," as either may appear as an abrupt termination of the ventral pancreatic duct. Pseudodivisum is concerning, as the etiology may be a focal pancreatic lesion (e.g., pancreatic adenocarcinoma), yet it can be mistaken for pancreas divisum.[65]

Pancreas divisum is detected at a greater frequency in patients with recurrent acute and chronic pancreatitis (25%–30%) than in healthy individuals.[66,67] However, in symptomatic patients, pancreas divisum is often coincident with genetic mutations (*CFTR*, *SPINK*) that also predispose to pancreatic disease. Studies and growing expert opinion now suggest that pancreas divisum is a complex condition that typically occurs in combination with

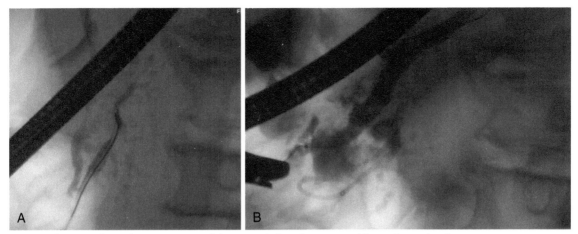

FIG 49.32 Complete pancreas divisum and chronic pancreatitis: radiograph of a pancreatogram showing pancreas divisum. **A,** Ventral duct fills via injection into the duct of Wirsung at the major papilla. **B,** Dorsal duct fills via injection into the duct of Santorini at the minor papilla. Pathologic findings include parenchymal calcifications, dilated side branches, dilated dorsal and ventral pancreatic duct, and dorsal duct leak with filling of pseudocyst(s) in the pancreatic head.

other etiologies and/or exposures (e.g., tobacco and alcohol abuse), rather than a stand-alone etiology for recurrent acute and chronic pancreatic disease.[68,69] For this reason, the precise role of endoscopic therapy for symptomatic patients with pancreas divisum remains an area of controversy.

OVERVIEW OF RADIOGRAPHIC PATTERNS OF PATHOLOGY SEEN DURING PANCREATOGRAPHY

During pancreatography, recognition of pathology requires differentiation between normal anatomy and patterns of abnormalities that suggest pathology. Categories of pathologic findings include (1) filling defects; (2) abnormalities in the main pancreatic duct or side branches (diameter and/or contour); (3) duct leaks, disruptions, or "disconnection"; and (4) filling of cystic spaces. Each abnormality has an associated differential diagnosis which should be considered carefully. Importantly, patients usually display multiple abnormalities that, in aggregate, offer a pattern that yields a diagnosis (e.g., chronic pancreatitis). Filling defects are often stones or mucus secreted by intraductal papillary mucinous neoplasm (IPMN). Ductal abnormalities include obstruction (partial or complete), duct dilation, and focal or diffuse contour irregularities, all of which may be secondary to benign inflammatory processes or malignancy. Leaks can be free, contained, or communicating with other organs as fistulas. They occur as a result of trauma, are iatrogenic (e.g., surgery, endoscopy), and/or occur as a local complication of acute or chronic pancreatitis (with or without necrosis). Filling of cystic spaces can be within or extrinsic to the pancreas, and may be associated with pseudocysts, pancreatic necrosis, or cystic neoplasms.

Features of Pancreatic Neoplasia

ERP can identify neoplastic lesions of the pancreas. However, diagnostic ERP has been supplanted by cross-sectional imaging, magnetic resonance (MR) ductography, and endosonography to detect, diagnose, and (with EUS) sample malignancy of the pancreas. Pancreatic carcinoma does have characteristic ductal abnormalities. Individually, these characteristics are nonspecific,

TABLE 49.5 Radiographic Features of Pancreatic Duct Strictures		
Attribute	Malignant	Benign (Chronic Pancreatitis, Autoimmune Pancreatitis)
Stricture length	Long (> 1–2 cm)	Long or short (focal)
Stricture contour	Blunt, abruptly pointed, or serrated	Smooth taper, concave (long), or web-like (focal)
Stricture severity	Usually complete with mass	Complete or partial
Side branches	Regionally absent	Present: dilated or ectatic
Upstream duct dilation	Always present	Present or absent
Multifocal strictures	Generally absent	Present

and overlap with ductal abnormalities caused by chronic and autoimmune pancreatitis. However, in aggregate, when taken as a pattern and interpreted in the proper clinical context, ERP ductal findings can elevate the suspicion for malignancy substantially and guide medical decision making (Table 49.5).

Again, the presence of concomitant neighboring strictures in both the pancreatic duct and the distal bile duct is highly suggestive of malignancy ("double duct" sign, see Fig. 49.24). The mechanisms for stricture of the neighboring, distal bile duct include: tethering by fibrosis, compression (mass or edema), and/or malignant effacement by a tumor, generally in the head, uncinate, or genu of the pancreas. Most often identified on preprocedure cross-section imaging, the presence of a double duct sign should substantially elevate suspicion for neoplasia.[70,71]

Of all the pancreatic neoplasms, ERP findings associated with main duct IPMN can be the most specific, but can also be difficult to identify.[72] The production of mucus by neoplastic epithelium lining the main pancreatic duct or side branches can be identified in the form of dilated ductal segments on cross-sectional imaging or through symptoms caused by intermittent obstruction (pancreaticobiliary pain or pancreatitis).[73] When IPMN involves the main pancreatic duct, pancreatography typically shows main duct dilation. Soft, bulky, or linear filling defects that can be stripped from the lumen with an occlusion balloon are considered specific, and are caused by layering mucin. Gross papillary changes of the duct lining mucosa are infrequently evident on pancreatography, but, when present, can be sampled with a transpapillary approach using biopsy forceps and brushings to diagnose IPMN. Fluid can also be aspirated from the main pancreatic duct during ERP for carcinoembryonic antigen (CEA) biomarker testing and to assess for cytologic atypia. However, pancreatic duct fluid analysis for the diagnosis of neoplasia, although specific (97%), has limited sensitivity (35%).[74]

To opacify branched duct IPMN lesions, a forceful injection of contrast agent may be required to displace mucus. Consequently, this maneuver is rarely justified, given the increased risk for pancreatitis. Moreover, for branched duct lesions, a work-up comprised of high-quality cross-sectional imaging (MRI/MRCP, contrast enhanced CT) and/or EUS-FNA with collection of fluid for biomarkers (e.g., CEA) and/or integrated molecular analysis is now the recommended diagnostic approach, given the superior accuracy and lower risk profile compared to ERCP.[75,76]

Transpapillary pancreatoscopy and intraductal ultrasound have been described as useful in preoperative staging of the longitudinal spread of main duct IPMN.[77,78] Endoscopic visualization of thick mucus plugs extruding from a dilated papillary duct is pathognomonic, and is considered highly specific (Fig. 49.33) for main duct IPMN of either the bile duct or the pancreatic duct.[32] The latter (pancreatic) disease is far more common. During pancreatoscopy, mucus markedly distorts endoscopic views; however, intraductal abnormalities such as papillary "fish-eggs" or villous, mass-like projections of epithelium along the wall of

the main pancreatic duct are considered diagnostic and afford targets for intraductal sampling. Wire-guided intraductal ultrasound identifies both the mucus and papillary changes. However, none of these endoscopic tools are highly sensitive for confirming invasive malignancy.[79]

Acute Pancreatitis, Recurrent Acute Pancreatitis, and Pancreatic Duct Disruption

Pancreatography during an episode of acute pancreatitis is generally not indicated. Pancreatogram findings in the setting of acute pancreatitis tend to be nonspecific, and endoscopic interventions during the acute phase of pancreatitis are generally not recommended. Nonspecific ductal findings include irregularity in the contours of the main duct and side branches, delayed filling of side branches, and unorganized parenchymal staining before side branch filling; this last finding is likely to be associated with early pancreatic necrosis.

Additional ERP findings during acute pancreatitis include strictures, duct leaks, and/or disruptions. These findings, when identified close to the onset of acute pancreatitis, are associated with pancreatic necrosis.[80,81] Leaks can also indicate complications from pancreatitis caused by an "internal" fistula (e.g., pancreatic ascites, pancreaticopleural fistula) or an external (e.g., cutaneous) fistula. In the absence of clinical findings that suggest the presence of a fistula, leaks during acute pancreatitis correlate poorly with late pathology and/or a disease state that requires an endoscopic intervention.[81] Overall, there are no data to support either early diagnostic or therapeutic pancreatography in "all comers" with acute pancreatitis with or without necrosis. The risk for introducing a secondary infection of unorganized necrotic tissue and/or fluid collections through the use of contaminating contrast injections further diminishes the utility of ERP during the acute phase of pancreatitis in the absence of symptomatic pancreatic duct disruption with fistula.[82]

However, if acute pancreatitis is associated with clinical evidence of internal/external fistula (e.g., pancreatic ascites, pancreaticopleural fistula, cutaneous fistula), a combination of medical intervention (pancreatic rest with enteral or parental nutrition, somatostatin, and/or large-volume paracentesis) and pancreatography with associated therapies may be beneficial.

The timing of onset for duct leaks from "disruption" of the pancreatic duct remains incompletely defined. Following acute pancreatitis, leaks occur frequently near the genu, a region of pancreatic anatomy that is particularly vulnerable to necrosis due to watershed blood supply. Leaks from disruptions of the pancreatic duct that are identified within the first few weeks tend to lead to unorganized collections in the retroperitoneum. Leaks identified after longer intervals enter more circumscribed spaces of maturing fluid collections. They are diagnosed as extravasation (or leak) of contrast from the main pancreatic duct on ERP (Fig. 49.34). ERCP is considered to be the most accurate method of identifying leaks and ductal disruption.[82–84] A main pancreatic duct disruption can be categorized as incomplete (visualization of the upstream pancreatic duct) or complete (nonvisualization of the upstream pancreatic duct or "disconnected" pancreatic duct).

Literature related to the effectiveness of endotherapy is limited to case series, and is reported in combination with drainage procedures, nutrition support, and medical interventions for associated pseudocysts and free intrabdominal/pleural fluid collections. Rates of therapeutic success for disruption and associated fistula approach 75%.[82,83]

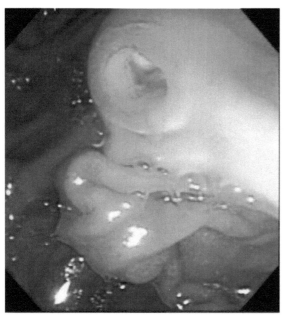

FIG 49.33 Endoscopic image of mucus extruding from the minor papilla in a patient with intraductal papillary mucin-producing neoplasm (IPMN) of the pancreas.

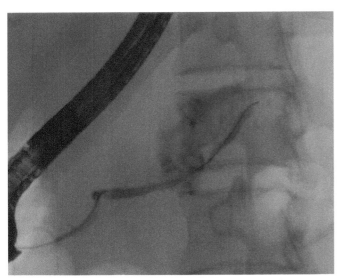

FIG 49.34 Pancreatogram showing a large pancreatic duct disruption with leak from the pancreatic duct in the region of the pancreas body. The pancreatic duct is in continuity, and the disruption is bridged with a guidewire. The patient presented with pancreatic ascites.

Smoldering pancreatitis is a disease state characterized by unrelenting pancreatic symptoms (> 7–10 days) in the setting of persistent pancreatic enzyme elevation and/or radiographic evidence of pancreatic/peripancreatic inflammation in the absence of pancreatic necrosis, pancreatic fluid collections, or organ failure. A single case series reported the use of therapeutic ERP in eleven patients. Eight of these patients demonstrated either duct irregularities or duct dilation on ERP. Pancreatic stent placement alleviated symptoms, resulting in discontinuation of parenteral nutrition and or narcotics, in 10/11 patients.[85] A review article by Das et al (2015) reported outcomes for ERP in patients with smoldering pancreatitis. Pancreatic stent placement resulted in successful management of symptoms in 83% of patients (10/12) when used as first-line therapy, and in 100% of patients as second-line therapy (n = 4) after pancreatic rest with nasojejunal feeds. However, the authors recommend that pancreatic stent placement should follow an attempt at management with post–ligament of Treitz feeds.[86]

Paraduodenal pancreatitis (also known as *groove* pancreatitis) is a disease entity characterized by persistent abdominal pain and biliary and/or gastric outlet obstruction from acute pancreatitis syndrome that has characteristic radiographic features. These include focal obstructing inflammation and/or fluid collections (linear or cystic) in the pancreaticoduodenal tissue interface (or groove) and in the apposing duodenal wall. A case series reported outcomes for 39 patients with paraduodenal pancreatitis managed with endoscopic therapy, which included varying combinations of pancreaticobiliary stenting and EUS-guided transduodenal drainage of periduodenal fluid collections with or without subcutaneous octreotide. A stricture of the main pancreatic duct and/or common bile duct was identified in 72.5% and 56.9% of patients, respectively. Features of chronic pancreatitis (calcifications, atrophy) were observed in more than 35% of patients. The authors reported a greater than 70% rate of clinical success with varying combinations of endoscopic and medical therapy. However, due to small numbers and heterogeneity in the authors' management of the cohort, a clear algorithm for endoscopic therapy remains unclear.[87]

With reference to recurrent, idiopathic pancreatitis, Venu et al (1989) reported results for ERCP and sphincter of Oddi manometry in 116 patients.[88] A treatable cause of pancreatitis was identified in 37% of cases, with patients having anatomic abnormalities, stones, and sphincter hypertension. We examined diagnostic findings at ERCP in patients with idiopathic pancreatitis at our center. In patients with recurrent idiopathic pancreatitis, sphincter of Oddi (SOD) dysfunction (45%), chronic pancreatitis (35%), and pancreatic divisum (22%) were the most common findings. Chronic pancreatitis was identified more often (35% vs. 17%, $p < 0.001$), and bile duct sludge and stones were identified less often (0.6% vs. 3.2 %, $p < 0.01$) in patients with idiopathic recurrent pancreatitis compared to those with a single episode of unexplained pancreatitis.[89] However, with the exception of SOD, the majority of morphologic and intraductal abnormalities can be identified using high-quality cross-sectional imaging, MR pancreatography, and EUS (alone or in combination).[90] This was elegantly demonstrated through a prospective study by Testoni et al (2009), in which patients with idiopathic pancreatitis underwent MRCP, EUS, and ERCP. Ultimately, the diagnostic yield of a non-ERCP approach was greater than 60%, and ERCP failed to identify pathology missed by the other two modalities. Hence, diagnostic ERCP for recurrent pancreatitis should be reserved for cases with a clear preprocedure intention for SOD manometry or a therapeutic maneuver (e.g., sphincterotomy, stone extraction, stricture therapy).[91] The approach to idiopathic pancreatitis will be covered in greater detail elsewhere in this volume (see Chapter 57).

Chronic Pancreatitis

The indications for pancreatography in the setting of chronic pancreatitis, in order of appropriateness, include: (1) to confirm pathology and characterize the anatomy, with preprocedure intention to perform endoscopic therapy; (2) to characterize anatomy before surgical management of pathology; and (3) to establish a diagnosis. With reference to the latter indications, ERP for many years was the gold standard for diagnosing chronic pancreatitis and for preoperative planning. However, diagnostic ERCP is no longer considered a first-line test for diagnosis of chronic pancreatitis. MR pancreatography with contrast and secretin-stimulated images, EUS, and secretin-stimulated pancreatic function testing should be performed prior to consideration of diagnostic ERCP, given that they have similar (or even superior) accuracy and a more favorable risk profile.[92–95]

The Cambridge classification has remained the most widely utilized system for characterizing the severity of chronic pancreatitis since its inception in 1983. This sequential gradation of both main pancreatic duct and side branch findings, combined with the weight given to discrete, specific ductal abnormalities (e.g., stones, strictures) has an established accuracy (Figs. 49.35 and 49.36).[94,96] However, it should be noted that there is significant risk of pancreatitis with pressurized injection for opacification of normal side branches. Fortunately, this system can be extrapolated for diagnosis of chronic pancreatitis using MRCP.[97]

The main challenges in the interpretation of pancreatography for the diagnosis of chronic pancreatitis are the differentiation of normal from early (minimal change) disease, and the differentiation of focal strictures associated with pancreatic carcinoma and chronic pancreatitis (see Table 49.5). Of note, mild changes on pancreatography—blunting, dilation, or shortening

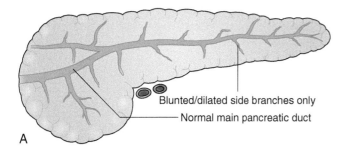

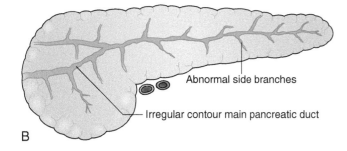

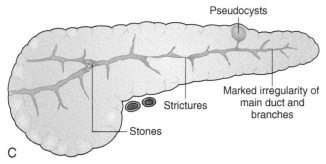

FIG 49.35 Cambridge classification of chronic pancreatitis. **A,** Mild. **B,** Moderate. **C,** Marked.

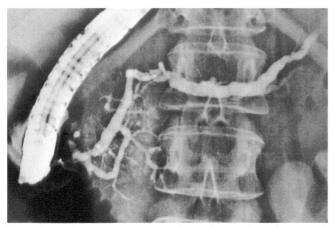

FIG 49.36 Pancreatogram showing advanced grade chronic pancreatitis.

of the side branches—are the least specific and most subjective observations, because they are highly dependent on technique and adequacy of filling, and can potentially be the result of age-related changes or transient effects of acute injury (e.g., acute pancreatitis, iatrogenic stent–induced changes).

Pancreatic duct morphology is best characterized by pancreatography (MRI or endoscopic), and this remains the procedure of choice for anatomic characterization before surgery and in patients with postsurgical pancreatic duct anatomy. With the exception of confirmation of fistula and leaks, MR pancreatography is now preferentially utilized for preoperative planning in patients with chronic pancreatitis. In patients with prior pancreatic surgery (e.g. pancreaticoduodenectomy, lateral pancreaticojejunostomy), MR pancreatography offers a distinct technical and safety advantage over diagnostic ERP, given the challenges of performing endoscopy in patients with altered anatomy.[76]

CHOLANGIOPANCREATOGRAPHY IN PATIENTS WITH SURGICALLY ALTERED ANATOMY

The clinical success of ERCP performed in patients with a history of Billroth II hemigastrectomy approaches 80% in large case series, which is lower than that reported in the setting of native anatomy.[98,99] We generally start with a standard side-viewing duodenoscope; however, a recent study suggests that an approach using an end-viewing gastroscope fitted with a transparent cap may have a lower risk for perforation (< 5% vs. 5%–18%) and comparable rates of therapeutic success.[100]

A 160-cm pediatric colonoscope or a 220-cm enteroscope can reach the bile duct in a significant proportion of patients with a long Roux-en-Y gastroenterostomy or a choledochojejunostomy. Single- and double-balloon enteroscopy is now considered the standard endoscopic approach for ERCP in patients without Roux-en-Y anatomy. However, rates of overall therapeutic success with balloon-assisted enteroscopy vary widely, even across expert centers, and generally remain significantly lower than in patients with conventional anatomy (> 70% vs. > 95%).[101–104] The lack of a catheter-deflecting elevator and the limited spectrum of compatible (long) ERCP accessories are a further hindrance for end-viewing endoscopy in this setting.[102] Although Roux-en-Y gastric bypass patients may have the lowest rates of therapeutic success for ERCP performed in surgically altered anatomy, they are and will remain a common type of patient encountered by the ERCP endoscopist.[104] Consequently, duodenoscopic ERCP through a surgical gastrostomy in the excluded stomach may be preferable for patients with Roux-en-Y gastric bypass anatomy. Rates of therapeutic success with this technique are greater than 95%, and it affords access to the full spectrum of endoscopic accessories. The gastrostomy tract can be maintained if repeat procedures are anticipated. The disadvantages of this approach relate to morbidity in the postprocedure setting, either associated with surgical complications and/or longitudinal management of the larger (greater than 30-Fr) surgical gastrostomy tract required to allow subsequent passage of the duodenoscope for repeat procedures.[105]

Cholangiography and biliary therapeutics are successful in 60% to 90% of patients with pancreaticoduodenectomy (Whipple) anatomy, with balloon-assisted enteroscopy enabling higher rates of success.[104,106,107] However, when taken as a subgroup, pancreatography and pancreatic therapeutics are met with much lower rates of diagnostic and therapeutic success (< 10%).[106,107] In most patients with post-Whipple anatomy, a pancreatogram is more likely to be successful via a transgastric EUS-guided duct puncture (Fig. 49.37). This maneuver is also used as either an adjunct to retrograde cannulation or as a prelude to EUS-guided transgastric stent decompression of obstructed ducts.[108]

TABLE 49.6 Approximate Frequencies of Complications From Endoscopic Retrograde Cholangiopancreatography (ERCP) and Sphincterotomy (%)

Complication	AVERAGE-RISK PATIENTS		HIGH-RISK PATIENTS*	
	ERCP	Sphincterotomy	ERCP	Sphincterotomy
Pancreatitis	3	5	8	12
Bleeding	0.2	1.5	0.4	3.5
Perforation	0.1	0.8	0.3	1.5
Infection	0.1	0.5	2	2
Sedation reaction or cardiopulmonary	0.5	0.5	2	2
Total[†]	3.9[‡]	8.3[‡]	12.7[‡]	21[‡]

*Certain patient characteristics and technical aspects of the procedure increase the risk of complications, including suspected sphincter of Oddi dysfunction, recurrent pancreatitis, difficult cannulation, precut sphincterotomy, coagulopathy, renal dialysis, cirrhosis, or advanced cardiopulmonary disease.
[†]Some patients have more than one complication.
[‡]Approximate severity of complications: mild, 70%; moderate, 20%; and severe, 10%.

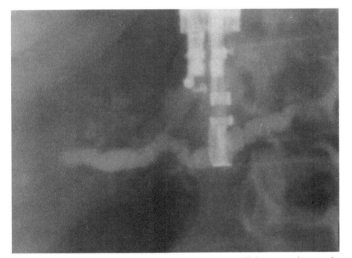

FIG 49.37 Transgastric pancreatogram utilizing endoscopic ultrasound.

COMPLICATIONS OF CHOLANGIOGRAPHY AND PANCREATOGRAPHY

The complications of diagnostic cholangiopancreatography include perforation, infection, bleeding, and pancreatitis, with the latter being a much more common complication (Table 49.6).[6]

Pancreatography during ERCP is one of the most consistently identified risk factors in studies on procedure-related pancreatitis. Further details regarding preprocedure and technical risk factors are now well-described.[109] Numerous studies have now established both temporary pancreatic duct stent placement and rectal indomethacin as effective interventions that reduce the incidence and severity of post-ERCP pancreatitis.[110,111] An in-depth discussion of this literature is beyond the scope of this chapter.

Infection in the form of cholangitis is a risk of cholangiopancreatography, and occurs in 2% to 3% of patients. However, studies evaluating the effectiveness of routine preprocedure antibiotics have yielded mixed findings, with summative literature in the form of meta-analyses and systematic reviews suggesting significant benefit in only select populations of patients.[112] Consequently, in the era of multidrug-resistant bacteria and the consequent need for antibiotic stewardship, the weight of evidence does not clearly establish a role for routine prophylactic antibiotics in the peri-ERCP period. Societal guidelines do support selective antibiotic prophylaxis in patients with pancreaticobiliary obstruction with the potential for incomplete drainage (e.g., PSC and cholangiocarcinoma), immunocompromised patients (e.g., liver transplant), and/or pancreatography cases with the potential for contamination of pancreatic/peripancreatic fluid collections.[113]

ACKNOWLEDGEMENTS

We would like to acknowledge Dr. Glen Lehman, Dr. Bret T. Petersen, Dr. Lee McHenry, and Dr. James L. Watkins for their contributions to prior editions of this chapter (Diagnostic Cholangiography and Diagnostic Pancreatography, Editions 1 and 2). Portions of their contributions to *Clinical Gastrointestinal Endoscopy* Editions 1 and 2, in the form of images and writing, were used to construct this chapter.

KEY REFERENCES

5. Freeman ML, DiSario JA, Nelson DB, et al: Risk factors for post-ERCP pancreatitis: a prospective, multicenter study, *Gastrointest Endosc* 54:425–434, 2001.
7. Cotton PB, Durkalski V, Romagnuolo J, et al: Effect of endoscopic sphincterotomy for suspected sphincter of Oddi dysfunction on pain-related disability following cholecystectomy: the EPISOD randomized clinical trial, *JAMA* 311:2101–2109, 2014.
18. Swan MP, Alexander S, Moss A, et al: Needle knife sphincterotomy does not increase the risk of pancreatitis in patients with difficult biliary cannulation, *Clin Gastroenterol Hepatol* 11:430–436.e1, 2013.
20. Choudari CP, Sherman S, Fogel EL, et al: Success of ERCP at a referral center after a previously unsuccessful attempt, *Gastrointest Endosc* 52:478–483, 2000.
23. Draganov PV, Forsmark CE: Prospective evaluation of adverse reactions to iodine-containing contrast media after ERCP, *Gastrointest Endosc* 68:1098–1101, 2008.
44. Navaneethan U, Jegadeesan R, Nayak S, et al: ERCP-related adverse events in patients with primary sclerosing cholangitis, *Gastrointest Endosc* 81:410–419, 2015.
46. Rizvi S, Eaton JE, Gores GJ: Primary sclerosing cholangitis as a premalignant biliary tract disease: surveillance and management, *Clin Gastroenterol Hepatol* 13:2152–2165, 2015.
47. Sinha R, Gardner T, Padala K, et al: Double-duct sign in the clinical context, *Pancreas* 44:967–970, 2015.
48. Navaneethan U, Njei B, Lourdusamy V, et al: Comparative effectiveness of biliary brush cytology and intraductal biopsy for detection of

malignant biliary strictures: a systematic review and meta-analysis, *Gastrointest Endosc* 81:168–176, 2015.

52. Sandha GS, Bourke MJ, Haber GB, et al: Endoscopic therapy for bile leak based on a new classification: results in 207 patients, *Gastrointest Endosc* 60:567–574, 2004.

53. Canena J, Horta D, Coimbra J, et al: Outcomes of endoscopic management of primary and refractory postcholecystectomy biliary leaks in a multicentre review of 178 patients, *BMC Gastroenterol* 15:105, 2015.

54. Samavedy R, Sherman S, Lehman GA: Endoscopic therapy in anomalous pancreatobiliary duct junction, *Gastrointest Endosc* 50:623–627, 1999.

69. Bertin C, Pelletier AL, Vullierme MP, et al: Pancreas divisum is not a cause of pancreatitis by itself but acts as a partner of genetic mutations, *Am J Gastroenterol* 107:311–317, 2012.

72. Venu RP, Atia G, Brown RD, et al: Intraductal papillary mucinous tumor of the pancreas: ERCP, EUS, and pancreatoscopy findings, *Gastrointest Endosc* 55:82, 2002.

74. Suzuki R, Thosani N, Annangi S, et al: Diagnostic yield of endoscopic retrograde cholangiopancreatography-based cytology for distinguishing malignant and benign intraductal papillary mucinous neoplasm: systematic review and meta-analysis, *Dig Endosc* 26:586–593, 2014.

75. Tanaka M, Fernandez-del Castillo C, Adsay V, et al: International consensus guidelines 2012 for the management of IPMN and MCN of the pancreas, *Pancreatology* 12:183–197, 2012.

82. Varadarajulu S, Rana SS, Bhasin DK: Endoscopic therapy for pancreatic duct leaks and disruptions, *Gastrointest Endosc Clin N Am* 23:863–892, 2013.

87. Arvanitakis M, Rigaux J, Toussaint E, et al: Endotherapy for paraduodenal pancreatitis: a large retrospective case series, *Endoscopy* 46:580–587, 2014.

89. Fischer M, Hassan A, Sipe BW, et al: Endoscopic retrograde cholangiopancreatography and manometry findings in 1,241 idiopathic pancreatitis patients, *Pancreatology* 10:444–452, 2010.

91. Cote GA, Imperiale TF, Schmidt SE, et al: Similar efficacies of biliary, with or without pancreatic, sphincterotomy in treatment of idiopathic recurrent acute pancreatitis, *Gastroenterology* 143:1502–1509.e1, 2012.

93. Conwell DL, Zuccaro G, Purich E, et al: Comparison of endoscopic ultrasound chronic pancreatitis criteria to the endoscopic secretin-stimulated pancreatic function test, *Dig Dis Sci* 52:1206–1210, 2007.

96. Axon AT, Classen M, Cotton PB, et al: Pancreatography in chronic pancreatitis: international definitions, *Gut* 25:1107–1112, 1984.

98. Bove V, Tringali A, Familiari P, et al: ERCP in patients with prior Billroth II gastrectomy: report of 30 years' experience, *Endoscopy* 47:611–616, 2015.

102. Inamdar S, Slattery E, Sejpal DV, et al: Systematic review and meta-analysis of single-balloon enteroscopy-assisted ERCP in patients with surgically altered GI anatomy, *Gastrointest Endosc* 82:9–19, 2015.

112. Brand M, Bizos D, O'Farrell P, Jr: Antibiotic prophylaxis for patients undergoing elective endoscopic retrograde cholangiopancreatography, *Cochrane Database Syst Rev* (10):CD007345, 2010.

A complete reference list can be found online at ExpertConsult .com

50

Difficult Cannulation and Sphincterotomy

Juergen Hochberger, Volker Meves, and Gregory G. Ginsberg

CHAPTER OUTLINE

INTRODUCTION

Endoscopic retrograde cholangiopancreatography (ERCP) requires several years of dedicated training and continuous refinement of knowledge and skill.[1–3] Selective ductal cannulation is the sine qua non for diagnostic and therapeutic ERCP. General issues on cannulation have already been highlighted in Chapter 40. In a 2017 consensus report, difficult papillary access is defined as the inability to achieve selective biliary cannulation by standard ERCP techniques within 10 minutes or up to five cannulation attempts.[4] This chapter concentrates on variations of standard techniques to overcome challenges to standard cannulation, including in patients with anatomic variations, gastric outlet obstruction, and surgically altered anatomy. With the development of endoscopic ultrasound (EUS) and magnetic resonance cholangiopancreatography (MRCP), ERCP has moved from a diagnostic to an almost purely therapeutic procedure.[5,6] When used as a diagnostic procedure, image-guided tissue sampling with forceps biopsy, brush cytology, or cholangiography are performed. For this reason sphincterotomy is necessary for most cases of diagnostic or therapeutic ERCP.

STANDARD ACCESSORIES

Standard Cannulas

Cannulation catheters range in size from 5 Fr (French) to 7 Fr. They are usually made of Teflon. The tip can be straight, tapered, or rounded, and accepts up to a 0.035-inch guidewire. Tapered tip catheters probably confer a higher risk of submucosal injection.

Sphincterotomes

Sphincterotome catheters are modified with an electrosurgical cutting wire at their distal end. Like cannulation catheters, they are usually made of Teflon. The cutting wire can be placed under tension to "bow" the tip of the catheter, providing another articulation to facilitate cannulation. The tensed wire is also used to perform sphincterotomy.

To facilitate cannulation, double- or triple-lumen sphincterotomes are available. They allow the introduction of a wire to accomplish a therapeutic task, and in the case of a triple-lumen sphincterotome, allow injection of contrast with a guidewire in place. Due to the small size of the injection channel, contrast flow is slow, and the use of a small syringe is recommended to facilitate injection.

In general, sphincterotomes require a higher level of coordination between the endoscopist and the assistant controlling flexure of the device. Short-wire systems, in which the guidewire can be stripped external to the catheter, allow the endoscopist to control and lock the guidewire, reducing the need for coordination between the assistant and endoscopist.

Catheter Versus Sphincterotome for Cannulation

A standard 6-Fr catheter with a 4-Fr tip accepting a 0.035-inch guidewire was the traditional first choice for cannulation. The advantage is high flexibility compared with a 6-Fr sphincterotome. The cannulation catheter could be used directly for deep cannulation (e.g., 0.035-inch J-tip with a hydrophilic Terumo guidewire [Terumo Medical Corporation, Tokyo, Japan]). For further intervention, the guidewire could be kept in place.

Sphincterotomes have largely supplanted the standard catheter in many institutions because they permit bowing of the catheter tip to facilitate alignment with the intraduodenal segment of the bile duct and because sphincterotomy is anticipated in the vast majority of ERCP procedures performed.

Data suggest an advantage of sphincterotome cannulation over standard catheter cannulation (84%–97% vs. 62%–75%),[7–9] but there is a great deal of heterogeneity in available studies, with variable criteria used to define cannulation failure.

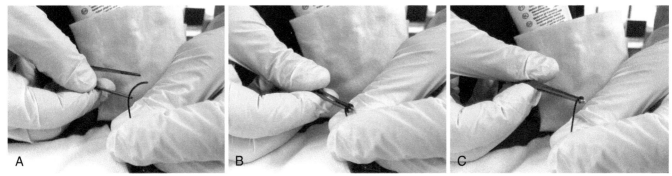

FIG 50.1 **A** to **C,** Reshaping of the distal end of a hydrophilic J-Tip of a 0.035-inch guidewire by means of an anatomical forceps in order to facilitate canulation of an angulated duct.

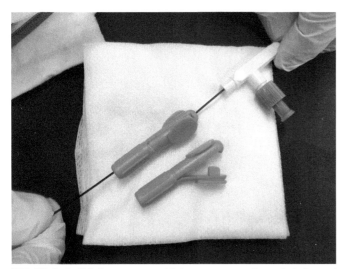

FIG 50.2 Self-fixing torque aid for easy steering of J-shaped guidewire.

Guidewires

Guidewires are frequently used for attaining and maintaining access to the biliopancreatic ducts.[10] Several studies have reported that wire-guided cannulation techniques increase cannulation success and may lower post-ERCP pancreatitis rates.[11–13]

The configuration of the guidewire tip can be straight or angled (J-shaped). Stiff shaft guidewires (e.g., monofilament guidewires) minimize lateral divergence and facilitate forward transmission of forces. To obtain access through biliary strictures, guidewires with activated hydrophilic coatings and flexible leading tips are generally recommended. For angulated accesses, the J-shaped distal end of a hydrophilic guidewire (e.g., Terumo 0.035-inch) can be customized by means of an anatomical forceps (Video 50.1 and Fig. 50.1). Guidewire tip steering is facilitated by a self-fixing torque aid (Terumo Corp.) (Fig. 50.2 and Video 50.2).

Currently available guidewire types include conventional, hydrophilic, and "hybrid," ranging from 0.018 to 0.035 inches in diameter and 260 to 480 cm in length. Enteroscopy length wires are available for balloon-assisted ERCP. Wire lengths greater than 400 cm are used for exchange of devices that are not compatible with the short-wire system. Only insulated (coated) wires should be used during electro-cautery applications to prevent aberrant transmission of electrosurgical energy.[14] Coated wires have a monofilament core of nitinol or stainless steel and an outer

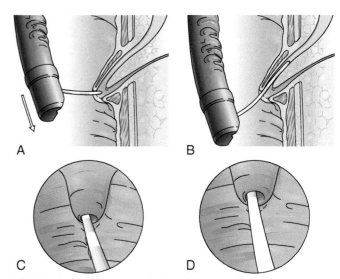

FIG 50.3 For primary cannulation of the common bile duct using a standard catheter and a therapeutic duodenoscope, it often helps to **A,** first intubate the papillary orifice with the catheter and then to **B,** change the angle of the catheter by gently advancing the endoscope. **C** and **D,** Alignment with the axis of the papilla is important for biliary cannulation. (Modified from Soehendra N, Binmoeller KF, Seifert H, et al: *Therapeutic Endoscopy: Color Atlas of Operative Techniques for the Gastrointestinal Tract.* New York, 1997, Thieme Medical Publishers.)

sheath of lubricious material (Teflon, polyurethane). Depending on the outer sheath, it is possible to improve radiopacity, slipperiness, and electrical insulation properties. To improve guidewire manipulation and accessory exchange, catheter lumens should be flushed with water to reduce friction with the guidewire.

DIFFICULTIES IN CANNULATION OF THE PAPILLA

One should develop and employ a pragmatic step-up approach to cannulation. Each escalating technique may be tried several times before moving up to the next method until success is achieved. One traditionally preferred progression begins with a sphincterotome flushed with contrast. The ampulla is inspected for its anatomic features in an attempt to localize the desired duct orifice and to determine the optimal angle of ductal traverse of the ampulla. For biliary cannulation, the catheter tip should be directed toward the 11 o'clock orientation with the catheter tip bowed to parallel duct alignment (Fig. 50.3). The surface of the ampulla should be gently stoked downward to the selected entry point (intended to deflect the fimbria separating the pancreatic and biliary orifices in the common channel) and the catheter tip advanced into the papillary meatus with an outward and upward deflection of the catheter. Gentle injection of contrast under fluoroscopic guidance will inform the catheter position as in the bile duct, pancreatic duct, common channel, or none of these. If the bile duct fills, further contrast should be injected and the catheter slid deeply into the common bile duct or, in the case of a triple-lumen catheter, the guidewire advanced. When the bile duct does not fill, bow the sphincterotome tip upward and tent the ampulla toward the endoscope and inject again. If still no filling, we employ a technique in which the sphincterotome is bowed and impacted into the papillary meatus at the 11 o'clock orientation, then the endoscopist deflects the endoscope toward and above the ampulla while slightly withdrawing the catheter within the accessory channel (so as to sustain a static depth of catheter tip entry into the papilla). This is performed concurrent with the assistant decreasing the tension on the bow of the sphincterotome. This maneuver helps direct the catheter into the location and orientation of the bile duct.

For selected pancreatic duct cannulation, the 5 o'clock papillary orientation is targeted, and with a straighter, as opposed to bowed, address (Fig. 50.4).

The guidewire cannulation technique is favored by many endoscopists. Herein, a straight or angled-tip guidewire is advanced to the tip of the catheter (standard or sphincterotome). The catheter tip is inserted into the desired location and angulation within the meatus, and the guidewire gently advanced under combined endoscopic and fluoroscopic guidance. Levels of resistance are appreciated, and we commonly "jiggle" the wire tip to seek out the desired ductal entry. Another approach is to advance the catheter into the papillary orifice with the guidewire tip extending slightly from the tip of the catheter. Lastly, the catheter can be set to hover just before the papilla and the guidewire advanced into the desired location within the papilla.

When there is repeated injection or guidewire advancement into the pancreatic duct, two techniques may be used to isolate it and facilitate selected bile duct cannulation. The first is to advance the guidewire into the pancreatic duct, exchange out the catheter, load it with another wire, and reinsert it alongside the pancreatic guidewire to attempt cannulation just above and to the left of the guidewire insertion point. This is known as the *double guidewire* technique. The second approach is to place a 3- to 5-Fr pancreatic duct stent and similarly cannulate just above and to the left. Both these approaches may be used to facilitate access prior to needle-knife sphincterotomy, detailed later.

Access Sphincterotomy in Difficult Papillary Cannulation

Standard cannulation techniques may fail even in the most experienced endoscopist's hands. A difficult anatomical position with inability to align the axis of the catheter and guidewire with the axis of bile or pancreatic duct may lead to failure of papillary cannulation. Other reasons may include impacted calculi, papillary stenosis, ampullary neoplasm, or duodenal inflammation.[15]

Access sphincterotomy (sometimes referred to as *pre-cut* sphincterotomy) commonly facilitates biliary cannulation safely and effectively in the hands of the experienced endoscopist. However, potentially severe complications may occur when performed by those who are inadequately trained.[16,17] The needle knife is the most common tool for access sphincterotomy (Fig. 50.5). Success rates vary widely according to the frequency of use and experience of the individual endoscopist, and range from 68.4% to 92.5%.[18,19]

There are two predominant access sphincterotomy techniques. For the conventional access sphincterotomy, the needle-knife tip is engaged within the papillary orifice and aligned with the presumed axis of the bile duct and papillary roof. Care has to be taken to modulate the cutting depth. Some advise beginning with a superficial cut of the papillary roof, starting at the papillary

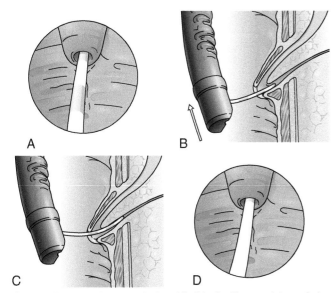

FIG 50.4 Pancreatic cannulation (**A–D**). **A,** Flat position of the catheter facing the papilla at the same level. **B** and **C,** If common bile duct cannulation was achieved first, pulling back the endoscope facilitates cannulation, as well as **D,** changing the direction of the catheter within the papilla. (Modified from Soehendra N, Binmoeller KF, Seifert H, et al: *Therapeutic Endoscopy: Color Atlas of Operative Techniques for the Gastrointestinal Tract.* New York, 1997, Thieme Medical Publishers.)

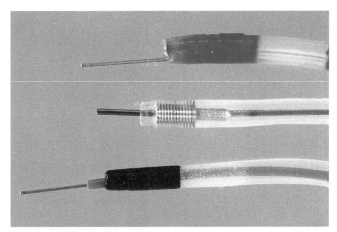

FIG 50.5 Different types of needle-knives. Diameter and length of the cutting wire influences cutting properties: the thinner the wire knife, the faster and sharper the cut; the longer the wire, the potentially deeper the cut, with relatively high risk of bleeding and perforation.

orifice, transecting first the mucosa and incrementally cutting until the muscle layer of the common sphincter is visualized. The round or point-like aspect of the biliary orifice may be seen and then selectively cannulated with a hydrophilic guidewire exiting 2 mm from a cannula or sphincterotome. Even if 11 o'clock is a common position of the biliary sphincter, this may vary, and careful identification of the round structure of the biliary orifice and distal biliary sphincter muscle is the most important pathfinder. In the case of failed pancreatic cannulation, a biliary sphincterotomy, using standard or needle-knife technique, may be performed to better expose the pancreatic orifice, which is typically found in the 5 o'clock position. After selective deep duct cannulation, a guidewire sphincterotomy is often performed to also open the biliary or pancreatic sphincter and to achieve an optimal permanent access and drainage.

The alternative techniques for access sphincterotomy are starting suprapapillary and cutting downward toward the papilla face, or direct puncture fistulotomy into the roof of the papilla.[20]

Access sphincterotomy is used in 3.8% to 19.2% of ERCP procedures, with a success rate ranging from 75% to 99% and complication rates from 1.9% to 30%.[18,21–24] Complications of precut sphincterotomy are similar to those with conventional sphincterotomy, such as bleeding, perforation, pancreatitis, and cholangitis.[25,26] The complication rates reported in international studies are in the range of 7% to 13.3%.[19,27,28] Risk factors for complications include young age, an inexperienced operator, periampullary carcinoma, diverticulum, sphincter of Oddi dysfunction, and nondilated common bile duct.[17,29]

The timing of and decision to perform access sphincterotomy should be individualized based on the indication for the procedure, the ampullary characteristics, and the endoscopist's training and experience, with a continuous weighing of the potential procedural expectations, risks, and benefits, including the risks associated with failed cannulation.

Periampullary Duodenal Diverticula

Duodenal diverticula are found in up to 15% of patients undergoing ERCP. They are defined as herniation of the mucosa or submucosa that occurs via a defect in the muscle layer. Some papillae are located on the edge of diverticula, others partially or completely within the diverticulum. Any of these locations may make access to the papilla for cannulation difficult or impossible. Due to the distortion, the pancreatic and biliary orifice locations can even be reversed. Depending on the position of the papilla and the distortion level, cannulation can be straightforward or extremely difficult. Thus, the challenge is to approach in the appropriate axis for access.

Success rates for cannulation in the context of periampullary diverticula versus no diverticulum are 62.4% versus 92.7%, respectively.[30] In contrast, Panteris et al (2008) reported similar success rates with or without diverticula, after excluding cases with undetectable papillae (94.9% vs. 94.8 %).[31]

The most common problem in patients with periampullary diverticula is the inability of the endoscopist to detect the orifice of the papilla.[31] In a review article by Altonbary et al (2016),[32] the following tips are presented:

1. In most cases, the papilla is located on the lower edge of the diverticulum or just inside, somewhere between the positions of 3 o'clock and 8 o'clock.
2. Very large diverticula are usually divided by a ridge-like septum. This ridge typically overlies the bile duct and terminates inferiorly at the papilla.

3. A catheter can be used to straighten and evert the folds to identify a hidden papilla within the diverticulum.
4. Advancement of the tip of the duodenoscope into the sac is also possible, but care must be taken to avoid perforation.
5. Due to the altered anatomy, the biliary duct is often not acutely angulated superiorly, but runs more directly. Thus, acute angulation of the sphincterotome is not necessary.
6. In some cases, air aspiration shows the side of the diverticulum.
7. Changing patients' position to the abdominal (prone) position or pushing the upper right abdominal quadrant of the patient can help.
8. Instillation of saline solution on the contralateral side of the diverticulum may cause the papilla to protrude.

Special Cannulation Techniques in Periampullary Duodenal Diverticula

Numerous techniques have been described to overcome difficulties in cannulation of an intra-diverticular papilla. Their use should be individualized based on specific indications and circumstances.

Two devices in one channel method. A biopsy forceps or thin caliber cannula is introduced through the working channel and used to retract the duodenal mucosa adjacent to the papilla. Thus, the papillary orifice can be drawn out of the diverticulum. Then a cannula or sphincterotome can be introduced alongside the forceps through the same working channel for cannulation.[32a]

Reversed guidewire method. A cannulation catheter loaded with a guidewire is introduced through the working channel of the duodenoscope. A second guidewire is introduced through the working channel in reverse (stiff end forward) alongside the catheter. This second guidewire is now used to push the mucosa next to the papilla toward the duodenum. This results in straightening of the duodenal folds and an acceptable direction for cannulation is achieved.[33] We recommend using this technique with caution, as perforation of the thin duodenal wall by the stiff guidewire can occur.

Endoscopic clip placement. Commercially available through-the-scope clips can be used to evert the ampullary orifice from within the diverticulum and fix it in an orientation that will better facilitate cannulation. With the clip in the opened configuration, the mucosa is gored with one arm of the open clip. The endoscope is then torqued to evert the papilla. When the orientation is deemed optimal, the other arm of the clip is engaged with tissue and the clip is closed to fix the configuration. Cannulation is then undertaken in the usual manner.[34]

"Clip and line"-assisted papillary cannulation (Video 50.3). We recently described this technique deriving from endoscopic submucosal dissection (ESD).[35] In ESD, the so-called "clip and line" technique or "traction-assisted ESD" uses a conventional hemoclip attached to dental floss or a nylon string to exert traction and facilitate dissection.[34] For exposure of the papilla during ERCP, the endoscope is first removed from the patient in case of a difficult intra-diverticular papilla. A standard single-use hemoclip is advanced though the working channel of the duodenoscope. The clip is then slightly opened and dental floss of approximately 2 m length tied to one arm of the clip. The clip is then withdrawn back into the endoscope channel. The endoscope is then reinserted with the dental floss on its outside. The clip is then reinserted the mucosa of the papillary roof at the desired location. Traction can now be exerted by gently pulling on the string extracorporeally to expose the papillary orifice (see Video 50.3). Care must be taken to avoid unintentionally dislodging the clip.

Double-endoscope method. First a conventional gastroscope is introduced into the diverticulum. This allows better visualization of the papilla. Through this endoscope a forceps is used to grasp tissue next to the papilla to achieve a better orientation. The gastroscope with the instrument is placed on the left side to prevent a relapse of the papilla after opening of the forceps. Then a conventional side-view duodenoscope is introduced next to the gastroscope and a cannulation of the papilla is possible. This technique is potentially associated with increased risk of perforation at the level of the upper esophageal sphincter and the level of the duodenal bulb.[36]

Balloon dilatation of the narrow diverticular neck. Balloon dilatation with a 15-mm stone-retrieval balloon can be used in case of a narrow-necked diverticulum with the papilla situated in the fundus of the diverticulum.[37]

Cap-assisted cannulation. A transparent cap is mounted on the tip of a conventional gastroscope for better exposure of the papilla. If cannulation through the papillary orifice fails, an endoscopic fistulotomy can be attempted. Fistulotomy is performed between the lower two-thirds and the upper one-third of the papillary roof. After needle puncture, a soft-tipped guidewire is advanced through the fistulotomy.[38]

Percutaneous transhepatic access and rendezvous. First a percutaneous ultrasound-guided or often purely radiologic transhepatic biliary puncture is performed. A long guidewire is advanced through the biliary duct and papilla into the duodenum. With a snare, the guidewire is then grasped and an over-the-wire cannulation is performed.[39]

A limitation to this technique is the difficulty to grasp the guidewire without distortion or kinking.[39] A coated guidewire with a hydrophilic tip (e.g., Jag Wire 450 cm, Boston Scientific, Marlborough, MA) is best used and captured at the level of its soft distal end.

A small study on the percutaneous ultrasound-guided rendezvous technique involving 14 patients showed success in 13/14 (success rate 93%) with 1 complication (retroperitoneal perforation; complication rate 7%).[39]

EUS-guided rendezvous technique. In 3% to 5% of cases ERCP is unsuccessful because of previous surgery (surgical bypass, gastrectomy, or Whipple resection) or duodenal stenosis, for example, because of periampullary tumor infiltration or hilar cholangiocarcinoma. In these cases the endoscopist may choose between percutaneous transhepatic cholangiography or an EUS-guided approach. Wiersema et al described the first case of EUS-guided transduodenal cholangiography in 1996.[40] EUS-guided hepatico-gastrostomy with stent placement was first performed by Burmester et al in 2000.[41] This technique is described in detail in Chapter 52.

ERCP in Surgically Altered Anatomy

In patients with surgically altered anatomy, access to the biliopancreatic orifices is usually more challenging than actual cannulation. ERCP in patients with surgically altered anatomy is associated with increased risk of perforation, particularly at the level of the anastomosis or the afferent limb.[41a]

Billroth I

In this anatomic variant, the major and minor papillae are located more proximally than usual. The papilla is presented in an exaggerated clockwise orientation relative to the endoscope in the short position. Without the pylorus, anchoring of the endoscope is challenging. Thus, a stable position for cannulation can be difficult. Sometimes working in the long-scope position is advantageous.

Billroth II

Due to the short distance to the papilla through the afferent loop, a standard duodenoscope may be used. Determining the afferent versus efferent limb may prove challenging, however. To access the afferent loop, the endoscope should follow the lesser curvature of the stomach. The upwardly oriented limb is usually the afferent loop. The efferent limb is usually easier to intubate because of the steep angle of fixation of the afferent loop that is sutured to the lesser curve.

In some cases the afferent loop is only visualized in the retroflexed position. In this case, suctioning gastric air may improve endoscope trajectory. Hand compression of the mid-abdomen or introducing a stiff guidewire or snare into the intended loop has been reported to possibly help.[42]

Once within the afferent loop and after advancing some distance, fluoroscopic confirmation that the scope has passed or is passing though the transverse duodenum is recommended. If it is found in the pelvis on fluoroscopy, then it is likely that the endoscope is in the efferent limb and should be withdrawn.[43]

Usually the major papilla is located near the duodenal stump at the 5 or 12 o'clock position. The minor papilla is usually located slightly further away from and to the left of the major papilla.[42] It is important to recognize that the orientation of the papilla will be inverted. The pancreatic duct is usually visualized at the 11 o'clock position.

A forward-viewing endoscope may be needed to identify and traverse the afferent loop in some cases. Most experienced biliary endoscopists prefer the conventional side-viewing duodenoscope to take advantage of the elevator lever. However, in a randomized trial of 45 patients in Korea, no difference was noted between the side-viewing and end-viewing endoscopes in success of cannulation and sphincterotomy.[44] Nevertheless, cannulation in the Billroth II situation is challenging. In a study involving 185 Billroth II ERCP procedures, the failure rate was 34%.[45] Even in a tertiary biliary center, failure to enter the afferent limb has been reported to be as high as 10%[45] (Figs. 50.6 and 50.7).

Sphincterotomy in BII cases. It is important to recognize the upside-down configuration of the papilla in these cases. Several techniques have been described to perform a BII sphincterotomy. One technique is to place a bile duct stent first and then use a needle-knife to cut over the stent. The cut should be performed toward the junction of the intramural segment and the duodenal wall, which translates to the 5 to 6 o'clock position.[46]

Another option is the use of a reverse-type sphincterotome. This BII (shark fin) sphincterotome has a diathermy wire that is positioned at 6 o'clock, allowing sphincterotomy in the direction of the biliary sphincter. Unfortunately, reverse sphincterotomes do not always align correctly. Rotatable sphincterotomes are preferred by some experts for this purpose. In some situations, there is a need for needle-knife fistulotomy with subsequent antegrade passage of a wire across the ampulla.[47]

Roux-en-Y Gastric Bypass

A very short blind stump and a long, efferent limb are present due to the end-to-side gastroenterostomy anastomosis. Usually the efferent limb extends approximately 40 cm before the jejunojejunostomy is encountered. At this point two or three lumens will be identified, depending on whether the two jejunal

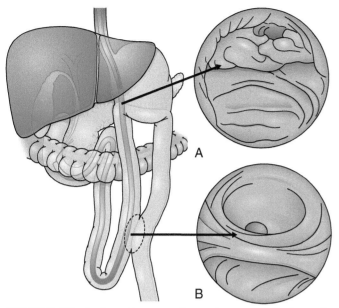

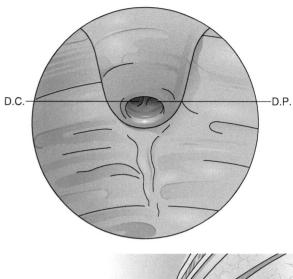

FIG 50.6 Billorth II anatomy: endoscopic access. Endoscopic view at **A,** the jejunal and **B,** enteroenteral (Braun) anastomosis. Intubate the afferent loop and stay to the same side of the enteral wall when you pass the enteroenteral anastomosis *(oval)*. (Modified from Soehendra N, Binmoeller KF, Seifert H, et al: *Therapeutic Endoscopy: Color Atlas of Operative Techniques for the Gastrointestinal Tract.* New York, 1997, Thieme Medical Publishers.)

limbs are connected end-to-side or side-to-side. If side-to-side, one of the three outlets is a short, blind stump. If the pancreaticobiliary limb is engaged, the endoscope will travel to the proximal jejunum, traversing the ligament of Treitz, the transverse duodenum, and finally the descending duodenum. This long distance makes it nearly impossible for a 125 cm-long duodenoscope to reach the major papilla. Many longer length endoscopes have been used to perform ERCP in this setting, including pediatric or adult colonoscopes and push enteroscopes, but it has most commonly been performed with balloon-assist enteroscopy.[47]

Thus, the challenges of performing ERCP in a Roux-en-Y gastric bypass are not just to traverse a great length of small bowel and to recognize the proper intestinal lumen (usually through trial and error), but finally to cannulate selectively the bile and/or pancreatic duct from the reverse of normal trajectory, with a forward-viewing instrument and using accessories not necessarily designed for these purposes.

The major papilla is located along the interior part of the duodenal C-loop. Thus, forward-viewing endoscopes have difficulty in identifying and cannulating the papilla. To evaluate and treat a pancreatic condition is particularly problematic and largely ineffective.[48,49]

Double-balloon enteroscopy for patients with Roux-en-Y anatomy.

End-viewing push enteroscopes or pediatric colonoscopes have often been reported to be inadequate in patients after partial or total gastrectomy such as Billroth II gastrojejunostomy, Roux-en-Y reconstruction, Whipple resection, or biliopancreatic reconstructions (pancreaticojejunostomy, choledocho-choledochostomy, hepaticojejunostomy).[49–51]

In a study by Raithel et al (2011), double-balloon enteroscopy (DBE)-ERCP was compared to push enteroscopy. DBE-ERCP

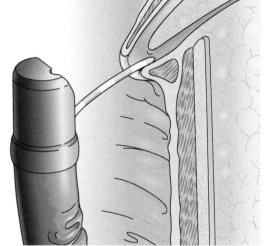

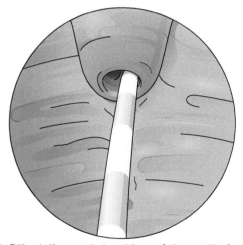

FIG 50.7 Billroth II cannulation. View of the papilla from below with inverted anatomy. Schematic illustration of cannulating the pancreatic duct. *D.C.,* Ductus choledochus; *D.P.,* ductus pancreaticus. (Modified from Soehendra N, Binmoeller KF, Seifert H, et al: *Therapeutic Endoscopy: Color Atlas of Operative Techniques for the Gastrointestinal Tract.* New York, 1997, Thieme Medical Publishers.)

was performed successfully in 74.1% of cases via the enteroscope, whereas push enteroscopy reached biliary anastomoses or papilla in only 16.2% of patients. These results were in good agreement with recently published data for the approach by double- or single-balloon enteroscopy.[50,52–54] The push-and-pull method by DBE proved to be markedly more effective, because pushing and stretching of small intestinal loops is reduced by regular retractions of the DBE cycle.

The threading of the small intestine onto the DBE and the option to block the balloons at the enteroscope provides the enteroscope tip with a greater possibility of movement for identifying the biliary or pancreatic anastomoses or the papilla. In addition, sliding back of the enteroscope may be prevented by inflated balloons.[53]

Biliary cannulation is performed similarly to the technique employed in the Bilroth II setting. Cannulation may be enhanced by placing a transparent cap on the tip of the endoscope to help anchor the papilla in place during attempts at cannulation. The enteroscope accessory channel length and small caliber limit the types and diameters of accessories and endoprostheses that can be used. Familiarity with these nuances is required for success. Only devices of 5 to 8 Fr may be passed through an operating channel of 2.8 mm.[52]

The double-balloon enteroscopy technique is successful in up to 70% of cases.[55] An alternative approach is intraoperative ERCP though a surgically created gastrotomy. This approach has a much higher success rate, albeit with the associated morbidity and cost of the operative approach.

Conventional Whipple Procedure

When an endoscope is passed into the mid-stomach, two small bowel orifices are seen in the conventional Whipple anatomy. One gastrojejunostomy opening ascends up the afferent limb and joins the bile duct and eventually the pancreatic duct. The other orifice leads to the efferent limb and the rest of the gastrointestinal tract. Fluoroscopy may occasionally be of benefit to confirm that the endoscope is within the afferent limb because it should be located in the right upper quadrant. Fluoroscopy may also help locate the pancreatic and biliary anastomoses, as they always come off the most cephalad portion of the bowel gas in the right upper quadrant.[56] A forward-viewing therapeutic channel gastroscope or colonoscope is commonly used to identify and access the choledocoenterostomy and pancreaticoenterostomy.

CANNULATION OF THE MINOR PAPILLA

Cannulation of the minor papilla is performed in cases of complete or incomplete pancreas divisum. Due to the small diameter of the minor papilla (it is typically a < 2-mm protrusion), cannulation is challenging. The usual position of the minor is 1.5 to 2 cm proximal and 5 to 10 mm to the right of the major papilla. We typically find that advancing the endoscope into the "long" position enables optimal visualization and access to the minor papilla. Cannulation is best achieved using a small atraumatic catheter or mini-sphincterotome (Glo Tip 3/5-Fr catheter and 3/5-Fr Minitome; Cook Medical, Winston-Salem, NC) in combination with an 18- or 25-inch hydrophilic guidewire (e.g., Terumo Medical or Visiglide, Olympus Optical, Tokyo, Japan). Needle tip catheters may prove valuable for cannulation and injection of contrast for diagnostic purposes, but are not capable of transmitting a guidewire. The minor papilla cannulation success rate is up to 90%.[57]

MAJOR PAPILLA SPHINCTEROTOMY

In most cases, a pull-type papillotome is used. Depending on the catheter used, the diathermy wire varies in length (range: 15–40 mm). A 25-mm cutting wire is most commonly used.[1] The aim of biliary sphincterotomy is to bisect the ampullary sphincter muscle as therapy for a number of conditions and to facilitate access for a variety of diagnostic and therapeutic accessories. Once free cannulation of the bile duct is achieved, the sphincterotome is positioned under endoscopic guidance within the papillary orifice. Maintenance of cannulation and precise positioning are enhanced by guidewire placement. The alignment of the cutting wire should parallel the intraduodenal segment of the common bile duct and the direction of the sphincterotomy should ideally seek the 11 to 12 o'clock orientation. We position the sphincterotome such that approximately 3 mm of cutting wire is in contact with the tissue. The catheter position, tension on the cutting wire, and length of cutting wire contact are incrementally adjusted during the sphincterotomy in response to observed effect and the intended extent of cut. So too, the sphincterotomy direction and speed are influenced by maneuvering of the elevator lever, endoscope tip deflections, and torque. The sphincterotomy should bisect the sphincter of Oddi and may extend to the junction of the papilla and duodenal wall.

For some time there had been debate as to the ideal electrosurgical current for sphincterotomy with regards to associated risks of bleeding and pancreatitis. It had been suggested that pure cutting current is associated with a lower risk of pancreatitis, and that a blended current is associated with a lower risk of bleeding.[58] However, a meta-analysis by Kerma et al (2007) showed that the type of current used for sphincterotomy (pure cut vs. blended) does not clearly influence the incidence or severity of pancreatitis.[63] This debate has since been quelled by the near universal adoption of microprocessor-controlled "auto-cut" or "endo-cut" currents that modulate the coagulation and cutting currents to optimal effect. In the microprocessor-controlled mode of these electrosurgical units, the generator will automatically shut on and off, which maintains the cut in short stages.[59,61,62]

Current should usually be applied for 1 or 2 seconds. If no effect is observed within this time, one should consider decreasing the length of cutting wire in contact with the tissue. Uncontrolled rapid cutting (*zipper effect*) may result if the force applied on the sphincterotome is great, although the microprocessor-controlled modes largely mitigate against this.[60]

PANCREATIC SPHINCTEROTOMY

The approach to pancreatic sphincterotomy is comparable to that of biliary sphincterotomy. A standard pull-type sphincterotome is typically used. An alternative is the use of a needle-knife after placement of a pancreatic duct stent.[64] The pancreatic duct is first cannulated with the pull-type sphincterotome with or without a guidewire. After confirmation of correct position with fluoroscopy, the incision is performed incrementally[65] toward the 1 to 2 o'clock position with the very distal extent of the cutting wire.[66,67] The cutting wire should not be inserted beyond 3 mm into the pancreatic duct to minimize the risk of perforation. In cases of larger duct diameter, longer cuts may be required.

In contrast to biliary sphincterotomy, in which the *cutting direction* is in the 11 to 1 o'clock position,[66] in pancreatic sphincterotomy the direction is more toward the right, along the floor of the papillary orifice.[68]

After pancreatic sphincterotomy, in addition to rectal indomethacin, prophylactic pancreatic stent placement has been shown to reduce the risk of procedure-related pancreatitis.[69,70]

In the needle-knife technique, after stent placement, the tip of the needle-knife is placed at the most proximal portion of pancreatic sphincter tissue that is overlying the top of the stent. The stent is used to direct the cut. The incision length is similar to the sphincterotomy in the pull-type style. Sometimes, a prior biliary sphincterotomy can help facilitate the needle-knife sphincterotomy.[71]

In a survey of 14 expert endoscopists in nine US centers, half "always" or "often" use the pull-type sphincterotome technique, whereas the other half "always" or "often" use the needle-knife technique.[70] Almost all endoscopists inserted a pancreatic stent after sphincterotomy. The type of stent (i.e., diameter, length, configuration, material, and duration of stenting) was not clearly defined.[69,70]

MINOR PAPILLOTOMY

Minor papillotomy, or more accurately septotomy,[52] in patients with pancreas divisum has been shown to decrease the rate of recurrent pancreatitis in selected patients.[72,73] Recent evidence pertaining to genetic mutations associated with acute recurrent pancreatitis in patients with incidental pancreas divisum should prompt thoughtful consideration before recommending minor duct septotomy. Any of the aforementioned papillotomy tools and techniques may be used. Some endoscopists prefer an ultra-tapered tip papillotome in this setting (e.g., 3-Fr). Others employ a standard papillotome, but always with guidewire access. Still others perform an over-the-wire–push sphincterotomy (0.75-Fr Minitome) cut with max 4-mm insertion (better, 2–3 mm) in the 11 to 12 o'clock direction. Often, a 2-mm pre-cut over-the-wire is necessary in the 11 to 12 o'clock position to allow advancement of the catheter into the duct. Blended current or pure cutting current may be used.[74] Typically, sphincterotomy is performed in the short position. To force the guidewire upward to the roof of papilla, bowing of the sphincterotome and use of the elevator are necessary in most cases. Sphincterotomy in the long position requires less bowing. After cannulation is achieved, the endoscopist can withdraw the sphincterotome to "tent" the minor papilla. Only 2 to 3 mm of the wire should be in contact with the papilla. The length of incision is based on the duct size, the surrounding anatomy, and indication, and is often in the range of 2 to 4 mm. The deeper the wire is in the papilla, the higher the risk of an uncontrolled zipper cut with retroperitoneal perforation.[75]

The needle-knife technique, as described earlier, may be performed over a previously placed pancreatic duct stent. The stent is generally maintained for 24 hours up to 2 weeks to reduce the risk of procedure-related pancreatitis. The overall complication rates are similar in those undergoing needle-knife and pull-type sphincterotomy.[76]

KEY REFERENCES

4. Liao WC, Angsuwatcharakon P, Isayama H, et al: International consensus recommendations for difficult biliary access, *Gastrointest Endosc* 85: 295–304, 2017.
28. Li G, Chen Y, Zhou X, Lv N: Early management experience of perforation after ERCP, *Gastroenterol Res Pract* 2012:657418, 2012.
32. Altonbary AY, Bahgat MH: Endoscopic retrograde cholangiopancreatography in periampullary diverticulum: the challenge of cannulation, *World J Gastrointest Endosc* 8(6):282–287, 2016.
33. Elmunzer BJ, Boetticher NC: Reverse guidewire anchoring of the papilla for difficult cannulation due to a periampullary diverticulum, *Gastrointest Endosc* 82(5):957, 2015.
38. Myung DS, Park CH, Koh HR, et al: Cap-assisted ERCP in patients with difficult cannulation due to periampullary diverticulum, *Endoscopy* 46(4):352–355, 2014.
53. Raithel M, Dormann H, Naegel A, et al: Double-balloon-enteroscopy-based endoscopic retrograde cholangiopancreatography in post-surgical patients, *World J Gastroenterol* 17(18):2302–2314, 2011.
58. Kogure H, Tsujino T, Isayama H, et al: Short- and long-term outcomes of endoscopic papillary large balloon dilation with or without sphincterotomy for removal of large bile duct stones, *Scand J Gastroenterol* 49:121–128, 2014.
76. Jamidar P, Kinzel J, Roberts K: Endoscopic Sphincterotomy: periprocedureal care, Dec 03 2015. Medscape Online.

A complete reference list can be found online at ExpertConsult.com

51

Endoscopic Ultrasound and Fine-Needle Aspiration for Pancreatic and Biliary Disorders

Jason B. Samarasena, Kenneth Chang, and Mark Topazian

CHAPTER OUTLINE

INTRODUCTION

Endoscopic ultrasound (EUS) is a powerful technique that is integral to the management of many patients with biliary and pancreatic disease. EUS provides detailed images of the extrahepatic biliary tree and pancreas with very little risk to the patient, and is useful in the evaluation of obstructive jaundice, biliary or pancreatic ductal dilation, pancreatic masses, and pancreatitis. EUS and endoscopic retrograde cholangiopancreatography (ERCP) can be performed during the same sedation session, with EUS identifying patients likely to benefit from therapeutic ERCP. EUS-guided therapeutic interventions have an evolving role in selected patients, including celiac plexus block (CPB), fiducial placement, drainage of pancreas fluid collections, and EUS-guided drainage of inaccessible biliary and pancreatic ducts. EUS is an increasingly important tool for the biliary and pancreatic endoscopist. This chapter reviews the technique of pancreaticobiliary EUS and discusses its role in selected diagnoses. The role of EUS in patients with pancreatic malignancies, pancreatic cysts, and cholangiocarcinoma is discussed in other chapters.

Linear Versus Radial Endoscopic Ultrasound Imaging

EUS imaging is currently available in two primary imaging planes: radial array and curved linear array. The imaging planes are determined by the orientation in which the individual piezoelectric crystals are arrayed on the echoendoscope. The radial echoendoscope has the imaging transducer in a plane perpendicular to the long axis of the endoscope, thus producing a circular image with the endoscope shaft located at the center. With linear echoendoscopes, the imaging transducer is oriented to produce a sector-shaped image parallel to the long axis of the endoscope.

A major advantage of linear array imaging over radial is that a therapeutic device (such as a biopsy needle) that is advanced through the therapeutic channel of the echoendoscope will remain within the imaging beam. As a result, the biopsy needle can be followed continuously as it is advanced through the bowel wall into adjacent structures of interest and placed precisely within targets (such as masses) imaged in real time on EUS.

Most early endosonographers learned EUS using radial devices, as it was often assumed that radial EUS was easier to learn than linear EUS due to the radial images more closely resembling standard computed tomography (CT) imaging. It was also argued that all EUS cases should be initially performed using a radial echoendoscope, reserving linear devices until a need for a biopsy is identified on the radial exam. This may have largely been due to superiority of radial imaging at the time. In the past decade, this practice has changed dramatically. It has become increasingly more common to perform a majority of EUS exams entirely with the linear array echoendoscope. This trend likely reflects an improvement in linear array imaging, an increasing acceptance of the clinical utility of EUS-guided tissue sampling, and an increase in percentage of cases in which a biopsy is needed. Furthermore, there are advantages to using linear EUS for pancreatic and biliary imaging. Because the linear echoendoscope visualizes tissues beyond the tip of the endoscope, the more proximal bile duct can be better visualized with a linear scope. In addition, a tandem study showed that linear EUS detects more pancreatic lesions than radial EUS in high-risk individuals undergoing pancreatic cancer screening.[1] At our institutions, the majority of pancreaticobiliary EUS examinations are performed solely with linear array imaging.

Preparation for EUS Examination

Patient preparation for endosonography with either the radial or linear system is similar to preparation for routine upper endoscopy. Patients should be positioned in the left lateral decubitus position, as for most upper endoscopy procedures. Moderate or deep sedation is recommended for EUS examination, and moderate sedation is typically sufficient. For some cases, water filling of the stomach and esophagus can help optimize imaging; if this is anticipated, performing the procedure with general anesthesia and airway intubation should be considered.

Esophageal Intubation

Prior to esophageal intubation, the balloon should be examined for air bubbles and water leakage to ensure optimal imaging during the examination. Lubricant gel should be avoided, as it may interfere with endoscopic or endosonographic imaging. Wetting the tip of the echoendoscope with water just prior to intubation is usually sufficient. If a lubricant gel is used, avoid the latex balloon and the optics of the scope. Intubation of the esophagus with an echoendoscope is similar to passing a duodenoscope, and is performed without endoscopic visualization. We often inflate the balloon slightly to aid with intubation and to minimize the risk for trauma and perforation. Placing the head in the sniffing position can aid in passage into the proximal esophagus.

Principles of Linear and Radial Pancreatic and Biliary Imaging

Endosonographic imaging of the pancreaticobiliary system and vascular structures is via the stomach and duodenum with both the radial and linear system. An understanding of the anatomic relationships of major blood vessels and the extraluminal organs of interest (primarily the gallbladder, liver, pancreas, bile duct, adrenal gland, and celiac axis) is essential for successful endosonography and EUS-guided fine-needle aspiration (FNA). The pancreas and the biliary system are best examined by beginning at three luminal stations: the proximal stomach, the duodenal bulb, and the second/third portion of the duodenum. The key principle in achieving efficient and complete linear EUS imaging in the pancreaticobiliary system is rapidly finding the "home base" anatomical landmarks, then using these locations to complete a systematic endosonographic examination.[2] Videos 51.1 and 51.2 detail the station-based technique for performance of pancreatic and biliary EUS using linear and radial imaging.

GALLBLADDER STONES, SLUDGE, AND POLYPS

EUS is useful for diagnosis of gallbladder sludge or stones missed by transabdominal ultrasound, and is more sensitive than bile microscopy in patients with these conditions (Fig. 51.1).[3,4] It may be especially useful in obese patients and patients with stones in the gallbladder neck, settings in which transabdominal ultrasound is less sensitive for diagnosis. Sludge is visualized as echogenic, nonshadowing, layering material. It should not be confused with gain artifact or "ring-down artifact," which appears as circular bright lines parallel to the transducer. A clear-cut sludge/bile interface is helpful for diagnosis of sludge. Cholesterol crystals have straight edges and are highly echogenic; they appear as bright flecks in bile, sometimes casting "comet tails." Calcium bilirubinate granules are rounded and much less echogenic, and can be missed by EUS unless they are present in sufficient quantity to form layering sludge.

EUS has been used for differential diagnosis of gallbladder polyps. The best clinical studies have been reported from Asia, and their applicability to Western populations has not been well studied. Most gallbladder polyps are readily imaged, although the fundus and cap of the gallbladder may be difficult or impossible to visualize in some patients. Adherent sludge can mimic a gallbladder polyp, but sludge can usually be distinguished from polyp by gently shaking the patient's abdomen or turning the patient to the right decubitus position during EUS to determine whether the lesion moves (Fig. 51.2).

The differential diagnosis of gallbladder polyps is listed in Table 51.1. The size of gallbladder polyps is the single most important consideration in differential diagnosis. Neoplasm is

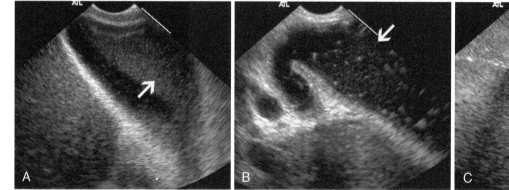
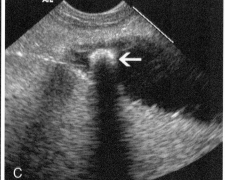

FIG 51.1 Gallbladder findings in patients with recurrent acute pancreatitis and previous normal transabdominal ultrasound. **A,** Layering sludge *(arrow).* **B,** Echogenic cholesterol crystals in the gallbladder neck *(arrow)* casting bright "comet tails." **C,** Stone *(arrow)* in the gallbladder neck.

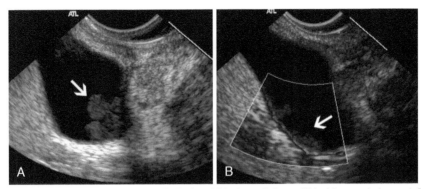

FIG 51.2 Polypoid gallbladder sludge. **A,** Polypoid lesion of the gallbladder neck *(arrow)*. **B,** When the patient is turned to the right decubitus position, the "lesion" moves to the gallbladder body and separates into several pieces *(arrow)*.

TABLE 51.1 Differential Diagnosis of Gallbladder Polyps	
Non-Neoplastic	**Neoplastic**
Cholesterol	Adenoma
Hyperplastic	Adenocarcinoma
Inflammatory	Adenosquamous carcinoma
Fibrous	Neuroendocrine tumor
Adenomyomatosis	

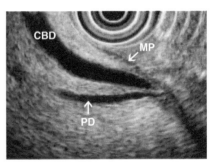

FIG 51.3 Normal bile duct viewed from the duodenal bulb with a radial echoendoscope. *CBD,* common bile duct; *MP,* muscularis propria of the duodenal wall; *PD,* pancreatic duct.

unlikely in polyps with a diameter of 5 mm or less, but is usually present in polyps greater than 15 mm in diameter, at least in Asian populations.[5-7] In patients with primary sclerosing cholangitis (PSC), neoplasia is likely in polyps of 8 mm diameter or greater, and cholecystectomy is recommended for gallbladder polyps in patients with PSC who have good liver function.[8] Particular ultrasound echofeatures that predict the type of polyp have been identified. Doppler evidence of vascularity has been associated with neoplasia in gallbladder polyps when evaluated by transabdominal ultrasound.[9] Neoplastic polyps may contain hypoechoic foci,[10] whereas cholesterol polyps often contain bright, echogenic spots or demonstrate comet tail artifacts caused by cholesterol crystals in the lesion. Adenomyomatosis typically appears as multiple small cystic or anechoic spaces, and may also show evidence of cholesterol deposits in the lesion. However, these features lack high predictive accuracy, particularly in polyps less than 10 mm in diameter.[11] When the distinctive findings of a non-neoplastic polyp are seen in a patient without risk factors for gallbladder cancer (such as stones or PSC), it may be reasonable to investigate larger gallbladder polyps, at least those that are less than 20 mm in diameter,[7] although neoplastic polyps containing EUS features of cholesterolosis or adenomyomatosis have been reported.[12] Neoplasm should be considered when the characteristic findings of a non-neoplastic lesion are absent and the lesion is greater than 5 mm, even in lesions confined to the mucosa. Loss of gallbladder wall architecture is suggestive of an invasive cancer.[13]

BILE DUCT STONES

EUS is highly accurate for the diagnosis of choledocholithiasis. EUS is especially useful in patients with a low or intermediate risk of bile duct stones, refining the use of ERCP and decreasing the overall risks of an endoscopic approach.

The accuracy of EUS for the diagnosis of bile duct stones and sludge relies on both endoscopic and patient factors. The common duct is best visualized from the duodenal bulb, where it can be followed from the common hepatic duct to the periampullary region. The biliary confluence is sometimes visualized from the bulb, more often with linear array echoendoscopes. The bile duct is distinguished from adjacent vessels by identifying its convergence with the pancreatic duct as both ducts taper into the duodenal wall (Fig. 51.3). The cystic duct insertion is another useful landmark. In addition, the bile duct wall has an inner hypoechoic mucosal layer that is not present in adjacent vessels. Imaging should also be performed with the endoscope opposite the ampulla in the second duodenum for detection of stones in the ampulla or periampullary bile duct.

Stones are identified as echogenic structures casting dark acoustic shadows (Fig. 51.4). Air bubbles in the duct also appear as echogenic, rounded structures, but cast hyperechoic acoustic reverberations instead of shadows. Sludge or cholesterol crystals can be visualized in the bile duct, much as they are visualized in the gallbladder (see Fig. 51.1).

Diagnosis of ductal stones is easiest when small stones are present in a dilated duct, the very situation in which cholangiography can miss stones. Conversely, sonographic diagnosis may be challenging when a diminutive duct is present or when the common duct is completely filled with stones, obliterating a visible ductal lumen. Care should be taken to visualize the entire bile duct, not skipping over portions. It is important to recognize a technically inadequate or incomplete EUS exam, and to consider

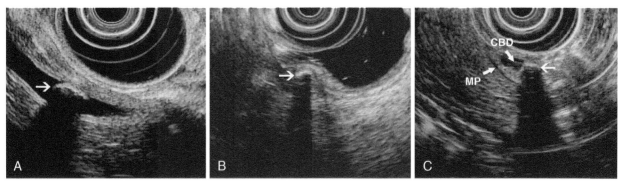

FIG 51.4 Bile duct stones *(arrows)* casting acoustic shadows. **A,** Common bile duct (CBD) stone. **B,** Ampullary stone. **C,** Ampullary stone with dilation of the obstructed intraampullary bile duct. *MP,* duodenal muscularis propria.

other imaging tests rather than concluding that no stones are present.

EUS (either radial or linear) has similar or superior sensitivity and overall accuracy for the diagnosis of bile duct stones compared to ERCP or magnetic resonance cholangiopancreatography (MRCP).[14–16] EUS appears to be more accurate for the diagnosis of stones less than 5 mm in diameter, and may also be preferable for the diagnosis of ampullary stones,[17] whereas MRCP diagnoses intrahepatic duct stones not visualized by EUS.

EUS can be used as the sole imaging study to exclude choledocholithiasis prior to laparoscopic cholecystectomy. When EUS showed no bile duct stones, recurrent symptoms due to ductal stones did not occur during almost 3 years of follow-up in a European cohort.[18] Several prospective randomized trials have compared clinical outcomes when either EUS or ERCP are used to evaluate the bile duct in patients at intermediate risk for bile duct stones, such as those with uncomplicated biliary pancreatitis or elevated serum liver tests.[19–22] Taken together, these studies show higher diagnostic accuracy, fewer overall complications, and less resource utilization in patients evaluated with EUS.[17] The majority of patients enrolled in the EUS arm of these studies did not have bile duct stones and did not require ERCP; those who did have ductal stones usually underwent ERCP immediately following EUS, under the same sedation. EUS has emerged as a preferred alternative to ERCP in patients at intermediate risk of bile duct stones, including many patients with a "positive" intraoperative cholangiogram.[23]

Biliary intraductal ultrasound (IDUS) is also accurate for diagnosis of bile duct stones and sludge. IDUS requires deep cannulation of the bile duct with the intraductal probe, which can be passed over a guidewire without sphincterotomy. Most investigators have performed IDUS after obtaining a cholangiogram during ERCP. To minimize trauma to the probe and extend its useful life, the operator should use as little elevator as possible and image only during slow probe withdrawal.

Because IDUS utilizes a high-frequency probe placed directly in the duct, it is probably the best available imaging technique for the diagnosis of small stones and ductal sludge. In one direct comparison of cholangiography and IDUS, the sensitivity of IDUS for stones was 97%, compared to 81% for ERCP.[24] Because it is performed during ERCP, IDUS is probably best used to clarify the diagnosis in patients with equivocal findings at cholangiography, such as small filling defects, possible air bubbles or polyps in the bile duct, or a dilated bile duct.[25] The use of IDUS improves diagnostic accuracy in approximately one-third

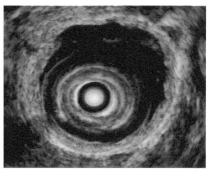

FIG 51.5 Layers of the bile duct wall as visualized by intraductal ultrasound. The inner, hypoechoic layer is markedly thickened in this patient with cholangitis. An outer hyperechoic layer is also visible. Small amounts of sludge are present in the bile duct lumen.

of these patients.[26] The need to diagnose and treat small (< 5 mm) stones detected only with IDUS has been questioned, however, because such stones often pass spontaneously.[27,28]

Direct cannulation of the papilla via a linear array echoendoscope with endosonographic confirmation of deep bile duct cannulation and subsequent sphincterotomy and stone extraction is technically feasible and appears to have similar efficacy and complications as standard ERCP for sphincterotomy and stone extraction in patients with small bile duct stones.[29] This technique may be desirable in pregnant patients, as it avoids use of fluoroscopy.

BILE DUCT STRICTURES

Biliary strictures may be of indeterminate etiology, particularly when cross-sectional imaging and intraductal biopsies and brushings obtained during ERCP are nondiagnostic. The cholangiographic appearance of a stricture and the patient's clinical history traditionally determined whether unexplained bile duct strictures should be resected on suspicion of malignancy. EUS and IDUS may be used to evaluate biliary strictures, and may aid clinical decision-making by suggesting a benign or malignant process. Endosonography can also be used for local staging of malignant biliary strictures.

The bile duct wall appears to have two or three layers on EUS and IDUS (Fig. 51.5). An internal, hyperechoic layer is sometimes seen, representing an interface echo. Deep to this layer is a hypoechoic layer corresponding to the mucosa, subepithelial connective tissue, muscularis propria, and the fibrous layer of the subserosa. The amount of muscularis varies, with little or no muscularis propria in the proximal bile duct. Deep to this hypoechoic layer is an outer hyperechoic layer formed by the adipose layer of the subserosa, the serosa, and the interface with surrounding tissue.[30] The normal bile duct wall is less than 1 mm thick on EUS,[31] although the presence of a stent or drain in the duct may lead to thickening of the wall up to 2.8 mm.[32]

The bile duct wall layers can be identified with either EUS or IDUS. IDUS probes can be passed into the central intrahepatic ducts, visualizing portions of the biliary tree not usually accessible to transduodenal EUS, and IDUS also provides high resolution images of the bile duct wall and adjacent vessels and tissue. EUS with a dedicated echoendoscope can image the extrahepatic biliary tree, including Klatskin tumors,[33] and its deeper penetration depth permits a thorough assessment of the gallbladder, pancreatic head, and regional nodes. The two techniques are complementary.

Endosonography has been used for differential diagnosis of indeterminate bile duct strictures. During IDUS, malignant strictures typically appear hypoechoic with a thickened wall and irregular margins, whereas postoperative strictures are usually relatively hyperechoic with smooth edges.[34] Importantly, both PSC and IgG4-related sclerosing cholangitis (IgG4-SC) can mimic malignant strictures on IDUS. IgG4-SC typically presents with diffuse thickening of the wall of long segments of the bile duct, including regions with no cholangiographic stricture. Studies have shown IDUS and EUS to be more accurate than ERCP and intraductal tissue sampling for the diagnosis of malignant bile duct strictures,[35–37] although these were retrospective studies that included few or no patients with PSC or IgG4-SC. In a large prospective study, IDUS was as useful as advanced cytology techniques (including fluorescent in-situ hybridization) for the diagnosis of indeterminate strictures.[38] The combination of ERCP and IDUS is reported to have superior diagnostic accuracy for indeterminate bile duct strictures compared to EUS or CT.[39] Indeterminate strictures are discussed in further detail in a later chapter of this book.

Both EUS and IDUS have been used to stage cholangiocarcinoma. The two techniques have a similar T stage diagnostic accuracy of approximately 80%, and can differentiate T1 lesions confined to the bile duct wall (involving the hypoechoic layer) from T2 lesions invading beyond the bile duct wall (with disruption of the outer hyperechoic layer) (Fig. 51.6).[30] IDUS is more useful than EUS for lesions of the proximal biliary tree. IDUS has also been used to estimate the longitudinal extent of cholangiocarcinoma because cholangiography often underestimates the longitudinal extent of ductal involvement. Unfortunately, nonspecific thickening of the bile duct wall due to the presence of a stent or drain limits the value of IDUS in previously drained patients.[40] Intravenous ultrasound contrast may improve the specificity of IDUS for malignancy, demonstrating hyperperfusion of inflammatory lesions and hypoperfusion of tumor.[41]

IDUS is probably a sensitive modality for the diagnosis of early cholangiocarcinoma in choledochal cysts. The technique should be considered in adult patients with choledochal cysts, especially if surgical resection of the cyst is not otherwise planned.

The diagnosis and staging of cholangiocarcinoma by EUS, IDUS, and EUS-FNA are discussed in detail in a later chapter.

AMPULLA OF VATER

EUS provides detailed images of the papilla of Vater. The papilla is best located during slow withdrawal of the echoendoscope from the third duodenum, using sonographic rather than endoscopic landmarks. The ventral pancreas is visualized, and the bile duct and/or pancreatic duct lumens identified. The ducts can then be traced to the duodenal wall and papilla. Administration of intravenous glucagon and instillation of water into the duodenum may improve visualization once the periampullary region has been located.

The submucosal apparatus of the papilla can be visualized as a round hypoechoic structure in the duodenal submucosa, composed of the sphincter of Oddi and the intramural ducts. This normal submucosal structure is usually 4 to 7 mm in transverse cross-sectional diameter. The lumens of the bile duct and the pancreatic duct are usually not visible within the papilla; they generally taper and disappear from view as they reach the duodenal wall. The finding of a visible ductal lumen in the papilla suggests obstruction of the papilla by a stone (see Fig. 51.3), stenosis, or tumor, but can also be seen in choledochocele (type 3 choledochal cyst) and intraductal papillary mucinous neoplasm.

IDUS has been used to study the ampulla, and may aid in the local staging of some ampullary tumors. It identifies the sphincter mechanism and permits accurate measurement of its length. Sonographic features do not distinguish normal from hypertensive sphincters.[42]

Ampullary Neoplasms

Adenomas of the papilla may occur on the duodenal surface of the papilla, within the papilla in the mucosa of the intraampullary ducts, or both. They may spread into or arise from the periampullary bile duct or pancreatic duct. EUS findings can include a mucosal mass on the duodenal surface of the papilla, enlargement of the submucosal ampullary apparatus due to intraampullary polyp, thickening of the periampullary duct walls, or the presence of an intraductal nonshadowing mass. These findings can be seen both in ampullary adenoma and in T1 ampullary cancer, and the two entities may be difficult or impossible to distinguish with EUS. We routinely perform EUS prior to ampullectomy to evaluate for intraductal extension.

The TNM staging of ampullary cancers is shown in Table 51.2 and illustrated in Fig. 51.7. T1 carcinoma may be limited to the mucosal surfaces of the ampulla and intraampullary ducts, but may also involve the sphincter mechanism of the ampulla. The presence of an irregular outer edge of the submucosal ampullary apparatus suggests a T2 lesion invading the duodenal submucosa or muscularis propria. T3 cancers invade the pancreas,

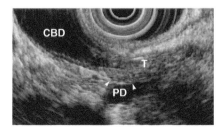

FIG 51.6 T2 distal cholangiocarcinoma. The tumor thickens the bile duct wall and focally disrupts the outer hyperechoic layer of the duct wall *(arrowheads)*. *CBD*, common bile duct; *PD*, pancreatic duct, *T*, tumor.

TABLE 51.2   Staging of Ampullary Carcinoma

TX	Primary tumor cannot be assessed		
T0	No evidence of primary tumor		
Tis	Carcinoma in situ		
T1	Tumor limited to ampulla of Vater or sphincter of Oddi		
T2	Tumor invades duodenal wall		
T3	Tumor invades pancreas		
T4	Tumor invades peripancreatic soft tissues or other adjacent organs or structures other than the pancreas		
NX	Regional lymph nodes cannot be assessed		
N0	No regional lymph node metastases		
N1	Regional lymph node metastases		
M0	No distant metastases		
M1	Distant metastases		
Stage 0	Tis	N0	M0
Stage 1A	T1	N0	M0
Stage 1B	T2	N0	M0
Stage 2A	T3	N0	M0
Stage 2B	T1–3	N1	M0
Stage 3	T4	Any N	M0
Stage 4	Any T	Any N	M1

Used with the permission of the American Joint Committee on Cancer (AJCC), Chicago, Illinois. The original source for this material is the *AJCC Cancer Staging Manual, Seventh Edition* (2009) published by Springer-Verlag New York, www.springer-ny.com.

extending either through the duodenal wall or else directly from the periampullary ducts. A T4 tumor extends into peripancreatic soft tissue or other adjacent structures. Regional lymph nodes include not only those adjacent to the pancreatic head but also the portal hepatic and celiac nodes.

In one large series, EUS accuracy for T staging of ampullary malignancies was 78%.[43] Adenomas were considered T1 lesions, highlighting the difficulty of distinguishing adenoma from T1 cancer with EUS. Most errors in staging involved overstaging of T2 lesions or understaging of T3 lesions, due to the difficulty of assessing the presence of invasion into the pancreas. The presence of peritumoral pancreatitis and edema, as well as shadowing and tissue thickening due to an indwelling biliary stent, were the major factors limiting the accuracy of EUS. Tumors may be difficult to distinguish from the normally hypoechoic ventral pancreas, and invasion of the duodenal muscularis propria may be difficult to detect because in normal anatomy the muscularis propria is interrupted by the ducts as they cross into the papilla. Despite these limitations, EUS is considerably more accurate than CT or magnetic resonance imaging (MRI).[43-45] Combined data from two centers reported the accuracy of ampullary tumor staging with multiple imaging modalities in patients with and without endobiliary stents.[46] Preoperative staging was performed in 50 consecutive patients with ampullary neoplasms by EUS plus CT (37 patients), MRI (13 patients), or angiography (10 patients) over a 3.5-year period. Of the 50 patients, 25 had a transpapillary endobiliary stent present at the time of EUS examination. EUS was shown to be more accurate than CT and MRI in the overall assessment of the T stage of ampullary neoplasms (EUS 78%, CT 24%, MRI 46%). No significant difference in N stage accuracy was noted between the

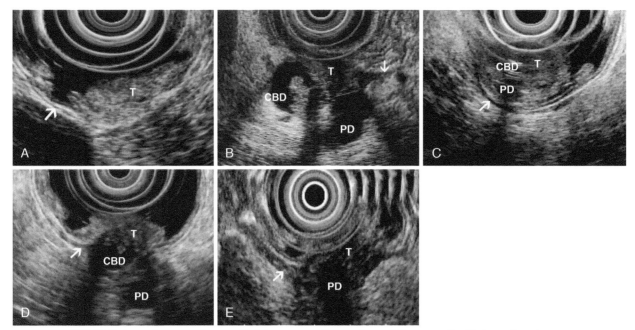

FIG 51.7 Ampullary neoplasms. **A,** Adenoma on the surface of the ampulla. **B,** Ampullary tumor extending into the distal bile duct. **C,** T1 ampullary carcinoma involving the sphincter of Oddi. This lesion was mostly adenoma but contained foci of invasive carcinoma. **D,** T2 ampullary carcinoma invading the duodenal wall. **E,** T3 ampullary carcinoma invading the pancreas. *Arrows* indicate the duodenal muscularis propria. *CBD,* common bile duct; *PD,* pancreatic duct; *T,* tumor.

three imaging modalities (EUS 68%, CT 59%, MRI 77%). EUS T stage accuracy was reduced from 84% to 72% in the presence of a transpapillary endobiliary stent. This was most prominent in the understaging of T2 and T3 carcinomas.

A study by Muthusamy et al (2001) demonstrated the role of EUS-guided FNA in the diagnosis and staging of ampullary lesions.[47] EUS-guided FNA was performed in 20 of 27 (74%) patients with suspected ampullary tumors, and made the initial ampullary tissue diagnosis in seven patients (adenocarcinoma in five patients, adenoma in one patient, neuroendocrine tumor in one patient). In addition, EUS-guided FNA resulted in a change of the diagnosis from adenoma to adenocarcinoma in one patient. In one patient, EUS-guided FNA detected a liver metastasis not seen on CT. Overall, EUS-guided FNA provided new histologic information in nine of 27 patients (33%). Another study of 35 patients who underwent EUS-guided FNA of ampullary lesions (with follow-up available in 27 patients) revealed 13 patients with adenocarcinoma, six with atypical cells (four suspicious for cancer and two consistent with reactive atypia), two with adenomas, one with carcinoid, and 13 with no evidence of malignancy. Three false-negative studies were identified, yielding a sensitivity of 82.4%, a specificity of 100%, a negative predictive value of 76.9%, and an overall accuracy of 88.8% for EUS-guided FNA in diagnosing ampullary lesions.[48]

A recent study by Ridtitid et al (2015) retrospectively evaluated 119 patients who underwent EUS for an ampullary lesion, 99 of whom had an adenoma or adenocarcinoma.[49] With surgical pathology used as the reference (n = 102), the sensitivity and specificity of EUS were 80% and 93%, respectively, and the sensitivity and specificity of ERCP were 83% and 93%, respectively; therefore they were comparable. The overall accuracy for EUS for local T and N staging was 90%.

IDUS is probably more accurate than transduodenal EUS for T staging of ampullary neoplasms. In one large series, IDUS had an overall accuracy of 89%.[44] IDUS visualized small tumors missed by EUS and was more accurate than endoscopic biopsies for diagnosis of ampullary neoplasm. IDUS was also accurate for the differentiation of adenoma from T1 carcinoma. These results were achieved by experienced endosonographers, using IDUS at the patient's initial ERCP and before sphincterotomy, stent placement, or biopsy, which is an optimal algorithm for tumor imaging, but difficult to replicate in most EUS referral centers.

ACUTE PANCREATITIS

Diagnostic EUS has two roles in patients with acute pancreatitis: the first is for timely diagnosis of common bile duct or ampullary stones in patients with acute gallstone pancreatitis, and the second is for differential diagnosis in patients with unexplained bouts of pancreatitis. In both cases, EUS can be used in place of diagnostic ERCP, and may identify those patients most likely to benefit from therapeutic ERCP.

The accuracy and cost effectiveness of EUS for the diagnosis of bile duct stones is discussed earlier in this chapter. When EUS is used to exclude ampullary stones, the ampulla must be examined from the second duodenum. A skilled examiner can perform a focused EUS of the extrahepatic bile duct in less than 10 minutes, and the patient can undergo therapeutic ERCP under the same sedation if a stone is demonstrated. This strategy allows patients with a suspected ductal stone to avoid the potential complications of ERCP if a stone is not present.

One prospective trial investigating EUS in gallstone pancreatitis reported that it was accurate for diagnosis of gallbladder and ductal stones, and predicted longer hospital stay in patients found to have peripancreatic fluid by EUS.[50] In another large series in which ERCP was used selectively on the basis of EUS findings, patient outcomes were favorable, and recurrent biliary pancreatitis was uncommon.[14]

EUS is also a useful tool in the evaluation of idiopathic pancreatitis, demonstrating abnormalities in the majority of patients.[51-53] Findings include missed biliary stones or sludge (see Fig. 51.1), chronic pancreatitis (CP), pancreas divisum, pancreatic or ampullary malignancy, and pancreatic duct stones. EUS does not diagnose pancreatic sphincter stenosis, but may nevertheless supplant ERCP by diagnosing or excluding previously unsuspected gallbladder pathology, CP, or pancreatic malignancy. EUS and MRCP appeared to have similar utility in one study, whereas others have suggested that EUS may be superior.[54-56] We feel it is best to wait until at least 4 weeks after an episode of acute pancreatitis, as acute inflammatory changes can make EUS interpretation and the detection of small tumors more challenging.

CHRONIC PANCREATITIS

The traditional endosonographic features of CP are listed in Table 51.3 and illustrated in Fig. 51.8. This list of consensus criteria uses minimal standard terminology adopted by an international working group,[57] and good interobserver agreement has been demonstrated for these criteria among experienced American endosonographers.[58] Investigators have also described other features not included in this list, including honeycombing (in which contiguous lobularity of pancreatic parenchyma forms a honeycomb pattern), heterogeneous echotexture, focal areas of hypoechogenicity, tortuous pancreatic duct, thickened pancreatic duct wall, and narrowing of the main pancreatic duct. The traditional EUS approach to the diagnosis of CP gives each feature equal weight, and sums the number of features present. The Rosemont criteria, proposed in 2009, offer an alternative approach to diagnosis based on major and minor criteria (Table 51.4).[59] The Rosemont criteria likely have higher specificity and lower sensitivity than the traditional scoring system.[60]

Definitions vary for some criteria. Hyperechoic foci have been defined greater than as g 3 mm by some investigators,[61] but as 1 to 2 mm by others.[62,63] Main pancreatic duct dilation has been variably defined, often as a diameter of greater than 2 mm in the body or greater than 1 mm in the tail.[58] The Rosemont criteria offer semiquantitative definitions for many criteria (see

TABLE 51.3 Traditional Endoscopic Ultrasound Features of Chronic Pancreatitis

Parenchymal Features	Ductal Features
Hyperechoic strands	Stones
Hyperechoic foci	Main duct irregularity
Lobularity	Hyperechoic main duct
Cysts	Visible side branches
	Main duct dilation

From The International Working Group for Minimal Standard Terminology in Gastrointestinal Endosonography: Minimal standard terminology in gastrointestinal endosonography. *Dig Endosc* 10(2):158–188, 1998.

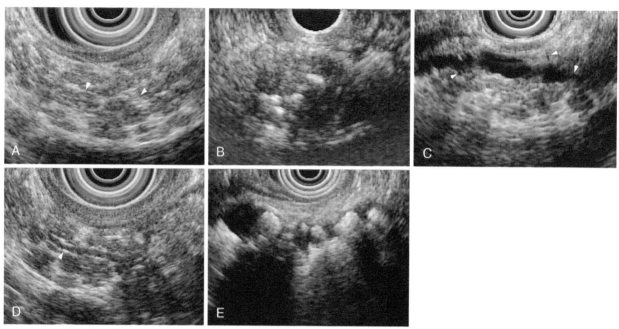

FIG 51.8 Chronic pancreatitis. **A,** Hyperechoic strands *(arrowheads)* and contiguous lobulation. **B,** Hyperechoic foci in a hypoechoic pancreas. **C,** Dilated, irregular main pancreatic duct with visible side branches *(arrowheads)*. **D,** Hyperechoic, irregular main duct wall *(arrowhead)*. **E,** Ductal stones.

TABLE 51.4   Rosemont Criteria for Diagnosis of Chronic Pancreatitis

Criterion		Definition	Criterion Weighting
Hyperechoic foci	With shadowing	Echogenic structures ≥ 2 mm in length and width that shadow	Major A
	Without shadowing	Echogenic structures ≥ 2 mm in length and width with no shadowing	Minor
Lobularity	With honeycombing	Well-circumscribed, ≥ 5 mm structures with enhancing rim and relatively echo-poor center, ≥ 3 contiguous lobules	Major B
	Without honeycombing	Well-circumscribed, ≥ 5 mm structures with enhancing rim and relatively echo-poor center, noncontiguous lobules	Minor
		Anechoic, round, or elliptical structures with or without septations	Minor
Stranding		Hyperechoic lines ≥ 3 mm in length in at least two different directions with respect to the imaged plane	Minor
MPD calculi		Echogenic structures within main pancreatic duct with acoustic shadowing	Major A
Irregular MPD contour		Uneven or irregular outline and ectatic course	Minor
Dilated side branches		≥ 3 tubular anechoic structures each measuring ≥ 1 mm in width, budding from the main pancreatic duct	Minor
MPD dilation		≥ 3.5-mm body or ≥ 1.5-mm tail	Minor
Hyperechoic MPD margin		Echogenic, distinct structure > 50% of entire main pancreatic duct in body and tail	Minor

Diagnostic Categories

Consistent with chronic pancreatitis	2 major A features, or 1 major A feature and major B feature, or 1 major A feature and ≥ 3 minor features
Suggestive of chronic pancreatitis	1 major A feature and < 3 minor features, or 1 major B and ≥ 3 minor features, or ≥ 5 minor features
Indeterminate for chronic pancreatitis	1 major B and < 3 minor features, or > 2 and < 5 minor features
Normal	< 3 minor features and no major features, dilated MPD and side branches, cysts

MPD, main pancreatic duct.
From Catalano M, et al.: EUS-based criteria for the diagnosis of chronic pancreatitis: the Rosemont classification. *Gastrointest Endosc* 69(7):1251–1261, 2009.

Table 51.4). Criteria have been considered abnormal when visualized at either 12 or 7.5 MHz by some investigators, but at only 7.5 MHz by others. Findings must be interpreted with considerable caution when imaging the pancreatic head because some features (such as hyperechoic strands, lobularity, and visible branch ducts) are often seen in the normal pancreatic head, whereas others (such as cysts and stones) are not. Diagnosis is best made based on features seen in the pancreatic body and tail. Visible duct side branches have been seen in the normal pancreatic body by some investigators.[61]

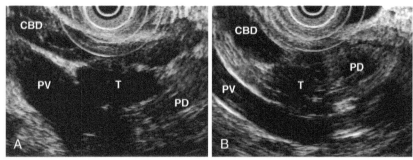

FIG 51.9 Focal pancreatitis versus pancreatic cancer. Both lesions (T) caused biliary obstruction and were resected. **A,** Focal pancreatitis. **B,** T1 pancreatic adenocarcinoma. *CBD,* common bile duct; *PD,* pancreatic duct; *PV,* portal vein.

There are caveats regarding the specificity of EUS criteria for the diagnosis of pancreatitis. EUS features of CP have been reported in members of pancreatic cancer kindreds, in whom lobularity may correlate with the presence of pancreatic intraepithelial neoplasia (PanIN) in pancreatic branch ducts.[64–66] Focal areas of pancreatic hypoechogenicity can be due to focal inflammation, but may also be due to neoplasm (Fig. 51.9). Acute pancreatitis may cause decreased parenchymal echogenicity (due to edema), accentuating the echogenicity of the pancreatic duct wall and the interlobular septa of the pancreas. When performed for diagnosis of CP, EUS should therefore be done after an acute episode of pancreatitis has resolved. Finally, some degree of ductal dilation and pancreatic fibrosis is common, and often occurs without clinical pancreatic disease.

Some EUS findings may be attributable to the effects of age, cigarettes, alcohol, and comorbidities on the pancreas, rather than CP. Although studies in healthy volunteers have generally demonstrated no parenchymal EUS abnormalities in young, asymptomatic people who do not use alcohol,[61,63,67] older patients with no history of pancreatic disease undergoing EUS for other indications had, on average, two EUS features of CP,[68] and EUS findings tend to correlate with the extent of alcohol ingestion and cigarette use.[69] Autopsy data show that pancreatic fibrosis is common in older persons, as well as in patients with diabetes, renal failure, or inflammatory bowel disease.[70,71] These histologic changes, which were termed *pancreatopathy* in the 1980s, are commonly found at autopsy in persons with no clinical history of pancreatic disease. In one small autopsy study, EUS showed CP in 90% of persons with no clinical history of pancreatic disease, and EUS findings were associated with histologic pancreatopathy.[72] A 2014 study of EUS elastography in persons with normal-appearing pancreases undergoing EUS for nonpancreatic indications found increasing pancreatic stiffness with increasing age, with overlap between age-related change and stiffness due to CP.[73] Improved methods of distinguishing pancreatopathy from CP are needed.

The accuracy of EUS for diagnosis of "early" or "minimal change" CP is debated, and EUS has been compared to pancreatography, functional tests, and histology. Early studies comparing EUS to pancreatography concluded that the presence of three or more traditional criteria was the best threshold for EUS diagnosis of CP.[61–63,74] These studies used pancreatography as a gold standard. However, the validity of pancreatography for the diagnosis of early CP is poorly established: the commonly used Cambridge criteria for pancreatogram interpretation are based on expert opinion, and autopsy studies have shown pancreato-

graphic abnormalities in the majority of persons without a clinical history of pancreatic disease.[71,75]

Histologic comparisons have reached conflicting conclusions, with retrospective studies of surgical specimens concluding that three or four EUS criteria are the best threshold for diagnosis,[76] and a prospective study of EUS fine-needle biopsy (FNB) concluding that histologic abnormalities were uncommon in persons with three or four traditional EUS criteria (see Fig. 51.9).[77] This discrepancy is most likely due both to differences in tissue sampling methods and differences in patient populations: the surgical studies included patients with pancreatic disease of sufficient magnitude to require surgery, some of whom had calcifications or pancreatic malignancies, whereas the EUS-FNB study enrolled patients with chronic abdominal pain and a paucity of other objective findings. More recently, a 2016 study of patients with presumed noncalcific CP treated with total pancreatectomy and islet autotransplantation demonstrated a poor correlation between preoperative EUS features and histologic extent of pancreatic fibrosis in the resected organ. Many subjects in that study had mild fibrosis that might be termed *pancreatopathy* rather than CP.[78]

EUS has also been compared to pancreatic function testing (PFT) and endoscopic PFT performed at the time of EUS. In populations of patients with either calcific CP or a low likelihood of CP, there is good overall correlation between the number of EUS features and the results of PFT; however, divergent results are common in patients with suspected minimal change CP. In those with divergent EUS and PFT results, it is unclear which test is more accurate.[63,79–81]

We conclude that, in some cases, EUS findings should be deemed indeterminate for CP. This category, introduced by the Rosemont criteria (which rate the presence of three or four minor criteria as indeterminate), reflects clinical and histologic realities and our current state of knowledge. In such cases, PFT, pancreatic biopsy, or repeat evaluation over time may be useful.

AUTOIMMUNE PANCREATITIS

Type 1 autoimmune pancreatitis (AIP) is a common manifestation of IgG4-related disease, and may have a variable EUS appearance. Type 1 AIP is often characterized by extensive parenchymal lymphoplasmacyctic infiltration, causing the pancreas to appear enlarged and hypoechoic on EUS, with loss of parenchymal lobulation and compression of the pancreatic duct. Long multifocal strictures of the pancreatic duct are common in Type I AIP, and may be apparent during EUS. In some cases, there is prominent infiltration around or within the main duct wall, causing a hypoechoic halo around the duct on EUS. Type 1 AIP may also present as solitary or multiple pancreatic mass lesions. Type 2 AIP, which is associated with inflammatory bowel disease and is often seen in younger patients than Type 1 AIP, may present as a focal pancreatic mass or as a diffusely abnormal pancreas, with hypoechoic enlargement of some regions and CP elsewhere. Diffuse bile duct wall thickening may suggest biliary involvement by IgG4-related disease, although this may be due to other processes, such as PSC, cholanogiocarcinoma, or the presence of a biliary stent.

EUS-guided tissue sampling is an important diagnostic tool for patients with suspected Type 1 AIP who do not otherwise meet clinical criteria for the diagnosis of IgG4-related disease. Although aspiration cytology has been deemed sufficient for diagnosis by some investigators, most favor core tissue biopsy, which allows histologic diagnosis using consensus pathologic criteria and includes quantitative analysis of tissue IgG and IgG4 immunostaining. EUS-FNB is also useful for the diagnosis of type 2 AIP, but the granulocyte epithelial lesion that is the pathognomonic histologic finding for this condition may be sparsely distributed in the lesion and missed by core biopsy samples.

EUS-GUIDED FINE-NEEDLE ASPIRATION AND BIOPSY TECHNIQUE

The technique of EUS-guided FNA has been well described in the literature.[82,83] In general, the area of interest is visualized by EUS and placed within the center (or just slightly left of center on the monitor) of the imaging field. Doppler imaging is used as needed to identify vascularity of the lesion and to assess adjacent vascular structures. A standard FNA needle, with the stylet slightly withdrawn to provide a sharp tip, is advanced into the lesion under direct ultrasound visualization, avoiding any possible intervening vascular structures. The central stylet is advanced to remove any tissue that may be present in the needle tip as a result of the transluminal puncture. The following section covers specific aspects of the FNA and biopsy technique, with a focus on pancreatic and biliary lesions.

Lesion Targeting

Generally, placing the FNA needle directly into the center of the targeted lesion is appropriate. However, this may not be the optimal technique for large tumors, especially tumors arising from the pancreas. The centers of large tumors may be necrotic, possibly from decreased oxygenation. If initial passes from the center show necrotic cells or acellular material, the endosonographer should realign the needle to target the periphery of the tumor. In addition, our experience suggests that targeting the precise site of obstruction of ductal structures provides a particularly high-quality cellular specimen.

Prioritizing Lesions for Fine-Needle Aspiration

There are situations when more than one lesion in a patient may be targeted for EUS-guided FNA. The priority and sequence for multiple lesions in a patient with a pancreatic primary are summarized in Table 51.5. The sequence priority is predicated on the principle of confirming the most advanced stage and economizing the number of passes.

If a patient has a pancreatic mass, a suspicious mediastinal lymph node, a suspicious celiac lymph node, and a lesion in the

TABLE 51.5 Sequence Priority for Endoscopic Ultrasound–Guided Fine-Needle Aspiration in a Patient With a Pancreatic Tumor

Target Site	Average Number of Passes	Sequence Priority
Mediastinal lymph nodes	2 (range 1–5)	1
Ascites or pleural fluid	1	2
Liver	2 (range 1–5)	3
Distant (e.g., celiac) lymph node	2 (range 1–10)	4
Proximal lymph node	2 (range 1–10)	5
Pancreatic tumor	3–5 (range 1–19)	6

left lobe of the liver (no ascites), the endosonographer should approach the mediastinal lesion first. If this lesion is positive for cancer, this would give the most advanced staging information (although the liver lesion would also lead to M_1 stage), and biopsy of the other lesions would not be needed. However, if this lesion is negative, biopsy of the liver lesion, followed by the celiac node, and then the pancreatic mass itself would be needed to make the diagnosis and confirm the most advanced disease stage. This sequence is also the most efficient from a technical standpoint. The most difficult lesions to obtain adequate cytologic samples from are pancreatic tumors and submucosal tumors. Lymph nodes and liver lesions are relatively easier because fewer passes are generally required to obtain an adequate sample.

Needle Selection

Needle selection for the endosonographer is often dictated by personal bias, but there are several guiding principles that should be kept in mind when decisions are being made about which needle to use for sampling a lesion. The first principle that should be considered, or the first question one should ask, is whether a good cytologic sample is desired, or if a histologic sample would better serve the patient. In most cases of pancreaticobiliary FNA, a sample that is sufficient for cytologic assessment is also sufficient to make a diagnosis and further direct the management of the patient. In several situations, however, cytologic assessment is not sufficient, and a sample that allows for assessment of both tissue architecture and cellularity is desired. Many have referred to this tissue acquisition technique as FNB, where a "core" specimen is achieved. EUS-guided FNB appears to allow improved diagnosis of AIP compared with standard EUS-FNA.[84–86] Other circumstances where using FNB to obtain a histologic core may be preferred over EUS-guided FNA include the diagnosis of well-differentiated neoplasms, lymphoma, subepithelial lesions, and neuroendocrine tumors.[84] Furthermore, it is increasingly apparent that histological core tissue is preferred over a cytological aspirate for the assessment of molecular markers that may facilitate risk stratification and tailored anticancer chemotherapy.

EUS-GUIDED FNA FOR CYTOLOGY

Needle Size

Studies regarding whether the choice of needle affects overall diagnostic yield or accuracy have had mixed results (Fig. 51.10). A study of 24 patients with solid pancreatic masses who underwent attempted tissue sampling with a 25-gauge, 22-gauge, and TruCut

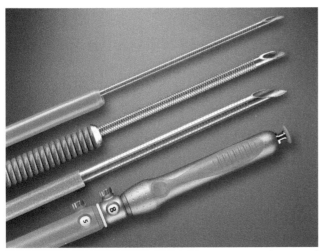

FIG 51.10 EchoTip Ultra with HD-FNA (high-definition fine-needle aspiration) (Cook Medical, Bloomington, IN). From top to bottom: 25-gauge, 22-gauge, 19-gauge, and handle. (Courtesy of Cook Medical, Bloomington, IN.)

Biopsy (TCB) (Becton, Dickinson and Company, Franklin Lakes, NJ) needle (discussed subsequently) showed similar diagnostic accuracy rates of 91.7%, 95%, and 91.7%, respectively, when technical success was achieved with each needle. However, technical success rates were significantly lower (50%) with the TCB, owing to the difficulty in accessing head and uncinate lesions using this needle, which led to overall accuracy rates of 91.7%, 79.7%, and 54.1%, respectively. These findings suggested that there is no statistically significant difference in overall diagnostic accuracy between the 25-gauge and 22-gauge needles, although the authors commented that the 25-gauge needle was easier to use and was associated with significantly higher technical success rates for uncinate lesions compared with the 22-gauge needle.[87] A similar study of 12 patients with pancreatic masses who underwent FNA with both 25-gauge and 22-gauge needles found no difference in cellularity with either needle, but three needle failures were seen in the 25-gauge group. A diagnosis was made in all cases.[88]

In contrast to these data, two larger studies have found significant improvement with the use of a 25-gauge needle in the diagnosis of solid pancreatic masses via EUS-guided FNA. The first study comprised 842 patients with pancreatic masses on EUS over a 6-year period who underwent EUS-guided FNA with a 22-gauge (n = 540) or 25-gauge (n = 302) needle. The sensitivity, specificity, positive predictive value, and negative predictive value were 84%, 100%, 100%, and 49%, respectively, for the 22-gauge group and 92%, 97%, 98%, and 89%, respectively, for the 25-gauge group. No complications were seen in the 25-gauge group; pancreatitis was reported in 2% of the 22-gauge group.[89] Our group reported on 100 patients with pancreatic masses undergoing EUS-guided FNA in two distinct time groups. The 22-gauge needle had a sensitivity, specificity, positive predictive value, and negative predictive value of 88%, 100%, 100%, and 67%, respectively, compared with 99%, 100%, 100%, and 93%, respectively, for the 25-gauge needle. In patients ultimately diagnosed with a pancreatic malignancy, 95% achieved a diagnosis within two passes using a 25-gauge needle compared with only 88% achieving a diagnosis after six passes with a 22-gauge needle. No complications occurred in either group.[90]

Both these latter studies and the randomized controlled trial suggest an 8% to 10% enhanced diagnostic yield with a 25-gauge needle. The specificity of the 25-gauge needle seems to be superior to that of the 22-gauge needle because of a reduction in the number of false negative FNA results. One theory related to this superiority for increased cytologic yield may be less blood contamination of the specimen.

Number of Passes

Pancreatic adenocarcinoma, as compared to malignant lymph nodes or liver metastases, generally requires the greatest number of FNA passes to obtain an adequate specimen; typically, approximately three to five passes are required.[91] Pancreatic tumors may have extensive fibrosis (desmoplastic reaction) or necrosis, which decreases the cellularity of malignant cells. The number of passes required for pancreatic tumors may be related to the differentiation of the tumor. A study designed to assess prospectively whether any patient or EUS characteristics could predict the number of EUS-guided FNA passes needed for diagnosis of pancreatic malignancy has been performed.[92] Among 95 patients undergoing EUS-guided FNA of a pancreatic mass, the average number of needle passes into the mass (includes head, neck, body, and tail) was 3.44 ± 2.19 (range 1–10). Tumors that were well differentiated required an average of 5.5 passes to obtain an adequate specimen; this is significantly different from the 2.7 passes needed for moderately differentiated tumors and the 2.3 passes needed for poorly differentiated tumors ($p < 0.001$).

Based on this study, it was recommended that, without a cytopathologist in attendance, five to six passes should be made for pancreatic masses. However, this approach would still be associated with a 10% to 15% reduction in definitive cytologic diagnoses, extra procedure time, increased risk, and additional needles, compared with having "real-time" cytopathology interpretations. Lymph nodes and liver lesions generally require significantly fewer passes. In an earlier series of 171 patients, the median number of passes for lymph nodes was two (range 1–10).[83] One series showed that the average number of passes for liver lesions was also two (range 1–5).[93] Lymph nodes and liver metastases generally do not exhibit the desmoplastic or necrotic reaction that is common for primary tumors of the pancreas.

Ascites and pleural fluid on average require only a single FNA pass to obtain a specimen for cytologic diagnosis.[94] The endosonographer should try to obtain as much fluid as possible (preferably > 10 mL). The fluid is spun down to concentrate the cells on a slide. Making the diagnosis of peritoneal metastasis from ascites fluid has a lower yield than solid lesions (approximately 50% false negative rate, especially with small amounts of fluid). However, a positive cytology result is still very helpful in staging the tumor as unresectable. Ascites fluid, if present, should be aspirated first before any other abdominal lesions, especially given the possibility of contamination of the ascites from other lesions if they were to undergo FNA first. In the presence of ascites, FNA of the primary pancreas tumor, lymph node metastasis, or liver metastasis theoretically could contaminate the fluid. In addition, the process of preparing cytology slides from ascitic fluid requires an additional step of concentrating the cells by centrifugation. To obtain the most relevant staging information and maximize the efficiency of FNA passes, the priority sequence for FNA is: suspicious mediastinal adenopathy, ascites, liver metastases, distant and local lymph nodes, and primary pancreatic tumor.

Needle Insertion and Fanning

The technique of needle advancement can vary considerably from very fine motion of the needle handle using only the fine motor pincher muscles of the thumb and index finger, to very large motions using a full hand grasp on the needle handle with gross motor elbow and shoulder movements similar to a downward thrust with an ice pick. The optimal technique of advancing the needle varies according to three factors: (1) the consistency of the gastrointestinal (GI) wall (wall parameter), (2) the size and consistency of the lesion targeted (lesion parameter), and (3) the proximity of surrounding vessels (vessel parameter). Table 51.6 summarizes the needle advancement technique with respect to these parameters.

The "fanning" technique for EUS-guided FNA involves sampling multiple areas within a lesion with each pass. The needle is positioned at different areas within the mass using the "up-down" dial of the echoendoscope with minimal use of the elevator. In a study by Bang et al (2013), 54 consecutive patients with solid pancreatic mass lesions were randomized to undergo EUS-FNA using either the standard or the fanning technique. There was no difference in diagnostic accuracy (76.9% vs. 96.4%; $p = 0.05$), technical failure, or complications. There was a significant difference in both the number of passes required to establish the diagnosis and the percentage of patients in whom a diagnosis was achieved on the first pass (57.7% vs. 85.7%; $p = 0.02$) between the standard and fanning groups, respectively.[95] In alignment with this study, fanning is a technique that we routinely strive for when performing FNA of pancreaticobiliary lesions.

Suction Methods

Two methods of needle suction are widely employed: syringe suction and the "slow pull" method. For syringe suction, typically, a 10-mL syringe is attached to the hub of the needle, and 5 cc of suction is applied as the needle is moved back and forth within the lesion (with typically 10–20 to-and-fro cycles used). The suction is slowly released, the needle is retracted into the catheter, and the entire assembly is removed from the biopsy channel.

Recently, a slow pull or "capillary" technique has emerged. With this technique, the slow withdrawal of the stylet from the needle serves to create negative pressure within the needle. The stylet is withdrawn by the assistant at the same distance as the needle throw of the to-and-fro action of the endosonographer. Typically, to-and-fro movements are continued within the lesion until approximately two-thirds of the entire stylet has been removed from the needle.

A recent study by Nakai et al (2014) compared the slow pull and suction techniques in patients with solid pancreatic lesions.[96] A total of 367 passes (181 by suction and 186 by the slow pull technique) were performed during 97 EUS-FNA procedures for 93 patients with solid pancreatic lesions. The slow pull technique resulted in lower scores for cellularity, but scores for contamination with blood were also lower. The sensitivity for diagnosing malignancy was higher for the slow pull technique (90.0 % vs. 67.9 %, $p < 0.01$) when a 25-gauge FNA needle was used. There were no significant differences between the two techniques when a 22-gauge needle was used.

Another technique recently described is the wet suction technique (WEST). WEST is carried out by flushing the needle with 5 mL of saline solution to replace the column of air within the lumen of needle with saline solution before needle aspiration. Attam et al (2015) conducted a study comparing the conventional technique with WEST on 117 lesions.[96a] All lesions were sampled with the same needle by using alternating techniques. Patients were randomized to WEST versus the conventional technique for the first pass. If the first pass was made with WEST, the second pass was made with the conventional technique, and subsequent passes were made in an alternating manner using the same sequence. All FNAs were performed using 22-gauge needles. WEST yielded significantly higher cellularity in a cell block compared with the conventional technique, with a mean cellularity score of 1.82 ± 0.76 versus 1.45 ± 0.768 ($p < 0.0003$). The WEST cell block resulted in a significantly better specimen adequacy of 85.5% versus 75.2% ($p < 0.035$). There was no difference in the amount of blood contamination between the two techniques.

One important strategy to keep in mind when performing FNA is to adjust technique through the course of the passes to optimize the sample. After the first pass, one should assess the gross specimen and make adjustments based on the appearance of the sample yielded. For a specimen that is too bloody, consider using the slow pull technique or no suction at all. For a specimen that has too few cells, consider more to-and-fro movements, attempt more of a fanning technique, or switch to WEST.

TABLE 51.6 Needle Advancement Technique for Endoscopic Ultrasound–Guided Fine-Needle Aspiration

Wall Parameter	Lesion Parameter	Vessel Parameter	Needle Advancement Technique	Difficulty Level
Thin wall, taut (e.g., esophagus)	Small (e.g., lymph node)	Vessel immediately behind lesion	Very fine, slow pincer movements	Moderate
Thin wall, taut	Large (e.g., tumor)	No adjacent vessel	Slow, moderate movements	Easy
Thick wall, elastic (e.g., gastric fundus)	Small lesion or scant fluid	Vessel immediately behind lesion	Consider puncturing through stomach first (adjacent to lesion) with a very quick dartlike motion (or use spring-loaded device), then fine pincer movements to target lesion	Difficult
Thick wall, elastic	Large	No adjacent vessel	Very quick dartlike motion using wrist action directly into lesion	Moderate
Duodenum	Small	Adjacent vessel	Quick, pincer movement to avoid pushing scope tip away	Difficult
Duodenum	Large, firm tumor	No adjacent vessel	Very quick, hand grasp with elbow and shoulder "ice pick" motion	Difficult

Rapid On-Site Evaluation and Macroscopic On-Site Evaluation

The importance of dynamic Real-Time On-Site Evaluation (ROSE) for cytologic interpretation has been debated recently. Earlier studies have emphasized its importance,[83,97–99] and showed that centers with an attendant cytopathologist had higher cytologic yield and diagnostic accuracy compared with centers that performed passes on an empiric basis. Increasing the number of empiric passes may increase cytologic accuracy, but at the expense of performing unnecessary passes with associated cost, time, and safety issues. One study described the experience of a single endosonographer practicing in two clinical sites, one with an attendant cytopathologist and one without.[99] In the site without an attendant cytopathologist, 17% of patients required repeat procedures, compared with 2% of patients requiring repeat procedures at the site where a cytopathologist was present ($p = 0.015$). Recently, Wani et al (2015) conducted a multicenter randomized controlled trial in which 241 consecutive patients with solid pancreatic masses underwent randomization to EUS-FNA with or without ROSE. The number of FNA passes in the ROSE+ arm was dictated by the on-site cytopathologist, whereas seven passes were performed in ROSE– arm. There was no difference between the two groups in terms of the diagnostic yield of malignancy (ROSE+ 75.2% vs. ROSE– 71.6%, $p = 0.45$) or the proportion of inadequate specimens (9.8% vs. 13.3%, $p = 0.31$). Although procedures in ROSE+ group required fewer EUS-FNA passes (medians: 4 vs. 7, $p < 0.0001$), there was no significant difference between the two groups with regard to the quality of the specimens, overall procedure time, adverse events, number of repeat procedures, or costs.[100]

A more recent concept for on-site evaluation of an FNA specimen is Macroscopic On-Site Evaluation (MOSE). With MOSE, the tissue adequacy is determined based on the macroscopic appearance of the specimen obtained, usually by the endoscopist. There is no cytology technologist needed, and there is no staining or microscopy performed in the room (as is done for ROSE). MOSE has the potential to decrease cost and time. Studies evaluating the feasibility of MOSE have yielded mixed results. A study by Nguyen et al (2009) evaluated MOSE performed by both experienced EUS technologists and cytotechnologists of 22-gauge FNA specimens of pancreatic tumors.[101] Only fair agreement was observed between cytotechnologists and EUS technologists versus final cytopathologic assessment of adequacy (κ0.20 and 0.19, respectively). More recently, however, Iwashita et al (2015) conducted a study to assess the efficacy of MOSE in estimating the adequacy of histologic core specimens obtained by EUS-FNA using a standard 19-gauge needle in 111 solid lesions. MOSE revealed macroscopic visible core (MVC) in 91.1% of lesions with a median length of 8 mm. Histologic core was confirmed in 78.9%. Comparisons of per-pass diagnostic yields showed significantly superior histologic, cytologic, and overall diagnostic yields in MVCs greater than 4 mm in length as compared to cores of less than 4 mm.[102] The difference in the results from these studies may be due to the different needles used and the ability of the larger needle to obtain a specimen where macroscopically visible cores were identified. Further study of MOSE is warranted.

Specimen Handling

There is significant variation in how FNA specimens are processed. In general, for a cytologic specimen, the aspirated material is expressed onto glass slides using an air-filled syringe or by reintroducing the stylet back into the needle. For each pass, a set of two slides is processed: a few drops of specimen are expressed onto a slide and smeared with a second slide. One slide is air-dried and evaluated using a Diff-Quik/modified Wright-Giemsa stain by a nearby cytopathologist in centers where ROSE is available. The other slide is wet-fixed in alcohol for later evaluation using the Papanicolaou stain. Residual material that is present within the needle is then expressed into a formalin container, which is collected and later processed into a cell block.

EUS-FNB FOR HISTOLOGY

Needle Type

The needles discussed thus far have been judged based on their ability to provide cytologic yield. In 2002, a new needle entered into the armamentarium: the TCB needle (Becton, Dickinson and Company) (Fig. 51.11). This needle, which contains an 18-mm tissue tray, allows for histologic, rather than cytologic, analysis owing to the ability of EUS-guided TCB to obtain tissue cores. Overall, EUS-guided TCB performance for pancreaticobiliary lesions has been poor, largely due to difficulties with deployment. As mentioned earlier, a comparative study of 25-gauge, 22-gauge, and TCB needles in 24 patients with solid pancreatic lesions showed that EUS-guided TCB achieved the lowest accuracy rates, a result almost entirely due to the fact that EUS-guided TCB was deployed successfully in only 11 of 24 patients and in only one of 12 patients with head or uncinate lesions.[87] The most recent and largest study (2009) of 113 patients undergoing EUS-guided TCB of pancreatic lesions also showed that EUS-guided TCB had a relatively poor sensitivity and overall diagnostic accuracy of 62% and 67.5%, respectively.[103]

To overcome some of the limitations encountered with the TCB design, new dedicated FNB needles have been developed. One such design includes reverse-bevel technology (ProCore; Cook Endoscopy, Bloomington, IN), and is currently available in three gauges: 19, 22, and 25 (Fig. 51.12). The needle has a lateral opening of varying lengths (depending on the gauge) in its shaft, as well as a reverse bevel that hooks and cuts the tissue and traps it in the needle during the FNA motion. However, unlike the TCB needle, the ProCore design does not rely on an

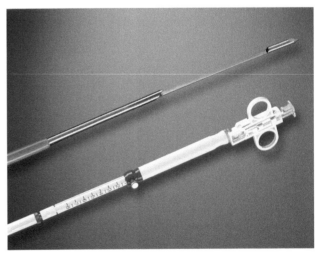

FIG 51.11 Quick-Core (Cook Medical, Bloomington, IN) 19-gauge needle (tip, above; handle, below). (Courtesy of Cook Medical, Bloomington, IN.)

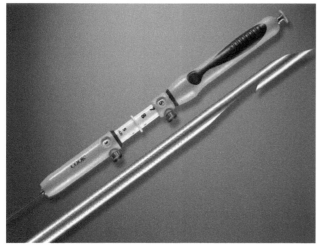

FIG 51.12 ProCore (Cook Medical, Bloomington, IN) 19-gauge needle (handle, above; tip below). (Courtesy of Cook Medical, Bloomington, IN.)

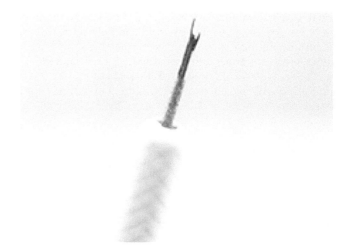

FIG 51.13 SharkCore needle (Medtronic, Dublin, Ireland). (Courtesy of Medtronic, Dublin, Ireland.)

in-built cutting mechanism, and is therefore less stiff and more maneuverable when performing FNA, especially within the duodenum. It was hypothesized that the ProCore needle design would yield a large piece of core tissue with preserved morphological (histological) architecture that would have significant advantages over the standard FNA (cytological) needle by resulting in superior diagnostic accuracy with possibly fewer passes.

A 2016 prospective multicenter randomized controlled trial evaluated the histologic diagnostic yield comparing a standard 25-gauge FNA needle with a 25-gauge ProCore needle for pancreatic masses.[104] Two hundred and fourteen consecutive patients with solid pancreatic masses who presented to eight Japanese referral centers for EUS-FNA were randomized to undergo sampling with a 25-gauge needle with a core trap (ProCore) or a standard 25-gauge needle. Tissue samples were fixed in formalin and processed for histologic evaluation. For the purposes of the study, only samples obtained with the first needle pass were processed for evaluation of diagnostic accuracy of malignancy, preserved tissue architecture adequate for histologic evaluation, and sample cellularity. Compared to the first pass with a standard needle (n = 108), the first pass with the ProCore needle (n = 106) provided samples that were more often adequate for histologic evaluation (81.1% vs. 69.4%; $p = 0.048$) and had superior cellularity (rich/moderate/poor, 36%/27%/37% vs. 19%/26%/55%; $p = 0.003$). There were no significant differences between the two needles in terms of sensitivity (75.6% vs. 69.0%, $p = 0.337$) and accuracy (79.2% vs. 75.9%, $p = 0.561$) for the diagnosis of malignancy.

A recent systematic review and meta-analysis was conducted by Bang et al (2016) to compare the performance of the ProCore and standard FNA needles when performing EUS-guided tissue acquisition of mostly pancreatic lesions, and showed slightly less favorable results.[105] Nine studies (including a total of 576 patients) met the inclusion criteria. There was no significant difference in diagnostic adequacy (75.2% vs. 89.0%, odds ratio [OR] 0.39, $p = 0.23$), diagnostic accuracy (85.8% vs. 86.2%, OR 0.88, $p = 0.53$), or rate of histological core specimen acquisition (77.7% vs. 76.5%, OR 0.94, $p = 0.85$) between the ProCore and standard FNA needles, respectively. The mean number of passes required for diagnosis, however, was significantly lower when using the

ProCore needle (standardized mean difference: −1.2, $p < 0.001$). Criticisms of the meta-analysis included the small number of studies that met the inclusion criteria, the heterogeneity in the definitions and design of the studies selected, and the inclusion of studies that did not use the 19-gauge ProCore needle.

More recently, another histology needle with a novel fork-tip needle, the SharkCore (SC) (Medtronic Corp., Dublin, Ireland), has been released for clinical use (Fig. 51.13). This needle does not have a side bevel, and its unique design is largely related to the six cutting edges on its tip. Early studies show promising results with improved histologic yield compared to standard FNA needles. Kandel et al (2016) conducted a retrospective case-control study whereby consecutive samples from EUS-FNB-SCs were matched in a 1 : 3 ratio by lesion site (e.g., pancreatic head) and needle gauge (i.e., 19-guage, 22-gauge, 25-gauge) to recent random samples taken by EUS-FNA. The procedures were performed with ROSE. For study purposes, the specimen slides were evaluated by two cytopathologists for histologic yield using a standard scoring system (0 = no material, 1–2 = cytologic, 3–5 = histologic). The main objectives were to assess the histologic yield of the samples and to compare the median number of passes required to obtain core tissue by using EUS-FNB-SC and EUS-FNA needles. Of the 156 patients included in the study, 39 were in the EUS-FNB-SC group, and 117 were in the EUS-FNA group. According to standard scoring criteria for histology, the median histology score for EUS-FNA was 2 (sufficient for cytology but not histology), and the median histology score for EUS-FNB-SC was 4 (sufficient for adequate histology). Ninety-five percent of the specimens obtained from the EUS-FNB-SC group were of sufficient size for histologic screening, compared with 59% from the EUS-FNA group ($p = 0.01$). The median number of passes required to achieve a sample was significantly lower in the EUS-FNB-SC group compared with the EUS-FNA group (two passes vs. four passes, $p = 0.001$). There was a significant difference in the median number of passes made at all lesion sites and with all needle gauges.[106]

EUS-FNB Technique

The optimal technique for acquiring a histologic sample using EUS-FNB is different from what has been described thus far for cytologic sampling. When a pancreatic lesion undergoes EUS-FNB, based on our experience, we believe the following technical aspects should be kept in mind. The initial forward thrust into the lesion is very important and should be rapid and deliberate, whereas the repetitive to-and-fro movements may be of less importance. Fanning is often more difficult with EUS-FNB, and should not be the goal for EUS-FNB. Both high dry suction and WEST appear to be more effective than the slow pull technique for EUS-FNB.

Complications of EUS-Guided FNA of Pancreaticobiliary Lesions

An important part of maximizing the yield of EUS-guided FNA is being aware of and avoiding potential complications. These complications include pancreatitis, bleeding, infection, seeding of malignant cells, and bile peritonitis. Initial data on the overall complication rates of EUS-guided FNA came from three large published series comprising more than 1000 patients.[83,107,108] One multicenter trial showed that complications associated with the procedure (457 patients) seem to arise predominantly from infectious or hemorrhagic events after puncturing pancreatic cystic lesions.[83] Five nonfatal complications occurred, for a rate of 0.5% (95% confidence interval [CI] 0.1%–0.8%) in solid lesions versus 14% (95% CI 6%–21%) in cystic lesions ($p <$ 0.001). Another single-institution study of 333 patients who underwent EUS-guided FNA reported only one complication (0.3%): streptococcal sepsis after puncture of a cystic pancreatic lesion.[109] A small risk (1 in 121 patients) of developing pancreatitis after EUS-guided FNA of the pancreas has been reported.[110] The overall risk with FNA is extremely low. Several more recent studies have reported on the specific risks of FNA of pancreaticobiliary lesions, and are discussed in the following sections.

The overall risk of pancreatitis from EUS-guided FNA appears to be less than 1%. A large retrospective series of 4909 patients undergoing EUS-guided FNA of solid pancreatic lesions from 19 centers over a 4-year period showed a 0.29% risk of pancreatitis.[111] This risk was 0.64% from the two centers that prospectively collected data and 0.26% from the 17 centers that retrospectively collected data, suggesting an underreporting of complications in the latter group. A subsequent prospective single-center study by the same lead author revealed a pancreatitis rate for solid pancreatic lesions of 0.85% (3 in 355).[112] The rates of pancreatitis are similarly low for cystic lesions; a large study of 603 patients with 651 pancreatic cysts undergoing EUS-guided FNA revealed only six cases of pancreatitis (0.92%) and an overall complication rate of only 2.2%.[113] Similarly, the complication rate from EUS-guided TCB is less than 2%, and is not significantly different from that for EUS-guided FNA.

Hemorrhage is a rare complication of EUS and EUS-guided FNA. Gress et al (1997)[110] initially reported two cases of hemorrhage (resulting in one death) in 208 patients who underwent 705 FNA passes using both radial and linear echoendoscopes. In both cases, EUS was performed using a radial echoendoscope, which precluded visualization of the needle tip during FNA. In one case, bleeding extended into the gastric lumen, whereas bleeding occurred in the pancreatic head region in the other case.

A 2005 study from Denmark reported on 3324 consecutive patients who underwent EUS procedures using curvilinear echoendoscopes over an 11-year period, of which 670 underwent EUS-guided FNA and 136 received EUS-guided interventions.[114] Only a single case of GI bleeding was reported in a patient with widespread pancreatic cancer who died 6 hours after EUS-guided FNA from massive GI bleeding. However, at autopsy, the FNA

puncture site showed no signs of bleeding and no vessels in the puncture route, and the cause of bleeding could not be established.

Limited data on extramural hemorrhage exist. One study reported that 3 of 227 patients (1.3%) undergoing FNA had extraluminal hemorrhage at the site of aspiration.[115] The bleeding lesions included a large pancreatic islet cell tumor, a benign lymph node in a patient with esophageal cancer, and a recurrent benign pancreatic cyst in a patient with a history of a mucinous cystadenoma that had been surgically resected. The authors described the bleeding as an expanding echo-poor region adjacent to the sampled lesions, although no clinically recognized sequelae of bleeding were noted. No predictive factors for bleeding were identified. The investigators applied pressure at the puncture site via balloon inflation and echoendoscope tip deflection for 15 to 25 minutes, although it is unclear if this had a tamponade effect on the extraluminal bleeding.

A case of self-limited retroperitoneal bleeding after EUS-guided FNA of the pancreas has also been reported.[116] Self-limited intracystic hemorrhage after EUS-guided FNA of pancreatic cysts has been reported to occur in 6% (3 of 50) patients in one series,[117] and clinically evident hemosuccus pancreaticus has also been observed after EUS-guided FNA of a pancreatic cyst.[118] However, a more recent and larger series of 651 cysts undergoing EUS-guided FNA revealed only a single retroperitoneal bleed.[113] These data indicate that clinically significant bleeding after EUS-guided FNA of solid or cystic pancreaticobiliary lesions is extremely uncommon with current techniques.

As stated previously, EUS-guided FNA seems primarily to be associated with infectious complications when cystic lesions are aspirated. Initial studies reported infectious complications in 14% (3 of 22) of patients undergoing EUS-guided FNA of pancreatic cystic lesions.[83] As a result, routine preprocedure and postprocedure antibiotic prophylaxis was adopted for FNA of such lesions. A single case of streptococcal sepsis after EUS-guided FNA of a pancreatic cystadenoma was reported in a large single-center report of 317 patients undergoing FNA of 327 sites[107]; this infection occurred despite the use of prophylactic antibiotics, and corresponded to an infectious complication rate of 0.3%. Fever, although infrequent, has also been reported in several studies after EUS-guided FNA. Chang et al (1997) reported one patient out of 44 (2%) undergoing EUS-guided FNA for pancreatic lesions who developed fever after sampling of a pancreatic cystic lesion.[119] This patient did not receive antibiotics before FNA.

Another series showed that two patients developed fever and infection out of 355 patients with solid pancreatic masses undergoing EUS-guided FNA, yielding an infectious complication rate of 0.56%.[112] One of these patients had cystic spaces within a pancreatic adenocarcinoma, and the other, who required surgical débridement, had acute pancreatitis with a focal lesion in the pancreatic tail. Bournet et al (2006)[120] reported 1 patient out of 224 undergoing EUS-guided FNA (0.45%) who developed fever and abdominal pain after aspiration of a mucinous cystadenoma, despite administration of antibiotics before the procedure. Similarly, Lee et al (2005)[113] reported 1 out of 603 patients undergoing aspiration of 651 pancreatic cysts who developed fever, pain, and leukocytosis, although it is unclear if this patient received antibiotics before the procedure. As a result of these data, current guidelines recommend the use of antibiotic prophylaxis for planned FNA of any cystic lesion, but not for solid pancreaticobiliary lesions.

The risk of malignant seeding from EUS-guided FNA is also believed to be very low. However, a case of focal gastric intramural recurrence at the site of an EUS-guided FNA of a pancreatic tail lesion that underwent distal pancreatectomy was reported 21 months after a surgical resection with negative margins.[121] Although seeding may occur with this technique, EUS-guided FNA seems to have a significantly lower potential for peritoneal seeding (2.2% vs. 16.3%) compared with CT-guided FNA, as mentioned earlier in the section on EUS-guided FNA of pancreatic lesions.[122]

Conclusions

EUS-guided FNA is extremely useful in the diagnosis and staging of pancreaticobiliary lesions such as pancreatic cancers (with associated lymph nodes, liver metastasis, and ascites), cystic tumors, neuroendocrine neoplasms, ampullary cancers, and cholangiocarcinomas. In addition, this technique has been extended via techniques such as EUS-guided fine-needle injection (FNI) into therapeutic modalities such as celiac plexus or ganglion block, cyst gastrostomy, achieving pancreaticobiliary access and drainage, assisting in or delivering radiation therapy, and delivering antitumor agents.

EUS-GUIDED FINE-NEEDLE THERAPY

The advent of linear EUS in the 1990s transformed EUS from a purely diagnostic modality into a platform for advanced diagnostic and therapeutic applications. EUS-FNA has brought us the ability to access countless anatomic sites to sample tumors and lymph nodes, as well as drain cysts and fluid collections. The development of EUS-guided celiac ganglion neurolysis (CGN) started a new era in EUS-guided techniques, where the fine needle has become the vehicle for delivery of various ablative agents, chemotherapeutic agents, radio-opaque markers, and miniature devices. The following is a brief overview of some of the mainstream and upcoming applications of EUS-guided fine-needle therapy for pancreatic and biliary disease.

EUS-Guided Celiac Plexus and Ganglia Interventions

Chronic abdominal pain is a common and debilitating symptom for patients with CP and pancreatic cancer. The etiology of pancreatic pain is multifactorial, and can be attributed to multiple causes, such as increased intrapancreatic pressure, pancreatic ischemia, fibrosis, pseudocysts, and neurogenic inflammation, as well as the invasion of pancreatic perineural space by cancer cells.[123] The current pharmacologic management for pancreatic pain involves starting with nonopioid analgesics, such as nonsteroidal antiinflammatory drugs, and progressing to increasing doses of opioid analgesics.[124] However, opioids often provide suboptimal pain relief, and their use is limited by side effects such as constipation, nausea, confusion, somnolence, addiction, and impaired immune function.[125,126] Sympathetic nerves innervating the pancreas pass through the celiac plexus, and celiac plexus neurolysis (CPN) can be performed with the goal of improving pain control, increasing quality of life (QOL), and reducing the risk of drug-induced side effects.

Relevant Anatomy

The celiac plexus is comprised of a dense network of ganglia and interconnecting fibers, is located caudal to the diaphragm (in an antecrural position), and surrounds the origin of the celiac trunk. Celiac ganglia vary in number (usually 1–5), size (0.5–4.5 cm) and location (T12–L2).[127] The celiac plexus transmits pain sensations from the pancreas and most of the abdominal viscera, except for the left colon, rectum, and pelvic organs.[128] The neurons that innervate the pancreas can receive nociceptive stimulation and then transmit this pain information to the celiac plexus.[125]

Non-EUS Methods for Celiac Plexus Neurolysis and Celiac Plexus Block

CPN and CPB can be performed percutaneously, surgically, or under EUS guidance. The retrocrural approach involves injecting the solution, which diffuses over the splanchnic nerves. The anterocrural approach, or "true" CPN, involves injection anterior to the diaphragm, thereby causing the solution to diffuse over the celiac ganglia.

Efficacy studies on percutaneous guided celiac plexus neurolysis (PQ CPN) for patients with pancreatic cancer have shown mixed results, but overall have demonstrated some benefit with fairly low risk. A 2011 Cochrane meta-analysis evaluated six randomized trials of 358 patients undergoing PQ CPN for pancreatic cancer pain.[129] At both 4 weeks and 8 weeks, patients in the treatment arm had significant improvement in pain compared with the control arm. Furthermore, opioid consumption was significantly lower in the treatment arm. In another meta-analysis by Eisenberg et al (1995) of 24 studies with 1145 patients treated with PQ CPN for palliation of cancer pain (of which 63% were pancreatic cancer patients), good to excellent pain relief was noted in 70% to 90% of patients up to 3 months after the procedure, regardless of which type of percutaneous technique was used.[130]

Patient Preparation and Technique for the EUS-Guided Approach

Early on, linear array echoendoscopic imaging from the proximal posterior stomach was shown to demonstrate superb visualization of the aorta and the take-off of the celiac artery, which is often regarded as "home base" for novice endosonographers, given its reproducibility as a landmark in nearly all patients. As a result, development of an EUS-guided technique for celiac neurolysis became a logical next step.

EUS-guided CPN is usually performed in the outpatient setting, and sometimes during the index examination conducted for the purpose of pancreatic cancer diagnosis and staging. Contraindications to CPN in our practice include uncorrectable coagulopathy (international normalized ratio > 1.5), thrombocytopenia (platelets < 50,000/L), inadequate hydration, and altered anatomy prohibiting visualization or access to the celiac plexus/ganglia. Patients are initially hydrated with 500 to 1000 mL of normal saline to minimize the risk of hypotension. The procedure is performed with the patient in the left lateral decubitus position under moderate sedation or anesthesia. Continuous monitoring is necessary during and for 2 hours after the procedure. Before discharge, the blood pressure is rechecked in a supine and erect position to assess for orthostasis.[125] There is little evidence to support the administration of prophylactic antibiotics after CPN, thus we do not routinely administer postprocedure antibiotics in our practice.

The most widely performed approach to EUS-guided CPN involves diffuse injection into the region of the celiac plexus.[131] Linear array endosonographic imaging from the posterior lesser curve of the gastric fundus allows identification of the aorta, which appears in a longitudinal plane. The aorta is traced distally to the celiac trunk, which is the first major branch below the diaphragm. Targeting with CPN is based on the expected location of the celiac plexus relative to the celiac trunk, and Doppler

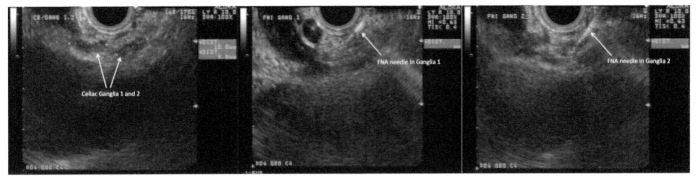

FIG 51.14 EUS-guided direct injection of alcohol and Marcaine (Hospira, Inc., Lake Forest, IL) solution into two celiac ganglia in a patient with pancreatic cancer. *FNA,* fine-needle aspiration.

should be used to clearly delineate vascular structures. In our practice, a standard 22-gauge needle without stylet is primed with the injectate, advanced through the scope working channel, and affixed at the inlet. The needle is inserted under EUS guidance immediately adjacent and anterior to the lateral aspect of the aorta at the level of the celiac trunk. An aspiration test is performed to rule out vascular penetration prior to each injection. For patients with pancreatic cancer, typically a premixed 10 to 20 mL solution of 98% dehydrated alcohol and 0.75% Marcaine (Hospira, Inc., Lake Forest, IL) in a 70:30 ratio is injected (see Table 51.1). When performing CPN, we inject bilaterally with a modified technique, with half the volume on the left side of the celiac take-off and the remainder at the midline of the take-off. Our rationale for the modified technique is that the right side of the celiac artery is not as accessible, given the slight tilt of the artery relative to the scope position. Therefore left and midline are the preferred areas for injection. Some prefer to inject at a single site, usually midline. The practice of bilateral injection has been supported by several studies, including a 2009 meta-analysis that reported the proportion of patients with initial pain relief as 84.5% with bilateral injection compared to 45.9% for unilateral (midline) injection.[132,133] However, a 2013 study including 53 patients showed no difference in efficacy with bilateral versus unilateral injection.[134]

An alternative approach that has been described, which may be more applicable to advanced abdominal cancer, is EUS-guided broad plexus neurolysis (BPN). In this technique, the injection is performed at the level of the superior mesenteric artery, resulting in a broader distribution of neurolysis. A study by Sakamoto et al (2010) of 67 patients showed that BPN had significantly better 7-day and 30-day pain relief scores as compared to conventional EUS-CPN.[135]

EUS-Guided Direct Celiac Ganglion Neurolysis

Recently, it has been recognized that the individual celiac ganglia can be visualized and accessed by EUS, allowing for direct injection into the individual celiac ganglia to perform CGN. The celiac ganglia are typically oval or almond-shaped, range in size from 2 to 20 mm, and are most readily detected to the left of the celiac artery, anterior to the aorta. Compared to the surrounding retroperitoneal fat, the ganglia are echo-poor and often display similar echogenicity to the left adrenal gland. Central echo-rich strands and foci are often present within the ganglia, and the margins of the ganglia are irregular. Color Doppler demonstrates little to no flow within these structures. Ganglia are detected by

EUS in 81% to 89% of patients.[136] Our approach is to always perform CGN rather than CPN if ganglia are visualized.

All aspects of the procedure, including patient candidacy, sedation, antibiotic use, and follow-up, are the same as for standard CPN. The technique for CGN and the volume of solution injected have not been standardized. Our approach is to target as many ganglia as possible by injecting a total of 10 to 20 mL of premixed alcohol and bupivacaine (mixture as outlined previously) among all the ganglia in amounts relative to their size (Fig. 51.14). For example, if there are three ganglia visualized (small, medium, and large), we would typically inject 5 mL in the largest ganglion, 3 mL in the medium-sized ganglion, and 2 mL in the small ganglion. For larger ganglia, we typically advance the needle tip into the deepest point within the ganglion and then inject while slowly withdrawing the needle, creating an even distribution of injectate throughout the ganglion. For smaller ganglia, we usually target the ganglion's center. During injection, a clear "ballooning" of the ganglia should be visualized; otherwise, needle placement is considered suboptimal. Each ganglion can be injected until injectate is seen spilling from the ganglion into adjacent soft tissue. After injecting each visualized ganglion, the remaining injectate can be injected adjacent to the celiac or superior mesenteric arteries, as described earlier.

Clinical Trial Data

The clinical trial data for CGN and CPN for patients with pancreatic cancer are summarized in Table 51.7. There is great variability among studies in terms of injection technique, type of injectate and volume, definition of pain relief, and follow-up. Most studies are small retrospective studies with short follow-up.

For CPN, partial pain relief has been reported in 50% to 78% of patients within the first 4 weeks.[133,135,137–139] A meta-analysis including 119 patients found that EUS-CPN alleviated abdominal pain in 73% of patients.[140] In a randomized trial, 96 patients with inoperable pancreatic cancer were randomized to conventional pain management or EUS-CPN. At 3 months, patients treated with CPN had greater pain relief with a trend toward lower morphine consumption, although no difference was observed in QOL.[141]

For CGN, partial pain relief has been reported in 65% to 94% of patients.[142–144] In the only prospective trial to date comparing CGN to CPN, 68 patients with upper abdominal cancer (over 85% had pancreatic cancer) were randomly assigned to treatment using either EUS-CGN or EUS-CPN with one midline

TABLE 51.7   Clinical Trial Data for Endoscopic Ultrasound-Guided Celiac Neurolysis

Study	Design	n	Injection Site	Injectate	Pain Relief (% of Patients)	Complications
Doi et al. 2013[142]	Prospective	68	Ganglia vs. plexus	1–2 mL bupivacaine 0.25–0.5% 10–20 mL alcohol	73.5% vs. 45.5% Partial 50% vs. 18.2% Complete	Hypotension 2.9% vs. 6.0% UGI Bleed 2.9% vs. 0% Pain exacerbation 29.4% vs 21.2%
Seicean et al. 2013[139]	Retrospective	32	Plexus	10 mL bupivacaine 1% 10–15 mL alcohol	75%	None stated
LeBlanc et al. 2011	Prospective	50	Plexus 1 vs. 2 injections	20 mL bupivacaine 0.75% 10 mL alcohol 98%	69% vs. 81%	Hypotension 2% Pain exacerbation 33%
Iwata et al. 2011	Retrospective	47	Plexus	2–3 mL bupivacaine < 20 mL alcohol	68%	Hypotension 17% Diarrhea 23% Transient inebriation 9%
Ascunce et al.[144]	Retrospective	64	Ganglia vs. plexus (bil)	10 mL lidocaine 1% 20 mL alcohol 98%	65% vs. 25%	Hypotension 2% Pain exacerbation 2% Diarrhea 23%
Sakamoto et al. 2010	Retrospective	67	Plexus (bil) vs. broad plexus (around SMA)	3 mL lidocaine 1% 9 mL alcohol 1 mL contrast	50% vs. 76%	No major complications
Sahai et al. 2009	Prospective	160	Plexus (central) vs. plexus (bil)	10 cc bupivacaine 0.5% 20 cc alcohol	50.7% vs. 77.5%	Retroperitoneal bleed 0.7%
Levy et al. 2008	Retrospective	17	Ganglia	8 mL bupivacaine 0.25% 12 mL alcohol 99%	94%	Hypotension 35% Pain exacerbation 41%
Gunaratnum et al 2001	Prospective	58	Plexus (bil)	6–12 mL bupivacaine 0.25% 20 mL alcohol 98%	78%	Hypotension 20% Pain exacerbation 9% Diarrhea 17%

SMA, superior mesenteric artery; *UGI,* upper gastrointestinal.

injection. The positive response rate was significantly higher in the EUS-CGN group (73.5%) than in the EUS-CPN group (45.5%). The complete response rate was also significantly higher in the EUS-CGN group (50%) than in the EUS-CPN group (18.2%). There was no difference in adverse events or duration of pain relief between the groups.[142] Follow-up was only 7 days, and much longer-term follow-up studies are needed, as well as comparison with bilateral EUS-CPN injections.

Complications

Most complications related to CPN and CGN are transient, and serious complications are rare. The most common side effects reported are transient hypotension (up to 35%), diarrhea (up to 20%), and transient exacerbation of pain following the procedure, which are consistent with rates seen with the PQ approach.[130] Hypotension and diarrhea are related to sympathetic blockade and the relative unopposed visceral parasympathetic activity. Hypotension generally responds to intravenous fluid administration. The diarrhea related to this procedure is usually self-limiting, and typically resolves in less than 48 hours. CPN via a PQ approach has been associated with a 2% rate of serious complications, including neurologic complications (lower extremity weakness, paresthesia, paralysis), pain (pleuritic chest, shoulder), pneumothorax, and hiccupping.[130] A very small number of serious complications (≤ 0.6%), including fatalities and paralysis (mainly with alcohol injection), have been reported with the EUS approach in case report and abstract form.[145,146] Serious infections including retroperitoneal abscess and empyema have occurred, as well as severe ischemic damage to abdominal organs.

EUS-Guided Radiofrequency Ablation

Image-guided radiofrequency ablation (RFA) is a well-recognized minimally invasive treatment modality in oncology, one that utilizes the generation of high-frequency electrical alternating current through target tissue to induce ion agitation and tissue friction, ultimately leading to thermal injury and consequent coagulative necrosis. Effective ablation is achieved by optimizing heat production and minimizing heat loss, with the objective of generating a clear tumor ablation margin while reducing potential side effects. The availability, safety, efficacy, and low cost of percutaneous RFA have facilitated its common utilization, in conjunction with ultrasound, CT, or MRI guidance, in the management of a variety of solid tumors, most commonly hepatocellular carcinoma, renal cell carcinoma, non–small cell lung cancer, and osteoid osteoma.

RFA has also been used to treat pancreatic cancer during exploratory laparotomy or laparoscopy; a 2014 systematic review identified five studies including 158 patients with a median survival after RFA of 3 to 33 months, 0% to 19% mortality, 10% to 43% overall morbidity, and 4% to 37% RFA-related morbidity, much of which was related to collateral injury to adjacent tissues.[147] Given its minimally invasive nature and superior imaging capabilities of the pancreas, EUS potentially provides an ideal vehicle for delivering RFA to pancreatic cancer, as well as other percutaneously inaccessible tumors.

Animal Studies

Using a modified 19-gauge needle electrode connected to a monopolar radiofrequency generator, Goldberg et al in 1999 first demonstrated the feasibility of EUS-guided RFA of the pancreas in 13 pigs.[148] The maximum diameter of the ablated area was 10 to 15 mm by EUS and 12 mm by histology. Correlation between EUS or CT and gross pathologic findings for size of the ablated region was excellent for all areas larger than 5 mm; the size of the ablated zone at pathologic examination was within 2 mm of that visualized on imaging. Complications included three transmural gastric wall burns, an intestinal serosal burn, and an asymptomatic pancreatic fluid collection.

In an attempt to improve ablation efficiency while reducing collateral thermal injury, Carrara et al (2008)[149] used a hybrid cryotherm probe combining bipolar radiofrequency current with carbon dioxide cryotherapy to ablate the body of the pancreas in 14 pigs; they achieved a larger ablation zone (18 mm vs. 10 mm) with a 300-second application than that obtained with a 360-second application using the monopolar system from the Goldberg et al study. However, similar side effects (most reflecting longer application duration) were encountered, including two cases of pancreatitis (one necrotizing and the other asymptomatic), a gastric wall burn, and four cases of adhesions between the pancreas and the gut. The same group demonstrated the feasibility of using the CT probe in EUS-guided RFA of the liver and spleen in porcine models with no reported complications.[150] Ultrasound-guided RFA with the CT probe of 16 explanted human pancreatic tumors with a mean diameter of 29 mm produced ablation zone diameters of 10 to 20 mm, with the size of the ablated area correlating with the duration of ablation.[151]

Varadarajulu et al (2009) used an EUS-guided umbrella-shaped retractable monopolar electrode array to ablate five porcine livers, generating ablation zone diameters of 23 mm at EUS and 26 mm at histology without any complications.[152] Gaidhane et al (2012) deployed a 1-Fr RFA probe through a 19-gauge needle to ablate five porcine pancreata without complications; only histological evidence of focal pancreatitis was documented.[153] Kim et al (2012) used an 18-gauge saline pump–cooled RFA electrode to ablate the body or tail of the pancreas of 10 pigs; ablation zone diameters of 14.5 mm at EUS and 23 mm at histology were achieved.[154] Complications included three cases of asymptomatic retroperitoneal fibrosis or pancreatogastric adhesions.

Human Studies

Human studies of EUS-guided RFA are limited. Arcidiacono et al (2012) ablated 16 unresectable stage 3 pancreatic cancers with a mean diameter of 35.7 mm using the CT probe.[155] RFA could not be deployed in six additional patients because of gastroduodenal wall or tumor stiffness. Complications included mild abdominal pain in three patients, one of whom had pancreatitis; a duodenal bleed requiring endotherapy; two cases of obstructive jaundice requiring stenting; a duodenal stricture treated with stenting; and an asymptomatic pancreatic cystic collection. Median postablation survival time was 6 months. CT imaging could clearly define the tumor margins in only 6 of 16 ablated patients, whereas no reduction or change in tumor size, however insignificant, was seen for up to 78 days.[155]

Song et al (2016) recently conducted a study to assess the technical feasibility and safety of EUS-RFA in six patients with unresectable pancreatic cancer using an 18-gauge RFA needle and the VIVA RF Generator system (STARmed, Koyang, Korea).[156] The length of the exposed tip of the RFA electrode was 10 mm. After insertion of the RFA electrode into the mass, the radiofrequency generator was activated to deliver 20 to 50 W ablation power for 10 seconds. Depending on the tumor size, the procedure was repeated to sufficiently cover the tumor. EUS-RFA was performed successfully in all six patients (median age 62 years, range 43–73 years). Pancreatic cancer was located in the head (n = 4) or body (n = 2) of the pancreas. The median diameter of masses was 3.8 cm (range 3–9 cm). Four patients had stage 3 disease, and two patients had stage 4 disease. After the procedure, two patients experienced mild abdominal pain, but there were no other adverse events, such as pancreatitis or bleeding.

Early studies of EUS-guided RFA for neuroendocrine tumors and pancreatic cysts have also been performed.[157–160]

At present, EUS-guided RFA remains a tool that requires further assessment, refinement, and validation of its safety and efficacy in well-designed randomized controlled studies before it can be formally recommended for use in clinical practice. In particular, future studies will need to address the development of sharper probe designs, possibly equipped with cutting current to facilitate transluminal access; the appropriate radiologic modality and time interval for assessing tumor response; and the optimal settings for treatment duration, generator power, and gas coolant pressure for effective ablation of pancreatic cancer as opposed to healthy pancreatic tissue.

EUS-Guided Fiducial Marker Placement

Fiducial markers are radiopaque coils or rods that assist in the targeting of cancer radiation therapy. Traditionally placed intraoperatively or percutaneously under radiology guidance, in more recent years EUS placement via an FNA needle has been preferred as a less invasive method for fiducial marker placement in GI malignancies, including esophageal tumors, cholangiogiocarcinomas, gastric cancers, and malignant lymph nodes.[161–163] In esophageal cancer, where there is a malignant lymph node far from the tumor, it is our practice to place fiducial markers into the lymph node to ensure radiation treatment to this region as well. There may be particular advantages for placement into the pancreas, with possibly a lower likelihood of peritoneal seeding, although recent protocols for pancreatic cancer have moved away from radiation therapy.[122,164]

Placement of fiducial markers allows accurate demarcation of the location and peripheral extent of the tumor in real time by image-guided radiotherapy (IGRT), which is a prerequisite to facilitating stereotactic body radiotherapy. The visualization of fiducial markers allows multiple beams of radiation to be delivered with extreme accuracy and consistency by quantifying respiratory motion and tumor extent, therefore maximizing radiation delivery to the tumor and minimizing collateral damage to the normal surrounding parenchyma.[165] This technique has also been used for intraoperative localization of small neuroendocrine tumors to allow parenchymal-sparing resections.[166,167]

Fiducial Characteristics

Fiducial markers can be made of gold, carbon, or polymer.[168] Gold markers are more commonly used, as they are most easily visualized and provide the highest level of contrast. Gold fiducial markers can also produce more artifact, but fortunately this can be minimized by employing the metal artifact reduction methods to improve CT image quality.[169]

The size of fiducial markers can vary. The length is anywhere from 2.5 to 10 mm, and the diameter can range between 0.35 to 0.8 mm, which dictates the gauge of needle used for delivery. The shape of fiducials can be cylindrical (rod) or coiled. A 2012 comparison study demonstrated that rod-shaped fiducials were significantly more visible than the coiled variety, without significant differences in the rate of migration.[170]

Technique for Fiducial Marker Placement

Fiducial markers can be delivered via a 19- or 22-gauge needle. The advantage of the 22-gauge delivery system is ease and success of deployment, especially when targeting more technically difficult locations such as the head or uncinate process of the pancreas. DiMaio et al (2010)[163] reported a 97% technical success rate with the 22-gauge system for GI-related malignancies, and Ammar et al (2010)[162] reported a 100% technical success rate in tumors and lymph nodes.

Up until recently, the technique for placement involved a single loading system whereby the sterile fiducial marker is loaded at the needle tip either anterograde[162] or retrograde[171] and secured with sterile bone wax placed at the very end of the needle. Once the lesion of interest is punctured, the stylet is pushed completely into the needle to deploy the fiducial marker. Saline flush is sometimes required instead of the stylet in situations where difficult stylet maneuverability is anticipated (e.g., uncinate process targets).[172] In general, this technique produces very high success rates of deployment with normal anatomy, but in the setting of altered or postsurgical anatomy, success rates decrease to 73%.[173] A new multifiducial system, the BNX needle aspiration system (Covidien, Dublin, Ireland), has been released for clinical use. It is engineered to improve the clinical workflow by facilitating the passage of multiple needles through a single delivery system without removing the delivery system between needle passages. It allows rapid exchange of the needles while keeping the needle sheath and catheter in the echoendoscope. Therefore having two or three preloaded needles can allow rapid deployment of multiple fiducials (this system allows placement of multiple fiducials through a single delivery system). This system was demonstrated to have a 95% success rate in porcine models, with four fiducials placed sequentially in under 1 minute.[174] This device has a narrowing or waist near the tip to provide the endoscopist tactile feedback indicating successful deployment of each individual fiducial marker. Cook Medical (Bloomington, IN) also manufactures a dedicated EUS needle, the EchoTip Ultra fiducial needle, which has four preloaded gold fiducial markers within a 22-gauge FNA needle.

Ideal Fiducial Geometry

Ideal fiducial geometry (IFG) is defined as having a minimum of three fiducials at least 2 cm apart and with interfiducial angles greater than 15 degrees (Fig. 51.15). Surgical placement has achieved IFG more consistently than EUS-guided methods, although IFG may not be necessary, as both surgical and EUS-guided methods achieve high visibility under Cyberknife (Accuray Inc., Sunnyvale, CA) imaging.[175] Placement protocols vary among centers, particularly regarding the actual number of fiducials placed. In most centers, three to four fiducial markers are inserted between 1.5 and 2 cm apart around the periphery of the tumor. The goal is to aim for IFG if the tumor is large enough to allow adequate spacing of the fiducials, regardless of the type of tumor. Smaller lesions may only allow one or two fiducials to be inserted.

Complications

Complications related to fiducial marker placements are rare. The most common is migration at 1 week postplacement, when IGRT typically commences. The median migration distance has been reported to be 1.3 mm[170]; however, total migration to the

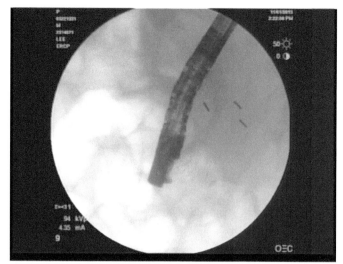

FIG 51.15 Fluoroscopic image of all three fiducial markers at the head of pancreas with a metal biliary stent coursing through the cancer.

extent whereby the fiducial marker is not seen at IGRT and the quality of IGRT is compromised has been reported in up to 7% of cases.[173]

Other reported complications include infection in two patients[163,164] who were managed without intravenous antibiotics or hospital admission. Given the overall low risk of infection with this procedure, we do not routinely administer antibiotic prophylaxis following EUS-guided fiducial marker placement for GI malignancy in our practice. There has been one report of postprocedural abdominal pain, which was ultimately diagnosed as mild pancreatitis.[173] Bleeding occurred on one occasion, although this was minor and did not require blood transfusion.[172]

In summary, fiducial markers play an integral role in the precise delivery of high intensity radiotherapy by Cyberknife. EUS-guided placement is particularly useful in deeper targets, particularly the pancreas, and has proven to be very safe and effective.

EUS-Guided Antitumor Agents

With CGN, EUS-guided FNI has demonstrated feasibility and safety in the delivery of a medication into a localized region and structure. As a result, EUS-FNI has received attention as a method for antitumor agent delivery, particularly for intratumoral and combination therapy for esophageal and pancreatic cancer. The evidence supporting the feasibility of EUS-FNI of antitumor agents has been expanding, with promising results. This topic is outside of the scope of this current chapter, but we feel it is important to mention that many remain optimistic that EUS-FNI will play an important role in future cancer therapy.

KEY REFERENCES

1. Shin EJ, Topazian M, Goggins MG, et al: Linear-array EUS improves detection of pancreatic lesions in high-risk individuals: a randomized tandem study, *Gastrointest Endosc* 82:812–818, 2015.
11. Cheon YK, Cho WY, Lee TH, et al: Endoscopic ultrasonography does not differentiate neoplastic from non-neoplastic small gallbladder polyps, *World J Gastroenterol* 15:2361–2366, 2009.
16. De Castro VL, Moura EG, Chaves DM, et al: Endoscopic ultrasound versus magnetic resonance cholangiopancreatography in suspected

choledocholithiasis: a systematic review, *Endosc Ultrasound* 5:118–128, 2016.

21. Lee Y, Chan F, Leung W: Comparison of EUS and ERCP in the investigation with suspected biliary obstruction caused by choledocholithasis: a randomized study, *Gastrointest Endosc* 67:660–668, 2008.

37. Vazquez-Sequeiros E, Baron TH, Clain JE, et al: Evaluation of indeterminate bile duct strictures, *Gastrointest Endosc* 53:372–379, 2002.

38. Levy M, Baron T, Clayton A, et al: Prospective evaluation of advanced molecular markers and imaging techniques in patients with indeterminate bile duct strictures, *Am J Gastroenterol* 103:1263–1273, 2008.

49. Ridtitid W, Schmidt SE, Al-Haddad MA, et al: Performance characteristics of EUS for locoregional evaluation of ampullary lesions, *Gastrointest Endosc* 81:380–388, 2015.

53. Tandon M, Topazian M: Endoscopic ultrasound in idiopathic acute pancreatitis, *Am J Gastroenterol* 96:705–709, 2001.

58. Wallace MB, Hawes RH, Durkalski V, et al: The reliability of EUS for the diagnosis of chronic pancreatitis: interobserver agreement among experienced endosonographers, *Gastrointest Endosc* 53:294–299, 2001.

65. Canto M, Goggins M, Hruban R, et al: Screening for early pancreatic neoplasia in high-risk individuals: a prospective controlled study, *Clin Gastroenterol Hepatol* 4:766–781, 2006.

72. Bhutani MS, Arantes VN, Verma D, et al: Histopathologic correlation of endoscopic ultrasound findings of chronic pancreatitis in human autopsies, *Pancreas* 38:820–824, 2009.

78. Trikudanathan G, Vega-Peralta J, Malli A, et al: Diagnostic performance of endoscopic ultrasound (EUS) for non-calcific chronic pancreatitis (NCCP) based on histopathology, *Am J Gastroenterol* 111:568–574, 2016.

82. Chang KJ, Wiersema MJ: Endoscopic ultrasound-guided fine-needle aspiration biopsy and interventional endoscopic ultrasonography. Emerging technologies, *Gastrointest Endosc Clin N Am* 7:221–235, 1997.

92. Erickson RA, Sayage-Rabie L, Beissner RS: Factors predicting the number of EUS-guided fine-needle passes for diagnosis of pancreatic malignancies, *Gastrointest Endosc* 51:184–190, 2000.

95. Bang JY, Magee SH, Ramesh J, et al: Randomized trial comparing fanning with standard technique for endoscopic ultrasound-guided fine-needle aspiration of solid pancreatic mass lesions, *Endoscopy* 45:445–450, 2013.

100. Wani S, Mullady D, Early DS, et al: The clinical impact of immediate on-site cytopathology evaluation during endoscopic ultrasound-guided fine needle aspiration of pancreatic masses: a prospective multicenter randomized controlled trial, *Am J Gastroenterol* 110:1429–1439, 2015.

102. Iwashita T, Yasuda I, Mukai T, et al: Macroscopic on-site quality evaluation of biopsy specimens to improve the diagnostic accuracy during EUS-guided FNA using a 19-gauge needle for solid lesions: a single-center prospective pilot study (MOSE study), *Gastrointest Endosc* 81:177–185, 2015.

105. Bang JY, Hawes R, Varadarajulu S: A meta-analysis comparing ProCore and standard fine-needle aspiration needles for endoscopic ultrasound-guided tissue acquisition, *Endoscopy* 48:339–349, 2016.

133. Sahai AV, Lemelin V, Lam E, et al: Central vs. bilateral endoscopic ultrasound-guided celiac plexus block or neurolysis: a comparative study of short-term effectiveness, *Am J Gastroenterol* 104:326–329, 2009.

137. Gunaratnam NT, Sarma AV, Norton ID, et al: A prospective study of EUS-guided celiac plexus neurolysis for pancreatic cancer pain, *Gastrointest Endosc* 54:316–324, 2001.

142. Doi S, Yasuda I, Kawakami H, et al: Endoscopic ultrasound-guided celiac ganglia neurolysis vs. celiac plexus neurolysis: a randomized multicenter trial, *Endoscopy* 45:362–369, 2013.

155. Arcidiacono PG, Carrara S, Reni M, et al: Feasibility and safety of EUS-guided cryothermal ablation in patients with locally advanced pancreatic cancer, *Gastrointest Endosc* 76:1142–1151, 2012.

156. Song TJ, Seo DW, Lakhtakia S, et al: Initial experience of EUS-guided radiofrequency ablation of unresectable pancreatic cancer, *Gastrointest Endosc* 83:440–443, 2016.

170. Khashab MA, Kim KJ, Tryggestad EJ, et al: Comparative analysis of traditional and coiled fiducials implanted during EUS for pancreatic cancer patients receiving stereotactic body radiation therapy, *Gastrointest Endosc* 76:962–971, 2012.

173. Sanders MK, Moser AJ, Khalid A, et al: EUS-guided fiducial placement for stereotactic body radiotherapy in locally advanced and recurrent pancreatic cancer, *Gastrointest Endosc* 71:1178–1184, 2010.

A complete reference list can be found online at ExpertConsult .com

52

Endoscopic Ultrasound–Guided Access and Drainage of the Pancreaticobiliary Ductal Systems

Takao Itoi and Marc Giovannini

CHAPTER OUTLINE

INTRODUCTION

Endoscopic retrograde cholangiopancreatography (ERCP) has traditionally represented the optimal approach to the bile duct and the pancreatic duct. However, ERCP is not always successful because of the inability to achieve selective cannulation or because of inaccessibility of the papilla owing to gastric outlet obstruction (GOO) and surgically altered anatomy (e.g., Roux-en-Y gastric bypass). Recently, new endoscopic drainage techniques guided by endoscopic ultrasonography (EUS) have been developed, mainly for use in failed ERCP patients. However, such techniques are not yet fully established, and their usefulness is still debated. Herein, we focus on EUS-guided pancreaticobiliary drainage by describing the technique and its algorithm from the viewpoint of an interventional EUS expert.

EUS-GUIDED BILIARY DRAINAGE (EUS-BD)

Percutaneous transhepatic biliary drainage (PTBD) is routinely used worldwide as an alternative biliary drainage technique in the case of failed ERCP. At present, EUS-BD is considered to be a viable second-line option for biliary decompression in case of failed ERCP, particularly at institutions with interventional expertise. This is because of its high technical success rate of 80% to 90% and its low adverse event rate of 10% to 20%,[1,2] and because its efficacy and safety are similar to those of PTBD.[3,4]

Technical Considerations

Anatomically, the EUS-BD approach can be classified into two types: extrahepatic bile duct (EHBD) drainage and intrahepatic bile duct (IHBD) drainage.[5] EUS-guided hepaticogas-trostomy (EUS-HGS) and EUS-guided choledochoduodenostomy (EUS-CDS) are typical transmural EUS-BD techniques. Other options, such as EUS-guided rendezvous (EUS-RV) and EUS-guided antegrade stenting (EUS-AS), have also been reported.

EUS-Guided Extrahepatic Bile Duct Drainage

Puncture of the EHBD via the duodenum (EUS-CDS) (Fig. 52.1 and Video 52.1) is a common approach in EUS-guided EHBD drainage. The EHBD is visualized from the duodenal bulb using EUS in a long scope position. The direction of the needle in the long scope position is toward the hilar bile duct. A 19-guage needle that has been prefilled with contrast medium is used to puncture the EHBD. After injection of contrast medium to delineate the IHBD, a 0.025-inch or 0.035-inch guidewire is placed. Tract dilation is performed using a standard ERCP catheter, a 6-Fr cautery dilator (Cyst-Gastro set, Mediglobe, Germany), and/or a 3- to 4-mm dilating balloon. Using a needle knife may increase the risk of adverse events. With regard to current, a high-frequency electrocautery setting such as AutoCut mode (100 W, effect 4, ICC200, ERBE Elektromedizin GmbH, Tübingen, Germany) is used. It is very important to keep the endoscope pressed against the duodenal wall (endoscopically, the so-called red spot) while taking ultrasonography images of the long axis of the bile duct and guidewire. It is also important to maintain the optimal scope position during radiography. In addition, it is critical to arrange the equipment that will be needed in advance to complete the procedure appropriately and in a short time. Finally, the type of stent used, such as a plastic stent (PS) or a self-expandable metal stent (SEMS) (including fully covered and partially covered SEMS), depends on the preference of the endosonographer, although SEMS appears to be more suitable for avoiding bile leakage and postprocedure bleeding.

Thus far, conventional tubular biliary stents have been used for EUS-CDS. Recently, dedicated stents for EUS-BD have also been developed. The new, commercially available biflanged lumen-apposing metal stent AXIOS (Boston Scientific Corp., Natick, MA) (Fig. 52.2) is a safe and useful SEMS for EUS-CDS.[6,7] Furthermore, the Hot AXIOS stent (Boston Scientific Corp.), a cautery-enhanced delivery system for single-step EUS-guided

puncture and delivery of a lumen-apposing stent for EUS-CDS, has also been developed[8] (Fig. 52.3). When we use this one-step delivery system, freehand EUS-CDS can be performed without any needle puncture or tract dilation, although the bile duct must be dilated to a diameter great than 2 cm for safe stent deployment.

EUS-Guided Intrahepatic Bile Duct Drainage

Puncture of the IHBD via the stomach (EUS-HGS) (Fig. 52.4 and Video 52.2) is a common approach to EUS-guided IHBD drainage. Although rare, transjejunal IHBD drainage is possible in patients with altered anatomy such as total gastrectomy and Roux-en-Y reconstruction. The IHBD is small compared with the EHBD. If the IHBD is not dilated adequately, the use of a 22-guage needle is also an option. However, in such cases, guidewire manipulation following puncture is not easy to perform.

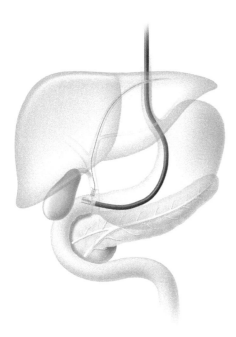

FIG 52.1 Schema of EUS-guided choledochoduodenostomy using a lumen-apposing stent.

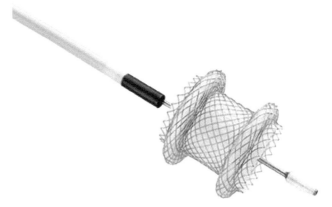

FIG 52.2 Lumen-apposing biflanged metal stent (Hot AXIOS). (Courtesy Boston Scientific, Marlborough, MA.)

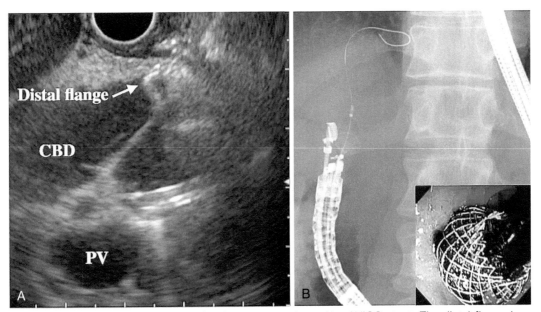

FIG 52.3 EUS-guided choledochoduodenostomy using a Hot AXIOS stent. The distal flange is deployed in the common bile duct (CBD) as an anchor, under **A,** EUS guidance and **B,** fluoroscopic guidance. Finally, the proximal flange (endoscopic image, right lower corner) is deployed under endoscopic guidance in the duodenum *(inset)*. PV, portal vein.

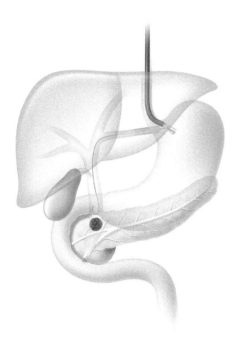

FIG 52.4 Schema of EUS-guided hepaticogastrostomy using a metal stent.

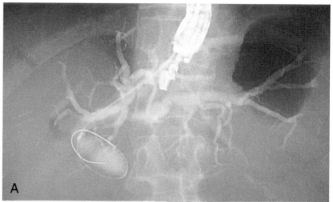

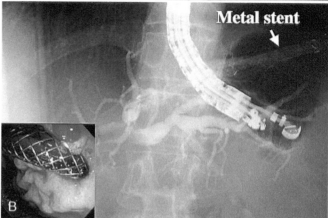

FIG 52.5 EUS-guided hepaticogastrostomy using a partially covered metal stent. In this case, needle puncture was performed via the B2 intrahepatic bile duct. **A,** After tract dilation using a cautery dilator, a partially covered metal stent was placed (**B,** fluoroscopy; lower endoscopic image, *inset*).

After needle puncture, it is important to insert the guidewire into the bile duct as far as possible. Tract dilation of the fistula is achieved by basically the same procedure as is EUS-guided EHBD drainage. Finally, a PS or SEMS is placed in the IHBD. Similar to EUS-CDS, dedicated PSs[9] and SEMSs (including partially or fully covered SEMSs[10]) have been developed for EUS-HGS (Fig. 52.5).

When selecting the IHBD to puncture, is it better to puncture intrahepatic bile duct 2 (B2) or bile duct 3 (B3)? Although this depends on the patient's anatomy, B2 puncture may provide easier guidewire manipulation and stent delivery system insertion because the puncture is performed smoothly in a downstream direction toward the EHBD compared with B3 puncture. However, the B2 puncture site tends to be close to the esophagogastric junction, and stent deployment or re-intervention may be difficult. Moreover, there is a possibility of transesophageal puncture, leading to mediastinitis.

EUS-Guided Rendezvous[11]

There are three puncture routes for EUS-RV. The first route is transmural puncture of the IHBD, known as the IHBD puncture route. For the IHBD puncture route, transesophageal puncture of B2 and transgastric puncture of B2 or B3 can be performed; in addition, transjejunal puncture is possible in patients who have undergone reconstruction after total gastrectomy. B2 puncture appears to be the preferable puncture route for EUS-RV because guidewire manipulation is easier than in the case of B3 puncture. On the other hand, there are two methods for transduodenal puncture of the EHBD: EHBD puncture via the proximal duodenum (D1) and EHBD puncture via the second portion of the duodenum (D2). For EHBD puncture via D1, the scope is in a push position (long position), whereas for EHBD puncture via D2, the scope is in a short position. When performing the EHBD puncture via the duodenum, the stomach antrum is rarely punctured.

After needle puncture, an angled tip hydrophilic-coated guidewire is passed into the duodenum as far as possible through the stenosis and papilla. Then, the EUS scope is switched to a duodenal scope for standard ERCP, leaving the guidewire in place. Biliary cannulation by ERCP is performed alongside the guidewire emerging from the papilla (parallel rendezvous), or the guidewire is grasped with snare or biopsy forceps and passed through the accessory channel, and the ERCP catheter is then advanced into the bile duct over the guidewire.

EUS-Guided Antegrade Stenting

EUS-AS (Fig. 52.6) is usually performed via the EUS-guided IHBD route. After needle puncture, an angled tip hydrophilic-coated guidewire is passed into the duodenum as far as possible through the stenosis and papilla, similar to EUS-RV. After the tract is dilated to the size needed for the stent delivery system (6-Fr to 8-Fr), a covered or uncovered metal stent is inserted antegrade and placed across the stenosis through to the duodenum via or above the papilla (Fig. 52.7). Some endoscopists perform simultaneous stent placement via the EUS-HGS route to avoid bile leakage in case of possible antegrade stent dysfunction.

Clinical Outcomes

Numerous studies have reported on the success of EUS-BD to date. The outcomes for each procedure type are summarized in Table 52.1.[12] The technical success rates of EUS-CDS (n = 340),

EUS-HGS (n = 153), EUS-RV (n = 267), and EUS-AS (n = 39) were 92%, 95%, 81%, and 77%, respectively, and the adverse event rates were 15%, 17%, 11%, and 5%, respectively. These results suggest that transmural drainage provided a high technical success rate, whereas transpapillary procedures showed a low adverse event rate. Regarding stent selection for EUS-HGS, a previous review showed that the technical success, clinical success, adverse event rates, and mortality rates did not differ significantly between PS (n = 26, 100%, 94.7%, 15.4%, and 0.038%, respectively) and SEMS (n = 147, 95.2%, 91.6%, 91.6%, 16.3%, and 0.007%, respectively. There was no significant difference of clinical outcomes between PSs and SEMSs. Based on these data, the use of either type of stent seems safe, but there could be publication bias because most of these data were collected retrospectively and from centers that perform a high volume of interventional EUS procedures. Notably, a Spanish survey showed that the technical success rates of EUS-HGS and EUS-CDS performed by various skilled endoscopists were 64.7% (22/34) and 86.3% (19/26), respectively.[13]

Although PTBD is the standard method used for draining a malignant biliary obstruction after failed ERCP, a 2016 randomized clinical trial comparing PTBD and EUS-BD showed that

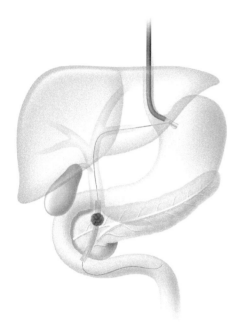

FIG 52.6 Schema of EUS-guided antegrade stenting using a metal stent.

TABLE 52.1   Summary of EUS-Guided Biliary Drainage

| | TRANSMURAL PROCEDURES | | TRANSPAPILLARY PROCEDURES | |
	EUS-CDS	EUS-HGS	Rendezvous	Antegrade
No. of cases	340	153	267	39
Technical success (%)	92	95	81	77
Early adverse events (%)	15	17	11	5

EUS-CDS, endoscopic ultrasound–guided choledochoduodenostomy; *EUS-HGS*, endoscopic ultrasound–guided hepaticogastrostomy.

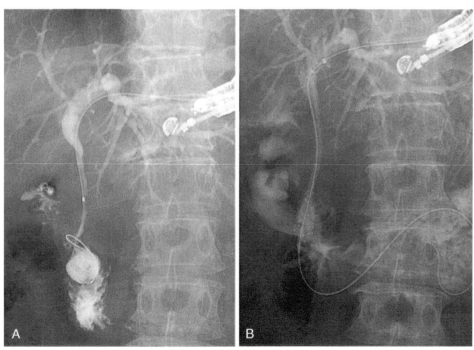

FIG 52.7 EUS-guided antegrade stenting using a metal stent. **A,** The guidewire was advanced into the duodenum across the stricture and papilla. **B,** After tract dilation, an uncovered metal stent was placed.

both techniques had similar levels of efficacy in patients with unresectable malignant distal biliary obstruction and inaccessible papilla, based on technical and functional success rates and quality of life.[14]

The use of EUS-guided right IHBD drainage has been reported in patients with complicated hilar obstruction.[15] Although its application is limited, EUS-guided right IHBD drainage should be considered as an alternative to PTBD in selected patients.

Clinical Algorithm

Which of the several EUS-BD techniques that have been developed thus far is the optimal procedure? The technique selected depends on the endoscopist's preference and experience. At present, the real issue is the unavailability of a perfect technique that can accomplish biliary drainage in a wide range of patients. For example, the intrahepatic (IH) approach is difficult or impossible in the case of a nondilated IHBD. In contrast, the extrahepatic (EH) approach can be used in the case of a distal bile duct stricture, but is not possible in cases of complete GOO or nearly complete blockage of the EH bile duct. Therefore, selection of the EUS-BD technique must be flexible and based on patients' anatomies, such as those who have undergone Whipple resection or the Roux-en-Y procedure, as well as patient conditions, such as GOO.[16]

Tyberg et al (2016) proposed a novel algorithm for individualizing technique selection based on patient anatomy.[17] Patients with a dilated IHBD, as determined by cross-sectional imaging and confirmed by EUS visualization, received an IH approach with AS or HGS stent placement if anterograde placement was not feasible. Patients with a nondilated IHBD, as determined by cross-sectional imaging and confirmed by EUS visualization, underwent an EH approach with an RV technique, or a transenteric stent placement if RV was not feasible. If the IHBD approach was attempted but unsuccessful, an EH approach was performed. A similar algorithm for guidewire manipulation was proposed by Park et al in 2013.[18] These two algorithms suggest that guidewire manipulation is the most difficult part of the procedure, and is a key factor for performing a successful EUS-BD procedure. An optimal algorithm for EUS-BD is thus required, with the progressive development of dedicated devices in the near future. Until then, all techniques (i.e., EUS-HGS/-CDS/-RV/-AS) should be adequately learned to be able to accommodate various patient situations.

The timing for performing EUS-BD is not clear. We recommend obtaining consent for possible EUS-BD at the time of ERCP in patients at high risk for failed biliary cannulation.[19] This means that the endoscopist must ensure that adequate time, as well as skilled staff and appropriate back-up staff, is available for performing EUS-BD and managing its possible complications. Obtaining consent for possible EUS-BD at the time of ERCP avoids the need for repeated endoscopic interventions, as well as allowing for timely biliary drainage and the initiation of chemoradiation, if needed.

Conclusion

EUS-BD is an effective alternative to PTBD or surgery in patients with failed ERCP as evidenced by previous data. Nevertheless, we advocate that this procedure should only be performed in appropriately selected patients and by experienced endoscopists trained in both EUS and ERCP, together with an available, well-trained radiologic and surgical back-up staff, after obtaining informed consent.

INTERVENTIONAL EUS-GUIDED PANCREATIC DUCT DRAINAGE

The development of interventional EUS has provided better access to the pancreas. Just as pancreatic fluid collections (such as pseudocysts) can be successfully drained from the stomach or duodenum by endoscopic cystenterostomy or cystgastrostomy, the same technique can be used to access a dilated pancreatic duct in cases where the duct cannot be drained by conventional ERCP because of complete obstruction.

The main indications are stenosis of the pancreaticojejunal or pancreaticogastric anastomosis after Whipple resection (which induces recurrent acute pancreatitis [AP]), main pancreatic duct (MPD) stenosis due to chronic pancreatitis (CP), post–acute pancreatitis, or post–pancreatic trauma after ERCP failure. The pain associated with CP is caused, at least in part, by ductal hypertension. Both surgical and endoscopic treatments can relieve pain by improving ductal drainage. Endoscopic drainage requires transpapillary access to the pancreatic duct during ERCP. EUS-guided pancreaticogastrostomy (Fig. 52.8) or bulbostomy (Fig. 52.9) offers an alternative to surgery. Despite the advances in endoscopy, EUS-guided pancreatic duct drainage remains a technically challenging procedure. Technical success rates are greater than 70%; however, the average rate of adverse events is nearly 20%, and increases to 55% when stent migration is included. Until recently, a significant challenge associated with this technique was the absence of dedicated devices.

Technical Considerations

The dilated MPD is visualized using a linear interventional EUS scope. Endoscopic papillosphincterography (EPG) is then performed under combined fluoroscopic and ultrasound guidance, with the tip of the echoendoscope positioned such that the inflated balloon is in the duodenal bulb while the accessory channel remains in the antrum. A 19-gauge needle is inserted transgastrically or through the bulbus into the proximal pancreatic duct, and contrast medium is injected. Opacification is verified via a pancreatogram. A guidewire (0.025- or 0.035-inch) is introduced through the needle. At this point in the procedure, there are two options.

Option 1: The guidewire passes the stenotic area and goes through the papilla into the duodenum. A rendezvous technique (Fig. 52.10) should be performed by exchanging the EUS scope for a duodenoscope, and "classic" pancreatic endotherapy can then be performed. This technique should be the first choice when the patient's anatomy is intact because the complication rate is very low.

Option 2: The guidewire does not pass the stenotic area, or the patient has had a previous surgery (Whipple or gastrectomy). The needle is passed over a guidewire (0.025- or 0.035-inch) with a 6.5-Fr or 8-Fr diathermic sheath (prototype Cysto-Gastro set, EndoFlex, Voerde, Germany), which is then used to enlarge the tract between the stomach and the MPD. The sheath is introduced using cutting current. After exchange over a guidewire (rigid, 0.035-inch diameter), a 7-Fr, 8 cm–long pancreaticogastric stent is positioned. This stent is then changed for two 7-Fr or one 8.5-Fr stents 1 month after the first procedure. This EUS-guided MPD technique was first reported by François et al (2002).[20] Other authors have reported different techniques that have similar first steps (i.e., puncture of the MPD, pancreatogram, and guidewire insertion)[21,22] but a balloon dilatation is used instead of a cystostome, as reported in the original study,[20] and also by Tessier et al (2007).[23]

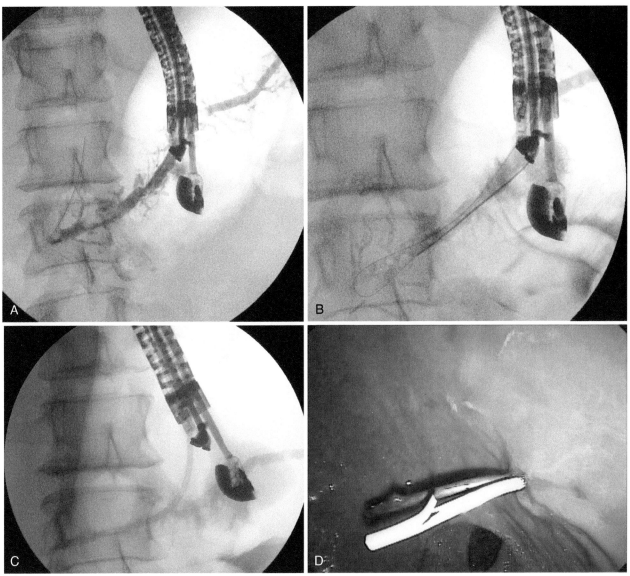

FIG 52.8 A to **D,** Pancreaticogastrostomy. Stenosis of the wirsungojejunostomy after Whipple surgery for a pancreatic neuroendocrine tumor of the head of the pancreas. **A,** Endoscopic ultrasonography–guided pancreatic ductography. **B,** Guidewire insertion. **C,** Stent placement to create a pancreatogastrostomy. **D,** Endoscopic view of plastic stent.

More research is needed on how to prevent pancreatic juice leakage using a diathermic technique versus balloon dilation. In our experience, peripancreatic collection occurs more frequently when we use balloon dilation than when we use the diathermic catheter, which prevents the leakage of pancreatic juice by creating fibrosis around the puncture tract.

Clinical Outcomes

The results from several published case series[21–27] do not recommend wider use of EPG (Table 52.2), which in any case should be restricted to tertiary centers specializing in biliopancreatic therapy. Pain relief was achieved in 70% of cases. However, the complication rate is high (approximately 15%); adverse events include bleeding, pancreatic collection, and perforation. Nevertheless, the possibility of draining the MPD into the digestive tract through an endoscopically created fistula, with patency maintained by stent placement, might be interesting as an alternative method

of drainage without the complication of stent occlusion that is associated with transpapillary drainage.

The first large series (of 36 patients) was published by Tessier et al (2007)[23]. Indications were CP with complete obstruction (secondary to tight stenosis, a stone, or MPD rupture) in patients with inaccessible papilla or impossible cannulation (n = 20); anastomotic stenosis after a Whipple procedure (n = 12); complete MPD rupture after AP; or trauma (n = 4). EPG or endoscopic pancreatic biopsy was unsuccessful in three patients; one was lost to follow-up. Major complications occurred in two patients, and included one hematoma and one case of severe AP. The median follow-up was 14.5 months (range: 4–55 months). Pain relief was complete or partial in 25 patients (69%, intention-to-treat). Eight patients had no improvement of their symptoms (four were subsequently diagnosed with cancer). Stent dysfunction occurred in 20 patients (55%) and required a total of 29 repeat endoscopies.

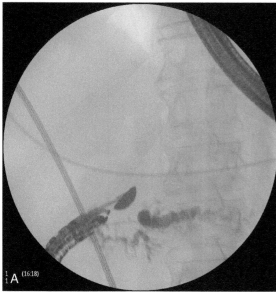

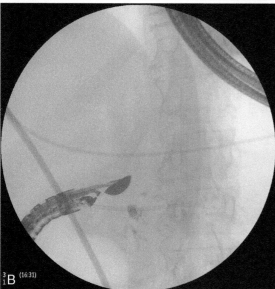

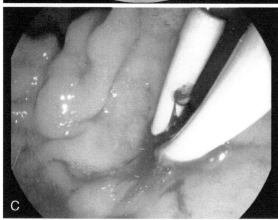

FIG 52.9 A to C, Pancreaticobulbostomy/chronic pancreatitis with a high degree of stenosis of the main pancreatic duct in the head of the pancreas, ERCP failure. **A,** Endoscopic ultrasonography–guided pancreatic ductography. **B,** Guidewire insertion. **C,** Endoscopic view of two plastic stents creating the pancreatogastrostomy.

Fujii et al (2013)[22] reported their experience with 45 patients, 37 of whom had undergone failed ERCP, and 29 of whom had surgically altered anatomy. Median follow-up after initial EUS-guided intervention was 23 months. Two underwent EUS for stent removal, and EUS-guided MPD stent placement was attempted in 43. Technical success was achieved in 32/43 (74%), with antegrade (n = 18) or retrograde (n = 14) stent insertion. Serious adverse events occurred in 3 patients (6%). Patients underwent a median of 2 (range: 1–6) follow-up procedures for revision or removal of stents, without complications. Complete symptom resolution occurred in 24/29 patients (83%) while stents were in place, including all six with nondilated ducts. Stents were removed from 23 patients, who were then followed for an additional 32 months (median); four had recurrent symptoms. Among the 11 failed cases, most had persistent symptoms or required surgery.

A larger study was reported by Will et al (2015).[28] This study enrolled 94 patients who underwent EUS-guided pancreatography and subsequent placement of a drain. In all, 94 patients underwent 111 interventions with one of three different approaches: (1) EUS-guided endoscopic retrograde drainage with a rendezvous technique; (2) EUS-guided drainage of the pancreatic duct; and (3) EUS-guided internal, antegrade drainage of the pancreatic duct. The technical success rate was 100%; in all cases, puncture of the pancreatic duct was accomplished successfully with the aid of pancreatography. Initial placement of a drain was successful in 47/83 patients (56.6%) requiring drainage. Of these, 26 patients underwent transgastric/transbulbar positioning of a stent for retrograde drainage; plastic prostheses were used in 11, and metal stents in 12. A ring drain (antegrade internal drainage) was placed in three of these 26 patients because of anastomotic stenosis after a previous surgical intervention. The remaining 21 patients with successful drain placement had transpapillary drains placed using the rendezvous technique; the majority (n = 19) received plastic prostheses, and only two received metal stents (covered SEMSs). Clinical success, as indicated by reduced or no pain after the EUS-guided intervention, was achieved in 68/83 patients (81.9%), including several who improved without drainage, but with manipulation of the access route.

In 2015, Fujii-Lau and Levy (2015)[29] summarized the current literature on EUS-guided pancreatic duct drainage, reviewing the published experience of 222 patients. Including both antegrade and rendezvous techniques, technical success was achieved in 170/222 patients (76.6%). A similar review by Itoi et al[30] in 2013 reported a technical success rate of more than 70% in 75 patients using the antegrade technique, and a range of success rates from 25% to 100% in 52 patients with the rendezvous technique.

More recently, Oh et al (2016)[31] reported the use of pancreatic fully covered self-expanding metal stents (FCSEMS). Twenty-five consecutive patients with painful obstructive pancreatitis underwent EUS-guided MPD drainage with a FCSEMS after failed ERCP. EUS-guided MPD drainage was successful in all 25 patients (technical success rate: 100%), and symptoms improved in all patients (clinical success rate: 100%). EUS-guided pancreatico-gastrostomy (n = 23), pancreaticoduodenostomy (n = 1), and pancreaticojejunostomy (n = 1) were performed. Pain scores improved significantly after FCSEMS placement (p = 0.001). Early mild-grade adverse events occurred in five patients (20%): four had self-limited abdominal pain, and one had minor bleeding. No other adverse events related to FCSEMS, including stent migration, stent clogging, pancreatic sepsis, and stent-induced ductal stricture, were observed during follow-up periods. The

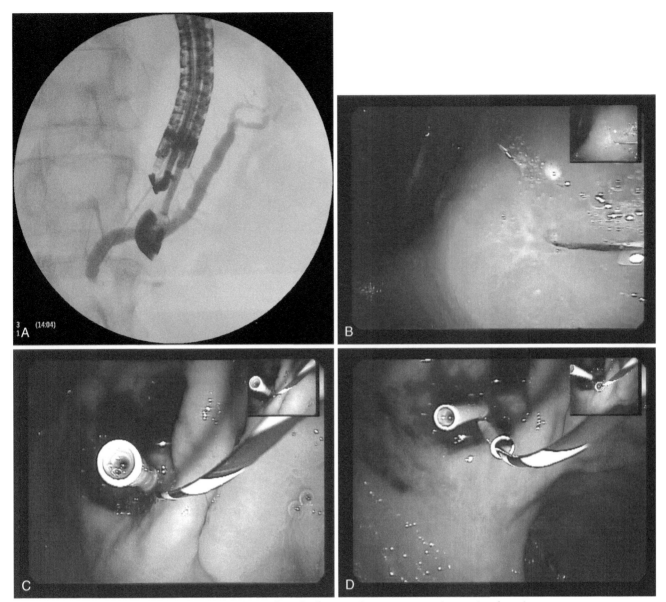

FIG 52.10 Rendezvous technique. **A** to **D,** Pancreaticogastrostomy/stenosis of a wirsungogastrostomy anastomosis after Whipple resection for benign cystic lesion of the head of the pancreas. **A,** Endoscopic ultrasonography–guided pancreatic ductography. **B,** Endoscopic view of a guidewire emerging from anastomosis. **C,** Endoscopic view of the first plastic stent. **D,** Endoscopic view of both plastic stents creating the pancreatogastrostomy.

TABLE 52.2   Studies of EUS-Guided Pancreaticogastrostomy

Authors	No. of Patients	% Success	% Complication	Median Follow-Up
Tessier et al, *Gastrointest Endosc*, 2007	36	70%	11%	16.5 months
Kahaleh et al, *Gastrointest Endosc*, 2007	13	92%	16%	14 months
Barkay et al, *Gastrointest Endosc*, 2010	21	48%	2%	13 months
Ergun et al, *Endoscopy*, 2011	20	90%	10%	37 months
Fujii et al, *Gastrointest Endosc*, 2013	45	74%	6%	32 months
Will et al, *World J Gastroenterol*, 2015	94	81,9%	8%	28 months
Oh et al*, *Gastrointest Endosc*, 2016	25	100%	20%	5 months

FCSEMS, Fully covered self-expanding metal stent

mean duration of stent patency was 126.9 days during a mean follow-up period of 221.1 days.

Clinical Algorithm

Regarding the three techniques, rendezvous[26] should be used preferentially because the complication rate is very low. EUS-guided pancreaticobulbostomy is recommended for stenosis of the MPD in the head of the pancreas because the EUS scope position is very stable. EUS-guided pancreaticogastrostomy is indicated when the patient's anatomy is altered (Whipple or gastrectomy), and mainly in the case of stenosis of the wirsungojejunostomy anastomosis, but this technique is the most difficult, with a high percentage of complications due to the instability of the EUS scope in the stomach.[25]

CONCLUSION

Therapeutic EUS-guided pancreaticogastrostomy and EUS-guided biliary drainage represent an alternative to surgery or percutaneous biliary drainage when ERCP fails or is impossible due to previous surgery (such as gastrectomy or Whipple resection). Although data have demonstrated that the procedure can be safe and effective, EUS-guided pancreatic duct drainage remains one of the most technically challenging therapeutic EUS interventions, as evidenced by the multiple considerations required for device selection and the risk of severe complications. At this time, we recommend that this procedure should only be performed in appropriately selected patients by experienced endoscopists trained in both EUS and ERP with well-trained surgical back-up available.

KEY REFERENCES

1. Giovannini M, Moutardier V, Pesenti C, et al: Endoscopic ultrasound-guided bilioduodenal anastomosis: a new technique for biliary drainage, *Endoscopy* 33:898–900, 2001.

4. Lee TH, Choi JH, Park DH, et al: Similar efficacies of endoscopic ultrasound-guided transmural and percutaneous drainage for malignant distal biliary obstruction, *Clin Gastroenterol Hepatol* 14(7):1011–1019.e3, 2016.

6. Itoi T, Binmoeller KF: EUS-guided choledochoduodenostomy by using a biflanged lumen-apposing metal stent, *Gastrointest Endosc* 79:715, 2014.

8. Teoh AY, Binmoeller KF, Lau JY: Single-step EUS-guided puncture and delivery of a lumen-apposing stent for gallbladder drainage using a novel cautery-tipped stent delivery system, *Gastrointest Endosc* 80:1171, 2014.

9. Umeda J, Itoi T, Sofuni A, et al: A newly designed plastic stent for endoscopic ultrasonography-guided hepaticogastrostomy: a prospective preliminary feasibility study (with videos), *Gastrointest Endosc* 82: 390–396, 2015.

10. Park do H, Lee TH, Paik WH, et al: Feasibility and safety of a novel dedicated device for one-step EUS-guided biliary drainage: a randomized trial, *J Gastroenterol Hepatol* 30:1461–1466, 2015.

11. Tsuchiya T, Itoi T, Sofuni A, et al: Endoscopic ultrasonography-guided rendezvous technique, *Dig Endosc* 28(Suppl 1):96–101, 2016.

12. Ikeuchi N, Itoi T: EUS-guided biliary drainage: an alternative to percutaneous transhepatic puncture, *Gastrointest Interv* 4:31–39, 2015.

15. Park SJ, Choi JH, Park do H, et al: Expanding indication: EUS-guided hepaticoduodenostomy for isolated right intrahepatic duct obstruction (with video), *Gastrointest Endosc* 78:374–380, 2013.

16. Mukai S, Itoi T: How should we use endoscopic ultrasonography-guided biliary drainage techniques separately? *Endosc Ultrasound* 5:65–68, 2016.

17. Tyberg A, Desai AP, Kumta NA, et al: Endoscopic ultrasound-guided biliary drainage (EUS-BD) after failed ERCP: a novel algorithm individualized based on patient anatomy, *Gastrointest Endosc* 84(6):941–946, 2016.

18. Park do H, Jeong SU, Lee BU, et al: Prospective evaluation of a treatment algorithm with enhanced guidewire manipulation protocol for EUS-guided biliary drainage after failed ERCP (with video), *Gastrointest Endosc* 78:91–101, 2013.

19. Khashab MA, Levy MJ, Itoi T, Artifon ELA: Endoscopic ultrasonography guided biliary drainage, *Gastrointest Endosc* 82:993–1001, 2015.

20. François E, Kahaleh M, Giovannini M, et al: EUS-guided pancreaticogastrostomy, *Gastrointest Endosc* 56(1):128–133, 2002.

21. Barkay O, Sheman S, McHenry L, et al: Therapeutic EUS-assisted endoscopic retrograde pancreatography after failed pancreatic duct cannulation at ERCP, *Gastrointest Endosc* 7:1166–1173, 2010.

22. Fujii LL, Topazian MD, Abu Dayyeh BK, et al: EUS-guided pancreatic duct intervention: outcomes of a single tertiary-care referral center experience, *Gastrointest Endosc* 78(6):854–864, 2013.

23. Tessier G, Bories E, Arvanitakis M, et al: EUS-guided pancreatogastrostomy and pancreatobulbostomy for the treatment of pain in patients with pancreatic ductal dilatation inaccessible for transpapillary endoscopic therapy, *Gastrointest Endosc* 65(2):233–241, 2007.

24. Kahaleh M, Hernandez AJ, Tokar J, et al: EUS-guided pancreaticogastrostomy: analysis of its efficacy to drain inaccessible pancreatic ducts, *Gastrointest Endosc* 65(2):224–230, 2007.

25. Kurihara T, Itoi T, Sofuni A, et al: Endoscopic ultrasonography-guided pancreatic duct drainage after failed endoscopic retrograde cholangiopancreatography in patients with malignant and benign pancreatic duct obstructions, *Dig Endosc* 25(Suppl 2):109–116, 2013.

26. Takikawa T, Kanno A, Masamune A, et al: Pancreatic duct drainage using EUS-guided rendezvous technique for stenotic pancreaticojejunostomy, *World J Gastroenterol* 19(31):5182–5186, 2013.

27. Ergun M, Aouattah T, Gillain C, et al: Endoscopic ultrasound-guided transluminal drainage of pancreatic duct obstruction: long-term outcome, *Endoscopy* 43:518–525, 2011.

28. Will U, Reichel A, Fueldner F, Meyer F: Endoscopic ultrasonography-guided drainage for patients with symptomatic obstruction and enlargement of the pancreatic duct, *World J Gastroenterol* 21(46):13140–13151, 2015.

29. Fujii-Lau LL, Levy MJ: Endoscopic ultrasound-guided pancreatic duct drainage, *J Hepatobiliary Pancreat Sci* 22:51–57, 2015.

30. Itoi T, Kasuya K, Sofuni A, et al: Endoscopic ultrasonography-guided pancreatic duct access: techniques and literature review of pancreatography, transmural drainage and rendezvous techniques, *Dig Endosc* 25:241–252, 2013.

31. Oh D, Park do H, Cho MK, et al: Feasibility and safety of a fully covered self-expandable metal stent with antimigration properties for EUS-guided pancreatic duct drainage: early and midterm outcomes (with video), *Gastrointest Endosc* 83:366–373, 2016.

A complete reference list can be found online at ExpertConsult .com

53

Gallstone Disease: Choledocholithiasis, Cholecystitis, and Gallstone Pancreatitis

Daniel K. Mullady and Christopher J. DiMaio

INTRODUCTION

Symptomatic gallbladder disease is one of the most common conditions encountered by the gastrointestinal endoscopist. It accounts for over 225,000 hospital discharges per year and over 2 billion health care dollars spent per year.[1] Whereas gallbladder disease can manifest itself in a variety of forms, it is the development and presence of gallstones which is responsible for the majority of disease. Typically, the presence of gallstones can result in intermittent and acute obstruction of the cystic duct, resulting in distention of the gallbladder, ischemia, inflammation, and infection. In addition, gallstones may enter the common bile duct (CBD) via the cystic duct, leading to symptomatic biliary obstruction. Impaction of stones at the level of the major papilla, or passage across it, can result in infectious complications such as ascending cholangitis, as well as induce pancreatitis, presumably via obstruction of flow of pancreatic ductal secretions.

The development of endoscopic retrograde cholangiopancreatography (ERCP) was spurred by the need for a minimally invasive approach to manage diseases of the biliary tree. The proven safety and efficacy of ERCP led to widespread adoption of this modality as a first-line approach for biliary interventions, and has nearly eliminated the need for complex surgical approaches for managing benign biliary tract disease. As such, on a global level, management of choledocholithiasis and gallstone pancreatitis remains the most common indication for ERCP. Traditionally, surgery has been the mainstay for management of gallbladder disease. However, advances in ERCP techniques and accessories have led to the ability to safely access the gallbladder itself, thus allowing for transpapillary drainage of

the gallbladder in select patients who may not be candidates for surgery. Further advances in endoscopic ultrasound (EUS)-guided transmural access to the gallbladder have gained attention in the past 5 years and are allowing the gastrointestinal (GI) endoscopist an opportunity to be all things for all biliary disease.

This chapter will focus on the endoscopic management of cholecystitis, choledocholithiasis, and gallstone pancreatitis.

BILIARY STONE DISEASE

Cholelithiasis refers to gallbladder stones and choledocholithiasis refers to stones in the bile ducts. Choledocholithiasis can be further classified as either primary stones, which develop within the bile ducts, or secondary stones, which occur as a result of passage from the gallbladder into the bile duct. Stones come in a variety of forms. Non-crumbling concretions greater than 2 mm in diameter are considered stones, whereas particles less than 2 mm in diameter are typically referred to as microlithiasis. Biliary sludge is a suspension of cholesterol monohydrate crystals or calcium bilirubinate granules in bile and has been implicated to act as a causative factor in acute pancreatitis and other biliary stone–related disease.[2]

Stone Types

Cholesterol stones are the most common type of stone encountered in the biliary system, accounting for approximately 80% of gallstones.[3] These stones form through an interplay of altered gallbladder absorption and secretion, bile stasis related to gallbladder dysmotility, cholesterol supersaturation in bile, and precipitation of calcium. Cholesterol stones are typically yellow in color and nodular (Fig. 53.1). There are numerous well-established risk factors for the development of cholesterol stones. Modifiable risk factors include diet, sedentary lifestyle, rapid weight loss, obesity, and dyslipidemia, whereas nonmodifiable risk factors include ethnicity, genetics, advanced age, and female gender. In addition, certain medications have been associated with increased risk of cholesterol stones due to their effect of increasing bile concentrations of cholesterol (e.g., oral contraceptives, estrogen, clofibrate) or by leading to biliary stasis by inhibiting gallbladder contraction (e.g., octreotide). Cholesterol stones typically present as cholelithiasis or secondary choledocholithiasis.

Pigment stones account for approximately 20% of gallstones.[3] Pigment stones can be further classified into brown pigment stones or black pigment stones (Fig. 53.2). Brown pigment stones

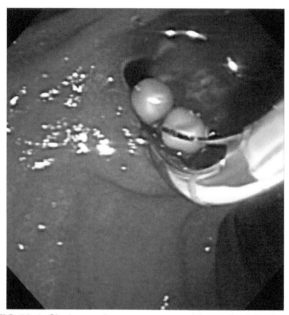

FIG 53.1 Cholesterol stones removed from the bile duct.

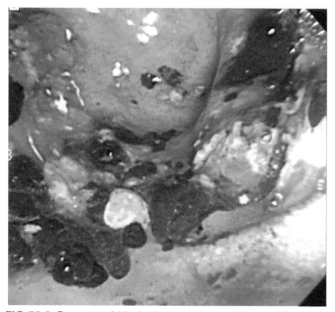

FIG 53.2 Brown and black pigment stones removed from bile duct.

are largely composed of calcium bilirubinate, and contain cholesterol and fatty acid soaps as well. Major risk factors that can precipitate the formation of brown pigment stones include any process resulting in biliary stasis and/or an infectious process. Examples include primary sclerosing cholangitis (PSC), chronic biliary obstruction from non-PSC strictures, and bacterial infections of the biliary tree, such as seen in recurrent pyogenic cholangitis. Other risk factors include conditions allowing for colonization of the biliary tree with enteric bacteria, such as indwelling biliary stents, prior biliary sphincterotomy, biliary-enteric anastomosis, and periampullary diverticula. As such, brown pigment stones typically present as primary choledocholithiasis. Black pigment stones consist of calcium bilirubinate with mucin glycoproteins. They form in the gallbladder and thus present as either cholelithiasis or secondary choledocholithiasis. Major patient risk factors include a history of hemolytic disease, such as sickle cell disease, or chronic liver disease.

CHOLECYSTITIS

The vast majority of patients with cholelithiasis will be asymptomatic, with the stones being found incidentally on imaging studies performed for other reasons. When symptomatic, gallstones typically exert symptoms by becoming lodged in the cystic duct, thereby preventing emptying of the gallbladder. Gallbladder obstruction in and of itself may produce symptoms of postprandial right upper quadrant pain in a crescendo-decrescendo pattern, otherwise known as biliary colic. The classical presentation is a few hours after eating, at the time when the gallbladder is stimulated to contract by cholecystokinin. Acute cholecystitis occurs when the cystic duct obstruction does not spontaneously resolve, leading to the development of subsequent inflammation and infection of the gallbladder, manifesting as right upper quadrant pain, fever, and leukocytosis.

Approximately 10% of cases of cholecystitis are actually acalculous cholecystitis, in which gallstones are not implicated as the cause, and there is no cystic duct obstruction. Acalculous cholecystitis typically presents in patients who are hospitalized and severely ill. Other comorbidities associated with this disease include diabetes mellitus, end-stage renal disease, immunocompromised states, coronary artery disease, congestive heart failure, cardiac surgery, and history of trauma. Acalculous cholecystitis typically occurs as a consequence of gallbladder stasis and ischemia, leading to local inflammation, followed by secondary infection by enteric flora. In approximately 50% of cases, gallbladder necrosis and gangrene can develop with subsequent perforation, occurring in as many as 10% of patients.[4] Given these risks and the associated underlying comorbidities, acalculous cholecystitis is associated with mortality rates as high as 33% to 41%.[4,5]

Patients with gallstones may also present with choledocholithiasis and subsequent bile duct obstruction, cholangitis, and pancreatitis. These topics will be covered later in this chapter.

Diagnosis

The clinical presentation of acute cholecystitis typically manifests as right upper quadrant abdominal pain with associated fever and leukocytosis. The classic physical exam finding is that of Murphy's sign. To assess for Murphy's sign, the examiner places their hand at the patient's right upper quadrant and palpates deeply, in the region of the gallbladder fossa under the liver edge. The patient is then asked to inspire deeply. As the diaphragm descends on inspiration, the inflamed gallbladder will approach the examiner's hand, resulting in increased pain and discomfort and typically resulting in the patient quickly halting the inspiratory effort.

No one piece of clinical, physical, or laboratory finding is sufficient to make a diagnosis of acute cholecystitis.[6] Thus, imaging is typically utilized to support the clinical suspicion and diagnosis of acute cholecystitis. Transabdominal ultrasound (TAUS) is an easy, noninvasive, and cost-effective tool in the evaluation of patients with suspected cholecystitis. Typical findings of acute cholecystitis on TAUS include gallbladder wall thickening and edema, pericholecystic fluid, and distention or hydrops of the gallbladder. In addition, a sonographic Murphy's sign can be elicited with the ultrasound transducer. A large systematic review reported a sensitivity for TAUS in diagnosing acute cholecystitis 88%.[7] TAUS is particularly sensitive in detecting the presence of cholelithiasis, with reported sensitivity as high as 98%.[8] Another imaging modality commonly employed in the evaluation for possible acute cholecystitis is a nuclear scintigraphy test called cholescintigraphy. In this test, technetium-labeled hepatic iminodiacetic acid (HIDA) in injected intravenously and acts as a radiolabeled tracer. The HIDA is taken up by hepatocytes and excreted in the bile. The tracer can then be visualized as it fills the bile ducts and gallbladder. Failure of the gallbladder to fill implies cystic duct obstruction, as would be expected when cholecystitis is suspected. Multiple studies demonstrate the superiority of cholescintigraphy to TAUS in diagnosing acute cholecystitis, with reported sensitivities ranging from 90% to 97%.[7,9–11]

Other Gallstone-Related Conditions

Aside from cholecystitis, gallstones can result in a number of other gallbladder conditions. When gallstones are impacted in the gallbladder neck or cystic duct, they may cause extrinsic compression of the adjacent common hepatic duct. The resulting bile duct obstruction typically presents as obstructive jaundice, with dilation of the upstream biliary tree (common hepatic duct and intrahepatic bile ducts), a condition referred to as Mirizzi syndrome. Type I Mirizzi syndrome occurs when there is external compression on the common hepatic duct, whereas Type II Mirizzi occurs when the impacted stone erodes through the gallbladder wall, creating a cholecysto-choledochal fistula (Figs. 53.3 and 53.4). Recognition or suspicion of Type II Mirizzi syndrome is key, as this condition requires surgical repair of the bile duct injury in addition to a cholecystectomy, and thus traditionally is managed via an open surgical approach.

Large gallstones (typically ≥2 cm) that erode into the luminal GI tract by means of a cholecysto-enteral fistula can lead to mechanical intestinal obstruction. Bouveret syndrome is a rare condition characterized by a large, often single, gallstone eroding through the gallbladder wall into the proximal duodenum by way of a cholecysto-duodenal fistula. Once present in the lumen, the stone can result in a mechanical gastric outlet obstruction (Fig. 53.5). Furthermore, should the stone subsequently dislodge and pass to the deep small bowel, it may again become impacted at the ileocecal valve with subsequent small bowel obstruction, thus resulting in a condition termed *gallstone ileus*. These conditions whereby cholecysto-enteral fistulas form are classically preceded by cholecystitis, with formation of adhesions between the gallbladder and small bowel, followed by pressure necrosis of a large gallstone, resulting in fistula formation and erosion of the stone in the GI lumen. In fact, there are numerous case

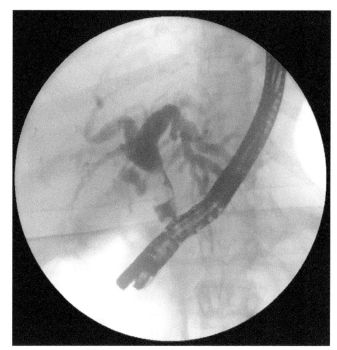

FIG 53.3 Type 1 Mirizzi syndrome.

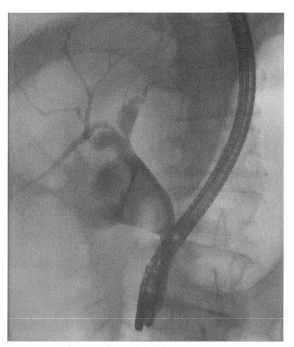

FIG 53.4 Type 2 Mirizzi syndrome.

reports of cholecysto-colonic fistula development resulting in gallstone erosion directly into the colon, with subsequent colonic obstruction.

The presence of cholelithiasis has long been recognized as a risk factor for the development of gallbladder cancer. Gallstones are present in up to 90% of cases of gallbladder cancer. Numerous epidemiologic studies demonstrate that the presence of gallstones can increase the risk for subsequent gallbladder cancer.[12–14] Fortunately, the incidence of gallbladder cancer remains quite low (approximately 1%) in patients with a history of cholelithiasis.[15] Factors that confer an increased risk of developing

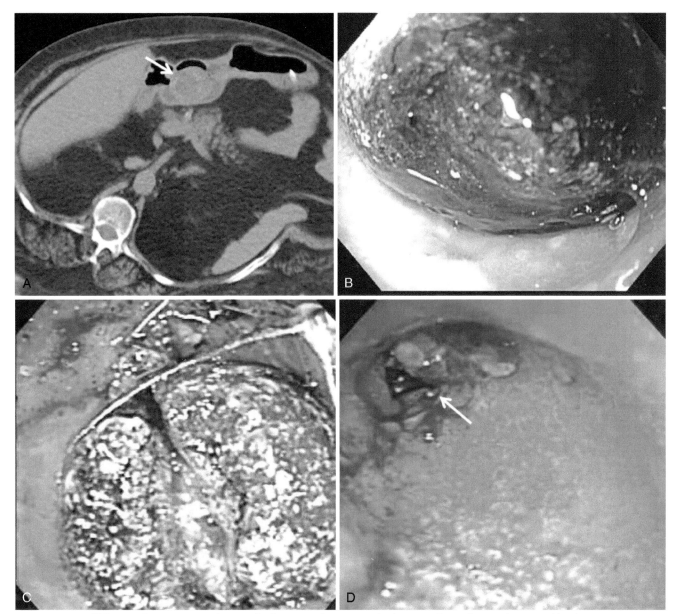

FIG 53.5 Bouveret syndrome. **A,** Computed tomography image of a gallstone impacted in the duodenal bulb *(arrow)*. **B,** Endoscopic image of the impacted stone. **C,** Partial fragmentation of the stone following mechanical lithotripsy with basket wires around stone. **D,** Cholecystoduodenal fistula *(arrow)*.

gallbladder cancer include stones larger than 3 cm and longer duration of cholelithiasis.[16–18] However, given the high prevalence of gallstones and very low incidence of gallbladder cancer, screening is currently not recommended.

Therapy for Cholecystitis and Symptomatic Cholelithiasis

The mainstay of treatment for the vast majority of patients with cholecystitis and symptomatic cholelithiasis is surgical cholecystectomy. Since its introduction in the mid 1980's, laparoscopic cholecystectomy has become the standard first-line treatment for cholecystitis. Laparoscopy allows for a less invasive approach, with associated fewer overall adverse events, reduced cost, decreased length of hospital stay, and increased patient satisfaction, compared to its predecessor of open surgical resection.

In the subset of patients who may not be suitable for surgery, such as those with sepsis, hemodynamic instability, or other comorbidities precluding safe administration of anesthesia, a nonsurgical approach to managing cholecystitis is required. Percutaneous drainage of the gallbladder is a technique that is widely available and effective for rapid drainage of an inflamed and/or infected gallbladder. Two percutaneous approaches exist. Percutaneous cholecystostomy involves the use of radiologic imaging (either TASU or computed tomography [CT]) to locate the gallbladder, identify an avascular window for puncture, and allow for the placement of a percutaneous drainage catheter directly into the gallbladder. Technical success rates are typically at or near 100% and clinical success rates of 78% to 95% have been reported.[19–25] Percutaneous drainage placement does have a number of associated downsides. Major procedural-related adverse events include bleeding, pneumothorax, bile peritonitis, and inadvertent displacement of the drainage catheter occur in up to 12% of patients.[19–27] Lastly, long-term indwelling drainage catheters are associated with diminished quality of life in patients unfit for surgery.[28] An alternative percutaneous approach involves simple aspiration of the gallbladder, without placement of a drainage catheter, and thus avoidance of its attendant risks. This has the advantage of being able to be performed bedside, with smaller gauge needles, fewer adverse events, and the ability to repeat the intervention if necessary. Overall, the percutaneous approach to emergent drainage of the gallbladder allows for stabilization of the severely ill patient, as well as resolution of local inflammation in severe cases, thus potentially avoiding the need for emergency surgery in high-risk individuals and/or avoidance of open surgical resection in patients with extensive pericholecystic inflammation.

A number of endoscopic options exist as an alternative to the traditional surgical or percutaneous approaches to managing cholecystitis and symptomatic cholelithiasis. These include transpapillary drainage of the gallbladder, EUS-guided transmural drainage of the gallbladder, and natural orifice transluminal endoscopic surgery (NOTES).

Endoscopic transpapillary nasogallbladder drainage involves the use of ERCP to gain transpapillary wire access to the gallbladder, followed by placement of a nasogallbladder tube, allowing for both drainage and irrigation of the infected gallbladder. The technique involves standard biliary cannulation, followed by selective guidewire cannulation of the cystic duct and the gallbladder. Given the varied locations of the cystic duct take-off, as well as the small caliber and tortuosity of the cystic duct, a variety of tools and techniques have been described to successfully achieve gallbladder access. These include the use of standard cannulating catheters, standard sphincterotomes, and sphincterotomes with the ability to rotate and/or "swing" in opposite directions to

allow for directed wire placement both into the cystic duct orifice, as well as navigating the wire across the cystic duct.[29–31] There is no favored guidewire size, as the use of 0.035-, 0.025-, and 0.018-inch guidewires with a hydrophilic tip have been reported.[29–32] Itoi et al (2010) reported using either a 0.025- or 0.018-inch guidewire in patients with left-sided distribution or deformation of the cystic duct.[29] Once gallbladder access is achieved, a 5-Fr or 7-Fr nasogallbladder drain can be placed over the wire. Multiple large retrospective series have been published, reporting a technical success rate of 71% to 89% and a clinical success rate of 69% to 89%.[33–38] Two prospective series demonstrated a technical success of 82% to 91.9% and a clinical success of 70.6% to 87%.[39,40] Overall, adverse events associated with endoscopic transpapillary nasogallbladder drainage occur in up to 14% of cases.[36] Reported adverse events associated with this technique include cystic duct perforation, gallbladder perforation, cholangitis, sepsis, inadvertent removal of the nasogallbladder drain, as well as post-ERCP pancreatitis, and sphincterotomy-related bleeding.[28,29,33–40]

Endoscopic transpapillary gallbladder stenting is similar to nasogallbladder drainage, with the exception that it has the advantages of internal placement of drainage tubes, allowing for physiologic drainage, and no risk of inadvertent dislodgement of the drain (Fig. 53.6). Wire guided cannulation technique is similar to that for nasogallbladder drainage. Most series report the use of 5-Fr or 7-Fr double-pigtail plastic stents. Glessing et al (2015) described the use of the Johlin pancreatic wedge stent (Cook Medical, Bloomington, IN), which is made of a softer polyurethane material compared to standard double-pigtail stents.[41] In addition to being softer, these stents are fenestrated, available in 8.5-Fr and 10-Fr sizes, as well as lengths up to 22 cm. Multiple large retrospective series report technical success rates ranging from 90% to 100%, and clinical success rates of 64% to 100%.[30,32,41–45] Lee et al (2011) reported their prospective

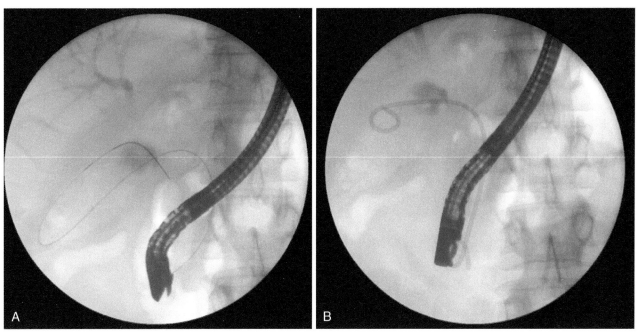

FIG 53.6 A, Endoscopic transpapillary gallbladder drainage by selective cannulation and placement of a guidewire across the cystic duct into the gallbladder lumen, followed by **B,** placement of a transpapillary double pigtail stent.

experience of transpapillary gallbladder stent placement in 29 patients, using a 7-Fr × 15-cm double pigtail stent. Technical success was 79% and clinical success was 100% in the group with successful stent placement.[46] Median follow-up was 586 days, during which time 20% of patients developed late adverse events including distal stent migration, cholangitis, and recurrent biliary pain. Overall, adverse events associated with gallbladder stenting have been reported in up to 16% of cases.

Two prospective randomized trials compared endoscopic transpapillary nasogallbladder drainage to transpapillary gallbladder stenting in patients with acute cholecystitis. Itoi et al (2015) studied 73 patients, reporting a clinical success of 86.5% in the nasogallbladder drain group compared to 77.8% in the stenting group (p > 0.05, nonsignificant [NS]), in their intention-to-treat analysis.[39] Adverse events included one postsphincterotomy bleed and one post-ERCP pancreatitis in the nasogallbladder drain group, and one post-ERCP pancreatitis in the stent group. The authors did note patients receiving the gallbladder stent reported a significantly lower patient discomfort score compared to those receiving the nasobiliary drain. Yang et al (2016) studied 35 patients, demonstrating a clinical success rate of 70.6% in the nasogallbladder drain group compared to 83.3% in the stenting group (p > 0.05, NS), in their intention-to-treat analysis.[40] Adverse events included one cystic duct perforation, one severe post-ERCP pancreatitis, and one inadvertent drain pull in the nasogallbladder drain group, and one mild post-ERCP pancreatitis in the stent group.

Overall, in expert hands, endoscopic transpapillary nasogallbladder drain placement and gallbladder stent placement appear to be equivalent in terms of technical and clinical success rates. One potential downside to gallbladder stenting is that gallbladder irrigation to dissolve/remove blood and debris is not feasible, unlike in nasogallbladder drain placement. As such, this can potentially increase the risk of subsequent recurrence of cholecystitis and biliary symptoms. Recurrent cholecystitis after transpapillary gallbladder stenting has been reported to occur in 0% to 11.8% of patients.[36,42–49] One potential strategy to minimize this risk is to place a nasogallbladder drain at initial endoscopy to allow for optimal drainage, irrigation, and possibly clearance of debris in the gallbladder, and then convert this drain to a stent once the acute inflammation resolves.

One advantage of transpapillary gallbladder stents is that they can remain in place indefinitely. In contrast to plastic CBD stents, which should be changed every 3 months to decrease the risk of cholangitis secondary to stent occlusion, there is no evidence that routine drainage of transpapillary gallbladder stents decreases the risk for recurrent biliary type pain or acute cholecystitis. Our practice has been to change the stents on an as-needed basis for the recurrence of symptoms regardless of etiology (calculous vs. acalculous). Additionally, despite lack of prospective data demonstrating an advantage of biliary sphincterotomy, we routinely perform biliary sphincterotomy in conjunction with stent placement with the thought that this may facilitate biliary drainage around the stent even in the setting of stent occlusion.

One potential challenge with attempting transpapillary gallbladder drainage pertains to the potential difficulty in achieving gallbladder access in the setting of cholecystitis. This may be secondary to the inability to identify the cystic duct on cholangiogram, and/or due to cystic duct obstruction and inability to advance a wire into the gallbladder. An emerging solution to this conundrum is the use of direct cholangioscopy to identify

the cystic duct takeoff and simultaneously guide placement of a wire across the cystic duct into the gallbladder. A handful of case reports and one case series have demonstrated the feasibility and success of this technique using single-operator cholangioscopy systems.[31,50–52]

The next evolutionary step in the endoscopic management of cholecystitis has been the development of EUS-guided transmural gallbladder drainage (EUS-GBD). First described in 2007, this technique mirrors that of EUS-guided transmural pseudocyst drainage and has the advantages of placement of internalized, larger diameter stents.[53] EUS is used to first locate the gallbladder, followed by EUS-guided puncture of the gallbladder, typically with a 19-gauge needle in a transgastric or transduodenal approach. A guidewire can be placed through the needle into the gallbladder lumen. Once the needle is removed, various devices such as bougies, balloons, or electrosurgical knives can be placed over the guidewire to dilate the newly created cholecysto-gastric fistula or cholecysto-duodenal fistula. Finally, biliary endoprostheses such as double pigtail stents, covered metal biliary stents, or dedicated lumen-apposing metal stents (LAMS) can be placed across the tract to allow for gallbladder drainage into the GI lumen.

Initial reports described the placement of nasogallbladder drains and/or plastic double-pigtail stents across the fistulous tract.[53–55] One early concern with this technique however, is that unlike most pancreatic pseudocysts that are amenable to transmural endoscopic drainage, the gallbladder is typically not adherent or apposed to the GI lumen wall. This poses the potential risk of leakage of pus and bile around the stents into the peritoneum, as well as risk of stent migration as the two lumens move away from each other with peristalsis and respiration. As such, to mitigate this risk, the use of covered metal biliary stents has become the favored approach. Widmer et al (2014) described the use of a fully covered self-expanding metal stent with antimigratory fins in three patients with symptomatic gallbladder obstruction secondary to underlying pancreatic cancer.[56]

The true breakthrough in EUS-GBD drainage came with the development of dedicated endoprostheses designed specifically for transmural drainage. These devices, dubbed LAMS, are short (1 cm long) and have dumbbell shaped flanges. Upon expansion, the two flanges catch and appose their respective lumen walls, allowing for fistula development. Currently available LAMS are fully covered, thus preventing spillage of luminal contents across the tract. In addition, they are specifically designed to fit through the working channel of a therapeutic linear echoendoscope. Lastly, the lumen of the LAMS is wide enough (10 mm or 15 mm) to allow insertion of standard endoscopes through the stent and into the gallbladder lumen, facilitating further intervention such as irrigation, debridement, and stone removal.

In 2011, Jang et al reported their experience with a modified covered self-expandable metal stent (SEMS) (BONA-AL Standard Sci Tech Inc, Seoul, Korea).[57] This stent is a partially covered metal stent, 10 mm in diameter, and 4 to 7 cm in length. The flares on the end of each stent were modified by enlarging them to 22 mm external diameter and placing them at a 90-degree angulation to prevent migration once in place. In 15 patients with acute cholecystitis, technical success rate was reported in 10/10 cases from a transgastric approach, and 5/5 cases from a transduodenal approach. All patients had a clinical response as well. Two patients experienced pneumoperitoneum. Choi et al (2014) reported long-term outcomes in 63 patients who underwent gallbladder drainage with this device.[58] Technical and clinical success was reported in 98% of cases. Adverse events included one patient with a perforation, and two patients with pneumo-peritoneum. Long-term outcome data was available in 56 patients, with a median follow-up of 275 days. There was no recurrence of biliary symptoms or cholecystitis in 54/56 (96%) cases over this time frame. Late adverse events were encountered in four (8.4%) patients, which included stent migration and stent occlu-sion. Overall, cumulative stent patency was 86% at 3 years. The authors concluded that EUS-GBD with a SEMS for acute cho-lecystitis showed excellent long-term outcomes and may be considered a viable definitive treatment in patients who are not surgical candidates or are suffering from advanced malignancy. Of note, the BONA-AL stent used in these two studies is not available in the Unites States.

The Axios stent (Boston Scientific, Marlborough, MA) is the only LAMS device available in the Unites States. The standard "cold" Axios device comes preloaded on an EUS needle-like delivery catheter. The standard technique for transmural gallblad-der stent placement involves the identification of the gallbladder on EUS, transduodenal or transgastric puncture of the gallbladder using a 19-gauge needle, followed by passage of a 0.035-inch Jagwire through the needle and into the gallbladder lumen (Fig. 53.7). The needle is then exchanged over the wire, leaving the wire in the gallbladder. The cholecysto-enteric fistula in then dilated, typically with a 6-Fr bougie dilator and/or a 4 to 6 mm biliary dilating balloon. Finally, the Axios delivery catheter is advanced over the wire, through the accessory channel of the therapeutic linear echoendoscope, and locked into place, similar to a standard EUS needle. The delivery catheter is then advanced across the fistulous tract under EUS guidance, followed by stepwise deployment of the inner distal flange, and then the outer proximal flange. Following deployment, the stent can be dilated to its final diameter using standard CRE dilating balloons (Boston Scientific); however this step is not always necessary, as the LAMS is a self-expanding type stent (Video 53.1).

Small, retrospective case series have been published describing the use of the Axios stent for EUS-GBD. A 2013 report demon-strated technical success in 11/13 (84%) and clinical success in 11/11 (100%) patients.[59] Ten of the eleven cases were transgastric. In 4/11 (36%) of patients, a tubular SEMS was placed in a coaxial fashion through the LAMS to ensure adequate drainage. During the same session, an endoscope was inserted through the stent lumen into the gallbladder to perform lavage and/or stone

extraction. A total of two adverse events were noted in this series, one patient with hematochezia and another with right upper quadrant abdominal pain. There was no recurrence of cholecystitis during a median follow-up of 100 days. Irani et al reported on a multicenter experience in 15 patients.[60] In this series, a trans-duodenal approach was favored in 14 cases, compared to one transgastric deployment. Technical success was 14/15 (93%) and clinical success 100%. One adverse event (fever) was noted. During a median follow-up of 160 days there was recurrence of chole-cystitis in this group. It is noted that in six patients, an additional double-pigtail plastic stent was deployed through the LAMS to decrease the risk of hyperplastic tissue overgrowth at either end of the stent.

Walter et al (2016) reported the results of a multicenter prospective trial of the Axios stent in 30 patients with acute cholecystitis.[61] Technical success was achieved in 27/30 (90%) of patients and clinical success in 26/27 (96%) patients. Recurrent cholecystitis due to stent obstruction was encountered in 7% of patients. Adverse events were encountered in 15/30 (50%) of patients, but the authors state that only 4 (13%) were possibly related to the stent or procedure. The 30-day mortality was 17% and the overall mortality was 23%. The authors state that 30-day mortality rate is comparable with that of percutaneous gallbladder drainage (15%). Their conclusion was that the high overall rate of adverse events was attributable to the overall morbid patient population of their study, as none of the patients were considered surgical candidates due to underling comorbidities.

In 2015, a modified version of the Axios stent was released with an electrocautery-enhanced tip. By allowing for direct puncture across lumen walls without the need for prior tract dilation, this "hot" Axios device allows for essentially a one-step delivery system without the need for multiple device exchanges (Video 53.2). As such, the electrocautery-enhanced Axios can be placed without a guidewire.

Given the relatively widespread adoption of EUS-guided transmural pancreatic fluid collection drainage, the prospect of routine EUS-GBD with LAMS holds promise. However, the gallbladder is a hollow organ rather than a collection and thus once the inflammatory/infectious issues are resolved it will not shrink or collapse as would be expected in a pancreatic fluid collection. As a result, there are unique issues related to LAMS use. One issue is that of impaction of the gallbladder and/or stent with food, particularly when a transgastric approach is

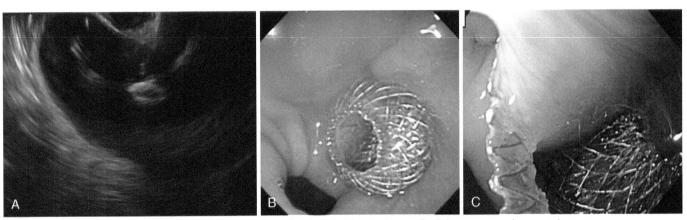

FIG 53.7 Endoscopic ultrasound-guided gallbladder drainage. **A,** A lumen-apposing metal stent is inserted under EUS-guidance into the gallbladder via **B,** a transgastric approach, with **C,** subsequent drainage of purulent bile.

utilized. Mechanical friction of the LAMS against the mucosal surface of the gallbladder can induce bleeding (Todd Baron, personal communication). Epithelial overgrowth of the intraluminal portion of the LAMS has been reported as well.[62,63] This "buried LAMS" phenomenon can result in stent occlusion and recurrent cholecystitis. In addition, this may result in technical difficulty in removing the buried stent.[62] It is postulated that buried LAMS is most likely to occur when the stent is placed in the prepyloric antrum, as gastric motility in this location may result in traction on the stent and a hypertrophic tissue reaction, similar to that seen with the formation of inflammatory polyps of the stomach.[63] One maneuver that has become adopted at some centers to minimize the risk of buried LAMS is to place one or two double pigtail stents inside the lumen of the LAMS. This may also decrease the risk of bleeding or food impaction.

Perhaps the biggest question remaining regarding the technique of EUS-GBD with LAMS is whether the creation of a cholecysto-duodenal fistula or cholecysto-gastric fistula will have a major impact on future cholecystectomy in any one patient.[64] It has been shown that the transmural placement of a small caliber 5-Fr drainage tube did not result in any significantly higher need for open cholecystectomy (9%) compared to patients undergoing percutaneous gallbladder drainage (12%, NS).[65] However, LAMS are much larger in diameter (10 mm or 15 mm) and will produce a larger fistula. As such, it remains unclear if the creation of a larger fistula will lead to difficulties in performing laparoscopic resection, or if new, unanticipated challenges will be created. Baron et al (2015) reported a case of a patient with end-stage liver disease who underwent transduodenal placement of a 10-mm LAMS for management of acute cholecystitis.[66] Five months later, when the patient underwent liver transplantation, a large duodenal defect was encountered upon take-down of the fistula and stent. Despite oversewing the defect, placing an omental patch, leaving in surgical drains, and keeping the patient on nasogastric tube suction for 2 weeks, a leak and abscess developed at the site. Ultimately, a large hepatic artery pseudoaneurysm developed at the site of the abscess necessitating aggressive vascular intervention and ultimately surgery.[67]

EUS-GBD remains an emerging technique. Regardless of whether plastic stents, SEMS, or LAMS are chosen, the overall adverse event rate remains moderate at 12%.[68] In a 2016 multicenter retrospective study involving 90 patients with acute cholecystitis, EUS-GBD had similar technical and clinical success with percutaneous transhepatic gallbladder drainage.[69] It should be emphasized that EUS-GBD should be reserved as an option for nonsurgical candidates. Optimal patient selection—ideally within a multidisciplinary approach involving surgeons, endoscopists, and interventional radiologists—remains key in predicting the overall success of this intervention.

The final frontier in the minimally invasive approach to acute cholecystitis is that of natural orifice transluminal endoscopic surgery, or NOTES. In this technique, the abdominal cavity is accessed through a small incision of an internal organ, such as the stomach, rectum, or vagina, and the endoscopic surgical tools are advanced through this incision. Thus far, this technique has been performed in a limited number of centers throughout the world, with the majority being performed via a hybrid transvaginal approach with the use of a small transumbilical port to facilitate visualization. The major potential advantages of a NOTES approach are less pain, faster recovery time, and decrease in risk of wound healing, as well as the avoidance of a visible scar.[70] However, two prospective trials comparing NOTES cholecystectomy to laparoscopic cholecystectomy failed to demonstrate any advantage to NOTES in terms of postoperative pain, recovery, length of stay, or complications.[71,72] Further studies are needed to better identify the role of NOTES in the management of gallbladder disease.

CHOLEDOCHOLITHIASIS

Epidemiology/Incidence/Risk Factors/Pathophysiology

Choledocholithiasis refers to the presence of stones within the extrahepatic bile duct. This is a common clinical problem, with an estimated incidence of 5% to 20% at the time of cholecystectomy in patients with cholelithiasis.[73] Choledocholithiasis can be primary or secondary. Secondary stones are those that originate within the gallbladder and migrate into the CBD via the cystic duct. In Western countries, secondary stones are much more common than primary bile duct stones. Primary stones refer to stones that form directly within the bile duct. Risk factors for primary bile duct stones include IgA deficiency, chronic infections of the biliary tree, and biliary dyskinesia. Primary bile duct stones can also occur in patients who have undergone biliary sphincterotomy, particularly in patients who have sphincterotomy stenosis. In this setting, duodenal contents can reflux into the bile duct and serve as a nidus for stone formation. Primary bile duct stones are usually soft and brown.

Symptoms

Patients with choledocholithiasis can be asymptomatic. Symptomatic patients can present with liver function test abnormalities, jaundice, cholangitis, or gallstone pancreatitis, with severity ranging from mild abdominal pain to sepsis.

Choledocholithiasis can cause ascending cholangitis, or bacterial infection within the biliary tree which develops behind an obstructing stone in the distal bile duct. The classic presentation for cholangitis is Charcot's triad (fever, right upper quadrant pain, and jaundice) and Reynold's pentad (renal dysfunction and mental status changes) which indicates more severe disease.

The Tokyo Guidelines (TG) for the management of cholangitis provide diagnostic criteria consisting of signs of systemic infection (fever, rigors, laboratory evidence of inflammatory response), cholestasis, and imaging findings consistent with biliary obstruction (biliary duct dilation, stone, stricture). The diagnosis of cholangitis is "suspected" in patients with evidence of systemic infection and either abnormal liver enzymes or imaging suggesting biliary obstruction. The diagnosis of cholangitis is considered "definite" in patients with evidence of systemic infection and both laboratory and imaging evidence for biliary obstruction. These were initially reported in 2007 and then revised in 2013. Within the retrospective cohort of patients with ascending cholangitis, Charcot's triad had excellent specificity (95%) but poor sensitivity (26%) for the diagnosis of cholangitis. This compared to TG13 criteria, which were 92% sensitive and 78% specific for the diagnosis of ascending cholangitis.[74]

Chronic or recurrent choledocholithiasis is frequently associated with chronic infection and inflammation within the bile ducts. This can predispose an individual to strictures within the biliary tree, or secondary biliary cirrhosis. It is also a risk factor for cholangiocarcinoma, presumably due to chronic inflammation progressing to neoplasia. Choledocholithiasis can also cause gallstone pancreatitis, which will be discussed in more detail later in this section.

Diagnosis

The diagnosis of choledocholithiasis can be suspected on the basis of abnormal liver enzymes. Early in the course of the disease, patients with choledocholithiasis may have elevations in transaminases only. Later in the course, patients may develop an obstructive pattern with elevations in direct bilirubin and alkaline phosphatase. A meta-analysis revealed that elevated bilirubin was 69% sensitive and 88% specific for choledocholithiasis, and elevated alkaline phosphatase was 57% sensitive and 86% specific.[75] Given the wide range of liver enzyme abnormalities which can occur in patients with choledocholithiasis, abnormal liver function tests (LFTs) are not specific for the diagnosis. However, the negative predicative value for bile duct stones in patients with normal liver enzymes is 97%.[76]

In cases of suspected choledocholithiasis, the least expensive and most available imaging modality is TAUS. TAUS is very specific for choledocholithiasis, but sensitivity is limited. In a meta-analysis of five studies, the sensitivity and specificity for choledocholithiasis was 73% and 91%, respectively.[77] The distal CBD may be obscured by intervening bowel and artifact from bowel gas or not visualized at all due to body habitus, which further decreases the sensitivity of the test. CBD stones appear as round, shadowing structures within the bile duct. In the setting of nonvisualization of the distal bile duct, the presence of bile duct dilation of greater than 6 mm is suggestive of distal obstruction, and the probability of a stone increases with increasing duct diameter.[78]

A strategy to assign risk of choledocholithiasis was created based on laboratory and TAUS parameters was proposed by the American Society for Gastrointestinal Endoscopy (ASGE) in a 2010 guideline.[78] The presence of a CBD stone on US, bilirubin greater than 4, and clinical signs and symptoms of cholangitis are considered "very strong" predictors. "Strong" predictors include a dilated CBD (> 6 mm with gallbladder in situ) and bilirubin 1.8–4. "Moderate" predictors include age greater than 55 or any abnormal liver biochemistry. Patients are considered high risk for choledocholithiasis in the presence of any very strong predictor or presence of both strong predictors. Patients are considered low risk if none of the predictors is present. All others are considered intermediate risk.

Patients who are considered intermediate risk should undergo additional studies prior to therapy directed at biliary drainage. The most commonly used modality for intermediate risk patients is magnetic resonance cholangiopancreatography (MRCP). MRCP allows for three-dimensional reconstruction of the bile ducts and is very sensitive and specific for choledocholithiasis; however, the sensitivity of MRCP decreases for stones greater than 6 mm.[79] EUS is the most sensitive test for the detection of choledocholithiasis with greater than 95% sensitivity and 100% specificity[80] (Fig. 53.8). A decision analysis suggested that for patients with low (< 40%) probability of choledocholithiasis, MRCP should be the test of choice, but in cases where choledocholithiasis is suspected despite a negative MRCP, EUS should be performed; for patients with a 40% to 91% probability, EUS should be performed, preferably in a setting where same-session ERCP can be performed if EUS is positive. Patients with a higher probability should undergo ERCP.[81] However, there are data suggesting that this guideline overexposes patients to ERCP with an overall accuracy of 63%.[82,83] Therefore it is important to recognize that current guideline lacks accuracy and should not replace clinical judgment. Additionally, large, multicenter studies are needed to

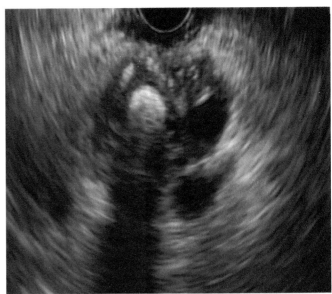

FIG 53.8 Endoscopic ultrasound identification of a common bile duct stone, represented by a bright, hyperechoic focus with shadowing.

further clarify appropriate risk stratification in patients suspected of choledocholithiasis.

In patients with an intact gallbladder suspected of having choledocholithiasis, cholecystectomy with intraoperative cholangiogram (IOC) or intraoperative ultrasound (IOUS) can be performed instead of MRCP or EUS, though practice varies among surgeons and institutions. These modalities can be useful in the detection of retained CBD stones and for bile duct injury. Data from a randomized controlled trial suggest that initial cholecystectomy with IOC may be preferred to endoscopic bile duct assessment and clearance (via EUS or ERCP) in patients with intermediate probability of having common duct stones with regard to length of stay, number of bile duct evaluations, without change in morbidity.[84] A prospective blinded study among patients with a positive IOC found that EUS had a positive predictive value (PPV) of 95% in detecting choledocholithiasis, and only 65% of patients who had a suspicious IOC had CBD stones at the time of ERCP.[80] Thus, in patients referred for a "positive" IOC, a reasonable approach, particularly in asymptomatic patients, is to perform an EUS to confirm the presence of choledocholithiasis prior to performing ERCP.

There is an approximate 5% to 15% incidence of silent choledocholithiasis at the time of cholecystectomy. Routine evaluation for choledocholithiasis intraoperatively, either with IOUS or IOC, is institution-dependent. However, data from a cost-analysis study, with a set incidence of choledocholithiasis of 9%, found that IOUS was more cost-effective than IOC or a watchful waiting approach.[85] Additionally, even among patients who undergo preoperative ERCP, approximately 12% will have retained stones on IOC during subsequent cholecystectomy.[86]

In select patients, especially in an increasingly cost-conscious environment, there may also be a role for no biliary imaging. In a study of 668 patients presenting with elevated but downtrending LFTs who did not undergo pre- or intraoperative biliary imaging and underwent same-admission cholecystectomy, only 38 required postoperative imaging and only 22 had definite choledocholithiasis.[87]

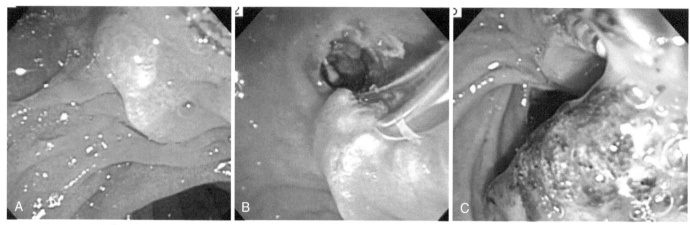

FIG 53.9 **A,** Image of normal papilla followed by **B,** large biliary sphincterotomy to facilitate **C,** balloon extraction of bile duct stones.

Treatment
ERCP

Patients with documented choledocholithiasis or those at high risk for choledocholithiasis based on the criteria described previously should have an ERCP for further evaluation. Typically, this is performed in conjunction with biliary sphincterotomy and stone extraction. For smaller stones, it is possible to perform ERCP with biliary sphincteroplasty instead of biliary sphincterotomy,[88] but this is generally discouraged due to the concern for possible higher risk for post ERCP pancreatitis (PEP).

In the majority of cases of choledocholithiasis, biliary sphincterotomy followed by use of an extraction balloon or retrieval basket is sufficient treatment (Fig. 53.9). Biliary sphincterotomy treats the principal barrier keeping the stone within the bile duct. Sphincterotomy should be complete, which decreases the risk for subsequent sphincterotomy stenosis and facilitates stone extraction. A blended current is usually used for biliary sphincterotomy, and there are no data to support the use of pure cut versus blended current. However, pure cut may increase the risk for postsphincterotomy bleeding but decrease the risk for PEP when compared to blended current. When performing extraction of multiple stones, the most distal stone should be removed first, progressing proximally. During stone extraction, it is useful to periodically inject contrast to identify the next stone to target for removal. Attempts at removing a stack of stones on one sweep can result in impaction of stones in the distal duct which can decrease the success of stone clearance and increase complications. There may be an advantage of using baskets instead of balloons in dilated bile ducts with multiple stones because balloons may slip by the stones.

For larger stones (generally > 15 mm) or in which a stone is larger than the distal duct, biliary sphincterotomy and sweep may be insufficient[89] (Fig. 53.10). There are several therapeutic options for larger bile duct stones, including large balloon sphincteroplasty,[90,91] mechanical lithotripsy, and cholangioscopy-directed stone fragmentation techniques such as electrohydraulic lithotripsy (EHL) and laser lithotripsy. Typically, these can and should be performed at the same setting, but one may choose the option of placing a biliary stent to ensure biliary drainage and refer to a tertiary care facility for more advanced techniques.

Balloon sphincteroplasty following biliary sphincterotomy is extremely effective and is the least labor- and time-intensive

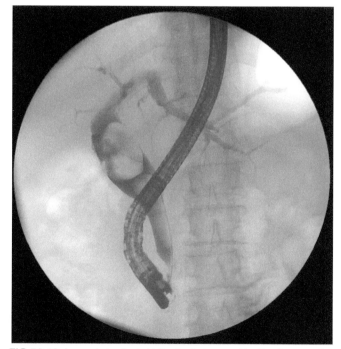

FIG 53.10 Large intraductal bile duct stone with distal narrowing of the common bile duct.

therapeutic maneuver for management of large bile duct stones. An over-the-wire dilation balloon should be used to ensure its proper placement within the bile duct. The choice of balloon size should be based on the diameter of the upstream duct and size of the stone. Dilation is performed under both endoscopic and fluoroscopic guidance to visualize both the apex of the sphincterotomy and waist of the balloon (Fig. 53.11). The balloon should be kept inflated until obliteration of the waist. There are data suggesting that for an intact papilla, the longer the balloon is inflated, the lower the risk for PEP,[92] though usually dilation to balloon effacement is sufficient. The balloon is then carefully deflated and withdrawn over the wire while evaluating for bleeding and perforation. The stones are then swept into the duodenum through the sphincteroplasty with an extraction balloon or basket (Video 53.3). A meta-analysis of six trials, including 835 patients,

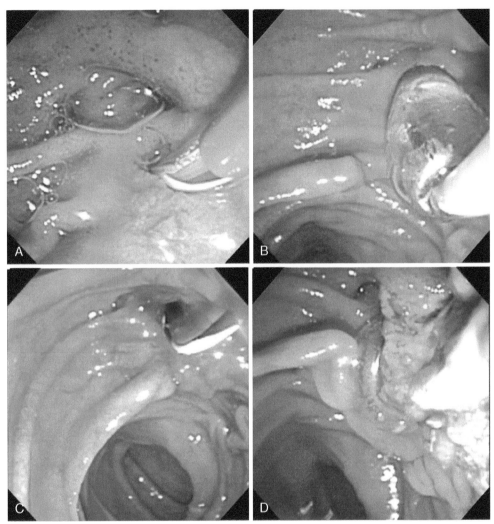

FIG 53.11 A and **B,** Performance of endoscopic papillary balloon dilation on a stenotic papilla to facilitate **C** and **D,** removal of large common bile duct stone burden.

concluded that biliary sphincterotomy plus large balloon sphincteroplasty was associated with fewer complications than biliary sphincterotomy alone.[93]

Usually, large balloon sphincteroplasty is performed following biliary sphincterotomy. However, a single retrospective study involving a small number of patients suggested that duct clearance could be achieved via balloon sphincteroplasty alone without biliary sphincterotomy, suggesting that biliary sphincterotomy is not mandatory, even in the management of large stones.[94] However, there are no prospective randomized data, and biliary sphincterotomy is routine for management of choledocholithiasis in clinical practice. Additionally, failure to perform sphincterotomy may increase the risk for PEP, which may be severe. In the setting of planned balloon sphincteroplasty for management of large bile duct stones, some experts recommend leaving room at the apex of the sphincterotomy prior to balloon sphincteroplasty. Doing so may decrease the risk of retroperitoneal perforation should there be extension of the sphincterotomy on performing balloon sphincteroplasty.

Mechanical lithotripsy involves use of large stone retrieval baskets attached to a crank mechanism. These are available either through the scope or outside of the scope, the former being used more commonly in clinical practice. Some retrieval baskets do not come prepackaged with the lithotripter components but are lithotripter compatible in situations in which a stone becomes impacted in a basket and cannot be extracted; this is known as *rescue lithotripsy*. Rescue lithotripsy, if needed, is an outside of the scope device. It is extremely important to recognize which baskets are lithotripter compatible and choose these baskets if lithotripsy is at all anticipated, because use of baskets that are not lithotripter compatible can lead to basket impaction and operative intervention.

Some baskets come prepackaged with a lithotripter setup. This is more labor-intensive to set up and use but can be very effective to fragment large stones, making them amenable to extraction through a biliary sphincterotomy. Hard stones can be very difficult to fragment and, not infrequently, wires of the basket can slip off the side of the stone, resulting in little to no fragmentation. Additionally, baskets tend to become easily misshapen and difficult to mold back into working condition.

In a single trial, 90 patients with large bile duct stones (12–20 mm) were randomized to mechanical lithotripsy or large balloon sphincteroplasty following sphincterotomy.[95] Overall, the rate of stone clearance was greater than 91% in both groups and without a statistically significant difference. However, there was a statistically significant increase in complications among

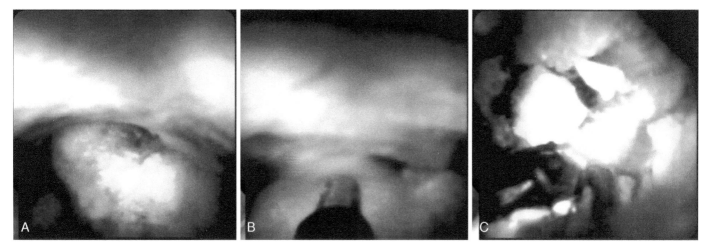

FIG 53.12 A, Use of single operator digital cholangioscopy to identify large common bile duct stone, and **B,** use of electrohydraulic lithotripsy to **C,** fragment to stone into smaller pieces.

the patients in the mechanical lithotripsy group (4.4% vs. 20%).[95] Thus, when possible, biliary sphincterotomy followed by large balloon sphincteroplasty should be attempted prior to mechanical lithotripsy for management of large bile duct stones.

Cholangioscopy directed stone fragmentation is another advanced technique for clearance of large bile duct stones. Common techniques include EHL and laser lithotripsy. Each requires direct visualization of the stone using cholangioscopy. Typically, cholangioscopy is performed using a mother-daughter scope system. A disposable digital cholangioscope is available in clinical practice. Direct peroral cholangioscopy can also be performed using an ultra-slim upper endoscope. Once the cholangioscope is within the duct, the duct is filled with sterile saline to improve visualization and serve as a medium for transmission of EHL. The EHL probe is then advanced close to, but not touching, the stone, and the energy is then delivered, initially at low power (Fig. 53.12). The power can be titrated up based on initial fragmentation. Once the stones are fragmented, standard retrieval with a basket or balloon is then performed. Patients should be given a dose of antibiotics intraprocedurally to decrease the risk of cholangitis. Cholangioscopy-guided laser lithotripsy is another option, but its use is dependent on operator expertise and availability varies by institution.

Biliary stenting may be required. The most common reason in the setting of choledocholithiasis is for incomplete stone clearance. This temporizes the condition, allowing for biliary drainage around the residual stones. Additionally, the stents may serve to fragment residual stones, making subsequent stone extraction easier, though there are no data to support this. Typically, plastic biliary stents are sufficient, but there are two situations where off-label use of fully covered biliary stents may be beneficial. One is for postsphincterotomy bleeding or suspected/confirmed retroperitoneal perforation. The other is to attempt progressive dilation of a narrow CBD with large stones proximally. Following complete stone clearance, there is no proven benefit for biliary stent placement to protect against biliary obstruction due to papillary edema, though anecdotally, this is not uncommon in clinical practice.

Percutaneous Transhepatic Biliary Drainage (PTBD)

Percutaneous transhepatic biliary drainage (PTBD) is an alternative to endoscopic management of choledocholithiasis. PTBD is performed by interventional radiologists and may be chosen in patients who have a contraindication for ERCP, who have had a failed ERCP, or in those with altered anatomy in whom ERCP is not attempted or unsuccessful. PTBD usually requires placement of a percutaneous transhepatic cholangiography drain. Approximately 6 weeks following initial drain placement, patients return for stone management. Techniques include antegrade balloon sphincteroplasty with a standard dilation balloon followed by attempts to push the stone into the duodenum. A "cutting balloon" may also be used to perform antegrade sphincterotomy. Additional devices including retrieval baskets, mechanical lithotripters, and choledochoscopes can be passed percutaneously through the PTBD tract to perform stone fragmentation and extraction (Fig. 53.13).

Surgery

In patients with concurrent choledocholithiasis and cholelithiasis with or without cholecystitis, the decision to perform ERCP pre- or postoperatively is largely institution- and provider-dependent. In most cases, patients with established choledocholithiasis undergo ERCP first, followed by cholecystectomy. Another option in these patients is to perform a laparoscopic CBD exploration (LCBDE) at the time of cholecystectomy, though data from a randomized controlled trial suggest that intraoperative ERCP is better than LCBDE at bile duct clearance.[96]

CBD exploration, either laparoscopic or open, is rarely performed. In patients undergoing laparoscopic cholecystectomy, meta-analysis revealed that single-stage cholecystectomy plus LCBDE was equivalent to two-stage cholecystectomy followed by ERCP.[97] Another study revealed that the surgical plus endoscopic approach was equivalent in morbidity and mortality, but that ERCP resulted in higher rates of duct clearance.[98] Although studies have demonstrated comparable efficacy between the two approaches, there are clinical scenarios in which the laparoscopic cholecystectomy and LCBDE may be a superior option, including patients presenting with choledocholithiasis and cholelithiasis with altered anatomy, particularly Roux-en-Y gastric bypass. This may be the preferred option to laparoscopic cholecystectomy followed by intraoperative ERCP, in which surgical access to the excluded stomach is obtained followed by transabdominal transgastric passage of the duodenoscope to the major papilla.

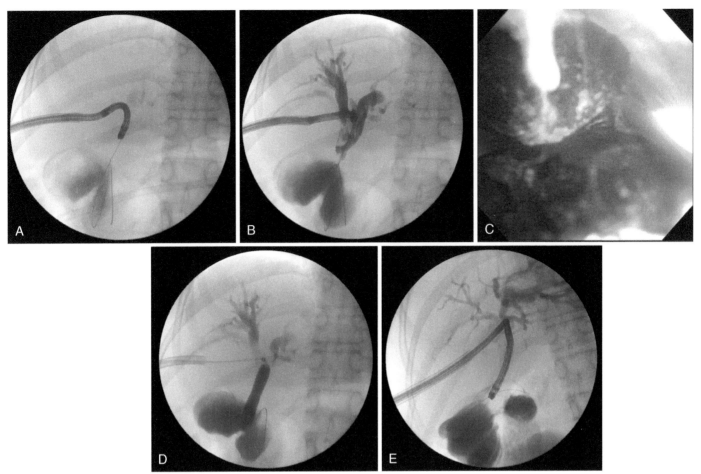

FIG 53.13 Percutaneous transhepatic cholangioscopy for management of bile duct stones in a patient with an inaccessible bilioenteric anastomosis in post Roux-en-Y hepaticojejunostomy anatomy. **A,** An endoscope with a 6-mm diameter is placed into the biliary tree via a mature percutaneous track. Multiple stones are visualized on both **B,** fluoroscopic and **C,** endoscopic examination. **D,** Papillary balloon dilation is performed via an antegrade approach, **E,** allowing for clearance of the biliary tree.

Special Situations
Cystic Duct Stones and Hepatolithiasis
Cystic duct stones and stones proximal to the common hepatic duct (hepatolithiasis) present a challenge for the endoscopist because treatment of these conditions usually requires more advanced ERCP techniques.

Cystic duct stones may masquerade as common duct stones, particularly given the limitations of fluoroscopy. A clue that one is dealing with a cystic duct stone and not a common duct stone is that the balloon or basket repeatedly slips by the stone. In reality, the stone is within the lumen of the cystic duct, which overlies the common duct on fluoroscopy. Rotation of the fluoroscopy unit (or patient) may splay the two ducts and delineate the problem. Once a cystic duct stone is identified, its retrieval can be problematic for several reasons. One is the limited space in the cystic duct in the postcholecystectomy patient; this may prevent balloon or basket passage proximal to the stone. In this situation, cholangioscopy with electrohydraulic or laser lithotripsy may be required. Another problem is the spiral valves of the cystic duct, which may impede retrieval of the stone. Again, lithotripsy may be required to fragment the stone prior to retrieval.

In extreme cases, extracorporeal shock wave lithotripsy (ESWL) may be utilized to fragment the stone, but a stent may be needed to localize the stone for targeting by ESWL if it is not radiopaque.

There are several considerations when dealing with hepatolithiasis. The first is whether ERCP is the best treatment modality. In patients with recurrent pyogenic cholangitis (formerly Oriental cholangiopathy) segmental hepatectomy may be the preferred option. The second is the reason the patient has hepatolithiasis. Is it due to a migrated stone or is there an underlying cholangiopathy or malignancy? When performing ERCP for hepatolithiasis, it is critically important to keep these questions in mind. Again, given its location proximal to the hilum, cholangioscopy with electrohydraulic or laser lithotripsy is often required.

Treatment of Choledocholithiasis in Surgically Altered Anatomy
Performing ERCP in patients with surgically altered anatomy is challenging. Knowledge of postoperative anatomy in general, and of each patient in particular, is crucial in determining choice of scope, instruments, and ultimately having a successful outcome. Additionally, developing a plan with a surgeon is important in

determining the best approach for these patients. For example, in patients with Roux-en-Y gastric bypass with concurrent choledocholithiasis and cholelithiasis, options include preoperative peroral ERCP followed by cholecystectomy, intraoperative ERCP through the excluded stomach, and cholecystectomy with bile duct exploration.

When performing peroral ERCP in patients with surgically altered anatomy, the choice of scope is usually determined by the type of surgery. In patients with Billroth II anatomy, advancement of a duodenoscope to the major papilla is often successful. In postpancreatoduodenectomy patients, a pediatric or adult colonoscope is usually utilized. In patients post-Roux-en-Y gastric bypass, the length of the Roux limb is critical in determining likelihood of success. For patients with short Roux limbs (< 75 cm), a colonoscope can usually be successfully advanced to the papilla. For patients with a long Roux limb, frequently balloon-assisted enteroscopy is required. It is important for the endoscopist to realize the limitations of non-duodenoscopes in performing ERCP, such as lack of an elevator and scope channel length and width, which will limit the types of instruments that can be used in the case (Fig. 53.14).

When peroral ERCP is unsuccessful or not pursued due to high likelihood of failure, EUS-guided biliary drainage (EUS-BD) is an alternative emerging technique for the management of choledocholithiasis. In this procedure, a therapeutic linear echoendoscope is used to visualize the intrahepatic ducts in the left lobe of the liver. A 19-gauge fine-needle aspiration needle is used to access an intrahepatic duct, followed by advancement of a standard ERCP wire through the needle, which is advanced antegrade across the papilla into the duodenum. A dilation balloon is then used to perform antegrade balloon dilation of the papilla (balloon sphincteroplasty) followed by pushing the stone(s) into the duodenum. Case series describing this technique have demonstrated high technical and clinical success rates with low complication rates comparable to PTBD and can be performed successfully during the same session as a failed ERCP. From a technical standpoint, it is more advantageous if the intrahepatic ducts are dilated, which facilitates biliary access.

Treatment of Choledocholithiasis in Pregnancy

Pregnancy is a risk factor for the development of cholelithiasis. The complications of gallstones, including cholecystitis, choledocholithiasis, and gallstone pancreatitis, appear to occur in the same incidence as patients who are not pregnant. Patients presenting with choledocholithiasis in the setting of pregnancy can safely undergo ERCP with particular attention to timing (delaying until the second trimester if possible), radiation exposure to the fetus, and sedation risks to the fetus.

Performing ERCP safely during pregnancy involves pre-, intra-, and postprocedural considerations. As with nonpregnant patients, the necessity of the procedure should be a strong preprocedure consideration. Diagnostic ERCPs should be avoided, and definitive documentation of a stone, usually by MRCP, should be obtained prior to performing ERCP. When possible, intervention should be delayed until the second trimester due to lower surgical risk and apparent lower risk for adverse radiation-associated complications in the fetus. Obstetric involvement should be sought and a plan for fetal heart rate monitoring during the procedure versus pre- and postprocedural documentation of fetal heart sounds should be discussed. Early in pregnancy, patients can be placed in a high prone position with the right leg bent significantly to take pressure off the uterus. Later in pregnancy, prone position is not possible and patients should be placed in a left lateral decubitus position.

Use of fluoroscopy during pregnancy appears safe, with no data suggesting adverse effects on the fetus from radiation exposure. Nonetheless, steps should be taken to limit radiation dosing to the fetus. The uterus should be shielded with lead aprons. Scout films and "hard copies" should be avoided due to higher radiation doses. Magnification should be avoided as this generally increases the radiation dose.

Despite the lack of evidence for fetal harm from radiation exposure during ERCP, there have been a number of studies looking at fluoroscopy-less ERCP. One technique involved wire-guided or free cannulation followed by aspiration in six patients. If bile was aspirated, the procedure was continued without the use of fluoroscopy.[99] In all six patients, there was resolution of jaundice and no maternal or fetal complications. Another technique involves EUS-guided ERCP. In a study involving 31 patients, EUS-guided cannulation and successful completion of the procedure was accomplished in 26 (84%) of patients.[100] Yet another technique involves cholangioscopy-assisted ERCP, not only to confirm entry into the bile duct without fluoroscopy but also to confirm duct clearance.[101]

Postprocedure considerations include documenting fetal heartbeat, standard approaches to fluid management, monitoring for complications, and surgical consultation regarding timing of cholecystectomy. Biliary sphincterotomy is usually protective against recurrent choledocholithiasis and gallstone pancreatitis through pregnancy such that cholecystectomy can be performed postpartum.

Posttreatment Recurrence

It is likely that a considerable proportion of recurrent choledocholithiasis is, in fact, not recurrence but failure to achieve duct clearance on the initial ERCP. Cholangiography alone has limited sensitivity for detection of duct stones, and the sensitivity decreases in larger caliber ducts where small residual stones can be missed. Use of dilute contrast may increase the sensitivity for detecting residual stones. Cholangioscopy is another modality to ensure complete ductal clearance, but this approach is costly and adds procedure time and complexity, so its use should be individualized.

The most important way to prevent recurrent choledocholithiasis is to ensure patients are referred promptly for cholecystectomy. In patients who do not undergo interval cholecystectomy, recurrent choledocholithiasis occurs in up to 11% patients.[102] However, there are data suggesting that elderly patients do not benefit from cholecystectomy,[103] so comorbidities and life expectancy should be considered when making recommendations regarding subsequent cholecystectomy in the elderly.

Some patients develop recurrent primary bile duct stones. Risk factors include sphincterotomy stenosis, biliary dyskinesia, IgA deficiency, and possibly the presence of a periampullary diverticulum.[104] Patients with recurrent primary bile duct stones have a higher rate of duodenal-biliary reflux.[105]

A variety of medical treatments, endoscopic treatments, and surgical treatments have been used to decrease the rate of bile duct stone reaccumulation. In a 2016 small randomized controlled trial, patients receiving ursodiol had a lower risk of recurrent choledocholithiasis; however, this was not statistically significant and the study was likely underpowered.[106] Additionally, case reports of ursodeoxycholic acid (UDCA) stones have been published suggesting that UDCA can exacerbate this problem

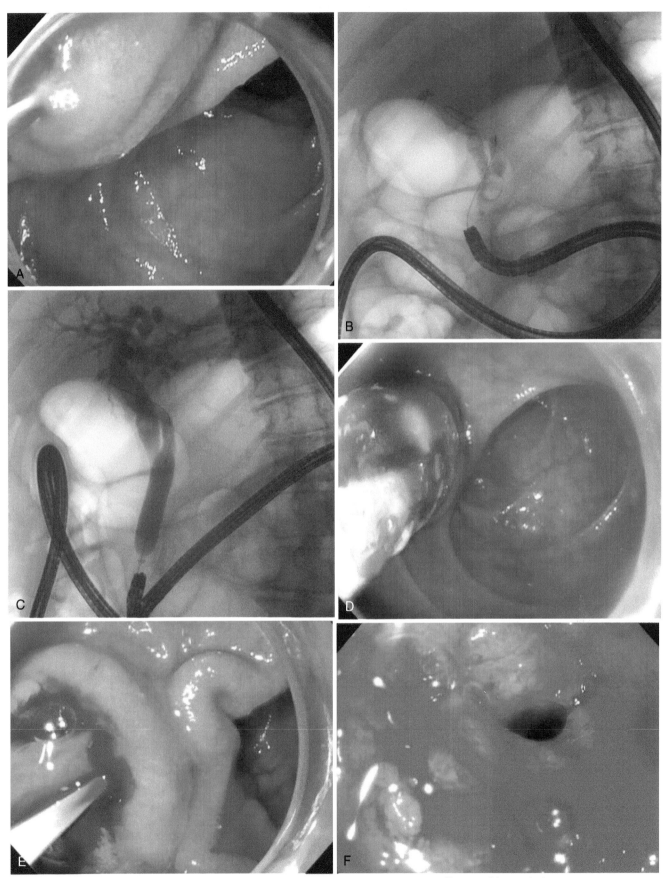

FIG 53.14 ERCP for choledocholithiasis in a patient status post Roux-en-Y gastric bypass. **A,** Endoscopic image of wire through major papilla which was reached via cap-assisted single balloon enteroscopy. **B,** Cholangiogram revealing choledocholithiasis with stones in the cystic duct and extrahepatic bile ducts. **C,** Fluoroscopic and **D,** endoscopic images of primary balloon sphincteroplasty to perform stone extraction; **E,** image of soft brown stone being extracted and **F,** biliary orifice following balloon sphincteroplasty and stone extraction.

in some patients.[107] However, UDCA is a reasonable option for those that have recurrent cholesterol or brown pigment stones given the relative safety profile despite the lack of data from large, randomized controlled trials. Likewise, there are no data regarding use of antibiotics, lipid-lowering agents, and biliary bypass in the prevention of recurrent primary bile duct stones.

Prophylactic biliary stenting and scheduled ERCPs with balloon sweep are options to manage recurrent primary bile duct stones. Data from a prospective comparison study suggest that patients with recurrent choledocholithiasis who undergo routine stent exchanges approximately every 3 months versus as-needed have a lower rate of cholangitis.[108] Another approach for which there is no data is to perform scheduled ERCPs periodically to clear the ducts. Our approach has been to perform ERCPs as-needed for signs and symptoms attributable to choledocholithiasis.

GALLSTONE PANCREATITIS

Incidence/Epidemiology

Gallstone, or biliary, pancreatitis is the most common cause of pancreatitis in the Western world, accounting for approximately 40% to 70% of all cases of acute pancreatitis.[109] However, only approximately 3% to 7% of patients with gallstones develop acute pancreatitis.[110] Additionally, a patient with acute pancreatitis and an intact gallbladder should not be assumed to have gallstone pancreatitis, particularly if the gallbladder is normal and if there is no significant elevation in liver enzymes.

Pathophysiology

The exact pathophysiologic mechanism of gallstone pancreatitis is unknown. Smaller stones are more likely than large stones to cause gallstone pancreatitis because smaller stones are more likely to traverse the cystic duct and enter the CBD. Additionally, smaller stones are more likely to migrate into the common channel or traverse the sphincter of Oddi than larger stones. It is thought that acute pancreatitis occurs by several possible mechanisms: a stone obstructs the common channel causing reflux of bile into the pancreatic duct, a stone obstructs the pancreatic duct causing ductal hypertension, or a stone causes periampullary inflammation.[111]

Diagnosis

The diagnosis of gallstone pancreatitis should be suspected in any patient presenting with acute pancreatitis and an intact gallbladder. However, not every patient with an intact gallbladder presenting with acute pancreatitis should be assumed to have gallstone pancreatitis. In patients with a normal-appearing gallbladder on TAUS, other etiologies for acute pancreatitis should be explored. In patients with recurrent unexplained pancreatitis with a normal-appearing gallbladder, performing empiric cholecystectomy or endoscopic biliary sphincterotomy are controversial and should be individualized.

The presence of sludge or gallstones within the gallbladder makes the diagnosis of gallstone pancreatitis more likely, particularly if associated with concurrent liver enzyme abnormalities or evidence for choledocholithiasis or recently passed stone (i.e., extrahepatic biliary duct dilation). Data from a meta-analysis revealed that elevated alanine aminotransferase (ALT) was the most useful predictor of gallstone pancreatitis with a value greater than 150 IU/L (> 3 × upper limit of normal) having a PPV of 95%.[112]

A TAUS should be a part of the work-up for any patient presenting with acute pancreatitis. However, additional cross-sectional imaging is usually not necessary unless there is a question of the diagnosis, complications associated with pancreatitis, or indeterminate probability of a retained stone. Patients with an indeterminate probability for choledocholithiasis (see earlier section on Choledocholithiasis diagnosis) should undergo MRI/MRCP or EUS.[113]

Treatment

The management of gallstone pancreatitis begins with conservative management that is standard for pancreatitis of any etiology. This includes goal-directed fluid resuscitation, monitoring of hemodynamics and standard laboratory parameters, pain management, and nil per os. Antibiotics are not recommended, unless there is concern for concurrent ascending cholangitis.

ERCP

Not all patients with suspected gallstone pancreatitis should undergo ERCP. Patients with pancreatitis and concurrent cholangitis should undergo ERCP, preferably within 24 hours of admission.[113] Patients with confirmed choledocholithiasis who do not have evidence for cholangitis can undergo ERCP for stone removal when stable from a pancreatitis standpoint. In the absence of cholangitis, the clinical course will be dictated by the evolution of pancreatitis that is not altered by performing an ERCP. Nearly 75% patients with biochemical or imaging evidence for choledocholithiasis on admission will spontaneously pass the stone into the duodenum within 3 days,[114] so rushing to perform ERCP in patients without cholangitis is ultimately unnecessary in a large majority of patients.

There have been several studies looking at whether ERCP with biliary sphincterotomy can reduce the severity, complications, and mortality of predicted severe acute pancreatitis. A study from the late 1980s looked at 121 patients with acute biliary pancreatitis and found a benefit of early ERCP (within 72 hours of admission) in decreasing complications associated with acute pancreatitis even when excluding the patients with obvious biliary obstruction.[115] However, there was no mortality benefit from early ERCP. Another study published several years later looked at another heterogeneous group of patients with biliary pancreatitis and showed a decrease in complications but no mortality benefit of early ERCP.[116] Another trial was performed several years later which excluded patients with a bilirubin greater than 5.[117] This study did not find a morbidity or mortality benefit of early ERCP with papillotomy in these patients.

Based on these studies and lack of subsequent data showing a mortality benefit from early ERCP with sphincterotomy in patients with severe biliary pancreatitis without concomitant biliary obstruction, ERCP should not be performed unless there is evidence of ongoing biliary obstruction. Performing ERCP with biliary sphincterotomy does not alter the mortality of acute biliary pancreatitis but may decrease the morbidity and mortality from concomitant cholangitis.

Patients with acute biliary pancreatitis and indeterminate evidence for choledocholithiasis (see earlier section on Choledocholithiasis) should undergo additional tests such as MRCP or EUS prior to ERCP. If such patients are not candidates for cholecystectomy, an ERCP with empiric biliary sphincterotomy should be performed to decrease the risk for recurrent biliary pancreatitis.

A validated protocol used five equally weighted parameters (CBD > 9, gamma-glutamyl transferase > 350, Alk phos > 250, direct bilirubin > 2, and total bilirubin > 3) to assign a score of 0 to 5 for each patient presenting with gallstone pancreatitis.[118] In this protocol, which enrolled 84 patients, patients with a score of 0 underwent cholecystectomy, patients with a score of 1 to 2 underwent cholecystectomy with IOC, patients with a score of 3 to 4 underwent MRCP, and patients with a score 5 underwent ERCP. This protocol had an overall accuracy of 88% for CBD stones and avoided unnecessary ERCPs in all patients in the protocol.

Cholecystectomy

Patients without ongoing biliary obstruction and uncomplicated biliary pancreatitis should undergo cholecystectomy during the same admission. A large, multicenter prospective randomized controlled trial (Pancreatitis of biliary origin: Optimal timiNg CHOlecystectomy [PONCHO]) from the Netherlands confirmed that failure to perform a same-admission cholecystectomy increases the risk for subsequent recurrent biliary pancreatitis, readmission, and pancreatitis-related complications.[119]

Patients with biliary pancreatitis undergoing ERCP with biliary sphincterotomy should fall into one of three groups: (1) patients who have documented, or a high suspicion for, choledocholithiasis and (2) those in whom cholecystectomy will be delayed or (3) those who are not candidates for cholecystectomy either due to comorbidities or refusal to undergo surgery.

In patients undergoing preoperative ERCP with biliary sphincterotomy, does this obviate the need for cholecystectomy? In these patients, the risk for development of recurrent pancreatitis appears to be similar to those undergoing cholecystectomy; in other words, biliary sphincterotomy appears to be similar to cholecystectomy in protecting against recurrent pancreatitis, particularly in elderly patients. The protective effect of biliary sphincterotomy is likely due to the disruption of the common channel and enlargement of the biliary orifice, which decreases the risk for pancreatic duct obstruction and increases the likelihood of atraumatic passage of gallstones. However, in young patients, biliary sphincterotomy should not be considered definitive therapy due to risk of sphincterotomy stenosis and biliary obstruction in the setting of a migrated gallstone and lifetime risk for acute cholecystitis.[120] Furthermore, patients who do not undergo interval cholecystectomy have a statistically higher mortality rate, incidence of biliary type pain, and cholecystitis.[120]

For patients who cannot undergo cholecystectomy or in whom cholecystectomy is going to be delayed, ERCP with empiric biliary sphincterotomy should be performed to protect against recurrent pancreatitis. Performance of neither cholecystectomy nor biliary sphincterotomy leads to the highest rate of readmission within 2 years from recurrent pancreatitis.[121,122]

Again, patients who lack gallbladder sludge or stones and significant liver enzyme abnormalities should not be assumed to have biliary pancreatitis, and cholecystectomy in these patients should not be uniformly recommended. Data suggest that patients with a normal gallbladder on ultrasound and lack of significant liver enzyme elevation had a 50% chance of developing recurrent pancreatitis following empiric cholecystectomy.[123] Given this finding, patients with unexplained recurrent acute pancreatitis with an intact, normal-appearing gallbladder should be counseled that cholecystectomy may not prevent recurrent pancreatitis and the decision to pursue cholecystectomy in this setting should be individualized.

KEY REFERENCES

11. Kiewiet JJ, Leeuwenburgh MM, Bipat S, et al: A systematic review and meta-analysis of diagnostic performance of imaging in acute cholecystitis, *Radiology* 264(3):708–720, 2012.

28. Penas-Herrero I, de la Serna-Higuera C, Perez-Miranda M: Endoscopic ultrasound-guided gallbladder drainage for the management of acute cholecystitis (with video), *J Hepatobiliary Pancreat Sci* 22(1):35–43, 2015.

29. Itoi T, Coelho-Prabhu N, Baron TH: Endoscopic gallbladder drainage for management of acute cholecystitis, *Gastrointest Endosc* 71(6): 1038–1045, 2010.

30. McCarthy ST, Tujios S, Fontana RJ, et al: Endoscopic transpapillary gallbladder stent placement is safe and effective in high-risk patients without cirrhosis, *Dig Dis Sci* 60(8):2516–2522, 2015.

34. Itoi T, Sofuni A, Itokawa F, et al: Endoscopic transpapillary gallbladder drainage in patients with acute cholecystitis in whom percutaneous transhepatic approach is contraindicated or anatomically impossible (with video), *Gastrointest Endosc* 68(3):455–460, 2008.

46. Lee TH, Park DH, Lee SS, et al: Outcomes of endoscopic transpapillary gallbladder stenting for symptomatic gallbladder diseases: a multicenter prospective follow-up study, *Endoscopy* 43(8):702–708, 2011.

48. Inoue T, Okumura F, Kachi K, et al: Long-term outcomes of endoscopic gallbladder stenting in high-risk surgical patients with calculous cholecystitis (with videos), *Gastrointest Endosc* 83(5):905–913, 2016.

51. Kedia P, Kuo V, Tarnasky P: Digital cholangioscopy-assisted endoscopic gallbladder drainage, *Gastrointest Endosc* 85(1):257–258, 2017.

60. Irani S, Baron TH, Grimm IS, Khashab MA: EUS-guided gallbladder drainage with a lumen-apposing metal stent (with video), *Gastrointest Endosc* 82(6):1110–1115, 2015.

61. Walter D, Teoh AY, Itoi T, et al: EUS-guided gall bladder drainage with a lumen-apposing metal stent: a prospective long-term evaluation, *Gut* 65(1):6–8, 2016.

63. Irani S, Kozarek RA: The buried lumen-apposing metal stent: Is this a stent problem, a location problem, or both? *VideoGIE* 1(1):25–26, 2016.

64. Khan MA, Atiq O, Kubiliun N, et al: Efficacy and safety of endoscopic gallbladder drainage in acute cholecystitis: Is it better than percutaneous gallbladder drainage? *Gastrointest Endosc* 85(1):76–87.e3, 2017.

68. Anderloni A, Buda A, Vieceli F, et al: Endoscopic ultrasound-guided transmural stenting for gallbladder drainage in high-risk patients with acute cholecystitis: a systematic review and pooled analysis, *Surg Endosc* 30(12):5200–5208, 2016.

74. Kiriyama S, Takada T, Strasberg SM, et al: New diagnostic criteria and severity assessment of acute cholangitis in revised Tokyo Guidelines, *J Hepatobiliary Pancreat Sci* 19(5):548–556, 2012.

78. ASGE Standards of Practice Committee, Maple JT, Ben-Meenachem T, et al: The role of endoscopy in the evaluation of suspected choledocholithiasis, *Gastrointest Endosc* 71(1):1–9, 2010.

80. Luthra AK, Aggarwal V, Mishra G, et al: A prospective blinded study evaluating the role of endoscopic ultrasound before endoscopic retrograde cholangiopancreatography in the setting of "positive" intraoperative cholangiogram during cholecystectomy, *Am Surg* 82(4):343–347, 2016.

84. Iranmanesh P, Frossard JL, Mugnier-Konrad B, et al: Initial cholecystectomy vs sequential common duct endoscopic assessment and subsequent cholecystectomy for suspected gallstone migration: a randomized clinical trial, *JAMA* 312(2):137–144, 2014.

88. Mathuna PM, White P, Clarke E, et al: Endoscopic balloon sphincteroplasty (papillary dilation) for bile duct stones: efficacy, safety, and follow-up in 100 patients, *Gastrointest Endosc* 42(5):468–474, 1995.

95. Stefanidis G, Viazis N, Pleskow D, et al: Large balloon dilation vs. mechanical lithotripsy for the management of large bile duct stones: a prospective randomized study, *Am J Gastroenterol* 106(2):278–285, 2011.

96. Poh BR, Ho SP, Sritharan M, et al: Randomized clinical trial of intraoperative endoscopic retrograde cholangiopancreatography versus

laparoscopic bile duct exploration in patients with choledocholithiasis, *Br J Surg* 103(9):1117–1124, 2016.

97. Prasson P, Bai X, Zhang Q, Liang T: One-stage laproendoscopic procedure versus two-stage procedure in the management for gallstone disease and biliary duct calculi: a systemic review and meta-analysis, *Surg Endosc* 30(8):3582–3590, 2016.

108. Di Giorgio P, Manes G, Grimaldi E, et al: Endoscopic plastic stenting for bile duct stones: stent changing on demand or every 3 months. A prospective comparison study, *Endoscopy* 45(12):1014–1017, 2013.

113. Tenner S, Baillie J, DeWitt J, et al: American College of Gastroenterology guideline: management of acute pancreatitis, *Am J Gastroenterol* 108(9):1400–1415, 1416, 2013.

119. da Costa DW, Bouwense SA, Schepers NJ, et al: Same-admission versus interval cholecystectomy for mild gallstone pancreatitis (PONCHO): a multicentre randomised controlled trial, *Lancet* 386(10000):1261–1268, 2015.

121. Nguyen GC, Rosenberg M, Chong RY, Chong CA: Early cholecystectomy and ERCP are associated with reduced readmissions for acute biliary pancreatitis: a nationwide, population-based study, *Gastrointest Endosc* 75(1):47–55, 2012.

A complete reference list can be found online at ExpertConsult .com

54

Postoperative Biliary Strictures and Leaks

Guido Costamagna and Andrés Cárdenas

CHAPTER OUTLINE

INTRODUCTION

Accidental injuries of the bile ducts leading to biliary leaks and strictures may occur during any surgical procedure involving the biliary tract. However, the main causes of injury of the bile ducts at the present time are laparoscopic cholecystectomy (LC) and after liver transplantation (LT). Although LC has proved to be superior to open cholecystectomy in terms of shorter hospitalization, lower overall morbidity, faster recovery, and better cosmetic outcome, the risk of bile duct injury during LC is two to six times greater compared with open cholecystectomy.[1,2] Bergman et al (1996)[3] described four types of postoperative bile duct injuries, as follows:

Type A: Cystic duct leaks or leakage from aberrant or peripheral hepatic radicles (minor lesions)

Type B: Major bile duct leaks with or without concomitant biliary strictures (major lesions)

Type C: Bile duct strictures without bile leakage (major lesions)

Type D: Complete transection of the duct with or without excision of some portion of the biliary tree (major lesions)

Biliary strictures in patients with LT are classified as anastomotic strictures (ASs) and nonanastomotic strictures (NASs). AS are by far the most common. In most centers, a biliary duct-to-duct anastomosis is preferred over a Roux-en-Y choledochojejunostomy as it offers the advantage of easy endoscopic access to the biliary system and preservation of the sphincter of Oddi. The type of LT and biliary reconstruction has some implications in the development of biliary strictures. Due to the small diameter of the anastomotic bile duct, biliary strictures are known to be more common in living-donor LT (LDLT) than in deceased-donor LT (DDLT). The type of biliary reconstruction (duct-to-duct choledocho-choledochostomy vs. Roux-en-Y choledochojejunostomy) in DDLT has been suggested as a risk factor for biliary complications; however, it is now generally agreed upon that the rate of complications is similar with the Roux-en-Y choledochojejunostomy.

EPIDEMIOLOGY

LC was first performed by Mouret in France in 1987. The technique was standardized by two other French surgeons, Dubois in Paris and Perissat in Bordeaux.[4,5] This new technique spread very rapidly around the world; in the United States, the percentage of cholecystectomies done laparoscopically grew from zero in 1987 to over 90% in 2010.[6] The advent of LC also induced an estimated increase of at least 25% in the overall number of cholecystectomies performed,[7,8] so that the likely number of cholecystectomies performed at the present time in the United States is 800,000 per year.[6,9] The number of iatrogenic injuries to the bile duct has increased accordingly.[10]

There are many reasons that may explain the increased incidence of biliary complications at the beginning of the laparoscopic era, most related to the new technical skills required to perform laparoscopically what had previously been done by open surgery: bidimensional vision, loss of tactile sensations, different visual approach of the hepatic pedicle, difficult hemostatic maneuvers, abuse of electrocoagulation, and lack of confidence with the new instrumentation.[11] The rate of injuries seemed to be related to the surgeon's learning curve and his or her personal experience. An inversely proportional relationship between the number of cholecystectomies performed and the rate of injuries was suggested by earlier reported series.[1,12] In a review of 77,604 LCs performed in the United States, the incidence of biliary injuries decreased from 0.6% to 0.4% ($p < 0.001$) for surgical teams having an experience of more than 100 LCs.[1] A Belgian survey[11] suggested the number of 50 LCs as the threshold of a completed learning curve; however, the same authors emphasized that one-third of the biliary injuries in their country had occurred with surgeons with an experience of more than 100 LCs. When reviewing several multicenter series published before 1995, totaling 198,267 LCs, the incidence of biliary injuries was 0.55% in 13 European series and 0.49% in 17 series outside Europe.[13]

In the mid-1990s, the incidence of biliary injury seemed to be three times higher for LC than for open cholecystectomy. However, these figures most likely underestimated reality because there was a tendency not to declare all the lesions, as revealed by the low rate of reply to most surveys and by the increasing number of reported lesions in direct proportion with the collected replies.[14] At the present time, the incidence of biliary injuries has not substantially changed, even if a trend toward reduction has been reported by some authors.[6,9,15] The estimated overall incidence is 0.25% to 0.74% for major biliary lesions (Table 54.1) and 0.1% to 1.7% for minor biliary lesions (Table 54.2).[16–18] These figures are only partially explained by the still increasing number of LCs performed around the world and by the activity of young surgeons at the beginning of their learning curve. However, at least one-third of biliary injuries may be ascribed to technical mistakes during surgery.[19] The learning curve is not the only risk factor for LC.

Bile duct strictures after LT account for approximately 40% to 50% of all biliary complications after LT.[20,21] The incidence of AS in various reports ranges between 10% and 15%.[22,23] Strictures that occur early after LT are mainly due to technical problems, whereas late strictures are mainly due to vascular insufficiency, ischemia, and problems with healing and fibrosis. Patients with Roux-en-Y choledochojejunostomy may also develop strictures at the anastomosis with the bowel, and in most cases

percutaneous therapy by interventional radiology is performed in these individuals. In some centers with experienced endoscopists, endoscopic retrograde cholangiopancreatography (ERCP) can be successfully performed in patients with a Roux-en-Y choledochojejunostomy with small bowel enteroscopy.[24]

PATHOGENESIS

An unintentional lesion of the bile duct also may occur during an "easy" cholecystectomy performed by an experienced surgeon. Intuitively, the likelihood of injuring the bile duct should increase when the cholecystectomy is difficult and the surgeon is inexpert. Any cholecystectomy may become unexpectedly difficult during surgery; however, clinical and morphologic criteria exist that may be useful in predicting a cholecystectomy at higher risk of bile duct injury. Clinical criteria are obesity; previous abdominal surgery; cirrhosis; portal hypertension; age of the patient; and previous cholecystitis, cholangitis, or pancreatitis. Morphologic criteria revealed by preoperative abdominal ultrasound (US) are related to the gallbladder status (scleroatrophic gallbladder, thickening of the gallbladder wall, gallbladder distention resulting from a stone in the infundibulum) and to the liver (hepatomegaly, atrophy or hypertrophy of the liver lobes). The presence of several criteria raises the chances of being confronted with a difficult cholecystectomy and the risk of concomitant common bile duct (CBD) stones.

In patients who have undergone LT, a number of factors play a role in the development of ASs and NASs. In most instances, the major underlying risk factor is ischemic due to problems with the hepatic artery, mainly stenosis or thrombosis (HAT). As the biliary system receives blood supply mainly via the hepatic artery, low flow of the hepatic artery can lead to complex ASs and hilar strictures. Hepatic artery stenosis can also lead to both ASs and NASs, particularly when associated with long, cold ischemia time.[25] T-tube placement in LT is controversial. Originally T-tubes were routinely placed as a prophylactic measure for AS development. However, the results of several comparative studies, systematic reviews, and meta-analysis suggest no major differences in the incidence of biliary complications, and the current trend has favored the abandonment of the use of T-tubes after LT in most centers.[26–28] Other factors include concomitant bile leak, technical factors during surgery (tight anastomosis, excessive dissection and electrocautery during the reconstruction, redundant bile duct), mismatched size between donor and recipient bile ducts, ischemia/reperfusion injury, presence of cytomegalovirus infection, donation after cardiac death, ABO blood group mismatch, older age of donor, graft, steatosis, prolonged cold and warm ischemia times, and primary sclerosing cholangitis.[29–34]

Unrecognized CBD stones are one of the major risk factors of cystic duct leakage after LC. The mechanism and the cause of a biliary injury remain unexplainable in at least one-third of cases.[13] In more than 50% of cases, the injury occurs during the dissection of the cystic duct or during separation of the gallbladder neck from the CBD. Misinterpretation of the cystic duct and the CBD is the most common cause of injury.[12] Excessive traction on the gallbladder neck, especially if the tissues are not inflamed, may facilitate the injury of the CBD. Conversely, when the area is acutely or chronically inflamed or when a stone is trapped in the gallbladder infundibulum, the risk of CBD injury is higher during the dissection of the gallbladder neck from the hepatic pedicle. Other common reasons for bile duct injury are related to incorrect hemostatic maneuvers in the case of bleeding from

TABLE 54.1 Incidence of Major Biliary Lesions (Bergman's Type B, C, and D) During Laparoscopic Cholecystectomy (LC) (Multicenter Surveys)

Author	Country	Year	No. LC	Major Biliary Lesions (%)
MacFayden et al[2]	United States	1998	114,005	0.5
Nuzzo[13]	Italy	2002	56,591	0.31
Russell et al[9]	United States	1996	15,221	0.25
Z'graggen et al[16]	Switzerland	1998	10,174	0.31
Gigot et al[11]	Belgium	1997	9959	0.5
Wherry et al[17]	United States	1996	9130	0.41
Adamsen et al[18]	Denmark	1997	7654	0.74
Richardson et al[15]	Scotland	1996	5913	0.33

TABLE 54.2 Incidence of Minor Biliary Lesions (Bergman's Type A) During Laparoscopic Cholecystectomy (LC) (Multicenter Surveys)

Author	Country	Year	No. LC	Minor Biliary Lesions (%)
MacFayden et al[2]	United States	1998	114,005	0.38
Nuzzo[13]	Italy	2002	56,591	0.1
Z'graggen et al[16]	Switzerland	1998	10,174	0.93
Wherry et al[17]	United States	1996	9130	0.53
Adamsen et al[18]	Denmark	1997	7654	1.7
Richardson et al[15]	Scotland	1996	5913	0.28

the cystic artery; inappropriate use of electrocautery; and other specific maneuvers, such as intraoperative cholangiography, which is used in cases of suspected CBD stones or difficult anatomy, cystic duct dilation, and transcystic CBD instrumental exploration.

An anatomic anomaly is often reported by the surgeon as having caused a biliary injury. Variations of the biliary anatomy, especially at the level of the main hepatic confluence, are present in 50% of patients (see the later section on interpretation of intrahepatic cholangiography). Surgeons must be aware of such variations and must keep in mind the danger of injuring aberrant ducts originating in the right liver during dissection of the gallbladder pedicle. Aberrant ducts must not be interpreted as accessory ducts because the biliary distribution within the liver parenchyma is of a terminal type; this implies that there are no intrahepatic anastomoses between the ducts and that every injury of an aberrant duct would determine functional exclusion of the corresponding liver area. Injury to a small aberrant duct may still be considered a minor lesion; however, it would cause a bile leak into the peritoneal space with all the related consequences. Another cause of injury is clipping or ligation of an aberrant duct. This injury does not involve a bile leak but entails the functional exclusion of the corresponding liver area leading to its progressive atrophy and hypertrophy of the remaining liver parenchyma. This possible event may be clinically totally asymptomatic and noted only by an increase in biochemical parameters of cholestasis and cytolysis (Fig. 54.1). Although there is no indication of treatment in asymptomatic cases, if the obstructed ducts become infected, recurrent cholangitis is the typical clinical manifestation often requiring operative reestablishment of an adequate bile flow.

CLINCIAL FEATURES

Schematically, three main clinical pictures are characteristic of a bile duct injury: (A) external biliary fistula, (B) choleperitoneum, and (C) cholestasis with or without the features of acute chol-

angitis. Various combinations of these clinical pictures may also be present. Most important, although some of the clinical manifestations, such as mild jaundice or well-drained external bile leakage, do not require any emergency treatment, the presence of infection must be regarded as an important criterion that requires intensive care and rapid decisions to treat sepsis. Septic complications are the main reason for mortality in these patients in the postoperative period. External biliary fistula and choleperitoneum are both typical features of the immediate postoperative period, whereas obstructive jaundice may occur either immediately after surgery or later, within days to several years. When symptoms arise late after surgery because of a slow progression from injury to stricture, overt jaundice may be absent, and the clinical picture is typically that of anicteric cholestasis, with or without itching, and recurrent bouts of acute cholangitis.

The suspicion of bile duct injury after LC injury is not always straightforward. When subtle symptoms such as dull abdominal pain, abdominal distention, low-grade fever, and nausea arise in the first days after LC, one should always suspect a possible complication. Intraperitoneal bile collections may initially produce very little or no specific symptoms, but they should be quickly suspected and eventually confirmed to identify the cause and to plan the best treatment for the individual patient. Hemobilia is a rare but alarming clinical presentation of a bile duct injury. The mechanism by which a biliary injury may be associated with hemobilia is often the perforation of a pseudoaneurysm of the right hepatic artery or one of its branches into the bile ducts. These pseudoaneurysms are the result of an inadvertent intraoperative injury of the artery produced by hemostatic maneuvers during a difficult cholecystectomy and cause hemoperitoneum. In patients with an external biliary drainage or fistula, the bleeding may become suddenly and massively apparent through the drain and may occasionally require emergency treatment.

In individuals who undergo LT, the clinical presentation is variable according to the type of lesion. In many cases, patients will have nonspecific symptoms such as malaise and anorexia. Others may present with pruritus, jaundice, or associated bile

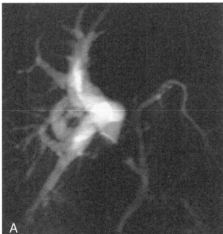
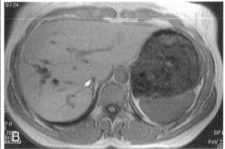

FIG 54.1 This patient presented 2 years after laparoscopic cholecystectomy (LC) with only occasional minor right upper quadrant pain and slightly elevated liver function tests. **A,** Magnetic resonance cholangiography shows complete obstruction and dilation of the right biliary ductal system with normal common bile duct (CBD) and left biliary ductal system. **B,** Abdominal magnetic resonance imaging shows hypotrophy of the right liver and compensatory hypertrophy of the left liver.

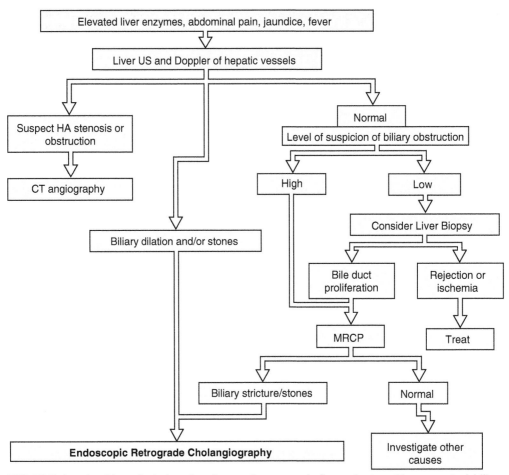

FIG 54.2 An algorithm depicting the diagnostic approach for patients with suspected biliary anastomotic strictures. *CT,* computed tomography; *HA,* hepatic artery; *MRCP,* magnetic resonance cholangiopancreatography; *US,* ultrasound.

ascites and abdominal pain. In most instances, a biliary stricture is usually first suspected in asymptomatic LT recipients who have elevations of serum bilirubin, alkaline phosphatase and/or gamma-glutamyl transferase levels. Although strictures usually present as asymptomatic cholestasis, some patients can present with cholangitis, especially if the patient has concomitant bile duct stones.

DIAGNOSTIC APPROACH AND DIFFERENTIAL DIAGNOSIS

In all cases of a suspect biliary stricture, the initial evaluation should include an abdominal US. In those with LT, a Doppler evaluation of the hepatic vessels to rule out hepatic artery thrombosis or stenosis and/or portal or hepatic vein occlusion must also be performed. Unfortunately, abdominal US may not be sufficiently sensitive (sensitivity 40% to 66%) to detect biliary obstruction in many patients.[35] Thus, the absence of bile duct dilation on US should not preclude further evaluation with more sensitive tests if there is clinical suspicion of a biliary stricture. In such cases, a magnetic resonance cholangiopancreatography (MRCP) is considered an optimal noninvasive diagnostic tool for the assessment of the biliary strictures. Although ERCP or percutaneous transhepatic cholangiography are the gold standard, MRCP has gained acceptance as the most reliable noninvasive

study for the evaluation of the bile ducts, particularly in patients after LT (sensitivity 96%, specificity 94%).[36] The preferred approach is to perform an MRCP first; however, proceeding with a diagnostic invasive procedure such as ERCP without an MRCP can be an acceptable clinical strategy in some patients because of the high likelihood that a therapeutic intervention will be required.[37] An algorithm depicting the diagnostic approach for patients with suspected AS is shown in Fig. 54.2.

Strictures occurring long after surgery may need to be distinguished from malignant strictures and other benign conditions such as primary sclerosing cholangitis, autoimmune cholangitis, or sclerosing cholangitis in critically ill patients among others. The clinical history may be helpful only in cases in which the biliary injury had been recognized and eventually treated at the time of surgery. In this setting, the stricture is usually the result of progressive scarring at the site of surgical repair. In all other circumstances, the relationship with cholecystectomy or LT should be questioned. However, clinical presentation may be helpful in discriminating postoperative and malignant stenoses; painless jaundice is in favor of a malignant disease, whereas development of overt jaundice in benign strictures is often heralded by a long period of anicteric cholestasis and relapsing attacks of mild to severe acute cholangitis. Stricture morphology may be very helpful in discriminating scars from neoplastic involvement of the bile duct. Postoperative strictures are usually short, with sharp, often

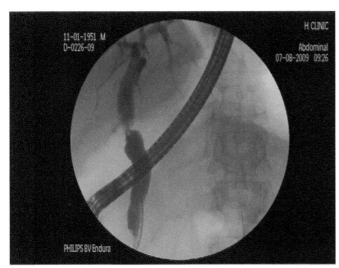

FIG 54.3 Biliary anastomotic stricture after liver transplantation. The structure is quite short and in the area of the anastomosis. These strictures are amenable to endoscopic therapy with biliary dilation and subsequent plastic stent placement across the stricture.

asymmetric edges, close to the cystic duct stump, and clips may be seen lying over the bile duct or located medially to it. ASs after LT are defined as a dominant short narrowing at the anastomotic site without free or effective passage of contrast material as demonstrated by cholangiography (Fig. 54.3).

TREATMENT

In recent years, ERCP has acquired a pivotal role in the management of postsurgical biliary complications. Both the major typical clinical presentations occurring in this setting may be addressed by ERCP: (A) biliary leak into the peritoneal cavity or external leak and (B) obstructive syndrome with cholestasis, cholangitis, or jaundice. ERCP confirms the clinical suspicion of biliary injury and provides detailed morphologic information of the lesion. ERCP is currently considered a first-line therapeutic tool in complications that are amenable to endoscopic treatment.

Endoscopic Retrograde Cholangiopancreatography and Biliary Leak

The presence of a bile leak invariably indicates a break in the continuity of the biliary system. However, the severity of the injury (i.e., ranging from simple leakage of the cystic stump to complete transection of the bile duct) and the complexity of its repair are extremely variable. The magnitude of the bile output of abdominal drains does not usually help in identifying the origin and the size of the leak. A direct cholangiogram is of utmost importance for accurate anatomic depiction and to classify the type of injury to plan therapy. The usefulness of MRCP in the delineation of postoperative biliary leaks[38] and of iatrogenic strictures[39] has been reported. However, in contrast to ERCP, MRCP has no therapeutic capability. MRCP may be recommended in anatomic situations in which the endoscopic approach is presumably difficult or occasionally impossible, such as in patients with a Billroth II anatomy and with Roux-en-Y hepaticojejunostomy. In LT recipients, bile leaks occur in 2% to 25% of patients.[20,21,40] An important thing to consider is that the presence

of a bile leak is an independent risk factor for the development of early or late strictures and requires prompt therapy.[31]

ERCP provides a detailed morphologic picture of the biliary tree and, when indicated, offers immediate therapeutic options during the same procedure. In cases of biliary leaks, ERCP is usually required in the early postoperative period when the patient has fresh surgical scars (which are potentially painful, especially if surgery has been converted to laparotomy) and has one or more external abdominal drains placed during surgery or in the postoperative period under US or computed tomography guidance; this is why the supine position is often preferred to the usual left lateral or prone position in performing ERCP. The supine position, although a little more demanding for the operator, is also preferable for interpretative purposes, especially in the case of complex hilar lesions. The anteroposterior radiologic projection, with the liver lying on the spine, substantially helps in identifying the anatomy of the main biliary confluence and of the segmental intrahepatic ducts. Use of the supine position also allows for the changing of the patient's position obliquely in the case of superimposition of the biliary branches, which may create difficulties in interpretation.

In the case of an external biliary fistula through an abdominal drain, it is not advisable to start the procedure by injecting contrast medium through the drain (fistulography). In most instances, especially in minor lesions, the contrast medium freely flows into the peritoneal space without depicting the biliary tree. The presence of contrast medium overlapping the area involved by the lesion may hinder the correct interpretation of subsequent cholangiography and occasionally disguise the picture entirely. In contrast, fistulography is indicated whenever endoscopic cholangiography shows an incomplete filling of the biliary system resulting from a complete transection of the main bile duct or lack of visualization of a sectorial or segmental intrahepatic branch. As an alternative to contrast medium, which occasionally might not fill the missing branch, air or CO_2 may be used to obtain a pneumocholangiogram.[41]

The technique of ERCP in the setting of a suspected biliary injury does not substantially differ from the routine examination. Special attention should be paid to the injection of contrast medium, however, which should be slow and careful to allow precise delineation of the lesions. Massive injection of the biliary tree should be avoided. Minimal injection and early filling x-ray films are also important in detecting small residual CBD stones, which are present in 13% to 20% of patients with biliary leakage originating from the cystic duct stump.[42] If the suspected lesion is located in an intrahepatic biliary branch, it is of paramount importance to obtain a complete intrahepatic cholangiogram, and to achieve an adequate pressure of injection, especially if a sphincterotomy has been previously performed, in which case the use of an occlusion balloon catheter is advisable. Intrahepatic biliary anatomy is better shown by multiple x-ray films taken in different projections. Percutaneous transhepatic cholangiography and MRCP should be reserved for patients in whom ERCP fails technically or fails to show the intrahepatic biliary anatomy because of proximal ductal disruption.[43]

Interpretation of Intrahepatic Cholangiography

The main biliary confluence is formed by the union of the right and left hepatic ducts, which drain the bile originating in the right hemiliver and the left hemiliver. The main confluence is often incorrectly called *bifurcation* in the English literature; actually, although the portal vein and the hepatic artery carrying

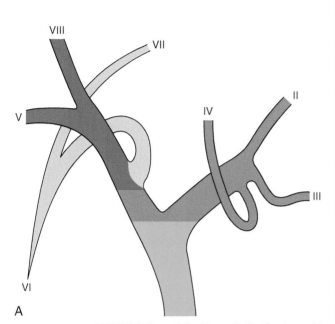

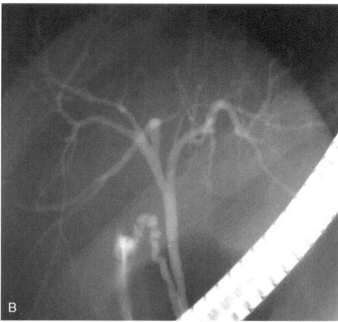

FIG 54.4 **A** and **B,** Normal distribution of intrahepatic bile ducts: common hepatic duct *(light green)*, left hepatic ducts *(blue)*, right hepatic duct *(dark green)*, right anteromedial duct *(red)*, and right posterolateral duct *(yellow)*.

the blood to the liver have bifurcations, the fusion of ducts collecting the bile from the liver with a flow directed toward the CBD generates a confluence. According to the segmental liver anatomy described by Couinaud,[44] the left hepatic duct collects the bile originating from segments II and III (left anatomic liver lobe or left lateral sector) and from segment IV (quadrate lobe). One or more small ducts originating from segment I (caudate lobe) also join the left hepatic duct close to the main confluence. The anatomic variations occurring in the left hepatic system are rare and are irrelevant in this perspective. The right hepatic duct is shorter than the left hepatic duct and follows the same axis of the common hepatic duct. The right hepatic duct originates from the confluence of the right anteromedial sectorial duct (segments V and VIII) and of the right posterolateral sectorial duct (segments VI and VII). The right anteromedial duct is recognizable thanks to its orientation, which follows the same axis of the right hepatic duct, whereas the right posterolateral duct joins the right anteromedial duct on its medial aspect with a typical umbrella handle-like shape.

This normal anatomy (called *modal* by Couinaud) is present in approximately 60% of the population (Fig. 54.4).[44,45] The main hepatic confluence is usually located high in the hilar region. A lower position at the level of the hepatic pedicle may also occur, causing a much closer proximity to the insertion of the cystic duct into the hepatic duct (Fig. 54.5). The main variations of the main hepatic confluence are the absence of the right hepatic duct with the anteromedial and posterolateral right ducts joining independently to the left duct to form the confluence (Fig. 54.6), or with one of the two right sectorial ducts joining the main bile duct at a more distal level closer to the insertion of the cystic duct (Fig. 54.7). More rarely, an isolated segmental or subsegmental duct may join the CBD away from the main confluence, usually on the lateral aspect of the CBD close to the insertion of the cystic duct. Most aberrant ducts arise from the right liver and drain into the common hepatic duct or cystic duct within

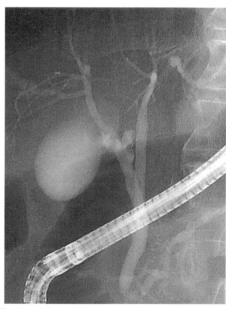

FIG 54.5 Endoscopic retrograde cholangiopancreatography (ERCP) shows low main confluence with the cystic duct joining the right hepatic duct on its medial aspect.

30 mm of the hepatocystic angle.[46] These are the most dangerous anatomic variations for the surgeon during the dissection of the gallbladder pedicle. Apart from complete transection of the CBD (type D of the Bergman classification) (Fig. 54.8), which is typically an indication for open surgical repair, an attempt at endoscopic treatment may be envisaged in all other circumstances of biliary injury with concomitant bile leak.

The basic principle of endoscopic treatment is diminishing the transpapillary pressure gradient, equalizing the bile duct and

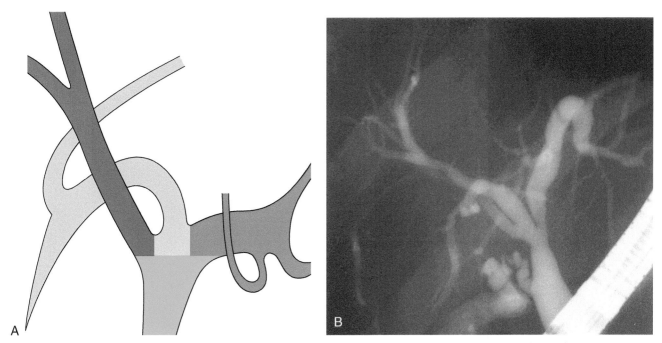

FIG 54.6 A and **B,** Absence of the right hepatic duct. *Light green,* common hepatic duct; *blue,* left hepatic ducts; *red,* right anteromedial duct; *yellow,* right posterolateral duct.

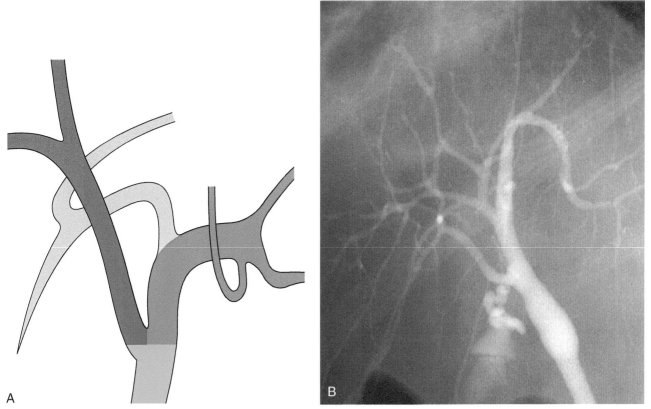

FIG 54.7 A and **B,** Absence of the right hepatic duct. On endoscopic retrograde cholangiopancreatography (ERCP), the cystic duct joins the right anteromedial duct on its lateral aspect. *Light green,* common hepatic duct; *blue,* left hepatic ducts; *red,* right anteromedial duct; *yellow,* right posterolateral duct.

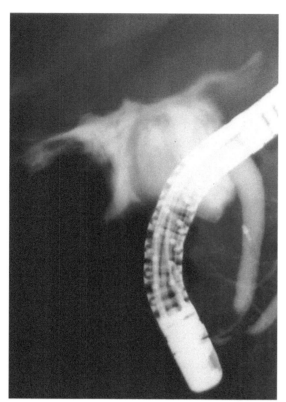

FIG 54.8 Endoscopic retrograde cholangiopancreatography (ERCP) shows complete transection of the common bile duct (CBD) with contrast medium freely flowing into the subhepatic peritoneal space.

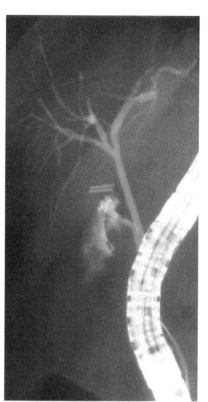

FIG 54.9 Postoperative endoscopic retrograde cholangiopancreatography (ERCP) after laparoscopic cholecystectomy (LC), with leakage of contrast medium from the cystic duct stump.

TABLE 54.3   Endoscopic Management of Biliary Leaks From Minor Lesions (Type A) After Cholecystectomy

Author, Year	n	LC (%)	Cystic (%)	Luschka (%)	Other (%)	CBDS (%)	ES (%)	ES + EP (%)	EP Only (%)	Success (%)
Bourke, 1995	85	62	79	6	15	18	33	67	0	95
Barkun, 1997	52	58	77	15	8	22	48	23	15	88
Ryan, 1998	50	78	72	8	20	22	12	26	62	100
Hourigan, 1999	53	85	68	17	15	11	15	15	70	96

CBDS, common bile duct stones; *EP,* endoprosthesis or nasobiliary drain; *ES,* endoscopic sphincterotomy; *LC,* laparoscopic cholecystectomy.

duodenal pressures, and allowing preferential flow of bile into the duodenum.[47]

Endoscopic Treatment of Minor Lesions

The largest part of biliary leaks from minor lesions originates from the cystic duct stump (Fig. 54.9), or the biliary anastomosis in the case of LT recipients. Bile leakage from the cystic duct stump may be due to stump dehiscence resulting from defective technique in clips positioning, inadvertent injury to the cystic wall below the closure, or partial disruption of the cystic duct implantation into the bile duct resulting from excessive traction. Biliary hypertension resulting from temporary impaction of a residual bile duct stone into the sphincter of Oddi in the early postoperative period is most likely the cause of cystic duct stump dehiscence in almost one-fifth of patients. Bile leakage in LT recipients can occur from the anastomosis, the cystic duct, the T-tube tract, or (in the case of living-donor or split liver LT)

from the cut surface of the liver. Many bile leaks can be resolved nonoperatively with early endoscopic intervention. Bile leaks after LC can also originate from severed ducts of Luschka (small peripheral ducts connecting the intrahepatic system with the gallbladder lumen) (Fig. 54.10), small subsegmental ducts running in the gallbladder bed, and segmental or subsegmental aberrant branches joining the CBD in the proximity of the cystic duct.

Treatment of these latter leaks does not differ from treatment employed when the leak arises from the cystic duct stump or the biliary anastomosis (Table 54.3). The transpapillary pressure gradient can be equalized by endoscopic sphincterotomy (ES) alone,[48,49] ES and stent or nasobiliary drain (NBD) placement,[50] and stent[51,52] or NBD placement alone[53] without prior ES (Fig. 54.11). All methods seem to be equally effective in facilitating the closure of the biliary leak, usually within 1 to 2 weeks of treatment in cases of LC[48–54] and 4 to 6 weeks in cases of LT.[21,55] If stones are present in the CBD, ES and stone extraction with

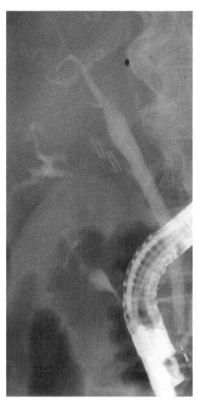

FIG 54.10 Postoperative endoscopic retrograde cholangiopan-creatography (ERCP) after laparoscopic cholecystectomy (LC) in a case of subhepatic bile collection. The common bile duct (CBD) is normal. Two clips are visible on the cystic artery and the cystic duct. A leak of contrast medium into the gallbladder bed originates from a duct of Luschka connecting a subsegmental branch that joins the CBD lower than the main confluence.

TABLE 54.4 Endoscopic Options to Treat Postoperative Bile Leaks (Type A According to Bergman)

Procedure	Advantages	Disadvantages
ES	Treatment of associated CBD stones	Complications
Nasobiliary drain (days)	Avoids ES Allows check cholangiography	Uncomfortable Prolongs hospitalization
Stent placement (wks)	Avoids ES	Repeat ERCP required Clogging, dislocation

CBD, common bile duct; *ERCP*, endoscopic retrograde cholangiopancreatography; *ES*, endoscopic sphincterotomy.

or without stent or NBD placement seems the preferred approach. However, each option has specific limitations. ES is associated with inherent immediate and potential long-term complications; stent placement requires a second procedure to remove the stent, which can also become clogged or can migrate; and NBD requires a prolonged hospital stay, is uncomfortable for the patient, and may be accidentally displaced. Advantages and disadvantages of the different options are summarized in Table 54.4.

To select the optimal endoscopic therapy, Sandha et al (2004)[56] proposed classifying the bile leaks after LC by ERCP into two categories: low-grade (identified only after intrahepatic opacification) and high-grade (observed before intrahepatic opacification). Of 104 low-grade leaks, 75 were treated by ES alone with a success rate of 91%. Of 100 high-grade leaks, 97 were treated by stent insertion with a final success rate (4 patients had to undergo retreatment) of 100%. The investigators concluded that this simple, practical endoscopic classification system might be clinically relevant in the choice of endoscopic therapy. Endoscopic local injection of botulinum toxin in a canine model (Botox) to decrease the transpapillary bilioduodenal pressure gradient has also been reported.[57] Injection of 100 IU of botulinum toxin into the sphincter of Oddi was shown to lower CBD pressure significantly within 24 hours. This effect lasted for 2 weeks on average in the animal model. Postoperative bile leaks from minor lesions (type A) are usually amendable to endoscopic management with plastic stents and biliary sphincterotomy with a very high success rate. All methods seem to be equally effective in facilitating the closure of the leak within a few days.

In cases of LT, bile leaks in the first month after LT usually occur at the anastomotic site and are usually related to technical problems of the surgery or severe HAT.[21] Late bile duct leaks are usually related to the removal of the T-tube, resulting from delay in T-tube tract maturation due to immunosuppression. A bile leak should be suspected in patients who develop pain when the T-tube is removed. In cases where a T-tube is in place, small anastomotic leaks can be diagnosed with a T-tube cholangiogram and can be managed by leaving the tube open without further intervention. In patients without a T-tube, endoscopic retrograde cholangiography (ERC) is considered the gold standard diagnostic method in detecting bile leaks. Therapy also includes placement of a plastic stent with or without sphincterotomy, as described earlier.[21,55,58–60]

Endoscopic Treatment of Major Lesions

Bile leakage in major lesions originates from a tear on the CBD or on one of the biliary branches that form the main hepatic confluence (type B). In both instances, ES alone may be inadequate to diminish the leak. It is preferable to insert at least one large-bore plastic stent (10-Fr to 11.5-Fr), long enough to bypass the site of injury. The secondary intent of stent placement is to prevent the development of stricture at the site of the injured bile duct wall. For this purpose, the stent should be left in place for at least 8 to 12 weeks to allow the healing process to stabilize. In case of secondary stricture formation at the site of injury, the presence of a stent already in place facilitates successive endoscopic maneuvers to dilate the stricture. Therapeutic success may be obtained in 71% to 90% of cases (Fig. 54.12 and Video 54.1).[3,61,62]

Biliary stents have also been successfully used to reestablish the continuity of disrupted segmental branches at the level of the main hepatic confluence[41] and for leaks from aberrant bile ducts.[43,63] In major biliary injury with bile leakage, the primary therapeutic objective, if there is no transection, is to bypass the leak with the stent to divert bile flow to the duodenum and convert an acute problem into a stable condition. The high efficacy of the endoscopic approach in this setting justifies its use as a first-line treatment whenever possible. Treatment of postoperative bile duct strictures in the prelaparoscopic era was traditionally surgical. The role of ERCP was limited to the diagnostic phase and particularly to the definition of the level and extent of the lesion (Video 54.2).

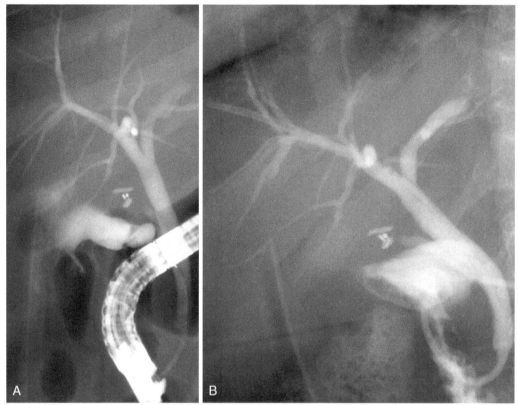

FIG 54.11 Postoperative endoscopic retrograde cholangiopancreatography (ERCP) after laparoscopic cholecystectomy (LC) in a case of external biliary fistula through a subhepatic drain. **A,** Leak of contrast medium originating in the gallbladder bed (duct of Luschka) is seen. **B,** Check cholangiography performed 3 days after endoscopic sphincterotomy and nasobiliary drain placement. The leakage is no longer visible.

In LT recipients, placement of a plastic biliary stent (10-Fr to 11.5-Fr), with or without biliary sphincterotomy, across the leak is successful in treating 90% to 95% of bile leaks.[21,55,58–60] As a result, if there is a strong clinical suspicion, ERC is the treatment of choice. In contrast to postcholecystectomy leaks, where the stent can be removed in 4 weeks, in post-LT leaks it is preferred that the stent be left in place for approximately 2 months because of problems with delayed healing that may arise due to immunosuppression.[21,60] Stents are not changed during this period unless there is a clinical suspicion of obstruction. At the end of this period, the leak has typically healed and no other stent is needed.

Aside from this approach (sphincterotomy with plastic stent placement), some authors now advocate the use of fully covered self-expandable metal stents (FCSEMS) for patients with bile leaks (mainly postcholecystectomy leaks) given the high resolution rates (93%-95%).[64,65] It is the clinical experience that FCSEMS are useful in some LT recipients with large or refractory bile leaks. However, information is limited.

BILIARY STRICTURES

Along with the increasing use of ERCP in the evaluation and treatment of acute complications of LC and LT, therapeutic ERCP has been increasingly employed to manage postoperative biliary strictures. The first nonoperative alternative in the management of bile duct strictures was the percutaneous transhepatic approach.

After establishment of percutaneous access to the intrahepatic bile ducts, the stricture is crossed with a guidewire, and pneumatic balloon dilation is performed. Although instantly very effective, this approach has a very limited value in the longterm because of the high rate of stricture recurrence.[66] Approximately one-third of patients undergoing this treatment modality experience complications, and stricture recurrence develops in at least 25% of cases during follow-up.[67,68] In another series published by the group at The Johns Hopkins University, the success rate of these procedures was only 55%, with 20% of patients having significant hemobilia.[69] The high recurrence rate after percutaneous pneumatic dilation is most likely due to the forceful disruption of the scar, which can add further traumatic damage to the tissue and consequential development of new local fibrogenic reaction.

The percutaneous approach has been progressively replaced by the endoscopic approach. The endoscopic approach avoids the need for liver puncture, which is the main cause of complications of the percutaneous approach; it is not more difficult when the intrahepatic bile ducts are not dilated or only slightly enlarged, which is often the case in postoperative strictures; and it is also feasible in case of liver cirrhosis, ascites, or coagulopathy. The endoscopic approach avoids the need for long-standing percutaneous internal-external catheters, improving the patient's comfort and compliance. At the present time, the endoscopic approach is considered the first-line, nonoperative alternative to surgical treatment; in addition, it never hinders the option of a surgical

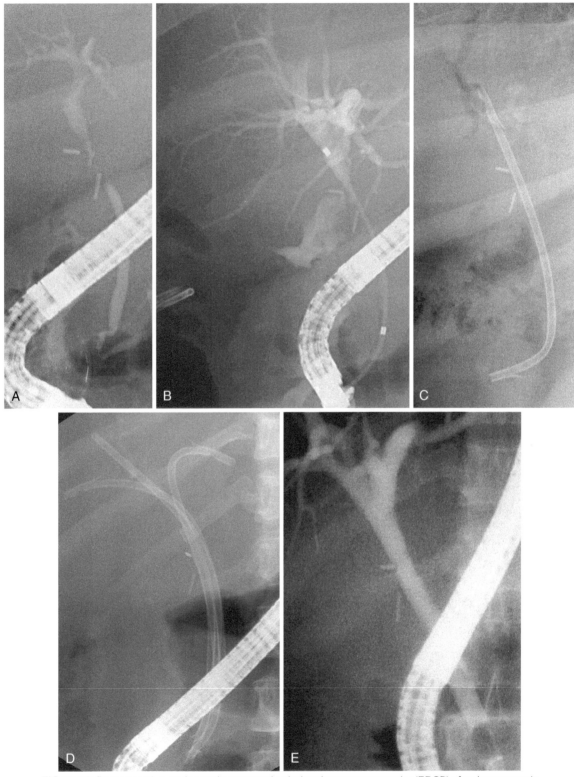

FIG 54.12 Postoperative endoscopic retrograde cholangiopancreatography (ERCP) after laparoscopic cholecystectomy (LC) in a case of peritoneal bile collection and cholestasis. **A,** Stricture of the common bile duct (CBD) with clips overlapping. **B,** A catheter has been passed over the stricture using a guidewire; injection of contrast medium through the catheter clearly shows the site of biliary injury and the correspondent leak. **C,** A 10-Fr plastic stent has been placed. **D,** During the following months, three 10-Fr stents were inserted to dilate the stricture, one in each main biliary territory (anteromedial right, posterolateral right, and left biliary ducts). **E,** Balloon-occluded check cholangiography after removal of the three stents. The stricture has completely disappeared.

approach as a rescue therapy in case of failure.[70] Both surgery and endoscopic treatment may obtain good results. However, the two alternatives have never been systematically compared in a prospective randomized trial. It is also very unlikely that such a study will ever be conducted in the future because of the relatively low incidence of this pathology, its dispersion in several centers, and the heterogeneity of its clinical and morphologic presentation, which would make it very difficult to gather cases in homogeneous groups large enough for any comparison.

Description of Technique

Endoscopic treatment of postoperative biliary strictures is based on three steps: (A) traversing the stricture, (B) dilation of the stricture, and (C) stent placement.

Traversing the Stricture

The morphologic requirement that allows the traversing of the stricture is the continuity of the CBD. In the case of complete transection or complete obstruction of the bile duct, the endoscopic option alone is applicable in only a very few cases. A combined percutaneous and endoscopic approach with an aim at reconstructing the missing segment of the bile duct can be performed.[71] A similar combined approach has also been described in the case of complete obstruction of the distal biliary stump; percutaneous puncture of the distal stump was performed under radiologic guidance with a device designed for nonbiliary use (a set marketed for placing transjugular intrahepatic portosystemic shunts).[72] However, because of the lack of standardization, these approaches cannot be recommended on a routine basis.

In most cases, and especially when symptoms develop a long time after surgery, the CBD is accessible by endoscopy, and the stricture is incomplete, traversing the stricture is the mandatory and preliminary step before performing dilation. This maneuver is often much more difficult in postoperative strictures than in neoplastic strictures because the stenosis, even if commonly very short, may be asymmetric and irregular. The fibrosis makes it especially thin and tightened. It is often necessary to use thin hydrophilic guidewires (0.021 inch or 0.018 inch) with a straight or J-type extremity; their manipulation requires patience, skill, and optimal x-ray control.

The morphology of the stenosis has to be respected, and forceful maneuvers with stiff guidewires that may create false routes leading to the failure of the procedure should be strictly avoided. Changing the position of the patient may help in radiologically identifying the right pathway to follow with the guidewire. Pulling on a stone retrieval balloon inflated under the stricture may help in stretching the bile duct and in modifying the axis of the guidewire. Manipulation of bendable catheters or papillotomes may also be used to change the direction of the guidewire. When the stricture is passed, the hydrophilic guidewire is exchanged for a stiffer and more stable one to proceed to dilation.

Dilation of the Stricture

Dilation of the stricture has two objectives: (A) to reopen the bile duct to achieve a regular bile flow, and (B) to secure a larger diameter to avoid restricture in the long-term. In the beginning of endoscopic treatment, only the first objective was pursued; in the percutaneous approach, the mainstay of treatment was pneumatic dilation alone.[73] However, it soon became clear that even if immediately very effective, pneumatic dilation alone was ineffective in granting good results in a long-term follow-up. At the present time, pneumatic dilation is mainly used as a preliminary step before placement of one or more plastic stents (Fig. 54.13). The role of stent placement is to keep the stricture open for a long time (months to years, according to different treatment strategies), while allowing scar modeling and its consolidation.[74]

Strictures After LC

Typically, two 10-Fr stents are placed, exchanged every 3 months to avoid cholangitis resulting from stent occlusion, and left in place for 1 year. In a retrospective study from the Amsterdam group reporting on the multidisciplinary experience obtained during a decade (1981–1990), the long-term results of endoscopic treatment were compared with the long-term results of surgery.[75] Surgery (Roux-en-Y hepaticojejunostomy) was performed in 35 patients, and endoscopic treatment was performed in 66 patients. Patient characteristics, type of initial injury, and level of obstruction were not significantly different in the two groups. At a mean follow-up of 50 months and 42 months for the surgical and the endoscopic groups, 83% of patients in both groups had an excellent (asymptomatic patient with normal or stable laboratory parameters) or good (single episode of cholangitis) result. Immediate complication rate was in favor of endoscopic treatment (8% vs. 26% for surgical treatment), whereas 21% of the patients had at least one episode of cholangitis resulting from stent malfunction during the stent period (two 10-Fr stents for 1 year with stent exchange every 3 months).[75]

When analyzing the long-term results, it becomes immediately evident how the time interval between the end of treatment and the symptomatic recurrence of the stricture is much shorter in the group with endoscopic treatment compared with the surgical group (on average 3 ± 11 months vs. 40 ± 11 months), indicating possible undertreatment in the endoscopy group.[75] However, this important study showed that endoscopic treatment may be considered at least as effective as surgical treatment in terms of long-term results, having the major advantage of not hindering any further surgery if necessary. Several other experiences of endoscopic treatment with plastic stents of postoperative biliary strictures have been published in recent years.[3,76–85] From the analysis of the available data, however, this treatment modality still seems far from standardized; the published experiences differ in terms of number of stents placed, their caliber, exchange intervals, and definition of treatment objectives and of outcomes. Examples of two different methodologic approaches follow:

- The treatment protocol used by the Amsterdam group (74 patients) is the classic one, entailing placement of two 10-Fr stents, exchanged every 3 months for 1 year (the period of stent placement).[80] Preliminary pneumatic dilation had been performed in approximately one-fourth of the patients before stent insertion. A combined percutaneous-endoscopic approach to bypass the stricture with a guidewire was required in only three cases. Stents were removed after 1 year.
- The protocol described by the Italian group (55 patients)[79] involved the placement of the maximum possible number of stents (ideally 10-Fr) in relation to the tightness of the stricture and diameter of the CBD at every treatment session with a trimonthly interval. Treatment was continued until complete morphologic disappearance of the stricture at cholangiography (Fig. 54.14).

Preliminary balloon dilation was performed in 40% of the patients, almost always at the first treatment session. A combined percutaneous-endoscopic approach was required in three cases.

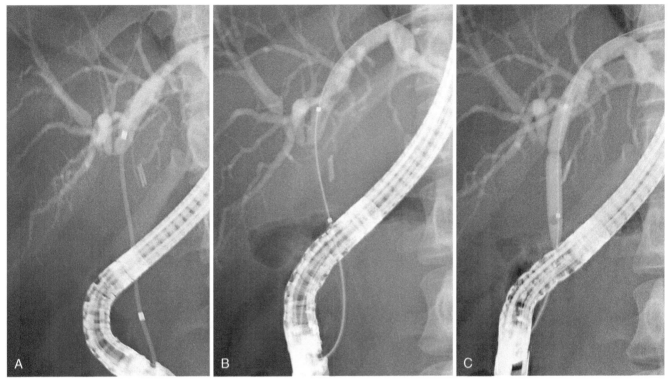

FIG 54.13 Postoperative stricture after laparoscopic cholecystectomy (LC) converted to open cholecystectomy. **A,** At the level of the main confluence, a very tight stricture has been overcome by a catheter and guidewire. **B,** A balloon dilator has been passed through the stricture over the guidewire. **C,** Balloon dilation is performed. Notice the waist on the balloon indicating high stricture firmness.

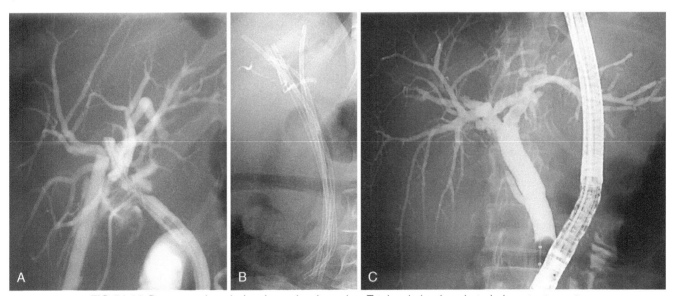

FIG 54.14 Postoperative cholangiography through a T-tube drain placed at cholecystectomy to repair complete transection of the common bile duct (CBD) at the hilum. **A,** Stricture and leak of contrast medium around the CBD are visible. **B,** At the end of the fifth treatment, 10-Fr stents have been placed. **C,** Balloon-occluded cholangiography after stent removal. The stricture has disappeared completely.

The mean number of stents inserted was 1.7 (range 1 to 4) at the first session and 3.2 (range 1 to 6) at the end of the treatment. Disappearance of the stricture was checked 24 to 48 hours after removal of the stents by check cholangiography through NBD. Early complications developed in four (9%) patients (three cholangitis, one pancreatitis), and stent occlusion that required early stent exchange occurred in eight (18%) patients. Mean duration of treatment was 12.1 ± 5.3 months (range 2 to 24 months). Follow-up included clinical evaluation, laboratory parameters, and liver US every 3 months during the 1st year and every 6 months in the following years.[79]

- In the Amsterdam series,[75] the technical success of stenting was 80%; however, only 44 patients (59% of the initial cohort and 75% of patients in whom an initial technical success had been obtained) concluded the 12-month stent period for different reasons. At a median follow-up of 9 years, 9 out of 44 patients (20%) developed recurrent strictures. In eight of nine cases, recurrent strictures developed within the first 6 months of follow-up (median 2.6 months). On an intention-to-treat basis, this protocol was able to resolve definitively the bile duct stricture in 47% of the initial cohort. The results of this study suggest that endoscopic stent placement is not the best treatment option for patients with low compliance to repeated treatment sessions. Similar results, with 81% of patients symptom-free at a mean follow-up of 9.5 years, were reported in an abstract form by the Toronto group by using the same treatment protocol.[78]

- In the Italian study, 42 out of 55 patients initially considered were evaluable at a mean follow-up of 49 months after the end of treatment.[79] Ten patients were excluded from the protocol because of complete CBD section (n = 5) or use of self-expandable metallic stents (SEMSs) (n = 5). Another three patients were not evaluable for different reasons. Two patients died of unrelated causes during follow-up. Among the remaining 40 patients, there was no recurrence of symptoms caused by relapsing biliary stricture. One patient sustained two episodes of cholangitis but without stricture recurrence. By an intention-to-treat analysis, the success rate was 89% (40 of 45). Although the follow-up period in this series is shorter compared with the Amsterdam series, it is longer than the typical period during which all the recurrences after endoscopic treatment have been described (2 years). This more aggressive approach to endoscopic treatment with stents seems to improve long-term results for patients with postoperative biliary strictures. The authors reported on the very long-term results of this aggressive approach in the same cohort of patients[86]; of 35 evaluable patients after a mean follow-up of 13.7 years, seven (20%) had recurrent cholangitis owing to relapse of the stricture in four patients (all successfully retreated with stents) and newly formed bile duct stones in three patients. The remaining 28 patients remained completely asymptomatic with normal liver function tests and abdominal US.

At the present time, multiple stent placement is a well-accepted strategy adopted for postoperative bile duct strictures.[85-89] According to the published data, endoscopic treatment with stents of major bile duct injuries and strictures is at least as effective as surgical treatment. The advantages of endoscopic treatment are its simplicity, reversibility, and minimal invasiveness. Endoscopic treatment should always be considered, whenever available, in the therapeutic algorithm of most patients with major bile duct injuries. For most patients, it may be the only treatment required. Endoscopy and surgery should be considered as complementary

treatments. This complex and difficult pathology is best managed in centers in which a multidisciplinary approach is available.

STRICTURES AFTER LT

The majority of ASs occur within the first year after LT.[90] ASs identified within the first 6 to 12 months after LT usually have a good response to stenting every 3 months.[91] However, patients require long-term surveillance because strictures often recur. One study demonstrated that patients with biliary strictures after LT and who were initially treated endoscopically with balloon dilation and plastic stents had a recurrence rate of 18% with a mean time to recurrence of 3.7 months.[92] In a second study, the recurrence rate following endoscopic treatment was 34%, with a mean time to recurrence of 14.5 months.[90]

The characteristic cholangiographic appearance of an AS is that of a thin narrowing in the area of the biliary anastomosis (see Fig. 54.3). In some patients, a transient narrowing of the anastomosis may become evident within the first 1 to 2 months after LT due to postoperative edema and inflammation. This type of narrowing responds to endoscopic balloon dilation and plastic stent placement; in most patients, it will resolve within 3 months, and the anastomosis will remain patent without further intervention.[60]

Most patients with ASs after LT require ongoing ERC sessions every 3 months with balloon dilation and long-term stenting (for 12 to 24 months). This technique consists of placing a guidewire across the stricture (Fig. 54.15), followed by a dilation of the AS using balloon diameters of 6 to 8 mm, and, finally, placing 10-Fr to 11.5-Fr plastic stents with an increasing diameter and number if possible in each session (see Fig. 54.15). The standard technique requires sphincterotomy of the papilla before stent placement. Plastic stents need to be exchanged every 3 months to avoid occlusion and bacterial cholangitis. This approach has been reported to be more effective than dilation alone.[93] Increasing the number of stents in each session improves success rates and thus placing the maximal number of stents possible in each session is recommended; in general up to 5 or 6 stents are needed. In a retrospective study of 83 LT recipients with ASs, treatment success was associated with the number of stents placed (8 in the success group vs. 3.5 in those in whom treatment failed).[94] Another study found that among 56 patients at a large academic hospital who underwent ERC for LT-related biliary complications between July 1994 and March 2012, resolution of AS was seen in 50 out of 51 patients (98%), and mean duration of endoscopic treatment was 11.5 months, with a median of 4 ERCs per patient.[95] After a median follow-up of 5.8 years from stent removal, 3 out of 50 patients (6%) had recurrence of ASs. All three were successfully treated again endoscopically and were asymptomatic after a further median follow-up of 5.6 years. This approach usually requires several interventional sessions (mean of 3 to 5 sessions per patient) in order to achieve long-term success rates of 70% to 100%.[93–102] Table 54.5 describes the findings of different studies evaluating the outcome of dilation and plastic stent placement of biliary ASs.

There is some clinical experience in temporary (approximately 3 to 12 months) placement of covered SEMS to reduce the need for repeated stent exchanges. In a systematic review that included 200 patients treated with SEMS, stricture resolution rates of 80% to 95% were seen when the stent duration was 3 months or longer.[103] However, the stent migration rate was 16%. By comparison, the stricture resolution rate was 94% to 100% for patients

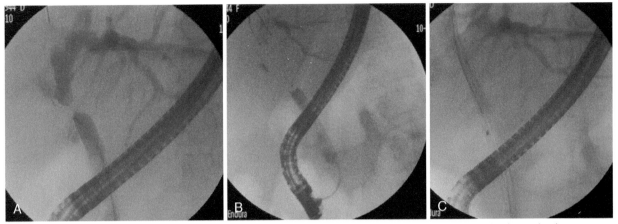

FIG 54.15 Biliary anastomotic stricture after liver transplantation (LT). **A,** A guidewire is pushed across the anastomotic stricture. **B,** The guidewire allowed the dilation of the stricture and afterward, **C,** The placement of two plastic stents across the stricture. Once placed, the stents allow drainage of bile and contrast.

TABLE 54.5 Studies in Liver Transplant Recipients Treated With Stricture Dilation and Multiple Plastic Stents

Authors: (Number of Patients Who Underwent ERC After LT) / Year	Number of Patients With AS	Age (Mean)	Time to Diagnosis of AS (Months)	Technical Success Rate (%)	Number of Stents (Mean)	Number of Procedures Per Patient (Mean)	Follow-Up in Months (Mean)	Resolution n (%)	AS Recurrence	Recurrence Treatment
Rerknimitr et al, 2002, USA (N=121) /	43	36.5	8.3	43/43 (100)	3.6	3.7	39.6	43/43 (100)	0	0
Morelli et al, 2003, USA (N=25)	25	48	4.5	24/25 (96)	3	3	54	22/25 (88)	2/22 (9)	1 ERCP
Alazmi et al, 2006, USA (N=148)	148	–	2.1	143/148 (97)	2–4	3	28	131/148 (89)	24/131 (18)	1–4 ERCP
Pasha et al, 2007, USA (N=25)	25	46.7	2	25/25 (100)	2-3	3.5	21.5	18/25 (72)	4/18 (22)	2 ERCP 2 Surgery
Holt et al, 2007, UK (N=53)	53	48.5	30.5	49/53 (92)	3	3	18	34/53 (64)	1/34 (3)	1 ERCP
Morelli et al, 2008, USA (N=38)	38	52.6	2.9	38/38 (100)	0.5	3.45	12	33/38 (89)	5/33 (15)	4 ERCP 1 Surgery
Tabibian et al, 2010, USA (N=83)	69	52.5	20	69/69 (100)	3 max.	4.2 ± 2.8	11	65/69 (94)	2/65 (3)	ERCP
Sanna et al, 2011, Italy (N=94)	45	–	–	34/34 (100)	–	2.5 ± 1.2	88.8	22/34 (65)	6/34 (18)	Surgery
Hsieh et al, 2013, USA (N=38)	32	–	2.1	32/32 (100)	3	4	74.2	32/32 (100)	8 (21)	8 ERCP
Poley et al, 2013, Netherlands (N=A) /	63	61	–	31/31 (80.6)	4	5	28	25/31 (80.6)	6 (19.4)	1 ERCP (SEMS) 5 Surgery
Tringali et al, 2016, Italy (N=119) /	56	51	6.8	50/51 (98)	4	4	5.8 years	50/51 (98)	3/50 (6)	3 ERCP

ERCP, endoscopic retrograde cholangiopancreatography; *SEMS,* self-expandable metal stent.

who were treated with plastic stents for 12 months or more.[103] A 2014 multicenter prospective study that included 187 patients with benign strictures analyzed the role of FCSEMS. In the study, 42 LT recipients with ASs were treated with FCSEMS. There was a resolution rate of only 68% with a significant complication rate (38%), mainly due to cholangitis.[104] Finally, a randomized trial with 112 patients with benign biliary strictures (from LT, chronic pancreatitis, or other postoperative injury) found a resolution rate by 12 months of 93% with SEMS and 85% for plastic stents.[105] Stricture recurrence was seen in 14% of the patients treated with SEMS and 5% of patients treated with plastic stents. However, in the subgroup of 73 patients with biliary strictures after LT, there was no difference in stricture resolution rates (95% each) or number of days (371 SEMS vs. 367 plastic) to resolution among both groups. Currently, there are not enough data to support the systematic use of SEMS over plastic stents in the treatment of ASs. The use of SEMS may be beneficial in patients who fail therapy with plastic stents and dilatation; however, data are scarce, and migration rates in this setting are also high.[106,107]

COMPLICATIONS

Complications may occur during the first treatment session and are related to ES (acute pancreatitis, retroperitoneal perforation, and bleeding), which is usually performed to gain access to the bile ducts, or occur during the stent period. ES-related complications in this setting do not differ in frequency, severity, and management from complications encountered in other, more common situations, such as treatment of CBD stones. In LT recipients, the rate of these complications is not very different from that of the general population. There is up to a 9% complication rate per procedure.[108] The most common complications are pancreatitis, cholangitis, and postsphincterotomy bleeding. Other complications include bile leak, subcapsular hematoma, perforation, and stent migration. Complications arising during the stent period are mostly due to stent dysfunction (i.e., obstruction, migration, dislocation, and impaction). Acute cholangitis is the typical clinical manifestation of stent dysfunction. Cholangitis is usually mild and often self-limited in this setting, but requires prompt endoscopic evaluation and reestablishment of correct bile drainage by stent repositioning.

A typical complication of long-term stent placement is the development of biliary sludge and stones above the stricture. This condition may cause cholangitis, but it may also be totally asymptomatic. In addition, liver function tests may be completely normal. The lack of symptoms and normal liver function tests may lead to unintentional prolongation of the planned stent period. Removal of all stones and sludge by basket or balloon extraction or both is mandatory before placement of a new stent or stents to avoid potential early reocclusion. To avoid stone formation, the trimonthly time schedule of stent replacement should not be prolonged. Patient compliance is crucial when dealing with postoperative bile duct stricture, and patients should always be fully informed of the inherent risks of not following the planned treatment program.

FUTURE TRENDS

The main limitation of endoscopic treatment of postoperative bile strictures with the current method of multiple plastic stent placement is the need for repeat interventions over a long time

(1 year on average). The ideal stent would allow progressive dilation of the stricture during weeks or months and would dissolve once the goal had been reached. Uncovered SEMS have proved to be a bad alternative to plastic stents for several reasons. First, SEMS invariably induce a hyperplastic response of the inflammatory tissue at the level of the stricture. This hyperplastic reaction ultimately leads to occlusion of SEMS, on average less than 1 year after their placement. Second, SEMS are usually not removable; treatment of secondary stricture resulting from hyperplastic reaction requires repeated balloon dilations and plastic stent placement. Third, biliary SEMS have been developed to produce abrupt recanalization of a stricture resulting from neoplastic invasion; the radial force exerted by the stent is much higher than the force desirable to induce progressive dilation of a scar, such as the scar of postoperative bile duct strictures.

Partially covered SEMS have the advantage of avoiding ingrowth of hyperplastic tissue at the level of the stricture and of often being removable; however, no clinical experience is available. The advent of fully covered, removable SEMS has raised new interest concerning their potential use in benign conditions. These stents, although effective, are not superior to plastic stents, and there is not enough information to recommend the systematic use of SEMS over plastic stents in the initial treatment of biliary strictures. The use of SEMS may be beneficial in patients who fail therapy with plastic stents and dilatation; however, data are scarce, and migration rates in this setting are also high.[103–107,109] Drug-eluting, self-expandable stents have been used in the vascular system to inhibit endothelial growth; it is conceivable that this technology might become available for use in the biliary system.[110,111] Local release of antiinflammatory drugs able to control the fibrogenetic process that occurs during healing of a biliary injury may be valuable in this setting.

KEY REFERENCES

1. Deziel DJ, Millikan KW, Economou SG, et al: Complications of laparoscopic cholecystectomy: a national survey of 4,292 hospitals and an analysis of 77,604 cases, *Am J Surg* 165:9–14, 1993.

3. Bergman JJ, van den Brink GR, Rauws EA, et al: Treatment of bile duct lesions after laparoscopic cholecystectomy, *Gut* 38:141–147, 1996.

8. Shea JA, Healey MJ, Berlin JA, et al: Mortality and complications associated with laparoscopic cholecystectomy: a meta-analysis, *Ann Surg* 224:609–620, 1996.

15. Richardson MC, Bell G, Fullarton GM: Incidence and nature of bile duct injuries following laparoscopic cholecystectomy: an audit of 5913 cases. West of Scotland Laparoscopic Cholecystectomy Audit Group, *Br J Surg* 83:1356–1360, 1996.

20. Pfau PR, Kochman ML, Lewis JD, et al: Endoscopic management of postoperative biliary complications in orthotopic liver transplantation, *Gastrointest Endosc* 52:55–63, 2000.

21. Thuluvath PJ, Atassi T, Lee J: An endoscopic approach to biliary complications following orthotopic liver transplantation, *Liver Int* 23:156–162, 2003.

23. Fernández-Simon A, Díaz-Gonzalez A, Thuluvath PJ, Cárdenas A: Endoscopic retrograde cholangiography for biliary anastomotic strictures after liver transplantation, *Clin Liver Dis* 18(4):913–926, 2014.

36. Jorgensen JE, Waljee AK, Volk ML, et al: Is MRCP equivalent to ERCP for diagnosing biliary obstruction in orthotopic liver transplant recipients? A meta-analysis, *Gastrointest Endosc* 73:955–962, 2011.

43. Mehta SN, Pavone E, Barkun JS, et al: A review of the management of post-cholecystectomy biliary leaks during the laparoscopic era, *Am J Gastroenterol* 92:1262–1267, 1997.

47. Bjorkman DJ, Carr-Locke DL, Lichtenstein DR, et al: Postsurgical bile leaks: endoscopic obliteration of the transpapillary pressure gradient is enough, *Am J Gastroenterol* 90:2128–2133, 1995.

54. Adler DG, Papachristou GI, Taylor LJ, et al: Clinical outcomes in patients with bile leaks treated via ERCP with regard to the timing of ERCP: a large multicenter study, *Gastrointest Endosc* 85(4):766–772, 2017.

60. Londoño MC, Balderramo D, Cárdenas A: Management of biliary complications after orthotopic liver transplantation: the role of endoscopy, *World J Gastroenterol* 14(4):493–497, 2008.

75. Davids PH, Tanka AK, Rauws EA, et al: Benign biliary strictures: surgery or endoscopy?, *Ann Surg* 217:237–243, 1993.

79. Costamagna G, Pandolfi M, Mutignani M, et al: Long-term results of endoscopic management of postoperative bile duct strictures with increasing numbers of stents, *Gastrointest Endosc* 54:162–168, 2001.

86. Costamagna G, Tringali A, Mutignani M, et al: Endotherapy of postoperative biliary strictures with multiple stents: results after more than 10 years of follow-up, *Gastrointest Endosc* 72:551–557, 2010.

91. Thuluvath PJ, Pfau PR, Kimmey MB, Ginsberg GG: Biliary complications after liver transplantation: the role of endoscopy, *Endoscopy* 37:857–863, 2005.

95. Tringali A, Barbaro F, Pizzicannella M, et al: Endoscopic management with multiple plastic stents of anastomotic biliary stricture following liver transplantation: long-term results, *Endoscopy* 48:546–551, 2016.

101. Poley JW, Lekkerkerker MN, Metselaar HJ, et al: Clinical outcome of progressive stenting in patients with anastomotic strictures after orthotopic liver transplantation, *Endoscopy* 45:567–570, 2013.

105. Coté GA, Slivka A, Tarnasky P, et al: Effect of covered metallic stents compared with plastic stents on benign biliary stricture resolution: a randomized clinical trial, *JAMA* 315:1250–1257, 2016.

108. Balderramo D, Bordas JM, Sendino O, et al: Complications after ERCP in liver transplant recipients, *Gastrointest Endosc* 74:285–294, 2011.

A complete reference list can be found online at ExpertConsult .com

55

Infections of the Biliary Tract

Zaheer Nabi, Andrew Korman, Nageshwar Reddy, and David Carr-Locke

CHAPTER OUTLINE

INTRODUCTION

The word *cholangitis* is a pathologic term that means "inflammation of bile ducts." It is a broad term and does not imply any specific diagnosis. In clinical practice, cholangitis is defined on the basis of symptoms and signs of systemic sepsis originating in the biliary tract.[1]

The most important predisposing factor for infections of the biliary tract, including the common bile duct (CBD) and gallbladder, is obstruction to the flow of bile. By far, gallstones remain the most common cause of obstruction and infection of biliary tract (cystic duct or CBD). Other causes of cholangitis include biliary strictures (benign or malignant), recurrent pyogenic cholangitis (RPC), iatrogenic (post-endoscopic retrograde cholangiopancreatography [ERCP]), parasitic (Ascaris, liver flukes, echinococcal), viral (HIV cholangiopathy), etc. (Box 55.1). In this chapter, we shall discuss biliary tract infections (cholangitis and cholecystitis) due to various etiologies and their management.

ENDOSCOPIC RETROGRADE CHOLANGIOPANCREATOGRAPHY

Indications

The primary indication for ERCP in infectious cholangitis is to decompress the obstructed biliary system.

Contraindications

Contraindications to ERCP in biliary tract infections are similar to other endoscopic procedures. Patients who are unable to tolerate conscious sedation because of cardiopulmonary disease require an anesthesia assessment. The risk of adverse reaction to iodine containing contrast media is very low, and prophylactic premedication for contrast allergy is usually not required.[2]

ERCP in pregnancy is apparently safe for both the mother and the fetus compared with the risk of delay in definitive treatment of cholangitis, which may be life-threatening.[3]

Radiation to the fetus can be minimized by external shielding with a lead apron placed under the lower abdomen, limiting fluoroscopy time, collimating the beam to the area of interest, using brief "snapshots" of fluoroscopy, and avoiding hard copy x-ray films.[4]

Equipment

To perform ERCP, a side-viewing endoscope (duodenoscope) and fluoroscopy are required. Cannulation with a sphincterotome is recommended because most cases of biliary tract infection require a sphincterotomy. A guidewire is essential for selective cannulation of the intrahepatic ducts and the cystic duct and for accessing the biliary tree proximal to a stricture. To extract intraluminal debris, a biliary extraction basket and/or balloon

BOX 55.1 Conditions Associated With Cholangitis

Intraluminal Obstruction

Choledocholithiasis and hepatolithiasis
Biliary stent occlusion
Mirizzi's syndrome
Biliary parasites
Fungal ball
Hemobilia
Sump syndrome
Choledochal cyst

Nonneoplastic Stricture

Primary sclerosing cholangitis
Chronic pancreatitis
Pancreatic cyst or pseudocyst
Papillary stenosis
Recurrent pyogenic cholangitis
AIDS cholangiopathy
Ischemic stricture
Anastomotic stricture
Liver transplant

Bilioenteric anastomosis
Radiation
Postchemoinfusion
Tuberculosis

Neoplastic Stricture

Cholangiocarcinoma
Pancreatic carcinoma
Ampullary adenoma or carcinoma
Duodenal carcinoma
Carcinoid tumor
Small intestinal lymphoma
Kaposi's sarcoma
Metastatic disease

Iatrogenic

Post-ERCP
Postsphincterotomy
Posthepatojejunostomy
Posttranshepatic cholangiography
Post–T-tube cholangiography

AIDS, acquired immunodeficiency syndrome; *ERCP,* endoscopic retrograde cholangiopancreatography.

TABLE 55.1 Acute Cholangitis and Sepsis After ERCP: Risk Factors and Mechanisms

	Risk Factors	Mechanism
1. Disease-related	Complex hilar strictures, PSC, post liver transplant	Incomplete biliary drainage
2. Instrument-related	Contaminated duodenoscopes/accessories Faulty scope design	Improper scope disinfection
3. Host defense	Immunocompromised patient	Impaired host defense

PSC, primary sclerosing cholangitis.

must be available. Mechanical lithotripsy may be necessary before extraction of larger stones. Dilating catheters or a biliary dilation balloon, or both, and a selection of plastic and metal biliary stents are required to manage cholangitis secondary to a biliary stricture. A cytology brush and biopsy forceps are used to sample the stricture before stent insertion. Nasobiliary tubes are needed for biliary instillation therapy in certain forms of parasitic cholangitis. Duodenoscope-assisted cholangioscopy may be required to identify completely obstructed intrahepatic ducts, place a guidewire across a stricture, perform directed biopsies of a biliary stricture, and perform electrohydraulic lithotripsy (EHL) or laser lithotripsy (LL).

Preparation

The patient should be kept nothing per mouth (NPO) after midnight the day before ERCP. In urgent situations this may not be possible. Coagulopathy should be corrected if possible. A decision to discontinue anticoagulants or antiplatelet agents should be individualized. There is insufficient evidence to support routine discontinuation of aspirin and nonsteroidal antiinflammatory drugs before therapeutic ERCP procedures. Antibiotics should be administered for prophylaxis of post-ERCP cholangitis if indicated, but patients with established cholangitis will already be receiving antibiotics.

Postprocedure Care

If complete endoscopic drainage is not achieved during the initial procedure, antibiotics should be continued until definitive therapy is performed by repeat endoscopic, percutaneous, or surgical biliary decompression. Biliary obstruction resulting from hilar strictures and intrahepatic duct strictures, particularly multiple strictures as seen in sclerosing cholangitis, often require antibiotics after the procedure. Antibiotics, however, are not a substitute for adequate biliary drainage.

The duration of antimicrobial therapy for acute cholangitis is a subject of debate. As per the Tokyo guidelines, patients with

moderate or severe acute cholangitis (see later sections in this chapter) should receive a minimum duration of antibiotics for 5 to 7 days. In patients with mild cholangitis or after successful endoscopic therapy, a duration of 2 to 3 days is sufficient.[5,6]

Complications

Complications of ERCP include the complications inherent to any endoscopic procedure, including reactions to medications, cardiopulmonary complications, infection, perforation, hemorrhage, and complications specific to ERCP, such as pancreatitis, postsphincterotomy hemorrhage, and biliary infection. Infectious complications of ERCP are post-ERCP cholangitis and long-term postsphincterotomy cholangitis. However, delayed and unsuccessful ERCP are the two major factors associated with complications and worse outcomes in patients with acute cholangitis.[7] Endoscopic sphincterotomy may be avoided in patients with acute severe cholangitis due to increased risk of bleeding.[8]

ERCP AND BILIARY TRACT INFECTIONS (IATROGENIC CHOLANGITIS)

ERCP is the mainstay of endoscopic drainage of the biliary tract. Asymptomatic bacteremia is common after diagnostic or therapeutic ERCPs. However, it is rarely significant clinically and routine antibiotic prophylaxis is not recommended after ERCP. Biliary tract infections after ERCP include acute cholangitis, acute cholecystitis, and cholangitic abscesses (Table 55.1).

The most important risk factor for acute cholangitis after ERCP continues to be incomplete drainage of an obstructed biliary system. ERCP in patients with complex hilar strictures (Bismuth type III/IV), post live donor liver transplant, and primary sclerosing cholangitis (PSC) are associated with higher risks of incomplete biliary drainage and subsequent cholangitis. Therefore, antibiotic prophylaxis should be considered in these situations.

Another important risk factor for post-ERCP sepsis is improper reprocessing of the endoscopes. Failure of adherence to the endoscope disinfection guidelines along with difficulty in cleaning the elevator of the duodenoscope has resulted in recent outbreaks of multidrug resistant organisms like *E. coli, Klebsiella,* and *pseudomonas.*[9,10] Therefore, newly designed endoscopes should be subjected to strict premarketing validation of the reprocess ability and post-marketing surveillance.[11]

Acute cholecystitis may occur in 1.9% to 12% of patients after ERCP.[12] It is usually associated with metal stent placement for malignant biliary obstructions. Obstruction of the cystic duct orifice by the stent, tumor involvement of the cystic duct, and introduction of nonsterile bile or contrast agent are the proposed factors that predispose to acute cholecystitis in these patients.[13]

Prevention

Iatrogenic cholangitis after ERCP should be prevented when possible. Delineation of biliary anatomy with prior magnetic resonance cholangiopancreatography (MRCP) will provide an anatomical road map for ERCP. Prophylactic antibiotics should be used in patients at high risk of incomplete biliary drainage. Contrast agents must not be instilled into obstructed segments prior to securing a guide wire beyond obstruction. The use of air cholangiogram is an attractive strategy to prevent cholangitis in hilar strictures and deserves further evaluation in randomized trials.[14]

In the case of incomplete drainage, biliary drainage with an alternate modality (percutaneous, endoscopic ultrasound [EUS]-guided, or surgical) should be promptly carried out to avoid morbidity and mortality. Adequate reprocessing of duodenoscopes and strict adherence to the guidelines for disinfection are mandatory.

ACUTE CHOLANGITIS

Acute cholangitis is a clinical syndrome defined by the triad of right upper quadrant pain, fever, and jaundice (Charcot's triad). The presence of altered sensorium and hypotension in addition defines Reynold's pentad. Although the presence of this pentad is uncommon, it portends a poor prognosis in these patients. The basic predisposing factors of cholangitis include stasis (due to biliary obstruction) and disruption of the anatomical barrier (i.e., sphincter of Oddi) due to previous surgery, sphincterotomy, or placement of biliary endoprostheses. This leads to bacterial infection of the biliary tract. Infected bile with elevated intrabiliary pressure, exceeding the cholangiovenous reflux pressure leads to translocation of bacteria into systemic circulation, eventually leading to sepsis. Choledocholithiasis, biliary strictures, and previous biliary instrumentation are relatively common causes of cholangitis (see Box 55.1). In contrast, cholangitis is relatively uncommon in malignant biliary strictures due to complete obstruction, which limits the chances of ascending infection.

Diagnosis and Grading of Severity

The Tokyo guidelines for the diagnosis and management of acute cholangitis were initially published in 2007 and updated in 2013. The diagnosis of cholangitis is based on the presence of systemic inflammation (clinical, laboratory data), cholestasis (abnormal liver function tests), and imaging (biliary dilatation/stone/stricture, etc.). Ultrasonography is a reasonable initial imaging modality in patients with suspected acute cholangitis. The sensitivity of ultrasonography is only 50% for detection of CBD stones due to the proximity of the duodenum and interference with bowel gas. In the authors unit, EUS or MRCP is performed prior to ERCP if the clinical suspicion of cholangitis is not strong. Unnecessary ERCPs and associated complications can be avoided with this approach. Moreover, MRCP can provide an anatomical road map for subsequent ERCP, which may be especially useful in the case of hilar or intrahepatic obstruction. However, ERCP is performed without delay in cases of strong suspicion of severe cholangitis based on clinical and laboratory features.

Three grades of severity of cholangitis in the Tokyo guidelines are based on the presence or absence of organ dysfunction, age, and laboratory parameters (white blood cell count, bilirubin level, serum albumin). In moderately severe cholangitis, at least two of the following conditions are present: abnormal leucocyte count ($> 12,000/mm^3$ or $< 4000/mm^3$), fever ($\geq 39°C$), age (> 75 years old), high bilirubin (> 5 mg/dL), and low albumin ($< 0.7 \times$ lower limit of normal). Presence of at least one organ dysfunction defines severe cholangitis.[15]

Management

Irrespective of the underlying etiology of cholangitis, the mainstay of management is drainage of the infected biliary system. However, initial stabilization of the patient is of paramount importance before any therapeutic intervention is contemplated. Intravenous antibiotics should be administered as per the local antimicrobial sensitivity trends. Antibiotic coverage against anaerobes should be considered in cases with prior history of bilioenteric surgery.

The modalities of drainage include endoscopic (ERCP and EUS-guided), percutaneous, and surgical. Initial medical treatment may be sufficient for patients with mild cholangitis, whereas urgent biliary drainage is indicated for those with moderate or severe cholangitis (organ dysfunction/elderly)[16] (Fig. 55.1).

Endoscopic biliary drainage is the preferred modality in most patients. ERCP may be performed with a palliative intent initially in patients with severe cholangitis. After resolution of cholangitis, a more definitive ERCP can be performed. Initial aspiration of infected bile under pressure before instilling contrast in the bile duct is a wise practice, and repeated injections of contrast into the bile duct should be avoided. Excessive injection of contrast into an obstructed biliary system may further increase the intrabiliary pressure leading to cholangiovenous reflux and aggravation of sepsis. The aspirated bile may be sent for culture and sensitivity. In the author's unit, a nasobiliary tube (NBT) is placed initially to drain the infected bile. In the subsequent days, a cholangiogram is obtained and definitive ERCP is carried out. Plastic biliary stents may also be used instead of NBT to avoid discomfort to the patient. Both approaches are equally effective in relieving acute cholangitis.[17,18] Initial stent placement may also be accomplished in experienced hands in the intensive care unit setting without fluoroscopy in those patients too sick for transport.

In the following section, we shall discuss the endoscopic management of acute cholangitis caused by different etiologies.

Postoperative Cholangitis

Various surgical procedures which are potentially associated with postoperative cholangitis include postcholecystectomy bile duct injury, hepatojejunostomy, post liver transplant biliary strictures, afferent limb syndrome, and choledochoduodenostomy (sump syndrome).

The endoscopic management of postoperative benign biliary strictures includes either serial placement of multiple plastic stents or a fully covered metal stent for optimal results (Fig. 55.2). Balloon or catheter dilatation may be required to facilitate stent placement. In a multicenter randomized trial, the stricture resolution was higher with covered metal stents as compared to multiple plastic stents (92.6% vs. 85.4%).[19]

In afferent limb syndrome, long-standing afferent loop obstruction (stricture, kinking, or adhesions) results in pancreaticobiliary obstruction and may present as obstructive jaundice, cholangitis,

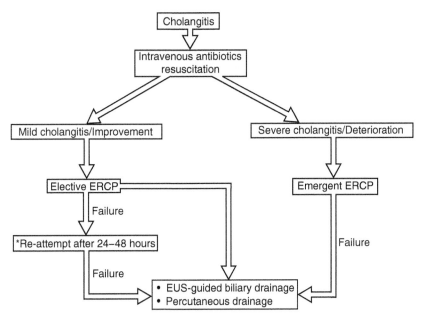

FIG 55.1 Algorithm for management of cholangitis. *ERCP*, endoscopic retrograde cholangiopancreatography; *EUS*, endoscopic ultrasound.

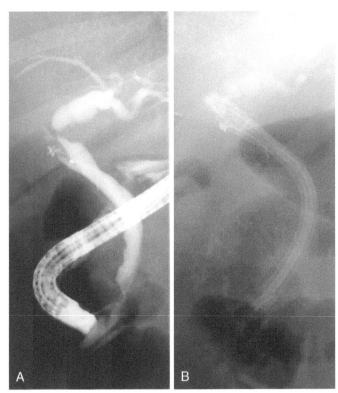

FIG 55.2 **A** and **B,** Patient with cholangitis resulting from a benign postoperative bile duct stricture shown by endoscopic retrograde cholangiopancreatography (ERCP) (**A**) and after placement of three 10-Fr plastic stents (**B**).

or liver abscess.[20] It usually occurs after subtotal gastrectomies, Billroth II surgeries, or other gastrojejunotomies. The management options include endoscopic, surgical, and percutaneous. Endoscopic treatment includes balloon dilatation and stenting across the afferent loop stricture. Limited data suggests that endoscopic management is safe and effective in these patients.[20]

Sump syndrome is an uncommon entity that occurs after creation of choledochoduodenostomy to manage retained CBD stones in a dilated bile duct. The distal bile duct between the papilla and the anastomosis becomes a stagnant reservoir or sump into which sludge, calculi, and food can accumulate. The clinical presentation includes recurrent pain, cholangitis, hepatic abscess, or pancreatitis. Management with endoscopic sphincterotomy (ES) and extraction of debris from the bile duct is successful in most patients.[21] However, a repeat sphincterotomy may be required in some cases due to restenosis of the sphincter.[22,23]

ERCP may be difficult in patients with bilioenteric strictures like hepatojejunostomy (Fig. 55.3). Treatment options include balloon enteroscopy–assisted ERCP, EUS-guided biliary drainage, and percutaneous biliary drainage.[24–26]

Biliary Strictures (Chronic Pancreatitis Related and Malignant)

Chronic pancreatitis related biliary strictures are often resistant to standard endoscopic management. However, stricture resolution of up to 90% has been reported with multiple plastic stents or covered metal stents.[27] Therefore, endoscopic treatment should be the preferred initial treatment in such patients and surgery should be reserved for refractory cases.

Malignant biliary strictures are usually not associated with cholangitis unless previous instrumentation has been done. If present, cholangitis is a definite indication for preoperative biliary drainage in these patients. Metal stents provide superior results and are preferred over plastic stents irrespective of the resectability status.[28]

In hilar strictures (Type III), bilateral stenting should be done (Y or parallel) with the goal of draining greater than 50% of liver volume.[29] In patients with duodenal narrowing due to tumor infiltration or altered anatomy, EUS-guided biliary drainage is often successful.

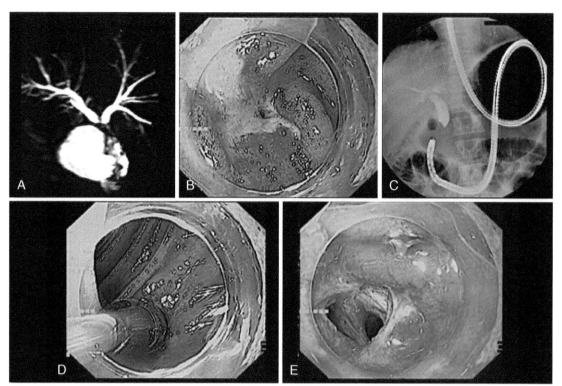

FIG 55.3 Patient with cholangitis and stricture at hepatojejunostomy anastomosis site. **A,** Magnetic resonance cholangiopancreatography (MRCP) image revealing stricture at hepatojejunostomy site with upstream dilatation of biliary tree. **B,** Endoscopic image of stricture site. **C,** Enteroscopy assisted cholangiography showing anastomotic stricture with upstream dilatation. **D,** Endoscopic dilatation of anastomotic stricture with balloon. **E,** Endoscopic image of stricture site after dilatation (**A** to **D,** Courtesy of Dr. Hrushikesh P. Choudhary, Hyderabad, India.)

Choledocholithiasis

CBD stones remain the most common cause of cholangitis. CBD stones act as nidus for the colonization of bacteria. More than 90% of CBD stones can be removed with standard ERCP techniques. In a sicker patient, the biliary system may be drained first by placing a biliary stent or NBT, followed by a more definitive procedure of clearing the bile duct (Fig. 55.4). A wire-guided approach is preferred for biliary cannulation to reduce the chances of post-ERCP pancreatitis. In cases of difficult biliary cannulation (> 5 attempts at cannulation, > 5 minutes spent at cannulation, or > 1 unintended pancreatic duct cannulation or opacification), the double wire technique or precut fistulotomy can be utilized to facilitate the cannulation.[30]

An endoscopic sphincterotomy is required for removal of CBD stones. Primary balloon dilation (often incorrectly termed *sphincteroplasty*) may be preferred for patients with coagulopathy as it is associated with a lower risk of bleeding. Recently, partial sphincterotomy followed by balloon sphincteroplasty has been successfully used, especially for large stones (> 1.5 cm). The procedure time was significantly shorter and the requirement of mechanical lithotripsy significantly lower in the combined technique as compared to endoscopic sphincterotomy alone in one study.[31] The rate of post-ERCP pancreatitis is not higher with this approach as the direction of papillary tearing is directed away from the pancreatic sphincter due to prior biliary sphincterotomy.[32]

Extraction devices include a balloon or basket and depends on the operator's preference. Other approaches for large CBD stones that are difficult to remove by standard techniques include mechanical lithotripsy, EHL, LL, and extracorporeal shock wave lithotripsy (Fig. 55.4).

RECURRENT PYOGENIC CHOLANGITIS

RPC is characterized by the triad of biliary calculi (intrahepatic and/or extrahepatic), biliary strictures, and recurrent cholangitis. The presence of biliary calculi, which are typically intrahepatic, and strictures result in biliary stasis and predispose the patient to recurrent bouts of cholangitis (Fig. 55.5). The pathogenesis of RPC is incompletely understood. The disease predominantly occurs in middle-aged individuals (4th decade) residing in Southeast Asia. Low socioeconomic status and biliary parasitosis (*Ascaris lumbricoides* and *Clonorchis sinensis*) are thought to predispose one to the development of RPC. Therefore, the disease is more prevalent in countries where gastrointestinal parasitoses is endemic.[33]

RPC typically involves intrahepatic ducts with focal stricturing and dilatation of the intrahepatic biliary tree along with intrahepatic pigmented stones. The left hepatic duct is involved more often than the right because of the more acute angulation of the former. The clinical presentation can be quite variable. RPC can present as acute cholangitis with right upper quadrant pain, fever, and jaundice. However, often the symptoms are subtle and the disease goes unrecognized in the initial period for months to several years. The long-term complications of RPC include cholangiocarcinoma (3% to 5%) and secondary biliary cirrhosis (7%) with portal hypertension.[34]

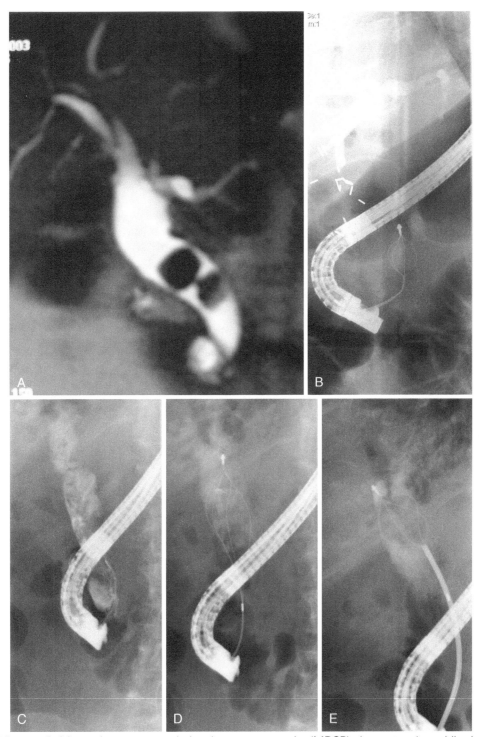

FIG 55.4 A, Magnetic resonance cholangiopancreatography (MRCP) shows two large bile duct stones in a patient with cholangitis. **B,** Endoscopic retrograde cholangiopancreatography (ERCP) in the same patient with basket extraction of one of the stones. **C,** ERCP shows dilated bile duct packed with stones. **D,** Basket extraction. **E,** Mechanical lithotripsy.

Diagnosis

The diagnosis of RPC relies on a combination of clinical features and imaging. Abdominal sonography is often the initial imaging modality revealing dilated intrahepatic ducts with calculi. It may also reveal associated cholangitic abscesses if present. Other imaging modalities include computed tomography (CT), ERCP, and MRCP. However, MRCP remains the imaging modality of choice for the initial evaluation of patients with RPC. The advantages of MRCP over ERCP include the ability to reveal ductal anatomy proximal to stricture or stone, its noninvasive nature, and no risk of aggravating biliary sepsis.[35]

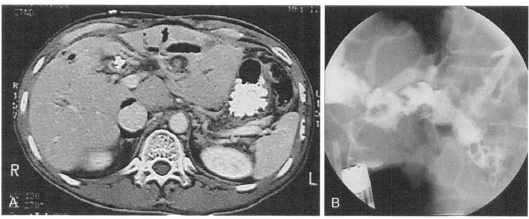

FIG 55.5 Patient with recurrent pyogenic cholangitis. **A,** Computed tomography (CT) scan shows dilated air-filled left intrahepatic ductal system with stones and two stents. **B,** Endoscopic retrograde cholangiography (ERC) shows multiple lucent stones in the same system.

Several classification systems have been proposed to characterize the phenotype of disease in patients with RPC.[36–38] These classifications broadly classify the disease into several grades of severity based on laterality of the disease (unilateral or bilateral), order of bile ducts involved (first, second, or third order) and presence or absence of concomitant parenchymal liver disease. Unfortunately, none of these classification systems have been validated in subsequent studies.

Management

The goal of treatment is not only to relieve cholangitis, but also to prevent or minimize the long-term consequences of the disease (e.g., biliary cirrhosis and cholangiocarcinoma).

The management of RPC includes drainage of obstructed biliary ducts by endoscopic, percutaneous, and surgical approaches. Often a combination of these modalities is required to achieve optimum biliary drainage. There has been no direct comparison among these modalities to demonstrate the superiority of any one approach over the other. A multidisciplinary approach involving gastroenterologists, interventional radiologists, and hepatobiliary surgeons appears to be rewarding in these patients.

Endoscopic Management

The primary goal is to relieve acute cholangitis by administering broad-spectrum antibiotics and placing a biliary plastic stent or NBT. Subsequently, a more definitive management is planned after the stabilization of the patient, which includes dilatation of the stricture and clearance of biliary calculi.

It is of paramount importance to select appropriate candidates for endotherapy. Strictures or stones in the CBD or main intrahepatic ducts can be managed with ERCP. A percutaneous approach may be more appropriate when the strictures/stones are located in peripheral biliary ducts, whereas surgery is more appropriate for patients with predominantly left-sided disease along with atrophy of the left lobe of the liver.

The endoscopic management of RPC can be divided into the following steps:
a. Biliary decompression and control of sepsis by placing a stent or nasobiliary drainage catheter
b. Accurate localization of the disease (stones and strictures) by cholangiogram

c. Securing the guidewire across the stricture
d. Dilatation of the stricture using biliary balloons
e. Brush cytology of suspicious strictures
f. If required: breaking the stone with either mechanical lithotripsy/EHL or laser probe
g. Retrieval of stones and placement of plastic biliary stent, if required

As a rule, broad-spectrum antibiotics should be administered in all patients undergoing endotherapy for RPC. Aggressive injection of contrast into the obstructed intrahepatic ducts should be avoided, and a prior MRCP should help in guiding through the location of strictures or stones.

Several sessions of endoscopic treatment are often required to achieve complete clearance of bile ducts. Regular follow-up is mandatory, as intrahepatic strictures and stones frequently recur after initial resolution.[39]

The major limitation of ERCP is its inability to achieve complete ductal clearance in a significant proportion of cases. Recurrent cholangitis is obviously more common in patients with residual intrahepatic stones. In a retrospective series, complete ductal clearance could be achieved in only 18 out of 57 patients (32%).[40] However, complete clearance of intrahepatic stones was achieved in approximately 67% of patients in two recently published series.[39,41]

The factors associated with negative outcomes include tortuous or sharply angulated duct, presence of intrahepatic stricture, and multiple stones scattered in many ducts.[42]

Role of Cholangioscopy

Cholangioscopy plays an indispensable role in the management of hepatolithiasis. With the recent availability of digital cholangioscopy, high-quality images of the biliary tract can be obtained. Moreover, any suspicious biliary stricture can be biopsied to rule out malignancy.

Therapeutic cholangioscopy can be performed perorally, via the percutaneous route, or intraoperatively via choledochotomy. In general, peroral cholangioscopy (POCS) is appropriate for stones in main intrahepatic ducts, whereas the percutaneous approach may be required for more peripheral disease. In some cases, a combination of both routes is required for complete ductal clearance.

In POCS, endoscopic sphincterotomy is performed and a cholangioscope is advanced through the accessory channel of a therapeutic duodenoscope. Calculi are then extracted via balloon or a basket. Large intrahepatic stones can be fragmented by either EHL or LL (Nd:YAG). Intrahepatic strictures are dilated with a balloon or biliary dilating catheters, followed by stent placement. In one study, POCS was found to be safe and effective for management of hepatolithiasis with complete and partial ductal clearance in 64% and 11% of patients, respectively.[43]

Percutaneous Approach

In the percutaneous approach, initially a percutaneous transhepatic drainage (PTBD) is performed. Subsequently the tract is dilated up to 18 Fr to facilitate the passage of a cholangioscope and the removal of stones. Intrahepatic strictures can be dilated by balloon or dilating catheters. Complete stone clearance is achieved in 80% to 85% of patients with percutaneous transhepatic cholangioscopy.[44,45] Complete clearance of stones is hampered by the presence of severe intrahepatic strictures, as with the endoscopic approach.

Role of Surgery

Surgery can provide definitive treatment for patients with unilateral disease (usually left-sided). Both stones and strictured segments of the biliary tree can be removed. The major advantages of surgery are a lower recurrence of intrahepatic stones and a significantly less incidence of complications (biliary cirrhosis, cholangiocarcinoma) as compared to nonoperative treatment.[34] The laparoscopic approach has been utilized with promising results in patients with hepatolithiasis, with the advantage of a shorter hospital stay.[46,47]

In patients with bilateral disease, a combined approach is useful (i.e., removing the more severely affected lobe and creating a hepaticojejunostomy in the remaining lobe for endoscopic management in future)[48] (Fig. 55.6). A Hutson access jejunal loop between the skin and the hepatic ducts has been used in the past to provide access for repeated interventions.

In patients who are not candidates for hepatectomy, laparoscopic bile duct exploration in conjunction with choledochoscopic lithotripsy has been shown to be safe and effective.[49]

PARASITIC CHOLANGITIS

Ascaris lumbricoides is a nematode or roundworm that matures within the small intestine and causes cholangitis by entering the bile duct across the major papilla. The trematodes *Opisthorchis sinensis, Opisthorchis viverrini, Opisthorchis felineus,* and *Fasciola hepatica* mature to adulthood within the human bile duct and are collectively known as liver flukes. *A. lumbricoides* and liver flukes cause inflammation of the bile duct and secondary bacterial cholangitis by allowing ascending bacterial contamination of bile, obstructing the bile duct and stimulating choledocholithiasis. Hepatic infection by *Echinococcus* species frequently involves the biliary tract by hydatid cyst compression or rupture and direct extension of alveolar echinococcosis.

Ascaris Cholangitis

A. lumbricoides exists worldwide but is most prevalent in Asia, Africa, and South America as a result of the crowded living conditions and poor sanitation. Ova are passed in human feces and are ingested on contaminated fruits or vegetables. Hepatobiliary ascariasis (HBA) may manifest as biliary colic, cholangitis, cholecystitis, liver abscess, and, rarely, hemobilia. Previous cholecystectomy, sphincterotomy, sphincteroplasty, choledochostomy, or biliary enteric anastomosis favor biliary tract migration, whereas low insertion of cystic duct facilitates gallbladder involvement.[33] *A. lumbricoides* causes inflammation of the bile duct and secondary bacterial cholangitis by allowing ascending bacterial contamination of bile, obstructing the bile duct, and stimulating pigment stone formation. Therefore, it is not surprising that HBA predisposes to RPC as well. Over 5% of patients with HBA develop RPC, and 10% of patients with RPC have a definite evidence of ascariasis.[50]

Ultrasound is the imaging modality of choice for diagnosis and follow-up of patients with HBA. Characteristic sonographic findings include thick echoic stripe with a central, longitudinal anechoic tube (gastrointestinal tract of the worm, inner tube sign), thin nonshadowing strip without an inner tube (strip sign), overlapping longitudinal interfaces in the main bile duct (spaghetti sign), and the characteristic movement of these long echogenic structures within the bile duct.[51]

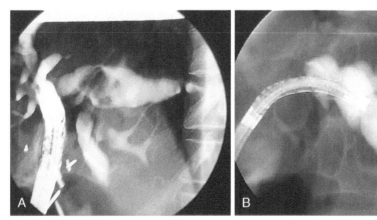

FIG 55.6 Patient with recurrent pyogenic cholangitis, previously treated surgically with the creation of a cutaneous-jejunal-hepatic duct conduit. **A,** Gastroscope passed through the conduit shows a large left intrahepatic duct stone. **B,** After electrohydraulic lithotripsy and extraction of fragments.

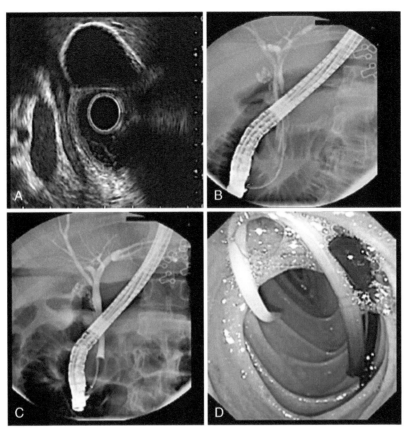

FIG 55.7 A, Endoscopic ultrasound image shows *Ascaris lumbricoides* as a hyperechoic linear structure within the bile duct. **B,** Endoscopic retrograde cholangiography in the same image shows a long linear filling defect in the common bile duct and left hepatic duct. **C,** Cholangiogram after balloon sweep and clearance of the bile duct. **D,** Endoscopic view of extracted adult *Ascaris.* (**A,** Courtesy of Dr. Sundeep Lakhtakia, Hyderabad, India; **B** to **D,** Courtesy of Dr. Zaheer Nabi, Hyderabad, India.)

In cases where ultrasonography is nondiagnostic, EUS and MRCP may be performed. On EUS, the worms appear as long linear hyperechoic structures without acoustic shadowing (single-tube sign) or with a central hypoechoic tube (double-tube sign)[52] (Fig. 55.7).

Indications of ERCP
Conservative management (intravenous fluids, antibiotics, anthelminthic medications, and analgesics for pain) is successful in 60% to 80% of cases.[53,54]

ERCP is indicated in severe cholangitis, failure of conservative management, and persistence of worms in the bile duct (indicating dead worms). Dead worms can incite inflammatory reaction leading to stricture formation or can act as nidus for stone formation. Therefore, dead worms should be extracted as well.[55]

Preparation. All patients with *Ascaris* cholangitis should receive antibiotics and anthelminthic therapy. Close contacts of infected individuals should submit stool specimens for analysis and be treated if positive.

Procedure. The goal of therapy is complete removal of the parasite and secondary stones or strictures if present. At duodenoscopy, the adult worm is seen as a long pale white or reddish yellow tubular structure, either within the lumen of the duodenum or crossing the major papilla. Worms across the papilla can be grasped with a biopsy forceps and then withdrawn along the endoscope by holding the worm near the accessory channel of the scope.

Worms located completely within the biliary tract appear as a tubular filling defect with tapered ends and may show the erratic motility pattern typical of *A. lumbricoides* on real-time fluoroscopy (see Fig. 55.7). Injection of contrast material may stimulate the worm to migrate distally into the duodenum. Otherwise, intrabiliary worms can be removed with a biliary extraction balloon or basket. Major papilla is often patulous in these patients due to frequent worm migrations, facilitating worm extraction and avoiding the need for a sphincterotomy. Moreover, sphincterotomy facilitates future biliary tract involvement by the worm and should be avoided when possible. Instead, papillary balloon dilatation can be done if required.[56]

The worm should be brought to the papillary orifice and grasped using the biopsy forceps as described previously. Polypectomy snares should be avoided as they are liable to transect the worm and complicate extraction.

Complications. In addition to infecting the biliary tree, *A. lumbricoides* parasites also burrow through the bile duct wall into the liver parenchyma to form hepatic abscesses. Acute pancreatitis has been reported secondary to worms obstructing the pancreatic duct.[57]

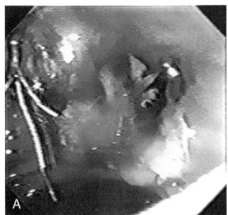
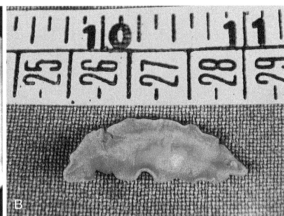

FIG 55.8 A, *Fasciola hepatica* being extracted at endoscopic retrograde cholangiopancreatography (ERCP). **B,** Adult worm after extraction. (**A,** Courtesy of Dr. Claudio Navarette, Santiago, Chile; **B,** courtesy of Dr. Alok Gupta, Kanpur, India.)

Outcomes. Endoscopic extraction of biliary *A. lumbricoides* is successful and safe in 99% of patients.[46] Approximately 15% of patients will experience symptomatic reinvasion of biliary tree, and 4% to 5% may develop biliary lithiasis in endemic regions.[58,59]

Therefore, antihelminthic therapy should be repeated at regular intervals in endemic zones. The indications of surgery include cholecystitis, failure of endoscopic bile duct clearance, and intrahepatic strictures or stones.

Liver Fluke Cholangitis

The most important liver fluke species include Clonorchis sinensis, *Fasciola* spp., and Opisthorchis spp. More than 750 million people across the globe are at risk of infection. Liver flukes are endemic in Southeast Asia and the Western Pacific region.[60]

Human infection occurs from eating uncooked or undercooked freshwater fish or plants such as watercress, alfalfa, and parsley that harbor the infective metacercarial cysts of liver flukes. *Opisthorchis* enter the biliary tree through the major papilla, whereas *Fasciola* penetrate the intestinal wall into the peritoneal cavity and enter the biliary tree transhepatically. Adult liver flukes most commonly reside in the intrahepatic branches but may be observed in the distal biliary tract.

Indications for ERCP

The hepatic phase of Fascioliasis can be managed with the antiparasitic drug triclabendazole (10 mg/kg body weight) alone. Praziquantel is the drug of choice for clonorchiasis (75 mg/kg in three divided doses). ERCP is indicated for the diagnosis and management of liver fluke cholangitis and associated secondary bile duct strictures and stones. ERCP enables the sampling of bile to show the presence of ova, which may be more sensitive than stool microscopy.[61]

Procedure. The goals and techniques of the endoscopic treatment of liver fluke cholangitis are similar to *Ascaris* cholangitis. The most characteristic cholangiographic finding of hepatic clonorchiasis in ERCP is filamentous or elliptic filling defects of the biliary tract.[61] Cholangiographic findings in patients with biliary phase fascioliasis include radiolucent, crescent-shaped shadows in the bile ducts with or without dilatation.[62] Other cholangiographic findings include diffuse saccular dilation of the intrahepatic ducts with blunted terminal ends.[63]

Endoscopic sphincterotomy is usually required for liver fluke extraction. Extraction of flukes is undertaken with a biliary extraction basket or balloon. Because liver flukes frequently inhabit the proximal biliary tree, complete clearance can be challenging. Placement of a NBT to perform biliary infusion of povidone-iodine has been described in the management of *F. hepatica* cholangitis.[64] At duodenoscopy, flukes appear as brownish, flat, leaf-shaped organisms 1 to 2 cm long and usually less than 1 cm wide[65] (Fig. 55.8).

Complications. The major hepatobiliary diseases associated with liver flukes include: cholangitis, cholecystitis, cholelithiasis, hepatocellular carcinoma, RPC, portal hypertension, and cholangiocarcinoma.[60]

Outcomes. Medical management with anti-parasitic drugs is sufficient for asymptomatic hepatobiliary fluke infections. Endoscopic extraction is required for patients with acute cholangitis and failure of conservative management. Surgical intervention is indicated for biliary or pancreatic obstruction after unsuccessful endoscopic therapy and for cholecystitis.

Echinococcal Cholangitis

Echinococcus granulosus accounts for up to 95% of all human echinococcal infections and is particularly prevalent in regions where dogs are used to raise livestock. *E. granulosus, Echinococcus vogeli,* and *Echinococcus oligarthrus* form a unilocular hydatid cyst within the liver. However, *Echinococcus multilocularis* cysts are not contained by an outer fibrous membrane and extend through the liver and into adjacent structures. The cyst is composed of three layers: an outermost layer of granulation and fibrous tissue, a middle layer of laminated membrane, and the innermost germinal layer of the parasite, which forms the daughter cysts and protoscolices. Biliary disease results from compression by the cyst or rupture of the cyst into the biliary tree. Larger cysts (> 7.5 cm) are more likely to harbor cyst-biliary communication.[66]

Indications for ERCP[67]

The indications for ERCP in biliary echinococcosis are listed in Box 55.2.

Procedure

The goals of ERCP are to document suspected *Echinococcus* cholangitis and treat biliary obstruction.

ERCP is performed in the usual manner. Duodenoscopy may show glistening, white membranes within the duodenum or protruding from the papilla, which can be removed with biopsy forceps (Fig. 55.9). On cholangiography, three patterns of filling defects have been reported. The membranes appear filiform, the daughter cysts round, and hydatid sand as debris.[68]

Endoscopic sphincterotomy is usually required prior to the removal of the filling defects with a biliary extraction balloon or basket.[69]

Saline irrigation facilitates the removal of hydatid cyst material.

In case of frank intrabiliary rupture, it is preferable to coil a hydrophilic guidewire into the cystic cavity, followed by the placement of a NBT. Subsequently, periodic irrigation of the cystic cavity with saline is carried out for several days, to ensure complete clearance of the cyst cavity.[67,70]

Some authors use a specially designed NBT (10-Fr) with additional holes on both duodenal and biliary ends.[67] Encouraging results with the NBT approach suggests that it should be attempted prior to surgery in the case of major intrabiliary ruptures.

Biliary strictures resulting from hydatid cyst compression or alveolar echinococcosis invasion can be managed with stent insertion.

Endoscopic therapy in the postoperative period may be required to manage external biliary fistulas, clear the hydatid remnants causing biliary obstruction, or biliary strictures from scolicidal agents.[67] In biliary fistulae, ERCP is indicated only if fistula output is high (> 300 mL/day), persistent, or rising each day. Endoscopic sphincterotomy alone may be sufficient in some cases. However, biliary stent placement may be required in cases of failure with ES alone or incomplete clearance of hydatid material in the bile duct. Stenting is also preferred to ES alone in those with chronic high output fistulae and if fistulae are accompanied by a biliary stricture.

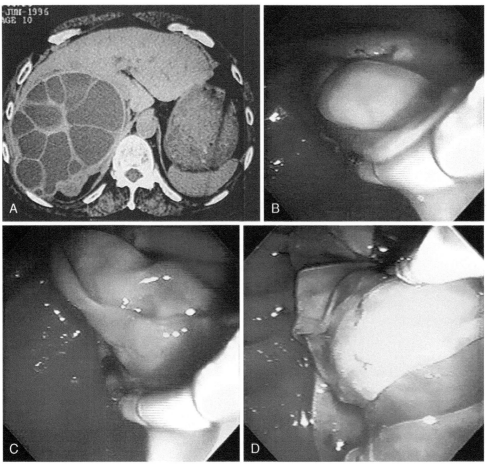

FIG 55.9 **A,** *Echinococcus* (hydatidosis) infection shown in right lobe of the liver on computed tomography (CT) scan. **B** to **D,** Sequence of cyst wall extraction at endoscopic retrograde cholangiopancreatography (ERCP) after sphincterotomy. (**A,** Courtesy of Dr. Nageshwar Reddy, Hyderabad, India; **B** to **D,** Courtesy of Dr. Claudio Navarette, Santiago, Chile.)

Complications

E. multilocularis may invade into the portal venous system resulting in portal hypertension.[71]

Outcomes of Endoscopic Therapy

Endoscopic management of biliary obstruction secondary to *E. granulosus* infection through extraction of hydatid debris or biliary endoprosthesis placement is successful at alleviating patient symptoms.[69] Endoscopic therapy alone is curative in approximately 25% of cases with frank intrabiliary rupture.[67]

In the postoperative period, endoscopic therapy is required for biliary fistulae, stricture, and remnant hydatid material in the bile duct. Overall, more than 80% of patients can be successfully managed with endoscopic therapy alone.[72] External biliary fistulae respond well to ES with or without placement of a biliary stent. In one study, 75% of biliary fistulae responded to ES alone.[73] In patients with high output external biliary fistulae, larger stents are preferable to ES alone or 7-Fr stents. In a multicentric study, the time to fistula closure was significantly shorter in the 10-Fr stent group as compared to ES alone and 7-Fr stent group.[74]

Other Therapies (Medical, Percutaneous, and Surgical)

Medical therapy with albendazole should be given for greater than 3 months and is curative in less than 60% of patients.[75] Small and simple cysts are more likely to get cured with medical therapy alone. Albendazole is also administered before surgery, as it results in a higher number of nonviable cysts and may decrease the risk of local recurrence or intraperitoneal seeding should spillage of cyst contents occur.[75]

Percutaneous evacuation with ultrasound-guided puncture-aspiration-injection-reaspiration (PAIR) is widely used to treat unilocular *E. granulosus* cysts. Scolicidal agents employed for PAIR include 95% ethanol and hypertonic saline. PAIR is equally effective, with fewer complications and shorter hospital stays as compared to surgery.[76]

Complications of PAIR include hypersensitivity reaction, infection, intraabdominal seeding, and fistula formation to adjacent organs. ERCP should be performed before protoscolicide administration to ensure there is no communication between the cyst and biliary tree because contact with protoscolicidal agents produces sclerosing cholangitis.

Surgical management, which includes excision by cystectomy, pericystectomy, or partial hepatic resection, is usually curative in *E. granulosus* infection. Surgical mortality is 1% to 2%.[77] Complications include infection, bile leak, and leakage of cyst contents with hypersensitivity reaction and dissemination of disease.

ACQUIRED IMMUNODEFICIENCY SYNDROME CHOLANGIOPATHY

AIDS cholangiopathy is a syndrome of right upper quadrant pain, elevated alkaline phosphatase, and typical cholangiography findings associated with the human immunodeficiency virus (HIV) infection. Elevation in serum bilirubin is minimal or absent in AIDS cholangiopathy unless a concomitant hepatobiliary disease is present. Opportunistic infections of the biliary tract implicated in AIDS cholangiopathy include *Cryptosporidium* (most commonly *Cryptosporidium parvum*),[78] *Microsporida*, cytomegalovirus, *Isospora*, *Cyclospora*, and *Mycobacterium*

avium intracellulare.[79,80] Cholangiopathy is the AIDS-defining illness in few patients, but most of these have had AIDS for at least 1 year.[81]

The characteristic bile duct abnormalities in AIDS cholangiopathy can be divided into four groups, including: (1) papillary stenosis, (2) sclerosing cholangitis involving extrahepatic and intrahepatic bile ducts, (3) combined papillary stenosis and sclerosing cholangitis, and (4) long extrahepatic strictures. AIDS cholangiopathy usually develops in patients with advanced disease and is rare in patients with CD4+ greater than 200. Therefore, its incidence has reduced after the introduction of highly active antiretroviral therapy (HAART). In fact, non–HIV-related biliary diseases (like choledocholithiasis, calculous cholecystitis, ampullary malignancies, etc.) may be more common in these patients.

Indications

ERCP is the gold standard in the diagnosis and management of AIDS cholangiopathy (Fig. 55.10). However, MRCP may be a good noninvasive alternative prior to ERCP for the evaluation of both the intrahepatic and extrahepatic biliary tree in these patients.[82] Bile duct abnormalities on MRCP in AIDS cholangiopathy include dilatation, dilatation with beading and strictures, distal stricture, and contrast enhancement.[83] Cholangiographic abnormalities may resolve with HAART and can be followed with MRCP. Therefore, with the availability of MRCP, ERCP should be reserved for carrying out therapeutic procedures like ES in papillary stenosis or balloon dilatation/stenting in symptomatic biliary strictures. The differential diagnosis of AIDS cholangiopathy and the management approach are shown in Box 55.3 and Fig. 55.11, respectively.

Precautions

Protease inhibitors decrease benzodiazepine metabolism and increase their serum levels, which may potentially cause respiratory depression.[84] Therefore, benzodiazepines such as diazepam and midazolam should be used cautiously for sedation in these patients.

Procedure

ERCP should be performed only in symptomatic patients with abdominal pain, cholestatic jaundice, or fever. The cholangiography findings in ERCP include papillary stenosis, with or without intrahepatic strictures (51%) (most common), and

---

BOX 55.3 Differential Diagnosis of Acquired Immunodeficiency Syndrome Cholangiopathy

Non–HIV-Related
Choledocholithiasis
Cholecystitis
Primary sclerosing cholangitis
Viral hepatitis
Chronic pancreatitis

HIV-Related
Medication hepatotoxicity
Opportunistic Infection

Acalculous cholecystitis
Peliosis hepatitis
Infectious pancreatitis
Mycobacterial (MAI, tuberculosis)
CMV
Opportunistic Neoplasm
Kaposi's sarcoma (papilla)
Lymphoma (papilla, pancreas, duodenum)
Adenoma/adenocarcinoma (papilla)

CMV, cytomegalovirus; *HIV*, human immunodeficiency virus; *MAI*, Mycobacterium avium-intracellulare.

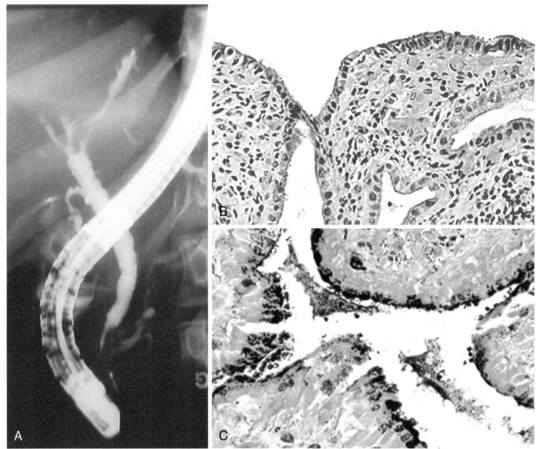

FIG 55.10 **A,** Acquired immunodeficiency syndrome (AIDS) cholangiopathy shown by endoscopic retrograde cholangiopancreatography (ERCP) with narrowed distal bile duct and irregular bile duct walls. **B,** Relatively normal bile duct epithelium on biopsy and standard hematoxylin and eosin staining. **C,** Microsporidia shown on the surface as black with silver staining. (Courtesy of Dr. Richard Tilson, Boston, MA.)

TABLE 55.2 Cholangiography Findings in Acquired Immunodeficiency Syndrome Cholangiopathy[79,81,88,89,93]

Finding	Frequency (%)
Papillary stenosis and intrahepatic duct strictures	33
Papillary stenosis alone	21
Papillary stenosis and intrahepatic and extrahepatic duct strictures	20
Intrahepatic duct strictures alone	12
Intrahepatic and extrahepatic duct strictures	8
Extrahepatic duct strictures alone	5
Papillary stenosis and extrahepatic duct strictures	1

isolated or combined intrahepatic and extrahepatic biliary strictures (25%)[79,81,85] (Table 55.2). Other reported cholangiography abnormalities include adherent polypoid filling defects; biopsy specimens of these defects show granulation tissue.[86]

Recently, single-operator cholangioscopy has been reported in a patient with AIDS cholangiopathy. Cholangioscopy showed fibrotic-appearing stricture of the common hepatic duct (CHD) with pseudodiverticula and multiple nonobstructing rings in the distal CHD.[87] Interestingly, pancreatography is abnormal in one-half of patients with AIDS cholangiopathy, revealing pancreatic duct strictures in the head of the pancreas.[79,88]

The standard ERCP procedure consists of an ES if papillary stenosis is present. ES is not beneficial in the absence of papillary stenosis. Dominant strictures should be sampled for cytology with a cytology brush or biopsy forceps to exclude cholangiocarcinoma or another malignant process. In a symptomatic patient, balloon or catheter dilation of the stricture may be performed, but long-term stent placement should be avoided to limit the migration of enteric pathogens into the biliary tract.

During ERCP, the duodenum should be inspected for mucosal abnormalities such as erosions or ulcerations that may indicate enteric infection. Duodenal/ampullary biopsy specimens and bile aspiration samples should be obtained and sent for microbiologic and cytologic analysis. Aspiration of bile for culture and multiple biopsy specimens of the duodenum and papilla reveal an underlying pathogen in up to 92% of cases.[88,89]

Complications and Outcomes

The complications of untreated non–HIV-related sclerosing cholangitis include secondary biliary cirrhosis and cholangiocarcinoma.

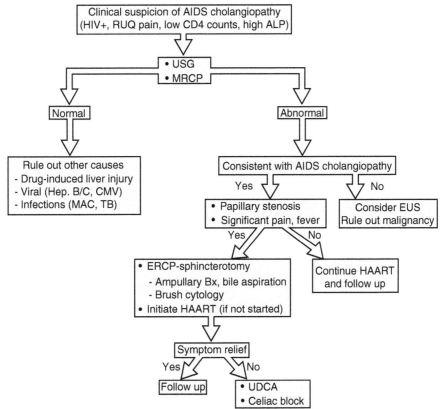

FIG 55.11 Algorithm for management of suspected acquired immunodeficiency syndrome (AIDS) cholangiopathy. *ALP*, alkaline phosphatase; *CMV*, cytomegalovirus; *ERCP*, endoscopic retrograde cholangiopancreatography; *EUS*, endoscopic ultrasound; *HAART*, highly active antiretroviral therapy; *Hep. B*, hepatitis B virus; *Hep. C*, hepatitis C virus; *HIV*, human immunodeficiency virus; *MRCP*, magnetic resonance cholangiopancreatography; *RUQ*, right upper quadrant; *UCDA*, ursodeoxycholic acid; *USG*, ultrasonography.

However, except for a rare case report of development of cholangiocarcinoma in a patient with AIDS cholangiopathy, these complications have not been reported in AIDS cholangiopathy.[90]

The mainstay of treatment in patients with AIDS cholangiopathy is restoration of immunity with HAART. The median survival in these patients has increased significantly after the introduction of HAART. In a 2010 series, the median survival was 34 months after the diagnosis of cholangiopathy as compared to 4 to 9 months in previous case series.[91] The development of cholangiopathy in patients on HAART is associated with a drop in CD4+ counts and may indicate resistance to antiviral drugs.

ERCP does not prolong survival in these patients and is intended only to provide symptom relief.[91,92] ES in patients with papillary stenosis results in improvement of abdominal pain in 32% to 100% of patients.[88,89,93]

Elevation in liver enzymes (especially ALP) may persist and should not be used as a criterion for successful endotherapy.[94] In patients with refractory pain after endotherapy, ursodeoxycholic acid (10 mg/kg) and celiac plexus block have been reported, with good results.[95,96]

Unfortunately, the treatment of pathogens implicated in AIDS cholangiopathy (cytomegalovirus, *C. parvum*, and *Microsporida*) has not been found useful in reducing patient's symptoms, liver enzymes, and cholangiography abnormalities.[78,89,97]

ROLE OF ERCP IN ACUTE CHOLECYSTITIS

Acute cholecystitis is an inflammatory injury to the gallbladder mucosa from bile stasis, ischemia, or infection. Bile stasis usually results from cystic duct obstruction by a gallstone or from decreased gallbladder motility. Less common causes of cystic duct obstruction are worms, hemobilia, and tumor. Decreased gallbladder motility and ischemia are implicated in the development of acalculous cholecystitis in critically ill patients. Infection of the gallbladder complicates cholecysitis in approximately 50% of cases but is not usually the causative factor, with the exception of parasitic and AIDS cholecystitis.

Indication

ERCP is indicated for gallbladder drainage in patients who are medically unfit for surgery and in whom percutaneous drainage is contraindicated or unsuccessful. The advantages of transpapillary drainage of gallbladder (EDGB) over percutaneous drainage are that coagulopathy and the presence of ascites are not contraindications, there is no risk of bile leak, there is less pain, and there is the option of removing coexisting bile duct stones.

Preparation

Antibiotic coverage is directed against *Enterobacteriaceae* and *Enterococcus* species until directed therapy can be instituted against specific organisms identified in blood or bile cultures.

Procedure[98]

ERCP is performed in the usual manner. EDGB is achieved by transpapillary placement of a NBT or double pigtail stent into the gallbladder (Fig. 55.12). Biliary sphincterotomy is not required unless coexisting bile duct stones are to be removed. After cannulating the bile duct, a hydrophilic guidewire (0.025- or 0.035-inch) is advanced into the cystic duct and subsequently into the gallbladder.

Either a sphincterotome or a flexible tip catheter can be used. A rotatable sphincterotome may be especially helpful in some patients with left-sided cystic duct takeoff. In case the cystic duct is not opacified by contrast due to cystic duct edema or calculus, a guidewire along with a catheter are gently manipulated to enter the cystic duct. An occlusion cholangiogram with balloon inflated just below the expected cystic duct takeoff may also help in opacifying the cystic duct. If the previous methods fail, cholangioscope can be used to place the guidewire under direct vision. Once the guidewire is in position, a NBT (5- or 6-Fr) or double pigtail stent (5- or 7-Fr) can be fashioned into the gallbladder. Nasobiliary lavage with saline or N-acetyl cysteine is carried out in case thick pus is aspirated from the gallbladder.

Outcomes

The outcomes of EDGB are encouraging and at par with percutaneous drainage. Technical and clinical success in recent studies range from 77% to 100% and 72% to 98%, respectively[99–103] (Table 55.3). There is no difference in success rates and adverse events between NBT or double pigtail stents.[101,102] The major reasons for technical failure are the inability to pass a 7-Fr stent or NBT due to impacted cystic duct stones or stenosis of cystic duct. Smaller catheters (5 Fr) may be useful in this situation but carry the risk of getting clogged readily due to the thick, purulent bile. However, the stent may act as a wick, and bile may flow within as well as alongside the stent into the duodenum. Therefore, the risk of recurrent cholecystitis appears small.[104]

The relapse of acute cholecystitis occurred in 20% of patients after a median follow-up of 17 months in one study.[105] Therefore, these patients should undergo cholecystectomy, once stabilized.

Complications

The incidence of procedure-related complications ranges from 0% to 14% and includes post-ERCP pancreatitis, perforation of the cystic duct or gallbladder, cholangitis, and sepsis[98] (see Table 55.3).

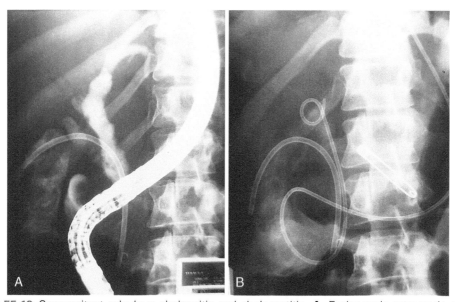

FIG 55.12 Concomitant calculous cholangitis and cholecystitis. **A,** Endoscopic retrograde cholangiopancreatography (ERCP) shows a plastic stent draining the gallbladder. **B,** Radiograph obtained after ERCP shows addition of a nasobiliary tube draining the common bile duct (CBD).

TABLE 55.3 Endoscopic Drainage of Gallbladder

Study	No. of Patients	Drainage Model	Technical Success (%)	Clinical Success (%)	Complications (%)
Pannala et al[99]	51	NBT	100	98	8
Maekawa et al[100]	40	7 Fr DPTS	77.5	72.5	None
Itoi et al[101]	73	NBT – 37	91.9	86.5	4.1
		DPTS – 36	86.1	77.8	
Yang et al[102]	35	NBT – 17	82.4	79.6	14.2
		DPTS – 18	88.9	83.3	
Widmer et al[103]	128	7 Fr DPTS	91	91	8

DPTS, double pigtail plastic stent; *NBT,* nasobiliary tube.

KEY REFERENCES

7. Khashab MA, Tariq A, Tariq U, et al: Delayed and unsuccessful endoscopic retrograde cholangiopancreatography are associated with worse outcomes in patients with acute cholangitis, *Clin Gastroenterol Hepatol* 10(10):1157–1161, 2012.

9. O'Horo JC, Farrell A, Sohail MR, Safdar N: Carbapenem-resistant Enterobacteriaceae and endoscopy: an evolving threat, *Am J Infect Control* 44:1032–1036, 2016.

10. Epstein L, Hunter JC, Arwady MA, et al: New Delhi metallo-β-lactamase-producing carbapenem-resistant Escherichia coli associated with exposure to duodenoscopes, *JAMA* 312(14):1447–1455, 2014.

11. Verfaillie CJ, Bruno MJ, Voor in 't Holt AF, et al: Withdrawal of a novel-design duodenoscope ends outbreak of a VIM-2-producing Pseudomonas aeruginosa, *Endoscopy* 47(6):493–502, 2015.

12. Saxena P, Singh VK, Lennon AM, et al: Endoscopic management of acute cholecystitis after metal stent placement in patients with malignant biliaryobstruction: a case series, *Gastrointest Endosc* 78(1):175–178, 2013.

15. Kiriyama S, Takada T, Strasberg SM, et al: TG13 guidelines for diagnosis and severity grading of acute cholangitis (with videos), *J Hepatobiliary Pancreat Sci* 20(1):24–34, 2013.

16. Takada T, Strasberg SM, Solomkin JS, et al: TG13: updated Tokyo Guidelines for the management of acute cholangitis and cholecystitis, *J Hepatobiliary Pancreat Sci* 20(1):1–7, 2013.

19. Coté GA, Slivka A, Tarnasky P, et al: Effect of covered metallic stents compared with plastic stents on benign biliary stricture resolution: a randomized clinical trial, *JAMA* 315(12):1250–1257, 2016.

27. Haapamäki C, Kylänpää L, Udd M, et al: Randomized multicenter study of multiple plastic stents vs. covered self-expandable metallic stent in the treatment of biliary stricture in chronic pancreatitis, *Endoscopy* 47(7): 605–610, 2015.

28. Walter D, van Boeckel PG, Groenen MJ, et al: Cost efficacy of metal stents for palliation of extrahepatic bile duct obstruction in a randomized controlled trial, *Gastroenterology* 149(1):130–138, 2015.

30. Testoni PA, Mariani A, Aabakken L, et al: Papillary cannulation and sphincterotomy techniques at ERCP: European Society of Gastrointestinal Endoscopy (ESGE) Clinical Guideline, *Endoscopy* 48(7):657–683, 2016.

33. Rana SS, Bhasin DK, Nanda M, Singh K: Parasitic infestations of the biliary tract, *Curr Gastroenterol Rep* 9(2):156–164, 2007.

36. Cheon YK, Cho YD, Moon JH, et al: Evaluation of long-term results and recurrent factors after operative and non-operative treatment for hepatolithiasis, *Surgery* 146(5):843–853, 2009.

42. Mori T, Sugiyama M, Atomi Y: Gallstone disease: management of intrahepatic stones, *Best Pract Res Clin Gastroenterol* 20(6):1117–1137, 2006.

45. Huang MH, Chen CH, Yang JC, et al: Long-term outcome of percutaneous transhepatic cholangioscopic lithotomy for hepatolithiasis, *Am J Gastroenterol* 98:2589–2590, 2003.

58. Khuroo MS, Zargar SA, Mahajan R: Hepatobiliary and pancreatic ascariasis in India, *Lancet* 335(8704):1503–1506, 1990.

63. Leung JW, Sung JY, Banez VP, et al: Endoscopic cholangiopancreatography in hepatic clonorchiasis—a follow-up study, *Gastrointest Endosc* 36:360–363, 1990.

70. Dzirlo L, Wasilewski M, Poeschl E, et al: Liver cyst of Echinococcus granulosus with rupture into the biliary tree—successful endoscopic and pharmaceutical treatment, *Am J Gastroenterol* 101:1674–1675, 2006.

81. Cello JP: AIDS-related biliary tract disease, *Gastrointest Endosc Clin N Am* 8:963, 1998.

94. Cello JP, Chan MF: Long-term follow-up of endoscopic retrograde cholangiopancreatography sphincterotomy for patients with acquired immune deficiency syndrome papillary stenosis, *Am J Med* 99:600–603, 1995.

98. Itoi T, Coelho-Prabhu N, Baron TH: Endoscopic gallbladder drainage for management of acute cholecystitis, *Gastrointest Endosc* 71(6):1038–1045, 2010.

A complete reference list can be found online at ExpertConsult.com

56

Sphincter of Oddi Disorders

Peter B. Cotton and Paul Tarnasky

"It is a riddle, wrapped in a mystery, inside an enigma"
Winston Churchill 1939

INTRODUCTION

Functional disorders of the biliary tree and pancreas are controversial topics, with insufficient scientific evidence to provide clear guidelines for clinical practice. This chapter attempts to summarize what is known, what is unclear, and what studies need to be done. One author (PBC) was recently involved in the comprehensive Rome IV process, conclusions from which have been published.[1] One recommendation was to change the names of the clinical syndromes, to functional biliary sphincter disorder (FBSD), and functional pancreatic sphincter disorder (FPSD).

THE SPHINCTER: STRUCTURE AND FUNCTION

The anatomy and physiology of the sphincter zone have been well described in standard texts. It is a complex of muscle fibers 4 to 10 mm in length, surrounding the distal bile and pancreatic ducts (Fig. 56.1). Although often subdivided into three sections (biliary, pancreatic and ampullary), the fibers are intertwined and the distinction probably has little clinical significance. The sphincter has a resting basal pressure, and phasic contractile activity, closely associated with the migratory motor complex. Its role is to control the flow of bile and pancreatic secretions into the duodenum, under both neural and hormonal control.

FUNCTIONAL BILIARY SPHINCTER DISORDER (FBSD)

The concept that disordered function of the sphincter can cause pain is based on the fact that many patients have "biliary" pain in the absence of recognized organic causes, and that some apparently are cured by ablation of the sphincter. The hypothesis is that it fails to relax sufficiently when the bile is flowing, thereby causing the pressure to rise in the bile duct to a level sufficient to produce biliary pain.

Postcholecystectomy Pain

FBSD is commonly considered in the 10% to 20% of patients who have persistent or recurrent pains after cholecystectomy. Loss of the gall bladder reservoir aggravates the increase in intrabiliary pressure when the sphincter is closed. There is also evidence that sphincter dynamics are altered after cholecystectomy.[2] Animal studies have shown a cholecysto-sphincteric reflex with distention of the gallbladder that results in sphincter relaxation.[3] Interruption of this reflex could affect sphincter behavior by an altered response to cholecystokinin (CCK), or because the loss of innervation unmasks the direct contractile effects of CCK on smooth muscle. Abnormalities in both basal pressure and responsiveness to CCK have also been described in humans.[4]

The simple concept that the pain in these patients is wholly or partly due to increased ductal pressure is now under challenge. Another explanation stems from the concept of nociceptive

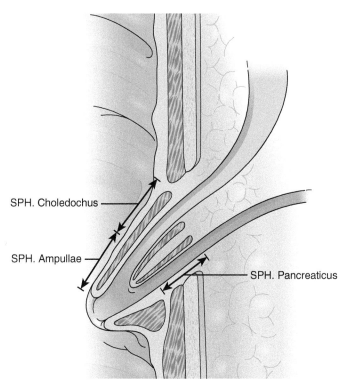

SPH. Choledochus

SPH. Ampullae

SPH. Pancreaticus

FIG 56.1 The sphincter of Oddi. *SPH,* sphincter.

BOX 56.1   **Definition of Biliary Pain in Rome IV**

Pain located in the epigastrium and/or right upper quadrant and *all* the following:
1. Builds up to a steady level and lasts 30 minutes or longer
2. Occurs at different intervals (not daily)
3. Severe enough to interrupt daily activities or lead to an emergency department visit
4. Not significantly (< 20%) related to bowel movements
5. Not significantly (< 20%) relieved by postural change **or** acid suppression

Supportive Criteria

The pain may be associated with the following:
1. Nausea and vomiting
2. Radiation to the back and/or right infra subscapular region
3. Waking from sleep

From Cotton PB, Elta GH, Carter CR, et al: Gallbladder and sphincter of Oddi disorders. *Gastroenterology* 150(6):1420–1429, 2016.

sensitization.[5] Significant tissue inflammation such as cholecystitis will activate nociceptive neurons acutely and, if it persists, also result in sensitization, and the gain in the entire pain pathway is increased. In most patients with gallbladder disease, cholecystectomy removes the ongoing stimulus and the system reverts back to its normal state. However, in a subset of patients, the "gain" stays at a high level. In such patients, even minor increases in biliary pressure within the physiological range can trigger nociceptive activity and the sensation of pain, a concept called *allodynia.*

A relevant related phenomenon is cross-sensitization. Many viscera share sensory innervation, and it is difficult to distinguish pain originating in one organ from that in another. Persistent sensitization in one organ can lead to sensitization of the nociceptive pathway from an adjacent organ. Thus, an entire region can be sensitized with innocous stimuli (such as duodenal contraction after a meal) leading to pain that was indistinguishable from that associated with the initial insult. Evidence for this was provided by an important study in which patients with postcholecystectomy pain were found to have duodenal, but not rectal, hyperalgesia.[6] A strong case can be made for nociceptive sensitization to be the principal cause of pain in these patients. Motor phenomena such as sphincter hypertension may still be relevant, but more as a marker for the syndrome rather than the cause.

There are many reasons why patients may have pains after cholecystectomy. The first task is to exclude organic causes. Possibilities include early postoperative complications (such as a bile leak or duct stricture), retained stones or partial gallbladder, other intraabdominal disorders such as pancreatitis, fatty liver disease, peptic ulceration, functional dyspepsia and irritable bowel syndrome, musculoskeletal disorders, and other rare conditions.

Nonbiliary findings are more likely when the symptoms are atypical and long-standing, similar to those suffered preoperatively and without a period of relief postoperatively, and when the removed gallbladder did not contain stones.[7–9] The concept and management of "functional gallbladder disorder" is equally controversial.[1]

Whether the pain appears to be "biliary" is a crucial clinical question because it focuses the approach to diagnosis and treatment. The Rome process has provided a consensus definition of biliary pain, which is unchanged in the IVth iteration (Box 56.1).[1] It must be said that few, if any, of the stated criteria are sufficiently based on evidence, and more data would be helpful.

Initial Investigation

When the pain appears to be biliary, and is sufficiently troublesome to warrant investigation, initial testing should include liver and pancreatic enzymes (preferably taken shortly after a pain episode) and transabdominal ultrasound, supplemented with computed tomography (CT) scan or magnetic resonance cholangiopancreatography (MRCP). The goal of imaging is to rule out other pancreatic and biliary pathology and to determine the size of the bile duct. Equivocal findings are best evaluated further by endoscopic ultrasound (EUS). Upper endoscopy is usually performed to rule out mucosal diseases, especially if the pains are meal-related.

How to proceed further will depend on the findings of these initial tests. In the past, patients have been classified into 3 categories.
- Type I: dilated bile duct and elevated liver enzymes
- Type II: dilated duct or elevated liver enzymes, but not both
- Type III: no abnormalities

Rome IV concluded that this classification is now outdated and should be abandoned.[1] Patients with both dilated ducts and elevated liver enzymes have an organic problem (sphincter fibrosis or microlithiasis) rather than functional pathology, and they benefit from biliary sphincterotomy.[7,10] Thus the term *sphincter of Oddi (SOD) I* is no longer appropriate; we prefer sphincter of Oddi stenosis. Equally, the term *SOD III* should be abandoned.

TABLE 56.1   Results of the EPISOD Randomized Trial, and the EPISOD 2 Observational Study, in Which Patient's Treatment Was Determined by the Results of Manometry

Study	Sphincter Treatment	N	Pain Relief at 1 Year
EPISOD	None (sham)	73	27 (37%)
	Any sphincterotomy	141	32 (23%)
EPISOD 2	Biliary sphincterotomy	21	5 (24%)
	Dual sphincterotomy	39	12 (31%)
	None	12	2 (17%)

Modified from Cotton PB, Elta GH, Carter CR, et al: Gallbladder and sphincter of Oddi disorders. *Gastroenterology* 150(6):1420–1429, 2016.

The 2014 randomized sham-controlled effect of endoscopic sphincterotomy for suspected sphincter of Oddi dysfunction on pain-related disability following cholecystectomy (EPISOD) trial showed that those patients do not have sphincter dysfunction because the results of sphincterotomy were no better than sham (Table 56.1).[11] The conclusions remained valid in the 99 subjects who were followed for 3 years. Contrary to widespread clinical belief, the EPISOD patients (even those who also had irritable bowel syndrome) had psychosocial profiles no different from population norms.[12] We recognize that these patients are often seriously disabled with pain, but the trial strongly suggests exploring other causes, and less dangerous methods of management.

With SOD types I and III eliminated as functional sphincter disorders we are left only with patients with postcholecystectomy pain and some objective findings (the prior SOD type II, now called *suspected functional biliary sphincter disorder*).

Our main task now is to guide these patients and their advisors through the clinical minefield into optimal management. Additional methodologically rigorous studies are needed to better define the characteristics of patients who may benefit from intervention.

Clinical Predictors of Biliary Sphincter Hypertension

Faced with a symptomatic patient with some evidence for biliary obstruction (a dilated bile duct or elevated liver enzymes) and no other determined cause, the clinician will need to assess the likelihood that the sphincter is the culprit, and that sphincterotomy may be helpful. What are those predictors? Even for bile duct size and liver enzymes, there are devils in the details. To start with, the definition of a *dilated duct* is arbitrary. It is widely believed that the bile duct enlarges normally after cholecystectomy, and radiologists often report "dilation consistent with prior cholecystectomy." However, many careful studies have shown no change, and others only a slight increase. There is a gradual increase with age.[13–16] Regular narcotic use can cause biliary dilation, although usually associated with normal liver enzymes. The main reason why the average size of the duct is bigger after cholecystectomy than the usual norm of 6 to 7 mm is because some of the patients had duct disease at the time of surgery. The original Milwaukee classification of SOD proposed 12 mm as the acceptable upper limit,[17,18] which seems high; the Rome III panel used 8 mm.[7] The EPISOD study used 9 mm.[11] It would

seem likely that a bile duct that is known to have dilated considerably since surgery would be a good sign of obstruction, but that has not been studied. In clinical practice, it is unusual to have access to perioperative imaging to make that assessment in an individual case.

Similar questions arise when considering elevated liver enzymes. Which ones, how high, how often, and when? The standard criteria state that transaminases should be more than twice normal on at least two occasions, and normalize between pain attacks. None of these are firmly evidence-based. Furthermore, as clinicians dealing with many of these patients, we know that these data elements are not always available. Patients are sometimes asked to obtain liver tests shortly after a pain episode, but the evidence that peaking transaminases predict the outcome of sphincterotomy is limited.[19] It is important to remember that elevation of transaminases above the usually accepted normal limits is common in the US population.

There are few data on predictors other than duct size and enzymes. Freeman et al (2007) showed that delayed gastric emptying, daily opioid use, and age less than 40 predicted a poor outcome.[20] They also showed no difference in outcomes between patients classified as SOD types I, II, and III. It has also been reported that patients are more likely to respond if their pain was not continuous, if it was accompanied by nausea and vomiting, and if there had been a pain free interval of at least 1 year after cholecystectomy.[21]

Further research is needed to establish more precisely which clinical features and investigations can best identify those who are likely to respond (or not) to sphincter ablation. Among other possible predictors that have not been investigated fully are: the reason for the cholecystectomy (stones or "gall bladder dyskinesia," another controversial diagnosis), the response to surgery, the presence of other digestive, functional or psychiatric problems, and details about the pain (classical "biliary" or not, its severity and frequency, whether it is the same as before surgery, and whether it subsided for a while). A survey of 164 members of the American Society of Gastrointestinal Endoscopy (ASGE) showed little consensus about predictors other than duct size and enzyme elevations.[22]

Further Investigation for Suspected FBSD

Further investigation is warranted if there are objective pointers to biliary obstruction, if organic disease has been ruled out as far as possible, and if symptoms are severe enough to move on when simple dietary advice and medications (e.g., antispasmodics) have not been helpful.

We recommend more widespread use of EUS in patients with only a dilated duct. It is the best method to detect and exclude relevant organic causes of pain, especially small stones, tumors and pancreatitis.[23]

Several noninvasive techniques have been developed to assess the drainage dynamics of the bile duct. A major problem with assessing their value is the lack of a gold standard. Manometry was previously believed to be an accurate measure of sphincter function, but the gold is increasingly looking tarnished, as discussed later. One could argue that the only proof that the sphincter is (or was) the cause of the pain is if patients are satisfied by the results of sphincter ablation, albeit recognizing the strong placebo effect of ERCP intervention.[11] There are very few studies with such objective assessments and only small randomized trials. Thus, our comments on the value of these various tests are not based on solid evidence.

Hepatobiliary Scintigraphy (HBS)

HBS involves intravenous injection of a radionucleotide, and deriving time-activity curves for its excretion thorough the hepatobiliary system. This technique has been used to assess the rate of bile flow into the duodenum and to look for any evidence for obstruction. Interpretation of the literature is difficult due to the use of different test protocols, diagnostic criteria and categories of patients, and whether the results are compared with manometry (usually) or the outcome of sphincterotomy. Various parameters are used: time to peak activity, slope values, and hepatic clearance at predefined time intervals, the disappearance time from the bile duct, the duodenal appearance time, and the hepatic hilum-duodenum transit time (HHDTT).[24–27] One study in asymptomatic postcholecystectomy subjects showed significant false positive findings and intraobserver variability.[28] The reported specificity of HBS was at least 90% when manometry was used as the reference standard, but the level of sensitivity is more variable.[29] Although HBS with HHDTT was shown to be predictive of the results of sphincterotomy in type I and II patients,[30] it is not widely used currently. The ASGE survey found that very few used HBS regularly.[22] Further studies of dynamic biliary imaging are needed.

Other Noninvasive Tests

Drainage dynamics have also been tested by measuring any dilatation of the duct with standard or endoscopic ultrasound after stimulation with a fatty meal or injection of CCK. The value of these tests was questioned when the results did not correlate with sphincter manometry. These techniques deserve further evaluation, and there is potential for studying dynamic parameters with contrast agents during MRCP[31] and CT scanning.[32]

ERCP

ERCP was widely applied to patients with postcholecystectomy pain in the past. Modern sophisticated imaging (CT, MRCP, and EUS) have eliminated its prior role in the diagnosis of structural problems, but it is still used to measure sphincter pressures. It is essential for practitioners and patients to appreciate that ERCP in this context is associated with a very high risk of pancreatitis. The rate is 10% to 15%, even in expert hands using pancreatic stent placement and/or rectal nonsteroidal antiinflammatory drugs (NSAIDs). Contrary to widespread belief, manometry does not add to the pancreatitis risk of ERCP alone in patients with suspected SOD.[33] ERCP should nowadays be applied only after careful reflection, and with the consent of patients who are fully informed of the potential benefits, risks, limitations and alternatives.

Sphincter Manometry

ERCP allows measurement of both the biliary and pancreatic sphincters. It is commonly performed with a pull-back technique, using a water-perfused catheter system (Video 56.1). The assessable variables at sphincter of Oddi manometry (SOM) include the basal sphincter pressure and the phasic wave amplitude, duration, frequency, and propagation pattern. Based on a few studies in volunteers and data from patients thought not to have sphincter pathology, the normal basal biliary pressure is approximately 17 mm Hg[34] (Fig. 56.2). The acceptable upper limit was defined at 35 to 40 mm Hg, by taking three standard deviations. The same value is accepted for basal pancreatic pressure, with less supporting data. There is considerable overlap between biliary and pancreatic sphincter hypertension.[35,36]

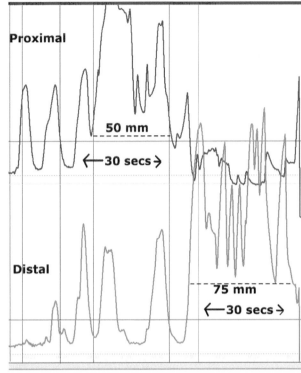

FIG 56.2 Abnormal sphincter of Oddi manometry tracing. Pull-through showing persistent elevation of the basal pressure in both proximal and distal leads above the accepted upper limit of normal (40 mm Hg, shown by the *red line*).

The belief that manometry results have clinical significance is based mainly on three small sham-controlled trials, which all showed that elevated basal biliary pressures predicted the outcome of biliary sphincterotomy in patients with SOD type II.[37–39] As a result, the use of manometry in SOD type II (and type III) patients was recommended by the panel of the National Institutes of Health ERCP state of the science conference in 2002.[10] However, confidence in the value of sphincter manometry has declined in recent years. The relevance of measurements taken when free of pain, and while under anesthetic, must be questioned. Recording periods are short and subject to movement artifact. Data showing poor reproducibility add to the concerns.[40,41] The ASGE survey mentioned earlier showed that most endoscopists now treat type II patients by empiric biliary sphincterotomy without manometry.[22] Sales of manometry catheters by the main supplier have declined progressively in recent years.[22]

Solid-state manometry catheters have also been used, with results identical to those of the water-perfused system.[42] A technique using a sleeve device also showed similar results, with the advantage of reducing movement artifacts, but is not commercially available.[43]

Nonmanometric ERCP Diagnostic Approaches

Trial placement of a biliary stent to predict response to subsequent sphincterotomy has been proposed as an alternative method for diagnosing SOD, but should be avoided due to the documented very high risk of inducing pancreatitis.[44] Injection of Botulinum toxin (BTX) has been shown to relax the sphincter complex temporarily[45] and appears to be safe. Most reporters have applied

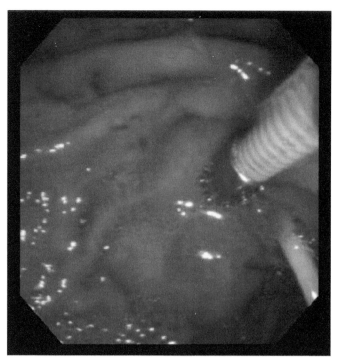

FIG 56.3 Injecting Botox into the sphincter.

25 units in each of four quadrants into or close to the papilla (Fig. 56.3). Temporary relief of pain is claimed to predict which patients would benefit from sphincterotomy.[46,47] The authors' own unpublished experience with this method has been confusing. Many patients appear to respond, but for varying periods (even years in some cases), but temporary benefit has not been a consistent predictor of response to subsequent sphincterotomy. The placebo effect must be strong.

Treatment of FBSD

Current recommendations for management of patients with suspected FBSD are based on expert consensus, with inadequate evidence. Many patients are disabled with pain and desperate for assistance. The placebo effect of intervention is strong, with more than one-third of sham-treated patients claiming long-term benefit in blinded randomized studies.[11,37–39]

Medical Therapy

Because of the risks and uncertainties involved in invasive approaches, it is important to explore conservative management initially. Nifedipine, phosphodiesterase type-5 inhibitors, trimebutine, hyoscine butylbromide, octreotide, and nitric oxide have been shown to reduce basal sphincter pressures in patients with suspected SOD and asymptomatic volunteers.[48,49] H2 antagonists, gabexate mesilate, ulinastatin, and gastro kinetic agents also showed inhibitory effects on sphincter motility. Amitriptyline, as a neuromodulator, has also been used, along with simple analgesics. A small open-label trial of duloxetine had encouraging results. Only 10 of the 18 enrolled patients completed the 3-month trial, mainly due to side effects of the drug, but 9 of the 10 had a successful outcome.[50] A French group was able to avoid sphincterotomy in 77% of patients with suspected SOD using treatment with trimebutine and nitrates.[51] None of these drugs are specific to the sphincter and therefore may also have positive effects in patients with nonbiliary dysfunctional syndromes. Transcutaneous electrical nerve stimulation[52] and acupuncture[53] also have been shown to reduce SOD pressures, but their long-term efficacy has not been evaluated.

Endoscopic Sphincterotomy

Consensus opinion remains that a patient with definite evidence for biliary obstruction (former biliary SOD type I) should be treated with endoscopic sphincterotomy, without manometry.[1,7] Reported results are good[54–56]; some patients probably had small stones undetected by prior testing methods. The evidence base for biliary sphincterotomy in patients with FBSD (prior SOD type II) is not strong; most studies have been retrospective, unblinded, and have not used objective assessments. Readers interested the details of the many published cohort studies are referred to comprehensive reviews by Petersen[57] and by Squoros and Periera,[58] and to the SOD chapter in the 2nd edition of this book. One large study claimed success in approximately three-quarters of patients simply because the others did not return to the treatment site for further intervention.[59] The best data come from three small randomized studies of suspected type II patients which showed that biliary sphincterotomy was more effective than a sham procedure in patients with elevated basal biliary sphincter pressures.[37–39] Although convincing, these studies were small, and performed before modern imaging; some patients may have had small stones or microlithiasis. The authors did not study pancreatic pressures or their treatment. One important issue, often overlooked, is that those early studies used the original definition for bile duct dilation (i.e., > 12 mm), a very unusual finding nowadays. The Rome III panel changed that to greater than 8 mm to "make it more applicable to clinical practice and, whenever possible, to avoid the invasive ERCP procedure."[7] It has had the opposite result as it brings in to play many other patients with minimally dilated ducts.

No study has claimed a high percentage of success, which emphasizes the need to understand the predictors, to be able to focus invasive treatment where it is most needed.

In addition to the 10% to 15% risk of postprocedure pancreatitis, sphincterotomy can cause bleeding and retro-duodenal perforation. Both occur in approximately 1% of cases, and can have devastating consequences. Late stenosis of the pancreatic orifice can occur after biliary and pancreatic sphincterotomies, and is difficult to manage.

Other ERCP Treatments

As mentioned previously, attempts to test or treat SOD by balloon dilation or by temporary stent placement are not recommended because of the very high risk of producing pancreatitis. Injection of BTX into the sphincter is another treatment option. It can be applied without doing an ERCP (relying on prior imaging to rule out any pathology) apparently without risk of pancreatitis.[47] Concern has been raised about possible scarring, especially with repeat injections. Stringent prospective studies are needed before this technique can be recommended.

Surgical Therapy

Surgical sphincteroplasty is more complete than endoscopic sphincterotomy and can be performed primarily, or following failed endoscopic therapy. Case series and one small, randomized study (published in abstract) suggest good outcomes in most patients[60–63] but less-invasive endoscopic intervention is currently preferred.

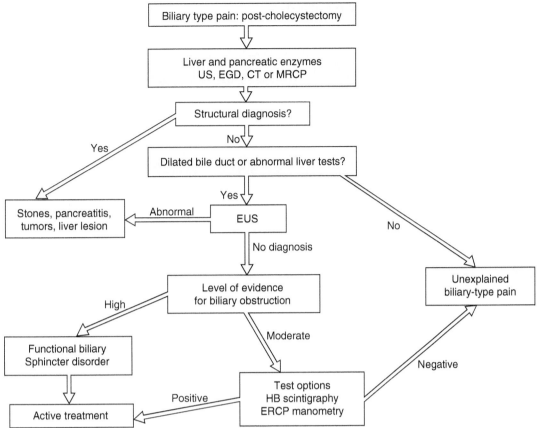

FIG 56.4 Management algorithm for patients with postcholecystectomy biliary pain. *CT,* computerized tomography; *EGD,* upper endoscopy; *ERCP,* endoscopic retrograde cholangiopancreatography; *EUS,* endoscopic ultrasound; *HB,* hepatobiliary; *MRCP,* magnetic resonance cholangiopancreatography; *US,* ultrasound.

FBSD in Patients With an Intact Gallbladder

Very few studies have addressed the role of sphincter dysfunction in patients with biliary-type pain in the presence of the gallbladder. One old small retrospective case series showed a lower chance of clinical response to biliary sphincterotomy in patients with an intact gallbladder than in those with prior cholecystectomy,[64] whereas a more recent one (2011) claimed more than 89% response in both groups.[65] Another earlier study performed biliary sphincterotomy on 35 patients with intact gallbladders and elevated biliary sphincter pressures.[66] Only half of them claimed improvement after a mean of 1 year. Eleven went on to cholecystectomy, and 8 improved. At this time, the data are not sufficient to recommend ERCP, manometry, or sphincterotomy in patients with intact (stone free) gallbladders. Some experts do perform sphincterotomy in this context if a patient has impressive intermittent pains with fluctuating liver enzymes, but only after complete review and discussion of the options and possible outcomes. More information is needed on how to manage these patients.

Summary of Functional Biliary Sphincter Disorder

Postcholecystectomy pain is a common complaint, the cause of which often remains obscure after careful enquiry and standard investigations. This is a clinical minefield, which patients and physicians should enter only with extreme caution, especially when considering the use of ERCP and sphincterotomy, with or without sphincter manometry. The EPISOD trial showed the strength of the placebo effect of intervention, which bedevils the assessment of all types of treatment.

We recommend the approach constructed in 2016 by the Rome IV consensus as shown in Fig. 56.4. Further stringent trials are needed to better inform clinical practice.

FUNCTIONAL PANCREATIC SPHINCTER DISORDER (FPSD)

Sphincter dysfunction has been proposed as a cause of pancreatitis, and indeed also pancreatic pain without pancreatitis. Proof is lacking, and the clinical approach is currently speculative. As recommended by Rome IV, this concept is now named FPSD.

Idiopathic Acute Recurrent Pancreatitis (IRAP)

The general approach to patients with unexplained recurrent acute pancreatitis is discussed in Chapter 57. Clearly it is essential to exclude all the known possible causes by comprehensive investigations, including genetic testing, before focusing on the possible role of FPSD. Obstruction at the level of the sphincter is a well-known cause of pancreatitis in animal experiments and in several clinical situations; for example, tumors of the papilla and intermittent obstruction of the sphincter due to passage of stones, or mucus plugs in intraductal papillary mucinous neoplasm. It is therefore reasonable to postulate that an overactive sphincter muscle could cause pancreatitis. Opiates can increase sphincter pressure and have been implicated in attacks of pancreatitis.[67] However, the evidence that sphincter hypertension is a common cause of pancreatitis is not strong.[68-70] Proof would require the demonstration of abnormal sphincter activity relative to controls, along with resolution of the attacks after sphincter ablation. Whether sphincter ablation is curative (or at least helpful) is obviously the key question. The limited data are given in the following sections.

Assessing Sphincter Dysfunction in IRAP

Measuring the size of the pancreatic duct by MRCP (or EUS) before and after an intravenous injection of secretin is an attractive method for detecting functional obstruction at the sphincter. One report suggested that the results do not correlate with those produced by sphincter manometry, but that they may predict the outcome of sphincterotomy.[71] This test deserves further assessment.

Manometry of both pancreatic and biliary sphincters at ERCP has been used widely in this context. Elevated pancreatic (and biliary) sphincter pressures have been found 25% to 78% of patients with IRAP.[72,73] One 2012 study also showed a 3.5-fold greater likelihood of recurrent attacks (without treatment) in patients with elevated pressures, compared to those with normal pressures.[73] The downside of ERCP in this context is the risk (at least 15%) of inducing pancreatitis.

Injection of BTX into the sphincter as a test of the effects of temporary sphincter ablation, as described previously in the biliary section, has been applied to patients with IRAP.[74] Temporary pancreatic stenting has also been used as a test of sphincter dysfunction, but concerns about stent-induced duct damage have eliminated this practice.

Treating FPSD in IRAP

Assessment of treatments in this context is difficult because any recurrences may be long delayed. Patients should be counseled to avoid factors (e.g., alcohol, tobacco, opiates) that may precipitate attacks. Certain medications, such as antispasmodics and calcium channel blockers, are known to relax the sphincter, but there have been no trials of their value in this context.

Whether to offer sphincterotomy to patients with IRAP is currently a difficult decision because the evidence base is thin and there are significant short- and long-term risks. It will be influenced by the frequency and severity of the attacks, the completeness of prior investigations, and by the patient's wishes when fully informed about the available data. The status of the gall bladder is also relevant. Empiric cholecystectomy is often advocated when gallbladder disease is still suspected despite negative investigations (e.g., in a nondrinking woman with elevated liver tests in attacks), and is probably safer than sphincterotomy.

Pancreatic sphincter ablation was initially performed by an open trans-duodenal approach. Small case series reported resolution of episodic pancreatitis in the majority of patients.[75] Endoscopic therapy quickly replaced surgical sphincteroplasty, with the assumption that the results would be equivalent.[76-78] Early small-cohort studies with short follow-up periods suggested a benefit when recurrence was reported in less than one-third of patients after pancreatic sphincterotomy.[72,76-78] Wehrmann (2011) reported a 51% recurrence rate after a 10-year follow-up

of 37 patients[79] and the recent trial by Coté et al (2012) reported a similar proportion after a mean of 6 years.[73]

Whether these reports indicate that sphincterotomy is beneficial is difficult to interpret in the absence of any untreated controls. A retrospective study suggested that patients who underwent dual endoscopic sphincterotomy had less recurrence than those who had either biliary or pancreatic sphincterotomy alone.[79] However, the Coté trial failed to show the superiority of dual sphincterotomy over biliary sphincterotomy alone.[73]

A confounding issue is the difficulty in performing a complete (and permanent) pancreatic sphincter ablation endoscopically. Repeat examinations in the Coté and EPISOD studies showed persistent hypertension or re-stenosis in many cases.[41,73] The actual incidence is uncertain as asymptomatic subjects were not studied.

Some experts perform ERCP with empiric biliary sphincterotomy initially without manometry in patients with IRAP, but the benefit is unproven.

Conclusion

In the absence of hard data, it is currently possible to argue that sphincter ablation does not alter the natural history of IRAP and that the finding of apparent sphincter abnormality is an epiphenomenon, the result of previous attacks, or due to a different, unexplained cause.

Additional randomized trials are required to determine whether any sphincter treatment is effective and, if so, to establish the preferred approach (biliary, pancreatic, or dual sphincterotomy), and indeed whether it can be achieved adequately and safely endoscopically when compared with surgery.

At the present time, clinicians and their patients will need to make individual treatment decisions in the full knowledge of the gaps in our knowledge.

SOD as a Cause of Pancreatic Pain Without Pancreatitis?

In the past, it was proposed that SOD can cause pancreatic pain without enzyme elevation or other evidence for pancreatitis, and a categorization of pancreatic SOD types similar to that used previously in suspected biliary SOD has been suggested.[72] However, there is currently no strong evidence that SOD can cause pancreatic pain in the absence of pancreatitis. Given the risks of ERCP with manometry and the short- and long-term risks of pancreatic sphincterotomy, evaluation of possible pancreatic SOD should be restricted to patients with IRAP.

SOD and Chronic Pancreatitis?

SOD as determined by manometry has been described in 50% to 87% of patients with chronic pancreatitis of many etiologies.[80] This high frequency in patients with a known etiology suggests that SOD is the result of chronic inflammation rather than its cause. Endoscopic pancreatic sphincterotomy was reported to improve pain scores in short-term uncontrolled studies in 60% to 65% of chronic pancreatitis patients with pancreatic SOD.[81,82] Whether ERCP with SOM should be offered to chronic pancreatitis patients with unexplained recurrent episodes of acute inflammation remains to be determined.

Summary of FPSD

At this time, there is no role for ERCP with manometry in patients with suspected pancreatic pain without evidence for pancreatitis, unless they are enrolled in a clinical trial.

Patients with a single episode of unexplained acute pancreatitis should not subject themselves to the risks of ERCP and manometry, because a second episode may never occur or be long delayed.

Patients with recurrent acute pancreatitis that remains unexplained after exhaustive investigation and appropriate medical treatments can be considered for a therapeutic intervention. Empiric cholecystectomy should be offered in some cases. It is reasonable to discuss ERCP with manometry, with a view to sphincterotomy if the pressures are elevated, while acknowledging the lack of supporting evidence. Biliary sphincterotomy alone appears as effective as dual sphincterotomy and likely lowers the procedural risk. There is currently no clear role for ERCP, manometry, or pancreatic sphincterotomy to treat postulated SOD in patients with chronic pancreatitis.

MANAGING FAILURES OF ENDOSCOPIC TREATMENT FOR FBSD AND FPSD

Managing patients with recurrent problems after endoscopic treatment for these controversial conditions is a common and challenging problem in tertiary centers. ERCP is usually applied to look for and treat any persisting functional sphincter hypertension. Stenosis of the biliary orifice is unusual after biliary sphincterotomy, but can be managed with balloon dilation and temporary stenting. The pancreatic orifice is more often the focus of concern. Biliary sphincterotomy alone can cause functional stenosis of the pancreatic orifice.[83] Five of fifteen individuals with initially normal pancreatic pressures became abnormal after only biliary sphincterotomy in the EPISOD trial.[41] Pancreatic sphincterotomies are rarely complete in the context of SOD, when the duct is not dilated, and scarring is probably common. A 2012 review of pancreatic sphincterotomy for IRAP revealed that 48% of the patients had a re-intervention.[73] Three of the nine pancreatic sphincterotomies were found to be incomplete in patients undergoing repeat procedures in the EPISOD trial.[41] Some endoscopists rely on repeat manometry to detect problems at the pancreatic orifice; most will go directly to balloon dilation and temporary stenting. The results of these maneuvers are unpredictable. It is a slippery slope; some patients eventually proceed to surgical sphincteroplasty,[63] and even pancreatic resections, with uncertain results.

Managing patients who return sometime after apparently gaining substantial benefit from earlier endoscopic treatment for SOD III is especially challenging, in view of the EPISOD data showing that the results are no better than sham. They are understandably reluctant to accept a nihilistic approach, and are often dismissive of medical management with neuromodulators. Most will demand and receive another ERCP, if only to check for restenosis.

CONCLUSION

It is clear that clinical confidence in the role of SOD, and sphincterotomy, in patients with postcholecystectomy pain and with unexplained recurrent pancreatitis has declined in recent years. The evidence is weak and there is increasing appreciation of other possible causes. The fact that ERCP carries significant hazards in the short- and long-term adds weight to our plea for clinicians to broaden their perspectives in dealing with these challenging patients, and for researchers to strengthen the evidence base to better inform our practice.

ACKNOWLEDGEMENTS

We are indebted to Rome co-authors Elta, Carter, Pasricha and Corazziaro for their input, and also to Sherman, Fogel, Watkins, McHenry and Lehman, for their comprehensive review and erudite discussion of this topic in the 2nd edition of this book, and for their permission to use some of their illustrations.

KEY REFERENCES

1. Cotton PB, Elta GH, Carter CR, et al: Gallbladder and sphinter of Oddi disorders, *Gastroenterology* 150(6):1420–1429, 2016.
6. Desautels SG, Slivka A, Hutson WR, et al: Postcholecystectomy pain syndrome: pathophysiology of abdominal pain in sphincter of Oddi type III, *Gastroenterology* 116(4):900–905, 1999.
7. Behar J, Corazziari E, Guelrud M, et al: Functional gallbladder and sphincter of oddi disorders, *Gastroenterology* 130(5):1498–1509, 2006.
8. Berger MY, Olde Hartman TC, Bohnen AM: Abdominal symptoms: do they disappear after cholecystectomy?, *Surg Endosc* 17(11):1723–1728, 2003.
10. Cohen S, Bacon BR, Berlin JA, et al: National Institutes of Health State-of-the-Science Conference Statement: ERCP for diagnosis and therapy, January 14–16, 2002, *Gastrointest Endosc* 56(6):803–809, 2002.
11. Cotton PB, Durkalski V, Romagnuolo J, et al: Effect of endoscopic sphincterotomy for suspected sphincter of Oddi dysfunction on pain-related disability following cholecystectomy: the EPISOD randomized clinical trial, *JAMA* 311(20):2101–2109, 2014.
12. Brawman-Mintzer O, Durkalski V, Wu Q, et al: Psychosocial characteristics and pain burden of patients with suspected sphincter of Oddi dysfunction in the EPISOD multicenter trial, *Am J Gastroenterol* 109(3):436–442, 2014.
13. Majeed AW, Ross B, Johnson AG: The preoperatively normal bile duct does not dilate after cholecystectomy: results of a five year study, *Gut* 45(5):741–743, 1999.
17. Sherman S, Lehman GA: Sphincter of Oddi dysfunction: diagnosis and treatment, *JOP* 2(6):382–400, 2001.
20. Freeman ML, Gill M, Overby C, Cen YY: Predictors of outcomes after biliary and pancreatic sphincterotomy for sphincter of oddi dysfunction, *J Clin Gastroenterol* 41(1):94–102, 2007.
21. Topazian M, Hong-Curtis J, Li J, Wells C: Improved predictors of outcome in post-cholecystectomy pain, *J Clin Gastroenterol* 38(8):692–696, 2004.
22. Suarez AL, Cotton PB, Pauls Q, et al: Sphincter of Oddi dysfunction: a survey of current practice in USA, *Gastrointest Endosc* 83(5):AB 251, 2016.
29. Corazziari E, Cicala M, Scopinaro F, et al: Scintigraphic assessment of SO dysfunction, *Gut* 52(11):1655–1656, 2003.
37. Toouli J, Roberts-Thomson IC, Kellow J, et al: Manometry based randomised trial of endoscopic sphincterotomy for sphincter of Oddi dysfunction, *Gut* 46(1):98–102, 2000.
38. Geenen JE, Hogan WJ, Dodds WJ, et al: The efficacy of endoscopic sphincterotomy after cholecystectomy in patients with sphincter-of-Oddi dysfunction, *N Engl J Med* 320(2):82–87, 1989.
39. Sherman S, Lehman G, Jamidar P, et al: Efficacy of endoscopic sphincterotomy and surgical sphincteroplasty for patients with sphincter of Oddi dysfunction (SOD); randomized, controlled study, *Gastrointest Endosc* 40:A125, 1994.
41. Suarez AL, Pauls Q, Durkalski-Mauldin V, Cotton PB: Sphincter of Oddi manometry: reproducibility and effect of sphincterotomy in the EPISOD study, *J Neurogastroenterol Motil* 22(3):477–482, 2016.
47. Murray W, Kong S: Botulinum toxin may predict the outcome of endoscopic sphincterotomy in episodic functional post-cholecystectomy biliary pain, *Scand J Gastroenterol* 45(5):623–627, 2010.
57. Petersen BT: An evidence-based review of sphincter of Oddi dysfunction: part I, presentations with "objective" biliary findings (types I and II), *Gastrointest Endosc* 59(4):525–534, 2004.

58. Squoros SN, Pereira SP: Systematic review: sphincter of Oddi dysfunction; non-invasive daignostic methods and long-term outcome after endoscopic sphincterotomy, *Aliment Pharmacol Ther* 24(2):237–246, 2006.

66. Choudhry U, Ruffolo T, Jamidar P, et al: Sphincter of Oddi dysfunction in patients with intact gallbladder: therapeutic response to endoscopic sphincterotomy, *Gastrointest Endosc* 39(4):492–495, 1993.

68. Wilcox CM, Varadarajulu S, Eloubeidi M: Role of endoscopic evaluation in idiopathic pancreatitis: a systematic review, *Gastrointest Endosc* 63: 1037–1045, 2006.

70. Wilcox CM: Endoscopic therapy for sphincter of Oddi dysfunction in idiopathic pancreatitis: from empiric to scientific, *Gastroenterology* 143:1423–1426, 2012.

72. Petersen BT: Sphincter of Oddi dysfunction, part 2: evidence-based review of the presentations, with "objective" pancreatic findings (types I and II) and of presumptive type III, *Gastrointest Endosc* 59:670–687, 2004.

73. Cote GA, Imperiale TF, Schmidt SE, et al: Similar efficacies of biliary, with or without pancreatic, sphincterotomy in treatment of idiopathic recurrent acute pancreatitis, *Gastroenterology* 143:1502–1509.e1, 2012.

79. Wehrmann T: Long-term results (>/= 10 years) of endoscopic therapy for sphincter of Oddi dysfunction in patients with acute recurrent pancreatitis, *Endoscopy* 43:202–207, 2011.

A complete reference list can be found online at ExpertConsult .com

57

Recurrent Acute Pancreatitis

Tyler Stevens and Martin L. Freeman

CHAPTER OUTLINE

INTRODUCTION

Acute pancreatitis (AP) has an excellent prognosis if the severity is limited, and if the underlying cause can be identified and treated. However, AP may recur if the underlying causes are not eliminated or modified. Patients with recurrent AP (RAP) endure frequent emergency room (ER) visits and hospitalizations, costly testing, potentially risky interventions, and may eventually develop chronic pancreatitis (CP) and related functional impairment. Thus, RAP has a detrimental impact on quality of life and places a tremendous cost burden on health care systems. The central clinical objective is to evaluate and treat the causes of RAP to interrupt the disease process. In this chapter, the evaluation and treatment of RAP are reviewed, with an emphasis on the appropriate role of endoscopy.

DEFINITIONS

The diagnosis of AP can be established based on two of the following: (1) typical pancreatic pain, (2) elevation in serum lipase and/or amylase levels to greater than 3 times the upper limit of normal, and (3) confirmatory imaging findings.[1] The term *RAP* is found in the literature dating back seven decades.[2] RAP is defined as "two or more episodes of AP." Reasonable stipulations have been imposed on this basic definition, including full resolution of symptoms between attacks,[3] the absence of imaging changes indicating CP, and a period of at least 3 months between the initial and recurrent episode(s).[4] The latter criterion is used to distinguish true recurrence from a complication from the initial attack or an exacerbation related to dietary advancement. The term *idiopathic RAP* (IRAP) is used when the cause is not immediately recognized based on history, physical examination, basic laboratory testing (e.g., serum triglyceride and calcium), and imaging tests (transabdominal ultrasound [TAUS] and/or computed tomography [CT] scan).[5] Patients with IRAP are at risk for further attacks and progression to CP. In efforts to find obscure causes and cure the disease, they may undergo second-line imaging tests, endoscopic retrograde cholangiopancreatography (ERCP), and genetic testing. Even after these advanced tests have been performed and thousands of dollars have been spent, the cause may remain unexplained or unmodifiable, and attacks or persistent intractable pain may persist with or without morphologic evidence of CP. The term *true idiopathic recurrent acute pancreatitis* (TIRAP) has been coined for such unfortunate patients.[6] An axiom of RAP and CP is that the symptom burden, especially chronic pain, correlates poorly with morphologic changes.[7,8] Some patients with frequent attacks or intractable pain between attacks even undergo total pancreatectomy with autologous islet cell transplantation as a last resort, despite the absence of morphologic or functional evidence of CP.[9]

EPIDEMIOLOGY

The incidence of AP ranges from 13 to 45/100,000.[10] In 2012, AP accounted for 330,561 ER visits and 275,170 hospitalizations, with a related aggregate cost of $2.6 billion.[11] Multiple observational studies have included consecutive patients followed after an index bout of AP to ascertain the rates of RAP and progression to CP. A 2015 meta-analysis showed a pooled recurrence rate of 22% (95% confidence interval [CI] 18%–26%) in 11 studies.[12] The pooled rate of progression from RAP to CP was 36% (CI 20%–53%) in five studies. The prevalence rates of RAP and CP were higher in alcohol-related compared to biliary pancreatitis.

The results for other etiologies and idiopathic pancreatitis are not always reported. However, some studies have shown higher recurrence and progression rates in those with idiopathic compared to biliary etiology.[13,14]

CAUSES

The causes of RAP and CP overlap, and have been categorized as toxic and metabolic, genetic, autoimmune, and obstructive (Table 57.1).[15] Several etiologies particularly relevant to endoscopists are discussed in the following sections.

Biliary Microlithiasis

Biliary microlithiasis is a common cause of IRAP in patients who have an intact gallbladder, particularly those with risk factors such as pregnancy, rapid weight loss, critical illness, prolonged fasting, ceftriaxone use, octreotide use, bone marrow or organ transplant, and prolonged fasting.[16] Microlithiasis refers to small gallstones (e.g., < 3 mm)[17] that are not easily visible on TAUS but may easily traverse the cystic duct and impact at the ampulla of Vater. Recurrent passage of small stones may produce an inflammation and fibrosis cycle resulting in ampullary stenosis, which increases susceptibility to obstructive AP episodes. Though microlithiasis is "invisible" on TAUS, it may coincide with the presence of biliary

sludge, which is more easily seen on TAUS, repeat TAUS,[18] and endoscopic ultrasound (EUS). Biliary sludge is a mixture of particulate matter, mucous, and bile, and is visible as nonshadowing echogenic material that forms layers in the dependent portion of the gallbladder.[16] Sludge visible on EUS may not always contain stones, but may be a reasonable biomarker to guide treatment. Two studies showed high rates of sludge or biliary crystals (67%–74%) in patients with IRAP and intact gallbladders.[18,19] In general, we consider both findings of microlithiasis or sludge visible on TAUS/EUS or the presence of crystals in the bile to indicate biliary pancreatitis, caused by passage of particulate material that causes transient ampullary obstruction.

The diagnostic workup for microlithiasis and the threshold for an empiric cholecystectomy have been sources of some controversy. EUS may be more sensitive for detecting sludge and microlithiasis than TAUS, CT, and magnetic resonance cholangiopancreatography (MRCP)[20,21] (Fig. 57.1). Some use cholecystokinin stimulation with endoscopic collection of expressed bile and polarized microscopy to check for crystals.[22] This method is performed infrequently because of questionable specificity and reproducibility.

Cholecystectomy is the definitive and currently preferred treatment for suspected microlithiasis. A practical approach advocated by many experts is to proceed to empiric cholecystectomy in those

TABLE 57.1	**TIGAR-O* Classification of Causes of Pancreatitis**	
Etiology		**Clinical Clues/Risk Factors**
Toxic	Alcohol	Heavy regular or binge alcohol consumption
	Cigarette smoking	
	Cannabis	
Metabolic	Hypertriglyceridemia	Familial lipid disorders, poorly controlled diabetes, obesity, excess estrogen, hypothyroidism, alcohol abuse
	Hypercalcemia	Hyperparathyroidism
Obstructive	Cholelithiasis/choledocholithiasis	Rapid weight loss/gain, pregnancy, obesity, preceding biliary colic
	Microlithiasis	Elevated liver function tests during episode
	Sphincter of Oddi dysfunction	Postcholecystectomy, use of opiates
	IPMN	Most common with main duct involvement
	Pancreatic cancer	New onset of RAP, age > 40 years, weight loss
	Chronic pancreatitis	Presence of ductal stones/strictures
	Upper GI Crohn's disease	History of Crohn's disease
	Pancreas divisum	Dorsal duct dilation or Santorinicele on imaging
	Duodenal duplication cyst	
	Juxtapapillary diverticulum	
Genetic	*CFTR*	Recurrent sinusitis/bronchitis, male infertility
	SPINK-1	
	PRSS1	Multiple family members in consecutive generations with pancreatitis and/or pancreatic cancer
Infectious	Ascariasis	
	Viral (mumps, coxsackie A)	
Autoimmune/Vascular	Type 1 AIP (IgG4-related sclerosing disease)	Typical imaging findings (pancreatic enlargement, capsular enhancement, ductal strictures)
		Other organ involvement (salivary glands, retroperitoneal fibrosis, renal cortical lesions, etc.)
		Elevated IgG4
	Type 2 AIP	History of IBD
	Lupus-associated pancreatitis	
Medications	Azathioprine, furosemide, valproic acid	Short latency from onset of medication to onset of attack, literature supportive of relationship, positive rechallenge

***T**oxic and Metabolic, **I**diopathic, **G**enetic, **A**utoimmune, **R**ecurrent and Severe Acute Pancreatitis Associated Chronic Pancreatitis, **O**bstructive.
AIP, autoimmune pancreatitis; *GI,* gastrointestinal; *IBD,* inflammatory bowel disease; *IPMN,* intraductal papillary mucinous neoplasm; *RAP,* recurrent acute pancreatitis.

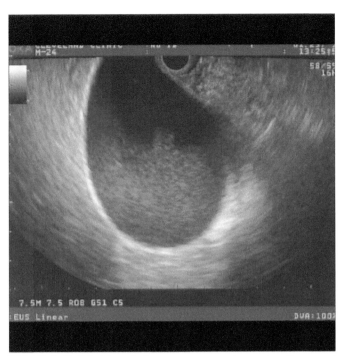

FIG 57.1 Gallbladder sludge seen on endoscopic ultrasound (EUS) in a 25-year-old woman with recurrent acute pancreatitis (RAP). She had slight alanine transaminase (ALT) elevations during the most recent bout. Transabdominal ultrasound (TAUS) was read as negative for stones. The attacks ceased after cholecystectomy was performed.

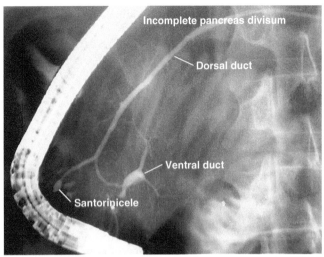

FIG 57.2 Endoscopic retrograde cholangiopancreatography (ERCP) performed on a patient with recurrent acute pancreatitis (RAP) shows incomplete pancreas divisum. The ventral duct and dorsal duct are connected by a small branch duct. At the most distal portion of the dorsal duct, a cystic outpunching (called a Santorinicele) is also seen. This patient responded to endoscopic minor papillotomy. (Image courtesy of Adam Slivka and Michael K. Sanders.)

with TIRAP and intact gallbladder. Some have even advocated this intervention after a first attack.[23] A 2015 interventional trial randomized patients experiencing their first attack of idiopathic AP to empiric cholecystectomy versus watchful waiting.[24] Baseline TAUS was negative for stones in all patients. The cholecystectomy group had significantly lower rates of recurrence compared to the observation group (8/39 vs. 23/46, $p = 0.016$) after a mean of 36 months of follow-up. The number-needed-to-treat with cholecystectomy to prevent one patient from having a recurrence was five. The use of empiric cholecystectomy in IRAP should be considered carefully based on the patient's clinical presentation and risk factors. For example, in a young, thin patient with IRAP who has normal liver function tests and whose gallbladder appears normal on ultrasonography, it would be prudent to first obtain genetic testing for pancreatitis-causing mutations. The finding of a significant high penetrance mutation (e.g., in *PRSS1*) may obviate cholecystectomy.

Endoscopic biliary sphincterotomy (EBS) is an effective alternative for selected patients. The rationale for performing EBS is that it separates the biliary and pancreatic orifices, allowing crystals and stones to pass into the duodenum with less chance of causing pancreatic duct obstruction or biliary reflux. In observational studies, EBS has been shown to decrease the rate of recurrence of biliary pancreatitis in patients with intact gallbladders to 2% to 6%.[25-27] EBS can be considered for very elderly patients, those with comorbidities increasing operative risk, those refusing cholecystectomy, or as a temporizing strategy if cholecystectomy is delayed. The use of EBS has waned since the advent of laparoscopic cholecystectomy, which may be safer than ERCP in this cohort of patients.

Pancreas Divisum

Pancreas divisum (PD) is a relatively common embryological anatomic variant that has been postulated to impair drainage of the pancreatic duct, contributing to obstructive pancreatitis. The pancreas begins as dorsal and ventral buds, each with separate ductal drainage into the foregut. Within the first trimester, the ventral bud rotates axially and fuses with the dorsal part. In most cases, the dorsal and ventral ducts likewise fuse, allowing redundant drainage of the entire pancreas through both minor and major papillae. In cases of PD, the ductal systems do not fuse, leading to separate drainage of the dorsal and ventral ducts, or only partially fuse (incomplete divisum), resulting in the presence of a thread-like connection between the systems (Fig. 57.2). Because the minor papilla is a smaller opening, patients with PD may suffer RAP affecting the dorsal pancreas (superior head, body, and tail of pancreas). Patients with PD are protected from biliary pancreatitis due to lack of continuity between the biliary and pancreatic ducts. As such, the diagnosis of PD may obviate empiric cholecystectomy in patients with IRAP. A rare exception is focal ventral gallstone pancreatitis, which may still occur in PD patients.[28]

The traditional gold standard for diagnosing PD has been ERCP. Cannulation and injection of the ventral pancreatic duct via the major papilla reveals a short, arborized ventral duct (Fig. 57.3). It is important to recognize that the finding of a short ventral duct may also indicate a benign or malignant pancreatic duct stricture.[29] Observance of ventral duct arborization may prompt subsequent endoscopic cannulation and injection of the minor papilla to define the dorsal duct anatomy and allow endoscopic therapy. ERCP is now rarely needed for diagnosis of PD since the advent of MRCP, secretin-enhanced MRCP, and EUS.[30] In most cases, endoscopists have a diagnostic MRCP available and undertake ERCP with therapeutic intent.

The decision to intervene in cases of PD must be considered carefully. PD is common, and its presence does not always indicate that it is a cause of or cofactor in IRAP. A comprehensive analysis of autopsy, ERCP, and MRCP studies suggest that the prevalence of PD in the general Western population is 8%.[31] PD is less common in African Americans (1%–2%)[32] and Asians (1.5%).[33] Whether this common anomaly is a true cause of IRAP continues to be debated. Favoring causation are ERCP studies that show increased rates of PD among those with IRAP and CP compared to controls.[34] However, a 2011 review highlights several biases that may explain these differences.[35]

Multiple retrospective and prospective studies have suggested that endoscopic therapy consisting of minor papillotomy or transpapillary dilation decreases the frequency of RAP or improves pain (Table 57.2).[36–49] However, many of these studies are limited by significant patient heterogeneity, small sample size, limited duration of follow-up, and lack of comparison groups. Recent studies have also found that genetic mutations may confound the relationship of PD and pancreatitis. In a case-control study, patients with idiopathic pancreatitis had the same prevalence of PD as controls (7%), whereas the prevalence of PD was significantly higher in IRAP/CP patients with serine protease inhibitor Kazal type-1 (*SPINK-1*) (16%) and cystic fibrosis transmembrane conductance regulator (*CFTR*) mutations (47%). The authors concluded there was an association of PD with these genetic defects in patients with IRAP and CP,[50] and that PD was acting as a "partner" in the genesis of pancreatitis. This latter argument (that PD is a cofactor) has been questioned by some who believe that PD does not cause pancreatitis.[51] They have argued that PD may be an "innocent bystander" in what is really a genetic problem. In light of these controversies, deciding which patients are most likely to benefit from endoscopic treatment is a frequent clinical conundrum. Signs of impaired dorsal duct drainage (e.g., dorsal duct dilation, the presence of a Santorinicele, which is a saccular dilation of the terminal duodenal portion of the dorsal pancreatic duct [Fig. 57.4], focal inflammation or fibrosis of the dorsal pancreas, and decreased duodenal filling after secretin), may favor causation.

Endoscopic therapy for PD involves minor papillotomy to enhance dorsal duct drainage (Fig. 57.5). After minor papillotomy, a temporary pancreatic stent is usually placed to maintain patency

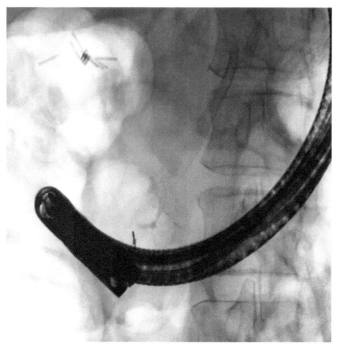

FIG 57.3 This 33-year-old female had presumed gallstone pancreatitis, but continued to have recurrent acute pancreatitis (RAP) following cholecystectomy. Endoscopic retrograde cholangiopancreatography (ERCP) with contrast injection of the ventral duct via the major papilla showed an arborized appearance, consistent with pancreas divisum.

TABLE 57.2 **Results of Endoscopic Therapy in Patients With Pancreas Divisum**

Author (Year)	Study Design	No.	Mean Follow-Up (mo)	Intervention	NP	ARP	CP	CAP	Restenosis	Chronic Duct Changes
Russell et al. (1984)[36]	Retro	5	8	MES	1/5	2/2	4/4		NP	
Soehendra et al. (1986)[40]	Retro	6	3	MES		5/8			NP	
Liquory et al. (1986)[39]	Retro	8	24	MES					3/8	
McCarthy et al. (1988)[38]	Retro	19	6–36	Stent	17/19					2/19
Prabhu et al. (1989)[37]	Retro	18	12–60	Stent		15/18				NS
Siegel et al. (1990)[42]	Retro	31	24	Stent	26/31					NS
Lans et al. (1992)[41]	RCT	10 (9 controls)	29	Stent		9/10				0/10
Sherman et al (1994)[43]	RCT	16 (17 controls)	25	MES				7/16	NP	
Lehman et al. (1993)[44]	Retro	52	20	MES		13/17	3/11	6/24	10/18	
Coleman et al. (1994)[48]	Retro	34	23	Stent		7/9	12/20	2/5	NP	NS
Kozarek et al. (1995)[45]	Retro	39	26	MES and/or stent		11/15	6/19	1/5	3/26	10/39
Boerma et al. (2000)[46]	Prosp	16	51	Stent		5/16				NS
Ertan (2000)[47]	Prosp	25	24	Stent		19/25				21/25
Heyries et al. (2002)[49]	Prosp	24	39	MES or Stent		22/24	NS			16/16

ARP, acute recurrent pancreatitis; *CAP*, chronic abdominal pain; *CP*, chronic pancreatitis; *mo*, months; *MES*, minor papilla endoscopic sphincterotomy; *NP*, not provided; *NS*, not significant; *Prosp*, prospective uncontrolled trial; *RCT*, randomized controlled trial; *Retro*, retrospective review.

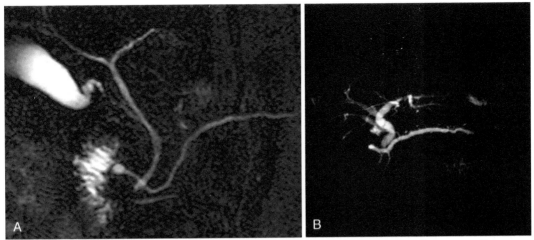

FIG 57.4 Magnetic resonance cholangiopancreatography (MRCP) examples of pancreas divisum with Santorinicele in two patients with recurrent acute pancreatitis (RAP). **A,** A 15-year-old boy with RAP. There is a normal caliber duct with a Santorinicele. Attacks ceased after endoscopic minor papillotomy. **B,** A 45-year-old man with RAP and chronic abdominal pain. MRCP shows a Santorinicele and a dilated dorsal duct with dilated side branches, indicating outflow obstruction and possible chronic pancreatitis. This patient had no further acute pancreatitis episodes after minor papillotomy, but continued to suffer with chronic daily pain.

of the orifice during healing and as prophylaxis against post-ERCP pancreatitis. Minor papilla localization and cannulation to achieve dorsal duct access can be challenging. The minor papilla is situated proximally and to the right of the major papilla, and is often best visualized from a long scope position. The minor papilla sometimes appears as a small mound or "mini-papilla," but in other cases is quite flat with an almost invisible orifice. Localization of the orifice may be aided by intravenous secretin injection, which stimulates pancreatic juice production, causing the orifice to open.[52] Methylene blue sprayed over the surrounding mucosa can be a useful adjunct.[53] After secretin is administered, the brisk pancreatic flow washes clear the blue dye surrounding the orifice, producing a visible blush for targeted cannulation. Smaller tapered catheters loaded with hydrophilic 0.021-inch wires are best for these cases. It is best to cannulate with the wire because probing with the catheter may cause trauma and bleeding, which can impair localization. After the duct is engaged successfully with a wire and then with the catheter, great care must be taken in passing the wire to the pancreatic tail. If the wire enters a side branch and force is applied, side branch perforation can easily occur, increasing the risk of pancreatitis. As with all pancreatic duct work in the era of MRCP, limited or no contrast injection is needed for guidewire passage. Once the guidewire is positioned, a minor papillotomy can be accomplished with the traction sphincterotome. If the catheter cannot be advanced over the wire because of stenosis, a needle-knife incision can be made over the wire. When wire access fails, precut needle-knife papillotomy may be needed to achieve access. This maneuver should only be performed carefully and incrementally when there is certainty regarding the location of the papillary orifice. Another common technique for minor papillotomy is to place a stent and then perform needle-knife sphincterotomy over the stent. Limited data suggest that the pull-type (traction) and needle-knife-over-stent techniques have similar safety and restenosis rates.[54] Video 57.1 demonstrates several techniques relative to minor papilla access.

Sphincter of Oddi Disorders

Elevated basal sphincter tone or spasm and ampullary stenosis may obstruct the flow of pancreatic secretions or cause bile reflux into the pancreatic duct, triggering episodes of pancreatitis. Sphincter of Oddi disorders (SODs) are sometimes considered as a possible cause of IRAP in postcholecystectomy patients. Pancreatic SOD is included in the well-known Milwaukee classification, with most IRAP patients falling into the type 2 category (pancreatic pain, recurrent elevations in amylase or lipase, and normal pancreatic duct).[55] There is ongoing debate over the relationship between SOD and pancreatitis, but evidence is mixed regarding a causative relationship. Multiple studies using manometry have shown elevated sphincter pressures ranging from 15% to 72% in patients with IRAP, although the significance of elevated sphincter pressures remains unclear, and hypertension may not translate to a clinical syndrome that responds to biliary and or pancreatic sphincter ablation.[56–64]

There are no evidence-based guidelines regarding the role of ERCP in diagnosis and treatment of SOD in IRAP. Relief from recurrent attacks occurs in 52% to 89% of patients with manometrically confirmed pancreatic SOD who undergo endoscopic therapy with sphincterotomy or botulinum toxin.[60,61,64–67] In prospective studies, the rates of RAP after endoscopic therapy range from 14% to 48% over a mean follow-up period of 29 to 78 months.[60,64,65] The decision to intervene in type 1 pancreatic SOD (i.e., IRAP and a dilated pancreatic duct) is fairly clear-cut. However, most patients fall into the type 2 category, and lack ductal dilation to implicate outflow obstruction. Because of the inherent risk and uncertain effectiveness of endoscopic therapy, it is preferred that the endoscopist meet the patient prior to performing the procedure. This preprocedure consultation allows the establishment of trust and a rapport between the physician and patient, and enables the physician to communicate realistic expectations regarding the risks of the procedure and the likelihood of a response. The risk of post-ERCP pancreatitis is elevated

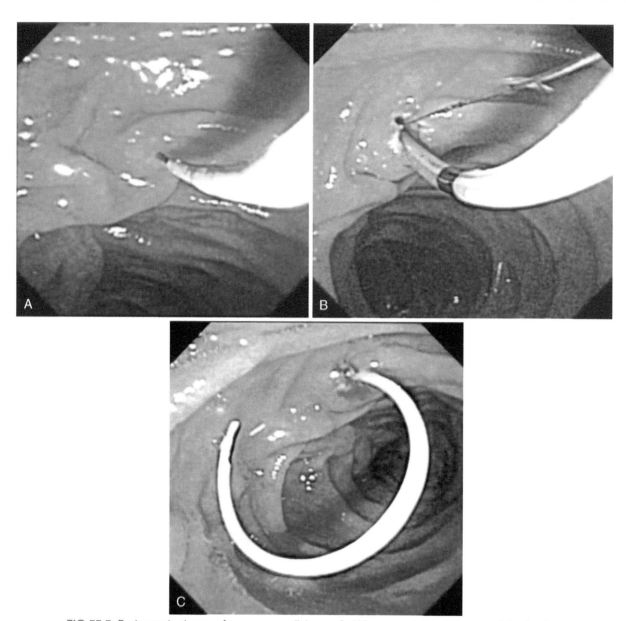

FIG 57.5 Endoscopic therapy for pancreas divisum. **A,** Wire cannulation is accomplished using a tapered-tip catheter with a 0.021-inch wire. **B,** After deep wire access is achieved, a minor papillotomy is performed using a traction sphincterotome and blended current. **C,** A 5-Fr single pigtail stent is placed to prevent post-endoscopic retrograde cholangiopancreatography (ERCP) pancreatitis.

in this group compared to other indications (10% vs. 4%),[68] and is highest for those with pancreatic sphincter hypertension.[69] Many additional patients will require admission for postprocedure abdominal pain, with or without modest enzyme elevations.

Endoscopic approaches to SOD have been heterogeneous, and there are few randomized trials to define the optimal technique and the efficacy of the intervention. Furthermore, outcomes in most studies of endoscopic therapy for IRAP have been variably defined, and many studies have suboptimal follow-up.[70] A common practice has been to perform empiric sphincterotomy (without manometry) in RAP, citing the increased time and risk and lack of precision of sphincter of Oddi manometry (SOM) measurements. However, many experts suggest SOM as a guide for sphincterotomy, especially in cases of suspected

pancreatic sphincter hypertension, given the increased risk of pancreatic sphincterotomy. The main argument in favor of SOM is that patients with high pressures have better response rates, whereas those with normal pressures can be spared the additional risk of sphincter ablation because they are unlikely to respond. In addition, it appears that SOM does not add significantly to the risk of the procedure.[71] Indirect tests (e.g., secretin-stimulated EUS, nuclear scintigraphy) have not shown sufficient sensitivity to be alternatives to SOM in ruling out SOD.[72,73]

Another question is what type of sphincterotomy to perform. The sphincter of Oddi is comprised of three components: common, biliary, and pancreatic sphincter fibers. An EBS may suffice to treat patients with type 2 pancreatic SOD, rather than an endoscopic dual sphincterotomy (EDS), as pancreatic sphincter hypertension is often primarily due to the common fibers rather than the pancreatic fibers. As such, cutting the common fibers may sufficiently decrease pancreatic sphincter pressure to prevent further attacks. Past observational studies have yielded mixed conclusions regarding the necessity of EDS rather than EBS in type 2 pancreatic SOD.[74,75] A 2012 randomized controlled trial compared EBS and EDS in patients with pancreatic sphincter hypertension. Patients with manometrically confirmed pancreatic sphincter hypertension were randomized to EBS (n = 33) or EDS (n = 36) and followed for a mean of 78 months (interquartile range 23–108 months).[64] There was no difference in the rate of RAP during follow up (48.5% vs. 47.2%, p = 0.20). The rates of RAP following both EBS/EDS were notably high compared to retrospective studies of pancreatic SOD. This interesting finding suggests that sphincter hypertension may not always be the true pathogenic factor in pancreatic SOD, and that underlying genetic factors or other unknown variables may be at play. The investigators also randomized patients with normal SOM (n = 20) to EBS or sham treatment. There was no difference in the rate of RAP observed during follow-up between these two groups (11% vs. 27%, p = non-significant). The results of this study call into question the role of manometry in directing sphincterotomy, and perhaps even the value of a sphincterotomy in RAP. Although sphincter ablation may still be considered on an individualized basis, we believe a prudent strategy is to selectively cannulate the bile duct and perform EBS without preceding manometry. In patients who recur following EBS, pancreatic manometry with or without EDS can be considered as a "salvage" procedure.

Ampullary and Pancreatic Neoplasms

A high suspicion for underlying cancer should be maintained in patients with RAP, especially in those over the age of 40 who have developed RAP in the past several months. Cancers of the duodenum, ampulla,[76] and pancreas may obstruct the pancreatic duct, leading to AP episodes (Fig. 57.6). In a consecutive series of 124 patients with pancreatic carcinoma, AP was the presenting symptom in 13.8%.[77] Though they do not arise from the pancreatic duct, neuroendocrine tumors may also occasionally cause AP.[78] Intraductal papillary mucinous neoplasm (IPMN) involving the main and branch ducts may be associated with pancreatitis in 7% to 43% of patients, though many of these reports are from surgical series that are enriched with symptomatic patients[79–82] (Fig. 57.7). The pathogenesis of pancreatitis is likely related to ductal plugging by mucous secretion. Patients with IPMN presenting with AP tend to be younger, and have greater odds of harboring malignancy compared to those without AP.[83] AP is more commonly observed with main-duct and mixed-type variants, but may also be seen in branch-duct IPMN.[82] In cases of branch-duct IPMN, it may be difficult to prove that the cyst is causing pancreatitis, as incidental IPMNs are common (Fig. 57.8).

Autoimmune Pancreatitis

RAP is rather unusual in type 1 autoimmune pancreatitis (AIP), with obstructive jaundice, diabetes, and weight loss being more common presentations. When AP does occur, the likely explanation is pancreatic duct stricturing. A systematic review of nine studies published in 2008 (140 patients with AIP) reported the occurrence of recurrent pain or pancreatitis.[84] The overall rate of recurrent pain or pancreatitis was only 10.1%. RAP appears to be a more common presentation in the type 2 rather than type 1 histological variant. Type 2 AIP is more difficult to diagnose than type 1 because of the lack of a serological marker and the greater difficulty in obtaining diagnostic histology. An international survey reported RAP in 5% of type 1 AIP cases and 34% of type 2 AIP cases.[85] The largest US study of type 2 AIP (n = 43) reported an even higher RAP rate of 58.1%.[86] In that series, type 2 AIP patients presenting with AP were younger (mean age 28 years vs. 47 years), less apt to have obstructive jaundice (16% vs. 50%), less apt to have a pancreatic mass (12% vs. 67%), and more likely to have inflammatory bowel disease (IBD) (60% vs. 22%). Though still a rare cause of AP, type 2 AIP should be considered in patients with IRAP who fit this clinical profile. Carefully selected patients (especially those with IBD) may warrant core biopsy or empiric corticosteroid trials (Fig. 57.9).

Choledochocele

Choledochoceles are cystic dilations of the intraduodenal portion of the common bile duct (CBD). They are classified as type 3 choledochal cysts, the least common subtype.[87] RAP is a common clinical presentation among patients with symptomatic choledochoceles, and likely occurs as a result of biliary reflux into the pancreas.[88] The incidence of malignancy arising from choledochoceles is thought to be much lower than from other types of choledochal cysts, though rare cases have been reported.[89] EBS is the current standard of care for choledochoceles (Fig. 57.10).[90] EBS unroofs the cyst and separates the biliary and pancreatic duct drainage. Outcome studies are lacking; however, available evidence suggests that EBS usually resolves pancreatitis.[91]

EVALUATION AND TREATMENT

The evaluation and treatment of RAP can be divided into three phases. In the primary evaluation, simple and obvious causes are sought through a careful history, laboratory testing, ultrasound with or without CT imaging, and careful review of the records from past attacks. In the secondary evaluation, advanced imaging is performed and laboratory testing is obtained to look for "occult" biliary, structural, and genetic causes. In the tertiary evaluation,

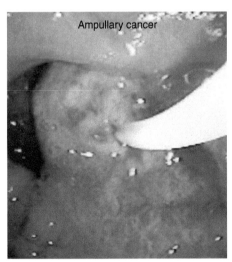

FIG 57.6 This 70-year-old patient presented with a single unexplained bout of acute pancreatitis. Subsequent endoscopic examination revealed ampullary cancer. (Image courtesy of Adam Slivka and Michael K. Sanders.)

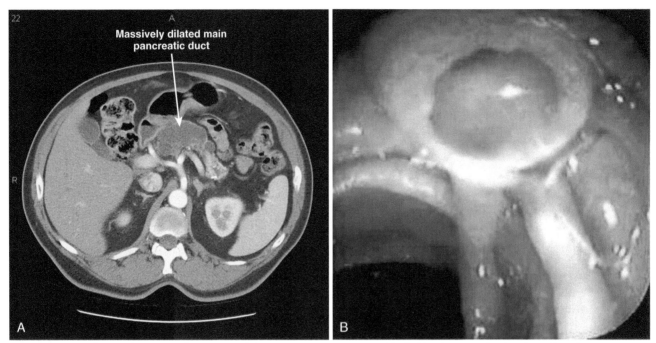

FIG 57.7 Example of a patient with recurrent acute pancreatitis (RAP) due to main duct intraductal papillary mucinous neoplasm (IPMN). **A,** CT scan shows hugely dilated pancreatic duct. **B,** Side-viewing endoscopy reveals gaping papilla with mucin extrusion. (Images courtesy of Adam Slivka and Michael K. Sanders.)

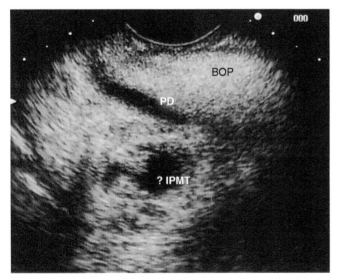

FIG 57.8 This 55-year-old patient had three unexplained bouts of acute pancreatitis. On EUS examination, a cyst was found in the uncinate process that communicated with a side branch suggestive of a branch-type IPMN. *BOP,* bleeding on probing; *EUS,* endoscopic ultrasound; *IPMN,* intraductal papillary mucinous neoplasm; *IPMT,* intraductal papillary mucinous tumor; *PD,* pancreas divisum. (Courtesy of Dr. Kevin McGrath, University of Pittsburgh Medical Center.)

endoscopic testing and empiric endoscopic or surgical approaches may be offered to identify causes or prevent attacks. The primary evaluation is often performed during hospitalization for AP, whereas the secondary and tertiary evaluations are often performed in an outpatient setting. A number of multidisciplinary "Pancreas Centers of Excellence" have been developed throughout the country to provide a comprehensive evaluation of patients with complex pancreatic disorders like IRAP.[92]

Primary Evaluation
Careful History
The evaluation of RAP starts with taking a careful history to ascertain risk factors. Heavy daily or binge alcohol consumption may suggest alcohol as the cause. However, alcohol-related pancreatitis may be overdiagnosed in moderate regular drinkers.[93] Alcohol may not be the primary driver in these patients, and other potentially treatable causes should not be missed. Smoking has long been known to be a risk factor for CP and pancreatic cancer, but until recently has been ignored in AP. Several studies now implicate smoking as a cause or cofactor in AP as well.[94] Case reports from 2012 implicate cannabis as a trigger.[95] Preceding biliary colic may suggest gallstones. New prescription medications started within 1 to 2 months of the index episode or class I or II medications that are known to be associated with pancreatitis may suggest medication-induced pancreatitis.[96] The past medical history is also important to review. A personal history of high triglycerides or poorly controlled diabetes may suggest hypertriglyceridemia-mediated AP. A history of cholecystectomy suggests the possibility of SOD. A history of parathyroid issues or renal failure may suggest hypercalcemia-induced AP. A history of recurrent bronchitis or sinusitis, asthma, or male infertility may implicate a *CFTR* polymorphism. A family history of pancreatitis or cystic fibrosis (CF) may suggest genetic causes.

Basic Laboratory Evaluation
The primary laboratory evaluation of AP includes serum amylase, lipase, liver function tests, calcium, and triglyceride levels. Serum

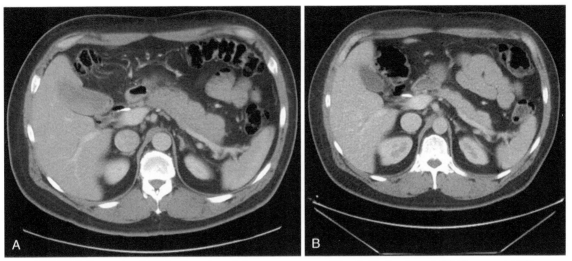

FIG 57.9 Example of CT findings in autoimmune pancreatitis. **A,** Pretreatment CT. The pancreatic body and tail are diffusely enlarged, with loss of normal contour. **B,** Posttreatment with corticosteroids. The previous pancreatic enlargement has resolved. (Images courtesy of Adam Slivka and Michael K. Sanders.)

alcohol levels may also be useful to detect surreptitious alcohol use. In recurrent episodes, it is helpful to obtain and review laboratory data from as many of the past attacks as possible. This serves to confirm whether significant lipase elevations are truly present to confirm the diagnosis of RAP. In addition, the presence of concomitant alkaline phosphatase and/or alanine transaminase (ALT) elevations may implicate gallstones, microlithiasis, or sphincter of Oddi dysfunction.[97] The admitting serum triglyceride level may help detect hypertriglyceridemia as a cause. A triglyceride level of more than 1000 mg/dL at the time of presentation strongly supports triglyceride-mediated AP; whereas a level of greater than 500 mg/dL should raise a high degree of suspicion.[98] If the triglyceride level was assessed later during the admission (after days of fasting), it may have decreased substantially. In these cases, repeating the serum triglyceride once the patient has returned to his or her usual diet may be warranted.

Imaging With TAUS and CT

The best initial imaging modality for detecting biliary causes of pancreatitis is TAUS. The results of all previous ultrasounds should be reviewed for findings that may implicate a biliary cause (e.g., sludge or stones in the gallbladder, biliary dilation) and suggest the need for cholecystectomy. CT scans have a limited role during an AP attack, and are performed primarily to detect local complications (necrosis, fluid collections, etc.). To detect necrosis, CT scans are optimally performed 3 days after symptom onset in patients who demonstrate signs of clinical severity.[99] If CT scans were performed during past attacks, it is useful to review them to ascertain the presence, severity, and location of inflammation. Most commonly, inflammation is diffused throughout the pancreas. However, inflammation that is focal in one area of the gland may help elucidate a structural cause. For example, inflammation confined to the tail of the pancreas may indicate a pancreatic duct tumor or stricture and indicate the need for further advanced imaging with MRCP or EUS.

Secondary Evaluation

In up to 90% of cases of AP, the primary evaluation reveals treatable causes (ongoing alcohol use, gallstones/sludge, liver function tests or biliary duct abnormalities indicating SOD, high triglycerides, culprit medications, etc.).[100] The underlying factors can thus be eliminated or treated, and patients observed for recurrence. However, a subset of cases remains undiagnosed. These cases are properly termed IRAP, and may require "second-line" testing to look for autoimmune, genetic, and structural causes.

Autoimmune Testing

Serum total IgG and IgG4 levels may be obtained to "screen" for AIP. However, proper diagnosis of AIP is usually more complicated than simply ordering a lab test. Serum IgG4 exhibits only approximately 76% sensitivity for type 1 AIP,[101] and levels are normal in patients with type 2 AIP. Additionally, IgG4 may be mildly elevated in the absence of AIP. Several scoring systems have been devised to diagnose AIP, including the HISORt (histology, imaging, serology, other organ involvement and response to therapy) criteria, which include a combination of laboratory, imaging, and histological features.[102] It is useful to review pancreatic imaging with an abdominal radiologist to look for features of AIP, such as diffuse pancreatic enlargement, capsular enhancement, or diffuse/multiple pancreatic duct stricturing. If past imaging is not optimal or is confounded by significant acute inflammation, then obtaining a contrast-enhanced MRCP may be useful to check for ductal and parenchymal features of AIP.

Genetic Testing

Testing for genetic causes may be considered in IRAP. There has been an explosion in knowledge regarding the genetics of pancreatitis. Genetic testing for certain pancreatitis-associated mutations is now commercially available, and may be considered in selected patients with IRAP. Important genetic causes include mutations of the cationic trypsinogen (*PRSS1*), CFTR, *SPINK-1*, and chymotrypsin C (*CTRC*) genes.

Mutations in *PRSS1* cause hereditary pancreatitis (HP). HP is an autosomal dominant disease with high penetrance, so patients will often have multiple family members in consecutive generations affected with pancreatitis. These patients classically

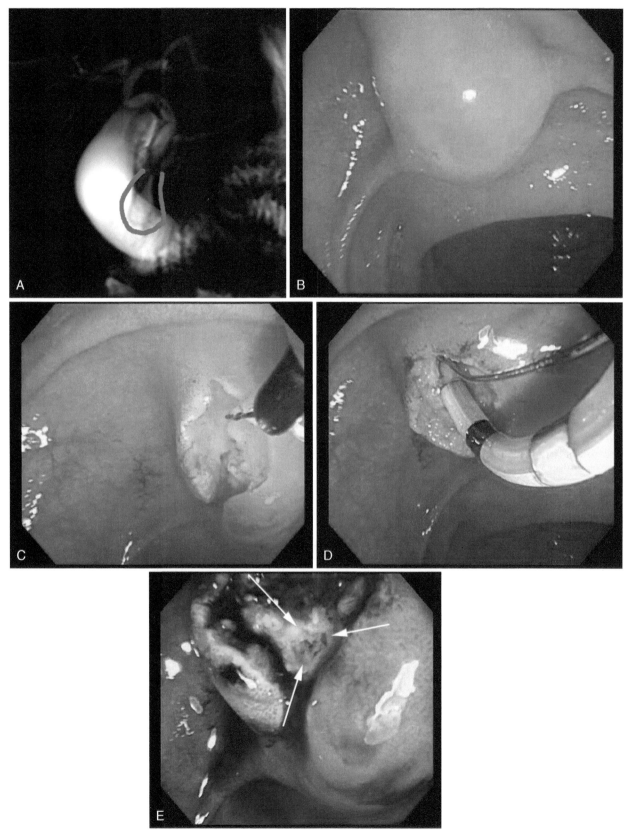

FIG 57.10 Example of choledochocele diagnosis and endoscopic treatment. An 8-year-old boy presented with idiopathic acute recurrent pancreatitis (IRAP). **A,** Secretin-enhanced magnetic resonance cholangiopancreatography (MRCP) shows a large saccular choledochocele with separate entry of common bile duct and pancreatic duct (outlined in red). **B,** Endoscopic view showing prominent choledochocele. Endoscopic therapy consisted of **C,** needle-knife unroofing of the lumen and **D,** biliary cannulation and extension of the biliary sphincterotomy. **E,** Methylene blue spray after secretin injection showing exposed pancreatic sphincter *(arrows)* without injury.

develop RAP in childhood and progress to CP in the teen years, and have a 40% lifetime risk of pancreatic cancer.[103] CF is a genetic disorder caused by impaired function of the CFTR protein that regulates chloride secretion in the pancreatic duct cells. CF is a heterogeneous disorder, likely because there are over 1200 known mutations that result in a range of problems with CFTR production, transport, and function. When the genetic defects are severe, pancreatic secretions are inspissated and plug the ductules, resulting in rapid and severe fatty replacement and atrophy of the pancreas. Children with severe mutations are often recognized promptly through newborn screening, and their pancreatic, pulmonary, and other problems are quickly and aggressively managed in CF centers. Adults may harbor milder or single allele *CFTR* defects that do not produce pancreatic insufficiency, but are recognized later in life with atypical manifestations including bronchitis, asthma, and RAP. Mutations in *SPINK-1* are unlikely to solely cause RAP, but may promote the development of CP, and sometimes present as a cofactor with other genetic or environmental causes.[104,105]

Genetic testing may be considered in patients with a family history of pancreatitis and in young patients with IRAP. This testing should be ordered with caution and should be accompanied by appropriate pretest counseling. There are several conceivable benefits of genetic testing, including obtaining insight into the cause and providing further motivation to avoid alcohol use and smoking. Although opponents counter that the results do not meaningfully affect management, this is not always the case. For example, the finding of a *PRSS1* mutation may prompt yearly imaging tests because of its associated risk of pancreatic cancer.[106] Finding a pancreatitis-associated mutation may also prevent empiric interventions like ERCP with sphincterotomy and cholecystectomy. Genetic mutations in patients with frequent RAP episodes may even prompt consideration of total pancreatectomy.[107] A major downside of testing is its high cost, and sometimes the lack of insurance coverage for testing.

Second-Line Imaging Tests

Some structural causes of RAP may be missed on ultrasound and CT performed at the time of the attack(s), and require more advanced imaging for diagnosis. Occult pancreatic cancer is a major concern, especially in those over age 40 who developed IRAP in the past several months. Pancreatic inflammation or necrosis may mask small cancers on initial imaging. Sometimes, only slight pancreatic duct dilation indicating downstream obstruction is present. In such patients, it is wise to repeat a contrast-enhanced pancreatic protocol CT or magnetic resonance imaging (MRI), or to consider EUS. The findings of these advanced tests often help guide subsequent treatment (see Fig. 57.7). Such testing is best performed 4 to 6 weeks after discharge, once inflammation has improved.

Additional obstructive causes include PD, pancreatic duct stricture, IPMN, ampullary neoplasm, and duodenal pathology. In years past, ERCP was frequently employed as a second-line evaluation in patients with RAP. Typically, ERCP would include a cholangiogram to look for biliary stones and a diagnostic pancreatogram to check for ductal pathology. Though ERCP has significant therapeutic potential in RAP, it has since fallen out of favor as a purely diagnostic test because of the advent of MRCP and EUS. Both provide excellent detail of the pancreatic duct and parenchyma, and have been used extensively in the

workup of patients with IRAP. However, each has its own advantages and limitations.

Magnetic Resonance Cholangiopancreatography

MRCP provides complete imaging of the pancreatic parenchyma and duct. MRCP protocols include heavily T2 (fluid)-weighted imaging to generate an "ERCP-like" image of the pancreatic duct. In young patients with IRAP, MRCP is an invaluable tool for screening for PD, and helps stratify its significance based on the presence or absence of dorsal duct dilation and Santorinicele. The addition of secretin administration improves ductal imaging resolution and has higher diagnostic accuracy for PD than standard MRCP (pooled sensitivity 86%; pooled specificity 97%).[30,108] The assessment of duct compliance and drainage following secretin administration has been used as a diagnostic test for outflow obstruction from SOD and PD and as a decision point for subsequent ERCP therapy.[109] In addition, MRCP detects pancreatic tumors, pancreatic duct strictures, and branch-type and main-duct IPMN. The main limitation of MRCP in the workup for IRAP is the lack of ampullary and luminal visualization.

Recent evidence (2015) suggests that secretin MRCP may be quite accurate in detection of underlying CP, which may always be present in patients with RAP.[110] In fact, secretin MRCP may be more accurate than EUS in detecting histologically less advanced forms of CP.[111]

Endoscopic Ultrasound

EUS is also frequently used in the secondary evaluation of IRAP and may help guide subsequent evaluation and therapy (Fig. 57.11). It is similar to MRCP in that it provides exquisite imaging of the pancreas. Its advantages over MRCP include luminal visualization, greater detection of biliary sludge and stones, tissue and fluid acquisition, and the ability to detect parenchymal changes indicative of CP. EUS may also be superior to CT for detecting small masses.[112] Some observational studies have compared the yield of EUS and MRCP in patients with IRAP.[113,114] One included 38 patients with IRAP who underwent both EUS and MRCP. A higher yield was observed for EUS than for MRCP (29% vs. 10.5%). MRCP was superior for detecting ductal abnormalities like PD, whereas EUS was better for biliary causes. The two tests had a combined 50% yield, suggesting that they may be complementary.

Linear EUS is most commonly used for pancreaticobiliary examinations, but radial EUS can also suffice, based on physician preference. It is usually best to delay EUS until 3 or 4 weeks after recovery from the last AP episode to maximize the diagnostic yield, as views of the pancreas can be obscured by pancreatic inflammation and peripancreatic fluid. When performing EUS to evaluate RAP, the endoscopist should have the following 7-point "checklist" in mind:

1. Is there duodenal or ampullary pathology? Generally, a screening endoscopy is advisable to look for duodenal inflammation or neoplastic pathology. The ampulla should be examined and photodocumented, with careful inspection for adenomas, masses, mucin extrusion, and diverticulae. Satisfactory ampullary views can often be obtained using the oblique view of the echoendoscope; however, a side-viewing duodenoscope should be passed if necessary.

2. Are biliary stones or sludge present? The bile duct should be carefully traced from the hilum to the ampulla, looking for layering echogenic sludge or echogenic rounded structures

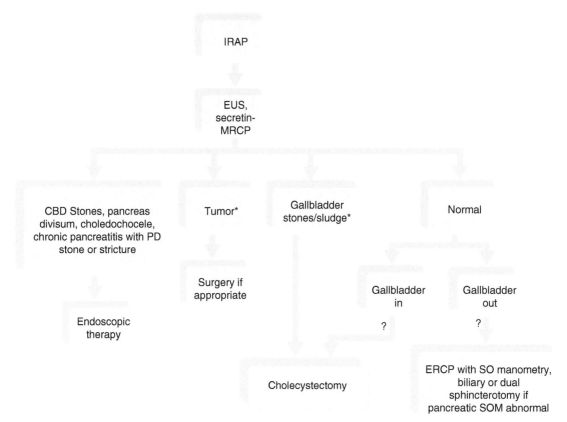

FIG 57.11 Treatment algorithm for unexplained recurrent pancreatitis. *Indicates conditions for which EUS appears to be superior to MRCP in terms of diagnosis. *CBD*, common bile duct; *ERCP*, endoscopic retrograde pancreatography; *EUS*, endoscopic ultrasound; *IRAP*, idiopathic acute recurrent pancreatitis; *MRCP*, magnetic resonance cholangiopancreatography, *PD*, pancreas divisum; *SO*, sphincter of Oddi; *SOM*, sphincter of Oddi manometry.

with shadowing indicating stones. Striving to achieve complete ampullary imaging from both the duodenal bulb (long position) and the second portion (short position) decreases the chance of missing small stones. In patients with their gallbladder *in situ*, the gallbladder fundus, body, and neck should be carefully scrutinized for stones and layering sludge.

3. Are there pancreatic tumors or strictures affecting the pancreatic duct? The pancreas should be viewed in its entirety, looking for masses or focal hypoechoic regions that indicate possible occult cancer. Fine-needle aspiration (FNA) should be performed of any suspicious lesions. The duct should be carefully traced into the stomach and duodenum to detect obstructing tumors, strictures, or stones, which may result in proximal duct dilation.

4. Is PD present? EUS can have similar or even superior accuracy as MRCP for diagnosing PD,[115] but is more operator-dependent. Various EUS findings have been reported as useful in diagnosing pancreas divisum, including a crossed appearance of the bile and pancreatic duct, absence of a "stack sign" (i.e., appearance of portal vein, pancreatic duct, and bile duct in single image), and separate insertion of bile and pancreatic ducts into the duodenal wall. In our experience, the best approach is to trace the pancreatic duct from the point of its insertion with the bile duct at the ampulla into the dorsal pancreas (Video 57.2). A sensitivity of 95% and specificity

of 97% have been reported using this approach; however, this study excluded 22% of patients in whom the ductal anatomy could not be adequately assessed.[116] We find EUS to be most useful to rule out PD when the duct can be successfully traced. The inability to trace the duct from ampulla to dorsal pancreas may suggest pancreas divisum, but might also indicate technical limitations preventing continuous visualization of the duct. In those with pancreas divisum, the Santorini duct can sometimes be traced to the minor papilla, and inspection can be made for a Santorinicele indicating functional outflow obstruction.

5. Are the pancreatic and/or bile ducts dilated? It is good practice to measure the CBD and pancreatic ducts to assess for dilation indicating ampullary outflow obstruction. Most experts agree a normal CBD diameter is 6 mm or less in patients with a gallbladder and 9 mm or less in those who are postcholecystectomy. The normal diameter of the pancreatic duct is 3 mm in the head, 2 mm in the body, and 1 mm in the tail.[117] Dilation of the ducts may help support a diagnosis of SO dysfunction, ampullary stenosis, or impaired drainage from PD.

6. Is CP present? The EUS diagnosis of CP is discussed in detail elsewhere in the text (see Chapter 59). The presence of CP helps to stage RAP and explains abdominal pain that persists between attacks. The finding of ductal obstruction related to CP (stones and strictures) may also indicate an obstructive

cause of ongoing RAP that could benefit from endoscopic or surgical management. CP findings are often observed in RAP, with prevalence in early series ranging from 0% to 65%.[23] Anecdotally, we find that many patients with IRAP ultimately found to possess genetic mutations have significant CP changes on EUS.

7. Is there evidence of AIP? The EUS appearance of AIP is typically a diffusely enlarged and hypoechoic-appearing gland, sometimes with interspersed hyperechoic lines or foci (Video 57.3).[118] Pancreatic duct dilation is typically absent. Focal hypoechoic masses may also be observed. In such cases, FNA is indicated to help rule out malignancy.[119] In patients with characteristic EUS features of AIP, FNA might also be considered to make a "tissue diagnosis" of AIP, but obtaining a satisfactory tissue sample that is able to confirm histology may be challenging. Cytological specimens obtained using 22- and 19-gauge needles have shown mixed results for obtaining lymphocytes and plasma cells suitable for IgG4 staining.[120,121] It is unusual to detect the more confirmatory finding of obliterative phlebitis using typical EUS needles, suggesting the need for needles that would provide larger tissue specimens with preserved tissue architecture. The use of the Tru-cut biopsy needle has fallen out of favor due to technical difficulties and complications, and is no longer commercially available. However newer, more flexible and easy-to-use fine-needle biopsy (FNB) needles are emerging, which may be able to obtain tissue "cores," facilitating the endoscopic diagnosis of AIP.

Tertiary Evaluation

After these primary and secondary evaluations, endoscopic and surgical approaches may be carefully considered to diagnose or provide targeted or empiric treatment. ERCP is the primary tool in the tertiary evaluation of RAP. As detailed previously, ERCP helps to diagnose and treat SOD, PD, ampullary pathology, and pancreatic duct strictures. Surgical approaches that are selectively employed in the tertiary evaluation of RAP include cholecystectomy; partial pancreatectomy in patients with masses, IPMNs, or strictures; major and minor sphincteroplasty; and total pancreatectomy with autologous islet cell transplant (TP/AIT) for those with genetic or "true" IRAP. In a case series of 49 patients with IRAP without evidence of CP on structural and/ or function testing, improvement in narcotic utilization and quality of life was observed after TP/IAT.[9] In addition, 45% of patients were insulin-independent after 1 year of follow-up, with a mean hemoglobin A1C of 6.0%. Further outcome studies are needed to determine if this intervention also decreases hospitalization and health care utilization by eliminating AP attacks.

KEY REFERENCES

1. Tenner S, Baillie J, DeWitt J, Vege SS: American College of Gastroenterology guideline: management of acute pancreatitis, *Am J Gastroenterol* 108:1400–1415, 2013.
9. Bellin MD, Kerdsirichairat T, Beilman GJ, et al: Total pancreatectomy with islet autotransplantation improves quality of life in patients with refractory recurrent acute pancreatitis, *Clin Gastroenterol Hepatol* 14: 1317–1323, 2016.
10. Yadav D, Lowenfels AB: The epidemiology of pancreatitis and pancreatic cancer, *Gastroenterology* 144:1252–1261, 2013.
13. Lankisch PG, Breuer N, Bruns A, et al: Natural history of acute pancreatitis: a long-term population-based study, *Am J Gastroenterol* 104:2797–2805, 2009.
15. Etemad B, Whitcomb DC: Chronic pancreatitis: diagnosis, classification, and new genetic developments, *Gastroenterology* 120:682–707, 2001.
19. Lee SP, Nicholls JF, Park HZ: Biliary sludge as a cause of acute pancreatitis, *N Engl J Med* 326:589–593, 2002.
23. Wilcox CM, Varadarajulu S, Eloubeidi M: Role of endoscopic evaluation in idiopathic pancreatitis: a systematic review, *Gastrointest Endosc* 63: 1037–1045, 2006.
24. Raty S, Pulkkinen J, Nordback I, et al: Can laparoscopic cholecystectomy prevent recurrent idiopathic acute pancreatitis? A prospective randomized multicenter trial, *Ann Surg* 262:736–741, 2015.
30. Rustagi T, Njei B: Magnetic resonance cholangiopancreatography in the diagnosis of pancreas divisum: a systematic review and meta-analysis, *Pancreas* 43:823–828, 2014.
50. Bertin C, Pelletier A, Vullierme M, et al: Pancreas divisum is not a cause of pancreatitis by itself but acts as a partner of genetic mutation, *Am J Gastroenterol* 107:311–317, 2012.
52. Devereaux BM, Lehman GA, Fein S, et al: Facilitation of pancreatic duct cannulation using a new synthetic porcine secretin, *Am J Gastroenterol* 97:2279–2281, 2002.
59. Gregg JA, Carr-Locke DL: Endoscopic pancreatic and biliary manometry in pancreatic, biliary and papillary disease, and after endoscopic sphincterotomy and surgical sphincteroplasty, *Gut* 25: 1247–1254, 1984.
63. Cotton PB, Durkalski V, Romagnuolo J, et al: Effect of endoscopic sphincterotomy for suspected sphincter of Oddi dysfunction on pain-related disability following cholecystectomy: the EPISOD randomized clinical trial, *JAMA* 311:2101–2109, 2014.
68. Masci E, Mariani A, Curioni S, Testoni PA: Risk factors for pancreatitis following endoscopic retrograde cholangiopancreatography: a meta-analysis, *Endoscopy* 35:830–834, 2003.
73. Corrazziari E, Cical M, Scopinaro F, et al: Scintigraphic assessment of sphincter of Oddi dysfunction, *Gut* 52:1655–1656, 2003.
77. Kohler H, Lankisch PG: Acute pancreatitis and hyperamylasemia in pancreatic carcinoma, *Pancreas* 2:177–179, 1987.
86. Hart PA, Levy MJ, Smyrk TC, et al: Clinical profiles and outcomes in idiopathic duct-centric chronic pancreatitis (type 2 autoimmune pancreatitis): the Mayo Clinic experience, *Gut* 65:1702–1709, 2016.
93. Coté GA, Yadav D, Slivka A, et al: Alcohol and smoking as risk factors in an epidemiology study of patients with chronic pancreatitis, *Clin Gastroenterol Hepatol* 9:266–273, 2011.
110. Trikudanathan G, Walker SP, Munigala S, et al: Diagnostic performance of contrast-enhanced MRI with secretin-stimulated MRCP for non-calcific chronic pancreatitis: a comparison with histopathology, *Am J Gastroenterol* 110:1598–1606, 2015.
111. Trikudanathan G, Vega-Peralta J, Malli A, et al: Diagnostic performance of endoscopic ultrasound (EUS) for non-calcific chronic pancreatitis (NCCP) based on histopathology, *Am J Gastroenterol* 111:568–574, 2016.
118. Farrell JJ, Garber J, Shahani D, et al: EUS findings in patients with autoimmune pancreatitis, *Gastrointest Endosc* 60:927–936, 2004.

A complete reference list can be found online at ExpertConsult .com

58

Pancreatic Fluid Collections and Leaks

Andrew Nett and Kenneth F. Binmoeller

INTRODUCTION

Pancreatic fluid collections (PFCs) and leaks develop due to main or secondary pancreatic ductal disruption caused by acute or chronic pancreatitis, trauma, or pancreatic surgery. PFCs include acute fluid collections, acute necrotic collections, pseudocysts, and walled-off necrosis.[1] Most nonnecrotic PFCs resolve spontaneously without need for drainage. Fluid collections that have become infected, or those that cause persistent symptoms, warrant drainage. Drainage of PFCs has historically been performed by open surgical approaches, but less invasive interventions have replaced open surgery over time. Whereas appropriate management of PFCs entails a multidisciplinary approach involving interventional endoscopy, interventional radiology, and minimally invasive surgery, endoscopic therapy of PFCs and pancreatic leaks has become a predominant initial therapeutic modality. Endoscopic transmural drainage of symptomatic pseudocysts has replaced surgical intervention as first-line therapy due to similar efficacy, less morbidity, shorter recovery, and greater cost-efficacy.[2–4]

PANCREATIC FLUID COLLECTION CLASSIFICATION AND CHARACTERIZATION

Appropriate classification of PFCs helps guide management. The revised Atlanta criteria categorize PFCs as either acute or chronic based upon their presence less than or more than 4 weeks

following an episode of pancreatitis. Categorization further depends on the presence or absence of necrosis.[1] Acute collections without significant necrosis are termed *acute fluid collections*. These may occur in up to 40% of cases of acute pancreatitis. Most of these acute collections remain sterile, are asymptomatic, and spontaneously resolve without intervention. Approximately 30% to 50% of acute fluid collections, however, may persist.[5,6] Acute fluid collections that persist longer than 4 weeks may evolve into pancreatic pseudocysts, which have a well-defined wall comprised of fibrous or granulation tissue containing no to minimal necrotic material.

Acute collections arising from necrotizing pancreatitis contain necrotic tissue and are termed *acute necrotic collections* (ANC). Mature, encapsulated collections of pancreatic necrosis may sometimes develop from acute necrotic collections, typically after 4 or more weeks following onset of necrotizing pancreatitis. These collections, called *walled-off necrosis* (WON), are comprised of a wall of fibrous or granulation tissue separating internal necrotic material from normal pancreatic parenchyma. WON has a well-defined enhancing wall of reactive tissue present on imaging. Approximately 15% of patients with acute pancreatitis will develop pancreatic necrosis, 33% of whom will develop infected necrosis.[7] The rate at which ANCs develop into WON is not clear.

In general, intervention on PFCs is unnecessary because they typically remain sterile and regress spontaneously. Due to the absence of a mature, noncompliant wall, acute fluid collections rarely cause mass-occupying effects such as gastric outlet or biliary obstruction.[6] Conservative observation is thus pursued, monitoring for symptoms or signs of infection. In the absence of infection, most ANCs are also managed conservatively with observation. If sepsis with suspicion of secondary infection of acute fluid and necrotic collections occurs, however, intervention is warranted. Whereas percutaneous drainage through small-diameter catheters may facilitate clinical improvement in some patients, persistent sepsis necessitates more aggressive débridement using either percutaneous necrosectomy or video-assisted ret-roperitoneal débridement (VARD).[6,8,9]

Once maturation of PFCs has occurred, indications for drainage include the presence of infection, gastric outlet or biliary obstruction, radiographic or clinical manifestations of vascular compression, or persistent symptoms such as anorexia, early satiety, weight loss, and refractory pain. In patients with mild symptoms or those with early pseudocysts or WON, medical supportive therapy with observation may still be appropriate to allow time for pseudocyst/WON regression. When indication for drainage is present, the maturity of the collection and differentiation of fluid versus necrotic collections helps to determine the most appropriate approach. Necrotic collections may require more intensive or multistep drainage techniques. Furthermore, the proportion of a WON that is comprised of solid debris may determine the outcome of standard endoscopic drainage, the number of therapeutic sessions required, and the need for direct endoscopic necrosectomy.[10] Significant complications may occur if WON is inappropriately managed as a pseudocyst.[11]

Differentiation of pseudocysts and WON may be performed by noninvasive cross-sectional imaging or by endoscopic ultrasonography (EUS). Although imaging for assessment of organized fluid collections is not standardized, contrast-enhanced computed tomography (CT) is most commonly performed for diagnosis and interventional planning. The sensitivity for detection of solid debris has been reported to be as low as 17% to 25%.[12,13] A retrospective review of CT imaging performed in patients with PFCs showed that a radiographic scoring system could improve accuracy in differentiating WON from pseudocysts up to approximately 80%.[14] Magnetic resonance imaging (MRI) is more accurate in prediction of solid debris within pancreatic fluid collections, with sensitivity up to 100% reported.[12,13] MRI has higher sensitivity for detection of pancreatic duct disruption as well, which may predict the likelihood of spontaneous PFC resolution, as the presence of pancreatic duct disruption is associated with the development of chronic, mature collections.[15,16] EUS may also be used to detect the presence of pancreatic necrosis and has been shown to be the most accurate imaging modality for characterizing pancreatic fluid collections (Fig. 58.1).[17] Transabdominal ultrasound may also be beneficial. In a prospective comparison of EUS, MRI, or transabdominal ultrasound, transabdominal ultrasound had a sensitivity of 92% (vs. 100% for EUS or MRI) for detection of WON, though it was less sensitive in detection of venous collaterals around the collection compared to EUS.[13]

PSEUDOCYST ACCESS

Endoscopy-Guided (Without EUS)

Endoscopic drainage without EUS guidance may be performed when a bulge into the gastrointestinal (GI) lumen is present from extrinsic compression by the pseudocyst (Fig. 58.2). In this instance, use of a duodenoscope permits good visualization of

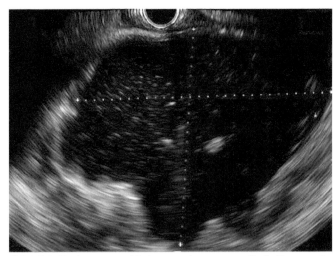

FIG 58.1 Endosonographic image of mature walled-off necrosis. (From Siddiqui AA, Adler DG, Nieto J, et al: EUS-guided drainage of peripancreatic fluid collections and necrosis by using a novel lumen-apposing stent: a large retrospective, multicenter US experience [with videos]. *Gastrointest Endosc* 83[4]:699–707, 2016.)

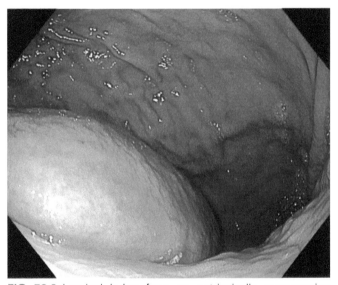

FIG 58.2 Luminal bulge from an extrinsically compressing pancreatic fluid collection (PFC).

the posterior gastric wall and the posteromedial duodenal wall. A 4.2-mm working channel will enable passage of 10-Fr stents. As described by Ballard and Coté (2012), optimal alignment ensures entrance of the pseudocyst at an area of maximal visible bulging of the gastric or duodenal wall.[18] The duodenoscope should be in a stable position with the ideal angle of needle puncture entry at 90 degrees to minimize the length of the GI wall that will be traversed. A cystotome or needle-knife catheter may be used to puncture across the gastric or duodenal wall and establish access into the pseudocyst. Electrocautery can be used to facilitate puncture across the wall and does not seem to affect bleeding complications.[19,20] Aspiration of a sample of pseudocyst contents and injection of contrast into the pseudocyst under fluoroscopy may be performed to confirm that access has been

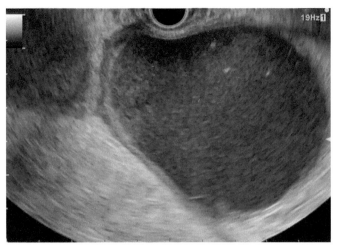

FIG 58.3 Endosonographic image of a mature pseudocyst.

achieved. A stiff guidewire can then be passed into the pseudocyst and coiled in the cyst under fluoroscopic visualization. The pseudocyst puncture tract is then dilated with a balloon and/or bougie catheter. Plastic or metal stents can then be deployed across the dilated cystgastrostomy or cystduodenostomy tract for drainage.

EUS-Guided

When EUS-guided pseudocyst drainage is performed, careful characterization of the pseudocyst is important. EUS imaging enables direct assessment of the distance separating the pseudocyst and GI tract wall, confirmation of a mature pseudocyst wall, and exclusion of interceding vessels (Fig. 58.3). As a general rule, the distance separating the pseudocyst and GI tract wall should not exceed 10 mm. Endosonographic visualization allows assessment for the presence of internal debris and/or necrosis that would warrant more aggressive drainage techniques.[21] Following endosonographic assessment, the next step in EUS-guided drainage involves puncture into the pseudocyst with a 19-gauge fine-needle aspiration (FNA) needle passed through a therapeutic echoendoscope. A 0.025- or 0.035-inch guidewire is passed through the needle and coiled within the pseudocyst. The needle is then exchanged over the guidewire for either a bougie catheter or dilating balloon, and dilation is performed to a size appropriate for stent delivery. Therapeutic linear echoendoscopes, which have a larger working channel (3.7 to 3.8 mm), enable pseudocyst puncture with a 10-Fr cystotome. The cystotome has an inner needle knife catheter used for initial cyst puncture and an outer 10-Fr sheath with a diathermy ring. After initial puncture, replacement of the inner needle knife catheter with a guidewire is followed by advancement of the 10-Fr outer sheath into the cyst using electrocautery, expanding the puncture site. Multiple guidewires may then be placed through the 10-Fr sheath. Plastic or metal stents may be placed across the tract for pseudocyst drainage.

EUS-Guided Versus Endoscopy-Guided

Though direct endoscopic pseudocyst access is possible when the fluid collection causes obvious extrinsic compression of the GI lumen, EUS-guided access has been shown to have higher success rates for pseudocyst drainage with similar adverse events.[18] A small, randomized, prospective trial comparing EUS-guided

versus endoscopy-guided transmural access showed higher technical success for EUS-guided access (94% vs. 72%). Furthermore, EUS-guided access was as successful as salvage crossover therapy in all cases where endoscopy-guided access failed because the pseudocysts were nonbulging. No significant difference existed in short-term clinical success rates (defined by cyst resolution) or long-term clinical outcomes.[21] Of note, the technical success of both approaches is similar except in cases when a luminal bulge is absent. Thus, the advantage of EUS-guided drainage seems to rest upon enhanced access specifically in cases of nonbulging pseudocysts. A meta-analysis performed by Panamonta et al (2012) examined two randomized-controlled trials and two prospective comparisons involving 229 patients.[22] This review confirmed that EUS-guided drainage had significantly higher technical success rates (relative risk [RR] 12.38, 95% confidence interval [CI] 1.39–110.22) and was a successful salvage therapeutic method in all patients with failed endoscopy-guided drainage due to lack of a luminal bulge. In those with technical success, short-term and long-term clinical success rates (defined as symptomatic relief and radiologic resolution of pseudocysts) were comparable (RR 1.03, 95% CI 0.95–1.11 and RR 0.98, 95% CI 0.76–1.25, respectively). Complication rates were also similar (RR 0.98, 95% CI 0.52–1.86), with the most common complications being bleeding and infection.

CYST DRAINAGE

Plastic Stents

Multiple studies have reported the use of single and multiple plastic stents ranging from 7- to 10-Fr size for drainage. No randomized controlled trial has compared the benefits of using a single stent versus multiple plastic stents. Retrospective studies have shown that insertion of even a single stent provides high rates of clinical resolution. Secondary infection does seem to be potentially more frequent in cases of single versus multiple-stent drainage, however.[23]

When using a plastic stent, a double pigtail design is preferentially used to reduce the risk of stent migration. Double pigtail stents also decrease delayed bleeding, as straight stents may erode into the pseudocyst wall with resultant hemorrhage.[24] Stents used for cyst drainage are 3 or 4 cm long. Multiple plastic stents are typically placed to enhance drainage by increasing the cumulative diameter of stent lumens, creating channel redundancy in the event one plastic stent occludes, and promoting drainage through the canals between stents. The placement of two stents is best accomplished by initially placing two guide wires. A 10-Fr catheter sheath (e.g., 10-Fr stent pusher tube, cytology brush sheath, multiport ramp catheter) is a helpful tool to accomplish this because the lumen is large enough to pass two 0.035-inch guidewires. Using a 10-Fr cystotome, two guidewires can be immediately inserted after entry into the cyst.

Of historic interest is the NAVIX device (NAVIX; Xlumena, Mountain View, CA), which enables exchange-free pseudocyst access, tract dilation, and placement of two guidewires with a single device.[25] This device helped streamline the otherwise laborious and time-consuming process of placing multiple plastic stents, and decreased opportunity for technical failure during multiple exchanges.

Fully Covered Self-Expanding Metal Stents (FCSEMS)

Compared to plastic stents, the appeal of FCSEMS is their larger lumens with resultant quicker pseudocyst drainage and decreased risk of stent occlusion. Procedure time may also be decreased because only a single stent needs deployment. Published studies, however, have not consistently shown an advantage in using FCSEMS. A retrospective comparison has shown improved rates of complete pseudocyst resolution at 1 year follow-up after endoscopic drainage using FCSEMS versus double pigtail plastic stents (98% vs. 89%, $p = 0.01$). Plastic stent usage also resulted in higher complication rates (odds ratio [OR] 2.9 after multivariate analysis).[26] Contrasting results, however, were obtained in a 2014 prospective randomized trial by Lee et al comparing the use of multiple plastic stents versus FCSEMS for PFC drainage. One caveat in this discussion of pseudocyst intervention is that results of this study were not necessarily stratified by fluid collection type. Drainage of WON will be discussed specifically later in this chapter.[27] Technical success was achieved for all cases regardless of stent type. Clinical success was achieved in 20 of 23 cases with FCSEMS and 20 of 22 cases with plastic stents ($p = 0.97$). No statistical difference was present in either adverse event rates or rate of recurrence during follow-up. One point of benefit from use of FCSEMS was shown, however, with achievement of a shorter median procedure time compared to use of plastic stents.

Lumen-Apposing Metal Stents (LAMS)

Whether plastic or metal, tubular stents have several limitations when applied to transluminal drainage. First, they do not impart lumen-to-lumen anchorage. This may result in leakage of contents if there is physical separation of the lumens. Second, stent migration may occur due to the absence of a stricture to hold it in place. Third, the length of tubular stents exceeds the anatomical requirement of a shorter transluminal anastomosis. The excess exposed stent ends may cause tissue trauma, resulting in bleeding or perforation. Placement of an internal plastic stent within a FCSEMS has been reported in an attempt to reduce migration and mitigate against erosion of the metal stent edge into the collapsed pseudocyst wall, but we have not found this method to prevent migration or tissue injury. Finally, the length of tubular stents predisposes to stent dysfunction. The longer the stent length, the more prone the stent is to clogging from food residue or cyst debris.[28]

A lumen-apposing metal stent (LAMS) designed for transluminal drainage was developed and first reported by Binmoeller in 2011.[5] The AXIOS stent (Boston Scientific, Marlborough, MA) is a nitinol braided FCSEMS with bilateral double walled flanges existing in a dumbbell configuration perpendicular to the lumen for the purpose of anastomosis creation (Fig. 58.4). Fully expanded, the flanges are either 20 mm or 24 mm in diameter, approximately twice that of the stent's mid-lumen diameter of either 10 mm or 15 mm. The bilateral flanges are designed to reduce stent migration and approximate structures in order to reduce rates of perforation and leak. Furthermore, the flanges are short in length and therefore have limited extension into the GI tract lumen and fluid collection cavity, potentially reducing the risk of stent erosion.

The AXIOS stent is deployed through a 10.8-Fr catheter delivery system. The delivery system is attached to the echoendoscope working channel port via a Luer-lock, similar to a standard FNA needle. The catheter is advanced into the fluid collection by manipulation of the distal catheter control hub and then locked into position. Retraction to a halfway point of the proximal stent deployment hub results in unsheathing of the distal stent flange within the collection cavity. The catheter

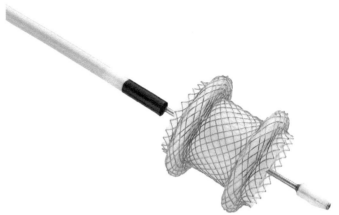

FIG 58.4 Fully covered, biflanged, lumen-apposing metal stent (AXIOS, Boston Scientific). (Courtesy Boston Scientific, Marlborough, MA. From Siddiqui AA, Adler DG, Nieto J, et al: EUS-guided drainage of peripancreatic fluid collections and necrosis by using a novel lumen-apposing stent: a large retrospective, multicenter US experience [with videos]. *Gastrointest Endosc* 83[4]:699–707, 2016.)

control hub is then unlocked and retracted until the point at which the distal stent flange starts to compress against the wall of the collection cavity. After relocking the catheter control hub, the stent deployment hub is then completely retracted and the proximal stent flange is unsheathed. To ensure that proximal flange deployment will occur within the GI lumen, catheter retraction until direct endoscopic visualization of the 2 to 3 mm of the black catheter shaft marker is advised prior to proximal flange deployment. Pulling back the echoendoscope to allow direct endoscopic visualization of this marker, however, risks excessive traction on the AXIOS stent, which may result in migration of the distal flange back into the GI lumen. To avoid excessive traction, the proximal flange may also be deployed inside the echoendoscope.[29] The unsheathed proximal flange may then be released from the echoendoscope by advancement of the catheter hub, again while pulling back the echoendoscope. Deployment may be performed under endoscopic, endosonographic, and fluoroscopic visualization to help ensure proper placement. With experience, however, deployment completely under endosonographic visualization is possible, and may be preferred as a way to avoid improper deployment due to excess traction on the deployment catheter (Figs. 58.5 and 58.6).

An electrocautery-enhanced delivery system ("hot AXIOS") enables placement of the AXIOS stent in a single step by obviating the need for initial 19-guage needle puncture of the collection cavity, guidewire insertion, and puncture tract dilation. The system has an electrocautery component comprised of two radially distributed diathermic wires that converge around the guidewire lumen at the catheter tip, allowing for direct cavity penetration and transmural advancement of the stent delivery catheter without tract dilation (Fig. 58.7). Thus, delivery can be performed in an exchange-free manner, which may make PFC drainage faster and safer.

A pilot study in 2012 using the AXIOS LAMS reported drainage of 15 symptomatic pseudocysts with achievement of a 100% therapeutic success rate and 0% recurrence rate at 11-month follow-up.[31] A subsequent multicenter trial reported achieving technical success in 91% of patients with either pseudocysts or

WON (n = 33) with use of the AXIOS LAMS.[32] Table 58.1 summarizes a published series involving LAMS placement for pseudocyst or WON management.

Plastic Versus Metal

A systematic review by Bang et al (2015) of seventeen studies involving 881 total patients compared outcomes of plastic versus metal stent placement for transmural drainage of PFCs.[33] Although this review included studies examining drainage of both pseudocysts and WON, subgroup analysis of each fluid collection

type was performed. No difference was found in treatment success, adverse event rates, or recurrence rates between FCSEMS or plastic stent drainage. It was concluded that available evidence did not support the routine use of metal stents for pseudocyst drainage, particularly given their higher price. Of note, the metal stent studies included in this review consisted of only a small number of patients (maximum n = 22).

A retrospective comparison of double pigtail plastic stents versus FCSEMS for pseudocyst drainage involved 230 patients. In this study, stent type was not associated with differences in technical success (92% vs. 98% for double pigtail plastic vs. FCSEMS, $p = 0.06$).[28] Placement of a FCSEMS, however, was associated with a significantly higher rate of complete pseudocyst resolution, which occurred in 98% of pseudocysts drained with a FCSEMS versus 89% drained with double pigtail plastic stents at 12-month follow-up ($p = 0.01$). FCSEMS placement also was

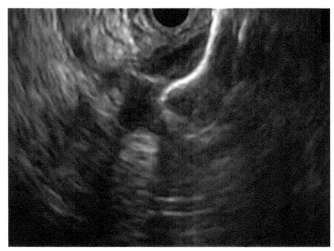

FIG 58.5 Lumen-apposing metal stent (LAMS) deployed into a pancreatic fluid collection (PFC). (From Rinninella E, Kunda R, Dollhopf M, et al: EUS-guided drainage of pancreatic fluid collections using a novel lumen-apposing metal stent on an electrocautery-enhanced delivery system: a large retrospective study [with video]. *Gastrointest Endosc* 82[6]:1039–1046, 2015.)

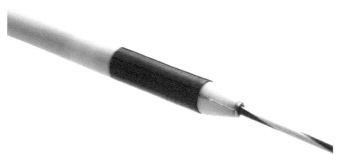

FIG 58.7 Electrocautery-enhanced delivery system (Hot AXIOS). (Courtesy Boston Scientific, Marlborough, MA. From Rinninella E, Kunda R, Dollhopf M, et al: EUS-guided drainage of pancreatic fluid collections using a novel lumen-apposing metal stent on an electrocautery-enhanced delivery system: a large retrospective study [with video]. *Gastrointest Endosc* 82[6]:1039–1046, 2015.)

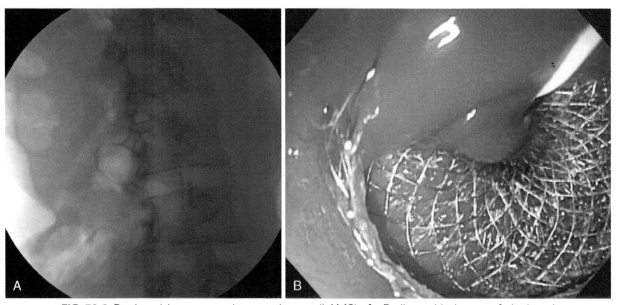

FIG 58.6 Deployed lumen-apposing metal stent (LAMS). **A,** Radiographic image of deployed LAMS. **B,** Endoscopic image of deployed LAMS with drainage of pseudocyst contents. (From Siddiqui AA, Adler DG, Nieto J, et al: EUS-guided drainage of peripancreatic fluid collections and necrosis by using a novel lumen-apposing stent: a large retrospective, multicenter US experience [with videos]. *Gastrointest Endosc* 83[4]:699–707, 2016.)

TABLE 58.1 Reported Outcomes From Published Series of Lumen-Apposing Metal Stent Placement for Management of Pancreatic Pseudocysts or WON

Author	Year	LAMS	N	PFC Type	Therapeutic Success	Clinical Success[‡‡]	Recurrence	Follow-up (mos)	Adverse Event
Sharaiha et al[28]	2016	AXIOS	124	WON	100%	86.3%	4.8%	4	18.5%
Siddiqui et al[51]	2016	AXIOS	14	PP	85.7%	85.7%	0%	8	7.1%
Siddiqui et al[51]	2016	AXIOS	68	WON	199%	88.2%	1.5%	9	5.9%
Rinninella et al[30]	2015	Hot AXIOS	93	PP/WON	98.9%	92.5%	0%	10.7	5.3%
Walter et al[57]	2015	AXIOS	61	PP/WON	98%	85%	NR	NR	9%
Shah et al[80]	2015	AXIOS	33	PP/WON	91%	85%	NR	NR	15.2%
Gornals et al[81]	2013	AXIOS	9	PP/WON	88.8%	88.8%	12.5%	12.5	11.1%
Itoi, et al[31]	2012	AXIOS	15	PP	100%	100%	0%	11.4	0%

[‡‡]Rate calculation incorporates cases of therapeutic failure as well.
LAMS, lumen-apposing metal stent; *NR,* not reported; *PFC,* pancreatic fluid collection; *PP,* pseudocyst; *WON,* walled-off necrosis.

associated with a reduced rate of adverse events at 30 days (31% vs. 16%, $p = 0.006$). With multivariate analysis, adverse events were 2.9 times more likely with use of double pigtail stents after adjustment for age, sex, number of endoscopy sessions, date of procedure, and original pseudocyst size. No difference occurred in long-term adverse event and recurrence rates.

Surgery Versus Endoscopic Drainage

A 2016 Cochrane review performed on management strategies for pancreatic pseudocysts examined four randomized control trials consisting of comparisons among open surgical drainage, EUS-guided drainage, endoscopic drainage, and EUS-guided drainage with nasocystic catheter drainage.[3] Short-term, health-related quality of life (at 4 weeks to 3 months) was worse following open surgical drainage versus EUS-guided drainage. The cost of surgery was also significantly higher. Statistically significant shorter hospital stays occurred following EUS-guided drainage with nasocystic drainage as opposed to EUS-guided drainage alone, endoscopic drainage, or open surgical drainage. Finally, EUS-guided drainage led to discharge faster than open surgical drainage, though hospital stay was the longest following endoscopic drainage alone.

A randomized trial has shown that endoscopic drainage has similar technical success and complication rates, but results in shorter stay, higher physical and mental health component scores, and lower costs compared to surgical cystgastrostomy.[2]

Endoscopic Versus Percutaneous Drainage

Endoscopic drainage has been found on a retrospective review to be favorable to percutaneous drainage with less need for repeat procedures, shorter hospitalization, and decreased need for follow-up imaging while having statistically equivalent rates of technical success, clinical success and adverse events.[34]

NECROSECTOMY

Surgical

Open surgical necrosectomy has been the traditional method for management of WON. Open necrosectomy, however, may cause significant morbidity and mortality. Mortality rates are particularly high within 14 days after onset of necrotizing pancreatitis, and early surgery within this time frame is not recommended.[35] Besselink et al (2007)[36] showed that surgery on day 30 or later following admission for necrotizing pancreatitis was associated with significantly lower mortality rates than earlier intervention (75% for days 1–14, 45% for days 15–29, 8% for day 30 or later). The mortality benefit that occurs with operative delay persists despite stratification for presence of preoperative organ failure and multiple organ failure.[36] A systematic review by the same authors of 11 studies with 1136 patients found a median mortality rate of 25% for open necrosectomy, with a range of 12% to 56%. This review confirmed the association between timing of intervention and mortality. Laparoscopic transperitoneal and retroperitoneal approaches are now preferred methods for surgical drainage.

Percutaneous

Percutaneous drainage serves as an alternative option for less invasive débridement of pancreatic necrosis, obviating the need for surgery in 30% to 100% of patients specifically with infected necrosis. In a series of 18 patients, Wronski et al (2013) reported complete resolution of infected necrosis by ultrasound-guided percutaneous catheter drain placement in 33% of patients, though the remaining patients eventually required surgical necrosectomy.[37] An overall mortality rate of 17% occurred with this management strategy. Another series of 34 patients with infected necrosis reported use of multiple large-bore percutaneous catheters with aggressive drainage. An average of three catheter sites with four exchanges were used. Surgery was avoided in 47% of patients with an overall mortality rate of 12%.[38] Bello and Matthews (2013) reviewed eight studies examining percutaneous drainage, involving a total of 286 patients.[39] Percutaneous access was performed via ultrasound or CT guidance, and drains were used with a diameter ranging from 10 to 28 Fr. Saline flush of the drains was typically performed every 8 hours. In this review, 44% of patients had successful therapy with avoidance of surgical necrosectomy. An overall mortality rate of 20% was reported and complications occurred in 28%, including multiple organ failure, colonic perforation, intraabdominal bleeding, and GI and pancreatic fistulae. Though percutaneous drainage is frequently inadequate for definitive management of pancreatic necrosis, a step-up approach, consisting of initial percutaneous drainage of a necrotic collection followed by minimally invasive retroperitoneal necrosectomy, if necessary, is now standard. The PANTER (Minimally Invasive Step Up Approach versus Maximal Necrosectomy in Patients with Acute Necrotizing Pancreatitis) trial found a decrease in the primary endpoint of death or composite of major complications with this step-up approach as compared to open necrosectomy (40% vs. 69%, $p = 0.0006$).[8]

Even if percutaneous drainage alone is adequate, significant morbidity may occur. Within the literature, a high rate of pancreaticocutaneous and pancreaticoenteric fistula formation occurs with pancreatic drainage approximately 20% of the time.[40] Furthermore, percutaneous drainage requires frequent catheter care, repeat procedures with upsizing of catheters, and frequent repeat cross-sectional imaging. WON may alternatively be managed endoscopically by direct endoscopic necrosectomy.

Endoscopic

Direct endoscopic necrosectomy was first reported by Seifert et al (2001) in three patients who had failed endoscopic plastic stent drainage of WON.[41] A stoma is created between the gastroenteric lumen and the walled-off collection for direct entry into the necrotic cavity with the endoscope. Débridement and removal of necrotic tissue is performed using various endoscopic accessories (Fig. 58.8, Video 58.1). A retrospective comparison by Gardner et al (2009) showed that direct endoscopic necrosectomy was superior to transmural endoscopic drainage, with successful resolution of necrotic cavities in 88% versus 45% of patients.[42] Direct endoscopic necrosectomy also resulted in decreased need for subsequent percutaneous drainage, standard surgical drainage, and collection recurrence.

Several publications depict endoscopic necrosectomy as a relatively favorable WON intervention. In 2011, Haghshenasskashani et al performed a systematic review of 260 patients in 10 series of patients with a total of 1100 endoscopic necrosectomy procedures.[43] Complete resolution of pancreatic necrosis was achieved 76% of the time, and the mortality rate was 5%. A median diagnosis to treatment interval of 6 weeks was present. In 2012, Bello and Matthews systemically reviewed 10 series involving endoscopic necrosectomy that reported success rates ranging from 59% to 100%.[39] Subsequent surgical necrosectomy was avoided in 78% of cases overall. Mortality ranged from 0% to 19% and was 5.6% overall. The mean complication rate reported was 28%.

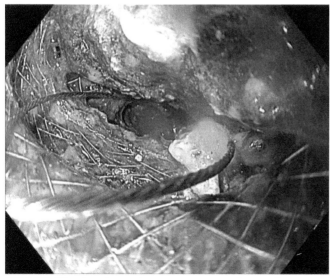

FIG 58.8 Direct endoscopic necrosectomy using a polypectomy snare.

A meta-analysis published in 2014 examined eight studies involving 233 patients with WON with a weighted mean necrotic cavity size of 12.9 cm.[44] A weighted mean of 4.1 procedures were necessary for necrotic cavity resolution. Endoscopic transmural necrosectomy had a pooled success rate of 82%. The pooled recurrence rate was 11% and complications occurred in 21%, consisting of bleeding, sepsis, and perforation. Surgery was ultimately required in 13% of patients.

Reported adverse event rates of EUS-guided treatment of WON ranges from 5% to 42%. The most significant adverse event rate associated with intervention of WON is infection, with an incidence of 15% to 26%. Additional complications include bleeding between direct endoscopic necrosectomy sessions, perforation/pneumoperitoneum, as well as stent migration, though stents are almost always retrieved successfully. Air and CO_2 embolisms are additional complications that may arise from blood vessel rupture with resultant direct insufflation into the bloodstream.[45] Air embolism has been reported to occur at a rate of 0.4%.[46]

Endoscopic Versus Surgical Necrosectomy

A 2016 Cochrane review of interventions for necrotizing pancreatitis examined eight randomized controlled trials, concluding that serious adverse events and adverse events were less frequent with an endoscopic-assisted minimally invasive step-up approach versus open necrosectomy. More adverse events occurred with the video-assisted minimally invasive surgery step-up approach group versus the endoscopic-assisted minimally invasive step-up approach group. The number of interventions, however, were less with the video-assisted versus endoscopic-assisted minimally invasive step-up approach.[4] The TENSION (transluminal endoscopic step-up approach versus minimally invasive surgical step-up approach in patients with infected necrotizing pancreatitis) trial is currently comparing endoscopic drainage followed by endoscopic necrosectomy, if necessary, versus percutaneous drainage followed by video-assisted necrosectomy, if necessary.

Bakker et al (2012) randomized patients with confirmed or suspected infected WON to endoscopic transgastric necrosectomy or surgical necrosectomy with either VARD, when possible, or open laparotomy if necessary.[47] The primary endpoint examined was level of interleukin 6 following necrosectomy as a measure of the postprocedure inflammatory response, which was lower following endoscopic necrosectomy ($p = 0.004$). A secondary endpoint of a composite of major complications or death was significantly lower with endoscopic necrosectomy versus surgery (20% vs. 80%, $p = 0.02$). Additionally, significantly less pancreatic fistulae occurred with endoscopic necrosectomy (10% vs. 70%).

Endoscopic Necrosectomy Versus Percutaneous Drainage

In 2014, a step-up approach with initial percutaneous drainage was compared to direct endoscopic necrosectomy in 24 patients. Resolution occurred in 92% of patients undergoing endoscopic necrosectomy versus 25% who underwent percutaneous drainage. The endoscopic necrosectomy group also had lower rates of antibiotic use, pancreatic insufficiency, and hospitalization.[48]

Endoscopic Necrosectomy Technique

Endoscopic necrosectomy requires the creation of a cystogastrostomy or cystoenterostomy tract that is large enough to allow the passage of an endoscope directly into the cavity. A tract of 15 to 20 mm diameter is usually created by balloon catheter dilation, but can also be created with a large diameter metal stent (see following section). Necrosectomy is performed using snares, forceps, baskets, and forceful irrigation. Intersession irrigation of the necrotic cavity with saline and/or hydrogen peroxide may be performed via a nasocystic catheter. Hydrogen peroxide irrigation of the collection cavity during endoscopy may decrease procedure duration, complication rates, and the total number of endoscopic necrosectomy sessions required.[40] Repeat necrosectomy sessions are performed until débridement of necrotic material within the cavity is complete.

Metal Stents (FCSEMS or LAMS) for WON

FCSEMS may enhance endoscopic drainage of WON. Esophageal FCSEMS have a lumen diameter that will permit endoscope advancement through the deployed, expanded stent. In 2014, two case series were published describing use of esophageal FCSEMS for WON drainage. One study consisted of 17 patients with a complete resolution rate of 88% over an average of five necrosectomy sessions.[49] The other involved 10 patients with a resolution rate of 90% after an average of three necrosectomy sessions.[50]

LAMS have large lumens, which can be immediately dilated following placement to enable direct endoscopic exploration and débridement of the necrotic cavity. The dumbbell structure of these stents allows for more aggressive manipulation without stent dislodgement during the index endoscopic session. The lumen-apposing nature of these stents intends to reduce rates of perforation and leak, particularly in cases where the mature necrotic fluid collection is not entirely adherent to the gastrointestinal wall.

In a large, US multicenter, retrospective study of patients who underwent EUS-guided drainage of PFCs using the AXIOS stent,[51] 68 of 80 patients had WON with a mean PFC size of 11.8 cm. Successful LAMS placement was achieved in 97.5% of patients. Endoscopic débridement was performed through the LAMS in 54 patients requiring a mean of 2.8 +/− 1.3 sessions. Stents remained patent in 98.7% of cases. Overall, endoscopic therapy with use of the LAMS was successful in 88.2% of patients with WON. One patient had PFC recurrence within the 3-month median follow-up. The procedure-related adverse event rate was 9.8%, with complications consisting of self-limiting bleeding, stent maldeployment (n = 2), and gastric perforation following stent maldeployment in one patient requiring surgical repair.

A retrospective comparison of LAMS versus FCSEMS has shown LAMS may facilitate complete resolution of WON in fewer procedures (p = 0.04).[52] Use of LAMS may cause more early adverse events, however, than either FCSEMS or plastic stents (OR 6.6, p = 0.02).

Flared-type biflanged metal stents that are not lumen-apposing have been used for the treatment of WON. In an ex vivo study, biflanged stents were found to have a higher migration rate than LAMS.[31] LAMS were also found to have a higher lumen-apposing force than the biflanged stent.[53]

It is unclear if metal stents should be removed after cavity resolution. Removal is typically pursued, however, given uncertainty regarding long-term adverse effects. Specifically, indefinite stent indwelling could potentially result in migration of food into the collection cavity, bleeding from tissue erosion, or, occasionally, stent burial. In a 2016 ongoing trial comparing LAMS and plastic stents for WON drainage, high rates of delayed complications due to persistent indwelling LAMS have been observed.[54] Stent-related bleeding, stent burial, and stent-induced

biliary obstruction occurred in 50% of patients receiving LAMS, whereas 0% of plastic stent participants had stent-related adverse events. As LAMS-related events all occurred over 3 weeks after placement, these complications prompted a change in protocol to earlier imaging assessment at 3 weeks followed by LAMS removal if WON resolution was demonstrated. The authors hypothesize that the stiff, immobile nature of LAMS, in contrast to flexible, mobile plastic stents, promotes tissue and vascular erosion and impingement upon WON cavity collapse. Nonetheless, other studies have not observed adverse event rates nearly as high when employing LAMS for WON management.[32,55–58]

Plastic Versus Metal Stents for WON

A two-center, retrospective comparison of EUS-guided drainage of PFCs with double pigtail plastic stents versus a flared-type biflanged FCSEMS (not lumen-apposing) showed that plastic stent use was associated with increased need for repeat drainage procedures (34.2% vs. 6.3% of patients).[59] This study is limited by the lack of stratified outcomes based upon the initial collection characteristics (pseudocyst or WON). Stent migration occurred in 18.4% of cases using plastic stents versus 6.3% of cases using the biflanged, but this difference was not statistically significant. Overall, this study did support a benefit to use of FCSEMS over plastic stents. Although technical success occurred in 100% of cases, inadequate drainage occurred in significantly more patients with plastic stents (26.3% vs. 0%). The initial clinical success rate was 92% in those with FCSEMS versus 65% in those with plastic stents (p = 0.074). Furthermore, though the overall cost of plastic stent use was lower in patients with noninfected pseudocysts, the advantage was not seen for infected pseudocysts or WON due to a reduced need for interventions using FCSEMS.

A single-center, retrospective series showed no difference between plastic stents and LAMS for treatment of WON in terms of technical success, clinical success, or adverse events, even though the plastic stent group had significantly larger WON.[60] Mean procedure times were shorter for the LAMS group for initial EUS-guided drainage and reintervention, however, and no difference in total cost was present between plastic stent and LAMS use.

As previously mentioned, a systematic review published by Bang et al in 2015 compared the use of FCSEMS versus plastic stents for PFC drainage.[33] No difference was detected in the pooled rate of overall treatment success for PFCs, specifically in patients with WON (78% vs. 70%). No difference occurred in either the rate of adverse events or fluid collection recurrence. No studies in this review were direct comparative studies, however. Siddiqui et al (2017) published a retrospective comparison of 313 patients with WON who underwent endoscopic intervention using either double pigtail plastic stents or 10-mm biliary metal stents (FCSEMS or LAMS).[52] Though therapeutic success was comparable regardless of stent type, long-term resolution of WON was more successful using metal stents (95% vs. 81%, p = 0.01). No prospective trials have compared the use of plastic versus metal stents in the management of WON. In some cases, initial placement of a LAMS for facilitation of direct endoscopic necrosectomy may be pursued followed by removal of the LAMS and long-term placement of multiple transmural plastic stents. This approach may be helpful in patients with a disconnected pancreatic tail that are poor surgical candidates. Exchange of the LAMS for plastic stents allows long-term management of the PFC, which may otherwise be expected to recur in the presence of duct disruption, and avoids complications of long-term LAMS indwelling, such as tissue erosions and hemorrhage.

Several questions exist regarding the role of FCSEMS and LAMS in drainage of WON. Further study is necessary to determine if the theoretical advantages of LAMS are borne out in clinical practice. In prospective trials, does single-step deployment decrease the rate of adverse events by improving the efficiency and simplicity of the procedure? If metal stents are advantageous compared to plastic stents, are LAMS more beneficial compared to FCSEMS? Does LAMS placement decrease the need for necrosectomy entirely? Is the use of LAMS cost-effective?[29] Other issues to address in the future are the role and duration of antibiotics following transmural endoscopic stent placement as well as the role of nasocystic catheter drainage. No studies have examined the role of nasocystic catheter drainage as adjunct therapy to transmural FCSEMS or LAMS in the management of PFCs. The larger stent lumen of an esophageal FCSEMS or 15-mm LAMS may reduce the need for nasocystic catheter irrigation and drainage. Consideration for nasocystic catheter drain placement should be made, however, particularly when infected necrosis is present.

TRANSPAPILLARY STENTING IN PFC MANAGEMENT

Questions have also surrounded the adjunct role of transpapillary pancreatic duct stenting in patients undergoing transmural drainage of PFCs. Pancreatic ductal leaks or disruption are the underlying mechanism of acute and mature PFCs. Spontaneous resolution of PFCs may occur in only 0% to 5% of patients with persistent ductal disruption compared to a normal pancreatic duct.[61] Acute pancreatic duct leaks are traditionally treated by transpapillary stent placement. In theory, treatment of persistent pancreatic ductal leaks or disruption may help promote resolution of pancreatic fluid collections, as well when applied as adjunct therapy to endoscopic transmural drainage.

Previous retrospective studies have suggested that transpapillary stenting may be an augmenting therapy for patients receiving endoscopic transmural drainage of PFCs.[62] Transpapillary drainage alone may be effective in the management of PFCs if the cavity communicates with the pancreatic duct, but there is concern for increased risk of PFC superinfection.[63] Transpapillary drainage alone could be considered in cases of small PFCs (< 4 cm) or when transmural drainage is not feasible. It is the practice at the author's institution to place two stents: one extending into the fluid collection, and the other across the area of pancreatic duct leak. As adjunct therapy, a 2016 multicenter, retrospective comparison of EUS-guided transmural drainage alone versus combined transmural and transpapillary drainage of pancreatic pseudocysts, showed no therapeutic benefit to adjunctive transpapillary drainage. Transpapillary drainage actually negatively affected the rate of long-term resolution of the pancreatic fluid collections (OR 0.11, 95% CI 0.02–0.8, $p = 0.03$).[64] Of note, the pancreatic duct stent traversed the site of ductal disruption in only 36.2% of cases. It is possible that bridging of the defect may have resulted in better outcomes, as bridging across the disruption has been associated with improved outcomes previously.[65] Nonetheless, in subgroup analysis of patients in which a pancreatic duct stent did successfully bridge the site of disruption, transpapillary drainage still added no benefit to transmural drainage.[66] Thus, at our institution, pancreatogram is only pursued in the setting of fluid collection recurrence to document the

presence of a disconnected duct. These patients would then require either surgical intervention or long-term stent placement with transmural plastic stents and possible transpapillary stent placement.

PANCREATIC DUCT LEAKS

Pancreatic leaks may result from trauma either from acute or chronic pancreatitis, direct pancreatic injury from abdominal trauma, or iatrogenic injury during endoscopy or surgery. Apart from manifesting as mature pancreatic fluid collections, pancreatic duct leaks may also result in external or internal fistulae. Magnetic resonance cholangiopancreatography (MRCP) and secretin-MRCP can delineate the ductal anatomy as a noninvasive method of diagnosing pancreatic duct leaks. Fluid aspiration of immature PFCs with amylase analysis can also be performed to diagnose pancreatic duct leaks. Endoscopic retrograde cholangiopancreatography (ERCP) with pancreatogram is the most sensitive method of detecting pancreatic duct leaks and disruption (Fig. 58.9).

Internal fistulae result from ductal disruption with the manifestation depending on the location of disruption. Anterior disruption may result in pancreatic ascites, whereas posterior disruption can lead to a mediastinal pseudocyst or pleural fistula.[67] Initial noninvasive management of pancreatic duct leaks may be pursued with bowel rest, deep enteral feeding, and use of octreotide. Conservative management is frequently ineffective, however, failing approximately 50% of the time. Failure occurs even more frequently in patients with advanced pancreatitis.[68]

Given the frequent inefficacy of noninvasive management, endoscopic therapy may be pursued as initial or second-line therapy. Transpapillary pancreatic duct stenting is effective in promoting leak healing by reducing the resistance of transpapillary flow by bypassing potential pancreatic duct strictures and stones and the sphincter of Oddi.[69] Tanaka et al (2013) reported on a series of six patients with internal pancreatic fistulae and associated downstream pancreatic duct stenosis.[67] Endoscopic therapy

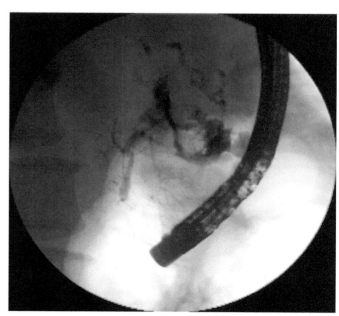

FIG 58.9 Pancreatic duct leak on pancreatogram. Completely disconnected pancreatic duct.

was performed with placement of a 5-Fr or 7-Fr plastic stent, with intention to perform stent exchange for a total duration of 1 year. Stent placement across the site of stenosis was successful in 100% of patients. Treatment was successful with resolution of leak in 66% of patients (four out of six), though one of these had recurrence refractory to further stenting. Despite endoscopic therapy, however, 50% eventually required surgery for definitive management (due to continuous pain with leak or intracystic bleeding). Bridging of the site of pancreatic duct disruption and long duration of stent therapy may enhance the efficacy of transpapillary stent therapy.[70] A more recent (2016) large series of 107 patients with pancreatic duct disruption showed that pancreatic duct stent placement resulted in healing of the leak in 75% of patients. Ninety-six percent had successful pancreatic duct stent placement, but bridging of the point of disruption was successful in only 44% of patients.[71] In cases where the disruption point was not bridged, treatment success was only 48%. In both these series, acute pancreatitis as the etiology of pancreatic duct disruption predicted poor response to pancreatic duct stenting. The presence of complete duct disruption was also predictive of failure of therapy.

In patients specifically with pleural fistulae, medical and endoscopic therapy is also typically advised prior to surgical intervention due to the latter's morbidity. Prior to intervention, pancreatic pleural fistulae can be differentiated from reactive pleural effusions that may develop in the setting of acute pancreatitis based upon the presence of a high amylase concentration within the pleural fluid. Imaging may also help diagnose a pancreatic pleural fistula. CT has a 47% sensitivity for detection of the fistulous tract, whereas MRCP and ERCP have roughly 80% sensitivity. For pleural fistulae, ERCP with transpapillary stenting is the standard endoscopic therapy. Following transpapillary stenting, diagnostic ERCP can be performed every 4 to 6 weeks for stent exchange or removal based upon assessment of fistula closure. The majority of patients with pleural fistulae that respond to endotherapeutic stenting have a stent that bridges the site of disruption. Endoscopic management fails in a significant proportion of patients, however.[72] Due to high failure rate, preintervention MRCP findings may be useful in guiding management strategies. Those with normal pancreatic ducts without downstream strictures may respond to conservative medical therapy. If a ductal stricture is present or disruption is noted in the head or body of the pancreas, endoscopic therapy may be the most appropriate first-line therapy. If there is complete ductal obstruction or both stricture and leakage from within the pancreatic tail, however, surgical treatment may be most appropriate due to the poor success of endoscopic stenting.[73]

The treatment of external pancreatic fistulae is similar to that of internal fistulae. In cases of conservative management failure, endoscopic transpapillary stenting may be pursued prior to surgical intervention. In addition, endoscopic fibrin glue injection has been reported for closure of pancreaticocutaneous fistula.[74]

Disconnected Duct Syndrome

Disconnected duct syndrome denotes the presence of a pancreatic leak resulting from complete transection of the pancreatic duct (see Fig. 58.9). Excretions from the upstream proximal pancreas thus drain entirely into the abdominal cavity. Surgical treatment has been the primary management modality for disconnected duct syndrome. Due to the inability to pass a guidewire into the disconnected duct, transpapillary placement of a pancreatic duct stent is typically not effective because bridging of the ductal

defect cannot be performed.[69] Varadarajulu et al (2005) have reported success in only 26% of cases with attempted transpapillary stent placement.[65]

As an alternative to surgery or endoscopic transpapillary stenting, endoscopic transmural stenting may be performed for creation of a fistula between the fluid collection and the GI tract. Permanent transmural stenting thus produces long-term drainage of the isolated pancreatic segment. Téllez-Ávila et al (2016) reported a series of 21 patients with confirmed disconnected duct syndrome (by MRCP or ERCP) who underwent transmural stent placement with two 7 Fr by 4 cm double pigtail stents.[75] Technical success was achieved in 100% of patients and clinical success in 81% after a median follow-up of 28 months. In those with clinical success, 20% had recurrence for which a second endoscopic treatment was successful, consisting of tract dilation with direct endoscopic necrosectomy followed by placement of two double pigtail stents. Reported complications included stent migration (10%), infection after drainage (5%), infection after stent migration (5%), and suspected stent migration with perforation (5%), though perforation was not actually confirmed after surgical exploration.[69]

As noted previously, if duct disruption results in formation of a mature fluid collection (pseudocyst or WON), transmural drainage is often adequate therapy and transpapillary pancreatic duct stenting does not seem to provide adjunct benefit.[64] Larsen and Kozarek (2014) have reported a combined endoscopic and percutaneous approach for patients with WON and disconnected duct syndrome. At their center, frequent development of external pancreaticocutaneous fistulae with solely percutaneous drainage prompted use of combined percutaneous and transmural drainage. In this scenario, plastic transmural stents were left in place indefinitely. This approach prevented development of cutaneous fistulae and successfully avoided need for surgery in more than 95% of patients.[69]

Postsurgical Acute Pancreatic Fluid Collections

Pancreatic duct leaks with resultant acute postoperative PFCs occur in approximately 30% of patients following pancreatic surgeries such as pancreaticoduodenectomy, pancreatic enucleation, and distal pancreatectomy. Spontaneous resolution typically will occur over days to weeks. Symptomatic collections may present with severe pain, gastric outlet obstruction, or intraabdominal infection and sepsis. Classic management consists of bowel rest, TPN, antibiotics, and possible intravenous octreotide. In approximately 20% to 40% of cases, further management may be necessary, at which time percutaneous drainage is traditionally pursued. Percutaneous drainage is effective, but presence of an external drain may decrease patient quality of life, requires monitoring of fluid output, catheter flushing, and possible catheter exchange. In cases of persistent leak, pancreatic duct stenting may also be indicated. Pancreatic duct stenting is not effective, however, if disrupted duct syndrome is present where there is complete transection of the pancreatic duct. Furthermore, large or infected peripancreatic fluid collections may not resolve quickly with a transpapillary stent. The risk of post-ERCP pancreatitis also detracts from the appeal of transpapillary stenting.

EUS-guided transmural drainage has been advocated as a possible therapeutic option for acute postoperative PFCs. In 2009, Varadarajulu et al reported a prospective series of 10 patients undergoing EUS-guided plastic stent drainage of PFCs after distal pancreatectomy with 100% technical success, and 90% therapeutic success, though it is unclear if any of these postoperative collections were acute.[76] A subsequent retrospective comparison of EUS-guided drainage (using one to three double pigtail stents) and percutaneous drainage of 23 patients with symptomatic PFCs following pancreatic enucleation or distal pancreatectomy showed 100% technical success with either method, but a higher rate of clinical success (defined as radiographic resolution of collection, stent, or removal, and symptomatic improvement) with EUS-guided drainage.[77] Necrosectomy was required in five patients with EUS-guided drainage, and two patients had concurrent ERCP with pancreatic duct stent placement. Most patients in this study were referred from an outside hospital with the possibility that varying surgical approaches, closure methods, and underlying histology may bias leak rates and subsequent clinical improvement. Furthermore, the maturity of fluid collections within this study were unknown and may not have been comparable between the two treatment groups.

In 2014, Tilara et al reported a retrospective analysis of 31 patients who underwent EUS-guided drainage of postoperative fluid collections developing following pancreatic resection.[78] A proportion of these patients had acute collections. The indications for PFC drainage were abdominal pain, infection, gastric outlet obstruction, and biliary obstruction. One to three double pigtail stents, 7 Fr or 10 Fr in diameter, were deployed. If symptoms persisted and PFC size did not improve on cross-sectional imaging 4 weeks postdrainage, repeated endoscopy with tract dilation, new stent insertion, and necrosectomy were performed, which was necessary in 19% of patients. Technical success was achieved in 100% of patients. PFC resolution on imaging with clinical improvement occurred in 93% of patients. Among all cases, 55% had successful early drainage within 30 days postoperatively. Forty-two percent of these patients had drainage performed within 2 weeks of surgery. Early drainage was not associated with increased complications. One complication occurred in patients undergoing early drainage: a bleed from a splenic artery stump.

Of note, the indication for drainage in patients undergoing early EUS-guided drainage was infection (fever, leukocytosis, or abscess formation) in 70% of cases. In those undergoing drainage within two weeks of surgery, the indication for drainage was infection or sepsis in all cases. Thus, most patients undergoing early EUS-guided drainage of postoperative collections had signs of sepsis necessitating drainage prior to maturation of the PFC. The authors propose that maturity of fluid collection may be less important for drainage of postoperative PFCs versus those that arise from pancreatitis adhesion formation; scarring may effectively compartmentalize the surgical bed and may limit intraperitoneal spillage. Further studies are necessary, however, to prove the safety of endoscopic transmural drainage of acute collections, particularly in the absence of preexisting infection necessitating early intervention.

CONCLUSION

Disruption of the main or secondary pancreatic ducts can result in pancreatic leaks and development of PFCs as a complication of pancreatitis, trauma, or iatrogenesis. In general, PFCs are best observed over time to allow for their likely spontaneous regression. When PFC drainage is indicated by persistent symptoms or evidence of infection, however, endoscopic transmural drainage has become a first-line therapy in lieu of surgical intervention. Appropriate management nonetheless rests on a multidisciplinary collaboration involving interventional radiology and surgery.

Overall, endoscopic management is an efficacious treatment modality for pancreatic pseudocysts. Further prospective trials are necessary to establish the benefits of metal stents over plastic stents, particularly given their increased cost. Further study is also required to determine ideal stent length, the need for nasocystic catheter placement, the need for dilation of FCSEMS after placement, the benefit of same-session pseudocyst exploration through the FCSEMS, and the benefit of internal plastic stent placement for metal stent anchoring.[79] The use of lumen-apposing metal stents over traditional stent design has the theoretical advantages of reducing stent migration and reducing stent erosion. LAMS design may be most useful, however, in cases of walled-off necrosis, in which the large stent diameter facilitates persistent drainage and the lumen-apposing flanges establish a more secure anastomosis that enables immediate direct endoscopic exploration and necrosectomy of the necrotic cavity.

KEY REFERENCES

1. Banks PA, Bollen TL, Dervenis C, et al: Classification of acute pancreatitis–2012: revision of the Atlanta classification and definitions by international consensus, *Gut* 62(1):102–111, 2013.
2. Varadarajulu S, Bang JY, Sutton BS, et al: Equal efficacy of endoscopic and surgical cystogastrostomy for pancreatic pseudocyst drainage in a randomized trial, *Gastroenterology* 145(3):583–590, e1, 2013.
3. Gurusamy KS, Pallari E, Hawkins N, et al: Management strategies for pancreatic pseudocysts, *Cochrane Database Syst Rev* (4):CD011392, 2016.
4. Gurusamy KS, Belgaumkar AP, Haswell A, et al: Interventions for necrotising pancreatitis, *Cochrane Database Syst Rev* (4):CD011383, 2016.
8. van Santvoort HC, Besselink MG, Cirkel GA, Gooszen HG: A nationwide Dutch study into the optimal treatment of patients with infected necrotising pancreatitis: the PANTER trial, *Ned Tijdschr Geneeskd* 150(33):1844–1846, 2006.
11. Baron TH, Harewood GC, Morgan DE, Yates MR: Outcome differences after endoscopic drainage of pancreatic necrosis, acute pancreatic pseudocysts, and chronic pancreatic pseudocysts, *Gastrointest Endosc* 56(1):7–17, 2002.
18. Ballard D, Cote G: Endoscopic (without endoscopic ultrasound guidance drainage of pancreatic fluid collections, *Techn Gastrointest Endosc* 14: 199–203, 2012.
21. Park DH, Lee SS, Moon SH, et al: Endoscopic ultrasound-guided versus conventional transmural drainage for pancreatic pseudocysts: a prospective randomized trial, *Endoscopy* 41(10):842–848, 2009.
28. Sharaiha RZ, Tyberg A, Khashab MA, et al: Endoscopic therapy with lumen-apposing metal stents is safe and effective for patients with pancreatic walled-off necrosis, *Clin Gastroenterol Hepatol* 14(12): 1797–1803, 2016.
31. Itoi T, Binmoeller KF, Shah J, et al: Clinical evaluation of a novel lumen-apposing metal stent for endosonography-guided pancreatic pseudocyst and gallbladder drainage (with videos), *Gastrointest Endosc* 75(4):870–876, 2012.
32. Shah RJ, Shah JN, Waxman I, et al: Safety and efficacy of endoscopic ultrasound-guided drainage of pancreatic fluid collections with lumen-apposing covered self-expanding metal stents, *Clin Gastroenterol Hepatol* 13(4):747–752, 2015.
33. Bang JY, Hawes R, Bartolucci A, Varadarajulu S: Efficacy of metal and plastic stents for transmural drainage of pancreatic fluid collections: a systematic review, *Dig Endosc* 27(4):486–498, 2015.
40. Tyberg A, Karia K, Gabr M, et al: Management of pancreatic fluid collections: a comprehensive review of the literature, *World J Gastroenterol* 22(7):2256–2270, 2016.
42. Gardner TB, Chahal P, Papachristou GI, et al: A comparison of direct endoscopic necrosectomy with transmural endoscopic drainage for the treatment of walled-off pancreatic necrosis, *Gastrointest Endosc* 69(6): 1085–1094, 2009.

48. Kumar N, Conwell DL, Thompson CC: Direct endoscopic necrosectomy versus step-up approach for walled-off pancreatic necrosis: comparison of clinical outcome and health care utilization, *Pancreas* 43(8): 1334–1339, 2014.

51. Siddiqui AA, Adler DG, Nieto J, et al: EUS-guided drainage of peripancreatic fluid collections and necrosis by using a novel lumen-apposing stent: a large retrospective, multicenter U.S. experience (with videos), *Gastrointest Endosc* 83(4):699–707, 2016.

52. Siddiqui AA, Kowalski TE, Loren DE, et al: Fully covered self-expanding metal stents versus lumen-apposing fully covered self-expanding metal stent versus plastic stents for endoscopic drainage of pancreatic walled-off necrosis: clinical outcomes and success, *Gastrointest Endosc* 85(4):758–765, 2017.

55. Itoi T, Binmoeller KF, Shah J, et al: Clinical evaluation of a novel lumen-apposing metal stent for endosonography-guided pancreatic pseudocyst and gallbladder drainage (with videos), *Gastrointest Endosc* 75(4):870–876, 2012.

57. Walter D, Will U, Sanchez-Yague A, et al: A novel lumen-apposing metal stent for endoscopic ultrasound-guided drainage of pancreatic fluid collections: a prospective cohort study, *Endoscopy* 47(1):63–67, 2015.

59. Ang TL, Kongkam P, Kwek AB, et al: A two-center comparative study of plastic and lumen-apposing large diameter self-expandable metallic stents in endoscopic ultrasound-guided drainage of pancreatic fluid collections, *Endosc Ultrasound* 5(5):320–327, 2016.

64. Yang D, Amin S, Gonzalez S, et al: Transpapillary drainage has no added benefit on treatment outcomes in patients undergoing EUS-guided transmural drainage of pancreatic pseudocysts: a large multicenter study, *Gastrointest Endosc* 83(4):720–729, 2016.

69. Larsen M, Kozarek R: Management of pancreatic ductal leaks and fistulae, *J Gastroenterol Hepatol* 29(7):1360–1370, 2014.

80. Shah RJ, Shah JN, Waxman I, et al: Safety and efficacy of endoscopic ultrasound-guided drainage of pancreatic fluid collections with lumen-apposing covered self-expanding metal stents, *Clin Gastroenterol Hepatol* 13(4):747–752, 2015.

81. Gornals JB, De la Serna-Higuera C, Sánchez-Yague A, et al: Endosonography-guided drainage of pancreatic fluid collections with a novel lumen-apposing stent, *Surg Endosc* 27(4):1428–1434, 2013.

A complete reference list can be found online at ExpertConsult .com

59

Chronic Pancreatitis

Uzma D. Siddiqui and Robert H. Hawes

CHAPTER OUTLINE

INTRODUCTION

Chronic pancreatitis (CP) is an inflammatory condition that results in fibrosis causing destruction of pancreatic parenchyma and ducts. These permanent structural changes can lead to impairment of exocrine and endocrine function, biliary strictures, and may increase the chances of developing pancreatic cancer.[1]

This disorder contrasts with acute pancreatitis in that the latter is non-progressive, and the gland returns to histologic and functional normalcy once the acute event subsides. There does exist overlap between the two conditions, and recurrent episodes of acute pancreatitis may lead to more permanent chronic changes. The most common clinical presentation of CP is abdominal pain, which is multifactorial in nature, and if associated with only minimal pancreatic fibrosis, can lead to confusion over the diagnosis.

The role of endoscopy has focused on relieving abdominal pain and managing complications, but interpretation of data on this topic remains challenging due to varied presentations, clinical courses, and etiologies. Given the limitations of medical therapy and the invasiveness of surgical options, endoscopic therapy has been widely employed in the treatment of CP, but long-term randomized trials are lacking and therefore its role continues to evolve.

ETIOLOGY

Alcohol

Alcohol accounts for 70% to 80% of cases of CP (Table 59.1); the mechanism by which this occurs is unclear. The risk seems to be related to the duration and amount of alcohol consumed rather than the type of alcohol or the pattern of consumption.[2] Only 5% to 10% of alcoholics develop CP, suggesting that other unidentified factors may be important in the pathogenesis of the disease.[3]

Smoking

More recently, smoking has emerged as an independent risk factor for CP, as demonstrated in two studies by the North American Pancreas Study Group.[4,5] Similar to alcohol, the effects of smoking on the development of CP appear to be dose dependent, with risk increasing for people smoking more than one pack per day.[6] Furthermore, in those with alcohol-induced acute pancreatitis, smoking appears to be the strongest risk factor for progression to CP.[7,8]

Genetic Causes

Several mutations associated with CP have been identified. Mutations in the cationic trypsin gene (*PRSS1*) that lead to premature trypsinogen activation have been suggested as the cause of hereditary pancreatitis.[9–11] *PRSS1* inheritance is autosomal dominant with high penetrance. Cystic fibrosis is caused by mutations in the *CFTR* gene. Most patients with cystic fibrosis develop progressive pancreatic damage as a result of defective ductular and acinar pancreatic secretion.[12] In some series, mutations in the *CFTR* gene have been identified in 13% to 37% of patients with idiopathic CP who have no clinical evidence of cystic fibrosis.[13,14] This percentage range could be an underestimation because currently available genetic screening tests identify only 18 to 23 of the most severe *CFTR* mutations that cause classic childhood cystic fibrosis.

TABLE 59.1 Etiology of Chronic Pancreatitis

Alcohol	70%
Idiopathic	10%–30%
Other	10%–15%
Pancreatic duct obstruction (trauma, divisum, tumor, fibrosis)	
Hereditary (*CFTR* gene mutation, trypsinogen gene mutation)	
Hyperlipidemia	
Tropical	

CFTR, Cystic fibrosis transmembrane conductance regulator.

SPINK1 is expressed on pancreatic acinar cells during an inflammatory response and codes for a trypsin inhibitor. A mutation in *SPINK1* is not an independent risk factor for CP, but has been implicated in the progression of recurrent acute pancreatitis to CP.[15] *SPINK1* mutations are strongly associated with tropical calcific pancreatitis.[16] Co-inheritance of *SPINK1* with *CFTR* mutations can increase the risk of CP.[17,18]

Ductal Obstruction

Obstruction of the pancreatic duct from any cause can lead to CP. The histologic abnormalities that are induced may persist after relief of the obstruction.

Idiopathic Chronic Pancreatitis

An etiology for pancreatitis cannot be determined in 10% to 30% of patients with CP despite extensive investigations. Concealed alcohol ingestion, hypersensitivity to small amounts of alcohol, unreported pancreatic trauma, and mutations in the *CFTR* and trypsinogen genes may be contributing factors in at least a small proportion of patients with idiopathic CP.[19,20] Although in the past patients with idiopathic CP were considered as a single group, data from the Mayo Clinic have defined an early- and late-onset form.[21] Age distribution at onset of symptoms showed a bimodal distribution of patients with early- and late-onset idiopathic CP with a median age of 19.2 years for early onset and 56.2 years for late onset. No gender differences were observed among patients in either group.

CLINICAL FEATURES

Abdominal pain and pancreatic insufficiency are the two cardinal clinical manifestations of CP.

Abdominal Pain

Abdominal pain in CP is typically centered in the epigastric area and frequently radiates to the back. The pain is worsened with eating and is sometimes associated with nausea and vomiting. Early in the course of CP, the pain may occur in discrete attacks; as the condition progresses, pain tends to become more continuous.

The mechanism for abdominal pain is poorly understood. Causes are likely multifactorial and include inflammation, duct obstruction, high pancreatic tissue pressure, fibrotic encasement of sensory nerves, and neuropathy characterized by both increased numbers and sizes of intrapancreatic sensory nerves, and by inflammatory injury to the nerve sheaths allowing exposure of the neural elements to toxic substances.[22,23] The view that chronic pain subsides in a substantial number of patients as the disease progresses to the point of organ failure has been widely accepted, but that process may take an unpredictable number of years or may never occur.[24]

Furthermore, there has been increasing interest in the central nervous system's role in mediating pain in CP patients. One small study of 22 patients compared patients with CP versus healthy controls and stimulated pain electrically.[25] Electroencephalograms were recorded from 64 surface electrodes, and event-related brain potentials were obtained. The results demonstrated that pain in CP patients leads to changes in cortical projections of the nociceptive system. This has also been demonstrated in other conditions resulting in neuropathic pain, and should be taken into account when considering treatment approaches.

Pancreatic Insufficiency

Patients with severe pancreatic exocrine dysfunction cannot properly digest complex foods or absorb digestive breakdown products. Nevertheless, clinically significant protein and fat deficiencies do not occur until more than 90% of pancreatic function is lost.[26] In a large natural history study, the median time for development of pancreatic insufficiency was 13.1 years in patients with alcoholic CP, 16.1 years in patients with late-onset idiopathic CP, and 26.3 years in patients with early-onset idiopathic CP.[21]

Steatorrhea usually occurs before protein deficiencies because lipolytic activity decreases more quickly than proteolysis.[27,28] Glucose intolerance occurs frequently in CP, but overt diabetes mellitus usually occurs late in the course of disease. Nearly 40% to 70% of patients with CP develop diabetes on prolonged follow-up. In one study, the median time to develop diabetes was 19.8 years, 11.9 years, and 26.3 years in patients with alcoholic, late-onset idiopathic, and early-onset idiopathic CP.[21] The nature of diabetes in this patient population is brittle, and management is more complicated than that of patients with type 1 diabetes.

DIAGNOSIS

Advanced CP is more easily diagnosed when compared with early or mild disease, which may require interpretation of clinical symptoms, pancreatic function testing, and expert interpretation of imaging studies such as MRCP and EUS. Tests for CP can be classified into tests that evaluate its exocrine function (Table 59.2) or the structure of the gland (parenchyma, ductal anatomy, or both). Noninvasive pancreatic function tests yield sufficient diagnostic accuracy only in the advanced stages of the disease, and their sensitivity for detection of early or moderate CP is low.[29] Tests that evaluate pancreatic structure, although limited by sensitivity, are advantageous in that they are more widely available, and attempts have been made to develop standardized criteria for clinical use.

Tests of Pancreatic Function
Invasive or Direct Pancreatic Function Tests (Secretin Stimulation Test)

The basis for the secretin simulation test is that secretin (with or without cholecystokinin) causes the secretion of bicarbonate-rich fluid from the pancreas. Intravenous secretin is administered, duodenal juice is collected every 10 minutes for 1 hour (either through a duodenal catheter the patient swallows or at endoscopy), and bicarbonate measured. Peak bicarbonate less than 80 mmol/L

TABLE 59.2	Diagnostic Tests for Chronic Pancreatitis	
	FUNCTIONAL TESTS	
Structural Tests	**Indirect**	**Direct**
X-ray	Serum enzymes (trypsinogen)	Secretin stimulation test
Ultrasound	Fecal tests (fat, elastase, chymotrypsin)	
CT	Urine tests (bentiromide, pancreolauryl)	
MRCP		
ERCP		
EUS		

CT, Computed tomography; *ERCP,* endoscopic retrograde cholangiopancreatography; *EUS,* endoscopic ultrasound; *MRCP,* magnetic resonance cholangiopancreatography.

is a widely accepted threshold consistent with pancreatic exocrine insufficiency. Sensitivity ranges from 74% to 97%, and specificity ranges from 80% to 90%.[30–35] Limitations of this test (time consuming, expensive, no standardized results) have prevented it from gaining widespread use.

Noninvasive or Indirect Pancreatic Function Tests

There has been great effort and interest to develop noninvasive tests for evaluating pancreatic function. These tests are designed to measure pancreatic enzymes in blood or stool, or the effect of pancreatic enzymes on an orally administered substrate by collection of metabolites in the blood or urine.

Serum enzymes. Because CP is a patchy, focal disease with significant parenchymal fibrosis, pancreatic serum enzyme levels (amylase and lipase) are within normal range or only minimally elevated. Very low levels of serum trypsinogen (< 20 ng/mL) are reasonably specific for CP, but levels as low as this are seen only in very advanced stages of the disease where there is accompanying steatorrhea.[26]

Fecal tests. Steatorrhea can be diagnosed qualitatively by Sudan staining of feces or quantitatively by determination of fecal fat excretion over 72 hours while the patient is consuming a 100 g/day fat diet for at least 3 days before the test. Excretion of more than 7 g of fat per day is diagnostic of malabsorption, although patients with steatorrhea often have values greater than 20 g/day. Stool fat analysis has limited sensitivity in CP because patients with mild and moderate disease would not be detected by this technique.

The low diagnostic value of fat malabsorption in CP led to the discovery of individual pancreatic enzymes in stool specimen that have increased diagnostic sensitivity. The fecal elastase assay exclusively detects the human enzyme form, and so no interference occurs with simultaneous pancreatic enzyme supplementation and is widely used in clinical practice due to ease of testing. Using a cutoff of 200 μg, fecal elastase concentrations greater than this have a sensitivity of 63% for mild, 100% for moderate, and 100% for severe disease. The sensitivity and specificity was 93% for all patients with exocrine pancreatic insufficiency.[36] However, this test has lower sensitivity and specificity in early disease and may be falsely abnormal in other diseases causing steatorrhea, such as short-bowel syndrome or small-bowel bacterial overgrowth syndrome.[37]

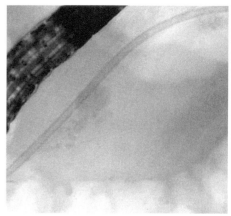

FIG 59.1 Chronic pancreatitis on digital radiography. Anteroposterior digital radiograph obtained as a scout image during endoscopic retrograde cholangiopancreatography (ERCP) shows multiple calcifications in the expected location of the pancreas with a plastic pancreatic duct stent.

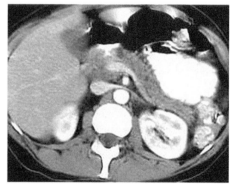

FIG 59.2 Chronic pancreatitis on computed tomography (CT). CT image shows diffusely decreased enhancement relative to the renal cortices.

Tests of Pancreatic Structure

Plain Abdominal Radiography

Calcifications within the pancreas are present on plain films in approximately one-third of patients with CP (Fig. 59.1). Calcifications occur late in the natural history of CP and may take 5 to 25 years to develop.[21,24] The finding of calcification is pathognomonic of CP, but the sensitivity of this test is very low.

Computed Tomography

The sensitivity and specificity of computed tomography (CT) for the diagnosis of CP is 75% to 90% and 85%, respectively.[31] The main advantage of CT is that it can be standardized and can visualize the entire pancreas. CT scan is the most sensitive test for detecting calcification, is accurate in detecting main pancreatic duct dilation, and can detect an irregular contour of the gland (Fig. 59.2).[31,38,39] These features are seen in advanced CP and CT is excellent in detecting these changes. However, CT is poor at detecting subtle abnormalities in pancreatic parenchyma or changes in side branches of the pancreatic duct, which are commonly seen in milder forms of the disease. CT has good specificity but lacks sensitivity for the diagnosis of CP. The newer multi-detector CT scanners may produce better sensitivity.

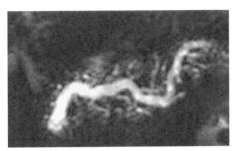

FIG 59.3 Chronic pancreatitis on magnetic resonance cholangiopancreatography (MRCP). Coronal two-dimensional MRCP shows diffuse, irregular side branch dilation and dilation of the main pancreatic duct.

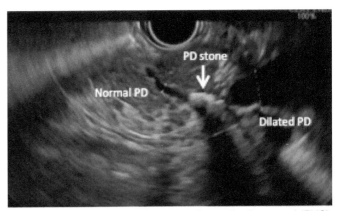

FIG 59.4 Chronic pancreatitis on endoscopic ultrasound (EUS). EUS shows the pancreatic duct (PD) becoming obstructed in the pancreatic head by a calcified intraductal stone causing upstream dilation.

Magnetic Resonance Cholangiopancreatography

Several small studies have reported on the utility of magnetic resonance cholangiopancreatography (MRCP) in assessing pancreatic duct morphology.[40,41] MRCP agrees with endoscopic retrograde cholangiopancreatography (ERCP) in 70% to 80% of findings, with higher rates of agreement in studies using the most advanced image analysis techniques (Fig. 59.3). In studies that compared MRCP findings with ERCP, MRCP visualized the main pancreatic duct in the head, body, and tail in 79%, 64%, and 53% of cases, respectively.[41] Correlation with ERCP with respect to main pancreatic duct dilation, narrowing, and filling defects was 83% to 92%, 70% to 92%, and 92% to 100%. The major disadvantage of MRCP compared with conventional cholangiography is that it has a lower spatial resolution, limiting its ability to detect subtle side branch changes, which are the earliest changes of CP.

Secretin-enhanced MRCP (SMRCP) involves administering intravenous synthetic secretin (0.2 μg/kg over 1 min) to stimulate pancreatic secretions and obtain heavily weighted T2 images of the pancreatic duct every 30 seconds over 10 minutes. This modality has recently been used to identify early changes of CP by detecting subtle abnormalities in duodenal filling, pancreatic duct compliance, and/or side branch ducts that may not be apparent on conventional MRCP.[42] However, due to the additional time, cost, and expertise required for the specialized protocol and interpretation of results, SMRCP is used mainly at specialized centers in select patients.

Endoscopic Ultrasound

Endoscopic ultrasound (EUS) provides a safe, minimally invasive method of obtaining detailed structural information of the pancreatic parenchyma and ducts. There are two main advantages for EUS that make it a very sensitive test for CP. First, the pancreas lies within a few millimeters of the duodenum and stomach, allowing use of higher frequencies that provide high-resolution images (but less penetration). Second, by positioning the EUS transducer at certain stations in the stomach and duodenum, complete visualization of the pancreas can be achieved.

Numerous EUS criteria for pancreatic disease have been described (Fig. 59.4). Lees et al (1986, 1979)[43,44] first described EUS findings in patients with clinical and radiologic evidence of CP and characterized EUS criteria that distinguish a normal from an abnormal pancreas. Wiersema et al (1993)[45] refined these definitions and found that abnormal EUS changes occurred frequently in patients with abnormal endoscopic pancreatograms

TABLE 59.3 **Endoscopic Ultrasound Criteria for Chronic Pancreatitis**	
Parenchymal Changes	**Ductal Changes**
Inhomogeneity	Ductal dilation
Hyperechoic foci	Hyperechoic main duct margins
Hyperechoic strands	Irregular main duct margins
Lobularity	Visible side branches
Pseudocysts	

and were absent in healthy volunteers. Criteria for CP that are specific to EUS can be divided into two groups (Table 59.3): parenchymal and ductal. Parenchymal criteria include inhomogeneity, hyperechoic foci, hyperechoic strands, cysts, and lobularity. Ductal criteria specific to EUS include obvious to more subtle ductal dilation (≥ 3 mm in the head, ≥ 2 mm in the body, ≥ 1 mm in the tail), hyperechoic main duct margins, irregular main duct margins, and visible side branches.

A quantitative analysis with nine possible criteria (hyperechoic foci, hyperechoic strands, lobularity, ductal dilation, ductal irregularity, hyperechoic duct margins, visible side branches, calcifications, and cysts) suggested that in a population at low-to-moderate risk of CP, EUS is most reliable only when it is either clearly normal (two or fewer criteria) or clearly abnormal (five or more criteria).[46] When the threshold for normal is set at two or fewer criteria and the threshold for abnormal is set at five or more criteria, the predictive values are 85%.[47]

Some of the controversy regarding the accuracy of EUS may be due to studies that use three or four criteria (i.e., mild abnormalities) as threshold values to distinguish normal from abnormal EUS. It is unclear whether minimal EUS changes reflect early CP disease. In a prospective study that compared EUS findings of the pancreas with surgical histopathology in 42 patients, there was a significant correlation between the number of EUS criteria and fibrosis score at histology ($r = 0.85$).[48]

As EUS provides higher resolution imaging than other imaging methods and provides information on both the ducts and the parenchyma, it is logical to assume that it can detect earlier changes of CP. Functional testing is said to become abnormal only after greater than 60% to 70% of pancreatic functional reserve is depleted.[49] If this is the case, it may also be reasonable to expect that EUS could detect subtle structural changes that predate functional abnormalities. Finally, even severe CP can be asymptomatic. EUS may show pancreatic abnormalities in asymptomatic individuals. It has been shown that alcohol consumption is often associated with asymptomatic abnormalities.[50,51]

Elastography measures tissue resistance (strain) resulting from compression and different tissue elasticity patterns are demonstrated as different colors in a qualitative analysis (blue = hard tissue and red = soft tissue). Normal pancreatic parenchyma typically has a homogenous yellow and green pattern, whereas CP has a heterogeneous green and blue pattern.[52] Quantitative elastography involves calculating the strain ratio between the strain in the region of interest and a reference area in surrounding soft tissue.[53] Recently, quantitative elastography has been compared with standard EUS criteria for diagnosing CP. A high correlation was found between the number of EUS criteria and the strain ratio.[54,55] Another study has shown a strong correlation between quantitative EUS elastography strain ratio and the probability of suffering from exocrine pancreatic insufficiency.[56] To date, the role of contrast-enhanced EUS for the diagnosis of CP has not been not been well studied.

Endoscopic Retrograde Cholangiopancreatography

In the past, ERCP with use of the "Cambridge criteria" was widely accepted as the most definitive method for interpreting pancreatography (Fig. 59.5). Studies cited a sensitivity of 70% to 90%, and specificity of 80% to 100% for diagnosing CP.[30–35] However, there are multiple limitations. CP can involve the pancreatic parenchyma per se and completely spare the radiographically visible portions of the pancreatic ductal system, leading to false-negative studies.[57,58] In addition, significant interobserver and intraobserver variability is noted in the interpretation of pancreatography.[59] Much of this variability is related to interpretation of mild pancreatographic changes rather than to severe abnormalities. Reliable interpretation of ERCP in the detection of early CP depends on adequate filling of side branches and this increases the risk of post ERCP pancreatitis.

Inadequate opacification of ducts, especially the secondary ducts, occurs in at least 30% of cases.[60]

ERCP is associated with a 3% to 7% chance of causing acute pancreatitis.[61] Therefore, due to the widespread use of EUS, limitations in pancreatography interpretation, and increased risk of pancreatitis, ERCP is no longer used solely for diagnostic purposes in CP.

ENDOSCOPIC MANAGEMENT

Major goals of treatment in CP and targets for endoscopic therapy are pain relief and managing associated complications. Pain is thought to result from ductal obstruction and/or nerve damage caused by chronic inflammation and fibrosis. There are three approaches to management: decrease pancreatic exocrine secretion, decompress the pancreatic duct, and, if the first two fail, perform partial or complete resection of the gland. Successful pain management can be clinically challenging and a multidisciplinary approach is warranted. A combination of medical, surgical, and endoscopic modalities are often utilized with varying success rates due to the significant heterogeneity in the clinical presentation and natural history of CP patients. In addition to pain, other associated complications such as pseudocysts, biliary strictures, and duodenal obstruction can occur. For the purposes of this chapter, treatment will focus solely on endoscopic therapies.

Pain Relief
EUS-Guided Celiac Plexus Nerve Block

Pancreatic pain is predominantly transmitted through the celiac plexus. Celiac plexus neurolysis, via a surgical or transcutaneous approach, has been used for many years to manage abdominal pain resulting from advanced malignancy.[62,63] These approaches have had complications such as paralysis, which might be overcome by better visualization of the region. The celiac artery is a landmark structure readily visualized on EUS (Fig. 59.6). Wiersema and Wiersema (1996) performed transgastric EUS-guided celiac plexus neurolysis and found that the success rate was similar to surgical or transcutaneous approaches.[64]

An injection of absolute ethanol that permanently destroys the plexus is referred to as a *celiac plexus neurolysis,* and an

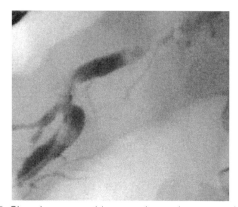

FIG 59.5 Chronic pancreatitis on endoscopic retrograde cholangiopancreatography (ERCP). ERCP image shows irregular narrowing and dilation of the main pancreatic duct and irregular side branch dilation, most prominent in the body and tail.

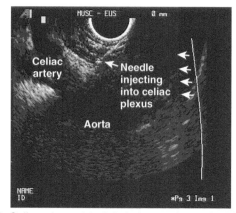

FIG 59.6 Celiac plexus block is being performed with the curvilinear array echoendoscope. The celiac artery is seen emerging from the aorta, and the needle is shown just above this point.

injection of local anesthetic and corticosteroids that temporarily blocks the plexus and reduces inflammation is referred to as a *celiac plexus block*. EUS-guided celiac plexus block and neurolysis are safe and well-tolerated procedures that can be performed in an outpatient setting with conscious sedation. Mild complications include transient diarrhea (4%–15%), transient orthostasis (1%), and transient increase in pain with neurolysis (9%). Major complications (2.5%) have included retroperitoneal bleeding and peripancreatic abscess.[65]

In a prospective study, Wiersema et al (1998) evaluated patients with pancreatic malignancy and CP treated by celiac plexus neurolysis, and found that the initial pain scores were similar between the two patient groups.[66] However, after 16 weeks of follow-up, the pain score improvement after celiac plexus neurolysis in patients with CP was not found to be significant. The malignant disease group had a mean pain score of less than baseline. Celiac plexus neurolysis is not recommended for the management of CP. Gress et al (1999)[67] compared EUS to CT-guided injection of triamcinolone in 22 patients with CP. At 8 weeks after the procedure, 50% of EUS patients had significant improvement in pain scores, whereas only 25% achieved this with the CT-guided approach. The corresponding results at 12 weeks were 40% and 12% for EUS and CT, respectively. In a prospective study of 51 patients with CP and pain who underwent celiac plexus block using either 1 or 2 injections, there was no significant difference in short-term pain relief between both cohorts.[68] Of patients, 57% who received a single injection had pain relief compared with 54% who received two injections.

Based on available data, the technique of performing celiac plexus block does not seem to affect treatment outcomes. Due to the complexity of pain associated with CP and the fact that most patients considered for celiac block have been on narcotics, it makes sense that this procedure is not a panacea for pain control in CP. It can be helpful to treat exacerbations of pain to avoid increasing narcotic dosages and sometimes it can be effective to move patients from an inpatient intravenous narcotic situation to an outpatient oral medical regimen.

ERCP Therapy

The goal of ERCP is to evaluate for an obstructive component to the pancreatopathy. Endoscopically treatable causes of obstruction can be at the level of the papilla (papillary stenosis) or along the course of the main pancreatic duct, primarily secondary to stones, strictures, or both.

Pancreatic duct stones. Approximately one-third of patients with CP have pancreatic stones. There is no close correlation between the presence of pancreatic duct stones and pain, and many patients with pancreatic duct stones report no pain. It is unclear if pancreatic calculi aggravate the clinical course of CP or are the consequence of ongoing glandular destruction from persistent disease processes. It is postulated that pain in CP is related to increased intrapancreatic pressure arising as a consequence of mechanical duct obstruction by stones with or without strictures.[69,70] This notion is supported by studies that show improvement in symptoms after ductal clearance of stones.[71–76]

Removal of pancreatic duct stones is recommended in patients with symptomatic CP and is most effective when applied to patients with chronic relapsing disease as opposed to those with chronic daily pain. More recently, treatment of obstructive pancreaticolithiasis in asymptomatic CP patients has been suggested to preserve pancreatic function and prevent gland atrophy. Given the limited data and risk of complications with endoscopic therapy, these authors would not currently endorse treatment in completely asymptomatic patients.

Pancreatic sphincterotomy, stricture dilation, and stone removal with balloons and baskets. The optimal conditions for successful endoscopic removal of pancreatic stones are a small number of mobile stones in the duct without significant strictures. Initial endoscopic management involves sphincterotomy, stricture dilation, and stone removal by baskets or balloons (Fig. 59.7 and Video 59.1). An impacted stone that impedes injection of contrast material into the pancreatic duct usually requires adjunctive therapy using extracorporeal shock wave lithotripsy (ESWL) or intraductal lithotripsy for clearance.

Removal of pancreatic stones requires an adequate opening of the pancreatic orifice. There is often thickening and fibrosis

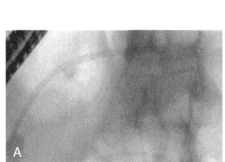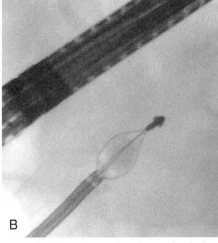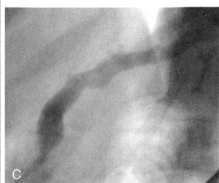

FIG 59.7 Pancreatic stone removal with endoscopic retrograde cholangiopancreatography (ERCP). ERCP images obtained before (**A**), during (**B**), and after (**C**) stone removal by lithotripsy. **A,** Scout ERCP image reveals a large stone within the main pancreatic duct. **B,** Second image was obtained during basket capture of the stone. **C,** Postprocedural ERCP image reveals absence of the stone within the duct and no evidence of residual obstruction.

or stenosis of the pancreatic orifice in CP. Cholangiography and pancreatography are performed initially, and the termination of both ducts is assessed. A biliary sphincterotomy may be performed first to improve access to the pancreatic orifice and to help expose the landmarks for completing a pancreatic sphincterotomy. Pancreatic sphincterotomy can be performed using either a standard pull-type sphincterotome (with or without a previous biliary sphincterotomy) or a needle-knife (usually over a previously placed pancreatic stent). In patients with pancreas divisum, a minor papilla sphincterotomy is required, which can be completed in the same way using a standard papillotome or a needle knife over a minor papilla stent. The ability to remove a stone by endoscopic methods alone depends on stone size and number, location inside the duct, presence of downstream stricture, and degree of impaction.[73] Downstream strictures may require dilation either with catheters or with hydrostatic balloons.

The conformation of the main pancreatic duct significantly influences the endoscopic approach to stones. If the duct makes a sigmoid turn or there is an ansa (360-degree turn within the head), it is almost impossible to get baskets or the single-operator cholangioscope around the turns. Negotiating around the genu can also be problematic if the turn is tight or there is a partial ansa. Soft-wire or wire-guided baskets may be necessary to navigate these tortuous areas of the pancreatic duct. Pancreatic stones are usually very hard because of the makeup of their crystalline structure. Careful assessment of the main pancreatic duct downstream of the stone is important prior to grasping stones to avoid basket impaction. In a grossly dilated duct, a "through-the-scope" mechanical lithotripsy device can be used, but this is often restricted to stones in the head of the pancreas with a straight line of approach to the stone. Otherwise, the rigidity of this device and its large diameter are restrictive. This device may also be used through a very dilated dorsal duct if it permits a straight approach.

Sherman et al (1991)[73] reported that endoscopic therapy was effective in 83% of patients presenting with chronic relapsing pancreatitis compared with 46% of patients presenting with continuous pain alone. Factors favoring successful endoscopic therapy included three or fewer stones, stones confined to the head or body of the pancreas, stone size less than 10 mm, absence of impacted stones, and absence of downstream strictures. After successful stone removal, 25% of patients had regression of ductographic changes of CP, and 42% had a decrease in the main pancreatic duct diameter. The only complication was pancreatitis encountered in 8% of patients. Studies have reported success rates with endoscopic therapy of 45% to 79% and improvement in symptoms of 60% to 90%.[71–74] One study reported clinical improvement in steatorrhea in 73% of patients after endoscopic management.[75]

Advanced Lithotripsy Techniques

Electrohydraulic lithotripsy. Electrohydraulic lithotripsy (EHL) may be an effective adjunct to endoscopic treatment of pancreatic stones.[76] In this technique, shocks are delivered in a fluid medium under direct visualization because inadvertent firing on tissue can cause perforation or bleeding. This technique requires the use of a small-caliber pancreatoscope (either a "baby" scope or single-operator disposable catheter; SpyDigital, Boston Scientific, Natick, MA) that is passed up the pancreatic duct to the stone.

Direct pancreatoscopy is mandatory to assure the EHL probe is against the stone and not the duct, manipulation within the main pancreatic duct remains difficult, and very limited smaller caliber baby scopes are fragile and have limited one-way tip deflection, which may hinder their utility. Additionally, the operating channel diameter is 0.75 to 1.0 mm and accepts only specialized, ultrathin accessories. The EHL probe is 1.9-Fr in diameter and can be used, but channels of 1.0 mm or less do not allow for much coaxial perfusion of saline necessary for lithotripsy. Saline is essential for transmission of the shock waves at the stone surface and for irrigation to clear debris.

Placement of a nasopancreatic tube (5-Fr) beyond the stone before pancreatoscopy is helpful for irrigation purposes, but requires that the main pancreatic duct is very dilated with no downstream strictures. Advancing the pancreatoscope requires an ample pancreatic sphincterotomy for insertion and may require a guidewire to advance through a tortuous pancreatic duct. A 450-cm wire is placed into the duct beforehand, and the proximal stiffer end is back-loaded into the baby scope. The stiff end of the wire should be slightly bent before back-loading to help negotiate the elbow junction of the accessory port and the scope body.

Laser lithotripsy. An alternative to EHL is laser lithotripsy. The most common laser used currently is the holmium laser (Lumenis VersaPulse Laser, Boston Scientific, Natick, MA). The holmium laser tends to pulverize stones into smaller particles when compared with EHL, which can be an advantage in the pancreas. The laser fiber is also more durable than the EHL probe. There are limited data available, but a multicenter US study of 28 patients achieved complete duct clearance in 79% (22 patients) and partial clearance in 11% (3 patients).[77] Even after treatment, pancreatic stones tend to recur, but this recurrence can be treated again endoscopically, whereas the rate of repeat surgery for recurrent pain is 20%, with a striking increase in morbidity and mortality after repeated surgery.[78]

Extracorporeal shock wave lithotripsy. ESWL has become almost indispensable to specialized centers treating many patients with advanced CP.[79] ESWL is considered a first-line therapy in Europe and Asia for the management of symptomatic chronic calcific pancreatitis. In the United States, it is not widely available, usually performed by urologists who are not experienced with the difference in treatment when compared with kidney stones, and insurance coverage is erratic. As a result, it is used more as a salvage procedure if endoscopic attempts fail. Stones are amendable to ESWL in almost all patients because the biochemical composition of the stones consists of 95% calcium carbonate on a protein matrix. The procedure is contraindicated only in patients who have coagulation disorders or who have calcified aneurysms or lung tissue in the shock wave path.

In some patients, a radiologic target is needed that can be provided by the placement of a stent. Fluoroscopic focusing of densely calcified stones can be achieved without pancreatography. In other patients, MRCP with secretin or CT can show pancreatic ductal obstruction related to stones. For very small stones or radiolucent stones, visualization can be improved by instillation of contrast material via a nasopancreatic catheter. Patients require sedation, which can range from conscious sedation to general anesthesia. Routine antibiotic prophylaxis is unnecessary.

Shock waves are focused first on the distal-most stone and then on other calculi moving from the head to tail, allowing stone fragments to drain downward through the papilla. In one treatment session, 3000 to 5000 shock waves using the highest possible energy levels are delivered. Pancreatic stones are hard and usually require a higher-powered shock wave (22–24 kV). Each session lasts approximately 45 to 60 minutes.

ESWL is an effective adjunct to the nonsurgical endoscopic approach in chronic calcifying pancreatitis with complete or partial relief of symptoms in 80% of patients, which is comparable to the surgical literature.[80,81] In one study, stones were successfully fragmented in 99% of patients, resulting in a decrease in duct dilation in 90%.[80] The main pancreatic duct was cleared of all stones in 59%. However, one of the challenges in pancreatic duct therapy is evaluating treatment efficacy. Disintegration of a stone can be considered successful when a decrease is seen in the radiographic density of the stone or the stone surface area. In addition, the ability to show relief of ductal obstruction at deep cannulation of the pancreatic duct during ERCP is an indicator of treatment efficacy. Using the aforementioned criteria, the success rate of fragmentation has been approximately 76% to 100% in most series, regardless of the shock wave system used.[80–83]

Most patients require endoscopic extraction of stone fragments after ESWL for complete clearance from the ductal system. Some authorities recommend that pancreatic sphincterotomy be performed before ESWL to facilitate stone passage.[71,84] With the exception of one report[73] in which successful treatment was more frequent in patients with solitary stones (74% vs. 43% for multiple stones), successful fragmentation and stone clearance was not correlated with the initial size or the number of main pancreatic duct stones by others.[84–86]

Repeat ESWL may be required if stones have not been adequately fragmented; this can be the case in patients with large, impacted, or multiple stones. The reported mean number of treatment sessions required to complete lithotripsy has ranged from 1.3 to 4.1 per patient in most reports.[71,83,84] The radiographic success of ESWL has been associated with clinical improvement (Table 59.4). Complete or partial pain relief was observed in 62% to 97% of patients in the largest series during a mean follow-up ranging from 7 to 44 months.[80,84,86–89] However, complete stone clearance was not required for symptom relief. Many patients gained weight because of a reduction in postprandial pain attacks, improvement in pancreatic function, or both. The number and location of stones, the presence of a stricture, or continued alcohol use did not seem to be associated with recurrent pain.[75,84] As a result, ESWL does not have to be restricted to patients without these unfavorable clinical characteristics.

One study[79] identified three independent predictors of pain relapse at long-term follow-up after ESWL therapy: (1) a high frequency of pain attacks before treatment (more than or at least two pain attacks during the 2 months before treatment), (2) a long duration of disease before treatment, and (3) the presence of a nonpapillary stenosis of the main pancreatic duct. This study suggests that ESWL in association with endoscopic therapy should be performed as early as possible in the course of CP. In another study, pain relapse was noted to occur more frequently in patients who had incomplete removal of stones than in patients in whom ductal clearance was complete.[76]

Early ductal decompression of the main pancreatic duct may also help prevent further fibrosis, which can lead to pancreatic insufficiency. In addition, it may improve pancreatic function in patients who have already developed pancreatic insufficiency. Although some studies investigating this issue found that exocrine pancreatic function improved more often after treatment compared with endocrine pancreatic function, others have shown progressive deterioration in both exocrine and endocrine functions at long-term follow-up.[78,80,86–88]

In a multicenter study, the rate of recurrence of pancreatic duct stones after ESWL was reported to be 20% to 30%.[88] Factors predictive of stone recurrence included ongoing alcohol use and the presence of pancreatic duct strictures. Complications in series using ESWL were primarily related to the endoscopic procedure.

Endoscopy Versus Surgery

Two prospective, randomized studies comparing surgical and endoscopic therapy in chronic calcific pancreatitis have been reported in the literature.[89,90] In the first study,[89] 140 patients with obstructive CP were treated either by endoscopic therapy or by surgical resection or drainage procedures. Although immediate relief of symptoms was identical in both groups (51.6% in the endotherapy group vs. 42.1% in the surgical group), at 5 years of follow-up complete absence of pain was more frequent after surgery (37% vs. 14%), with partial relief of pain being similar (49% vs. 51%). The increase in body weight was also greater by 20% to 25% in the surgical group, whereas new-onset diabetes mellitus developed with similar frequency in both groups (34% in the surgical group vs. 43% in the endotherapy group).

TABLE 59.4	Technical and Clinical Results of Extracorporeal Shock Wave Lithotripsy for Pancreatic Stones			
Reference	No. Patients	Complete or Partial Pain Relief (%)	Fragmentation (%)	Complete Clearance (%)
Dumonceau et al[78]	70	68	58	50
Sherman et al[73]	32	85	99	58
Delhaye et al[79]	123	85	99	59
Sauerbruch et al[80]	24	83	87.5	42
Farnbacher et al[81]	114	93	82	39
Adamek et al[82]	80	76	54	ND
Schneider et al[83]	50	62	86	60
Ohara et al[84]	32	86	100	75
Kozarek et al[87]	40	80	100	ND
Tadenuma et al[76]	117	97	97	56
Inui et al[88]	555	91.1	92.4	73

ND, Not determined.

In the second randomized trial of 39 patients with CP and pain, patients managed surgically had lower pain scores and better quality of life at 2-year follow-up.[90] In addition, although only 32% of patients randomly assigned to endoscopy had better or partial pain relief, 75% of patients randomly assigned to surgery had better pain relief. There was no difference in the complications, length of hospital stay, and pancreatic function between both groups; however, patients undergoing endotherapy required more interventions.

More recently, these studies have been included in two meta-analyses by the same Dutch group of Ahmed et al, published in 2012 and then updated in 2015, comparing endoscopic versus surgical intervention for painful obstructive CP.[91,92] The 2015 study also included an additional study examining surgery versus conservative management (no intervention) for a total of 143 patients.[92] This meta-analyses showed that compared with the endoscopic group, the surgical group had a higher proportion of participants with pain relief, both at long-term follow-up (≥5 years; relative risk [RR]: 1.56; 95% confidence interval [CI]: 1.18–2.05). Morbidity and mortality were similar between the two intervention modalities, but the small study sizes may have been underpowered to detect differences. Regarding the comparison of surgical intervention versus conservative treatment, this 2015 study suggested that surgical intervention in an early stage of CP should be considered in terms of managing both pain control and pancreatic function. Obviously, these results will need further validation in larger studies, but the limited available data suggest more durable success in terms of pain management with surgery over endoscopy in patients with obstructive chronic calcific pancreatitis.

Pancreatic Duct Strictures

Pancreatic duct strictures (Fig. 59.8) may be a complication of a previously embedded stone or a consequence of acute inflammatory changes around the pancreatic duct. Pancreatic duct strictures may contribute to pain, recurrent acute pancreatitis, and exocrine insufficiency. Strictures may also be associated with stones, pseudocysts, and pancreatic malignancy.[93–96] The mechanism of pain in patients with pancreatic strictures is poorly understood, but may be partly attributable to pancreatic duct hypertension. Pancreatic duct strictures may be present in association with biliary strictures, and liver function test abnormalities, jaundice, and cholangitis may be presenting symptoms.

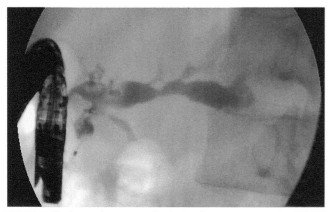

FIG 59.8 Endoscopic retrograde cholangiopancreatography (ERCP) shows changes of chronic pancreatitis with a stricture in the main pancreatic duct.

Endoscopic therapy for pancreatic duct strictures is primarily indicated for patients presenting with refractory abdominal pain, with or without upstream ductal dilation.

Stenting and Dilation

The technique for placing a stent in the pancreatic duct is similar to the technique used for inserting a biliary stent. A guidewire is first maneuvered beyond the stricture several centimeters. Hydrophilic, flexible-tip wires are generally helpful. Pancreatic stents are similar to biliary stents, except for side holes along their length to allow for flow from side branches. Generally, the diameter of the stent should not exceed the size of a normal downstream duct. In small ducts, 3-, 4-, and 5-Fr stents are used commonly, whereas 7-Fr and 10-Fr stents can be used in advanced CP with dilated pancreatic ducts. Occasionally, in patients with small duct disease who have recurrent strictures, we place multiple 3-Fr stents to dilate the stricture. We believe that stent-induced trauma could be obviated by this method, but data are still forthcoming. In addition, the severity of the stricture, location, and duct size influence the choice of stent.

Generally, the best candidates for stent treatment are patients with a distal stricture and upstream dilation. Other therapy, such as pancreatic or biliary sphincterotomy, pancreatic duct stone removal, and dilation of strictures, may be required concomitantly at the time of stent placement. Dilation to widen single or multiple strictures of the main pancreatic duct in CP can be performed successfully. Dilating catheters with graded tips and balloons are generally used. In strictures where only a guidewire can be passed, use of the 7- or 8.5-Fr Soehendra stent-retrieval devices (Cook Endoscopy, Winston-Salem, NC) can be a successful salvage technique. The device is slowly rotated clockwise while pressure is applied with the same technique as advancing a stent through a tight stricture. After dilation, stents of adequate size are left in place to facilitate drainage and to prevent recurrent stricture formation. If stents larger than 7-Fr are to be used, patients often require dual sphincterotomy followed by stricture dilation. For optimal results, therapy must address both the pancreatic duct stricture and duct stones, if any are present.

The appropriate duration of pancreatic stent placement is currently unknown. Most stents in diagnostic trials or for short-term therapy are left in place for 2 to 4 weeks. In contrast, stents for long-term therapy are left in place for several months. If the patient has improvement in symptoms, the stent can be removed and the patient can be followed clinically, stent therapy can be continued for a more prolonged period, or a surgical drainage procedure can be performed. The last option suggests that the results of endoscopic stent treatment would predict the surgical outcome. Two studies support this concept, but more data are warranted.[97,98] Quantifying the degree of improvement in pancreatic disorders is often poorly defined. Generally, partial or complete symptom improvement indicates that intraductal hypertension was an etiologic factor. Continued improvement in symptoms after stent removal indicates adequate dilation of the narrowing. The results of stent insertion for dominant pancreatic duct strictures (Table 59.5) have been favorable, with technical success in 72% to 99%, relief of pain in 75% to 94%, and good long-term outcomes in 52% to 81%. Average stent indwelling time ranged between 3 and 12 months.[90,99–101]

Although long-term symptom resolution has been reported in more than 60% of patients, endoscopic resolution of strictures has been documented in only approximately one-third of patients managed by endoscopic stent placement.[99–101] Although these

TABLE 59.5   Stent Therapy for Chronic Pancreatitis With Dominant Strictures

Reference	No. Patients	Technical Success	No. Patients Improved	Mean Follow-Up Duration (Months)
Cremer et al[93]	76	75	41	37
Ponchon et al[100]	28	23	12	26
Smits et al[101]	51	49	40	34
Binmoeller et al[102]	93	84	61	39
Costamagna et al[103]	19	19	16	38
Total	267	231 (94%)	154 (64%)	35

data suggest that stricture resolution is not a prerequisite for symptom improvement, other concomitant therapies at the time of pancreatic stent placement such as pancreatic sphincterotomy or pancreatic stone removal may account for successful outcomes. It is also likely that pain in CP tends to decrease over time as glandular destruction of the pancreas progresses in an uninhibited manner.[24]

In a study of 75 patients with pancreatic duct strictures and upstream dilation managed by placement of 10-Fr stents, Cremer et al (1991)[93] reported that 71 patients (94%) were improved over a follow-up of 3 years, with 40 patients (53%) symptom free. Improvement in symptoms was associated with a decrease in the pancreatic duct diameter. In addition, in a prospective study of 23 patients, Ponchon et al (1995)[100] reported that disappearance of stenosis at stent removal and a reduction in the pancreatic duct diameter by more than 2 mm were predictive of pain relief after pancreatic duct stent placement. Binmoeller et al (1995)[102] made a similar observation in their study of 93 patients with CP and dominant pancreatic duct strictures managed by pancreatic duct stent placement. Although 74% of the patients experienced complete or partial symptom relief, most patients were found to have a regression of ductal dilation after successful stent treatment.

Multiple Stents

Based on data demonstrating that placement of multiple stents results in successful obliteration of benign biliary strictures, the role of multiple stents in pancreatic duct strictures has been evaluated. In a study of 19 patients, 11 patients with a single main pancreatic duct stricture underwent balloon dilation (6–10 mm) followed by placement of multiple stents (8.5–11.5 Fr) across the stricture site.[103] All stents were retrieved at a mean follow-up of 7 months. The median number of stents placed per patient was three, and the most common stent diameters used were 10-Fr and 11.5-Fr. During a mean follow-up of 38 months, 84% of patients were asymptomatic, and 10.5% developed symptom recurrence.

Self-Expandable Metal Stents

Although all the previously described studies used conventional plastic stents, Cremer et al (1990),[104] in a pilot study, reported their experience with self-expandable metal stents (SEMSs) in

patients with CP. Stent placement through the major duodenal papilla was performed in 22 patients with relapsing dominant strictures of the main pancreatic duct. Successful placement, associated with an immediate decrease of pancreatic duct diameter and disappearance of pain, was noted in 100% of cases. Although no immediate complications were encountered, follow-up of these patients showed a high occlusion rate of these metal stents from mucosal hyperplasia.

Another pilot study evaluated the role of covered SEMSs (8-mm) in patients with refractory main pancreatic duct strictures.[105] The stents were retrieved by endoscopy 3 months after placement. Although the pain scores improved significantly, three out of six patients developed recurrent strictures warranting subsequent placement of large-caliber (10-mm) metal stents. Although this concept appears novel, more studies with a larger cohort of patients are needed to evaluate the role of covered metal stents in the management of benign pancreatic duct strictures. In addition, modification of these stents, which are designed for the biliary tree, will likely be needed before they are widely applied to the pancreatic duct. Direct comparative studies evaluating the efficacies of surgery and endoscopic therapy are required to identify a subset of patients who would benefit from either treatment modality.

Stent-Related Adverse Events

Pancreatic stent therapy is not without consequences. Adverse events related directly to stent therapy include acute pancreatitis, pancreatic infection, pseudocyst formation, duct injury, stone formation, and migration.[70,106] The rate of pancreatic stent occlusion appears similar to that of biliary stents.[99] Most of these occlusions are without adverse clinical events, however, because pancreatic juice may siphon along the sides of the stent. Morphologic changes of the pancreatic duct directly related to stent placement occur in more than 50% of patients.[107–110] It is uncertain what the long-term consequences of these stent-induced ductal changes are in most patients, although permanent new strictures are seen in a few patients. EUS identified parenchymal changes in 68% of patients who underwent short-term pancreatic stent treatment.[111] Although such changes may have significant long-term consequences in patients with a normal pancreas, the outcomes in patients with advanced CP seem less certain.

Associated Complications

CP may be associated with various complications. Splenic vein thrombosis, pseudoaneurysm formation, and common bile duct or duodenal strictures are occasionally encountered. Other complications such as pseudocyst formation and pancreatic ascites or pleural effusion are discussed in Chapter 58.

Benign Biliary Strictures

Intra-pancreatic common bile duct strictures have been reported in 2.7% to 45.6% of patients with CP.[112,113] Common bile duct strictures can have serious sequelae of cholangitis, cholelithiasis, choledocholithiasis, intrahepatic stones, and secondary biliary cirrhosis. Deviere et al (1990)[113] evaluated the use of biliary stent placement in patients with biliary strictures secondary to CP. They reported that endoscopic biliary drainage is an effective therapy for resolving cholangitis or jaundice in this patient subset. However, the long-term efficacy of this therapy was unsatisfactory because stricture resolution rarely occurred.

Preliminary results using metal stents for this indication suggest they could be an effective alternative to operative biliary diversion.

More than 90% of patients had no recurrence of strictures at 3 years, but longer follow-up and controlled trials are necessary to confirm these findings.[114,115] In a nonrandomized retrospective study that compared surgical drainage procedures with stent insertion, Pitt et al (1989)[116] found a significantly higher success rate of 88% in the surgically treated group compared with 55% for patients managed by stent insertion. More recently, Cote et al (2016) published their results comparing plastic stents versus fully covered self-expandable metal stents (FCSEMS) in the treatment of benign biliary strictures, including those encountered in the post-transplant setting (65% of study patients) and with CP (31% of study patients).[117] Unfortunately, the study was not adequately powered to conduct subgroup analyses between these two groups and therefore all patients were analyzed together. In this randomized, open-label trial, FCSEMS were shown to be noninferior to multiple plastic stents. However, the mean number of ERCPs to achieve biliary stricture resolution was lower for FCSEMS (2.14) versus plastic (3.24; mean difference: 1.10; 95% CI: 0.74–1.46; $p < 0.001$). Originally only approved for use in malignant disease, this study led to Food and Drug Administration approval of FCSEMS by Boston Scientific (Natick, MA) for use in benign biliary strictures. In our clinical practice, the FCSEMS is typically left in place for 2 to 3 months before being removed endoscopically using a snare or grasping forceps.

Duodenal Obstruction

Duodenal stenosis is seen in approximately 5% of patients with CP, particularly patients with alcoholic pancreatitis. Coexistent obstruction of the common bile duct may be seen. The diagnosis is made at upper endoscopy or barium swallow. Attempts to dilate the stricture endoscopically are generally futile. The simplest and safest approach is operative drainage via gastrojejunostomy; this may be combined with drainage of the bile duct or pancreatic duct, or both.

Enteral stents that are currently available have been used in malignant obstruction with similarly high success rates (> 90%) compared with surgical gastrojejunostomy. However, more than 50% of enteral stents become occluded after 6 months. In addition, currently available enteral stents are uncovered and thus not removable. For these reasons, they would not be suited for use in benign disease such as CP.[118–120]

FUTURE TRENDS

CP can be a difficult disease both from diagnostic and therapeutic aspects. Improvements in these areas could help prevent and manage long-term complications and perhaps reduce morbidity, mortality, and costs associated with this often debilitating disease.

Developments in Testing

The available diagnostic armamentarium for CP focuses exclusively on pancreatic structure and function with inability to diagnose the disease in its early stages.

CFTR Testing in Idiopathic Cases

The association between *CFTR* mutations and idiopathic CP raises the possibility of widespread use of genetic testing to evaluate idiopathic CP. The role of routine *CFTR* mutation testing is uncertain because no guidelines exist for genetic counseling or altered clinical management based on the results. As further research clarifies whether patients with idiopathic CP with *CFTR* mutations differ from other patients with idiopathic CP, this

information may lead to wider use of genetic testing during the evaluation of patients with idiopathic CP.

Micro-RNA for Early Diagnosis

Micro-RNAs (miRNAs) have been established as modulators that control fibrogenesis and inflammation. One 2017 study demonstrated that there were significant differences of serum miRNA expression in patients with early and late CP and healthy controls.[121] This type of testing would enable earlier diagnoses of CP and initiation of management strategies prior to the development of late-stage complications.

Advances in EUS Techniques
EUS-Guided Pancreatic Duct Drainage

EUS has been advocated more recently as a means to establish pancreatic ductal drainage in patients after failed ERCP.[122] EUS-guided pancreatic duct drainage (EUS-PDD) can be accomplished either by rendezvous stent placement after passage of a guidewire into the main pancreatic duct and through the ampulla under EUS guidance, or by transmural drainage of the main pancreatic duct via the stomach or duodenum (Fig. 59.9). Itoi et al (2013) published a retrospective review of the published literature on EUS-PDD with varying technical success rates.[123] Technical success using the transmural technique was greater than 70% in 75 patients, whereas success rates with the rendezvous technique ranged from 25% to 100% in 52 patients. A more recent 2015 review by Fujii-Lau and Levy included 222 patients.[124] Technical success was achieved in 170 out of 222 patients (76.6%) and included both rendezvous and transmural EUS-PDD techniques. Reported technical difficulties include difficulty with dilation, wire passage and stripping, and inability to deploy stents or their migration.[123,124] Adverse event rates of nearly 20% have been reported and include pancreatitis, perforation, bleeding, and peripancreatic abscess.[124–126] More data are needed on long-term success rates and adverse events related to this technique.

EUS-Guided Gastroenterostomy

In the past few years, various EUS-guided techniques that utilize lumen-apposing metal stents (LAMS) have been described as an endoscopic treatment of gastric outlet obstruction (off-label indication). The LAMS is placed between the stomach and bypassed small bowel, with different techniques described including direct puncture with cautery-enhanced LAMS or needle puncture of a fluoroscopically placed dilation balloon and then LAMS deployment (both cautery and non-cautery) over a guidewire (Fig. 59.10). Two recent cases series have been published on this technique as a treatment for both malignant and benign etiologies of gastric outlet obstruction. Khashab et al (2015) published the first American series of EUS-guided gastroenterostomy in 10 patients (7 with CP), and demonstrated high technical (90%) and clinical success rates (92%) with no adverse events.[127] Meanwhile, an international multicenter experience in 26 patients (9 with CP) reported similarly high technical (92%) and clinical success rates (85%), but did have significant adverse events in 11.5%.[128] These adverse events included peritonitis, perforation, and bleeding, with one death. EUS-guided gastroenterostomy is a promising technique that may obviate the need for invasive surgery in select patients. Currently, there are no data on optimal duration of LAMS placement. The goal would be a permanent anastomosis to allow for removal after a few months, but anecdotal reports have noted tract closure once the LAMS is removed. Therefore, some experts have advocated

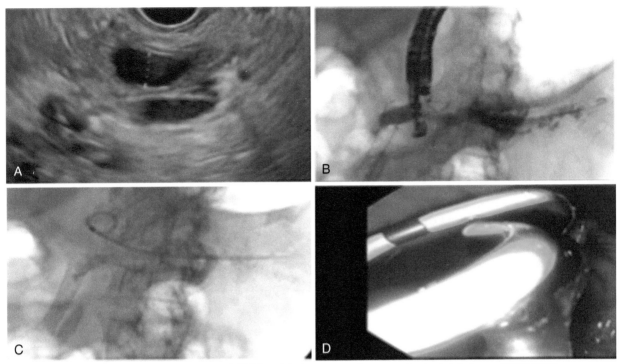

FIG 59.9 Endoscopic ultrasound (EUS)-guided transmural pancreatic ductal drainage (EUS-PDD). **A,** EUS view of dilated pancreatic duct (PD) of 7 mm. **B,** Radiographic view of pancreatogram (obtained from direct EUS puncture through the stomach) showing dilated PD with stricture in the head of the pancreas and guidewire placed into the pancreatic tail. **C,** Single pigtail plastic PD stent on radiographic view. **D,** PD stent on endoscopic view in the stomach.

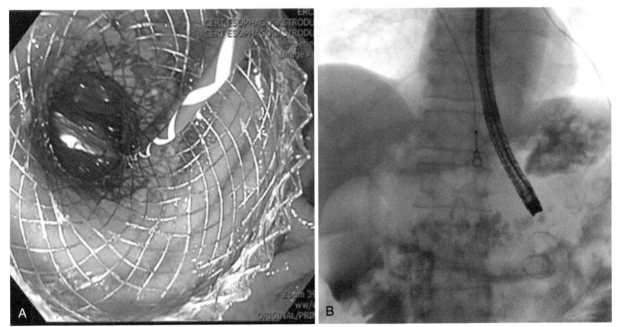

FIG 59.10 Endoscopic ultrasound (EUS)-guided gastroenterostomy using lumen-apposing metal stent (LAMS). **A,** Endoscopic view through LAMS in stomach showing small bowel. **B,** Radiographic view of LAMS with EUS scope.

leaving the LAMS in place indefinitely. Limited published data have shown that even in the hands of skilled endoscopists, this procedure can result in significant adverse events and should only be done in select patients at referral centers in collaboration with surgical colleagues. Similar to EUS-PDD, this therapeutic EUS maneuver warrants further study to establish the ideal technique and overall safety profile.

KEY REFERENCES

4. Coté GA, Yadav D, Slivka A, et al; for the North American Pancreatitis Study Group: Alcohol and smoking as risk factors in an epidemiology study of patients with chronic pancreatitis, *Clin Gastroenterol Hepatol* 9:266–273, 2011.

8. Majumder S, Chari ST: Chronic pancreatitis, *Lancet* 387:1957–1966, 2016.

13. Cohn JA, Friedman KJ, Noone PG, et al: Relation between mutations of the cystic fibrosis gene and idiopathic pancreatitis, *N Engl J Med* 339:653–658, 1998.

48. Varadarajulu S, Eltoum I, Tamhane A, et al: Histopathologic correlates of noncalcific chronic pancreatitis by EUS: a prospective tissue characterization study, *Gastrointest Endosc* 65:501–509, 2007.

52. Janssen J, Schlorer E, Greiner L: EUS elastography of the pancreas: feasibility and pattern description of the normal pancreas, chronic pancreatitis, and focal pancreatic lesions, *Gastrointest Endosc* 65: 971–978, 2007.

56. Dominguez-Munoz JE, Iglesias-Garcia J, Castineira Alvarino M, et al: EUS elastography to predict pancreatic exocrine insufficiency in patients with chronic pancreatitis, *Gastrointest Endosc* 81:136–142, 2015.

67. Gress F, Schmitt C, Sherman S, et al: A prospective randomized comparison of endoscopic ultrasound and computed tomography-guided celiac plexus block for managing chronic pancreatitis pain, *Am J Gastroenterol* 94:900–905, 1999.

76. Tadenuma H, Ishihara T, Yamaguchi T, et al: Long-term results of extracorporeal shockwave lithotripsy and endoscopic therapy for pancreatic stones, *Clin Gastroenterol Hepatol* 3:1128–1135, 2005.

77. Attwell AR, Patel S, Kahaleh M, et al: ERCP with per-oral pancreatoscopy-guided laser lithotripsy for calcific chronic pancreatitis: a multicenter U.S. experience, *Gastrointest Endosc* 82(2):311–318, 2015.

89. Dite P, Ruzicka M, Zboril V, et al: A prospective, randomized trial comparing endoscopic and surgical therapy for chronic pancreatitis, *Endoscopy* 35:553–558, 2003.

90. Cahen DL, Gouma DJ, Nio Y, et al: Endoscopic versus surgical drainage of the pancreatic duct in chronic pancreatitis, *N Engl J Med* 356: 676–684, 2007.

92. Ahmed AU, Pahlpalatz JM, Nealon WH, et al: Endoscopic or surgical intervention for painful obstructive chronic pancreatitis, *Cochrane Database Syst Rev* (3):CD007884, 2015.

98. Kwon RS, Young BE, Marsteller WF, et al: Narcotic independence after pancreatic duct stenting predicts narcotic independence after lateral pancreaticojejunostomy for chronic pancreatitis, *Pancreas* 45:1126–1130, 2016.

111. Sherman S, Hawes RH, Savides TJ, et al: Stent-induced pancreatic ductal and parenchymal changes: correlation of endoscopic ultrasound with ERCP, *Gastrointest Endosc* 44:276–282, 1996.

113. Deviere J, Devaere S, Baize M, et al: Endoscopic biliary drainage in chronic pancreatitis, *Gastrointest Endosc* 36:96–100, 1990.

115. Kahl S, Zimmermann S, Glasbrenner B, et al: Treatment of benign biliary strictures in chronic pancreatitis by self-expandable metal stents, *Dig Dis Sci* 20:199–203, 2002.

117. Cote G, Slivka A, Tarnasky P, et al: Effect of covered metallic stents compared with plastic stents on benign biliary stricture resolution a randomized clinical trial, *JAMA* 315(12):1250–1257, 2016.

118. Fukami N, Anderson MA, Khan K, et al: ASGE Standards of Practice Guidelines: the role of endoscopy in gastroduodenal obstruction and gastroparesis, *Gastrointest Endosc* 74(1):13–21, 2011.

119. Jeurnink SM, Steyerberg EW, Hof G, et al: Gastrojejunostomy versus stent placement in patients with malignant gastric outlet obstruction: a comparison in 95 patients, *J Surg Oncol* 96:389–396, 2007.

122. Gines A, Varadarajulu S, Napoleon B: EUS 2008 Working Group Document. Evaluation of EUS-guided pancreatic-duct drainage, *Gastrointest Endosc* 69(2 Suppl):S43–S48, 2009.

123. Itoi T, Kasuya K, Sofuni A, et al: Endoscopic ultrasonography-guided pancreatic duct access: techniques and literature review of pancreatography, transmural drainage and rendezvous techniques, *Dig Endosc* 25(3):241–252, 2013.

125. Fujii LL, Topazian MD, Abu Dayyeh BK, et al: EUS-guided pancreatic duct intervention: outcomes of a single tertiary-care referral center experience, *Gastrointest Endosc* 78:854–864, 2013.

126. Chapman CG, Waxman I, Siddiqui UD: Endoscopic ultrasound (EUS)-guided pancreatic duct drainage: the basics of when and how to perform EUS-guided pancreatic duct interventions, *Clin Endosc* 49(2):161–167, 2016.

127. Khashab MA, Kumbhari V, Grimm IS, et al: EUS-guided gastroenterostomy: the first U.S. clinical experience, *Gastrointest Endosc* 82:932–938, 2015.

128. Tyberg A, Perez-Miranda M, Sanchez-Ocana R, et al: Endoscopic ultrasound-guided gastrojejunostomy with a lumen-apposing metal stent: a multicenter, international experience, *Endosc Int Open* 4(3): 276–281, 2016.

A complete reference list can be found online at ExpertConsult .com

60

The Indeterminate Biliary Stricture

Amrita Sethi and Douglas A. Howell

INTRODUCTION

Indeterminate biliary stricture (IDBS) remains one of the biggest challenges that pancreaticobiliary endoscopists face. While a strict definition of IDBS is frequently not adhered to in the literature, this term refers to biliary strictures with no overt mass on noninvasive imaging such as computed tomography (CT) or magnetic resonance cholangiopancreatography, and that cannot be distinguished as malignant or benign after standard diagnostic procedures such as endoscopic retrograde cholangiopancreatography (ERCP) with tissue sampling (either brushing alone or in combination with biopsies). Surgical series demonstrate that 15% to 24% of patients who undergo resection for suspected malignant strictures based on preoperative imaging or ERCP will ultimately have a benign diagnosis on pathology.[1,2] This small but significant cohort of patients with benign strictures highlights the importance of accurate preoperative tissue diagnosis to avoid the morbidity and mortality of hepatobiliary surgery. For example, the two most common causes of malignant strictures are cholangiocarcinoma (CCA) and pancreatic cancer. Diagnosis of these malignancies at an early stage can allow curative surgical resection or even liver transplantation for early stage CCA. Tissue diagnosis of pancreaticobiliary malignancy via endoscopic approaches is well known to be limited due to poor cellular yield and often requires surgical exploration for definite diagnosis. This diagnostic dilemma ultimately serves as the driving force behind advances in biliary imaging, improvements in sampling techniques, and the identification of emerging molecular markers. This section will review the etiologies of biliary strictures, the initial clinical evaluation of IDBSs, the diagnostic yield of

ERCP-based sampling methods and recommended methods of improving acquisition and analysis, and the role of newer imaging tools in our approach to evaluating strictures.

ETIOLOGIES OF BILIARY STRICTURES

The leading causes of malignant biliary obstruction are pancreatic cancer and CCA.[3] CCA is a primary malignancy of the bile duct epithelium, and therefore can affect both intra- and extrahepatic ducts. It is the second most common primary liver malignancy after hepatocellular carcinoma.[4] When diagnosed in early stages, surgical resection can have an excellent prognosis.[5] The challenge, however, is in obtaining a histological diagnosis given the typically inadequate cellular yield from initial sampling methods such as ERCP with brush cytology and/or biopsy. Unfortunately, the differential for CCA includes a host of benign causes of biliary strictures that can radiographically mimic CCA.

Biliary strictures due to pancreatic cancer are most often found at the distal common bile duct and are due to extrinsic compression of the extrahepatic duct from a pancreatic head mass with or without biliary invasion. Diagnosis of biliary stricture in the setting of a pancreatic mass does not technically fall into the category of IDBS; however, early tumors may go undetected on cross-sectional imaging, and thorough evaluation of the pancreatic head in such strictures is a necessary part of the evaluation. This is in contrast to CCA, whose desmoplastic nature results in its growing in an infiltrative pattern along the length of the bile duct, making its early detection particularly difficult due to the lack of a visible growth or tumor on imaging. Other less common malignant causes of biliary strictures include intraductal

TABLE 60.1 Etiologies of Biliary Strictures

Malignant	Benign
Cholangiocarcinoma	Chronic pancreatitis
Pancreatic adenocarcinoma	Primary sclerosing cholangitis
Ampullary adenocarcinoma	Ig4 (autoimmune) sclerosing cholangitis
Gallbladder cancer	Postsurgical, anastomotic stricture
Hepatocellular carcinoma	Mirizzi syndrome
Metastatic disease	Fibrostenotic benign stricture
Lymphoma	Ischemic stricture
	Radiation-induced stricture
	Infectious (HIV-associated, parasitic cholangiopathy, tuberculosis)
	Vasculitis

hepatocellular carcinoma, metastatic lesion, and extrinsic compression of the biliary tree from an associated visible mass or lymphadenopathy (Table 60.1).

The varying forms of malignant biliary obstruction are pathologically distinct and represent special problems when attempting tissue sampling. The first major pathologic factor influencing biopsy or cytologic yield is tumor cellularity. Pancreatic carcinoma, in particular, often stimulates an intense desmoplastic and fibrotic reaction, making the tumor very dense and of low cellularity. Sampling often produces acellular or false-negative specimens.[6,7] Maximizing yield requires repeated, deep, or large specimen sampling. Occasionally, an immune response or relative ischemia produces ulceration, bleeding, exudate, or debris that can obscure the rare malignant cell recovered in an endoscopic specimen. CCA of the primary type begins in the mucosa of the primary or secondary bile ducts. It is a relatively cellular cancer, and cells are more often shed in bile and can be more readily collected by sampling the superficial epithelium. However, the intrahepatic location of these tumors poses difficult access issues, making endoscopic ultrasound fine-needle aspiration (EUS FNA) yields lower, although the procedure is technically possible in select patients.[6,8–10]

Hepatocellular carcinoma can often invade and extend intraductally. Superficial sampling generally obtains diagnostic cells in this setting as well. As with pancreatic cancer, gallbladder cancer and, especially, metastatic cancer, encase or compress the biliary tree, often while preserving intact benign biliary epithelium. Establishing a tissue diagnosis often requires sampling deeper than the surface epithelium.[6,8–10] Very well-differentiated tumors represent a significant minority of malignant pancreaticobiliary tumors and prove very difficult to diagnose by cytologic criteria. Large specimens are often necessary to permit the pathologist to examine and compare these tumors to differentiate them from normal tissue. This fact likely explains why no biopsy technique, even open surgical wedge biopsy, has a 100% yield. These pathogenetic factors demand refined techniques and devices if adequate specimens are to be obtained to permit a positive cytologic or histologic diagnosis to be made in most cases.

Causes of benign biliary strictures include a variety of diseases ranging from recurrent cholangitis, postsurgical causes (most commonly after cholecystectomy or liver transplantation) to cholangiopathy from autoimmune disease, HIV, and primary sclerosing cholangitis (PSC). A long-standing yet poorly understood impersonator of a malignant stricture is autoimmune or

Ig4-associated sclerosing cholangitis (IgG4-SC). The prevalence and pathogenesis of this disease remains largely unknown, but more than 80% of patients will have elevations of serum IgG4 above the upper limit of normal, and a similar percentage of patients will have an associated autoimmune pancreatitis.[11,12] On cholangiogram, hilar IgG4-SC strictures can be indistinguishable from CCA. Histologic sampling, which can be diagnostic, may demonstrate diffuse infiltration of IgG4-positive plasma cells with fibroinflammatory involvement of the submucosa of the bile duct wall.[11]

LABORATORY EVALUATION

The most common laboratory abnormality seen in patients with malignant biliary stricture is obstructive cholestasis. Direct hyperbilirubinemia is seen more commonly in patients with malignant obstruction than those with a benign etiology such as choledocholithiasis.[13] Hyperbilirubinemia also has a higher likelihood of being associated with malignancy than elevations in alkaline phosphatase.[13,14]

The most frequently used serologic markers for CCA are CA19-9 and possibly carcinoembryonic antigen (CEA). CEA has sensitivities and specificities that range from 33% to 84% and 50% to 87.8%, respectively.[15–17] Unfortunately, CA19-9 also has a wide range of sensitivity and specificity: 38% to 93% and 67% to 98%.[15–19] Furthermore, it can be undetectable in 7% of the general population due to absence of the Lewis antigen.[20] The variable diagnostic accuracies of CA19-9, therefore, limit its role in screening, and its greatest value may be in the surveillance of patients with PSC.

In response to this poor reliability of CA19-9, other serum tumor markers have been recently evaluated. For example, cytokeratin-19 fragments (CYFRA 21-1) get released into the bloodstream by malignant epithelial cells.[20] Several studies have demonstrated elevated CYFRA 21-1 expression in CCA, albeit with variable sensitivities depending on the cut-off value.[17,20,21] Specificities also vary given that elevation of CYFRA 21-1 expression has been reported in multiple other gastrointestinal (GI) and non-GI epithelial malignancies such as gastric, breast, and cervical. Similarly, high matrix metalloproteinase-7 (MMP-7) expression has been found to be associated with cancer invasion in esophageal,[22] colon,[23] and pancreatic[24] cancers. Given the lack of specificity for these individual markers, use of combinations of the markers may be the most useful, such as in multimarker panels. For example, a panel with the combination of these markers with CEA and CA19-9 demonstrated the highest diagnostic accuracy of 93.9%.[20]

Another serum marker, interleukin-6 (IL-6), which has been shown to be a biliary epithelial growth factor,[25] has demonstrated sensitivity as high as 100% in diagnosing CCA.[26] Like the other markers mentioned earlier, however, the specificities are limited due to its elevation in patients with hepatocellular carcinoma, benign biliary disease, and metastatic lesions.[27] Sperm-specific protein 411 (SSP411) is a protein that shows some promise in serving as a single serum-based biomarker given its elevation in the bile of CCA patients and use in distinguishing CCA from choledocholithiasis.[28]

Recent work has been performed evaluating the utility of measuring microRNAs (miRNAs) that are shed into the circulation in a free form when dysregulated in the setting of malignancies, compared to their stable protein-bound form.[29] The value of miRNAs lies in their tissue-specific patterns of expression.

MicroRNAs that are commonly upregulated in other epithelial cancers such as miR-192, 194, and 215 in colon, liver, pancreas, and stomach cancers,[30] are not altered in CCA. Conversely, CCA-specific miRNA expression profiles do exist, such as downregulation of miR-125a, -31,[31,32] or, alternatively, upregulation of some miRNA's such as miR-21.[33–35] The specificity is limited, however, given its upregulation in other cancers (gastric,[36] breast,[37] and colon[38]). As with tumor markers discussed earlier, perhaps the evaluation for miRNAs are best performed as part of a multimarker panels specific for CCA.

ERCP

History

While noninvasive imaging modalities such as magnetic resonance imaging/magnetic resonance cholangiopancreatography and computed tomography (CT) are an essential part of the baseline evaluation of biliary strictures, they carry low diagnostic accuracy in distinguishing benign from malignant causes of obstruction.[10] Furthermore, they provide no means by which to obtain tissue diagnosis and thus, when discussing IDBS, the gold standard remains ERCP.

ERCP was developed in the late 1960s as a diagnostic technique to provide detailed radiography of the biliary tree and pancreatic ducts. ERCP remained primarily a diagnostic tool until 1973, when endoscopic sphincterotomy was performed in Japan and Germany, specifically to allow for additional diagnostic and therapeutic maneuvers, such as performing forceps biopsies of proximal strictures.

Tissue Acquisition During ERCP

The goals of ERCP for a suspected malignant biliary stricture are to first obtain definite tissue diagnosis to obviate the need for exploratory surgery, and second, to provide palliation of biliary obstruction with stent placement. In fact, the constant quest for improved methods of tissue acquisition remains the focus of innovation in biliary technology. Initial efforts were limited to simple aspiration of bile and occasionally pancreatic juice when deep cannulation was achieved. While specificity in early reports was uniformly 100%, low sensitivities of only 6% to 32% in six published studies[39–44] have caused this technique to fall from practice.

Aspirating bile after brush cytology has occasionally been reported to increase yield using standard cell block preparation.[45] Combined methods of tissue sampling will be presented later in this chapter.

Finally, advanced molecular diagnostics in bile, including proteomic, lipidomic, and volatile organic compound analysis, may reopen bile aspiration as an accepted modality to determine a malignant diagnosis with sufficient specificity.

Brush Cytology Sampling Methods

Inadequate tissue acquisition at ERCP remains the most common reason for failing to establish an accurate pathologic diagnosis. Technical difficulty, time consideration, patient restlessness, and the need to proceed with the primary goal of biliary drainage all contribute to limit the time and thoroughness of tissue collection for many endoscopists. Because of these factors, brush cytology has been the universally adopted technique in clinical practice. Initially, standard nonwire guided endoscopic brushes were inserted, usually after sphincterotomy; however, negotiation through the stricture was often problematic. This factor and the

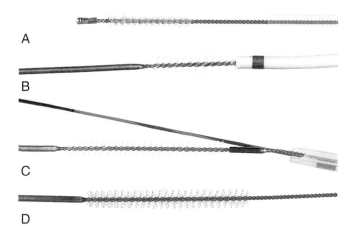

FIG 60.1 Brushes for endoscopic retrograde cholangiopancreatography (ERCP) brush cytology. *From top to bottom:* **A,** Standard metal-tipped brush, **B,** Geenen spring-nosed brush in a diagnostic catheter, **C,** Cytomax 8-Fr brush catheter over a 0.035-inch guidewire, **D,** large HBIB brush for use in the Howell biliary introducer (HBI).

very superficial nature of this technique of sampling produced disappointing yields, and it never became popular. Thus, a variety of cytology brushes, some of which could be inserted over a guidewire placed through the malignant-appearing stricture before attempted sampling, were developed and are the devices we currently use today. These brushes are housed in catheters with a variety of diameters and stiffnesses, and the brushes themselves range in configuration as well as bristle length (Fig. 60.1). Techniques for performing brushing have subtle varieties but are centered around the idea of advancing the brush and catheter over the guidewire through the stricture, followed by manipulation of the exposed brush through the stricture multiple times. Protection of the acquired cells is paramount and best achieved by withdrawing the brush back into the catheter before leaving the area of the stricture (Fig. 60.2). Some also advocate for simultaneous aspiration of bile immediately after brushing, thereby collecting loose cells in the milieu of the brushing into the catheter before removing the entire device from the duct.

Published yields of ERCP brush cytology devices vary widely for reasons that can only be speculated. Generally, series that have a higher proportion of pancreatic adenocarcinomas and, perhaps, earlier smaller tumors, have a much lower yield of positive results compared with series with more cholangiocarcinomas. Published overall sensitivities using these devices range from 8% to 57%.[43,46–51]

A 2013 review of ERCP brush cytology covered 16 studies over 10 years from 2002 to 2012, which included a total of 1586 patients.[52] The combined yield of brush cytology ranged from 6% to 64% with an overall sensitivity of only 41.6% +/− 3.2%, and did not appear to vary across new devices and techniques.

As discussed subsequently, many of these series are also flawed by including patients with "suspicious for malignancy" reports as positive results. A single center study of 142 patients with pancreatic or biliary cancer undergoing ERCP brushing reported in 2016 is such an example. The overall sensitivity was 58%, but actually only 50% in distal and presumably pancreatic cancer strictures. Adding "atypia" as a positive result increased yield to 65.5% but decreased specificity from 100% to 68.6%, clearly an unacceptable result.[53]

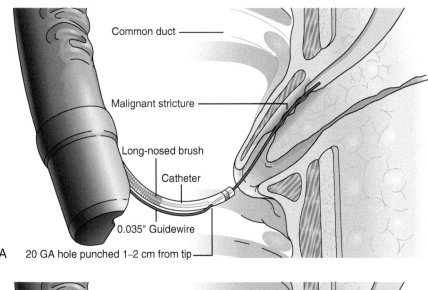

Common duct

Malignant stricture

Long-nosed brush

Catheter

0.035" Guidewire

A 20 GA hole punched 1–2 cm from tip

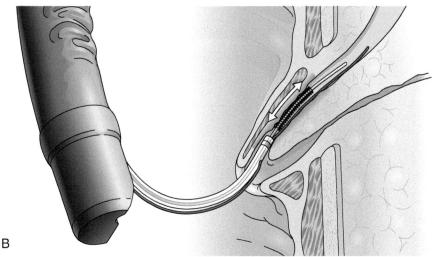

B

FIG 60.2 A, Monorail brush: a long-nosed brush is preloaded into a diagnostic catheter and passed with the catheter over a guidewire in a monorail fashion through the stricture. **B,** The monorail catheter has been passed over the end of the guidewire well above the stricture. Once off the guidewire, the long-nosed brush can be advanced to brush the stricture. The long nose maintains access. The guidewire remains in place.

A probable pathologic explanation for these varied yields relates to the observation that the interiors of malignant strictures are composed of benign epithelium compressed by surrounding neoplastic tissue, with the exception of CCA of the major bile ducts. This fact explains the low yield of simple bile aspiration for cytology because few, if any, malignant cells are in contact with the bile flow as previously discussed. When the stricture is traumatized by dilation, removing the benign epithelium, the yield of aspirating bile increases.[51]

The yield of brushing is lower with deeper and more remote encasing tumors. One would predict the lowest yield is in metastatic malignancy, followed by pancreatic cancer, with a much higher yield with primary CCA. Generally, this prediction has been confirmed in clinical practice.

The type of brush bristles, the overall brush length, and the amount of time spent brushing all affect yield. Rabinovitz et al (1990)[54] used three separate brushes at each ERCP and repeated the procedure with three new brushes when suspicious strictures

were initially negative. Positive yield continued to increase until diagnoses were eventually made by brushing alone in 62% of their patients. Two additional ERCP brushing studies have been performed in an attempt to increase yield. In a large number of patients, a newer long cytology brush with stiff angulated bristles was compared with the standard-length brushes described previously. The true-positive yields were uniformly disappointing—only 27% and 30%—and no advantage was observed with the new brush.[55] The second study compared brushing with a more traumatic technique of inserting a grasping basket through the suspicious stricture. Of 50 malignant strictures, the basket technique had a near doubling of yield to 80% compared with a brush yield of 48% ($p = 0.018$). The unexpected high yield of the brushing suggests some selection bias, and this technique requires additional study.[56]

Building on this concept of traumatizing the surface epithelium, a new scraping device was developed and trialed in Japan.[57] In 123 indeterminate stricture cases, 119 were eventually proven

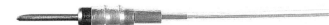

FIG 60.3 The Howell biliary aspiration needle (HBAN-22) is a 22-gauge Chiba-type needle mounted in a 7-Fr ball-tipped catheter, precurved for placement into the common bile duct (CBD) after sphincterotomy.

to be malignant. This device involves a three-leaf clover–type design of three nitinol loops, rather than bristles, that are compressed in guidewire-compatible catheters. The structure is roughly scraped and bile is aspirated using the device's side angled port. The yield was compared to a transpapillary forceps biopsy, and the device was also used in combination. The yields of forceps biopsy, the new scraping device, and both were 51%, 65%, and 75%, respectively. It is important to consider that 67% of their 119 cases had CCA and only 32% had pancreatic cancer. Furthermore, experience with this device is needed.

ERCP Needle Biopsy

Intraductal FNA during ERCP required the development of a specifically designed endoscopic accessory device. Howell et al (1992)[46] reported on such a device after developing a ball-tipped catheter with a retractable 22-gauge Chiba-type biopsy needle (HBAN-22; Wilson-Cook Medical, Bloomington, IN). The needle extends 7 mm beyond the ball tip when the catheter is placed within the duct, and permits deeper sampling than afforded by brushing (Fig. 60.3). Unlike transmural EUS-FNA, intraductal FNA cytology during ERCP traverses only tissue to be resected en bloc, and therefore there can be no contamination of the peritoneal cavity, including the lesser sac behind the stomach. The technique requires sphincterotomy, however, and proves to be technically challenging.

The initial relatively high yield of 62% (positive and suspicious samples) has not been reproduced in more recent series. The true-positive sensitivity has been reported to be 27% to 30% of cases in three series.[47,58,59] This technique has been used in combination with cytology and forceps biopsy, known as triple sampling, and is described later in the chapter.

Forceps Biopsy

Initially, there was only one method of performing intraductal forceps biopsies, known as fluoroscopically guided biopsies. Subsequently, with the development of cholangioscopy systems and accessories, directly visualized mini-biopsy forceps can be used as well. This method and its performance will be reviewed during the discussion of the role of cholangioscopy in indeterminate strictures. Initial efforts to perform fluoroscopically guided biopsies used gastroscopic forceps until special flexible-tipped duodenoscopic forceps (Olympus Medical, Center Valley, PA) were developed and proved to work better over the elevator. A large sphincterotomy was still required to pass these forceps retrograde up the duct.

The technique of forceps biopsy involves insertion of the device to the lower edge of the stricture. Using fluoroscopy, an accurate biopsy specimen can be obtained from the lower edge of the apparent tumor. Several passes of the forceps are required to produce an optimal yield. Reporting on their experience, Ponchon et al (1995)[9] suggested a minimum of three forceps bites.

For the technique to be practical, specialized forceps were developed. Several devices have been marketed to permit easier

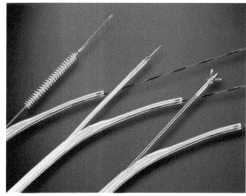

FIG 60.4 Howell biliary introducer (HBI; Wilson-Cook) with three tissue sampling devices advanced to biopsy or cytology position. Each device is placed sequentially to attempt to maximize yield at a single endoscopic retrograde cholangiopancreatography (ERCP) procedure. The HBI is placed over a prepositioned 0.035-inch guidewire.

insertion, including two devices that are purported not to need sphincterotomy. Easier to insert but still unguided, pediatric forceps of 5-Fr to 6-Fr work reasonably well but provide small specimens. Disposable 6-Fr pediatric forceps are now available, although they are relatively expensive. A device has been marketed to enable forceps placement over a guidewire. As previously discussed, the guidewire is generally placed early in therapeutic ERCP to ensure that the major goal of biliary stent placement is successful. It is logical to use the in-place guidewire for subsequent tissue sampling.

The guidewire-based device currently in use, developed by the author, is the Howell biliary introducer (HBI; Cook Medical). The 10-Fr device goes over a 0.035-inch or smaller guidewire while permitting the passage of a specially designed reusable 5-Fr long forceps (Fig. 60.4). Multiple passes of the forceps and other sampling devices can be quickly accomplished once the introducer is in position.

In a review published in two consecutive issues of *Gastrointestinal Endoscopy*, the journal of the American Society of Gastrointestinal Endoscopy (ASGE), de Bellis et al (2002)[60] tabulated all reports in the literature for the three major techniques, including forceps biopsy and ERCP tissue sampling, since 1989 (see Table 60.1). Complications of forceps biopsy have been reported but seem to be rare. Among the 502 patients tabulated in Table 60.1, major bleeding requiring transfusion in one cancer patient was reported,[61] and a significant perforation of a benign stricture required surgery in one additional patient.[50] The perforation may have been caused by the use of a large cup forceps and repeated biopsy sampling of the same location. Pediatric forceps produce a smaller specimen, but no complications were encountered in more than 200 cases. A review of the devices for endoscopic tissue sampling has been published by the ASGE Technology Assessment Committee.[62]

Combining Multiple Sampling Techniques

With the disappointing yields of single technique sampling as presented previously, endoscopists began to report their experience of combining techniques during the same ERCP procedure. Although this approach takes more time than a single technique, improved yields have made the combined approach the preferred sequence in many, particularly academic, centers. Using standard brushes and nonguidewire forceps, Ponchon et al (1995)[9] reported improved combined yields for diagnosing cancer at ERCP. Although brushing had a sensitivity of 43% and forceps biopsy had a sensitivity of 30%, their combined yield was increased to 63% (a 20% overall gain). A more comprehensive approach was studied by the Indiana University group. Researchers attempted to perform all three techniques of brush, FNA, and forceps sampling and submitted withdrawn indwelling stents for cytology when present. This demanding approach resulted in a positive diagnosis in 82% of patients at a single ERCP.[49] When the investigators analyzed their results, each technique contributed to making the diagnosis in at least some patients. In other words, many patients had only one of the techniques positive, and the other two or three techniques were negative or equivocal.

Despite this report and the logic of this approach, the technique of triple sampling has not become a standard practice during ERCP. Several explanations can be advanced. The first and probably most important reason was previously discussed: triple sampling is technically difficult, time-consuming, and ancillary to the main goal of the therapeutic procedure.

The second may be the delay in tissue diagnosis when specimens are submitted for processing. Most important has been the wider availability of EUS-guided FNA cytology with its high sensitivity and safety.[63] EUS procedures are often done before ERCP, or during the same setting, especially when anesthesia is being used. This approach can shorten the ERCP, have a higher yield with multiple needle passes, and permit immediate cytologic diagnosis when a cytologist is in-suite. However, in many patients, a role remains for ERCP tissue sampling, especially when advanced disease makes EUS less valuable for staging and a cytologist is not available. Finally, newer techniques for intraprocedural tissue diagnosis during initial ERCP have been developed and will be discussed later in this chapter.

As introduced earlier, the HBI 10-Fr device introducer was developed to enhance the ability of the average endoscopist to perform triple sampling with a minimum of time, expense, and risk. The goal was to permit maximum sampling at various depths to increase the chance of detecting all three types of malignancy and to do so without requiring a sphincterotomy if so desired. The details of the device and our initial procedural sequence, techniques, and yields were reported in 1996.[64] An overall sensitivity of 69%, despite a large proportion of small early pancreatic cancers, suggested the potential of the device. The HBI introducer is a double-lumen 10-Fr tapered dilator that contains a 0.035-inch channel for a standard ERCP guidewire and a 6-Fr large channel for the introduction of endoscopic accessories.

The device includes a biliary introducer needle, which is a 5-Fr ball-tip catheter with a 22-gauge needle (HBIN, Cook Medical), 5-Fr reusable forceps (HBI forceps, Cook Medical), and a spring-tipped, through-the-channel brush (HBIB, Cook Medical). This brush has extra-long, extra-stiff bristles and is mounted on a stiff braided-wire shaft resulting in an aggressive device (see Fig. 60.1D). Its use is illustrated in Fig. 60.5.

A comparative trial of the HBI device against standard brushing was reported.[65] For the purpose of their study, the authors considered any "positive," "suspicious," or "atypical or suggestive of malignancy" to be true-positive samples. The authors used only the HBIN 22-gauge needle and HBI brush and reported an 85% yield compared with a sensitivity of 57% for brushing alone. Presumably, if the HBI forceps had also been used, yield would have been greater.

Other Methods of Endoscopic Retrograde Cholangiopancreatography Tissue Sampling

Numerous, less productive or controversial techniques of tissue acquisition have been reported and warrant review. Leung et al (1989)[67] originally reported that examining indwelling plastic biliary stents on their removal may produce a positive cytologic specimen when the diagnosis had not been established at the initial ERCP placement. Since 1989, only one series[60] has approached the initial 70% yield of Leung and coworkers. Most centers report only 11% to 44% positive specimens.[43,68,69] The most recent report (1997) of stent cytology included withdrawn pancreatic stents and stents from biliary strictures.[70] The true-positive yield from pancreatic stents was 25% compared with only 11% from biliary stents. In addition, the investigators agreed with other authors that the technique had limited clinical value because of the long delay in diagnosis when positive results were obtained.

Another approach to tissue acquisition at ERCP has been to attempt to collect specimens from the adjacent stricture of the pancreatic duct. Collection of pancreatic juice has been advocated by a few authors.[71,72] The technique involves deep insertion of a standard ERCP catheter and aspiration of juice below a malignant-appearing stricture. Yields may increase to greater than 50% with the infusion of secretin. This approach has not become popular, perhaps because of its complexity and concern for inducing pancreatitis. Pugliese et al (1995)[50] concluded that pancreatic juice collection did not add to positive diagnosis when pancreatic duct strictures were directly sampled by brushing.

Brushing in the pancreatic duct has been reported since 1979.[73] More recent reports (1994–96) emphasize that yields increase very little when a biliary stricture is also present and can be sampled.[74-76] Most concerning has been the report of postprocedural pancreatitis after pancreatic ductal stricture brushing. Vandervoort et al (1999)[77] noted a 21.5% pancreatitis rate after such procedures in both benign and malignant cases, but noted a marked decrease in risk if pancreatic temporary plastic stents were placed. Other authors have also advocated stent placement after pancreatic brushing, but all studies do not outline the eventual management and outcome of these temporary stents. The utility of stents is likely outweighed by subsequent procedures for pancreatic stent removal and delayed stent obstruction with resulting pancreatitis or sepsis, and other approaches to tissue sampling are favored. At the present time, we sample from the pancreatic duct only when a pancreatic stent is clinically warranted to manage obstructing pancreatitis, fistula, or upstream pseudocyst. We prefer to use the over-the-guidewire technique for brushing as outlined previously, so that the guidewire, which was placed before tissue sampling, can remain in position.

Specimen Handling and Analysis

When intraprocedural diagnosis is not a goal or not available, specimens need optimal care. Improper handling of collected specimens remains a problem in many endoscopy units. A major cause of uninterpretable smears is an air-drying artifact that can occur rapidly after creation of appropriate thin smear.[6] Thick smears and specimens with excessive blood are other significant problems.[78] Slide preparation requires the time and attention of ERCP team members during a busy and often complex procedure. Preference should be given to depositing all collected specimens into transport media rather than preparing any smears or slides in the ERCP suite, unless an in-suite cytologist is present. Available transport media include 95% ethanol or commercially prepared

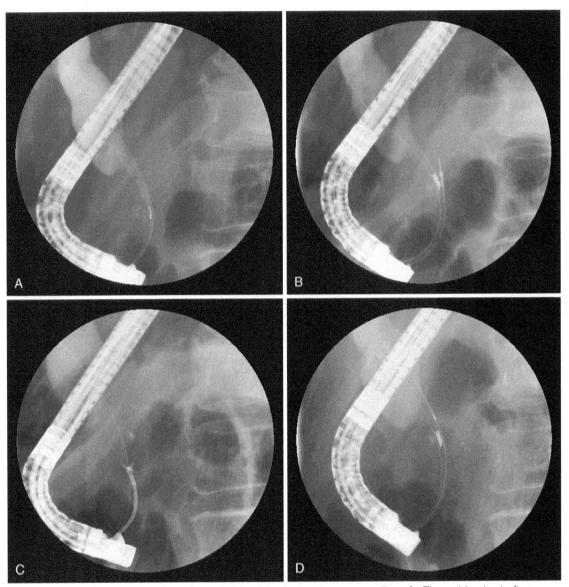

FIG 60.5 Howell biliary introducer (HBI) triple device tissue sampling. **A,** The guidewire is first negotiated through a malignant-appearing stricture. Sphincterotomy is optional. **B,** HBI preloaded with the 5-Fr, 22-gauge needle for fine-needle aspiration (FNA) is placed over the guidewire and positioned just beneath the lower edge of the stricture. The needle has been thrust into the tumor at 30 degrees from the axis of the guidewire. **C,** The 5-Fr reusable HBIN forceps is passed for repeat biopsies of the lower edge of the stricture. **D,** To perform brush cytology with the HBI, the introducer is advanced so that the metal port lies above the stricture. The special brush (HBIB) is advanced into the proximal duct. The introducer is pulled down into the stricture to permit vigorous brushing with adequate side pressure to maximize cellular collection.

solutions such as CytoLyt (Cytyc Corporation, Marlborough, MA) or CytoRich (UtoCyte, Burlington, NC). Papanicolaou-stained spun smears and, when applicable, hematoxylin and eosin-stained cell block sections are prepared for cytologic evaluation. In our institution, we prefer CytoLyt solution, which lyses red blood cells and minimizes obscuring debris, with smears prepared via the Thin Prep method (Cytyc Corporation).

Interpretation of specimens should follow accepted cytologic criteria to be clinically useful. Several such schemes exist with each accepting frankly positive (Fig. 60.6A) and negative (see Fig. 60.6B) features. Intermediate cytologic abnormalities present

on the slides may lead to interpretations such as "atypical," in which mild cellular abnormalities are usually associated with inflammation and reparative changes, and "suspicious," in which there are rare cells exhibiting cytologic features of malignancy, but they are present in insufficient numbers to render a definitive diagnosis of malignancy.

In patients with PSC or postbiliary irradiation, be aware that cytologic changes can result in occasional false-positive samples. A larger series noted only 80% specificity in this setting.[79]

The findings of "cellular atypia" should include criteria that make the diagnosis of malignancy unlikely and demand further

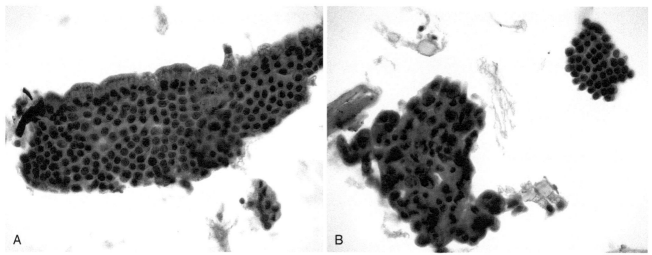

FIG 60.6 A, Benign biliary sample collected at endoscopic retrograde cholangiopancreatography (ERCP) by fine-needle aspiration (FNA). The specimen shows normal monolayer architecture with cells of high cytoplasm-to-nuclear ratio. The nuclei are smooth with fine chromatin and without obvious nucleoli. **B,** ERCP-collected specimen reveals malignant features diagnostic of adeno-carcinomas. Note the clusters of cells with nuclear crowding. The nuclei have irregular membranes, coarse chromatin, and prominent nucleoli. Finally, the nuclei are large, producing high nuclei-to-cytoplasmic ratio.

attempts at confirmation. We interpret all atypia findings as negative, understanding that many will turn out to be falsely negative. Finally, because of the inherent difficulties in ERCP tissue sampling, negative results can never be accepted as definitive.[7,11]

Sampling problems are often due to the relative hardness of pancreaticobiliary adenocarcinomas that may greatly resist needle puncture and forceps sampling. These desmoplastic tumors can be relatively hypocellular, resulting in inadequate numbers of cells for interpretation. A small fraction of adenocarcinomas are so well differentiated they can be diagnosed histologically only in the setting of an excisional biopsy to permit the recognition of invasion; this is also true of lymphoma, which does occasionally produce biliary obstruction. As previously discussed, metastatic lesions obstructing the biliary tree are relatively deep and cannot be readily accessed at ERCP from within the ductal stricture, except occasionally by intraductal FNA. These lesions are best approached with EUS FNA or the new core-type needles. All these factors result in a low negative predictive value in all series reporting techniques of tissue sampling. This low negative predictive value should not discourage endoscopists from developing a preferred sequence of tissue sampling at ERCP because specificity in most reports is generally 100% for true-positive samples except as noted previously. A false-negative result leads to additional invasive tests, procedures, or surgery,[80] the same result as when no effort is made. Using the outlined techniques of endobiliary sampling during ERCP, patients receive benefit at a minimum of expense and risk.

Intraprocedural Techniques at ERCP

A major development in indeterminate biliary stricture sampling has been the development of intraprocedural analysis of specimens obtained by EUS FNA, and ERCP specimens as well.

We have experimented with triple sampling as previously outlined and on occasion had ERCP FNA or brushings slides made and sent for immediate Papanicolaou staining and interpretation. With additional experience, we noted increasing yield with increased numbers of forceps biopsy without an increase in complications, but needed techniques for immediate processing and interpretation. ERCP-guided FNA has the disadvantages of technical difficulty, more shallow depth of puncture, and limited number of passes before needing to employ a new needle.

A new technique developed in our unit using a new cytologic preparation of forceps specimens at ERCP can permit direct intraprocedural diagnosis similar to the sequence used at EUS.[81] In neurosurgery, intraoperative samples of margins during brain tumor resection have been sampled by preparing quick fixed smears of brain tissue on dry slides. Termed *squash prep,* this technique evolved because frozen sections cannot be done on fat-rich brain tissue. Paralleling this established technique, our group prepared small 5-Fr or 6-Fr forceps biopsy specimens by vigorously smashing them between two dry glass slides to attempt to create a monolayer. These specimens are immediately stained by rapid Papanicolaou and read in suite. This new technique is termed *SMASH protocol* (Video 60.1).[81] At our center, experience with this approach added only an additional 10 to 20 minutes to the ERCP procedure and produced a definitive positive diagnosis in 49/66 (74%) of pancreaticobiliary cancers.[82] This high yield is in part produced by the cytopathologist who can request additional specimens similar to EUS. We generally halt at 10 specimens, in favor of collecting additional biopsy specimens for histology and a final one or two ERCP-guided FNA passes. This new approach at tissue sampling adds little time and little cost and avoids delay in tissue diagnosis in most patients. Immediate tissue diagnosis avoids additional efforts at biopsy, such as EUS-guided FNA or CT-guided FNA, and often shortens hospital stay.[81]

When in-suite cytopathology is not available and time permits, we have reported a further method of intraprocedural diagnosis. Forceps biopsies can be sent to most hospital pathology labs for frozen section analysis, often on short notice and at odd hours. Our initial technique was to send five rapidly obtained specimens from the lower edge of an indeterminate stricture using only

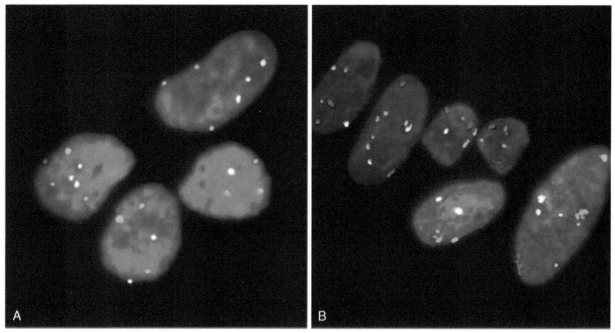

FIG 60.7 **A,** Trisomy of chromosomes 3,7,17 (3 copies of red, green, and aqua probes). **B,** Homozygous deletion of 9p21 (absence of gold probes in all but one normal cell). (Images courtesy of Dr. Tamas Gonda.)

fluoroscopic guidewire during ERCP. If negative, an additional five specimens could be sent. Noting no complications in greater than 50 cases using only 5-Fr or 6-Fr pediatric forceps, we now send 10 specimens and complete our sampling with two forceps specimens for H&E staining and do a single ERCP FNA sample.

Our experience suggests that the yield of the frozen section protocol is somewhat lower than SMASH protocol, likely due to the absence of the cytopathologist, but provides prompt, simple, and widely available interpretation with a true positive yield of 80+%.[83]

In the specific setting of CCA of the common bile duct, common hepatic duct, or bifurcation, these techniques of forceps tissue sampling by SMASH, frozen, or standard triple sampling established an overall true positive diagnosis in 87% of consecutive cases at our institution.[82,84] The intraprocedural diagnosis by SMASH or frozen was 79% and the addition of H&E and ERCP FNA added 8% to achieve the final total.

Advanced Specimen Analysis

Despite these advances in tissue sampling of indeterminate biliary strictures, false negative specimens still plague the goal of 100% diagnostic accuracy. After collection, specimens can undergo additional techniques of analysis in an attempt at increasing positive results, only their current status demands an update.

FISH

While improved methods of acquisition of tissue remains a challenge, developments in the methods of analysis of available tissue has made significant advancement. One promising tissue-based diagnostic tool that gained a prominent role in the diagnostic armamentarium for IDBS is the use of fluorescent in-situ hybridization (FISH) to detect chromosomal aneuploidy or polysomy. Positive findings are found in an estimated 80% of pancreaticobiliary malignancies.[85] FISH uses fluorescently

labeled chromosome-specific DNA probes to identify cells with an abnormal number of chromosomes or mutations. The four commercially available FISH probes target chromosomes 3 (CEP3), 7 (CEP7), 17 (CEP17), and the 9p21 locus of chromosome 9 (Fig. 60.7). While this method of molecular analysis is markedly different from the cytological methods used conventionally, its use adds no additional burden of sampling as these tests can be performed on cells obtained from routine brush cytology samples during ERCP. In fact, the same brush can even be used to provide both FISH results and cytology results with the use of a multipart brush, such as a brush with 3 separate clusters of bristles (Infinity Brush, US Endoscopy, Mentor, OH). The relative disadvantage is that centers that analyze FISH samples are limited and may require samples to be sent out. Another disadvantage is that FISH analysis typically can take up to 3 weeks to return, depending on the practices of the individual center, as many samples are run in batches and the evaluation for aneuploidy or polysomy is not an automated process.

Data regarding diagnostic yield has been variable and is dependent on the specific panel of probes included in individual studies. Early prospective data on the diagnostic yield of FISH in indeterminate strictures by Levy et al (2008), using CEP3, CEP7, and CEP 17 probes found that, in previously cytology-negative strictures, the sensitivity of FISH was 62%, with specificity of 79% for malignancy.[85] When a fourth probe to the 9p21 loci of chromosome 9 (associated with mutation of the p16 tumor suppressor gene) is added to the repertoire, the sensitivity of FISH can be improved significantly from 47% to 84%, with preserved specificity of 97%.[86] As discussed earlier with respect to combined sampling, Nanda et al (2007) demonstrated that triple modality sampling with brush cytology, fluoroscopically guided biopsies, and FISH resulted in significantly higher sensitivity of 82% versus 42% for brush cytology alone.[87] Individual modality results for cytology, biopsies, and FISH were 27%, 50%, and 59% respectively. Cost analysis in a study population, in which the respective sensitivity of cytology and FISH was 42% and 70% respectively, suggested that FISH testing be used as a second-line evaluation if cytology samples were negative given the significant additional cost for FISH analysis.[88] The main limitation of FISH is its reduced specificity in the setting of chronic inflammatory conditions such as PSC where polysomy can occur in the absence of CCA.[89] By adding trisomy-7 as a marker of malignancy in the combined cohort of both PSC and non-PSC patients, the overall sensitivity for diagnosing malignancy was 64%, specificity 82%, and diagnostic accuracy 72%. However, trisomy 7 in particular can be found in benign strictures of PSC patients and decreases the specificity of FISH for malignancy in that challenging cohort. This elevated rate of false positive results in the setting of PSC has resulted in recommendations suggesting FISH results be followed in surveillance sampling of PSC patients and that a positive FISH result alone not be considered positive.

Other molecular-based techniques that have been examined to improve the diagnostic yield include bile aspirate analysis for p53 and KRAS mutations, but these are not currently considered part of the routine workup and are still in the early phases of investigation.[90] One study has evaluated the value of combination testing of FISH and genetic analysis (KRAS mutation, LOH, tumor suppressor genes at 10 loci)[91] and found that adding both FISH and molecular profiling to cytology can increase sensitivity from 32% to 73% ($p < 0.001$). This supports that sampling methods and analysis should be performed in tandem to optimize diagnostic accuracies. Nevertheless, the proven performance of FISH in the evaluation of biliary strictures has earned the recommendation by cytologic societies that it be considered the only ancillary technique to biliary brushing with sufficient efficacy.[92]

Endoscopic Ultrasound-FNA

EUS FNA is another modality that has entered the algorithm of evaluation of IDBS as a complementary tool to ERCP. A discussion regarding its role and results in tissue sampling is discussed elsewhere. It is worthy to note, however, that the exact role of FNA in the setting of suspected proximal CCA remains controversial. This is mostly due to the theoretical potential for malignant peritoneal seeding via the needle access pathway. Data from a small number of case series of patients who underwent percutaneous biliary biopsies for CCA who developed carcinomatosis with rates as high as 83%[93,94] have driven most transplant centers to adopt protocols in which tissue sampling with EUS FNA of the primary lesion is a contraindication to liver transplantation of hilar CCA.[95] For those patients who are not going to be considered for transplant or who have extrahepatic disease and are being considered for resection only, the reported overall sensitivity of EUS FNA is 43% to 86% for the diagnosis of all malignant strictures.[96–98] EUS FNA is generally less reliable in the evaluation of proximal CCA, as its sensitivity decreases to 59% compared to 81% in distal CCA.[98] The presence of a previously placed biliary stent can also decrease its sensitivity for malignancy detection due to a combination of stent-related acoustic shadowing, image degradation, and difficult needle access.

Intraductal Ultrasound

If the infiltrative nature of CCA and other biliary strictures serves as an obstacle to adequate tissue acquisition, then having a method of investigating wall layers to identify and characterize that invasion might be helpful in providing a predictive diagnosis, as well as targeting tissue. One such intraductal imaging modality is intraductal ultrasound (IDUS), which enhances endobiliary imaging by the wire-guided placement of a high-frequency probe directly into the bile ducts. Technically, this is a simple maneuver to perform as the probe is a small-caliber catheter that is passed over a wire during ERCP, does not require a sphincterotomy, and is radiopaque, and thus the probe's exact location can be determined. The probe provides high-quality imaging of the periductal tissue along with limited tumor staging, such as mass size and periportal vascular invasion (full lymph node staging still requires EUS).[99] IDUS criteria for differentiating benign from malignant strictures have been established and include disruption of the normal triple layer wall architecture, eccentric wall thickening, presence of a hypoechoic mass with irregular margins or invasion of adjacent structures, papillary surface, and malignant-appearing periductal lymph nodes.[100] These criteria have been validated in multiple studies demonstrating diagnostic sensitivities of IDUS to be 80% to 90%, specificity 83%, and improvement in the accuracy of ERCP from 58% to 83%.[101,102] The disadvantage to IDUS is that it is solely an adjunctive imaging tool that helps direct evaluation of IDBSs but does not provide histopathology. This may explain the relatively rare use of this modality in the algorithm of evaluation. Furthermore, the probe itself is relatively fragile, and not disposable, and requires a separate processor, and therefore, it falls into the capital inventory of most endoscopy suites and limitations this incurs.

Optical Coherence Tomography

Another technology that allows for greater evaluation of the bile duct wall layers is optical coherence tomography (OCT), which was introduced over 20 years ago[103] and allows for high-resolution, cross-sectional, tomographic imaging of tissue. An earlier catheter version worked by measuring the interference of low-power infrared light (750–1300 nm) reflected from the tissue and light reflected from reference mirrors. In-vitro and in-vivo studies have demonstrated the feasibility of using this catheter to visualize multiple wall layers of the gut and pancreaticobiliary ducts, as well as visualizing microscopic structures, such as blood vessels, lymphoid aggregates, crypts, and glands.[104–108] Early animal and human studies of the pancreaticobiliary epithelium and sphincter of Oddi helped to demonstrate OCT findings that correlated to the three ductal wall layers, single layer epithelium, deeper fibromuscular layer, and an outer smooth muscle layer. The corresponding OCT images were an inner hyporeflective layer, a homogenous hyperreflective layer, and a less defined hyporeflective layer, respectively.[109] In addition, neoplastic and nonplastic tissue could be differentiated.[109–111]

Using two OCT criteria to diagnose malignancy, including unrecognizable layer architecture, and the presence of large, nonreflective areas compatible with tumor vessels, Arvanitakis et al (2009)[112] evaluated the feasibility of OCT in detecting malignant biliary strictures in 35 patients. Using the mid-focus OCT probe (PENTAX Corporation Tokyo, Japan/Lightlab Imaging Ltd, Boston, MA; outer diameter 0.75 mm, depth of penetration 1 mm, resolution 10 um) malignant strictures were diagnosed in 19/25 (54%) of patients compared to tissue as gold standard. The sensitivity of at least one or both OCT was 79% and 53%, respectively, and accuracy was 70% for both categories. When combining brushings and biopsies to at least one criteria, sensitivity increased to 84%.[112]

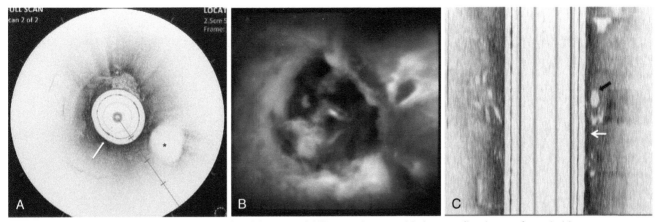

FIG 60.8 **A,** VLE cross-sectional image of biliary stricture with hyperreflective surface *(white arrow)*, and periductal vessel *(asterisk).* **B,** Spy image of corresponding biliary stricture to (**A**). **C,** Longitudinal image of biliary stricture with features of subepithelial glands *(black arrow)* and hyperreflective surface *(white arrow).* (Images courtesy of Dr. Doug Pleskow.)

A newer probe has just become commercially available in the United States that uses volumetric laser electromicrography to provide very similar images to the prior OCT catheter (NinePoint Medical, Cambridge, MA). Similar to its predecessor, the probe fits through the working channel of the ERCP scope, is not currently wire-guided, and requires a dedicated processor for imaging. Circumferential radial and 6-cm longitudinal images are provided with depth of 3 mm, lateral resolution of 40 microns, and axial resolution of 7 microns. Similar to prior OCT work, the principles of image interpretation come from data using the technology in setting of Barrett's epithelium, where features such as loss of wall definition, increased reflectivity, and glandular structures are indicative of dysplastic areas (Fig. 60.8). Data regarding the use of this low-profile catheter is currently being collected from select centers. Similar to its predecessor, it holds promise as an additional tool to increase the predictive value of imaging and targeting for further sampling of pancreaticobiliary strictures.

Cholangioscopy

Logically, the most direct way to diagnose a malignancy in the practice of any endoscopy is to directly visualize the epithelium to allow for a diagnostic impression and for precise targeted sampling. This technique, cholangioscopy, was first made possible in the 1970s with the use of the first generation "mother-baby" cholangioscopes. While newer versions of the video cholangioscopy systems provided outstanding imaging, widespread adoption was limited due to the need for two operators, scope fragility, limited tip maneuverability, and prolonged procedures.[113] The development of single-operator cholangioscopy (SOC), and the release of the Spyglass Direct Visualization System (Boston Scientific, Marlborough, MA) in 2005 have measurably changed the practice of cholangioscopy worldwide.

The Spyglass system (Boston Scientific, Marlborough, MA) consists of a 10-Fr access catheter (SpyScope) that can be inserted through the standard 4.2-mm working channel of a therapeutic duodenoscope, a reusable optical probe (SpyGlass) that fits through the SpyScope catheter, and disposable 3-Fr biliary biopsy forceps to allow visually-directed biopsies (SpyBite). The optical catheter provides 6000 pixel images and has tip maneuverability to allow 30-degree views in four directions.[114] A second-generation

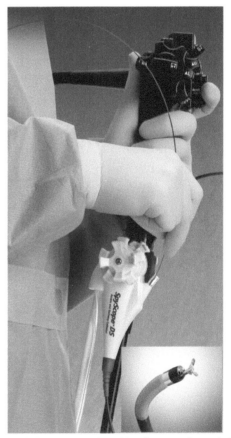

FIG 60.9 Spy DS scope and spybite forceps *(insert).* (Courtesy of Boston Scientific, Marlborough, MA.)

Spyglass system, known as Spyglass DS, has a digital chip embedded at the end of the SpyScope and thus eliminates the need for the optic fiber and the necessary preprocedural calibration required, while providing a wider field of view (Fig. 60.9). The accessory channel size is also slightly larger and thus facilitates passage of accessories such as forceps and lithotripsy probes. Last, there are dedicated individual irrigation and aspiration

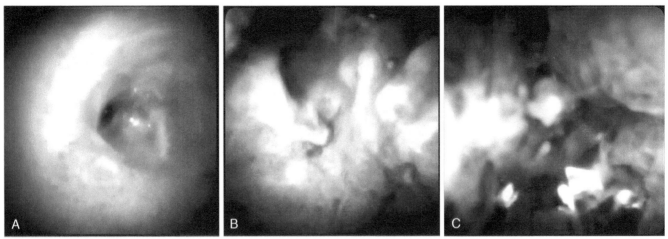

FIG 60.10 **A,** Spy image of benign biliary stricture. **B,** Spy image of malignant biliary stricture. **C,** Spy image of directly visualized biopsy. (Images courtesy of Dr. Amrita Sethi.)

channels that improve duct clearance of debris and visualization significantly.

At this stage, data regarding outcomes of the use of SOC in the evaluation of IDBSs reflect use of the first-generation system.

The largest prospective, multicentered, observational study of the operating characteristics of the SOC system by Chen et al (2011)[115] included 226 patients with biliary strictures (not all were cytology negative) with a sensitivity, specificity, positive predictive value, and negative predictive value for malignancy of 78%, 82%, 80%, and 80%, respectively, based on the visual impression criteria.[115,116] Visual impression had a higher sensitivity compared to visually targeted biopsies, which was only 47%, although biopsy specificity was much higher at 98%, with a positive predictive value of 100%. A smaller prospective series from Ramchandani et al (2011)[117] involving 36 patients with indeterminate strictures also found the sensitivity of the SOC visual impression to be 95%, and specificity of 79%, while sensitivity and specificity for SpyBite biopsies were lower at 82%. A comparison study of directly visualized (DV) biopsies versus both brush cytology and fluoroscopically guided biopsies in 26 patients demonstrated that despite adequate tissue quantity with all three modalities, the accuracy of the DV biopsies was 84.6%, which was significantly higher than brush cytology (38.5%) and standard forceps (53.8%).[118] By analysis in a systematic review, the sensitivity and specificity of cholangioscopy-directed biopsies' ability to detect malignancy in IDBS with prior negative findings in a total of four studies was 74.7% (95% confidence interval [CI], 63.3%–84.0%) and 93.3% (95% CI, 85.1%–97.8%).[119] Another systematic review found that the sensitivity and specificity of visual impression were 90% (95%CI, 73%–97%), and 87% (95% CI, 76%–94%), respectively.[120] In a more recent study evaluating the role of performing rapid on-site evaluation of touch imprints of DV biopsy specimens (ROSE-TIC), Varadarajulu et al (2016) studied 31 patients and with a mean of 3.3 biopsies, were able to achieve a sensitivity of 100% and accuracy of 93.5% in diagnosing malignancy in IDBS.[121]

The issue of visual impression remains an unanswered topic given the lack of validated criteria by which to diagnose malignancy. Early imaging with video cholangioscopy led to considerations for imaging criteria that have been proposed for the diagnosis of malignancy including dilated, tortuous blood vessels (also termed tumor vessels), intraductal nodules or masses,

---

BOX 60.1 Malignant Stricture Criteria for SOC Cholangioscopy

Dilated, tortuous blood vessels
Intraductal nodules or mass
Infiltrative or ulcerated stricture
Papillary or villous mucosal projections

SOC, single-operator digital cholangioscopy.
Data from Seo DW, Lee SK, Yoo KS, et al: Cholangioscopic findings in bile duct tumors. *Gastrointest Endosc* 52(5):630–634, 2000.

---

infiltrative or ulcerated strictures, and papillary or villous mucosal projections[122] (Fig. 60.10; Video 60.2). The strongest feature suggestive of malignancy has been the presence of dilated and tortuous vessels with a reported specificity and positive predictive value of 100%[123–125] (Box 60.1), as this was felt to represent underlying neovascularization of the malignant tumor. However, when viewed by first fiber optic and now digital cholangioscopy, and when removed from clinical context, it is not clear that these findings are validated. In two consecutive studies, interobserver agreement of SOC visual findings, using the fiber optic system, and final diagnosis, were only slight to fair and the accuracy was less than 50% on diagnosing malignancy.[126,127] Further attempts are being made by multiple groups to create a new classification system using the digital cholangioscopy system, with the hopes that clearer imaging and new tissue-correlated definitions may lead to a validated system. Ultimately, however, in this tissue-based era, it is unclear what role visual impression alone will play and whether the true benefit will be in the ability to target sampling and additional diagnostic methods.

A few considerations need to be made when performing cholangioscopy, namely, the need for biliary sphincterotomy to advance the system into the biliary tree and higher rates of complications due to sphincterotomy and cholangitis. Chen et al (2011)[115] reported serious procedural complication rates of 7.5%; a later study by Sethi et al (2011)[128] confirmed a complication rate of 7.0% versus the routine ERCP rate of 2.9%, with the difference attributed to higher incidence of cholangitis in the cholangioscopy group. Such findings have led to routine use of antibiotics when performing cholangioscopy in otherwise low-risk patients during ERCP.

Confocal Laser Endomicroscopy

Another method of direct evaluation of the biliary epithelium is probe-based confocal laser endomicroscopy (pCLE), which uses an optical probe during ERCP to allow real-time, microscopic level examination of the bile ducts.[129] The CholangioFlex probe (Maunakea Tech, Paris, France) fits into multiple ERCP accessory devices or the 1.2 mm-diameter working channel of the SpyGlass (Boston Scientific) cholangioscope. This probe provides images to a depth 40 to 70 μm below the tissue surface. An intravenous contrast agent, usually fluorescein, is used to delineate cellular features that have been determined to represent criteria of malignancy versus benign disease and inflammation. Identification of these criteria have been performed in a series of steps, the first iteration known as the "Miami Classification," which helped to distinguish malignant from benign features. This was prospectively studied in a multicentered, larger cohort of 89 patients with indeterminate pancreaticobiliary strictures by eight investigators (Table 60.2).[130,131] The sensitivity, specificity, positive predictive value, and negative predictive value of pCLE using the Miami criteria were 98%, 67%, 71%, and 97%; the accuracy of combination ERCP with pCLE was significantly higher than ERCP with tissue sampling alone (90% vs. 73%).[130]

In attempts to improve the specificity of these criteria, refinement with the Paris classification was conducted that allowed for identification of features that would predict inflammation from benign and malignant disease (Fig. 60.11). Addition of these

criteria did in fact improve specificity from 61% to 81.2% in lesions previously scored by the Miami classification system.[132] Prospective validation of the Paris criteria was performed by Slivka et al (2015)[133] in the FOCUS trial in which confocal diagnosis was added to ERCP imaging and sampling, as well as clinical history, and scored by two physicians. The results of this prospective study demonstrated that the additive value of all three diagnosis (pCLE, ERCP, and sampling) could provide an accuracy of 88% in the diagnosis of malignancy in indeterminate strictures.[133]

Practically, the low specificity of pCLE and the dedicated operator training needed (as has been demonstrated in interobserver agreement studies)[134] for accurate interpretation of confocal images remain the major limiting factors of its widespread use as a routine tool in the evaluation of indeterminate strictures. However, in expert centers with pCLE experience, it has become a valuable tool in the multimodality approach to the management of difficult cases of biliary stricture.

EVALUATION OF STRICTURES IN PSC

The caveat to the preceding discussion regarding IDBSs is the ever-elusive diagnosis of CCA in PSC. PSC is a chronic, progressive inflammatory condition of the intrahepatic and extrahepatic bile ducts, characterized by diffuse stricturing that can lead to biliary cirrhosis and increases patients' risk for CCA threefold.[135,136] Liver transplantation is the only curative treatment for both end-stage biliary cirrhosis and early-stage hilar CCA, with a posttransplant, 5-year survival of 65% to 88% when performed in expert centers under rigorous protocols.[137,138] However, due to the chronic stricturing nature of the disease, differentiating between benign and malignant strictures in this population is particularly difficult. Per guidelines, the presence of a dominant stricture prompts an endoscopic evaluation that often includes many of the modalities discussed earlier in this chapter. However, the diagnostic performance of these modalities from molecular analysis to advanced imaging appear to be even more challenged in PSC patients. A recent meta-analysis showed that FISH sensitivity for CCA in PSC is only 51%, although specificity is preserved at 93%.[139] Similarly, confocal endomicroscopy's reduced reliability in distinguishing chronic inflammatory benign changes from malignant transformation suggests that further refinement is needed for evaluation of PSC strictures by this modality. Cholangioscopy may be the most promising method, with some prospective studies suggesting sensitivity for CCA in PSC patients of 92%, specificity 93%, and overall accuracy

TABLE 60.2   Miami and Paris Classification of pCLE for Predicting Malignant Biliary Stricture

Criteria Suggestive of Malignancy	Criteria Suggestive of Inflammation	Criteria Suggestive of Benign Disease
Thick, dark bands (> 40 μm)	Thick reticular network	Thin, dark bands
Thick, white bands (> 20 μm)	Increased intraglandular space	Thin, white bands
Dark clumps	Vascular congestion	
Villous glands		
Fluorescein leakage		

pCLE, probe-based confocal laser endomicroscopy.

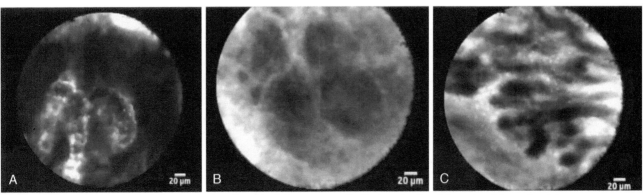

FIG 60.11 **A,** Miami criteria of epithelial structure. **B,** Paris criteria of increased intraglandular space or scales. **C,** Paris criteria of thickened reticulum. (Images courtesy of Dr. Amrita Sethi.)

of 93%, but in half of the patients a second cholangioscopy was needed for tissue diagnosis.[113] Furthermore, there is the theoretical increased risk of cholangitis when performing these advanced imaging modalities in patients with PSC. Thus, the literature suggests a multimodality approach in any PSC patient in whom there is a high clinical suspicion for malignancy, such as a persistently, markedly elevated CA19-9 despite biliary decompression, or new or symptomatic dominant stricture, is likely to offer the greatest diagnostic value.

CONCLUSION

IDBSs remain a challenge despite developments in imaging, tissue acquisition, development of additional tissue analysis methods, and even serum markers. There is no question, however, that a multimodality approach must be employed to optimize diagnostic results. The components of this combined approach will depend on local expertise and resources. First-line approach should include routine ERCP with brushings and FISH, and if nondiagnostic despite high clinical concern, consider an adjunct endobiliary imaging study, to either confirm clinical suspicions or to use for continued close surveillance. Proximal biliary strictures may be best imaged by IDUS, whereas EUS can evaluate for suspicious periductal lymph nodes. Practices in the use of cholangioscopy and confocal endomicroscopy will vary more widely depending on its availability, operator experience, and further definition and validation of diagnostic criteria. Ultimately, the future for endoscopic evaluation of biliary strictures will need to move toward developing a diagnostic algorithm that reconciles the cost-effectiveness of extensive and repeated evaluations for stable-appearing strictures with the potential for a missed malignancy and/or unnecessary surgical exploration. Ultimately, the inherent problem may not lie within the methods used, but rather the nature of the disease. And in this era of tissue-specific diagnoses, future efforts will likely focus on identifying the highest yield area for sampling and maximizing acquisition from this area. Indeed, the evaluation of IDBS remains a rich area for research and eventual change in practice as new tools are developed and their respective roles established.

KEY REFERENCES

9. Ponchon T, Gagnon P, Berger F, et al: Value of endobiliary brush cytology and biopsies for the diagnosis of malignant bile duct stenosis: results of a prospective study, *Gastrointest Endosc* 42(6):565–572, 1995.

46. Howell DA, Beveridge RP, Bosco J, Jones M: Endoscopic needle aspiration biopsy at ERCP in the diagnosis of biliary strictures, *Gastrointest Endosc* 38(5):531–535, 1992.

47. Jailwala J, Fogel EL, Sherman S, et al: Triple-tissue sampling at ERCP in malignant biliary obstruction, *Gastrointest Endosc* 51(4 Pt 1):383–390, 2000.

48. Lee JG, Leung JW, Baillie J, et al: Benign, dysplastic, or malignant—making sense of endoscopic bile duct brush cytology: results in 149 consecutive patients, *Am J Gastroenterol* 90(5):722–726, 1995.

58. Farrell RJ, Jain AK, Brandwein SL, et al: The combination of stricture dilation, endoscopic needle aspiration, and biliary brushings significantly improves diagnostic yield from malignant bile duct strictures, *Gastrointest Endosc* 54(5):587–594, 2001.

86. Gonda TA, Glick MP, Sethi A, et al: Polysomy and p16 deletion by fluorescence in situ hybridization in the diagnosis of indeterminate biliary strictures, *Gastrointest Endosc* 75(1):74–79, 2012.

87. Nanda A, Brown JM, Berger SH, et al: Triple modality testing by endoscopic retrograde cholangiopancreatography for the diagnosis of cholangiocarcinoma, *Therap Adv Gastroenterol* 8(2):56–65, 2015.

88. Boldorini R, Paganotti A, Andorno S, et al: A multistep cytological approach for patients with jaundice and biliary strictures of indeterminate origin, *J Clin Pathol* 68(4):283–287, 2015.

89. Bangarulingam SY, Bjornsson E, Enders F, et al: Long-term outcomes of positive fluorescence in situ hybridization tests in primary sclerosing cholangitis, *Hepatology* 51(1):174–180, 2010.

91. Gonda TA, Viterbo D, Gausman V, et al: Mutation profile and fluorescence in situ hybridization analyses increase detection of malignancies in biliary strictures, *Clin Gastroenterol Hepatol* 15(6):913–919.e1, 2017.

94. Nakamuta M, Tanabe Y, Ohashi M, et al: Transabdominal seeding of hepatocellular carcinoma after fine-needle aspiration biopsy, *J Clin Ultrasound* 21(8):551–556, 1993.

98. Mohamadnejad M, DeWitt JM, Sherman S, et al: Role of EUS for preoperative evaluation of cholangiocarcinoma: a large single-center experience, *Gastrointest Endosc* 73(1):71–78, 2011.

101. Stavropoulos S, Larghi A, Verna E, et al: Intraductal ultrasound for the evaluation of patients with biliary strictures and no abdominal mass on computed tomography, *Endoscopy* 37(8):715–721, 2005.

112. Arvanitakis M, Hookey L, Tessier G, et al: Intraductal optical coherence tomography during endoscopic retrograde cholangiopancreatography for investigation of biliary strictures, *Endoscopy* 41(8):696–701, 2009.

115. Chen YK, Parsi MA, Binmoeller KF, et al: Single-operator cholangioscopy in patients requiring evaluation of bile duct disease or therapy of biliary stones (with videos), *Gastrointest Endosc* 74(4):805–814, 2011.

116. Nishikawa T, Tsuyuguchi T, Sakai Y, et al: Comparison of the diagnostic accuracy of peroral video-cholangioscopic visual findings and cholangioscopy-guided forceps biopsy findings for indeterminate biliary lesions: a prospective study, *Gastrointest Endosc* 77(2):219–226, 2013.

119. Navaneethan U, Hasan MK, Lourdusamy V, et al: Single-operator cholangioscopy and targeted biopsies in the diagnosis of indeterminate biliary strictures: a systematic review, *Gastrointest Endosc* 82(4):608–614.e2, 2015.

120. Sun X, Zhou Z, Tian J, et al: Is single-operator peroral cholangioscopy a useful tool for the diagnosis of indeterminate biliary lesion? A systematic review and meta-analysis, *Gastrointest Endosc* 82(1):79–87, 2015.

121. Varadarajulu S, Bang JY, Hasan MK, et al: Improving the diagnostic yield of single-operator cholangioscopy-guided biopsy of indeterminate biliary strictures: ROSE to the rescue? (with video), *Gastrointest Endosc* 84(4):681–687, 2016.

122. Seo DW, Lee SK, Yoo KS, et al: Cholangioscopic findings in bile duct tumors, *Gastrointest Endosc* 52(5):630–634, 2000.

123. Itoi T, Neuhaus H, Chen YK: Diagnostic value of image-enhanced video cholangiopancreatoscopy, *Gastrointest Endosc Clin N Am* 19(4):557–566, 2009.

124. Kim HJ, Kim MH, Lee SK, et al: Tumor vessel: a valuable cholangioscopic clue of malignant biliary stricture, *Gastrointest Endosc* 52(5):635–638, 2000.

128. Sethi A, Chen YK, Austin GL, et al: ERCP with cholangiopancreatoscopy may be associated with higher rates of complications than ERCP alone: a single-center experience, *Gastrointest Endosc* 73(2):251–256, 2011.

131. Meining A, Shah RJ, Slivka A, et al: Classification of probe-based confocal laser endomicroscopy findings in pancreaticobiliary strictures, *Endoscopy* 44(3):251–257, 2012.

133. Slivka A, Gan I, Jamidar P, et al: Validation of the diagnostic accuracy of probe-based confocal laser endomicroscopy for the characterization of indeterminate biliary strictures: results of a prospective multicenter international study, *Gastrointest Endosc* 81(2):282–290, 2015.

139. Navaneethan U, Njei B, Venkatesh PG, et al: Fluorescence in situ hybridization for diagnosis of cholangiocarcinoma in primary sclerosing cholangitis: a systematic review and meta-analysis, *Gastrointest Endosc* 79(6):943–950.e3, 2014.

A complete reference list can be found online at ExpertConsult .com

61

Pancreatic Cystic Lesions

Anne Marie Lennon, Omer Basar, and William R. Brugge

Pancreatic cysts are relatively rare lesions, and their diagnosis has increased with the widespread availability and use of cross-sectional imaging. In many cases pancreatic cysts are detected on imaging performed for another indication; however, they can also be seen in patients with symptoms such as abdominal pain or jaundice. Pancreatic cysts are reported to be found in 3% of computed tomography (CT) scans and 20% of magnetic resonance imaging (MRI) scans, and an increased prevalence is reported with advancing age. Patients with intraductal papillary mucinous neoplasms (IPMNs) and mucinous cystic neoplasms (MCNs) are at higher risk of pancreatic malignancy compared to the general population. The majority of pancreatic cystic lesions are nonneoplastic cysts, which are predominantly pancreatic pseudocysts (PPs) and are mostly seen as a local complication of pancreatitis.[1] Neoplastic cysts of the pancreas are broadly categorized as mucinous and nonmucinous lesions, and the type of epithelial lining determines the risk of malignancy. Once a PP has been eliminated as a possibility, the next step is to determine the type of cyst based on cross-sectional imaging, aspiration cytology, and cyst fluid analysis (Box 61.1).

NONNEOPLASTIC CYSTS

Pancreatic Pseudocysts

PPs may occur secondary to acute or chronic pancreatitis or pancreatic trauma. They are inflammatory fluid collections and 10% to 20% of patients with acute pancreatitis develop a PP.[2] A pseudocyst is often diagnosed when cross-sectional imaging demonstrates an enhancing capsule surrounding a peripancreatic fluid collection 4 weeks from the onset of acute nonnecrotizing pancreatitis. The capsule does not contain an "epithelial lining,"[3] and a PP usually contains an opaque, dark, low-viscosity fluid free of epithelial cells. PPs are usually sterile collections, but may become infected or hemorrhagic. The majority of PPs are solitary, unilocular cysts ranging from 2 to 20 cm in diameter.[1,3,4] Abdominal pain, early satiety, and weight loss are common symptoms, and a PP is suspected when abdominal pain continues and serum amylase is consistently elevated after clinical resolution

of pancreatitis.[5] PPs may be complicated by intracystic hemorrhage, infection or rupture, which leads to pancreatic ascites. Symptoms of abdominal pain, fever, and chills suggest an infection in a patient with known PP.

Large PPs are well-circumscribed, oval or round, thick-walled fluid collections on abdominal ultrasound (US) and CT[1] (Fig. 61.1). CT imaging may also reveal signs of inflammation of the pancreatic tissue in the course of acute or chronic pancreatitis. MRI, magnetic resonance cholangiopancreatography (MRCP), and endoscopic retrograde cholangiopancreatography (ERCP) do not contribute much to the diagnosis. Currently, endoscopic ultrasound (EUS) is the most used modality for the differential diagnosis, and they appear as hypoechoic fluid collections surrounded by a thick rim (Fig. 61.2). Cysts can be aspirated by EUS-guided fine-needle aspiration (FNA) (EUS-FNA), and the cyst fluid is high in amylase and low in carcinoembryonic antigen (CEA)[6]; cytologic analysis shows histiocytes and inflammatory cells.

The majority of PPs resolve spontaneously.[7–9] Symptomatic and large PPs can be drained endoscopically or via a percutaneous route. With a high degree of success and low recurrence rate, EUS-guided transgastric or transduodenal endoscopic drainage is the current choice of treatment.[6] Furthermore, cystogastrostomy or cystoduodenostomy allows removal of debris and necrotic material in some patients. Surgical drainage is not preferred currently, except in the face of endoscopic drainage failure.[10]

NEOPLASTIC CYSTS

Neoplastic cysts of the pancreas can be broadly categorized as mucinous cystic lesions and nonmucinous cystic lesions. MCNs and IPMNs both produce mucin and are often combined and called either *mucin-producing neoplasms* or *mucinous neoplasms*. MCNs and IPMNs share similar cyst fluid features, and have the potential for transformation into pancreatic adenocarcinoma.[11,12] Nonmucinous neoplastic cystic lesions include serous cystic neoplasms, solid pseudopapillary neoplasms (SPNs), and cystic pancreatic neuroendocrine tumors (PNETs). The common features of pancreatic cystic neoplasms (PCNs) are summarized in Table 61.1.

Mucinous Cystic Neoplasm

MCNs are relatively rare, and account for 16% of surgically resected pancreatic cysts.[13] They occur almost exclusively in women, with men accounting for less than 5% of MCNs in large series.[14,15] Although over 70% of patients are symptomatic, most of the symptoms are nonspecific abdominal pain and unrelated to the cyst, with only 13% of patients who undergo surgical resection for MCNs presenting with symptoms related to their cyst. The most common of these is acute pancreatitis, which occurs in approximately 9%.[14,15] MCNs have some features that are very helpful in differentiating them from other types of pancreatic cysts; they are single, occur almost exclusively in women, and are located in the body and tail of the pancreas in over 97% of cases.[14,15] They can be uni- or multilocular and are classically well defined with a thin wall. Approximately 15% of MCNs have calcification, which is located at the edge of the cyst, in contrast to serous cystadenomas (SCAs) in which the calcification occurs in the center of the cyst (Fig. 61.3). The key-imaging feature used to differentiate IPMNs from MCNs, is that in MCNs, the main pancreatic duct is of normal diameter with no communication between it and the MCN.

Both MCNs and IPMNs are mucin-producing cysts and have very similar cyst fluid analysis features, namely, a high cyst fluid CEA and the presence of mucin on cytology. There is debate about the optimum CEA level to differentiate mucin from nonmucin-producing cysts, with all major studies defining

BOX 61.1   Common Types of Pancreatic Cysts

Neoplastic Pancreatic Cysts
Mucinous cystic lesions
Intraductal papillary mucinous neoplasm
Mucinous cystic neoplasm
Nonmucinous cystic lesions
Serous cystic neoplasm
Solid-pseudopapillary neoplasm
Pancreatic neuroendocrine tumors

Nonneoplastic Pancreatic Cysts
Pancreatic pseudocysts
Retention cysts
Squamoid cysts of the pancreatic duct
Lymphoepithelial cysts

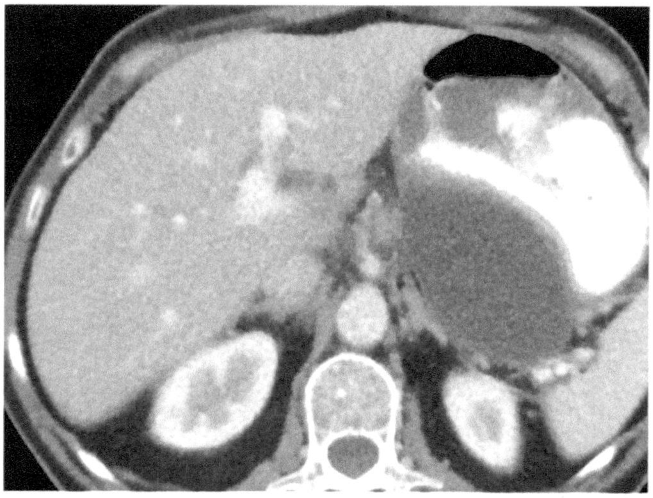

FIG 61.1 CT showing a pseudocyst measuring 5.7 × 7.6 × 5.0 cm.

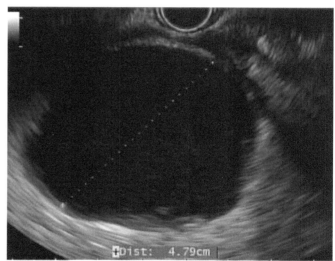

FIG 61.2 Endoscopic ultrasound (EUS) showing a 4.8 cm unilocular pseudocyst in the pancreatic body. The cyst is adjacent to the gastric wall and contains some debris.

TABLE 61.1   General Features of Pancreatic Cystic Neoplasms

Cysts Type	Sex	Median Age	Pancreatic Localization	Morphology	Communication with PD	Epithelium Type	Malignancy Risk
IPMN	♂/♀	65	Head	Unilocular, septated, associated dilated main pancreatic duct	Yes	Papillary mucinous	High
MCN	♀	40	Body & tail	Unilocular	No	Mucinous	High
SCN	♀	60	Entire pancreas	Microcystic	No	Serous (PAS-positive for glycogen)	Low
SPN	♀	30	Body & tail	Mixed solid and cystic	No	Endocrine-like	Low
PNET	♂/♀	50	Entire pancreas	Associated mass	No	Endocrine	Low

IPMN, Intraductal papillary neoplasm; *MCN,* mucinous cystic neoplasm; *SCN,* serous cystic neoplasm; *SPN,* solid-pseudopapillary neoplasm; *PD,* pancreatic duct; *PNET,* pancreatic neuroendocrine tumor.

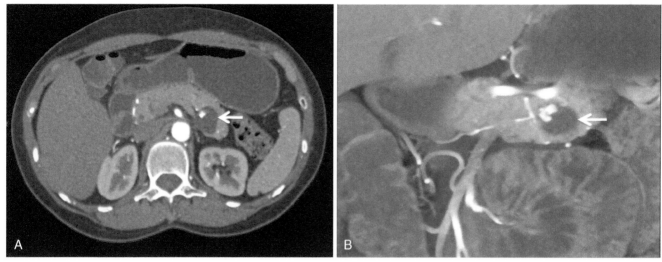

FIG 61.3 **A** and **B**, Cross-sectional CT scan demonstrating a mucinous cystic neoplasm (MCN) *(arrows)* in the body with a calcification in the wall.

mucin-producing cysts as those with a CEA greater than 192 ng/mL, which was derived from the 2004 prospective, multicenter cooperative cyst study by Brugge et al.[12] However, cyst fluid CEA alone is imperfect; a recent meta-analysis of 18 studies with 1438 patients found that cyst fluid CEA had 63% sensitivity and 88% specificity for identifying mucin-producing cysts.[16] Cyst fluid amylase levels are high in both MCNs and IPMNs, and cannot be used to differentiate MCNs from IPMNs.[17]

In both IPMNs and MCNs, columnar or cuboidal epithelial cells, as well as mucin, can be found. In addition, cytology can detect marked atypia (the cytological equivalent of high-grade dysplasia) or invasive adenocarcinoma. Although cytology has a high specificity of over 90%, it suffers from a low sensitivity of only 50% in the diagnosis of a mucinous cyst. In addition, over 60% of cases are found to have inadequate cellularity. On the other hand, the cyst fluid cytology rarely provides a definitive diagnosis. A needle-guided tissue micro forceps was approved recently for epithelial tissue acquisition in pancreatic cysts. In a study, the micro forceps provided a tissue sample that was sufficient for histological evaluation in 90% of patients. It also provided better information about the subgroup of PCN and the grade of dysplasia.[18] In surgically resected cysts, MCNs are differentiated from IPMNs by the presence of ovarian-like stroma.

There are no long-term studies examining the natural history of MCNs; thus the estimate of the risk of malignant transformation into pancreatic adenocarcinoma is based on retrospective surgical series in which the risk of invasive adenocarcinoma in modern series is between 4% to 13% at the time of resection.[14,19]

There is debate about whether MCNs can be watched or if all should undergo surgical resection.[20–23] There is an agreement that MCNs that are clearly causing symptoms, such as acute pancreatitis, have imaging features concerning for malignant transformation, such as a solid component or cytology showing marked atypia (the cytological equivalent of high-grade dysplasia), or invasive adenocarcinoma should undergo surgical resection. However authors, guidelines, and surgeons differ as to the management of presumed MCNs that measure less than 3 cm and have no concerning features. Some authors argue that all MCNs should be resected.[20] This is because (1) they occur in young women, who would otherwise require 30 to 40 years of surveillance, (2) they are single cysts which, in contrast to IPMNs, do not recur, and (3) they are located in the body or tail of the pancreas, which is technically easier to surgically resect than performing a Whipple. However, others argue that it is not always possible to differentiate MCNs from IPMNs preoperatively, that more recent data suggest that the risk of malignant transformation of MCNs is less than that of branch-duct IPMNs, and that although associated with a low mortality, a distal pancreatectomy has an approximate 25% morbidity rate, which includes a 15% to 20% risk of diabetes.[21,22] When caring for a patient with a presumed MCN, it is important to discuss these two differing views, the pros and cons of each approach, and ensure that the patient is reviewed by a multidisciplinary pancreatic cyst group.[24] Once patients undergo surgical resection for an MCN, in the absence of invasive adenocarcinoma, no further follow-up is required.

Intraductal Papillary Mucinous Neoplasm

IPMNs are the most common type of neoplastic pancreatic cyst encountered, and account for over 50% of surgically resected pancreatic cysts in modern series.[13] They can occur at any age, but usually present in patients in their late 60s or early 70s, with an equal distribution between men and women. IPMNs can cause symptoms including jaundice and acute pancreatitis; however, the vast majority of patients with IPMNs do not have pancreatic symptoms.

IPMNs can present with dilation of the main pancreatic duct alone (≥ 5 mm) which is called *main-duct IPMN* (Fig. 61.4A).[20] IPMNs can also present with a pancreatic cyst(s) termed *branch-duct* or *side-branch IPMNs* (see Fig. 61.4B). Finally, a small number of patients present with both a dilated main pancreatic duct and pancreatic cysts, which is referred to as a *mixed IPMN*. Up to 40% of IPMNs have multiple pancreatic cysts. This finding is useful; with the exception of pseudocysts, the majority of other types of cysts are single. Although they have a slight preponderance for the head and uncinate process, they can also occur in the body and tail. Thus, unlike MCNs, the location of IPMNs is not helpful. Branch-duct IPMNs can be uni- or multilocular, are typically well defined with thin walls, and have no calcification. The classic feature of a branch-duct IPMN is the presence of

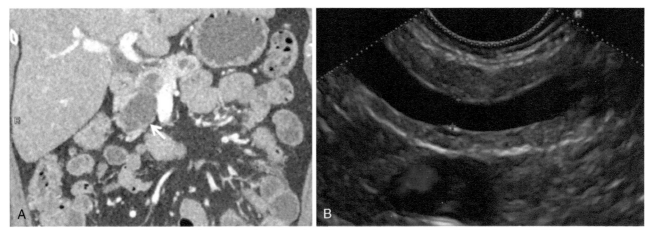

FIG 61.4 **A,** CT image of main-duct intraductal papillary mucinous neoplasm (IPMN) (*arrow* highlights a dilated main pancreatic duct in the head of the pancreas). **B,** Endoscopic ultrasound (EUS) image of main-duct IPMN.

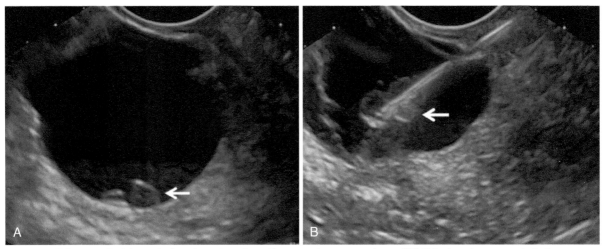

FIG 61.5 **A,** A branch-duct intraductal papillary mucinous neoplasm (IPMN) showing a mucin ball *(arrow)*. **B,** Endoscopic ultrasound fine-needle aspiration (EUS-FNA) of the lesion in Fig. 5A showing that the lesion *(arrow)* is not attached to the wall and is indeed mucin and not a mural nodule.

communication, or a connection, between the main pancreatic duct and the cyst. This feature of communication between the cyst and the main pancreatic duct is used to differentiate IPMNs from MCNs. This is best assessed with EUS or MRI/MRCP, which have a reported sensitivity of between 89% to 100%.[25]

IPMNs are neoplastic cysts and have the potential for progression to invasive adenocarcinoma. Imaging features that raise concern that an IPMN may have high-grade dysplasia or an associated invasive adenocarcinoma are the presence of a mural nodule (particularly if it is shown to enhance on CT or MRI), a dilated main pancreatic duct (especially if it is over 9 mm in diameter), and thick or enhancing cyst walls or an abrupt change in the diameter of the main pancreatic duct, particularly if there is evidence of upstream ductal obstruction. On EUS it can sometimes be difficult to differentiate a mural nodule from a mucin ball within the cyst (Figs. 61.5 and 61.6). Three features can be used to separate these two entities: (1) mucin will have a smooth edge whereas a mural nodule has an irregular edge, (2) mucin is hypoechoic compared with adjacent tissue, whereas a mural nodule is iso- or hyperechoic compared with surrounding

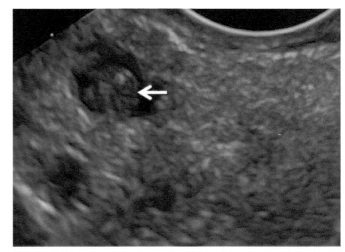

FIG 61.6 Mural nodule *(arrow)* within a branch duct intraductal papillary mucinous neoplasm (IPMN). The patient underwent surgery, and high-grade dysplasia was detected.

tissue, (3) mucin has a hyperechoic (bright) rim whereas a mural nodule has none. The presence of all three of these features can differentiate mucin from a mural nodule with 90% accuracy.[26] The second issue that endoscopists encounter is whether a slight protuberance of the wall of a cyst is significant or not. The first question is whether this area is enhancing on CT or MRI. The presence of an enhancing mural nodule is highly concerning for the presence of high-grade dysplasia or an associated invasive adenocarcinoma.

It is important to remember that the main pancreatic duct can be dilated for a number of reasons, such as a small pancreatic adenocarcinoma, ampullary adenoma, papillary stenosis, chronic pancreatitis, or main-duct IPMN, and can also increase with age. When referring a patient with a dilated main pancreatic duct, it is important to try to exclude these other entities. The presence of a "fish mouth" in which mucin is seen extruding from the ampulla, is highly suggestive of main-duct IPMN. On EUS the presence of mucin within the main pancreatic duct, or a thickened or irregular wall, are suggestive of main-duct IPMN. In cases where the diagnosis remains unclear, pancreatoscopy has been used to identify papillary projections and to determine the extent of involvement of the main pancreatic duct.

The cyst fluid analysis for IPMNs is identical to that of MCNs described previously. The presence of an elevated cyst fluid CEA or mucin is used to make the diagnosis of a mucin-producing cyst. The presence of marked atypia or invasive adenocarcinoma on cytology raises the concern for the presence of high-grade dysplasia or an associated invasive adenocarcinoma. Patients with these cytology findings should be seen by a multidisciplinary group and considered for surgical resection.

Several studies have focused on the underlying genetic mutations in pancreatic cysts, and have found that cysts have a unique molecular profile (Table 61.2).[27] MCNs and IPMNs share mutations in *KRAS*, *RNF43*, and *TP53*, whereas IPMNs have a unique mutation in *GNAS*, which is present in 58% of IPMNs and can be used to differentiate IPMNs from other types of cysts.[27] Preliminary studies examining the use of a combination of molecular markers in cyst fluid to identify different types of pancreatic cysts appears very promising, identifying SCAs with 100% sensitivity and 91% specificity, MCNs with 100% sensitivity and 75% specificity, and IPMNs with 76% sensitivity and 97% specificity.[28] The presence of a mutation in *GNAS* or *KRAS* is particularly helpful in identifying mucin-producing cysts, and is found in over 90% of IPMNs.[28,29] Recent studies (2016) have shown that the use of molecular markers is cost effective and alters patient management.[30,31] The final results of large, multicenter studies are expected to be published in 2017. If these studies confirm the findings of the smaller studies, it is likely that the use of molecular markers will be incorporated into clinical practice in cases in which the diagnosis is unclear. It is

important to note that not all techniques for identifying molecular markers are the same, with significant variations in the sensitivity for identifying a mutation. The results reported previously were performed using SafeSeq sequencing, which can detect a mutation that is present in 0.01% of alleles.

IPMNs are neoplastic pancreatic cysts with the potential to progress from low-, to intermediate-, to high-grade dysplasia, and ultimately invasive pancreatic adenocarcinoma.[11] It is currently impossible to know the exact grade of dysplasia present in an IPMN without sending the patient for surgical resection; however, certain imaging features are associated with a higher prevalence of high-grade dysplasia or invasive adenocarcinoma. The presence of a mural nodule or solid component within the cyst is associated with an odds ratio (OR) of 7.73, the presence of a dilated main pancreatic has an OR of 2.38, and cyst size greater than 3 cm is associated with an OR of 2.97 for high-grade dysplasia or invasive cancer. In contrast, there is accumulating evidence that the risk for developing invasive malignancy from suspected branch duct (BD)-IPMN without concerning features is low, about 0.72% per year, or 2% to 4% (average 2.8%, 95% confidence interval 1.8%–4%) over a period of 10 years.[32] Several different groups have developed guidelines for the management of IPMNs.[20-22] The most commonly used guidelines are the International Consensus Criteria (ICC), which will be reviewed here.[20] These guidelines recommend consideration of surgical resection in the presence of "high risk features," which are jaundice caused by an IPMN, an enhancing mural nodule, or main-duct IPMN measuring greater than 9 mm. "Worrisome features" are the presence of dilation of the main pancreatic duct between 5 to 9 mm, abrupt change in caliber in the main pancreatic duct, a nonenhancing mural nodule, thickened or enhancing wall, cyst size of 3 cm or more, or a recent history of acute pancreatitis. In the case of worrisome features, EUS should be performed; where there is clear evidence of main-duct IPMN, a definite mural nodule on EUS, or cytology showing marked atypia or invasive adenocarcinoma, surgical resection should be considered. In all other cases surveillance can be undertaken with the interval determined by the size of the cyst. The positive predictive value of worrisome, high-risk, or worrisome or high-risk features is 29%, 66%, and 36%, respectively, for the presence of high-grade dysplasia or invasive cancer.[33] The absence of any of these features has a negative predictive value of 90%.[33]

IPMNs affect the entire pancreas and can develop in the residual pancreas following resection. In addition, patients with IPMNs are also at risk of developing pancreatic adenocarcinoma in an area unrelated to a pancreatic cyst.[34] The remnant pancreas should therefore undergo surveillance following a Whipple or distal pancreatectomy.[20,21]

In cases that cannot tolerate or refuse surgery, or in asymptomatic BD-IPMN patients without risk factors, EUS-guided cyst ablation has emerged as a promising approach. The first well-demonstrated study showed a 33% rate of complete cyst ablation following EUS-guided cyst lavage with ethanol.[35] Infusing and leaving paclitaxel in the cyst after ethanol lavage raised the complete ablation rates to 60% to 79% in further studies.[35-37] EUS-guided radiofrequency ablation is another alternative treatment. In a preliminary study, the response ranged from complete resolution to a 50% reduction in size.[38]

Serous Cystic Neoplasm

SCNs are predominantly benign neoplasms that can arise anywhere in the pancreas, and malignant SCNs are extremely

TABLE 61.2 Genetic Profile of Pancreatic Cysts

Mutation	SCA	SPN	MCN	IPMN
KRAS			+	+
GNAS				+
RNF43			+	+
CTNNB1		+		+
VHL	+			

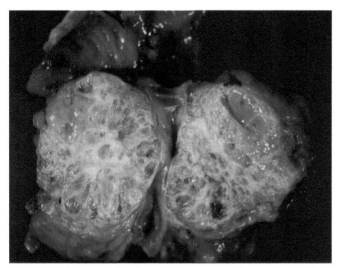

FIG 61.7 Macroscopic view of a serous cystic neoplasm. Note the stellate-shaped central scar and numerous small cysts.

rare[39] (Fig. 61.7). The degree of dysplasia categorizes these cysts into serous cystadenomas and serous cystadenocarcinomas. The typical clinical presentation of a SCN occurs mostly in women over the age of 60 years. SCNs are slow-growing tumors[40] and are usually incidentally detected on abdominal imaging for other unrelated conditions.[41,42] The *VHL* gene mutation plays an important role in the pathogenesis of SCNs[43,44] and, in contrast with mucinous cysts, *KRAS* mutations are not seen in SCN.[43]

Glycogen-rich cells that are stained periodic acid–Schiff (PAS)-positive arise from centroacinar cells of the pancreas and line SCNs. The SCN wall is thin and surrounds a thin nonviscous and bloody cyst fluid. SCNs contain a prominent fibrous stroma, glycogen-rich epithelial cells, and endothelial, as well as smooth, muscle cells.[44] Ultrastructurally, the fibrocollagenous stroma is composed of myofibroblasts and endothelial cells embedded in thick collagen bundles. Estrogen and progesterone receptors are not present.[45]

Histologic variants include macrocystic serous cystadenomas, solid serous adenomas, VHL-associated SCNs, and mixed serous neuroendocrine neoplasms.[39] The majority of SCNs are microcystic, and the classical appearance of a microcystic SCN is a cluster of numerous tiny cysts separated by a delicate fibrous septa, which resembles a "honeycomb-like appearance" on cross-sectional abdominal imaging or EUS. Microcystic lesions grow slowly; however, they may reach large diameters. Frequently the large lesions have a stellate-shaped central scar. Macrocystic (oligocystic) serous cystadenomas are composed of fewer and larger cysts[46–49] and can be difficult to distinguish from an MCN, BD-IPMN, and a pseudocyst. *VHL*-associated SCN consists of multiple SCNs that affect patients with the *VHL* syndrome. The mixed serous neuroendocrine neoplasms are rare and highly suggestive of *VHL* syndrome.[39]

Although most SCN patients present with abdominal pain and discomfort historically, many patients may present with a palpable mass when the cyst attains a large size. Currently, SCNs are mostly detected in asymptomatic patients during evaluation for another indication.

On CT and MRI, the diagnostic classical appearance is a solitary lesion composed of a central scar surrounded by multiple tiny cysts. Alternatively, the macrocystic serous cystadenomas

on cross-sectional imaging are usually indistinguishable from BD-IPMNs and MCNs.[49,50] As discussed previously, MCNs are solitary, thinly septated cysts and may have "eggshell" peripheral calcification, which is in contrast with central scar and calcification in SCNs. Pseudocysts are unilocular lesions with pancreatic parenchymal changes (calcification and atrophy). The presence of multiple, small, thin-walled cysts is suggestive of *VHL* syndrome.[51] Additionally, SCNs generally do not communicate with the pancreatic duct, which is best seen on MRCP. The typical appearance of SCNs on EUS is numerous anechoic small cysts with thin septations. EUS with Doppler may demonstrate the characteristic hypervascular central region. The cyst fluid is nonviscous and may be bloody (because of this hypervascular nature) during EUS-FNA. The cytology is negative for malignancy, but PAS-positive small cuboidal cells are diagnostic for SCNs.[52] However, diagnostic cytology for SCN is rare. A CEA level of less than 5 ng/mL is also highly suggestive of an SCN,[53] and SCNs are negative for both *KRAS* and *GNAS* mutations but positive for *VHL* mutations.[54–56]

Currently, with the available diagnostic studies, the differentiation of pancreatic cysts is sometimes challenging. Needle-based confocal endomicroscopy is a novel endoscopic technique that enables real-time optical biopsies and provides in vivo histopathological assessment during EUS-FNA. On confocal endomicroscopy, SCNs demonstrate a typical superficial vascular network, whereas IPMNs show papillary projections with an epithelial border and vascular core.[57,58]

The prognosis for SCNs is excellent.[39] Generally, SCNs should be followed by surveillance imaging. Previously large SCA size or rapid growth had been considered indications for surgical resection; however, a large, multicenter study in over 2500 patients with SCA found that the risk of serous cystadenocarcinoma was 0.1%.[59] Surgery should only be considered for symptomatic SCAs or when there is an uncertainty about the diagnosis and a concern for malignancy.[60]

Solid-Pseudopapillary Neoplasm

SPNs are rare neoplasms of the pancreas that typically affect women in their 30s. Microscopically, a mixture of solid (solid pseudopapillary) and cystic (hemorrhagic-necrotic pseudocystic) components is observed. SPNs are usually well-circumcised, single, round, and fluctuant masses and are most commonly found in the body and tail of pancreas.[61,62] The majority of SPNs were symptomatic in the past; however, currently incidental detection on cross-sectional imaging is becoming more common. The most common symptoms are abdominal pain, vomiting, nausea, and patients may have a palpable mass.[63]

Although the majority of SPNs demonstrate a benign behavior, they are generally considered as low-grade malignant neoplasms. Criteria for solid pseudopapillary carcinoma are defined as vascular invasion, perineural invasion, invasion of adjacent tissues, or metastases.[64] The most common site of metastases is the liver.

On CT and MRI, SPNs may appear as well-demarcated encapsulated pancreatic masses mixed with solid components without septa (Fig. 61.8). MRI reveals lower signal intensity on T1-weighted images and higher signal intensity on T2-weighted images. The capsule is usually thick, and sometimes internal calcifications may be observed.[65]

The typical appearance of SPN on EUS is a well-demarcated, hypoechoic, solid-appearing mass, which can also sometimes appear as a mixed cystic and solid lesion or purely cystic lesion.[66] The aspirated fluid is typically bloody, highly cellular, and CEA level is low, consistent with nonmucinous epithelium.[67]

SPNs are slow-growing neoplasms, and complete resection is the treatment of choice. Surgery is curative in most cases, and recurrence rates after resection are very low.[41,68] Prolonged survival is reported even in patients with recurrence and metastases.[64,69,70]

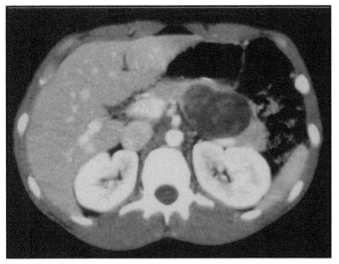

FIG 61.8 CT showing a solid-pseudopapillary neoplasm. Note the mixture of solid and cystic components.

Pancreatic Neuroendocrine Tumors

PNETs are rare neoplasms that account for less than 10% of all pancreatic neoplasms.[46,71] They are indolent tumors, which arise from both endocrine and nervous system cells with a variable malignant potential. 1% to 2% of pancreatic neoplasms are PNETs,[72] both sexes are equally affected, and the incidence of PNETs increases with age. The majority of PNETs are hormonally nonfunctional and are frequently sporadic; however, an association with von Hippel-Lindau syndrome (vHL), multiple endocrine neoplasia type 1, and neurofibromatosis type 1 may be seen.[73–76]

PNETs are well-circumscribed lesions, surrounded by a thick, fibrous capsule and may be unilocular or multilocular. Generally, they do not communicate with the pancreatic duct, and their size varies from small to large. The aspirated fluid is usually hemorrhagic, and the lesion appears like a hypoechoic mass after aspiration. A large hypervascular pancreatic mass on CT/MRI in a patient without producing hormonal symptoms is highly suspicious for nonfunctional PNETs.[77,78] To differentiate from malignant tumors of pancreas, EUS-FNA and scintigraphy are the most valuable tools (Fig. 61.9).

Surgery with complete resection is the only curative therapy for PNETs. Somatostatin analogs for functional tumors are recommended. Locoregional treatment is suggested for liver metastasis and chemotherapy is suggested for residual disease.[79] The prognosis is better than for pancreatic adenocarcinoma.[80]

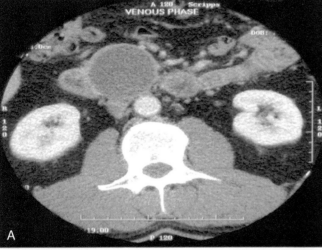

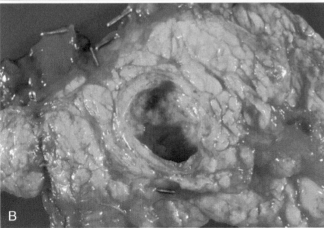

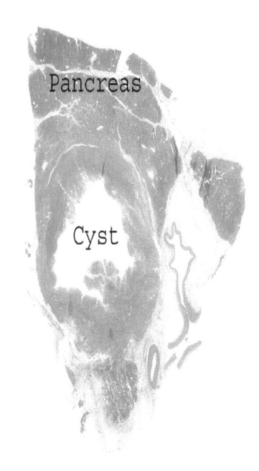

FIG 61.9 **A,** CT showing a thick-walled cystic lesion consistent with a cystic pancreatic neuroendocrine neoplasm. **B,** Macroscopic view of the same lesion. **C,** Histologic view of the same lesion.

APPROACH FOR A PATIENT WITH A PANCREATIC CYST

When a patient with a pancreatic cyst is seen, we review their cross-sectional imaging to determine the type of cyst, and to evaluate whether there are any features concerning for the presence of high-grade dysplasia or invasive carcinoma. In cases in which the diagnosis is unclear, or there are concerning features, then EUS +/− FNA is performed with cyst fluid sent for CEA, amylase (if there is concern for a pseudocyst), *KRAS*, *GNAS*, and cytology.

For patients with BD-IPMNs, there are several different guidelines available, including those developed by the American College of Gastroenterology[23] (ACG), the ICC,[20] the European Consensus Criteria (ECC),[21] and the American Gastroenterology Association (AGA).[22] Updated guidelines are expected from the ACG and ECC in 2017, as concerns have been raised about several aspects of the AGA guidelines.[81-86] We therefore currently follow the revised ICC with presumed BD-IPMNs measuring under 1 cm followed every 2 years, 1 to 2 cm BD-IPMNs followed yearly, and BD-IPMNs over 2 cm, or IPMNs with main duct involvement, followed every 6 months. Surveillance intervals can be increased if the cysts are stable in size and have no concerning features.

KEY REFERENCES

3. Brun A, Agarwal N, Pitchumoni CS: Fluid collections in and around the pancreas in acute pancreatitis, *J Clin Gastroenterol* 45:614–625, 2011.

5. Cannon JW, Callery MP, Vollmer CM, Jr: Diagnosis and management of pancreatic pseudocysts: what is the evidence? *J Am Coll Surg* 209: 385–393, 2009.

6. Brugge WR: Approaches to the drainage of pancreatic pseudocysts, *Curr Opin Gastroenterol* 20:488–492, 2004.

8. Brugge WR: The use of EUS to diagnose cystic neoplasms of the pancreas, *Gastrointest Endosc* 69:S203–S209, 2009.

11. Lennon AM, Wolfgang CL, Canto MI, et al: The early detection of pancreatic cancer: what will it take to diagnose and treat curable pancreatic neoplasia? *Cancer Res* 74:3381–3389, 2014.

12. Brugge WR, Lewandrowski K, Lee-Lewandrowski E, et al: Diagnosis of pancreatic cystic neoplasms: a report of the cooperative pancreatic cyst study, *Gastroenterology* 126:1330–1336, 2004.

13. Valsangkar NP, Morales-Oyarvide V, Thayer SP, et al: 851 resected cystic tumors of the pancreas: a 33-year experience at the Massachusetts General Hospital, *Surgery* 152:S4–S12, 2012.

16. Anand N, Sampath K, Wu BU: Cyst features and risk of malignancy in intraductal papillary mucinous neoplasms of the pancreas: a meta-analysis, *Clin Gastroenterol Hepatol* 11:913–921, quiz e59–e60, 2013.

17. Thornton GD, McPhail MJ, Nayagam S, et al: Endoscopic ultrasound guided fine needle aspiration for the diagnosis of pancreatic cystic neoplasms: a meta-analysis, *Pancreatology* 13:48–57, 2013.

20. Tanaka M, Fernandez-Del Castillo C, Adsay V, et al: International consensus guidelines 2012 for the management of IPMN and MCN of the pancreas, *Pancreatology* 12:183–197, 2012.

22. Vege SS, Ziring B, Jain R, et al: American gastroenterological association institute guideline on the diagnosis and management of asymptomatic neoplastic pancreatic cysts, *Gastroenterology* 148:819–822, 2015.

23. Khalid A, Brugge W: ACG practice guidelines for the diagnosis and management of neoplastic pancreatic cysts, *Am J Gastroenterol* 102: 2339–2349, 2007.

24. Lennon AM, Manos LL, Hruban RH, et al: Role of a multidisciplinary clinic in the management of patients with pancreatic cysts: a single-center cohort study, *Ann Surg Oncol* 21(11):3668–3674, 2014.

28. Springer S, Wang Y, Dal Molin M, et al: A combination of molecular markers and clinical features improve the classification of pancreatic cysts, *Gastroenterology* 149:1501–1510, 2015.

30. Singhi AD, Zeh HJ, Brand RE, et al: American Gastroenterological Association guidelines are inaccurate in detecting pancreatic cysts with advanced neoplasia: a clinicopathologic study of 225 patients with supporting molecular data, *Gastrointest Endosc* 83(6):1107–1117.e2, 2016.

32. Scheiman JM, Hwang JH, Moayyedi P: American Gastroenterological Association technical review on the diagnosis and management of asymptomatic neoplastic pancreatic cysts, *Gastroenterology* 148: 824–848 e22, 2015.

33. Goh BK, Tan DM, Ho MM, et al: Utility of the sendai consensus guidelines for branch-duct intraductal papillary mucinous neoplasms: a systematic review, *J Gastrointest Surg* 18:1350–1357, 2014.

36. Oh HC, Brugge WR: EUS-guided pancreatic cyst ablation: a critical review (with video), *Gastrointest Endosc* 77:526–533, 2013.

41. Yoon WJ, Brugge WR: Pancreatic cystic neoplasms: diagnosis and management, *Gastroenterol Clin North Am* 41:103–118, 2012.

46. Brugge WR, Lauwers GY, Sahani D, et al: Cystic neoplasms of the pancreas, *N Engl J Med* 351:1218–1226, 2004.

56. Kadayifci A, Brugge WR: Endoscopic ultrasound-guided fine-needle aspiration for the differential diagnosis of intraductal papillary mucinous neoplasms and size stratification for surveillance, *Endoscopy* 46:357, 2014.

67. Jani N, Dewitt J, Eloubeidi M, et al: Endoscopic ultrasound-guided fine-needle aspiration for diagnosis of solid pseudopapillary tumors of the pancreas: a multicenter experience, *Endoscopy* 40:200–203, 2008.

72. Halfdanarson TR, Rabe KG, Rubin J, et al: Pancreatic neuroendocrine tumors (PNETs): incidence, prognosis and recent trend toward improved survival, *Ann Oncol* 19:1727–1733, 2008.

74. Boninsegna L, Partelli S, D'Innocenzio MM, et al: Pancreatic cystic endocrine tumors: a different morphological entity associated with a less aggressive behavior, *Neuroendocrinology* 92:246–251, 2010.

79. Dimou AT, Syrigos KN, Saif MW: Neuroendocrine tumors of the pancreas: what's new. Highlights from the "2010 ASCO Gastrointestinal Cancers Symposium". Orlando, FL, USA. January 22-24, 2010, *J Pancreas* 11:135–138, 2010.

A complete reference list can be found online at ExpertConsult .com

62

Evaluation and Staging of Pancreaticobiliary Malignancy

Michael Levy and Mohammad Al-Haddad

EUS FOR THE EVALUATION AND STAGING OF PANCREATIC TUMORS

Introduction

Examination of the pancreas and biliary structures by endoscopic ultrasound (EUS) can be technically challenging to master due to the need to recognize patterns of normal, benign, and pathologic anatomy. However, once these skills are learned, EUS permits the most detailed nonoperative view of the pancreas and the bile ducts. This chapter summarizes the role of EUS for the evaluation of solid malignant pancreatic and biliary neoplasms.

EUS Detection of Pancreatic Tumors

EUS is the most sensitive imaging test for the detection of all pancreatic and periampullary lesions (Table 62.1).[1-8] In studies that compared EUS and computed tomography (CT), the sensitivity of EUS for mass detection was superior to CT.[1-8] EUS is clearly superior to conventional CT[1-3,6] and transabdominal ultrasound (US).[1-3,5] A few comparative studies between EUS and multidetector-row CT (MDCT) for pancreatic tumors have demonstrated the superiority of EUS for tumor detection. There are relatively sparse comparative data between EUS and magnetic resonance imaging (MRI) for tumor detection, with at least one study showing the superiority of EUS.[4] EUS is particularly useful for identification of small tumors that can go undetected by other imaging modalities.[1,4,7,8] For tumors of 30 mm or less in diameter (Fig. 62.1), EUS was found in early literature to have a sensitivity of 93% compared to 53% for CT and 67% for MRI.[4] Nowadays, with thinner slice imaging and precisely timed contrast administration coupled with multiplanar reconstruction, CT (often referred to as *pancreas protocol*) may now be able to identify small pancreatic masses that previously may have been undetected by conventional or even single-detector dual-phase imaging.[8] EUS remains the test of choice in all patients with obstructive jaundice or dual pancreatic and bile duct dilations in whom CT or MRI do not identify a lesion.

EUS has a few limitations including the potential failure to identify true pancreatic masses in patients with chronic pancreatitis, a diffusely infiltrating carcinoma, a prominent ventral/dorsal split, or after a recent episode (< 4 weeks) of acute pancreatitis. Therefore, a normal pancreas by EUS examination essentially rules out pancreatic cancer, although follow-up EUS or other studies should be undertaken in the setting of chronic pancreatitis due to impaired visualization. It is also important to remember that acoustic shadowing caused by an indwelling biliary or pancreatic stent may also impede visualization of a small pancreatic mass.

Due to the ability of EUS to provide high-resolution images, there has been increasing interest in using this technique to screen asymptomatic high-risk cohorts for early cancer detection. A consensus statement by the International Cancer of the Pancreas Screening Consortium recommended screening with EUS and/or MRI for the following groups: first-degree relatives (FDRs) of patients with pancreatic cancer from a familial pancreatic cancer kindred with at least two affected FDRs; Peutz-Jeghers syndrome; *p16* or *BRCA2* mutations; and hereditary nonpolyposis colorectal cancer mutation carriers with 1 or more affected FDRs.[9] A 2016 comparative analysis highlighted the complementary roles EUS and MRI play in screening these high-risk individuals.[10] MRI was found to be more sensitive for the detection of cystic lesions of any size; EUS, however, detected more solid lesions then MRI. The optimal screening modality, interval, need for

TABLE 62.1 Sensitivity (%) of EUS Compared to Other Imaging Tests for Detection of Pancreatic Masses

Author (yr)	No. Patients	EUS	CT	MRI	US
Rosch et al. (1991)[1]	102	99	77		67
Rosch et al. (1992)[2]	60	98	85		78
Palazzo et al. (1993)[3]	49	91	66		64
Muller et al. (1994)[4]	33	94	69	83	
Sugiyama et al. (1997)[5]	73	96	86		81
Gress et al. (1999)[6]	81	100	74		
Agarwal et al. (2004)[7]	71	100	86		
DeWitt et al. (2004)[8]	80	98	86		

CT, computed tomography; *EUS,* endoscopic ultrasound; *MRI,* magnetic resonance imaging; *US,* ultrasound.

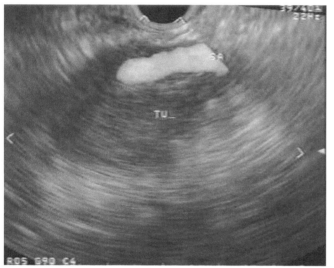

FIG 62.1 Endoscopic ultrasound images of a 2.9-cm hypoechoic, irregular pancreatic body mass encasing the splenic vessels. *SA,* Splenic artery; *TU,* tumor.

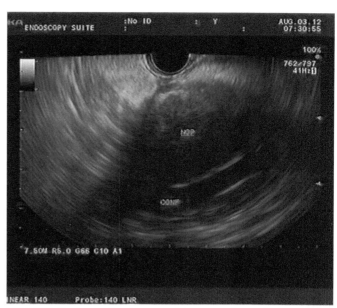

FIG 62.2 Endoscopic ultrasound images of autoimmune pancreatitis presenting as a hypoechoic mass in the head of the pancreas with dilation of the common bile duct. *CONF,* Portovenous confluence; *HOP,* head of pancreas.

fine-needle aspiration (FNA), and screening abnormalities of sufficient concern for surgery remain unknown, and further studies are required to answer these questions.

Autoimmune pancreatitis (AIP) may mimic pancreatic adenocarcinoma, and accurate preoperative detection may avoid unnecessary surgery. The EUS morphology of AIP may include diffuse pancreatic enlargement, a focal mass, focal hypoechoic areas, bile duct wall thickening, or peripancreatic lymphadenopathy (Fig. 62.2).[11] EUS-guided fine-needle aspiration (EUS-FNA) may demonstrate a nonspecific plasmacytic predominant chronic inflammatory infiltrate, but this finding has variable sensitivity and poor specificity. Diagnosis may be confirmed by EUS-guided core biopsies with staining for IgG4 plasma cells.[12,13]

Imaging-based technologies such as contrast-enhanced ultrasonography (CE-EUS) may be able to differentiate pancreatic adenocarcinoma from pancreatic neuroendocrine tumors (PNETs) and inflammatory pseudotumors, which can all present as a hypoechoic mass. Whereas ductal adenocarcinomas typically demonstrate hypoenhancement, PNET and inflammatory pseudotumors are hyperenhancing or isoenhancing. A recent

meta-analysis of 12 studies involving 1139 patients reported a pooled sensitivity, specificity, and receiver operating characteristic (ROC) of 94%, 89%, and 0.9732, respectively.[14] EUS elastography is another emerging technique based on the different stiffness of benign and malignant tissue. In a meta-analysis of 13 studies involving 1044 patients, the pooled sensitivity, specificity, and ROC was 95%, 67%, and 0.90.[15] However, several limitations to their routine use exist and include costs and the lack of both agent availability and expertise with the technique.

Staging of Pancreatic Adenocarcinoma

Staging of pancreatic malignancy is done according to the American Joint Committee for Cancer (AJCC) Staging TNM classification, which describes the tumor extension (T), lymph node (N), and distant metastases (M) of tumors, respectively. Reported accuracies of T-staging by EUS range from 62% to 94% (Table 62.2).[2–4,6,8,16–21] This wide variation may be due to improved detection of distant metastasis or vascular invasion by MDCT, resulting in less operative management for suspected locally advanced or metastatic disease. The exclusion of such patients may have resulted in the decreased T-staging accuracy of some recent studies compared to earlier ones. For the last decade, some tertiary referral centers will attempt to achieve negative surgical margins by surgical resection with or without reconstruction of the portal and/or superior mesenteric vein in patients with venous invasion without thrombosis or occlusion. Currently, only vascular invasion of the celiac or superior mesenteric arteries is classified as T4 cancer (Box 62.1).

Nodal (N) metastases have uniformly been classified as absent (N0) or present (N1) across all AJCC editions. The accuracy of EUS for N-staging of pancreatic tumors ranges from 50% to 86%.[2–4,6,8,17–19] Various criteria have been proposed for endosonographic features of metastatic lymph nodes including: size greater than 1 cm, hypoechoic echogenicity, distinct margins, and round shape. When all four features are present within a lymph node, there is an 80% to 100% chance of malignant invasion.[22] However,

TABLE 62.2 Accuracy of EUS for Tumor (T) and Nodal (N) Staging of Pancreatic Cancer

Author (year)	No. Enrolled Patients	No. Patients to Surgery With Pancreatic Cancer	T Stage	N Stage
Rosch et al. (1992)[2]	60	40	NR	72
Rosch et al. (1992)[18]	46	35	94	80
Palazzo (1993)[3]	64	49	82	64
Muller (1994)[4]	49	16	82	50
Midwinter et al. (1999)[17]	48	23	NR	74
Gress et al. (1999)[6]	151	75	85	72
Ahmad (2000)[16]	NA	89	69	54
Soriano et al. (2004)[19]	127	62	62	65
DeWitt et al. (2004)[8]	104	53	67	41
Shami et al. (2011)[21]	50	50	80	NR
Tellez-Avila et al. (2012)[20]	127	48	71*	NR

*Reported as accuracy for overall stage.
EUS, endoscopic ultrasound; *NA,* not applicable; *NR,* not reported.

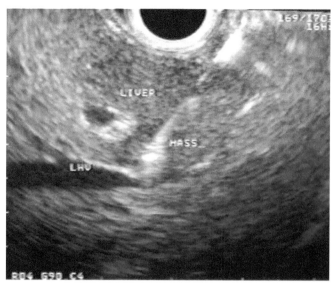

FIG 62.3 A 9-mm oval hypoechoic hepatic nodule in a patient with a pancreatic mass. Fine-needle aspiration of the liver nodule demonstrated metastatic adenocarcinoma of pancreatic origin. *LVH,* Left hepatic vein.

BOX 62.1 American Joint Committee on Cancer (AJCC) 2010 TNM Staging Classification for Pancreatic Cancer

Primary tumor (T)

TX: Primary tumor cannot be assessed
T0: No evidence of primary tumor
Tis: Carcinoma in situ
T1: Tumor limited to the pancreas, 2 cm or less in greatest dimension
T2: Tumor limited to the pancreas, more than 2 cm in greatest dimension
T3: Tumor extends beyond the pancreas but without involvement of the celiac axis or the superior mesenteric artery
T4: Tumor involves the celiac axis or the superior mesenteric artery (unresectable primary tumor)

Regional lymph nodes (N)

NX: Regional lymph nodes cannot be assessed
N0: No regional lymph node metastasis
N1: Regional lymph node metastasis

Distant metastasis (M)

MX: Distant metastasis cannot be assessed
M0: No distant metastasis
M1: Distant metastasis

AJCC Stage Groupings

Stage 0: Tis, N0, M0
Stage IA: T1, N0, M0
Stage IB: T2, N0, M0
Stage IIA: T3, N0, M0
Stage IIB: T1, N1, M0 or T2, N1, M0 or T3, N1, M0
Stage III: T4, any N, M0
Stage IV: Any T, any N, M1

From Edge SB, Byrd DR, Compton CC, et al (editors): *American Joint Committee on Cancer: AJCC Cancer Staging Manual,* 7th ed. New York, Springer, 2010, pp 241–250.

sensitivity of EUS for malignant lymphadenopathy is often lower, presumably for two reasons. First, most metastatic lymph nodes do not have all four endosonographic features described previously. Second, peritumoral inflammation and large tumor size may obscure visualization of adenopathy. The specificity of EUS alone for the diagnosis of metastatic adenopathy in pancreatic cancer is 26% to 100%,[3,4,17,19] with most reported specificities being above 70%. It is presumed that the addition of EUS-FNA of suspicious lymph nodes may increase specificity, although little data support this. For tumors involving the head of the pancreas, malignant lymph nodes are removed en bloc, with the surgical specimen and accurate detection of these lymph nodes not essential. However, as preoperative identification and EUS-FNA of celiac nodes may preclude surgery, meticulous survey of this region is critical during staging of all pancreatic tumors. Mediastinal lymph node metastases occur in a minority of patients and thus, a brief survey of this region may be helpful during staging of pancreatic lesions.

Although early studies found EUS to be superior to conventional CT for tumor[3,4] and nodal[2–4] staging of pancreatic cancer, more recent studies have found that the two are equivalent for both tumor[17,19] and nodal staging.[8,17,19] Similarly, early experience reporting on the superiority of EUS over MRI[3,4] have been replaced by more recent data that have found little to no difference.[19,21,23] Clearly, the initial advantage demonstrated by EUS over other imaging modalities for the staging of pancreatic tumors has narrowed considerably due to the rapid advancement in imaging technologies.

For detection of non-nodal metastatic cancer, CT and MRI are superior to EUS due to both the anatomic limitations of normal upper gastrointestinal anatomy and the limited range of EUS imaging. However, EUS still has an important role in the evaluation of hepatic metastasis in the left or caudate lobe and malignant ascites, both of which may be accessible by EUS-FNA (Fig. 62.3). Identification of liver metastases or malignant ascites by EUS-FNA may preclude surgical resection and is associated with poor survival following diagnosis.[24]

Assessment of Vascular Invasion

Interpretation of data regarding the accuracy of EUS for vascular invasion is difficult for several reasons. First, there is little histologic correlation with intraoperative findings regarding vascular invasion in most studies. Second, there is no established consensus among endosonographers for the optimal criteria to utilize for determination of vascular invasion. Consequently, multiple criteria have been proposed by various authors for this indication.

For overall vascular invasion, the accuracy of EUS ranges from 68% to 93%.[6,19,23,25] Sensitivity and specificity of EUS for malignant vascular invasion range from 42% to 91% and 89% to 100%, respectively.[6,19,23,25] Although some have reported EUS as more accurate[6] than CT for vascular invasion, others report the opposite.[19,23] Overall accuracy of MRI is reportedly equivalent[19] or superior[23] to EUS.

The sensitivity of EUS for tumor invasion of the portal vein (PV) or PV confluence is 60% to 100%[2,5,17,18,26] with most studies demonstrating sensitivities over 80% (Fig. 62.4). The sensitivity of EUS for PV invasion is consistently superior to that of CT.[2,5,17,18] For the superior mesenteric vein, superior mesenteric artery (SMA), and celiac artery, the sensitivity of EUS is only 17% to 83%,[25] 17%,[27] and approximately 50%,[2,18] respectively. The sensitivity of CT for staging of the SMA[17,27] and celiac artery[2,18] appear to be better than EUS. EUS staging of the superior mesenteric vessels may be difficult due to either the inability to visualize the entire course of the vessel or the obscuring of these vessels by a large tumor in the uncinate or inferior portion of the pancreatic head.[26] This is in contrast to the splenic artery and vein, which are generally easily seen and staged well by EUS.[18,26] Until further conclusive data become available, assessment of tumor resectability should be done by both EUS and CT (or MRI) rather than by EUS alone.

Several studies have attempted to describe the accuracy of various endosonographic features to assess vascular invasion by malignant pancreatic tumors. Using the criteria of abnormal contour, loss of hyperechoic interface, and close contact, Rosch et al (1992)[2] found a sensitivity, specificity, and accuracy of 91%, 96%, and 94%, respectively, for invasion of the PV. The same

authors later found that no single criterion was able to predict venous invasion with a sensitivity and specificity exceeding 80%.[26] However, they found that both complete vascular obstruction and the presence of collaterals demonstrated a specificity of 94% for vascular invasion. There exists a tradeoff between various criteria for sensitivity and specificity for vascular invasion. However, criteria with the highest specificity are needed to optimize selection of those most likely to benefit from surgical exploration. Therefore, the findings of an irregular vascular wall, venous collaterals and visible tumor within the vessel are the preferred criteria for assessment of vascular invasion.

Resectability of Pancreatic Tumors

Complete surgical resection of pancreatic cancer with negative histopathologic margins (R0 resection) is the only potentially curative treatment and is an independent predictor of postoperative survival.[28,29] Therefore, the main role of preoperative evaluation is to accurately identify patients with resectable disease who may benefit from surgery while avoiding surgery in patients with suspected unresectable disease (Fig. 62.5).

In a pooled analysis of 9 studies involving 377 patients, the sensitivity and specificity of EUS for resectability of pancreatic cancer was 69% and 82%, respectively.[6,8,16,19,23,25,30–32] Ranges of reported sensitivities and specificities were 23% to 91% and 63% to 100%, respectively. Overall EUS accuracy for tumor resectability was 77%.

Because most studies have reported that EUS is similar to both CT and MRI for assessment of resectability, some authors have proposed that optimal preoperative imaging of pancreatic cancer requires the use of multiple modalities. Using a decision analysis, Soriano et al (2004)[19] found that accuracy for tumor resectability was maximized and costs were minimized when CT or EUS was performed initially, followed by the other test in those with potentially resectable neoplasms. Ahmad et al (2000)[16] proposed that although EUS and MRI individually are not sensitive for tumor resectability, their use together may increase positive predictive value of resectability compared to either test alone. When surgery is performed only when MDCT and EUS agree on tumor resectability, DeWitt et al (2004)[8] reported a nonsignificant trend toward improved accuracy of resectability compared to either study alone. However, a study by Bao et al (2008)[33] found that MDCT was a better predictor of resectability than EUS, although the performance of EUS improved in patients without biliary stents. From a practical standpoint, the actual role of EUS in staging of pancreatic cancer will depend on its availability, referral patterns, and local expertise.

EUS-FNA of Pancreatic Cancer

EUS-FNA remains the preferred method to sample pancreatic mass lesions due to its high accuracy, well demonstrated by two meta-analyses that reported sensitivity and specificity in the range of 85% to 89% and 96% to 98%, respectively.[34,35] However, the diagnostic accuracy of EUS-FNA may be impaired in the setting of chronic pancreatitis. Fritscher-Ravens et al (2002)[36] found that in a series of 207 consecutive patients with focal pancreatic lesions, the sensitivity of EUS-FNA for the diagnosis of malignancy in patients with normal parenchyma (89%) was superior to those with parenchymal evidence of chronic pancreatitis (54%).

On-site cytopathology review is available currently at most referral centers to provide immediate feedback to the endosonographer about the quality of EUS-FNA specimens obtained. On-site

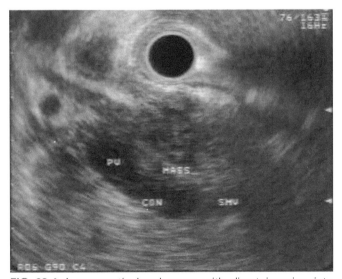

FIG 62.4 A pancreatic head mass with direct invasion into the portal vein (PV) and superior mesenteric artery (SMA). *CON,* Portovenous confluence.

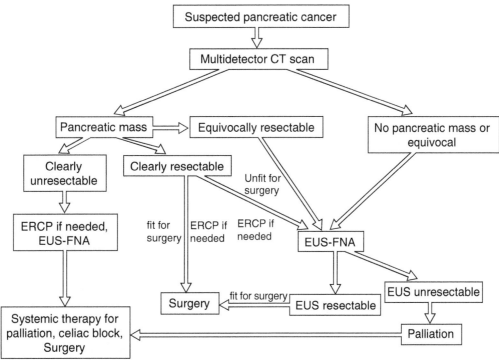

FIG 62.5 Endoscopic ultrasound based management algorithm for suspected pancreatic cancer. *CT,* computed tomography; *ERCP,* endoscopic retrograde cholangiopancreatography; *EUS,* endoscopic ultrasound; *FNA,* fine-needle aspiration.

review was found to correlate highly with the final diagnosis and can improve diagnostic certainty.[37] Occasionally, on-site cytology review of a suspected pancreatic cancer demonstrates insufficient tissue to confirm malignancy. This may be due to tumor necrosis, fibrosis, or hypervascularity. Yield may be increased by "fanning the lesion" using different angles of scope deflection in order to sample the peripheral parts of the lesion with a more viable tumor.[38] Increasing the number of passes may also overcome this problem, but the additional yield typically plateaus at 7 passes, and the amount of blood in the aspirate may increase with additional passes.[39] In this situation, avoiding suction and switching to a smaller-gauge needle could help limit the amount of blood in the specimen. Improving the yield of EUS-FNA by modifying the current sampling techniques has been the focus of several recent studies. Among the factors found to not increase the diagnostic yield include replacing the stylet after every pass.[40] Use of suction during FNA is generally recommended for pancreatic solid lesions but not for associated adenopathy due to increase in bloodiness of the sample.[40] Other novel techniques involving wet suction instead of vacuum, and the capillary stylet withdrawal technique showed superior diagnostic yield and cellularity and is discussed elsewhere in this book.[41,42]

The most commonly used commercially available EUS-FNA needles are 19-, 22- and 25-gauge needles. The impact of needle size on the diagnostic accuracy of EUS-FNA has been an area of uncertainty until recently. In a meta-analysis of 8 studies involving 1292 patients who underwent EUS-FNA with either a 22- or 25-gauge needle and had surgical histology or at least 6 months follow-up as the reference standard, Madhoun et al (2013)[43] reported that the sensitivity of the 25-gauge needle was superior to the 22-gauge (93% vs. 85%, $p = 0.0003$), although they have comparable specificity (97% and 100%, respectively).

Major complications following EUS-FNA of solid pancreatic masses occur in 0.5% to 2.5% of patients, including a 1.2% risk of pancreatitis and a 1% risk of severe bleeding.[44–46] In another prospective study, no delayed complications following EUS-FNA were reported in 127 patients with solid pancreatic masses followed for 30 days.[46] The risk of peritoneal seeding of tumor cells following EUS-FNA (2.2%) appears to be less than CT-guided FNA (16.3%) but requires further study.[47]

Despite excellent accuracy and a low incidence of major complications, EUS-FNA of pancreatic masses has several limitations. First, an on-site cytopathologist during EUS-FNA is recommended for assessment of specimen adequacy but is not available at some centers. Second, primary pancreatic lymphomas and well-differentiated ductal adenocarcinomas are often difficult to diagnose by use of cytology alone. Finally, the low negative predictive value of EUS-FNA does not permit exclusion of malignancy in negative specimens. To address these limitations, core biopsy devices have been developed to obtain histological tissue samples using a standard linear array echoendoscope. Two such devices include the Quick-Core and ProCore biopsy needles (Cook Medical, Bloomington, IN). In a multi-center cohort study of 109 patients with intestinal and extra-intestinal lesions (including 47 pancreatic tumors), the ProCore needle provided adequate histology and a correct diagnosis in 96% and 89% of cases, respectively.[49] However, a recent meta-analysis comparing the performance of the ProCore needle with standard FNA needles, including nine studies of 576 patients, demonstrated no difference in diagnostic adequacy (75% vs. 89%), diagnostic accuracy (86% vs. 86%) or rate of histological core specimen acquisition (78% vs. 77%) between the ProCore and standard FNA needles, respectively. The mean number of passes required for diagnosis, however, was significantly lower when using the ProCore needle (standardized mean difference 1.2, $p < 0.001$).[49] Nevertheless, ProCore biopsy needles will continue to have niche applications including autoimmune pancreatitis[12] and lymphoma,[50] where its superiority has been demonstrated. In addition, core biopsy needles could be used as a rescue technique when on-site FNA results are inconclusive or if this service is not available.

Some investigators have evaluated whether analysis of abnormal genes may increase the diagnostic yield of EUS-FNA of pancreatic masses. A meta-analysis of 8 prospective studies, involving 931 patients who had k-ras mutation, reported a pooled sensitivity and specificity of 77% and 93%, respectively.[51] When combined with EUS-FNA alone, the addition of k-ras mutation testing increased sensitivity from 81% to 89% but reduced specificity from 97% to 92%. Fluorescence in situ hybridization is another assay that was found to augment the sensitivity of cytology alone by 11%, according to Levy et al (2012).[52] Due to the high diagnostic accuracy of standard EUS-FNA, as well as the cost and limited availability of these genetic tests, it appears that use of genetic testing of EUS-FNA samples should be limited to inconclusive specimens and research protocols. Additional assays (like microRNAs and proteomics) are being evaluated on an experimental basis,[53] but clinical studies are needed to define its role in the diagnostic work-up of pancreatic tumors.

Pancreatic Neuroendocrine Tumors

PNETs are rare solid, cystic or mixed neoplasms that represent less than 10% of pancreatic tumors (Fig. 62.6). Approximately one-third of these tumors are classified as functional PNETs (FPNETs) in which excessive hormone secretion produces a distinct clinical syndrome. The two most clinically important FPNETs are gastrinomas and insulinomas. When PNETs do not produce a clinical syndrome, they are classified as nonfunctional (NFPNETs). Due to a lack of characteristic symptoms related to hormone excess, NFPNETs are usually recognized later, with larger tumors and nonspecific symptoms such as jaundice, weight loss, abdominal pain, or pancreatitis. Similar to primary ductal adenocarcinoma, surgical resection is the only cure for these tumors. Therefore, a high index of suspicion coupled with a stepwise preoperative evaluation for localization may optimize patient selection for potentially curative surgery.

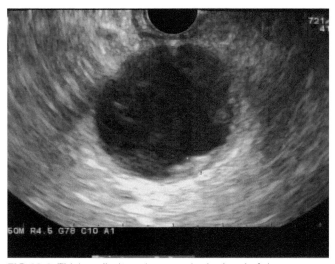

FIG 62.6 Thick-walled cystic tumor in the head of the pancreas diagnosed on fine-needle aspiration (FNA) as a neuroendocrine tumor.

In a series of studies that compared EUS to other imaging modalities, the sensitivity of EUS for detection of PNETs was 77% to 94%.[54–58] EUS appears especially useful for detection of small PNETs (< 2.5 cm) missed by other imaging studies. The sensitivity of transabdominal ultrasound for detection of PNETs is poor and only between 7% and 29%.[54,55,57] Similarly, early studies with CT demonstrated poor sensitivity that was generally less than 30%.[54,55,57] However, with ongoing improvements in CT scanners and the development of MDCT, the sensitivity of CT for PNETs has improved. In their study of 217 patients with 231 PNETs, Khashab et al (2011)[59] reported an overall sensitivity for MDCT of 84%. Factors associated with reduced sensitivity include small lesions less than 2 cm in diameter and insulinomas, which had a sensitivity of 54%. Among the 56 patients who had both CT and EUS, the sensitivity of EUS was far greater than CT (91.7% vs. 63.3%, $p = 0.0002$). Whereas MDCT is a suitable initial imaging modality for PNET, EUS provides cytologic confirmation and the detection of suspected CT negative PNET. In addition, EUS is the preferred initial imaging modality for insulinomas due to the low sensitivity of MDCT. In addition to their known role in assessing cystic lesions, MRI is an excellent imaging modality for PNET with sensitivity of 85% to 100%.[60,61]

The use of EUS-FNA permits tissue confirmation of a suspected PNET. In a retrospective study of 30 patients, Ardengh et al (2004)[62] reported a sensitivity, specificity, positive and negative predictive values, and accuracy of EUS-guided FNA of 82.6%, 85.7%, 95%, 60%, and 83.3%, respectively for tumor diagnosis. In a larger 2012 study of 81 patients, EUS-FNA correctly diagnosed a PNET in 73 out of 81 patients, with a diagnostic accuracy of 90.1%.[63] For cystic PNETs, the use of FNA was studied by Ridtitid et al (2015) in a case-controlled study comprising 50 patients with cystic PNETS compared to a cohort of 50 patients with solid PNETS over a 14-year period.[64] EUS-FNA accuracies for malignancy of cystic and solid PNETs were 89% and 90%, respectively; cystic PNETs were less associated with metastatic adenopathy (22% vs. 42%, $p = 0.03$) and liver metastasis (0% vs. 26%, $p < 0.001$). Cyst fluid analysis showed that benign cystic PNETs had low carcinoembryonic antigen, Ki-67 (< 2%). Immunocytochemistry staining for synaptophysin was seen in all 100 cases included in the study, whereas chromogranin A was positive in 90% and 88% of the cystic and solid PNETs, respectively.

Preoperative EUS-guided tattooing has been demonstrated to aid in intraoperative localization of an insulinoma,[65] and more recently demonstrated to be of utility for all small pancreatic lesions.[66] This information may confirm clinically suspected tumors and aid in appropriate planning of medical or surgical management.

Other Pancreatic Tumors

Primary pancreatic lymphoma (PPL) is rare and accounts for less than 0.5% of pancreatic tumors.[67] They are localized to the pancreas and peripancreatic lymph nodes and, by definition, do not involve other lymphoid tissue. PPL may present as a hypoechoic mass with poorly defined borders indistinguishable from pancreatic adenocarcinoma (Fig. 62.7). Whereas EUS and radiographic imaging alone may not confirm the diagnosis, EUS-FNA with flow cytometry is very accurate for PPL. In a case series of 16 patients with PPL, Khashab et al (2010)[68] reported a sensitivity and specificity of EUS-FNA with cytology and flow cytometry of 85% and 100%, respectively. This is in contrast to EUS-FNA with cytology alone, which had a sensitivity and

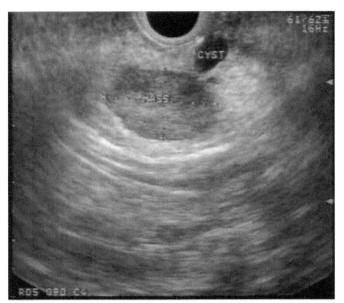

FIG 62.7 A well-delineated hypoechoic mass in the pancreatic tail adjacent to a cyst, diagnosed on FNA as a primary pancreatic lymphoma.

specificity of less than 30%. This diagnosis should be suspected based on clinical appearance, lack of definite malignancy, and abundance of abnormal lymphocytes on rapid cytological review.

Isolated pancreatic masses are usually due to focal chronic pancreatitis, benign neoplasms, or primary pancreatic malignancies. Rarely, metastasis to the pancreas from another primary malignancy occurs and has been reported in 2% to 3% of pancreatic resections.[69] Accurate identification of isolated pancreatic metastases is clinically important because aggressive surgical resection in selected patients may permit long-term survival. In other patients, however, proper diagnosis may avoid unnecessary surgery and permit triage to more appropriate nonoperative therapy.

EUS features of pancreatic metastases appear to be different from those observed in cases of primary pancreatic cancer. In 7 patients with metastatic pancreatic lesions, Palazzo et al (1996)[70] described homogeneous, round, well-circumscribed lesions in 15 out of 16 masses observed. Compared to patients with primary cancer (n = 80), DeWitt et al (2005)[71] found that pancreatic metastases (n = 24) were more likely to have well-defined borders compared to irregular margins. In another report of 11 patients with metastatic renal cell carcinoma (RCC),[72] ten had well-defined borders (Video 62.1). Therefore, it appears that EUS visualization of a well-defined pancreatic mass in a patient with a history of malignancy should raise suspicion for a metastatic lesion.

EUS-FNA permits an accurate cytologic diagnosis of metastatic lesions to the pancreas. In the largest series to date of 72 masses in 49 patients, El Hajj et al (2013)[73] reported metastatic lesions from the kidney (n = 21), lung (n = 8), skin (n = 6), colon (n = 4), breast (n = 3), small bowel (n = 2), stomach (n = 2), liver (n = 1), ovary (n = 1), and bladder (n = 1). Metastasis to the pancreas may occur many years (especially for RCC) after diagnosis of the primary tumor. In patients with a remote history of malignancy, obtaining additional cytological material for cell block and the use of immunocytochemistry may be helpful to confirm the diagnosis of pancreatic metastases and recurrent malignancy.

Conclusion

We can confidently state that EUS has passed the test of time as the modality of choice for the detection of pancreatic tumors, mainly small solid lesions. Although the competitive edge of EUS in the staging of pancreatic tumors appears to be eroding due to the rapid improvement in imaging technologies, the role that EUS plays in predicting their resectability remains obvious due to its ability to detect occult metastasis missed by other preoperative imaging studies. EUS-guided tissue acquisition is essential in the management of pancreatic tumors, mainly due to its high accuracy and low overall morbidity and mortality. Tissue confirmation is of particular importance in pancreatic cancer where the majority of patients are unresectable and tissue is needed prior to initiation of any systemic palliative therapies or neoadjuvant therapy in some potentially resectable patients. Finally, EUS-guided tissue helps triage the patients to the appropriate care in some conditions presenting as pancreatic cancer, such as pancreatic lymphoma and autoimmune pancreatitis.

EVALUATION AND STAGING OF CHOLANGIOCARCINOMA

Introduction

Cholangiocarcinoma (CCA) is rare tumor that is occurring with increasing frequency and develops from bile duct epithelium found within the intrahepatic and extrahepatic biliary tree, excluding the ampulla or gallbladder.[74] CCA is associated with a poor prognosis largely due to the tumor biology, late presentation, and difficulty in diagnosis. For hilar CCA, the 5-year survival after resection is 20% to 40%, largely dependent on tumor stage.[75–78] Liver transplantation of unresectable hilar CCA has a 5-year survival that approaches 75%.[79–81] Diagnostic and staging procedures must be improved to help identify patients most apt to benefit from these aggressive medical and surgical therapies, especially in regard to liver transplantation. This information helps direct resource utilization and allocation of scarcely available organs.

The limitations of diagnostic and staging modalities largely encouraged the new technology development. One such technology, EUS has seen a growing use for CCA due to its unprecedented imaging and tissue acquisition capabilities. However, there is some controversy regarding the role of EUS in CCA, especially as it pertains to the use of primary tumor FNA. Although FNA enhances diagnosis, it does so at the risk of tumor seeding. Whereas EUS findings help guide patient care and improve outcomes, misdirected use may result in iatrogenic upstaging and compromise patient care.

An aim of this section is to suggest a role for EUS in patients with suspected or known extrahepatic CCA based on published data. These data must be carefully considered because some investigators preselected patients with a suspected or confirmed CCA, versus others who evaluated a broader cohort having a "biliary stricture," "jaundice," or "pancreatic head mass"[82–87] (Table 62.3). Enrollment from a diverse patient cohort does help determine the role of EUS among patients with a given symptom or presentation. However, such studies often lack the ideal target enrollment population and often provide insufficient detail to establish the role of EUS in this setting (see Tables 62.3 and 62.4).[82–87] Another potential limitation when drawing any conclusion from existing studies of patients with CCA is the lack of clarity regarding the tumor location within the biliary tree. The

TABLE 62.3   Study Design, Inclusion Criteria, Enrollment, and Tumor Site for EUS Literature

Study	Design	Inclusion Criteria	Total Enrollment	Study Population	PRIMARY STRICTURE/TUMOR SITE AND NUMBER PER SITE	
Mohamadnejad (2011)[87]	Retrospective	Known cholangiocarcinoma	81	81	Proximal Distal	30 51
Rosch et al. (2004)[86]	Prospective	Indeterminate biliary stricture or pancreatic head mass	50	50	Hilar CBD	4 8
Eloubeidi et al. (2004)[85]	Prospective	Bile duct stricture Suspected cholangiocarcinoma[1]	28	25[3]	Proximal Distal	15 13
Lee et al. (2004)[84]	Retrospective	Known or suspected bile duct stricture Prior intraductal tissue sampling, if any, negative Prior CT and/or MRI failed to demonstrate the cause	42	40[4]	CHD CBD	1 39
Byrne et al. (2004)[83]	Retrospective	Bile duct mass or stricture with biliary EUS FNA	35	31[5]	CHD CBD	3 32
Fritscher-Ravens et al. (2003)[81]	Prospective	Clinical suspicion of hilar cholangiocarcinoma ERC[2] with nondiagnostic tissue sampling Fit for hepatic resection	44	44	Hilar	44
			280	271	"Perihilar"[6] "Distal"[7]	97 (40%) 143 (60%)

[1]Patients ultimately found to have pancreatic cancer or nodal metastasis were excluded.
[2]Endoscopic retrograde cholangiography.
[3]3 patients were excluded because the tumor could not be visualized with linear imaging.
[4]2 patients were excluded because of inadequate follow-up.
[5]4 patients were excluded because of the absence of a diagnostic gold standard.
[6]We employ the term *perihilar* to represent tumors designated as hilar, common hepatic duct, or proximal.
[7]We employ the term *distal* to represent tumors designated as distal or common bile duct.
CBD, common bile duct; *CHD,* common hepatic duct; *CT,* computed tomography; *EUS,* endoscopic ultrasound; *FNA,* fine-needle aspiration; *MRI,* magnetic resonance imaging.

TABLE 62.4   Tumor Type and EUS Stricture/Tumor Detection

Study	Benign Versus Malignant		Details Regarding Malignancy	Primary Stricture/Tumor Detection With EUS (Grouped Data)	Primary Stricture/Tumor Detection With EUS (CCA Patients Alone)
Mohamadnejad et al. (2011)[87]	Malignant Benign	81 0	Cholangiocarcinoma (n = 81)	N/A	76 of 81 (94%)[3]
Rosch et al. (2004)[86]	Malignant Benign	28 22	Cholangiocarcinoma (n = 12) Pancreatic (n = 16)	47 of 50 (94%)	11 of 12 (92%)
Eloubeidi et al. (2004)[85]	Malignant Benign	21 4	Cholangiocarcinoma (n = 21)	25 of 28 (89%)	~
Lee et al. (2004)[84]	Malignant Benign	24 16	Cholangiocarcinoma/Pancreatic (n = 23)[1] Metastatic (n = 1)	40 of 40 (100%)	~
Byrne et al. (2004)[83]	Malignant Benign	14 17	Cholangiocarcinoma/Pancreatic (n = 11)[1] Metastatic (n = 3)	(Preselected)[2]	~
Fritscher-Ravens et al. (2003)[82]	Malignant Benign	36 8	Cholangiocarcinoma (n = 30)[1] Metastatic (n = 6)	44 of 44 (100%)	~
Summary	Malignant Benign	204 (73%) 76 (27%)	Cholangiocarcinoma (n = 144-178)[1]	156 of 162 (96%) (excluding preselected)	87 of 93 (94%)

[1]Patients with cholangiocarcinoma cannot be reliably distinguished because the studies combine data from patients with other pathologies (e.g., pancreatic carcinoma, metastatic biliary lesions). Therefore, some of the following analyses are based on grouped data.
[2]The cited study included preselected patients whose enrollment necessitated endoscopic ultrasound (EUS) visualization and fine-needle aspiration (FNA). Therefore, the findings do not apply in terms of stricture/tumor detection.
[3]Tumor detection varied by site: Proximal 25/30 (83%) versus distal 51/51 (100%).
CCA, cholangiocarcinoma.

clinical presentation, diagnostic approach, and management vary for tumors within the proximal versus distal extrahepatic duct. Therefore, uncertainty regarding the tumor location leaves uncertainty as to how best to interpret and apply the data. Likewise, there are no published data to guide the use of EUS for intrahepatic CCA. To facilitate our discussion, we use the term *perihilar* to indicate tumors that studies designated as hilar, common hepatic duct, or proximal,[88] and use the term *distal* to represent tumors designated as distal or common bile duct (Video 62.2).

EUS Stricture/Tumor Detection

Studies indicate that EUS imaging (not necessarily with FNA confirmation), identified 156 of 162 (96%) biliary strictures or

TABLE 62.5 Details Regarding Performance of EUS FNA

Study	Number of FNA Performed	Onsite Review Available	Cytological Interpretations Indicative of a Positive FNA Test Result
Mohamadnejad et al. (2011)[87]	Median 5 Passes (range 1–12)	Yes	Positive or Suspicious
Rosch et al. (2004)[86]	≥ 2 passes with material sufficient for assessment[3] Mean 2.8 passes (range 2–4)	No	Only Positive
Eloubeidi et al. (2004)[85]	≥ 5 passes unless onsite review confirmed malignant cells Median 3 passes (range 1–7)	Yes	Dual Analyses[2]
Lee et al. (2004)[84]	Until adequate cellularity or ≥ 5 passes Mean 2.8 passes	Yes	Dual Analyses[2]
Byrne et al. (2004)[83]	Range 2–7 passes	Yes[1]	Dual Analyses[2]
Fritscher-Ravens et al. (2003)[82]	2 or 3 passes	No	Dual Analyses[2]

[1]On-site cytopathology review available in 32 of 35 patients.
[2]Data provided when considering "Positive" for malignancy as the only indicator of a positive test result. Authors also provided data when considering either a "Positive" or "Suspicious" interpretation as indicative of a positive test result.
[3]Based on gross inspection by the endosonographer who deemed the material sufficient when visible material was identified.
EUS, endoscopic ultrasound; *FNA*, fine-needle aspiration.

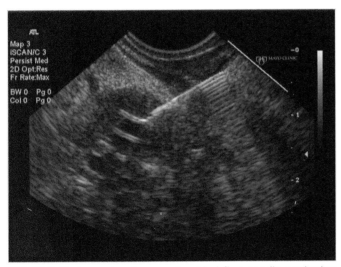

FIG 62.8 Endoscopic ultrasound guided fine-needle aspiration for sampling of a common hepatic duct cholangiocarcinoma.

TABLE 62.6 Diagnostic Sensitivity of EUS FNA

Study	"Positive" or "Suspicious" Interpretation Equates to Positive for Malignancy	Only "Positive" Interpretation Equates to Positive for Malignancy
Mohamadnejad et al. (2011)[87]	54/74 (73%)[1]	~
Rosch et al. (2004)[86]	~	3/11 (27%)
Eloubeidi et al. (2004)[85]	18/21 (86%)	17/21 (75%)
Lee et al. (2004)[84]	11/24 (47%)	7/24 (29%)
Byrne et al. (2004)[83]	9/14 (64%)	6/14 (43%)
Fritscher-Ravens et al. (2003)[82]	32/36 (89%) 124/169 (73%)	30/36 (83%) 63/106 (59%)

~ Indicates that data were not provided.
[1]The diagnostic sensitivity was significantly greater when sampling distal versus proximal CCA; 38 of 47 (81%) versus 16 of 27 (59%), *p* = 0.04.
EUS, endoscopic ultrasound; *FNA*, fine-needle aspiration.

tumors.[82,84–86] In the two studies that clearly and specifically reported their data for CCA patients, EUS imaging detected 87 of 93 (94%) primary tumors.[86,87] One study provided separate data for proximal versus distal tumors and noted that proximal CCA was identified less often than distal CCA; 25 of 30 (83%) versus 51 of 51 (100%), respectively.[87]

EUS-FNA Diagnostic Accuracy

One of the most beneficial yet potentially harmful applications of EUS in CCA patients is the use of FNA for primary tumor diagnosis (Fig. 62.8). The desmoplasia and tendency for longitudinal rather than radial growth associated with CCA can compromise efforts at a tissue diagnosis and result in a delayed or failed diagnosis. Endoscopic retrograde cholangiography and brush cytology with intraductal biopsy are the standard diagnostic approaches yielding a high specificity, but low diagnostic sensitivity of 20% to 60%.[89–91] The poor performance characteristics have led to the use of molecular markers, such as fluorescence in situ hybridization which increases diagnostic sensitivity by

10% to 30%, but in combination with standard cytology and biopsy still offer a composite sensitivity of only 60% to 70% in most series.[92–94]

Published reports show a diagnostic sensitivity for primary tumor EUS FNA between 29% and 89%, depending on the means by which cytological specimens were analyzed[82–87] (Tables 62.5 and 62.6). For studies that deemed a "positive" or "suspicious" cytological interpretation as indicative of malignancy, the diagnostic sensitivity was 124 of 169 (73%).[82–85,87] However, studies requiring a "positive" cytological interpretation reported a diagnostic sensitivity of only 63/106 (59%).[82–86] The diagnostic sensitivity of EUS FNA may be greater for distal versus proximal CCA; 38 of 47 (81%) versus 16 of 27 (59%), *p* = 0.04.[87] In contrast, one study reported a sensitivity of 32/36 (89%) for hilar strictures or tumors.[82] The diagnostic capabilities of EUS FNA are further demonstrated in studies employing FNA after either a negative or unsuccessful endoscopic retrograde cholangiography (ERC) sampling, yielding sensitivities of 77% and 89% for EUS FNA in these respective settings.[82,87]

Tumor Seeding

The perceived risk and implications of tumor seeding following EUS FNA for CCA is debated. There are insufficient data to meaningfully guide this discussion, but our views are largely based on those of transplant centers, for which the impact of any perceived risk of tumor seeding most substantially impacts patient management. Tumor seeding is often referred to as needle track seeding or implantation metastasis and has been reported following EUS-,[95–97] percutaneous ultrasound– or CT-guided FNA of various sites including the brain, eye, thyroid, breast, lung, tongue, liver, gallbladder, pancreas, colon, kidney, ureter, bladder, stromal tumor, bone and bone marrow, and bile duct among others.[98–103] Tumor seeding has also been associated with preoperative percutaneous drainage and ERC with stent placement.[104,105]

Limited data suggest that the risk of clinically apparent tumor seeding following FNA is 1/10,000–40,000.[106,107] However, there are a number of limitations in determining the incidence of tumor seeding and the cited rates likely significantly underestimate the occurrence. The high mortality, short survival, and obviated need for subsequent abdominal imaging in patients with unresectable cancer prohibit accurate determination of the tumor seeding rate. Even for patients who undergo potentially curative resection, tumor seeding may result in minute foci of occult cells undetected in the surgical specimen or result in deposition outside the field of resection. These occult reservoirs of tumor cells may ultimately result in apparent clinical disease that is falsely considered to represent tumor recurrence rather than disease progression of occult tumor cells deposited during needle track seeding. There is also controversy as to the implications of tumor seeding, with some finding a correlation with clinical outcomes including tumor stage, prognosis, resectability, surgical margin status, recurrence, and survival.[108–118] Other investigators have failed to discover a correlation with clinical outcomes.[119–122]

The potential of tumor cells to be displaced during FNA was been demonstrated.[123] In 140 prospectively enrolled patients who underwent EUS, luminal fluid that is typically aspirated via the accessory channel was instead submitted for cytological analysis. The cytology specimens from the aspirated luminal fluid were positive for malignancy in 48% of patients, who had a luminal cancer, which may be accounted for by cells shed from the luminal cancer. More concerning was the post-FNA luminal fluid cytology that was positive for malignancy in 3/26 patients with pancreatic adenocarcinoma. Among patients with extraluminal cancers one would not anticipate recovering malignant cells from the gastrointestinal luminal fluid. These findings may indicate that the process of FNA displaces some malignant cells from the original primary site to the needle track and even more distant locations, and may help explain the process of needle track seeding. This hypothesis is supported in a study that evaluated the rates of peritoneal carcinomatosis in matched pancreatic adenocarcinoma cohorts diagnosed by either EUS versus percutaneously guided FNA.[124] Peritoneal carcinomatosis developed in 1 in 7 patients (2.2% vs. 16.3%; $p < 0.025$) in the EUS FNA versus percutaneous FNA group, respectively. The findings indicate a potential difference in tumor seeding risk between biopsy approaches and potentially greater frequency of tumor seeding than historically appreciated. Similarly, a meta-analysis of 8 studies identified tumor seeding in 2.7% of patients following hepatocellular carcinoma biopsy.[125]

Another study evaluated the tumor seeding risk among 191 patients with hilar CCA who underwent primary tumor transperitoneal FNA as part of liver transplant evaluation for locally unresectable disease.[126] Among all 16 patients who underwent transperitoneal FNA (13 percutaneous, 3 EUS), the initial cytological specimens were interpreted as positive for malignancy (n = 6), negative for nine (n = 9), and one equivocal test result (n = 1). During intraoperative staging, peritoneal metastases were identified in 5/6 (83%) versus 0/9 (0%) patients who had an FNA interpretation of positive versus negative, respectively. In addition, peritoneal metastases were discovered in only 14/175 (8%) patients who did not undergo FNA versus 5/6 (83%), $p = 0.0097$, with a positive preoperative FNA. However, the study findings must be carefully considered. For instance, based on their data it is not possible to determine whether clinical or tumor-related features indicated more advanced disease, which might have removed concern for tumor seeding, thereby leading to FNA. In addition, whereas both study groups had similar CA 19-9 levels, frequency of mass detection, tumor size, and histology, precise staging information was not provided. A discrepancy in staging may itself explain the greater occurrence of peritoneal metastasis rather than performing FNA.

Based on our communications, most liver transplant centers consider primary tumor FNA of suspected CCA an absolute contraindication, which must not only be considered by colleagues within such centers, but also by referring clinicians given the medical implications. This philosophy places additional burden and exhaustive efforts to firmly establish a CCA. Caution is needed if proceeding to surgery without a tissue diagnosis because 10% to 20% of patients resected for presumed CCA are ultimately diagnosed with benign disease or alternate tumor type.[127–130] The challenges of CCA diagnosis leads some to advocate less stringent surrogate markers (e.g., CA 19-9 levels and imaging criteria alone) as means of a presumptive diagnosis setting. Whereas this practice may be questioned even for highly experienced clinicians, there is particular concern for false diagnosis that may result in inappropriate and often risky surgery. Proper patient counseling is required to convey the potential for extensive operative intervention (even transplantation) for benign disease. Patients often accept this approach once understanding the diagnostic challenges and the importance of avoiding delayed oncologic care, as well as the risks and implications of tumor seeding.

Staging and Resectability

Accurate tumor staging is needed to optimize clinical decision making. Several staging systems are utilized for CCA,[77,131,132] which differ in intended application and accuracy for determining prognosis and resectability, and when guiding the extent of resection. Common features employed by each staging system including the longitudinal tumor margins (proximal and distal), presence of nodal disease, vascular infiltration, parenchymal lobar atrophy, and distant metastasis. Improved preoperative staging reduces the need for isolated staging laparoscopy and rate of tumor upstaging at laparoscopy (Fig. 62.9).

Published data are limited and prohibit any meaningful effort to establish the utility of EUS for CCA staging. Existing studies provide few EUS staging details and the underlying aims and methodologies were insufficient to determine of EUS staging accuracy. One study did provide some useful staging data for the cohort of 81 patients, 75 of whom underwent evaluation for surgical candidacy.[87] Among the 15 patients ultimately designated as unresectable, EUS discovered the evidence of unresectable

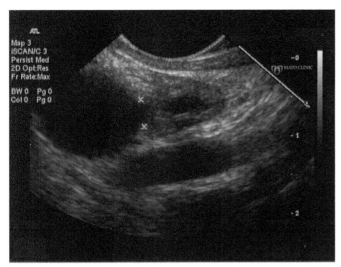

FIG 62.9 A cholangiocarcinoma infiltrating the portal vein on linear endoscopic ultrasound (EUS) exam. The X's delineate the interface between the bile duct and the portal vein.

disease in a greater number than CT; 8/15 (53%) versus 5/15 (33%), respectively. EUS identified six disease sites that were not discovered by CT/MRI including tumor infiltration of the PV (n = 2), hepatic artery, celiac lymph node, liver metastasis, and peritoneum. In contrast, the sites discovered by CT/MRI that were not identified by EUS included PV invasion (n = 2) and celiac lymphadenopathy (n = 1). Finally, 4 disease sites were confirmed only at surgery and failed prior EUS or CT/MRI detection including malignant infiltration of the hepatic artery, PV, celiac node, and longitudinal bile duct extension. Other key data were excluded from this report, thereby limiting firm calculation of EUS staging and resectability accuracy.

EUS Nodal Staging and Features of Malignant and Benign Lymph Nodes

Most published data do not thoroughly indicate the accuracy of EUS nodal staging.[87,133] Other studies only indicated if any nodes had been identified[82,84] or often ignored this issue.[83,85,86] For CCA, lymph node metastasis is a poor prognostic indicator,[134,135] and distant malignant nodal involvement precludes curative resection. However, the significance of locoregional lymph node metastasis is debated. Transplant centers uniformly view any nodal involvement as an absolute contraindication to liver transplant and for many centers even precludes attempted curative resection.

The accuracy of EUS FNA nodal staging was studied among 47 patients with locally unresectable hilar CCA undergoing liver transplantation evaluation.[133] Lymph nodes were seen at EUS in each patient, resulting in FNA of 70 lymph nodes with metastatic adenopathy diagnosed in 8 patients. Only 2/8 patients' malignant nodes were detected by CT and/or MRI. For the 22 patients who had benign lymph nodes at FNA cytology, 20 (91%) were confirmed benign at exploratory laparotomy. However, EUS failed to detect malignant lymph nodes in 2 patients. Data were also obtained to help determine EUS features to distinguish benign from malignant nodes in patients with CCA. Conventional EUS features that include long-axis length, roundness, echogenicity, and homogeneity both individually and collectively provided poor predictive value (Table 62.7; Figs. 62.10 and 62.11). Therefore, in our practice, in patients with CCA we biopsy all

TABLE 62.7   EUS Features for Malignant and Benign Lymph Nodes

Mean	Malignant LN	Benign LN	P Value
Long Axis (mm)	1.61 +/− 0.61	1.47 +/− 0.78	0.68
Roundness Score	2.5 +/− 1.55	2.9 +/− 0.81	0.32
Echogenicity Score	4.0 +/− 0.63	3.78 +/− 0.71	0.48
Homogeneity Score	3.0 +/− 1.1	3.32 +/− 0.84	0.41

EUS, endoscopic ultrasound.

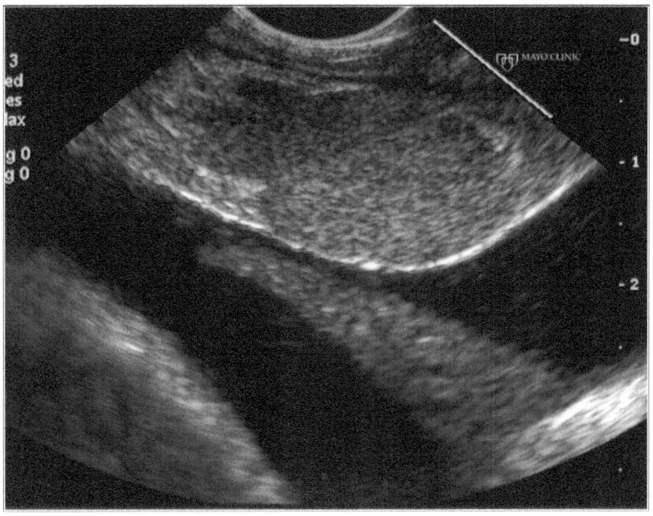

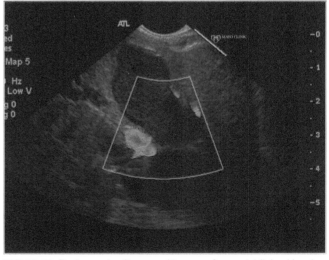

FIG 62.10 Endoscopic ultrasound image of a biopsy proven malignant lymph node.

FIG 62.11 Endoscopic ultrasound image of an established benign lymph node.

locoregional visualized lymph nodes regardless of the EUS appearance.

A separate study compared EUS and surgical nodal staging in 45 patients and reported an EUS diagnostic sensitivity of only 2/23 (9%). In this study, locoregional lymph nodes were not routinely sampled, which may have contributed to the low sensitivity.[87]

TABLE 62.8 Potentially Confounding Variables and Complications

Study	PSC[1] Present	Stent Present at time of EUS	Complications Related to EUS
Mohamadnejad et al. (2011)[87]	2 of 81 (2%)	64/74 (86%)[4]	1 (Hemobilia)
Rosch et al. (2004)[85]	~	~	0
Eloubeidi et al. (2004)[85]	1 of 28 (4%)	27/28 (96%)	0
Lee et al. (2004)[84]	3 of 40 (8%)[2]	40/42 (95%)[5]	0
Byrne et al. (2004)[83]	0 of 35 (0%)	~	~
Fritscher-Ravens et al. (2003)[82]	4 of 44 (9%)[3]	44 of 44 (Implied)	0
Summary	10/228 (4%)	131/146 (90%)	

~ Indicates that data were not provided.

[1] Primary sclerosing cholangitis.

[2] There was no evidence of PSC at the time of EUS. Cholangiographic features of PSC subsequently developed in 3 patients.

[3] EUS FNA was falsely negative in the 4 patients with PSC.

[4] The diagnostic sensitivity of EUS FNA was 45 of 64 (70%) versus 9 of 10 (90%) for patients with and without a stent, respectively.

[5] Stent data were given for the initial 42 patients evaluated, but not specifically for the 40 patients ultimately included in the overall analyses.

EUS, endoscopic ultrasound; FNA, fine-needle aspiration.

Potentially Confounding Variables and Complications

Primary sclerosing cholangitis (PSC) is a prime risk factor for developing CCA. Although details pertaining to PSC were typically limited or omitted among the 5 studies documenting this information, only 10/228 (4%) patients had PSC (Table 62.8).[82–87] This is important, as PSC is routinely associated with multiple and diffuse bile duct strictures, increased desmoplasia, and benign lymphadenopathy. Each of these features can negatively impact EUS imaging and FNA performance. Therefore, the low rate of PSC in the study cohort is likely to have artificially improved EUS imaging and FNA results from most practice settings.

Among the cited studies, a biliary stent was in place at the time of EUS in 131/146 (90%) patients (see Table 62.8). The presence of an indwelling biliary stent can impair EUS imaging due to stent-induced artifacts and stent-induced sludge. However, any impaired imaging is seldom of consequence except for diminutive biliary or pancreatic lesions. Imaging can be optimized by examination various locations, by limiting the amount of air insufflated that may pass through the stent into the duct, or by removing the stent prior to EUS. The presence of a stent can facilitate detection of a biliary mass, as the stent often courses through the lesion, aiding detection.

Conclusion

The proper management of patients with suspected CCA requires a definitive tissue diagnosis. EUS is increasingly being used to both diagnose and stage CCA largely due to the limitations of endoscopic bile duct sampling. Whereas studies indicate the utility of EUS in patients with CCA, there remains debate as to the accuracy and role in this setting. Although some perform bile duct EUS FNA for primary tumor diagnosis, we strongly discourage doing so because of the potential for tumor seeding and impact on transplant candidacy or standard resection.

One should also consider the high false-negative of primary tumor FNA.

We consider CCA data to most strongly support EUS FNA to evaluate lymphadenopathy when considering liver transplantation. Confirmation of malignant lymphadenopathy avoids unnecessary neoadjuvant therapy and staging laparotomy, and resulting quality of life and cost. We believe EUS is indicated irrespective of the CT and/or MRI findings due to their insufficient sensitivity for lymph node detection and poor discrimination of benign from malignant nodes. Likewise, extensive sampling is indicated regardless of the nodal appearance due to the poor predictive value of EUS imaging features. Patients with negative FNA cytology subsequently undergo staging laparotomy to verify N0 status. Additional data are needed to clarify the role of EUS regarding other staging criteria in patients being considered for liver transplantation. More research is also needed to determine the impact of EUS staging among patients considered for non-transplant forms of operative intervention. Finally, existing reports provide no information pertaining to the use of EUS for intrahepatic CCA.

KEY REFERENCES

8. DeWitt J, Devereaux B, Chriswell M, et al: Comparison of endoscopic ultrasonography and multidetector computed tomography for detecting and staging pancreatic cancer, *Ann Intern Med* 141(10):753–763, 2004.

9. Canto MI, Harinck F, Hruban RH, et al: International Cancer of the Pancreas Screening (CAPS) Consortium summit on the management of patients with increased risk for familial pancreatic cancer, *Gut* 62(3): 339–347, 2013.

11. Farrell JJ, Garber J, Sahani D, Brugge WR: EUS findings in patients with autoimmune pancreatitis, *Gastrointest Endosc* 60(6):927–936, 2004.

13. Iwashita T, Yasuda I, Doi S, et al: Use of samples from endoscopic ultrasound-guided 19-gauge fine-needle aspiration in diagnosis of autoimmune pancreatitis, *Clin Gastroenterol* 10(3):316–322, 2012.

19. Soriano A, Castells A, Ayuso C, et al: Preoperative staging and tumor resectability assessment of pancreatic cancer: prospective study comparing endoscopic ultrasonography, helical computed tomography, magnetic resonance imaging, and angiography, *Am J Gastroenterol* 99(3):492–501, 2004.

22. Catalano MF, Sivak MV, Jr, Rice T, et al: Endosonographic features predictive of lymph node metastasis, *Gastrointest Endosc* 40(4):442–446, 1994.

34. Hewitt MJ, McPhail MJ, Possamai L, et al: EUS-guided FNA for diagnosis of solid pancreatic neoplasms: a meta-analysis, *Gastrointest Endosc* 75(2):319–331, 2012.

42. Wani S, Muthusamy VR, Komanduri S: EUS-guided tissue acquisition: an evidence-based approach (with videos), *Gastrointest Endosc* 80(6): 939–959.e7, 2014.

51. Fuccio L, Hassan C, Laterza L, et al: The role of K-ras gene mutation analysis in EUS-guided FNA cytology specimens for the differential diagnosis of pancreatic solid masses: a meta-analysis of prospective studies, *Gastrointest Endosc* 78(4):596–608, 2013.

53. Frampton AE, Krell J, Jamieson NB, et al: microRNAs with prognostic significance in pancreatic ductal adenocarcinoma: a meta-analysis, *Eur J Cancer* 51(11):1389–1404, 2015.

58. van Asselt SJ, Brouwers AH, van Dullemen HM, et al: EUS is superior for detection of pancreatic lesions compared with standard imaging in patients with multiple endocrine neoplasia type 1, *Gastrointest Endosc* 81(1):159–167.e2, 2015.

59. Khashab MA, Yong E, Lennon AM, et al: EUS is still superior to multidetector computerized tomography for detection of pancreatic neuroendocrine tumors, *Gastrointest Endosc* 73(4):691–696, 2011.

64. Ridtitid W, Halawi H, DeWitt JM, et al: Cystic pancreatic neuroendocrine tumors: outcomes of preoperative

endosonography-guided fine needle aspiration, and recurrence during long-term follow-up, *Endoscopy* 47(7):617–625, 2015.

78. DeOliveira ML, Cunningham SC, Cameron JL, et al: Cholangiocarcinoma: thirty-one-year experience with 564 patients at a single institution, *Ann Surg* 245(5):755–762, 2007.

81. Rea DJ, Heimbach JK, Rosen CB, et al: Liver transplantation with neoadjuvant chemoradiation is more effective than resection for hilar cholangiocarcinoma, *Ann Surg* 242(3):451–458, discussion 458–461, 2005.

86. Rosch T, Hofrichter K, Frimberger E, et al: ERCP or EUS for tissue diagnosis of biliary strictures? A prospective comparative study, *Gastrointest Endosc* 60(3):390–396, 2004.

87. Mohamadnejad M, DeWitt JM, Sherman S, et al: Role of EUS for preoperative evaluation of cholangiocarcinoma: a large single-center experience, *Gastrointest Endosc* 73(1):71–78, 2011.

92. Moreno Luna LE, Kipp B, Halling KC, et al: Advanced cytologic techniques for the detection of malignant pancreatobiliary strictures, *Gastroenterology* 131(4):1064–1072, 2006.

93. Levy MJ, Baron TH, Clayton AC, et al: Prospective evaluation of advanced molecular markers and imaging techniques in patients with indeterminate bile duct strictures, *Am J Gastroenterol* 103(5):1263–1273, 2008.

114. Miyazono F, Natsugoe S, Takao S, et al: Surgical maneuvers enhance molecular detection of circulating tumor cells during gastric cancer surgery, *Ann Surg* 233(2):189–194, 2001.

123. Levy MJ, Gleeson FC, Campion MB, et al: Prospective cytological assessment of gastrointestinal luminal fluid acquired during EUS: a potential source of false-positive FNA and needle tract seeding, *Am J Gastroenterol* 105(6):1311–1318, 2010.

124. Micames C, Jowell PS, White R, et al: Lower frequency of peritoneal carcinomatosis in patients with pancreatic cancer diagnosed by EUS-guided FNA vs. percutaneous FNA, *Gastrointest Endosc* 58(5): 690–695, 2003.

126. Heimbach JK, Sanchez W, Rosen CB, Gores GJ: Trans-peritoneal fine needle aspiration biopsy of hilar cholangiocarcinoma is associated with disease dissemination, *HPB (Oxford)* 13(5):356–360, 2011.

131. Bismuth H, Nakache R, Diamond T: Management strategies in resection for hilar cholangiocarcinoma, *Ann Surg* 215(1):31–38, 1992.

133. Gleeson FC, Rajan E, Levy MJ, et al: EUS-guided FNA of regional lymph nodes in patients with unresectable hilar cholangiocarcinoma, *Gastrointest Endosc* 67(3):438–443, 2008.

A complete reference list can be found online at ExpertConsult .com

63

Palliation of Malignant Pancreaticobiliary Obstruction

Marco J. Bruno and Fauze Maluf-Filho

INTRODUCTION

Pancreaticobiliary malignancies comprise a mixed bag of cancers including pancreatic cancer, carcinoma of the ampulla of Vater, duodenal carcinoma, gallbladder carcinoma, and cholangiocarcinomas. When they are located at the level of the liver hilum, cholangiocarcinomas are referred to as *Klatskin's tumors*. Although there are marked differences in biologic behavior and clinical outcome, the overall prognosis of these tumors is dismal. At the time of presentation, more than 80% to 90% of patients have locally unresectable disease or distant metastases, leaving only a few patients suitable for curative resection. Other treatment modalities such as chemotherapy and radiotherapy have little to no effect on survival, although various multimodality schemes in a (neo)adjuvant setting to surgery are currently being explored. Hence many patients, sooner or later in their disease course, are in need of optimal palliative treatment directed toward relief of jaundice, pain, and gastric outlet obstruction.

More than 85% of patients with pancreaticobiliary malignancies develop obstructive jaundice, and often it is a presenting symptom. Endoscopic retrograde cholangiopancreatography (ERCP) with placement of plastic or metallic self-expandable biliary stents has become the standard of care to relieve jaundice and has largely replaced surgical treatment. In case of failure of ERCP, percutaneous transhepatic cholangiographic drainage (PTCD) or endosonographic guided (EUS) biliary drainage are alternative treatment options.

EPIDEMIOLOGY

Of all pancreaticobiliary malignancies, pancreatic adenocarcinoma has the highest incidence. It is the fourth leading cause of cancer death in the United States, and it is estimated that in 2016 approximately 53,070 people will be diagnosed with pancreatic cancer, and 41,780 will die as a result of the disease.[1] It is predicted to become the second leading cause of cancer death in the United States by 2030.[2] Only a minority of patients (10% to 20%) are suitable candidates for curative resection, although this number is increasing with the advent of (neo)adjuvant chemo(radiation) therapy. The overall 5-year survival rate is still less than 4%. For patients having undergone a surgical resection it is less than 20%. Tobacco smoking doubles the risk of pancreatic cancer.[3] Patients with chronic pancreatitis have an increased risk for developing pancreatic cancer that is estimated at 4% per 20 years.[4] The risk of developing pancreatic cancer in patients with hereditary pancreatitis is 20% to 40%, with smoking as an important risk modifier.[5]

The incidence of gallbladder carcinomas averages 1 per 100,000 person-years, but is considerably higher among Native Americans. Patients most likely to survive are those in whom early cancer is detected in a postcholecystectomy specimen, with a 5-year survival of 80% to 100% for early T1–T2 cancers.[6] For locally advanced T3/4 tumors, survival drops to 10% to 30%. Gallstone disease is the most important risk factor for gallbladder cancer.[7]

Hilar cholangiocarcinoma originates from the biliary epithelium at the hepatic confluence. Radical surgical resection of the tumor offers the only chance for long-term survival, with 5-year survival rates reported between 25% and 40%.[8,9] The median survival of patients with unresectable disease is only 12 to 15 months.[10] Neoadjuvant chemoradiation followed by orthotopic liver transplantation has been employed for the treatment of patients with unresectable, nonmetastatic, perihilar cholangiocarcinoma with encouraging results.[11] Established risk factors for cholangiocarcinoma include parasitic infection of the biliary tract, primary sclerosing cholangitis (PSC), bile duct cysts, hepatolithiasis, and toxins (e.g., Thorotrast).[12]

Duodenal cancer is a rare condition that may occur sporadically, but patients with multiple duodenal adenomas, such as those that occur in familial adenomatous polyposis (FAP) and Gardner syndrome, are at particularly high risk.[13,14]

Ampullary carcinoma is a rare condition with an incidence of 0.49 per 100,000 persons.[15] Biliary obstruction usually develops early in the course of the disease. As a result, tumors are often relatively small, and radical resection is possible in a large proportion of cases with an overall 5-year survival rate of 50%.[16]

CLINICAL FEATURES

The most common presenting symptoms of pancreaticobiliary malignancies are painless jaundice, anorexia, and weight loss. If pain occurs, it is most often located in the epigastric region or right upper quadrant and may radiate to the back. Back pain usually indicates retroperitoneal tumor infiltration and unresectability. Other symptoms related to obstructive jaundice include dark urine, pale stools, and pruritus. At the time of presentation, approximately 80% of patients with pancreatic cancer have impaired glucose tolerance or diabetes mellitus. Carcinoma of the body and tail of the pancreas manifests with similar features, although jaundice is usually absent or develops very late in the course of the disease.

PATHOLOGY

Approximately 90% of pancreaticobiliary malignancies are ductal adenocarcinomas (Fig. 63.1). Most tumors arise from the pancreatic head. Other exocrine malignancies are mucinous cystic adenocarcinoma and acinar cell carcinomas. Endocrine tumors include gastrinoma and insulinoma. Metastases of a primary tumor (mammary, lung, and melanoma) and lymphoma are rare but must be considered because of important treatment implications (e.g., chemotherapy) that influence prognosis. Mesenchymal tumors are extremely rare.

The definitive diagnosis of malignancy is dependent on acquiring a tissue diagnosis. Currently, with various means of tissue acquisition that all have proven to be safe procedures, it is advisable to always attempt to obtain a tissue diagnosis for diagnostic confirmation regardless of management consequences. Evidently it is a prerequisite when (neo)adjuvant or palliative chemo(radio) therapy is considered. If an ERCP is indicated for biliary drainage, one can attempt to obtain a tissue diagnosis by means of brush cytology, intraductal biopsies, or fluid collection from the bile duct or pancreas or both. Cytologic brushings are easy to obtain. Specificity approaches 100%, but sensitivity is relatively low, ranging from 30% to 45%.[17] The yield of intraductal

forceps biopsies is higher compared to brush cytology and approaches 50% to 60%.[17,18] Sampling of ductal fluid is a simple method that is not widely used, but may offer an additional way of obtaining a tissue diagnosis.[19] Several studies have shown that sensitivity can be increased by combining various techniques of tissue sampling. Endoscopic ultrasound (EUS)–guided fine-needle aspiration (FNA) or biopsy (FNB) has an excellent sensitivity of 85% to 90% and specificity that approaches 100%.[20] Although FNB provides the opportunity to obtain tissue cores with preservation of cellular architecture, thereby potentially increasing sensitivity and accuracy (including a better opportunity for advanced tissue processing, such as immunohistochemical analyses), that verdict is still out. Percutaneous computed tomography (CT)-guided FNA biopsy is another method for confirmation of malignancy, with a reported sensitivity of 60% to 90%. Some have argued that, because of the risk of needle tract seeding, this technique should only be used in cases of unresectable disease.

Single-operator digital cholangioscopy (SOC) and probe-based confocal laser endomicroscopy (pCLE) are recent additions for determining the nature of indeterminate biliary strictures. In a multicenter, observational study, SOC was performed in 44 patients with indeterminate biliary strictures.[21] The sensitivity and specificity of SOC visual impression for diagnosis of malignancy was 90% and 95.8%, respectively. All 44 patients underwent SOC-guided biopsies of which specimens were adequate for histologic evaluation in 43 patients (97.7%). The sensitivity and specificity of SOC-guided biopsies for diagnosis of malignancy was 85% and 100%. In a prospective, international, multicenter study, pCLE was investigated in 112 patients with indeterminate biliary strictures, of which 71 finally proved to be malignant. ERCP and pCLE had an 89% sensitivity, 71% specificity, and 82% accuracy rate for the correct diagnosis of the nature of the biliary stricture.[22]

DIFFERENTIAL DIAGNOSIS

Adequate discrimination between a benign or malignant nature of a pancreatic head lesion is pivotal, as management differs substantially. In the case of the former, surgery may not be indicated and even harmful to the patient. In the latter case, surgery is the treatment of choice, if a lesion proves to be resectable. An enlarged pancreatic head may be caused either by

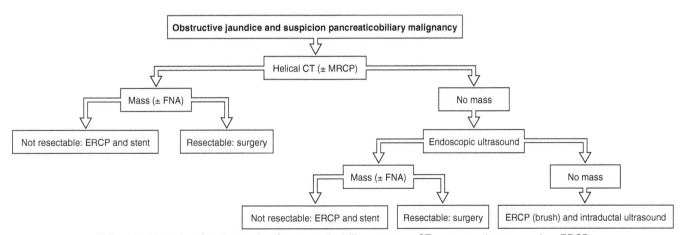

FIG 63.1 Algorithm for diagnosis of pancreaticobiliary cancer. *CT*, computed tomography; *ERCP*, endoscopic retrograde cholangiopancreatography; *FNA*, fine-needle aspiration; *MRCP*, magnetic resonance cholangiopancreatography.

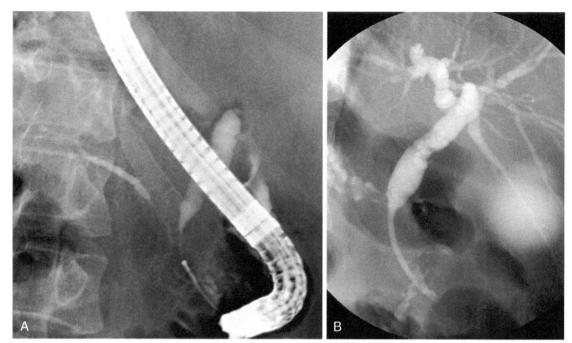

FIG 63.2 A, Stenosis of both the common bile duct and the pancreatic duct, also called a *double-duct sign,* caused by pancreatic adenocarcinoma. **B,** A 10-Fr, 9-cm plastic endoprosthesis inserted through a distal bile duct stricture.

pancreatitis or by carcinoma. Autoimmune pancreatitis is a condition that is increasingly recognized and may mimic a malignant tumor. Differential diagnosis is based on a distinct clinical picture with a diffusely enlarged pancreas with a non-dilated pancreatic duct, elevated IgG4 levels, and a prompt response to corticosteroid therapy with improvement of clinical symptoms, including jaundice, and resolution of morphologic abnormalities on cross-sectional imaging.[23]

Paraduodenal pancreatitis, also known as groove pancreatitis, may also mimic pancreatic adenocarcinoma.[24] This condition is associated with chronic pancreatitis, male gender, and alcohol abuse.[25] Cross-sectional imaging typically demonstrates an enhancing mass in the paraduodenal space, with medial duodenal wall thickening and multiple cysts.[26]

Cystic lesions of the pancreas may be benign (pancreatic pseudocyst or serous cystadenoma), premalignant (intrapancreatic mucinous neoplasm [IPMN] mucinous cystadenoma), or malignant (cystadenocarcinoma, malignant degenerated IPMN). Radiologic imaging is used to characterize these lesions, although differential diagnosis, as well as assessing the degree of neoplastic progression, is notoriously difficult and challenging. EUS in combination with FNA, fluid analysis, intracystic biopsy, and probe-assisted CLE may increase diagnostic accuracy.[27]

Whenever there is a suspicious stricture in the mid–bile duct or proximal bile duct, a gallbladder carcinoma should be considered. It is also important to exclude benign causes of strictures, such as Mirizzi's syndrome, primary and secondary sclerosing cholangitis, and postoperative conditions. An algorithm for the diagnosis of pancreaticobiliary cancer is presented in Fig. 63.2.

ENDOSCOPIC STENTING OF MALIGNANT BILIARY OBSTRUCTION

Since the introduction of endoscopic biliary stent therapy in 1980, the management of biliary obstruction due to pancreati-

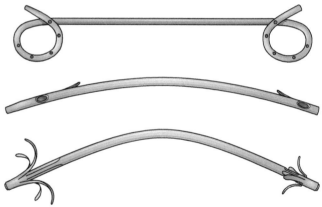

FIG 63.3 Different types of plastic endoprosthesis *(from top downward)*: double-pigtail stent, Amsterdam-type stent (one side hole and one side flap at each end), and Tannenbaum-type stent (without side holes and multiple side flaps at each end).

cobiliary malignancies has changed considerably. Nowadays, endoscopic stent placement is the preferred treatment to relieve jaundice (Fig. 63.3). Compared with percutaneous and surgical drainage, endoscopic biliary stent therapy is associated with lower morbidity and mortality rates.[28,29] A potential complication of endoscopic biliary drainage is late stent occlusion causing recurrent jaundice, or cholangitis, which necessitates stent exchange. The technical success rate of endoscopic biliary drainage is between 70% to 90% and is higher for distal tumors compared with proximal malignancies involving the bifurcation. The complication rate of therapeutic ERCP is 5% to 10%.[30]

Indications and Contraindications

Nowadays ERCP is almost exclusively a therapeutic procedure. Magnetic resonance imaging (MRI) and EUS have largely replaced it for diagnostic purposes. Clinical symptoms that prompt biliary drainage via ERCP include jaundice, fever, and pruritus. Biliary stent placement has been shown to improve symptoms of anorexia and quality of life.[31,32] It has also been suggested that preoperative biliary drainage may improve surgical outcome after pancreaticoduodenectomy, but this has not been substantiated in clinical trials.[33–35] In a randomized study comprising 202 patients with pancreatic head carcinoma comparing direct surgery with delayed surgery after biliary drainage, surgical outcome and complication rates were not affected by preoperative stent placement.[36] The overall complication rate in the delayed surgery group with preoperative stent placement was significantly increased, mainly owing to stent-related complications. The outcome of this study strongly argues against standard preoperative drainage in patients with pancreatic head cancer in whom immediate surgery is planned. Preoperative drainage is indicated, however, when operative resection is not imminent; for example, because serum bilirubin exceeds 14 mg/dL, or when patients need to undergo neoadjuvant chemotherapy. In such cases, biliary drainage should be accomplished by inserting a metal biliary stent, as stent-related complications (occlusion and exchange) are significantly lower (6% versus 31%) compared to plastic stenting.[37]

There are few absolute contraindications to perform ERCP. Coagulation disorders are a relative contraindication and should be corrected before ERCP.

Plastic Stents

The median patency of a conventional 10-Fr plastic stent is 3 to 6 months. The incidence of stent occlusion is 20% to 50%.[38–40] The initial event in stent blockage is adherence of proteins and bacteria to the inner wall of the stent and subsequent formation of a biofilm. Bacteria are introduced into the biliary system during transpapillary placement of the stent. Sludge forms from the accumulation of bacteria, which produce β-glucuronidase and form calcium bilirubinate and calcium palmitate.[40] Many efforts have been made to prolong stent patency, some of which are discussed in the following paragraphs.

Stent Diameter

The first biliary stents that were placed were only 7-Fr or 8-Fr in diameter because of limitations of the diameter of the working channel of the endoscope (2.8 mm). When side-viewing endoscopes with large-diameter working channels (4.2 mm) were introduced in 1980, it became possible to insert large-bore plastic stents. Larger stents (10-Fr) perform better than smaller stents (7- or 8-Fr) because of the higher flow rate, as predicted by Poiseuille's law, and because there is less stasis with larger diameter stents.[41] Theoretically, bile flow rate is proportional to the internal diameter raised to the fourth power; even a small increase in diameter results in a substantial increase in flow capacity. Contrary to this hypothesis, the use of even larger diameter plastic stents of 11.5-Fr or 12-Fr did not result in further improvements in stent patency.[42–44]

Stent Design

The first biliary stents had a pigtail configuration at the proximal end to provide better anchorage. Straight stents were developed because of their improved bile flow characteristics compared with pigtail stents (Fig. 63.4).[45–47] Huibregtse and Tytgat developed the Amsterdam-type stent—a straight design with two side holes to facilitate biliary drainage and two side flaps to prevent dislocation—which has been the standard type of stent since 1980.[48] Sludge in plastic stents mainly accumulates around side holes.[39,49] This accumulation seems to be the result of higher intraluminal flow turbulence and decreased flow rates.[45] Soehendra and others postulated that elimination of side holes might improve patency rates and designed the so-called Teflon Tannenbaum stent (a straight stent without side holes and with multiple

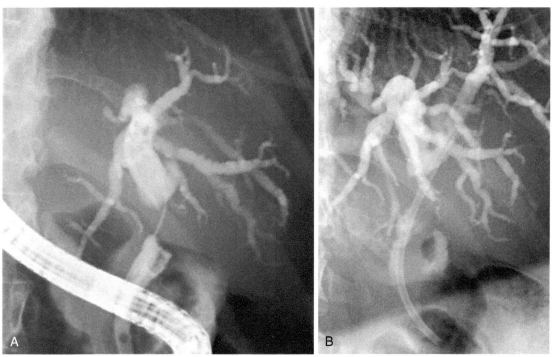

FIG 63.4 **A,** Mid–common bile duct stricture caused by gallbladder carcinoma. **B,** An 11-cm, 10-Fr plastic endoprosthesis has been inserted.

proximal and distal side flaps to prevent dislocation).[50,51] At first, uncontrolled results were encouraging, with patency rates comparable to metal stents, but randomized trials could not confirm these initial results.[52–54] Omitting side holes in a standard-design polyethylene stent also did not improve stent patency.[55]

Stent Material and Coating

Different materials have been used for stent construction, including polyethylene, polyurethane, and polytef (Teflon). In vitro studies have shown a direct relationship between the coefficient of friction and the amount of encrusted material. Teflon has the lowest friction coefficient and the best potential for preventing stent clogging. Initially, Teflon Tannenbaum stents showed a favorable patency rate.[50,51] A randomized study comparing Amsterdam-type stents made from polyethylene versus Teflon did not show a difference in stent patency.[56] Other controlled clinical trials also could not confirm the superiority of Teflon material in a Tannenbaum-design stent.[52–54] Scanning electron microscopy of out-of-package biliary stents has shown that the inner surface smoothness of plastic stents is highly variable. This variability is possibly a result of the manufacturing process of plastic stents by extrusion. Only the polyurethane stent was found to have an extremely smooth surface.[57] Two new polymers were introduced with an ultra-smooth surface, Vivathane and Hydromer. Both materials have been shown to reduce bacterial adherence in vitro. In addition, the Hydromer stent not only has a smooth texture but also a coating that absorbs water and provides a hydrophilic sheath. Because bacteria initially attach by hydrophobic interactions, this coating could potentially lower bacterial adhesion and increase stent patency. However, the encouraging results of in vitro studies could not be confirmed in prospective clinical trials.[58,59]

Priming the inner surface of a stent with a coating that comprises some form of antiadhesive property may reduce biofilm formation and stent clogging. Antibiotics, antithrombotics, silver, and hydrophilic coating all were effective in reducing bacterial colonization in vitro.[60–62] However, clinical studies using antibiotic-coated or hydrophilic-coated stents did not show any benefit.

Supra- Versus Transpapillary Plastic Stent Placement

Placing a plastic stent entirely within the common bile duct has the theoretical advantage of preserving the barrier function of the sphincter of Oddi; this prevents duodenal reflux of food and bacteria into the stent and biliary tree. This so-called inside stent approach can be performed only when a free margin of 1 to 2 cm is maintained between the distal end of the stricture and the papilla. With this parameter in mind, approximately one-third of patients with malignant obstructive jaundice are potential candidates for such treatment.[63] However, for plastic stents no difference was found in stent performance in a randomized trial. In the inside stent group, stent migration occurred significantly more often.[64]

Oral Antibiotics

Bacteria can enter the bile duct through the portal circulation, but more easily directly from the duodenum. When an endoprosthesis is placed, the barrier function of the sphincter of Oddi is lost, and bacteria enter the biliary tract freely. Sludge may form because these bacteria produce β-glucuronidase and form calcium bilirubinate and calcium palmitate. To prolong stent patency, prophylactic treatment with antibiotics seemed a logical step. In vitro studies showed that antibiotic treatment reduced

bacterial adherence to plastic stents.[65] In a prospective randomized study with ciprofloxacin, no difference in stent patency was found.[66] In another study, rotating antibiotics (cycles of 2 weeks of ampicillin, metronidazole, and ciprofloxacin) were combined with ursodeoxycholic acid, and no difference in stent patency was shown.[67] Only one small pilot study showed a reduced rate of stent blockage with norfloxacin plus ursodeoxycholic acid.[68] Other studies combining antibiotics and bile salts (ofloxacin and ursodeoxycholic acid, ciprofloxacin, and rowachol) did not show a longer duration of stent patency.[69,70] There is no compelling evidence that stent patency benefits from antibiotic prophylaxis.

Bile Salts

Bile salts have a potent antibacterial effect and may stimulate bile flow. Because bacteria attach by hydrophobic interactions, hydrophobic bile salts (deoxycholate, taurodeoxycholate) inhibit initial bacterial attachment, as was shown in experimental studies.[71] However, hydrophobic bile salts are not well tolerated. Hydrophilic bile salts such as ursodeoxycholate, which are better tolerated, have a minimal effect on bacterial adhesion. Except for one small pilot study, different prospective clinical studies using ursodeoxycholic acid alone or combining ursodeoxycholic acid with antibiotics could not show an improvement in stent patency.[67–70]

Aspirin

Animal studies in prairie dogs showed that aspirin inhibits mucous glycoprotein secretion by blocking prostaglandin synthesis.[72] In a clinical study, the use of aspirin reduced the content of all sludge components, although no effect was shown on stent patency.[73] No further studies using aspirin to prevent early stent clogging have been performed.

Elective Stent Exchange

Some endoscopists prefer to schedule patients for elective stent exchanges, usually every 3 to 4 months. The optimal time interval however, is unknown.[74,75] Prophylactic stent exchanges require multiple elective endoscopies over time. The risk and burden of such policy must be weighed against a policy of watchful waiting with a risk of (severe) cholangitis developing. Because many patients do not experience stent occlusion before dying of the underlying disease, some endoscopists favor an expectant management strategy.

Self-Expanding Metal Stents

The diameter of biliary stents was restricted by the size of the instrumentation channel of the endoscope until the development of self-expanding metal stents (SEMSs). All currently available expandable stents are made of metal. They differ in the way they are braided, the size of the mesh, the metal used, and their rigidity. One of the first available metal stents was the self-expanding Wallstent (Boston Scientific, Marlborough, MA). This stent is delivered in a collapsed configuration on an 8-Fr delivery system. When deployed, it expands to a final diameter of 30 Fr (approximately 10 mm) and foreshortens approximately 30% in length. The final diameter is achieved after 2 days to 1 week, when equilibrium is achieved between the dilating force of the stent and the resistance of the bile duct wall and tumor. These large-caliber SEMSs of 30 Fr remain patent for longer than plastic stents but do not prevent blockage indefinitely. Metal stents with a 6-mm diameter occlude significantly more frequently than 10-mm (30-Fr) metal stents, again showing that size is the most

TABLE 63.1 Results of Randomized-Controlled Trials Comparing Self-Expandable Stents With Plastic Stents

Reference	NO. PATIENTS		DRAINAGE (%)		OCCLUSION RATE (%)		MEDIAN STENT PATENCY (DAYS)	
	PE	SEMS	PE	SEMS	PE	SEMS	PE	SEMS
Davids et al[77]	49	56	95	96	54	33	126	273
Carr-Locke et al[79]	78	86	95	98	13	13	62	111
Knyrim et al[78]	31	31	100	100	43	22	140*	189*

*Mean.
PE, polyethylene stent; *SEMS,* self-expanding metal stent.

important determining factor for stent patency.[76] Because of their design, SEMSs have much less surface to which bacteria can adhere. The mechanism of stent blockage differs from that seen in plastic stents and includes tumor ingrowth through the interstices of the stent or overgrowth of the end of the stent and intima hyperplasia. Several studies have shown a median stent patency of approximately 6 to 9 months of uncovered metal stents (Table 63.1).[75,77–79]

Various types of SEMSs are available to date. The wire construction is made of Nitinol or platinol-cored Nitinol Platinol (Boston Sci, Natick, MA). Stents are available in uncovered, partially covered, and fully covered versions. The covering is intended to resist tumor ingrowth. Partially covered stents have noncovered parts at both stent ends. It was thought that the covering would reduce stent obstruction while fixation of the proximal stent end due to intimal hyperplasia would prevent stent migration. This, however, was not substantiated in a 2015 trial.[80] Nowadays, depending on the manufacturer, metallic expandable stents are available in 3 diameters (6, 8, and 10 mm) and various stent lengths ranging from 40 up to 120 mm. Most expandable metal stents foreshorten, and this should be taken into account when they are deployed. Stents with a slotted tube design like the Zilver biliary self-expandable stent (Wilson-Cook Medical, Winston-Salem, NC) have a particular advantage in that they do not foreshorten on expansion. Specially designed metal uncovered stents with a Y-type and T-type design are available for the treatment of hilar obstruction (see later section on Intrahepatic Biliary Obstruction).

Covered Metal Stents

Tissue ingrowth through the mesh of the stent is responsible for stent occlusion in approximately 22% to 33% of patients.[77,78] To overcome this problem, SEMSs have been covered with a polyurethane or silicone membrane. At first, many prospective cohort studies could not confirm a lower rate of tumor ingrowth while using covered metal stents.[81,82] However, in a prospective comparative study, stent obstruction owing to tumor ingrowth occurred significantly less frequently with covered stents compared with uncovered stents.[83] Data with regard to the risk of complications are limited, but stent migration, cholecystitis, and pancreatitis seem to occur at a slightly higher rate.[82–84] There seems to be no benefit from endoscopic papillotomy before deployment of covered metal stents with regard to the prevention of pancreatitis, whereas migration rates may increase.[85] Covered stents should not be used intrahepatically because of occlusion of hepatic side branches by the covering membrane. Taking into consideration the previously mentioned points, many endoscopists have more often used fully covered SEMS as the first-line stent to palliate malignant obstruction.

Supra- Versus Transpapillary Metal Stent Placement

No studies have compared endoscopic supra- versus transpapillary metal stent placement without a preceding sphincterotomy to reduce metal stent clogging. After percutaneous transhepatic SEMS placement, however, stent occlusions by tumor growth was more frequently observed after suprapapillary stent placement ($p = 0.007$), whereas stent occlusion by sludge incrustation was more frequently found after transpapillary stent placement.[86] Overall there was no significant difference in cumulative stent patency ($p = 0.401$). For more proximal strictures, our routine practice is to place metal stents not crossing the papilla (after sphincterotomy), ensuring that the distal stent ends aligns horizontally with the duct for easy recannulation in case of obstruction. However there is no evidence to preferentially support either approach (having stent(s) cross the papilla after sphincterotomy or not).

Plastic Versus Metal Stent

SEMSs have a longer duration of patency than plastic stents and ideally should be placed in all patients. The high initial costs have limited their use in different health care settings worldwide. In a cost-effective approach, the choice between a plastic and metal stent depends mainly on an estimate of patient survival. Tumor size seems to be a reliable predictor of survival. Prat et al (1998) claimed that in the case of a tumor greater than 30 mm, a polyethylene stent should be placed because of shorter expected survival.[87] The presence and number of liver metastases have also been shown to be independently related to prognosis.[88,89] Comparative studies did not show any benefit of SEMSs compared with polyethylene stents in the first 3 months after insertion.[75,77] Therefore, it seems reasonable to insert a polyethylene stent in patients with a life expectancy of less than 3 months (Fig. 63.5). If expected survival is 3 to 6 months, a SEMS should be considered (Fig. 63.6), as various authors have shown this strategy to be cost-effective.[77,90–93] Patients scheduled to undergo neoadjuvant chemo(radio) therapy in preparation of a surgical resection are immunocompromised and at particular risk of severe cholangitis and cholangiosepsis due to stent clogging. In these patients, a metal expandable stent should be inserted to minimize this risk.[37]

Technique of Biliary Stent Placement

A large-channel (4.2-mm) side-viewing therapeutic endoscope is introduced into the second portion of the duodenum. Standard cannulation of the papilla of Vater is performed by a ball-tip, cone-tip catheter or sphincterotome with or without a guidewire. Use of the latter device may aid in achieving an optimal angle for bile duct cannulation. If a sphincterotome is unsuccessful, a precut sphincterotomy is performed to obtain biliary access.

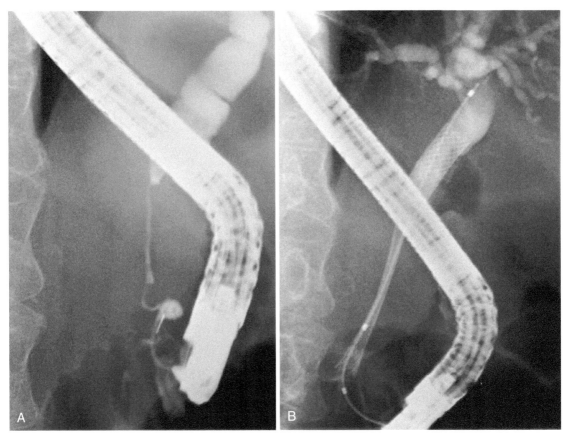

FIG 63.5 **A,** Distal common bile duct stricture caused by pancreatic adenocarcinoma. **B,** Self-expanding metal stent has been inserted.

With the use of all these different techniques, deep cannulation is achieved in up to 95% of patients. After the bile duct is selectively cannulated, a contrast agent is injected. It is important to define the exact anatomy, location, and nature of the stenosis. To avoid postprocedural cholangitis in patients with complex hilar strictures, contrast filling of segments that are not to be drained should be avoided as much as possible. A guidewire is used to pass strictures and to facilitate introduction of devices. Various guidewires are available with different flexibility, diameter, and tip shape. On the one hand, rigid guidewires facilitate the introduction of devices (e.g., an intraductal ultrasound probe) and small-diameter stents. On the other hand, very slippery guidewires with a hydropolymer coating are used to pass asymmetric strictures. After the guidewire is passed through the stricture, a catheter can be advanced, and selective contrast filling can be achieved. If only one biliary stent is inserted, a sphincterotomy is not routinely required.

Plastic Stents

Preferably, a guiding catheter is introduced over the guidewire through the stricture to ensure a more rigid introductory system to facilitate stent placement. This can be achieved by the conventional method using a long wire and a standard guiding catheter, as well as with the so-called short wire exchange technique in which the guidewire follows the devices only at its distal tip, making it possible to use a short guidewire which, during device manipulation, can be safely locked at the scope handle using a locking device. The endoprosthesis is positioned over the guiding catheter and inserted into the instrumentation channel. With a pusher tube, the stent is advanced farther toward the tip of the endoscope with the elevator bridge closed. When the prosthesis has reached the distal end of the instrumentation channel, the elevator bridge is opened, and the stent is pushed out of the endoscope under endoscopic and fluoroscopic control. During advancement of the stent, it is important to keep the endoscope tip close to the papilla. The stent should be pushed out the scope and into the common bile duct one step at a time to avoid looping and dislocation into the duodenal lumen. After the stent has been pushed out a little, the elevator bridge is closed, which raises and fixates the stent. The tip of the endoscope is moved closer to the papilla using the up-and-down knob, thus pushing the stent into the common bile duct. These steps are repeated until the distal side flap has reached the papilla. Finally, the assistant pulls out the guiding catheter and guidewire while the endoscopist keeps the endoprosthesis in position with the pusher tube. In most distal common bile duct and mid–common bile duct strictures, it is usually possible to insert a 10-Fr endoprosthesis without prior dilation. In proximal strictures, however, the stricture may need to be dilated to allow stent passage; this can be achieved with the use of dilating catheters that are introduced over a rigid guidewire or, more easily, with a dilation balloon. If it is still impossible to insert a 10-Fr stent, a smaller-caliber prosthesis (7-Fr) should be inserted that can be exchanged for a 10-Fr prosthesis at a later stage. When both right and left liver lobes have to be drained, it is usually more convenient to drain the left side first, followed by the right side, which is typically straighter and thus presents less challenge to stent insertion.

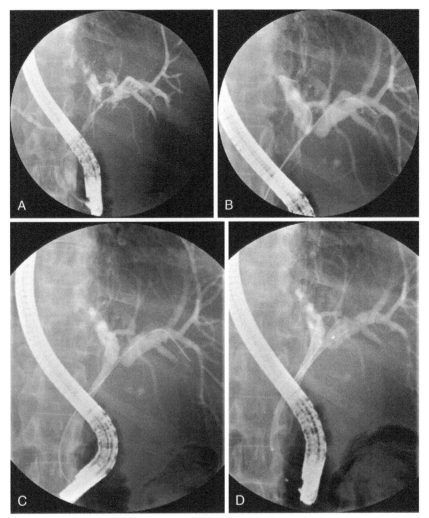

FIG 63.6 A, Klatskin type II tumor (unresectable because of vascular involvement). **B,** Guidewires inserted to both the left and the right biliary system. **C,** Self-expanding metal stent has been inserted into the left system and deployed. **D,** Bilateral self-expanding metal stent drainage.

The required length of the endoprosthesis can be determined by checking the predefined markers on the guidewire or by using the guidewire as a ruler. For this, the proximal tip of the guidewire is positioned under fluoroscopic control at the level at which the proximal tip of the endoprosthesis is intended. The guidewire is then fixed between index finger and thumb at the level where it exits the working channel. Subsequently, under fluoroscopic control, the guidewire is withdrawn from the catheter until the proximal tip reaches the duodenum. When using a short wire system, the distance between finger and thumb and the exit hole of the working channel is the required length of the endoprosthesis. When using a long wire system, the technician can obtain the same measurement at the end of the catheter. Biliary plastic stents are available in various diameters (range 5-Fr to 12-Fr) and lengths (range 5 to 20 cm).

Management of plastic stent occlusion. A clogged plastic stent can be removed with the use of a snare or basket. When a snare is used, the stent is caught in the snare and removed either by pulling out the scope or by pulling the stent through the instrumentation channel of the endoscope. When a basket is used, the stent is pulled close to the endoscope and, while the catheter of the basket is kept fixed at the scope handle, both the endoscope

and the stent are withdrawn. When massive tumor invasion is present in the duodenum, and difficult stent exchange is anticipated because of a nonoptimal scope position, it can be helpful to leave the occluded stent in place and use it as a guide for common bile duct cannulation and introduction of a second stent. Soehendra et al (1990) described a technique that enables the removal of a clogged stent while maintaining the original pathway into the bile duct.[94] A ball-tip catheter is positioned at the distal end of the stent, after which the stent is cannulated with the guidewire. A Soehendra retriever is introduced over the guidewire, and its tip is screwed into the distal end of the stent. The retriever is pulled out the scope along with the stent, leaving the guidewire in place to facilitate the placement of a new stent.

Self-Expanding Metal Stents (Video 63.1)

For introduction of a SEMS, a stiff guidewire is positioned through the stricture using standard techniques. The insertion device containing the constrained metal stent is inserted through the instrumentation channel over the guidewire. When the insertion device has been properly positioned across the stricture with the help of the radiopaque markers, the prosthesis can be released by removing the outer catheter while keeping the inner catheter in place. Deployment occurs gradually as the outer catheter is withdrawn and can be followed fluoroscopically. If deployment is not proceeding according to plan and repositioning is required, the stent may be constrained again by pushing the outer catheter inward, provided that the point of no return has not yet been passed. This point may vary with stent type but may extend up to 83% of total stent deployment and is indicated by a fluoroscopic marker and a marker on the handle of the insertion device. Deployment reduces the length of certain SEMSs up to approximately 30%. It is therefore important to constantly adjust the position of the expanding stent under fluoroscopic or endoscopic control, meaning that the endoscopist has to pull on the insertion device while deploying the stent. When the expanding metal stent needs to bridge the ampulla, for example in the case of a distal common bile duct stricture, the endoscopic image is used to keep a fixed distance of approximately 1 cm between the papillary orifice and the distal margin of the stent. The distal end of the stent can be checked either fluoroscopically (represented by the most distal radiopaque distal marker) or endoscopically (represented by a color indicator on the insertion catheter). Stent diameter ranges from 6 to 10 mm, and stent lengths are available from 40 mm to 120 mm.

There are two techniques for inserting dual metal stents in the intrahepatic biliary tree. The conventional technique consists of inserting stents side-by-side (SBS technique; Fig. 63.7).[95] The potential limitation of the SBS technique is failure to advance the second metal stent alongside the first metal stent that is already expanded. A 6-Fr delivery system made possible simultaneous introduction and positioning of two insertion devices with subsequent simultaneous deployment of metal stents in 85% to 100% of patients. Another technique is referred to as the "stent-in-stent" (SIS) technique. This technique makes use of a specially designed "Y" stent consisting of two uncovered Niti-S Y-type biliary stents (TaeWoong Medical Co. Ltd., Goyang, South Korea). The first SEMS has a radiologically marked segment with wider mesh holes in its middle part, through which the second stent is advanced into the contralateral liver lobe.[96] A more challenging approach for introducing a second stent through the wire mesh of a conventional metal stent using balloon dilation has also been described.[97] The slim 6-Fr delivery system seems particularly suited to pass the dilated metal mesh.[98,99] There are only retrospective reports comparing SBS and SIS techniques for the management of intrahepatic malignant obstruction. In one study, no

differences in stent patency or adverse event rates were observed.[100] In another study a higher adverse event rate (44% vs. 13%) but longer stent patency were reported in the SBS group (469 vs. 181 days, respectively).[101]

To facilitate reintervention in case of stent obstruction, it is important to either ensure that the ends of both metal stents cross the ampulla or to confirm that when located within the common bile duct, both distal metal stent ends are positioned at the same level.

Management of self-expanding metal stent occlusion. Covered metal stents can be removed by grasping the distal stent end with a snare or with a forceps in case a retrieval loop is present. An uncovered SEMS can only be removed early after its deployment. These stents quickly become embedded due to tumor ingrowth and formation of hyperplastic tissue through the stent mesh after which stent extraction becomes extremely difficult or impossible. Mechanical cleaning using a balloon and water flushing is effective only in cases of sludge formation. Placement of a polyethylene stent or a second SEMS through the occluded SEMS may resolve the obstruction but may not provide optimal drainage because the new stent may not expand to its intended size, leaving the patient at higher risk for reobstruction. A novel technique for removal of metal stents entails the so-called SIS technique.[102,103] With this technique, a fully covered stent is deployed through the obstructed stent (either an uncovered or a partially covered stent), making sure that both stent ends are covered. Tissue that has grown through the interstices or over the stent ends is entrapped by the newly placed fully covered stent and becomes necrotic. Two to four weeks after placement of the fully covered stent in the obstructed stent, it is pulled out, after which the original stent can usually be removed without much difficulty. This strategy proves particularly useful when an uncovered metal stent is inadvertently placed into an apparently malignant biliary stricture that ultimately proves to be benign.

Intrahepatic Biliary Obstruction

Strictures at the level of the hepatic confluence account for approximately 20% of malignant bile duct obstructions and mainly involve primary cholangiocarcinoma, gallbladder neoplasms, and metastatic spread to hilar nodes. Cholangiocarcinomas arising at the hilar level are also referred to as *Klatskin tumors* and are classified according to the degree of involvement of the intrahepatic bile ducts (Fig. 63.8).[104] Stent placement in case of a proximal stricture in the biliary tree is more challenging and

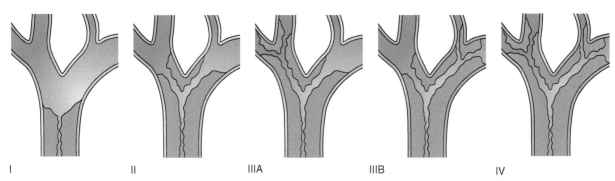

FIG 63.7 Bismuth classification. *I:* Stricture involving the common hepatic duct. *II:* Stricture involving both the right and the left hepatic duct. *IIIA:* Stricture extending proximally to the right secondary intrahepatic ducts. *IIIB:* Stricture extending proximally to the left secondary intrahepatic ducts. *IV:* Stricture involving secondary intrahepatic ducts bilaterally.

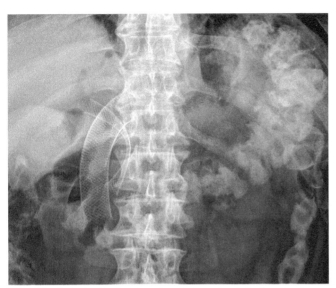

FIG 63.8 Pancreatic adenocarcinoma growing into the duodenum with a self-expanding metal stent (not yet fully deployed) in the biliary tract and a self-expanding metal stent in the duodenum.

associated with lower success rates than stent placement for distal common bile duct stenosis. Drainage can be achieved either endoscopically (retrograde) or percutaneously (antegrade). Procedure-induced cholangitis caused by contrast agent injection into undrained biliary branches is the main complication and occurs in 30% of cases.[105–107] The current management strategy (depending on local services available) is first to attempt endoscopic drainage. When this is unsuccessful, percutaneous drainage is attempted.[108–110] When internal drainage fails, an external drain can be left in situ, thus minimizing the risk of cholangitis. Based on consensus statements, some societies have suggested that the percutaneous route is the preferred option to drain patients with a Bismuth III and IV hilar strictures. As long as scientific data are not available, local expertise should guide individual patient management.[111]

Unilateral versus bilateral drainage. There is controversy regarding whether to drain one or both liver lobes in patients with a proximal cholangiocarcinoma (Klatskin tumor) with a Bismuth type II, III, and IV stricture. In Bismuth type I, one stent suffices because the left and right ducts communicate. An early study suggested that at least 25% of the liver volume should be drained to achieve biochemical improvement and relief of symptoms.[112] More recently, it has been suggested that drainage of more than 50% of liver volume of patients with malignant hilar strictures is predictive for lower cholangitis and higher survival rates.[110,113] Drainage of a dilated duct of an atrophic hepatic segment does not contribute to relief of jaundice and therefore should only be attempted in case of segmental cholangitis.

For patients with Bismuth III and IV strictures, this concept has important implications, as drainage of either the right or left lobe is usually not enough to achieve this goal. What seems undisputed based on the literature is that the worst treatment results are achieved in patients with cholangiographic opacification of both lobes, but drainage of only one.[114] Obviously, such practice promotes bacterial contamination with ensuing cholangitis in the undrained lobe. Indeed, in a prospective randomized trial comparing unilateral with bilateral hepatic duct drainage,

the latter procedure was associated with a significantly higher rate of complications because of early cholangitis.[115] Magnetic resonance cholangiopancreatography (MRCP)–guided endoscopic stent placement in Bismuth III and IV malignancies has been shown to be associated with lower morbidity and mortality rates in an uncontrolled study.[116] The intention was to place a unilateral stent in one lobe guided by MRCP findings, and to avoid guidewire entry and contrast agent injection in the contralateral lobe. In patients in whom, by accident, guidewire entry (50%) or contrast agent injection (20%) occurred in the contralateral liver lobe, stents were placed bilaterally. This treatment strategy resulted in a very low cholangitis rate of only 6%. In a 2003 study in which selective unilateral MRCP-targeted or CT-targeted drainage was evaluated, no episodes of cholangitis were observed.[117]

The message seems to emerge that unilateral drainage is appropriate when unilateral cannulation and opacification has been achieved. If the contralateral lobe is (unintentionally) opacified or probed, it should also be drained to avoid cholangitis. On the other hand, a 2015 meta-analysis suggests that bilateral stenting for malignant hilar strictures is not recommended because it does not reduce obstruction or 30-day mortality rates. A point of criticism is that most studies pooled in this meta-analysis included patients with Bismuth I hilar strictures for whom bilateral stents are not useful.[118]

It seems that clinical decision-making and future studies should focus on the following three factors: (1) Complete versus incomplete drainage based on MRCP findings with the aim to drain at least 50% of liver parenchyma; (2) Drainage of all endoscopically manipulated liver segments during ERCP (unintentional contrast injection, guidewire entry or cannulation); and (3) Avoiding drainage of massively dilated but atrophic intrahepatic segments.

Plastic versus self-expanding metal stents in hilar malignant strictures. By design, expandable stents may be more suitable than plastic stents for draining hilar tumors. The stent lumen is much wider, and, more importantly, intrahepatic side branches can drain through the metal mesh. SEMSs that were inserted via the percutaneous route showed a higher rate of treatment efficacy than plastic stents.[108,119] No randomized studies comparing endoscopic and percutaneous insertion of SEMSs in hilar strictures are available. Additional proof of the superiority of SEMSs over plastic stents is suggested by a retrospective series of patients with unresectable hilar cholangiocarcinoma in whom plastic stents were replaced by metal expandable stents during stent treatment.[120] Successful palliation without the need for further biliary reintervention was achieved in most patients (69%). In a prospective multicenter observational cohort study in patients with a malignant hilar biliary obstruction, metal stents were superior to plastic stent in terms of short-term outcomes (30 days), independent of disease severity, Bismuth class, or drainage quality.[121] A 2015 meta-analysis on the use of plastic versus metal stents for hilar strictures showed that for the latter, 30-day and long-term occlusion rates were lower with no impact on survival.[118]

Antibiotics before stent placement to avoid postprocedure cholangitis. The mainstay of therapy for patients presenting with a biliary obstruction caused by a malignancy with or without cholangitis is endoscopic drainage. There is controversy about the routine use of preprocedure antibiotic prophylaxis.[122–124] Preoperative administration of antibiotics should definitely be started in a patient with fever. Because failure to drain the entire biliary tree is the most important risk factor associated with occurrence of cholangitis after ERCP, in particular when contrast has been injected into segments that cannot be drained, antibiotic prophylaxis should also be administered in patients in whom incomplete drainage is anticipated, such as patients with a hilar malignancy or patients with PSC.[125,126] Prophylaxis can be commenced by a single intravenous dose shortly before the procedure and is usually continued orally for 3 to 5 days.

Gram-negative bacteria are consistently the most common organisms in bile (*Escherichia coli* and to a lesser extent *Klebsiella* species and gram-positive *Enterococcus* species). Antibiotics in these cases should be bactericidal and aimed at gram-negative bacteria with good penetration in liver tissue and bile. Ciprofloxacin is currently the first choice of antibiotic in our unit, with the caveat that it does not cover *enterococci*. In cases of fever despite ciprofloxacin, the addition of amoxicillin or a switch to piperacillin/tazobactam is advisable.

Duodenal Stenosis

Duodenal stenosis resulting from pancreaticobiliary malignancies occurs in 10% to 20% of patients.[127] Symptoms include nausea and vomiting resulting from gastric outlet obstruction. Duodenal stenosis is usually a late event in patients in poor general condition who have already undergone biliary drainage. Surgical bypass has a significant procedure-related mortality of 10% and related morbidity and prolonged hospital stay.[29,128,129] Placement of a duodenal stent has a high technical success rate without major procedure-related complications.[130–132] In a systematic review comprising 1281 patients from 19 studies early (< 30 days) and late (> 30 days), perforations occur in 0.7% and in 0.5% of patients, respectively.[133] Massive bleeding requiring urgent intervention was observed in 0.8% of cases.

Duodenal stent placement is performed under simultaneous endoscopic and fluoroscopic control. Immediately after stent placement patients are usually able to tolerate a liquid diet. Full stent expansion may take a few days, during which time soft foods are allowed. Uncovered duodenal stents seem to be associated with a higher occlusion rate, whereas partially covered duodenal stents seem to have a higher migration rate.[133] A retrospective study in 95 patients suggested that duodenal stent placement is associated with better short-term outcomes, whereas surgical gastrojejunostomy is associated with better long-term outcomes.[134] The choice of treatment modality may depend on the life expectancy of the patient. On the other hand, in patients with longer survival, duodenal stenting may still be considered a valid treatment modality, as endoscopic reintervention for stent dysfunction, albeit common (30%–40% of the cases), is clinically successful in most cases. Some recent small case series (2015–16) have reported promising results of EUS-guided gastrojejunostomy thanks to the advent of lumen apposing metal stents.[135–137]

Similar success rates have been reported for simultaneous endoscopic decompression of biliary and duodenal obstruction compared with duodenal stent placement alone.[138] In the former case, because of the difficulty accessing the biliary tree after duodenal stent placement, an expandable metal biliary stent should be placed first (Fig. 63.9). In case a plastic biliary stent is already in situ, it should be exchanged for a metal expandable stent. In expert hands, it may be feasible to drain the biliary tree endoscopically through the mesh of a metal duodenal stent, but this is a technically challenging procedure.[139] More recently, EUS-guided biliary drainage has been employed in the setting of a failed biliary drainage by means of ERCP in patients with

a duodenal stent in situ. In a small case series, this approach was successful in most of the patients using various strategies, including transmural hepaticogastrostomy or choledochoduodenostomy or even antegrade or "rendez-vous" transpapillary drainage.[140]

If endoscopic treatment of biliary obstruction after duodenal stent placement fails, remaining treatment options include percutaneous stent placement, combined percutaneous and endoscopic management, and surgical bypass.

Postprocedural Care

General measures after conscious sedation include observation in a day care unit for several hours monitoring blood pressure and oxygen saturation. When a patient develops fever after ERCP, blood samples should be obtained for culture, and antibiotics should be administered. If fever does not subside, the accuracy of biliary drainage should be reassessed, and migration and early stent occlusion should be excluded. In the case of a complex malignant hilar stricture, it is important to check for undrained dilated intrahepatic segments and to rule out abscesses by transabdominal ultrasound or CT. Depending on the findings, ERCP should be reattempted or percutaneous drainage performed.

Complications
Early Complications

Early complications are defined as complications that occur less than 1 week after the conclusion of the procedure. The rate of complications is 5% to 10% for therapeutic ERCP with a mortality rate of up to 1%.[30,141,142] Cotton et al (1991) introduced a classification system in which complications are graded as mild, moderate, and severe, and these guidelines are still widely used.[141] The most frequent early complication is cholangitis, probably resulting from introduction of bacteria into the biliary tract during the procedure. Cholangitis is reported in approximately 10% to 15% of patients in most series. It occurs more often after endoscopic procedures for complex hilar strictures when incomplete drainage is achieved. The same holds true for patients with PSC. In these high-risk procedures, antibiotics should be administered prophylactically and continued for a few days after the procedure.

Pancreatitis develops after ERCP in approximately 5% to 7% of patients. It is defined as new-onset or increased abdominal pain lasting at least 24 hours after ERCP, with associated elevation in serum amylase or lipase to at least three times normal, and a minimum of 2 days of hospital admission.[30,141] Most cases are mild and self-limiting, requiring only intravenous fluids and gut rest. Selected cases may evolve into (infected) necrotizing pancreatitis with multi-organ failure.

The rate of postsphincterotomy bleeding is approximately 0.2% to 5%, with an associated mortality rate less than 1%.[143] Bleeding usually occurs immediately after sphincterotomy but can be delayed for hours or several days. In our experience, most episodes of delayed bleeding are managed successfully by conservative measures and blood transfusions. Postsphincterotomy bleeding usually occurs at the apex of the sphincterotomy site and can be managed endoscopically with injection of epinephrine. When clipping or thermal coagulation are used to stop the bleeding, one should be cautious to avoid the pancreatic orifice for obvious reasons. When in doubt, or the site of hemostatic therapy is close to the pancreatic orifice, a protective pancreatic stent should be placed first. In some situations, the apex of the sphincterotomy can be clipped away from the pancreatic orifice with minimal risk of pancreatitis. In such cases, the risk of further

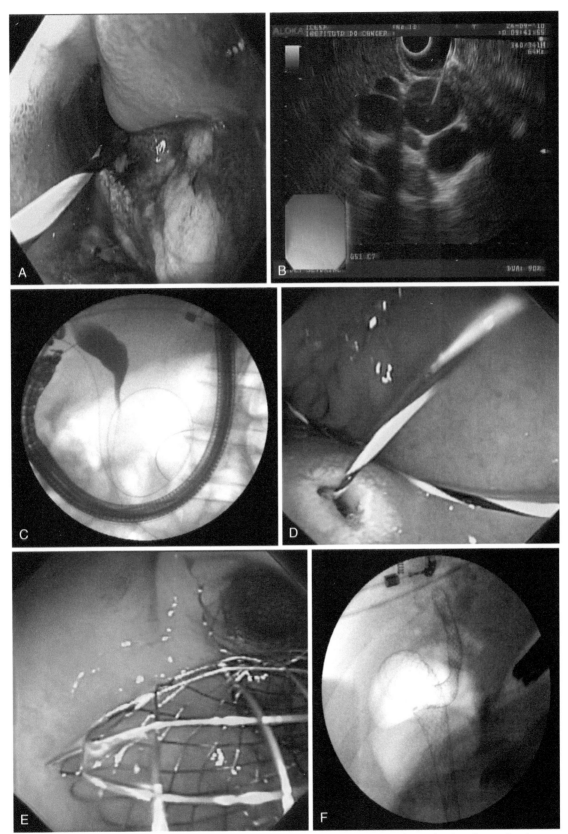

FIG 63.9 EUS-guided choledochoduodenal anastomosis with concomitant duodenal stenting in a patient with a malignant biliary and duodenal stricture due to advanced adenocarcinoma of the pancreas. **A,** Duodenal stenosis caused by advanced pancreatic adenocarcinoma, **B,** EUS-guided puncture of the dilated common bile duct with a 19-gauge needle, **C,** EUS-guided cholangiography revealing a long and tortuous malignant stricture of the distal common bile duct stricture, **D,** bulbo-choledochal fistula created with a cystotome with a guidewire positioned well into the biliary tree, **E,** Endoscopic image of the expanded biliary and duodenal stent, **F,** Radiologic image of the expanded biliary and duodenal stent.

manipulation of the pancreatic duct for prophylactic pancreatic stent insertion may not be justified.

Retroperitoneal perforation occurs in less than 1% of cases.[144] It may be caused by standard sphincterotomy, precut sphincterotomy, or guidewire manipulation. Most cases are diagnosed or suspected during ERCP. These retroperitoneal perforations mostly heal with conservative measures consisting of nil per mouth, intravenous antibiotics, and nasogastric suction. In cases of peritoneal perforation caused by the duodenoscope, prompt exploratory laparotomy, with repair or oversewing of the defect in the duodenal wall, has traditionally been deemed mandatory.[145] Recently, the use of large over-the-scope clips has been reported to successfully close duodenal perforations caused by side viewing endoscopes.[146]

Late Complications

The most common late complication of stent placement is occlusion of the endoprosthesis, which occurs in approximately 50% of cases.[77,78] These patients clinically present with recurrent jaundice, a flulike syndrome with cholestasis or frank cholangitis. Treatment consists of exchange of the occluded stent or, in the case of an occluded uncovered SEMS, of insertion of a polyethylene stent or second SEMS through the obstructed expanding stent. See also the earlier sections on Management of Plastic Stent Occlusion and Management of Self-Expanding Metal Stent Occlusion.

Future Trends
Photodynamic Therapy

Photodynamic therapy (PDT) involves the intravenous administration of a photosensitizer that is activated with a laser light, causing necrosis of the exposed tissue. Preliminary results suggest prolonged survival and stent patency for PDT in cholangiocarcinoma at the hilum.[147–149] There are, however, no prospective randomized controlled studies available. Previously, it was thought that metal stents and PDT were incompatible.[150] However, this does not seem to be a major issue as long as the light dose is adjusted to counteract the reduction of light transmittance caused by the metal.[151] PDT has also been used successfully to recanalize metal stents that were blocked by tumor ingrowth.[152]

Radiofrequency Ablation

Radiofrequency ablation (RFA) is a relatively simple low-cost procedure that is increasingly being studied for local treatment of biliary obstructive malignancies.[153] RFA can be performed via an antegrade route by means of PTC or a retrograde route using ERCP. With the use of a bipolar probe that is mounted on a catheter, coagulative necrosis of the intraductal tumor mass is achieved after which biliary stents are placed; generally plastic when multiple RFA sessions are planned. A retrospective study comparing 16 patients treated with RFA and 32 patients treated with PDT did not show a difference in median survival (9.6 vs. 7.5 months).[154] Some studies have successfully explored the use of RFA to de-obstruct metal expandable stents after they had become clogged with tumorous or hyperplastic tissue ingrowth.[155,156]

Drug-Coated Biliary Stents

Covering biliary stents with a chemotherapeutic agent, thereby delivering the drug directly into the tumor, may provide protection against tumor ingrowth and overgrowth. For an optimal therapeutic effect, these drugs should be released over a longer period with good penetration into the tumorous tissue and without causing systemic toxicity. Carboplatin and paclitaxel have been shown to inhibit cell proliferation in vitro.[157,158] Carboplatin-coated plastic stents have been used with promising preliminary results in a few patients.[158] In a small pilot study, placement of a metal stent covered with a paclitaxel-incorporated membrane in patients with malignant biliary obstruction proved feasible, safe, and effective.[159] Median patency was 270 days (range 68 to 810 days), and cumulative patency rates at 3 months, 6 months, and 12 months were 100%, 71%, and 36%. However, whether drug-eluting stents represent an advancement in the treatment of patients with malignant biliary strictures remains to be proven in prospective comparative trials.

Endoscopic Ultrasound–Guided Biliary Drainage

EUS-guided biliary drainage is being explored as an alternative to ERCP. The successful outcome of EUS-guided drainage of pancreatic pseudocysts and infected pancreatic necrosis, and the development of specially designed fully covered metal lumen apposing stents has accelerated its introduction for this novel indication. EUS-guided biliary drainage encompasses EUS-guided antegrade rendezvous drainage, EUS-guided choledochoduodenostomy, and EUS-guided hepaticogastrostomy.

In a retrospective study including 208 patients from multiple tertiary referral centers, a single session of EUS-guided biliary drainage (EUS-BD) after 1 or more failed ERCP attempts, either EUS-guided choledochoduodenostomy or EUS-guided antegrade rendezvous drainage, was compared to ERCP in patients with a distal common bile duct obstruction requiring placement of a SEMS.[160] SEMS was equally successful after both procedures (93.26% vs. 94.23%, $p = 1.00$). The frequency of adverse events in the ERCP and EUS-BD groups was comparable (8.65%), but postprocedure pancreatitis rates were higher in the ERCP group (4.8% vs 0%, $p = 0.059$).

EUS-guided hepaticogastrostomy has been reported by several groups as an alternative treatment to percutaneous biliary drainage or surgical bypass in the case of failed ERCP, in particular in the case of a bulboduodenal obstruction or a proximal stricture at the level of the hepatic hilum when EUS-guided choledochoduodenostomy is not possible.[161,162] For this, a dilated biliary branch in the left lobe is punctured by a 19-gauge needle under EUS guidance. Next, a guidewire is advanced, and the needle is removed. A cystotome is introduced over the wire to create a fistulous tract by the use of electrocautery. Successful long-term drainage has been reported with plastic stents and covered metal stents.

In conclusion, in case of ERCP failure, EUS-guided biliary drainage has emerged as a viable alternative to percutaneous tranhepatic drainage. Local expertise, logistics, and cost should be taken into consideration in the planning of the therapeutic algorithm in cases of ERCP failure.

KEY REFERENCES

1. American Cancer Society: Key statistics for pancreatic cancer. April 2016. Available at http://www.cancer.org/cancer/pancreaticcancer/detailedguide/pancreatic-cancer-key-statistics. (Accessed 26 October 2016).
11. Sapisochin G, Fernandez de Sevilla E, Echeverri J, Charco R: Liver transplantation for cholangiocarcinoma: current status and new insights, *World J Hepatol* 7(22):2396–2403, 2015.
17. Navaneethan U, Njei B, Lourdusamy V, et al: Comparative effectiveness of biliary brush cytology and intraductal biopsy for detection of

malignant biliary strictures: a systematic review and meta-analysis, *Gastrointest Endosc* 81(1):168–176, 2015.

21. Navaneethan U, Hasan MK, Kommaraju K, et al: Digital, single-operator cholangiopancreatoscopy in the diagnosis and management of pancreatobiliary disorders: a multicenter clinical experience (with video), *Gastrointest Endosc* 84(4):649–655, 2016.

23. Finkelberg DL, Sahani D, Deshpande V, Brugge WR: Autoimmune pancreatitis, *N Engl J Med* 355(25):2670–2676, 2006.

28. Speer AG, Cotton PB, Russell RC, et al: Randomised trial of endoscopic versus percutaneous stent insertion in malignant obstructive jaundice, *Lancet* 2(8550):57–62, 1987.

29. Smith AC, Dowsett JF, Russell RC, et al: Randomised trial of endoscopic stenting versus surgical bypass in malignant low bileduct obstruction, *Lancet* 344(8938):1655–1660, 1994.

30. Freeman ML, Nelson DB, Sherman S, et al: Complications of endoscopic biliary sphincterotomy, *N Engl J Med* 335(13):909–918, 1996.

32. Abraham NS, Barkun JS, Barkun AN: Palliation of malignant biliary obstruction: a prospective trial examining impact on quality of life, *Gastrointest Endosc* 56(6):835–841, 2002.

36. van der Gaag NA, Rauws EA, van Eijck CH, et al: Preoperative biliary drainage for cancer of the head of the pancreas, *N Engl J Med* 362(2): 129–137, 2010.

37. Tol JA, van Hooft JE, Timmer R, et al: Metal or plastic stents for preoperative biliary drainage in resectable pancreatic cancer, *Gut* 65(12):1981–1987, 2016.

42. Pereira-Lima JC, Jakobs R, Maier M, et al: Endoscopic biliary stenting for the palliation of pancreatic cancer: results, survival predictive factors, and comparison of 10-French with 11.5-French gauge stents, *Am J Gastroenterol* 91(10):2179–2184, 1996.

77. Davids PH, Groen AK, Rauws EA, et al: Randomised trial of self-expanding metal stents versus polyethylene stents for distal malignant biliary obstruction, *Lancet* 340(8834-8835):1488–1492, 1992.

78. Knyrim K, Wagner HJ, Pausch J, Vakil N: A prospective, randomized, controlled trial of metal stents for malignant obstruction of the common bile duct, *Endoscopy* 25(3):207–212, 1993.

79. Carr-Locke D, Ball TJ, Conners PJ: Multicenter randomized trial of Wallstent biliary prosthesis versus plastic stents, *Gastrointest Endosc* 39:310–316, 1993.

81. Yoon WJ, Lee JK, Lee KH, et al: A comparison of covered and uncovered Wallstents for the management of distal malignant biliary obstruction, *Gastrointest Endosc* 63(7):996–1000, 2006.

87. Prat F, Chapat O, Ducot B, et al: Predictive factors for survival of patients with inoperable malignant distal biliary strictures: a practical management guideline, *Gut* 42(1):76–80, 1998.

88. Kaassis M, Boyer J, Dumas R, et al: Plastic or metal stents for malignant stricture of the common bile duct? Results of a randomized prospective study, *Gastrointest Endosc* 57(2):178–182, 2003.

95. Dumas R, Demuth N, Buckley M, et al: Endoscopic bilateral metal stent placement for malignant hilar stenoses: identification of optimal technique, *Gastrointest Endosc* 51(3):334–338, 2000.

110. Paik WH, Park YS, Hwang JH, et al: Palliative treatment with self-expandable metallic stents in patients with advanced type III or IV hilar cholangiocarcinoma: a percutaneous versus endoscopic approach, *Gastrointest Endosc* 69(1):55–62, 2009.

111. Rerknimitr R, Angsuwatcharakon P, Ratanachu-ek T, et al: Asia-Pacific consensus recommendations for endoscopic and interventional management of hilar cholangiocarcinoma, *J Gastroenterol Hepatol* 28(4):593–607, 2013.

113. Vienne A, Hobeika E, Gouya H, et al: Prediction of drainage effectiveness during endoscopic stenting of malignant hilar strictures: the role of liver volume assessment, *Gastrointest Endosc* 72(4):728–735, 2010.

133. van Halsema EE, Rauws EA, Fockens P, van Hooft JE: Self-expandable metal stents for malignant gastric outlet obstruction: a pooled analysis of prospective literature, *World J Gastroenterol* 21(43):12468–12481, 2015.

136. Khashab MA, Kumbhari V, Grimm IS, et al: EUS-guided gastroenterostomy: the first U.S. clinical experience (with video), *Gastrointest Endosc* 82(5):932–938, 2015.

160. Dhir V, Itoi T, Khashab MA, et al: Multicenter comparative evaluation of endoscopic placement of expandable metal stents for malignant distal common bile duct obstruction by ERCP or EUS-guided approach, *Gastrointest Endosc* 81(4):913–923, 2015.

A complete reference list can be found online at ExpertConsult .com

INDEX

Page numbers followed by "*f*" indicate figures, "*t*" indicate tables, and "*b*" indicate boxes.